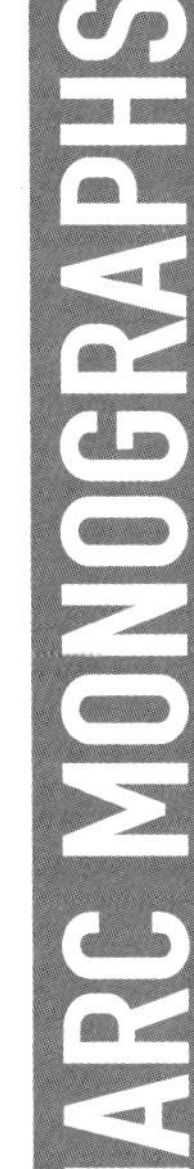

AF597900

PERSONAL HABITS AND INDOOR COMBUSTIONS

VOLUME 100 E

A REVIEW OF HUMAN CARCINOGENS

This publication represents the views and expert opinions of an IARC Working Group on the Evaluation of Carcinogenic Risks to Humans, which met in Lyon, 29 September-6 October 2009

LYON, FRANCE - 2012

IARC MONOGRAPHS ON THE EVALUATION OF CARCINOGENIC RISKS TO HUMANS

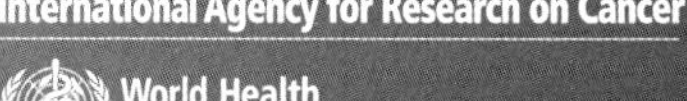
International Agency for Research on Cancer

World Health Organization

IARC MONOGRAPHS

In 1969, the International Agency for Research on Cancer (IARC) initiated a programme on the evaluation of the carcinogenic risk of chemicals to humans involving the production of critically evaluated monographs on individual chemicals. The programme was subsequently expanded to include evaluations of carcinogenic risks associated with exposures to complex mixtures, lifestyle factors and biological and physical agents, as well as those in specific occupations. The objective of the programme is to elaborate and publish in the form of monographs critical reviews of data on carcinogenicity for agents to which humans are known to be exposed and on specific exposure situations; to evaluate these data in terms of human risk with the help of international working groups of experts in chemical carcinogenesis and related fields; and to indicate where additional research efforts are needed. The lists of IARC evaluations are regularly updated and are available on the Internet at http://monographs.iarc.fr/.

This programme has been supported since 1982 by Cooperative Agreement U01 CA33193 with the United States National Cancer Institute, Department of Health and Human Services. Additional support has been provided since 1986 by the Health, Safety and Hygiene at Work Unit of the European Commission Directorate-General for Employment, Social Affairs and Equal Opportunities, and since 1992 by the United States National Institute of Environmental Health Sciences, Department of Health and Human Services. The contents of this volume are solely the responsibility of the Working Group and do not necessarily represent the official views of the U.S. National Cancer Institute, the U.S. National Institute of Environmental Health Sciences, the U.S. Department of Health and Human Services, or the European Commission Directorate-General for Employment, Social Affairs and Equal Opportunities.

This volume was made possible, in part, through Cooperative Agreement CR 834012 with the United States Environmental Protection Agency, Office of Research and Development. The contents of this volume do not necessarily reflect the views or policies of the U.S. Environmental Protection Agency.

Published by the International Agency for Research on Cancer,
150 cours Albert Thomas, 69372 Lyon Cedex 08, France
©International Agency for Research on Cancer, 2012

Distributed by WHO Press, World Health Organization, 20 Avenue Appia, 1211 Geneva 27, Switzerland
(tel.: +41 22 791 3264; fax: +41 22 791 4857; e-mail: bookorders@who.int).

Publications of the World Health Organization enjoy copyright protection in accordance with the provisions of Protocol 2 of the Universal Copyright Convention. All rights reserved.

The International Agency for Research on Cancer welcomes requests for permission to reproduce or translate its publications, in part or in full. Requests for permission to reproduce or translate IARC publications – whether for sale or for noncommercial distribution – should be addressed to WHO Press, at the above address (fax: +41 22 791 4806; email: permissions@who.int).

The designations employed and the presentation of the material in this publication do not imply the expression of any opinion whatsoever on the part of the Secretariat of the World Health Organization concerning the legal status of any country, territory, city, or area or of its authorities, or concerning the delimitation of its frontiers or boundaries.

The mention of specific companies or of certain manufacturers' products does not imply that they are endorsed or recommended by the World Health Organization in preference to others of a similar nature that are not mentioned. Errors and omissions excepted, the names of proprietary products are distinguished by initial capital letters.

The IARC Monographs Working Group alone is responsible for the views expressed in this publication.

IARC Library Cataloguing in Publication Data

A review of human carcinogens. Part E: Personal habits and indoor combustions / IARC Working Group on the Evaluation of Carcinogenic Risks to Humans (2009: Lyon, France)

(IARC monographs on the evaluation of carcinogenic risks to humans ; v. 100E)

1. Air Pollution, Indoor 2. Carcinogens 3. Food Preservation 4. Habits 5. Neoplasms – etiology
I. IARC Working Group on the Evaluation of Carcinogenic Risks to Humans
II. Series

ISBN 978 92 832 1322 2 (NLM Classification: W1)
ISSN 1017-1606

PRINTED IN FRANCE

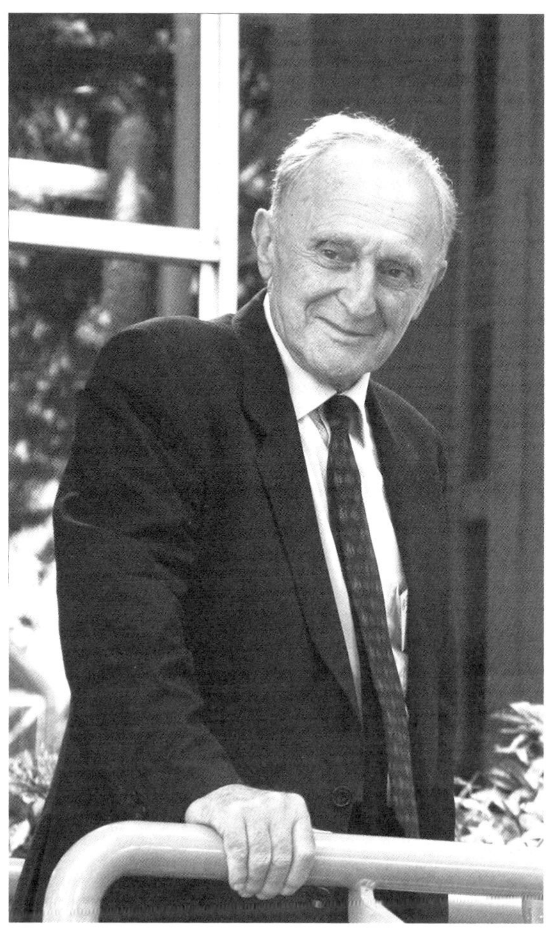

Lorenzo Tomatis (1929-2007)
Founder of the *IARC Monographs* Programme

Lorenzo Tomatis, MD, with other colleagues knowledgeable in primary prevention and environmental carcinogenesis, perceived in the 1960s the growing need to objectively evaluate carcinogenic risks by international groups of experts in chemical carcinogenesis. His vision and determination to provide a reliable source of knowledge and information on environmental and occupational causes of cancer led to his creating the *IARC Monographs* Programme for evaluating cancer risks to humans from exposures to chemicals. The first meeting, held in Geneva in December 1971, resulted in Volume 1 of the IARC Monographs on the Evaluation of Carcinogenic Risk of Chemicals to Man [1972], a series known affectionately since as the "orange books". As a champion of chemical carcinogenesis bioassays, Tomatis defined and promoted the applicability and utility of experimental animal findings for identifying carcinogens and for preventing cancers in humans, especially in workers and children, and to eliminate inequalities in judging cancer risks between industrialized and developing countries. Tomatis' foresight, guidance, leadership, and staunch belief in primary prevention continued to influence the *IARC Monographs* as they expanded to encompass personal habits, as well as physical and biological agents. Lorenzo Tomatis had a distinguished career at the Agency, arriving in 1967 and heading the Unit of Chemical Carcinogenesis, before being Director from 1982 to 1993.

Volume 100 of the *IARC Monographs* Series is respectfully dedicated to him.

(photo: Roland Dray)

CONTENTS

NOTE TO THE READER

The term 'carcinogenic risk' in the *IARC Monographs* series is taken to mean that an agent is capable of causing cancer. The *Monographs* evaluate cancer hazards, despite the historical presence of the word 'risks' in the title.

Inclusion of an agent in the *Monographs* does not imply that it is a carcinogen, only that the published data have been examined. Equally, the fact that an agent has not yet been evaluated in a *Monograph* does not mean that it is not carcinogenic. Similarly, identification of cancer sites with *sufficient evidence* or *limited evidence* in humans should not be viewed as precluding the possibility that an agent may cause cancer at other sites.

The evaluations of carcinogenic risk are made by international working groups of independent scientists and are qualitative in nature. No recommendation is given for regulation or legislation.

Anyone who is aware of published data that may alter the evaluation of the carcinogenic risk of an agent to humans is encouraged to make this information available to the Section of IARC Monographs, International Agency for Research on Cancer, 150 cours Albert Thomas, 69372 Lyon Cedex 08, France, in order that the agent may be considered for re-evaluation by a future Working Group.

Although every effort is made to prepare the *Monographs* as accurately as possible, mistakes may occur. Readers are requested to communicate any errors to the Section of IARC Monographs, so that corrections can be reported in future volumes.

LIST OF PARTICIPANTS

Members[1]

Michael Alavanja

Division of Cancer Epidemiology & Genetics
National Cancer Institute
Rockville, MD 20892
USA

Naomi Allen

Cancer Epidemiology Unit
University of Oxford
Headington
Oxford OX3 7LF
United Kingdom

Helmut Bartsch

Toxicology and Cancer Risk Factors
German Cancer Research Center
69120 Heidelberg
Germany

Rajani A. Bhisey

Mahim
Mumbai 400 016
India

[1] Working Group Members and Invited Specialists serve in their individual capacities as scientists and not as representatives of their government or any organization with which they are affiliated. Affiliations are provided for identification purposes only. Invited specialists are marked by an asterisk.
Each participant was asked to disclose pertinent research, employment, and financial interests. Current financial interests and research and employment interests during the past 3 years or anticipated in the future are identified here. Minor pertinent interests are not listed and include stock valued at no more than US$10 000 overall, grants that provide no more than 5% of the research budget of the expert's organization and that do not support the expert's research or position, and consulting or speaking on matters not before a court or government agency that does not exceed 2% of total professional time or compensation. All grants that support the expert's research or position and all consulting or speaking on behalf of an interested party on matters before a court or government agency are listed as significant pertinent interests.

Patricia A. Buffler

School of Public Health
University of California at Berkeley
Berkeley CA 94720
USA

Jenny Chang-Claude

Unit of Genetic Epidemiology
German Cancer Research Centre
69120 Heidelberg
Germany

David M. DeMarini

Integrated Systems Toxicology Division
US Environmental Protection Agency
Research Triangle Park, NC 27711
USA

Peter Eriksson

Department of Alcohol, Drugs and Addiction
National Institute for Health and Welfare
00271 Helsinki
Finland

Jeppe Friborg

Department of Epidemiology Research
Statens Serum Institute
2300 Copenhagen S
Denmark

Vendhan Gajalakshmi

Epidemiological Research Center
Chennai 600 010
Tamil Nadu
India

Prakash C. Gupta

Healis Sekhsaria Institute for Public Health
Navi Mumbai – 400 614
India

Stephen S. Hecht[2]

University of Minnesota Cancer Center
Minneapolis, MN 55455
USA

[2] Dr Hecht is serving as an expert witness for the plaintiff in a court case against a smokeless tobacco company. His fee is donated to a cancer center at his university.

Kirsti Husgafvel-Pursiainen

Biological Mechanisms and Prevention
of Work-Related Diseases
Finnish Institute of Occupational Health
00250 Helsinki
Finland

Hannu Norppa

New Technologies and Risks
Work Environment Development
Finnish Institute of Occupational Health
00250 Helsinki
Finland

Qing Lan

Occupational & Environmental
Epidemiology Branch
National Cancer Institute
Rockville, MD 20852
USA

Hiroshi Ohshima

Department of Food and Nutritional Sciences
University of Shizuoka
Shizuoka 422-8526
Japan

Joellen Lewtas

School of Public Health & Community
Medicine
University of Washington
Seattle, WA 98195
USA

Igor Pogribny

Division of Biochemical Toxicology
National Center for Toxicological Research
Jefferson, AR 72079
USA

Manabu Muto

Department of Gastroenterology
Kyoto University
Kyoto 606-8507
Japan

Vladimir Poznyak (absent during evaluations)

Department of Mental Health and Substance
Abuse
World Health Organization
1211 Geneva 27
Switzerland

Jerry M. Rice[3]

Georgetown University Medical Center
Lombardi Comprehensive Cancer Center
Washington, DC 20057
USA

Isabelle Romieu[4]

National Institute of Public Health
Cuernavaca, Morelos 62100
Mexico

Tore Sanner

Department of Environmental and Occupational Cancer
Institute for Cancer Research
0310 Oslo
Norway

Gary Stoner

Department of Internal Medicine
Ohio State University
Columbus, OH 43240
USA

Paul D. Terry

Department of Epidemiology
Rollins School of Public Health
Emory University
Atlanta, GA 30322
USA

Michael J. Thun[5]

Epidemiology & Surveillance Research
American Cancer Society
Atlanta, GA 30329
USA

Paolo Vineis

Department of Environmental Epidemiology
Imperial College
London W2 1PG
United Kingdom

Saman Warnakulasuriya

Department of Oral Medicine & Experimental Oral Pathology
Guy's, King's & St Thomas' Dental Institute
University of London
London SE5 9RS
United Kingdom

[3] Dr Rice is a partner in a winery. He receives no income from this investment.
[4] New address: IARC, Section of Nutrition and Metabolism.
[5] Dr Thun has served as an expert witness for the plaintiff in a court case against a tobacco company. His fee was donated to his employer.

Elisabete Weiderpass

Department of Etiological Research
The Cancer Registry of Norway
0310 Oslo
Norway

Deborah M. Winn

Division of Cancer Control & Population Sciences
National Cancer Institute
Bethesda, MD 20892
USA

Victor Wünsch Filho

Department of Epidemiology
University of São Paulo
CEP: 01246-904 São Paulo
Brazil

IARC Secretariat

Devasena Anantharaman
Robert Baan (*Rapporteur, Mechanistic and Other Relevant Data*)
Lamia Benbrahim-Tallaa (*Rapporteur, Cancer in Experimental Animals*)
Lubna Bhatti, WHO
Véronique Bouvard (*Rapporteur, Mechanistic and Other Relevant Data*)
Paul Brennan
Rafael Carel (*Visiting Scientist*)
Vincent Cogliano (*Head of Programme*)
Fatiha El Ghissassi (*Rapporteur, Mechanistic and Other Relevant Data*)
Crystal Freeman (*Rapporteur, Cancer in Humans*)
Laurent Galichet (*Editor for the Meeting*)
Yann Grosse (*Rapporteur, Cancer in Experimental Animals*)
Neela Guha (*Rapporteur, Cancer in Humans*)
Zdenko Herceg
Christian Herrmann
Farhad Islami
Gauri Khanna, WHO
Béatrice Lauby-Secretan (*Responsible Officer; Rapporteur, Cancer in Humans*)
Florence Le Calvez-Kelm
Maria León-Roux
Qian Li
Valerie McCormack
Aurélie Moskal
Richard Muwonge
Madlen Schütze (*Visiting Scientist*)
Chiara Scoccianti
Hai-Rim Shin
Kurt Straif (*Co-Responsible Officer; Rapporteur, Cancer in Humans*)
Lydia Voti
Nualnong Wongtongkam

Post-Meeting Scientific Assistance

Alice Kang
Berkeley, California
USA

Anthony B Miller (*Visiting Scientist, Editor*)
Toronto, Ontario
Canada

Dhirendra Narain Sinha
WHO SEARO
New Delhi
India

Administrative Assistance

Sandrine Egraz
Anne-Sophie Hameau
Michel Javin
Brigitte Kajo
Helene Lorenzen-Augros
Karine Racinoux

Production Team

Arthur Bouvard *(Reproduction of Graphics)*
Elisabeth Elbers
Sylvia Moutinho
Annick Papin
Dorothy Russell

PREAMBLE

The Preamble to the *IARC Monographs* describes the objective and scope of the programme, the scientific principles and procedures used in developing a *Monograph*, the types of evidence considered and the scientific criteria that guide the evaluations. The Preamble should be consulted when reading a *Monograph* or list of evaluations.

A. GENERAL PRINCIPLES AND PROCEDURES

1. Background

Soon after IARC was established in 1965, it received frequent requests for advice on the carcinogenic risk of chemicals, including requests for lists of known and suspected human carcinogens. It was clear that it would not be a simple task to summarize adequately the complexity of the information that was available, and IARC began to consider means of obtaining international expert opinion on this topic. In 1970, the IARC Advisory Committee on Environmental Carcinogenesis recommended '...that a compendium on carcinogenic chemicals be prepared by experts. The biological activity and evaluation of practical importance to public health should be referenced and documented.' The IARC Governing Council adopted a resolution concerning the role of IARC in providing government authorities with expert, independent, scientific opinion on environmental carcinogenesis. As one means to that end, the Governing Council recommended that IARC should prepare monographs on the evaluation of carcinogenic risk of chemicals to man, which became the initial title of the series.

In the succeeding years, the scope of the programme broadened as *Monographs* were developed for groups of related chemicals, complex mixtures, occupational exposures, physical and biological agents and lifestyle factors. In 1988, the phrase 'of chemicals' was dropped from the title, which assumed its present form, *IARC Monographs on the Evaluation of Carcinogenic Risks to Humans*.

Through the *Monographs* programme, IARC seeks to identify the causes of human cancer. This is the first step in cancer prevention, which is needed as much today as when IARC was established. The global burden of cancer is high and continues to increase: the annual number of new cases was estimated at 10.1 million in 2000 and is expected to reach 15 million by 2020 (Stewart & Kleihues, 2003). With current trends in demographics and exposure, the cancer burden has been shifting from high-resource countries to low- and medium-resource countries. As a result of *Monographs* evaluations, national health agencies have been able, on scientific grounds, to take measures to reduce human exposure to carcinogens in the workplace and in the environment.

The criteria established in 1971 to evaluate carcinogenic risks to humans were adopted by the Working Groups whose deliberations resulted in the first 16 volumes of the *Monographs* series. Those criteria were subsequently updated by further ad hoc Advisory Groups (IARC, 1977, 1978, 1979, 1982, 1983, 1987, 1988, 1991; Vainio *et al.*, 1992; IARC, 2005, 2006).

The Preamble is primarily a statement of scientific principles, rather than a specification of working procedures. The procedures through which a Working Group implements these principles are not specified in detail. They usually involve operations that have been established as being effective during previous *Monograph* meetings but remain, predominantly, the prerogative of each individual Working Group.

2. Objective and scope

The objective of the programme is to prepare, with the help of international Working Groups of experts, and to publish in the form of *Monographs*, critical reviews and evaluations of evidence on the carcinogenicity of a wide range of human exposures. The *Monographs* represent the first step in carcinogen risk assessment, which involves examination of all relevant information to assess the strength of the available evidence that an agent could alter the age-specific incidence of cancer in humans. The *Monographs* may also indicate where additional research efforts are needed, specifically when data immediately relevant to an evaluation are not available.

In this Preamble, the term 'agent' refers to any entity or circumstance that is subject to evaluation in a *Monograph*. As the scope of the programme has broadened, categories of agents now include specific chemicals, groups of related chemicals, complex mixtures, occupational or environmental exposures, cultural or behavioural practices, biological organisms and physical agents. This list of categories may expand as causation of, and susceptibility to, malignant disease become more fully understood.

A cancer 'hazard' is an agent that is capable of causing cancer under some circumstances, while a cancer 'risk' is an estimate of the carcinogenic effects expected from exposure to a cancer hazard. The *Monographs* are an exercise in evaluating cancer hazards, despite the historical presence of the word 'risks' in the title. The distinction between hazard and risk is important, and the *Monographs* identify cancer hazards even when risks are very low at current exposure levels, because new uses or unforeseen exposures could engender risks that are significantly higher.

In the *Monographs*, an agent is termed 'carcinogenic' if it is capable of increasing the incidence of malignant neoplasms, reducing their latency, or increasing their severity or multiplicity. The induction of benign neoplasms may in some circumstances (see Part B, Section 3a) contribute to the judgement that the agent is carcinogenic. The terms 'neoplasm' and 'tumour' are used interchangeably.

The Preamble continues the previous usage of the phrase 'strength of evidence' as a matter of historical continuity, although it should be understood that *Monographs* evaluations consider studies that support a finding of a cancer hazard as well as studies that do not.

Some epidemiological and experimental studies indicate that different agents may act at different stages in the carcinogenic process, and several different mechanisms may be involved. The aim of the *Monographs* has been, from their inception, to evaluate evidence of carcinogenicity at any stage in the carcinogenesis process, independently of the underlying mechanisms. Information on mechanisms may, however, be used in making the overall evaluation (IARC, 1991; Vainio *et al.*, 1992; IARC, 2005, 2006; see also Part B, Sections 4 and 6). As mechanisms of carcinogenesis are elucidated, IARC convenes international scientific conferences to determine whether a broad-based consensus has emerged on how specific mechanistic data can be used in an evaluation of human carcinogenicity. The results of such conferences are reported in IARC Scientific Publications, which, as long as they still reflect the current state of scientific knowledge, may guide subsequent Working Groups.

Although the *Monographs* have emphasized hazard identification, important issues may also involve dose–response assessment. In many cases, the same epidemiological and experimental studies used to evaluate a cancer hazard can also be used to estimate a dose–response relationship. A *Monograph* may undertake to estimate dose–response relationships within the range of the available epidemiological data, or it may compare the dose–response information from experimental and epidemiological studies. In some cases, a subsequent publication may be prepared by a separate Working Group with expertise in quantitative dose–response assessment.

The *Monographs* are used by national and international authorities to make risk assessments, formulate decisions concerning preventive measures, provide effective cancer control programmes and decide among alternative options for public health decisions. The evaluations of IARC Working Groups are scientific, qualitative judgements on the evidence for or against carcinogenicity provided by the available data. These evaluations represent only one part of the body of information on which public health decisions may be based. Public health options vary from one situation to another and from country to country and relate to many factors, including different socioeconomic and national priorities. Therefore, no recommendation is given with regard to regulation or legislation, which are the responsibility of individual governments or other international organizations.

3. Selection of agents for review

Agents are selected for review on the basis of two main criteria: (a) there is evidence of human exposure and (b) there is some evidence or suspicion of carcinogenicity. Mixed exposures may occur in occupational and environmental settings and as a result of individual and cultural habits (such as tobacco smoking and dietary practices). Chemical analogues and compounds with biological or physical characteristics similar to those of suspected carcinogens may also be considered, even in the absence of data on a possible carcinogenic effect in humans or experimental animals.

The scientific literature is surveyed for published data relevant to an assessment of carcinogenicity. Ad hoc Advisory Groups convened by IARC in 1984, 1989, 1991, 1993, 1998 and 2003 made recommendations as to which agents should be evaluated in the *Monographs* series. Recent recommendations are available on the *Monographs* programme web site (http://monographs.iarc.fr). IARC may schedule other agents for review as it becomes aware of new scientific information or as national health agencies identify an urgent public health need related to cancer.

As significant new data become available on an agent for which a *Monograph* exists, a re-evaluation may be made at a subsequent meeting, and a new *Monograph* published. In some cases it may be appropriate to review only the data published since a prior evaluation. This can be useful for updating a database, reviewing new data to resolve a previously open question or identifying new tumour sites associated with a carcinogenic agent. Major changes in an evaluation (e.g. a new classification in Group 1 or a determination that a mechanism does not operate in humans, see Part B, Section 6) are more appropriately addressed by a full review.

4. Data for the *Monographs*

Each *Monograph* reviews all pertinent epidemiological studies and cancer bioassays in experimental animals. Those judged inadequate or irrelevant to the evaluation may be cited but not summarized. If a group of similar studies is not reviewed, the reasons are indicated.

Mechanistic and other relevant data are also reviewed. A *Monograph* does not necessarily cite all the mechanistic literature concerning the agent being evaluated (see Part B, Section 4). Only those data considered by the Working Group to be relevant to making the evaluation are included.

With regard to epidemiological studies, cancer bioassays, and mechanistic and other relevant data, only reports that have been published or accepted for publication in the openly available scientific literature are reviewed. The same publication requirement applies to studies originating from IARC, including meta-analyses or pooled analyses commissioned by IARC in advance of a meeting (see Part B, Section 2c). Data from government agency reports that are publicly available are also considered. Exceptionally, doctoral theses and other material that are in their final form and publicly available may be reviewed.

Exposure data and other information on an agent under consideration are also reviewed. In the sections on chemical and physical properties, on analysis, on production and use and on occurrence, published and unpublished sources of information may be considered.

Inclusion of a study does not imply acceptance of the adequacy of the study design or of the analysis and interpretation of the results, and limitations are clearly outlined in square brackets at the end of each study description (see Part B). The reasons for not giving further consideration to an individual study also are indicated in the square brackets.

5. Meeting participants

Five categories of participant can be present at *Monograph* meetings.

(a) The Working Group

The Working Group is responsible for the critical reviews and evaluations that are developed during the meeting. The tasks of Working Group Members are: (i) to ascertain that all appropriate data have been collected; (ii) to select the data relevant for the evaluation on the basis of scientific merit; (iii) to prepare accurate summaries of the data to enable the reader to follow the reasoning of the Working Group; (iv) to evaluate the results of epidemiological and experimental studies on cancer; (v) to evaluate data relevant to the understanding of mechanisms of carcinogenesis; and (vi) to make an overall evaluation of the carcinogenicity of the exposure to humans. Working Group Members generally have published significant research related to the carcinogenicity of the agents being reviewed, and IARC uses literature searches to identify most experts. Working Group Members are selected on the basis of (a) knowledge and experience and (b) absence of real or apparent conflicts of interests. Consideration is also given to demographic diversity and balance of scientific findings and views.

(b) Invited Specialists

Invited Specialists are experts who also have critical knowledge and experience but have a real or apparent conflict of interests. These experts are invited when necessary to assist in the Working Group by contributing their unique knowledge and experience during subgroup and plenary discussions. They may also contribute text on non-influential issues in the section on exposure, such as a general description of data on production and use (see Part B, Section 1). Invited Specialists do not serve as meeting chair or subgroup chair, draft text that pertains to the description or interpretation of cancer data, or participate in the evaluations.

(c) Representatives of national and international health agencies

Representatives of national and international health agencies often attend meetings because their agencies sponsor the programme or are interested in the subject of a meeting. Representatives do not serve as meeting chair or subgroup chair, draft any part of a *Monograph*, or participate in the evaluations.

(d) Observers with relevant scientific credentials

Observers with relevant scientific credentials may be admitted to a meeting by IARC in limited numbers. Attention will be given to achieving a balance of Observers from constituencies with differing perspectives. They are invited to observe the meeting and should not attempt to influence it. Observers do not serve as meeting chair or subgroup chair, draft any part of a *Monograph*, or participate in the evaluations. At the meeting, the meeting chair and subgroup chairs may grant Observers an opportunity to speak, generally after they have observed a discussion. Observers agree to respect the Guidelines for Observers at *IARC Monographs* meetings (available at http://monographs.iarc.fr).

(e) The IARC Secretariat

The IARC Secretariat consists of scientists who are designated by IARC and who have relevant expertise. They serve as rapporteurs and participate in all discussions. When requested by the meeting chair or subgroup chair, they may also draft text or prepare tables and analyses.

Before an invitation is extended, each potential participant, including the IARC Secretariat, completes the WHO Declaration of Interests to report financial interests, employment and consulting, and individual and institutional research support related to the subject of the meeting. IARC assesses these interests to determine whether there is a conflict that warrants some limitation on participation. The declarations are updated and reviewed again at the opening of the meeting. Interests related to the subject of the meeting are disclosed to the meeting participants and in the published volume (Cogliano *et al.*, 2004).

The names and principal affiliations of participants are available on the *Monographs* programme web site (http://monographs.iarc.fr) approximately two months before each meeting. It is not acceptable for Observers or third parties to contact other participants before a meeting or to lobby them at any time. Meeting participants are asked to report all such contacts to IARC (Cogliano *et al.*, 2005).

All participants are listed, with their principal affiliations, at the beginning of each volume. Each participant who is a Member of a Working Group serves as an individual scientist and not as a representative of any organization, government or industry.

6. Working procedures

A separate Working Group is responsible for developing each volume of *Monographs*. A volume contains one or more *Monographs*, which can cover either a single agent or several related agents. Approximately one year in advance of the meeting of a Working Group, the agents to be reviewed are announced on the *Monographs* programme web site (http://monographs.iarc.fr) and participants are selected by IARC staff in consultation with other experts. Subsequently, relevant biological and epidemiological data are collected by IARC from recognized sources of information on carcinogenesis, including data storage and retrieval systems such as PubMed. Meeting participants who are asked to prepare preliminary working papers for specific sections are expected to supplement the IARC literature searches with their own searches.

For most chemicals and some complex mixtures, the major collection of data and the preparation of working papers for the sections on chemical and physical properties, on analysis, on production and use, and on occurrence are carried out under a separate contract funded by the US National Cancer Institute. Industrial associations, labour unions and other knowledgeable organizations may be asked to provide input to the sections on production and use, although this involvement is not required as a general rule. Information on production and trade is obtained from governmental, trade and market research publications and, in some cases, by direct contact with industries. Separate production data on some agents may not be available for a variety of reasons (e.g. not collected or made public in all producing countries, production is small). Information on uses may be obtained from published sources but is often complemented by direct contact with manufacturers. Efforts are made to supplement this information with data from other national and international sources.

Six months before the meeting, the material obtained is sent to meeting participants to prepare preliminary working papers. The working papers are compiled by IARC staff and sent, before the meeting, to Working Group Members and Invited Specialists for review.

The Working Group meets at IARC for seven to eight days to discuss and finalize the texts and to formulate the evaluations. The objectives of the meeting are peer review and consensus. During the first few days, four subgroups (covering exposure data, cancer in humans, cancer in experimental animals, and mechanistic and other relevant data) review the working papers, develop a joint subgroup draft and write summaries. Care is taken to ensure that each study summary is written or reviewed by someone not associated with the study being considered. During the last few days, the Working Group meets in plenary session to review the subgroup drafts and develop the evaluations. As a result, the entire volume is the joint product of the Working Group, and there are no individually authored sections.

IARC Working Groups strive to achieve a consensus evaluation. Consensus reflects broad agreement among Working Group Members, but not necessarily unanimity. The chair may elect to poll Working Group Members to determine the diversity of scientific opinion on issues where consensus is not readily apparent.

After the meeting, the master copy is verified by consulting the original literature, edited and prepared for publication. The aim is to publish the volume within six months of the Working Group meeting. A summary of the outcome is available on the *Monographs* programme web site soon after the meeting.

B. SCIENTIFIC REVIEW AND EVALUATION

The available studies are summarized by the Working Group, with particular regard to the qualitative aspects discussed below. In general, numerical findings are indicated as they appear in the original report; units are converted when necessary for easier comparison. The Working Group may conduct additional analyses of the published data and use them in their assessment of the evidence; the results of such supplementary analyses are given in square brackets. When an important aspect of a study that directly impinges on its interpretation should be brought to the attention of the reader, a Working Group comment is given in square brackets.

The scope of the *IARC Monographs* programme has expanded beyond chemicals to include complex mixtures, occupational exposures, physical and biological agents, lifestyle factors and other potentially carcinogenic exposures. Over time, the structure of a *Monograph* has evolved to include the following sections:

Exposure data
Studies of cancer in humans
Studies of cancer in experimental animals
Mechanistic and other relevant data
Summary
Evaluation and rationale

In addition, a section of General Remarks at the front of the volume discusses the reasons the agents were scheduled for evaluation and some key issues the Working Group encountered during the meeting.

This part of the Preamble discusses the types of evidence considered and summarized in each section of a *Monograph*, followed by the scientific criteria that guide the evaluations.

1. Exposure data

Each *Monograph* includes general information on the agent: this information may vary substantially between agents and must be adapted accordingly. Also included is information on production and use (when appropriate), methods of analysis and detection, occurrence, and sources and routes of human occupational and environmental exposures. Depending on the agent, regulations and guidelines for use may be presented.

(a) General information on the agent

For chemical agents, sections on chemical and physical data are included: the Chemical Abstracts Service Registry Number, the latest primary name and the IUPAC systematic name are recorded; other synonyms are given, but the list is not necessarily comprehensive. Information on chemical and physical properties that are relevant to identification, occurrence and biological activity is included. A description of technical products of chemicals includes trade names, relevant specifications and available information on composition and impurities. Some of the trade names given may be those of mixtures in which the agent being evaluated is only one of the ingredients.

For biological agents, taxonomy, structure and biology are described, and the degree of variability is indicated. Mode of replication, life cycle, target cells, persistence, latency, host response and clinical disease other than cancer are also presented.

For physical agents that are forms of radiation, energy and range of the radiation are included. For foreign bodies, fibres and respirable particles, size range and relative dimensions are indicated.

For agents such as mixtures, drugs or lifestyle factors, a description of the agent, including its composition, is given.

Whenever appropriate, other information, such as historical perspectives or the description of an industry or habit, may be included.

(b) Analysis and detection

An overview of methods of analysis and detection of the agent is presented, including their sensitivity, specificity and reproducibility. Methods widely used for regulatory purposes are emphasized. Methods for monitoring human exposure are also given. No critical evaluation or recommendation of any method is meant or implied.

(c) Production and use

The dates of first synthesis and of first commercial production of a chemical, mixture or other agent are provided when available; for agents that do not occur naturally, this information may allow a reasonable estimate to be made of the date before which no human exposure to the agent could have occurred. The dates of first reported occurrence of an exposure are also provided when available. In addition, methods of synthesis used in past and present commercial production and different methods of production, which may give rise to different impurities, are described.

The countries where companies report production of the agent, and the number of companies in each country, are identified. Available data on production, international trade and uses are obtained for representative regions. It should not, however, be inferred that those areas or nations are necessarily the sole or major sources or users of the agent. Some identified uses may not be current or major applications, and the coverage is not necessarily comprehensive. In the case of drugs, mention of their therapeutic uses does not necessarily represent current practice nor does it imply judgement as to their therapeutic efficacy.

(d) *Occurrence and exposure*

Information on the occurrence of an agent in the environment is obtained from data derived from the monitoring and surveillance of levels in occupational environments, air, water, soil, plants, foods and animal and human tissues. When available, data on the generation, persistence and bioaccumulation of the agent are also included. Such data may be available from national databases.

Data that indicate the extent of past and present human exposure, the sources of exposure, the people most likely to be exposed and the factors that contribute to the exposure are reported. Information is presented on the range of human exposure, including occupational and environmental exposures. This includes relevant findings from both developed and developing countries. Some of these data are not distributed widely and may be available from government reports and other sources. In the case of mixtures, industries, occupations or processes, information is given about all agents known to be present. For processes, industries and occupations, a historical description is also given, noting variations in chemical composition, physical properties and levels of occupational exposure with date and place. For biological agents, the epidemiology of infection is described.

(e) *Regulations and guidelines*

Statements concerning regulations and guidelines (e.g. occupational exposure limits, maximal levels permitted in foods and water, pesticide registrations) are included, but they may not reflect the most recent situation, since such limits are continuously reviewed and modified. The absence of information on regulatory status for a country should not be taken to imply that that country does not have regulations with regard to the exposure. For biological agents, legislation and control, including vaccination and therapy, are described.

2. Studies of cancer in humans

This section includes all pertinent epidemiological studies (see Part A, Section 4). Studies of biomarkers are included when they are relevant to an evaluation of carcinogenicity to humans.

(a) *Types of study considered*

Several types of epidemiological study contribute to the assessment of carcinogenicity in humans — cohort studies, case–control studies, correlation (or ecological) studies and intervention studies. Rarely, results from randomized trials may be available. Case reports and case series of cancer in humans may also be reviewed.

Cohort and case–control studies relate individual exposures under study to the occurrence of cancer in individuals and provide an estimate of effect (such as relative risk) as the main measure of association. Intervention studies may provide strong evidence for making causal inferences, as exemplified by cessation of smoking and the subsequent decrease in risk for lung cancer.

In correlation studies, the units of investigation are usually whole populations (e.g. in particular geographical areas or at particular times), and cancer frequency is related to a summary measure of the exposure of the population to the agent under study. In correlation studies, individual exposure is not documented, which renders this kind of study more prone to confounding. In some circumstances, however, correlation studies may be more informative than analytical study designs (see, for example, the *Monograph* on arsenic in drinking-water; IARC, 2004).

In some instances, case reports and case series have provided important information about the carcinogenicity of an agent. These types of study generally arise from a suspicion, based on clinical experience, that the concurrence of two events — that is, a particular exposure and occurrence of a cancer — has happened rather more frequently than would be expected by chance. Case reports and case series usually lack complete ascertainment of cases in any population, definition or enumeration of the population at risk and estimation of the expected number of cases in the absence of exposure.

The uncertainties that surround the interpretation of case reports, case series and correlation studies make them inadequate, except in rare instances, to form the sole basis for inferring a causal relationship. When taken together with case–control and cohort studies, however, these types of study may add materially to the judgement that a causal relationship exists.

Epidemiological studies of benign neoplasms, presumed preneoplastic lesions and other end-points thought to be relevant to cancer are also reviewed. They may, in some instances, strengthen inferences drawn from studies of cancer itself.

(b) Quality of studies considered

It is necessary to take into account the possible roles of bias, confounding and chance in the interpretation of epidemiological studies. Bias is the effect of factors in study design or execution that lead erroneously to a stronger or weaker association than in fact exists between an agent and disease. Confounding is a form of bias that occurs when the relationship with disease is made to appear stronger or weaker than it truly is as a result of an association between the apparent causal factor and another factor that is associated with either an increase or decrease in the incidence of the disease. The role of chance is related to biological variability and the influence of sample size on the precision of estimates of effect.

In evaluating the extent to which these factors have been minimized in an individual study, consideration is given to several aspects of design and analysis as described in the report of the study. For example, when suspicion of carcinogenicity arises largely from a single small study, careful consideration is given when interpreting subsequent studies that included these data in an enlarged population. Most of these considerations apply equally to case–control, cohort and correlation studies. Lack of clarity of any of these aspects in the reporting of a study can decrease its credibility and the weight given to it in the final evaluation of the exposure.

First, the study population, disease (or diseases) and exposure should have been well defined by the authors. Cases of disease in the study population should have been identified in a way that was independent of the exposure of interest, and exposure should have been assessed in a way that was not related to disease status.

Second, the authors should have taken into account — in the study design and analysis — other variables that can influence the risk of disease and may have been related to the exposure of interest. Potential confounding by such variables should have been dealt with either in the design of the study, such as by matching, or in the analysis, by statistical adjustment. In cohort studies, comparisons with local rates of disease may or may not be more appropriate than those with national rates. Internal comparisons of frequency of disease among individuals at different levels of exposure are also desirable in cohort studies, since they minimize the potential for confounding related to the difference in risk factors between an external reference group and the study population.

Third, the authors should have reported the basic data on which the conclusions are founded, even if sophisticated statistical analyses were employed. At the very least, they should have given the numbers of exposed and unexposed cases and controls in a case–control study and the numbers of cases observed and expected in a cohort study. Further tabulations by time since exposure began and other temporal factors are also important. In a cohort study, data on all cancer sites and all causes of death should have been given, to reveal the possibility of reporting bias. In a case–control study, the effects of investigated factors other than the exposure of interest should have been reported.

Finally, the statistical methods used to obtain estimates of relative risk, absolute rates of cancer, confidence intervals and significance tests, and to adjust for confounding should have been clearly stated by the authors. These methods have been reviewed for case–control studies (Breslow & Day, 1980) and for cohort studies (Breslow & Day, 1987).

(c) Meta-analyses and pooled analyses

Independent epidemiological studies of the same agent may lead to results that are difficult to interpret. Combined analyses of data from multiple studies are a means of resolving this ambiguity, and well conducted analyses can be considered. There are two types of combined analysis. The first involves combining summary statistics such as relative risks from individual studies (meta-analysis) and the second involves a pooled analysis of the raw data from the individual studies (pooled analysis) (Greenland, 1998).

The advantages of combined analyses are increased precision due to increased sample size and the opportunity to explore potential confounders, interactions and modifying effects that may explain heterogeneity among studies in more detail. A disadvantage of combined analyses is the possible lack of compatibility of data from various studies due to differences in subject recruitment, procedures of data collection, methods of measurement and effects of unmeasured co-variates that may differ among studies. Despite these limitations, well conducted combined analyses may provide a firmer basis than individual studies for drawing conclusions about the potential carcinogenicity of agents.

IARC may commission a meta-analysis or pooled analysis that is pertinent to a particular *Monograph* (see Part A, Section 4). Additionally, as a means of gaining insight from the results of multiple individual studies, ad hoc calculations that combine data from different studies may be conducted by the Working Group during the course of a *Monograph* meeting. The results of such original calculations, which would be specified in the text by presentation in square brackets, might involve updates of previously conducted analyses that incorporate the results of more recent studies or de-novo analyses. Irrespective of the source of data for the meta-analyses and pooled analyses, it is important that the same criteria for data quality be applied as those that would be applied to individual studies and to ensure also that sources of heterogeneity between studies be taken into account.

(d) Temporal effects

Detailed analyses of both relative and absolute risks in relation to temporal variables, such as age at first exposure, time since first exposure, duration of exposure, cumulative exposure, peak exposure (when appropriate) and time since cessation of exposure, are reviewed and summarized when available. Analyses of temporal relationships may be useful in making causal inferences. In addition, such analyses may suggest whether a carcinogen acts early or late in the process of carcinogenesis, although, at best, they allow only indirect inferences about mechanisms of carcinogenesis.

(e) Use of biomarkers in epidemiological studies

Biomarkers indicate molecular, cellular or other biological changes and are increasingly used in epidemiological studies for various purposes (IARC, 1991; Vainio *et al.*, 1992; Toniolo *et al.*, 1997; Vineis *et al.*, 1999; Buffler *et al.*, 2004). These may include evidence of exposure, of early effects, of cellular, tissue or organism responses, of individual susceptibility or host responses, and inference of a mechanism (see Part B, Section 4b). This is a rapidly evolving field that encompasses developments in genomics, epigenomics and other emerging technologies.

Molecular epidemiological data that identify associations between genetic polymorphisms and interindividual differences in susceptibility to the agent(s) being evaluated may contribute to the identification of carcinogenic hazards to humans. If the polymorphism has been demonstrated experimentally to modify the functional activity of the gene product in a manner that is consistent with increased susceptibility, these data may be useful in making causal inferences. Similarly, molecular epidemiological studies that measure cell functions, enzymes or metabolites that are thought to be the basis of susceptibility may provide evidence that reinforces biological plausibility. It should be noted, however, that when data on genetic susceptibility originate from multiple comparisons that arise from subgroup analyses, this can generate false-positive results and inconsistencies across studies, and such data therefore require careful evaluation. If the known phenotype of a genetic polymorphism can explain the carcinogenic mechanism of the agent being evaluated, data on this phenotype may be useful in making causal inferences.

(f) Criteria for causality

After the quality of individual epidemiological studies of cancer has been summarized and assessed, a judgement is made concerning the strength of evidence that the agent in question is carcinogenic to humans. In making its judgement, the Working Group considers several criteria for causality (Hill, 1965). A strong association (e.g. a large relative risk) is more likely to indicate causality than a weak association, although it is recognized that estimates of effect of small magnitude do not imply lack of causality and may be important if the disease or exposure is common. Associations that are replicated in several studies of the same design or that use different epidemiological approaches or under different circumstances of exposure are more likely to represent a causal relationship than isolated observations from single studies. If there are inconsistent results among investigations, possible reasons are sought (such as differences in exposure), and results of studies that are judged to be of high quality are given more weight than those of studies that are judged to be methodologically less sound.

If the risk increases with the exposure, this is considered to be a strong indication of causality, although the absence of a graded response is not necessarily evidence against a causal relationship. The demonstration of a decline in risk after cessation of or reduction in exposure in individuals or in whole populations also supports a causal interpretation of the findings.

Several scenarios may increase confidence in a causal relationship. On the one hand, an agent may be specific in causing tumours at one site or of one morphological type. On the other, carcinogenicity may be evident through the causation of multiple tumour types. Temporality, precision of estimates of effect, biological plausibility and coherence of the overall database are considered. Data on biomarkers may be employed in an assessment of the biological plausibility of epidemiological observations.

Although rarely available, results from randomized trials that show different rates of cancer among exposed and unexposed individuals provide particularly strong evidence for causality.

When several epidemiological studies show little or no indication of an association between an exposure and cancer, a judgement may be made that, in the aggregate, they show evidence of lack of carcinogenicity. Such a judgement requires first that the studies meet, to a sufficient degree, the standards of design and analysis described above. Specifically, the possibility that bias, confounding or misclassification of exposure or outcome could explain the observed results should be considered and excluded with reasonable certainty. In addition, all studies that are judged to be methodologically sound should (a) be consistent with an estimate of effect of unity for any observed level of exposure, (b) when considered together, provide a pooled estimate of relative risk that is at or near to unity, and (c) have a narrow confidence interval, due to sufficient population size. Moreover, no individual study nor the pooled results of all the studies should show any consistent tendency that the relative risk of cancer increases with increasing level of exposure. It is important to note that evidence of lack of carcinogenicity obtained from several epidemiological studies can apply only to the type(s) of cancer studied, to the dose levels reported, and to the intervals between first exposure and disease onset observed in these studies. Experience with human cancer indicates that the period from first exposure to the development of clinical cancer is sometimes longer than 20 years; latent periods substantially shorter than 30 years cannot provide evidence for lack of carcinogenicity.

3. Studies of cancer in experimental animals

All known human carcinogens that have been studied adequately for carcinogenicity in experimental animals have produced positive results in one or more animal species (Wilbourn *et al.*, 1986; Tomatis *et al.*, 1989). For several agents (e.g. aflatoxins, diethylstilbestrol, solar radiation, vinyl chloride), carcinogenicity in experimental animals was established or highly suspected before epidemiological studies confirmed their carcinogenicity in humans (Vainio *et al.*, 1995). Although this association cannot establish that all agents that cause cancer in experimental animals also cause cancer in humans, it is biologically plausible that agents for which there is *sufficient evidence of carcinogenicity* in experimental animals (see Part B, Section 6b) also present a carcinogenic hazard to humans. Accordingly, in the absence of additional scientific information, these agents are considered to pose a carcinogenic hazard to humans. Examples of additional scientific information are data that demonstrate that a given agent causes cancer in animals through a species-specific mechanism that does not operate in humans or data that demonstrate that the mechanism in experimental animals also operates in humans (see Part B, Section 6).

Consideration is given to all available long-term studies of cancer in experimental animals with the agent under review (see Part A, Section 4). In all experimental settings, the nature and extent of impurities or contaminants present in the agent being evaluated are given when available. Animal species, strain (including genetic background where applicable), sex, numbers per group, age at start of treatment, route of exposure, dose levels, duration of exposure, survival and information on tumours (incidence, latency, severity or multiplicity of neoplasms or preneoplastic lesions) are reported. Those studies in experimental animals that are judged to be irrelevant to the evaluation or judged to be inadequate (e.g. too short a duration, too few animals, poor survival; see below) may be omitted. Guidelines for conducting long-term carcinogenicity experiments have been published (e.g. OECD, 2002).

Other studies considered may include: experiments in which the agent was administered in the presence of factors that modify carcinogenic effects (e.g. initiation–promotion studies, co-carcinogenicity studies and studies in genetically modified animals); studies in which the end-point was not cancer but a defined precancerous lesion; experiments on the carcinogenicity of known metabolites and derivatives; and studies of cancer in non-laboratory animals (e.g. livestock and companion animals) exposed to the agent.

For studies of mixtures, consideration is given to the possibility that changes in the physicochemical properties of the individual substances may occur during collection, storage, extraction, concentration and delivery. Another consideration is that chemical and toxicological interactions of components in a mixture may alter dose–response relationships. The relevance to human exposure of the test mixture administered in the animal experiment is also assessed. This may involve consideration of the following aspects of the mixture tested: (i) physical and chemical characteristics, (ii) identified constituents that may indicate the presence of a class of substances and (iii) the results of genetic toxicity and related tests.

The relevance of results obtained with an agent that is analogous (e.g. similar in structure or of a similar virus genus) to that being evaluated is also considered. Such results may provide biological and mechanistic information that is relevant to the understanding of the process of carcinogenesis in humans and may strengthen the biological plausibility that the agent being evaluated is carcinogenic to humans (see Part B, Section 2f).

(a) Qualitative aspects

An assessment of carcinogenicity involves several considerations of qualitative importance, including (i) the experimental conditions under which the test was performed, including route, schedule and duration of exposure, species, strain (including genetic background where applicable), sex, age and duration of follow-up; (ii) the consistency of the results, for example, across species and target organ(s); (iii) the spectrum of neoplastic response, from preneoplastic lesions and benign tumours to malignant neoplasms; and (iv) the possible role of modifying factors.

Considerations of importance in the interpretation and evaluation of a particular study include: (i) how clearly the agent was defined and, in the case of mixtures, how adequately the sample characterization was reported; (ii) whether the dose was monitored adequately, particularly in inhalation experiments; (iii) whether the doses, duration of treatment and route of exposure were appropriate; (iv) whether the survival of treated animals was similar to that of controls; (v) whether there were adequate numbers of animals per group; (vi) whether both male and female animals were used; (vii) whether animals were allocated randomly to groups; (viii) whether the duration of observation was adequate; and (ix) whether the data were reported and analysed adequately.

When benign tumours (a) occur together with and originate from the same cell type as malignant tumours in an organ or tissue in a particular study and (b) appear to represent a stage in the progression to malignancy, they are usually combined in the assessment of tumour incidence (Huff *et al.*, 1989). The occurrence of lesions presumed to be preneoplastic may in certain instances aid in assessing the biological plausibility of any neoplastic response observed. If an agent induces only benign neoplasms that appear to be end-points that do not readily undergo transition to malignancy, the agent should nevertheless be suspected of being carcinogenic and requires further investigation.

(b) Quantitative aspects

The probability that tumours will occur may depend on the species, sex, strain, genetic background and age of the animal, and on the dose, route, timing and duration of the exposure. Evidence of an increased incidence of neoplasms with increasing levels of exposure strengthens the inference of a causal association between the exposure and the development of neoplasms.

The form of the dose–response relationship can vary widely, depending on the particular agent under study and the target organ. Mechanisms such as induction of DNA damage or inhibition of repair, altered cell division and cell death rates and changes in intercellular communication are important determinants of dose–response relationships for some carcinogens. Since many chemicals require metabolic activation before being converted to their reactive intermediates, both metabolic and toxicokinetic aspects are important in determining the dose–response pattern. Saturation of steps such as absorption, activation, inactivation and elimination may produce nonlinearity in the dose–response relationship (Hoel et al., 1983; Gart *et al.*, 1986), as could saturation of processes such as DNA repair. The dose–response relationship can also be affected by differences in survival among the treatment groups.

(c) Statistical analyses

Factors considered include the adequacy of the information given for each treatment group: (i) number of animals studied and number examined histologically, (ii) number of animals with a given tumour type and (iii) length of survival. The statistical methods used should be clearly stated and should be the generally accepted techniques refined for this purpose (Peto *et al.*, 1980; Gart *et al.*, 1986; Portier & Bailer, 1989; Bieler & Williams, 1993). The choice of the most appropriate statistical method requires consideration of whether or not there are differences in survival among the treatment groups; for example, reduced survival because of non-tumour-related mortality can preclude the occurrence of tumours later in life. When detailed information on survival is not available, comparisons of the proportions of tumour-bearing animals among the effective number of animals (alive at the time the first tumour was discovered) can be useful when significant differences in survival occur before tumours appear. The lethality of the tumour also requires consideration: for rapidly fatal tumours, the time of death provides an indication of the time of tumour onset and can be assessed using life-table methods; non-fatal or incidental tumours that do not affect survival can be assessed using methods such as the Mantel-Haenzel test for changes in tumour prevalence. Because tumour lethality is often difficult to determine, methods such as the Poly-K test that do not require such information can also be used. When results are available on the number and size of tumours seen in experimental animals (e.g. papillomas on mouse skin, liver tumours observed through nuclear magnetic resonance tomography), other more complicated statistical procedures may be needed (Sherman *et al.*, 1994; Dunson *et al.*, 2003).

Formal statistical methods have been developed to incorporate historical control data into the analysis of data from a given experiment. These methods assign an appropriate weight to historical and concurrent controls on the basis of the extent of between-study and within-study variability: less weight is given to historical controls when they show a high degree of variability, and greater weight when they show little variability. It is generally not appropriate to discount a tumour response that is significantly increased compared with concurrent controls by arguing that it falls within the range of historical controls, particularly when historical controls show high between-study variability and are, thus, of little relevance to the current experiment. In analysing results for uncommon tumours, however, the analysis may be improved by considering historical control data, particularly when between-study variability is low. Historical controls should be selected to resemble the concurrent controls as closely as possible with respect to species, gender and strain, as well as other factors such as basal diet and general laboratory environment, which may affect tumour-response rates in control animals (Haseman *et al.*, 1984; Fung *et al.*, 1996; Greim *et al.*, 2003).

Although meta-analyses and combined analyses are conducted less frequently for animal experiments than for epidemiological studies due to differences in animal strains, they can be useful aids in interpreting animal data when the experimental protocols are sufficiently similar.

4. Mechanistic and other relevant data

Mechanistic and other relevant data may provide evidence of carcinogenicity and also help in assessing the relevance and importance of findings of cancer in animals and in humans. The nature of the mechanistic and other relevant data depends on the biological activity of the agent being considered. The Working Group considers representative studies to give a concise description of the relevant data and issues that they consider to be important; thus, not every available study is cited. Relevant topics may include toxicokinetics, mechanisms of carcinogenesis, susceptible individuals, populations and life-stages, other relevant data and other adverse effects. When data on biomarkers are informative about the mechanisms of carcinogenesis, they are included in this section.

These topics are not mutually exclusive; thus, the same studies may be discussed in more than one subsection. For example, a mutation in a gene that codes for an enzyme that metabolizes the agent under study could be discussed in the subsections on toxicokinetics, mechanisms and individual susceptibility if it also exists as an inherited polymorphism.

(a) Toxicokinetic data

Toxicokinetics refers to the absorption, distribution, metabolism and elimination of agents in humans, experimental animals and, where relevant, cellular systems. Examples of kinetic factors that may affect dose–response relationships include uptake, deposition, biopersistence and half-life in tissues, protein binding, metabolic activation and detoxification. Studies that indicate the metabolic fate of the agent in humans and in experimental animals are summarized briefly, and comparisons of data from humans and animals are made when possible. Comparative information on the relationship between exposure and the dose that reaches the target site may be important for the extrapolation of hazards between species and in clarifying the role of in-vitro findings.

(b) Data on mechanisms of carcinogenesis

To provide focus, the Working Group attempts to identify the possible mechanisms by which the agent may increase the risk of cancer. For each possible mechanism, a representative selection of key data from humans and experimental systems is summarized. Attention is given to gaps in the data and to data that suggests that more than one mechanism may be operating. The relevance of the mechanism to humans is discussed, in particular, when mechanistic data are derived from experimental model systems. Changes in the affected organs, tissues or cells can be divided into three non-exclusive levels as described below.

(i) Changes in physiology

Physiological changes refer to exposure-related modifications to the physiology and/or response of cells, tissues and organs. Examples of potentially adverse physiological changes include mitogenesis, compensatory cell division, escape from apoptosis and/or senescence, presence of inflammation, hyperplasia, metaplasia and/or preneoplasia, angiogenesis, alterations in cellular adhesion, changes in steroidal hormones and changes in immune surveillance.

(ii) Functional changes at the cellular level

Functional changes refer to exposure-related alterations in the signalling pathways used by cells to manage critical processes that are related to increased risk for cancer. Examples of functional changes include modified activities of enzymes involved in the metabolism of xenobiotics, alterations in the expression of key genes that regulate DNA repair, alterations in cyclin-dependent kinases that govern cell cycle progression, changes in the patterns of post-translational modifications of proteins, changes in regulatory factors that alter apoptotic rates, changes in the secretion of factors related to the stimulation of DNA replication and transcription and changes in gap–junction-mediated intercellular communication.

(iii) Changes at the molecular level

Molecular changes refer to exposure-related changes in key cellular structures at the molecular level, including, in particular, genotoxicity. Examples of molecular changes include formation of DNA adducts and DNA strand breaks, mutations in genes, chromosomal aberrations, aneuploidy and changes in DNA methylation patterns. Greater emphasis is given to irreversible effects.

The use of mechanistic data in the identification of a carcinogenic hazard is specific to the mechanism being addressed and is not readily described for every possible level and mechanism discussed above.

Genotoxicity data are discussed here to illustrate the key issues involved in the evaluation of mechanistic data.

Tests for genetic and related effects are described in view of the relevance of gene mutation and chromosomal aberration/aneuploidy to carcinogenesis (Vainio *et al.*, 1992; McGregor *et al.*, 1999). The adequacy of the reporting of sample characterization is considered and, when necessary, commented upon; with regard to complex mixtures, such comments are similar to those described for animal carcinogenicity tests. The available data are interpreted critically according to the end-points detected, which may include DNA damage, gene mutation, sister chromatid exchange, micronucleus formation, chromosomal aberrations and aneuploidy. The concentrations employed are given, and mention is made of whether the use of an exogenous metabolic system in vitro affected the test result. These data are listed in tabular form by phylogenetic classification.

Positive results in tests using prokaryotes, lower eukaryotes, insects, plants and cultured mammalian cells suggest that genetic and related effects could occur in mammals. Results from such tests may also give information on the types of genetic effect produced and on the involvement of metabolic activation. Some end-points described are clearly genetic in nature (e.g. gene mutations), while others are associated with genetic effects (e.g. unscheduled DNA synthesis). In-vitro tests for tumour promotion, cell transformation and gap–junction intercellular communication may be sensitive to changes that are not necessarily the result of genetic alterations but that may have specific relevance to the process of carcinogenesis. Critical appraisals of these tests have been published (Montesano *et al.*, 1986; McGregor *et al.*, 1999).

Genetic or other activity manifest in humans and experimental mammals is regarded to be of greater relevance than that in other organisms. The demonstration that an agent can induce gene and chromosomal mutations in mammals in vivo indicates that it may have carcinogenic activity. Negative results in tests for mutagenicity in selected tissues from animals treated in vivo provide less weight, partly because they do not exclude the possibility of an effect in tissues other than those examined. Moreover, negative results in short-term tests with genetic end-points cannot be considered to provide evidence that rules out the carcinogenicity of agents that act through other mechanisms (e.g. receptor-mediated effects, cellular toxicity with regenerative cell division, peroxisome proliferation) (Vainio *et al.*, 1992). Factors that may give misleading results in short-term tests have been discussed in detail elsewhere (Montesano *et al.*, 1986; McGregor *et al.*, 1999).

When there is evidence that an agent acts by a specific mechanism that does not involve genotoxicity (e.g. hormonal dysregulation, immune suppression, and formation of calculi and other deposits that cause chronic irritation), that evidence is presented and reviewed critically in the context of rigorous criteria for the operation of that mechanism in carcinogenesis (e.g. Capen *et al.*, 1999).

For biological agents such as viruses, bacteria and parasites, other data relevant to carcinogenicity may include descriptions of the pathology of infection, integration and expression of viruses, and genetic alterations seen in human tumours. Other observations that might comprise cellular and tissue responses to infection, immune response and the presence of tumour markers are also considered.

For physical agents that are forms of radiation, other data relevant to carcinogenicity may include descriptions of damaging effects at the physiological, cellular and molecular level, as for chemical agents, and descriptions of how these effects occur. 'Physical agents' may also be considered to comprise foreign bodies, such as surgical implants of various kinds, and poorly soluble fibres, dusts and particles of various sizes, the pathogenic effects of which are a result of their physical presence in tissues or body cavities. Other relevant data for such materials may include characterization of cellular, tissue and physiological reactions to these materials and descriptions of pathological conditions other than neoplasia with which they may be associated.

(c) Other data relevant to mechanisms

A description is provided of any structure–activity relationships that may be relevant to an evaluation of the carcinogenicity of an agent, the toxicological implications of the physical and chemical properties, and any other data relevant to the evaluation that are not included elsewhere.

High-output data, such as those derived from gene expression microarrays, and high-throughput data, such as those that result from testing hundreds of agents for a single end-point, pose a unique problem for the use of mechanistic data in the evaluation of a carcinogenic hazard. In the case of high-output data, there is the possibility to overinterpret changes in individual end-points (e.g. changes in expression in one gene) without considering the consistency of that finding in the broader context of the other end-points (e.g. other genes with linked transcriptional control). High-output data can be used in assessing mechanisms, but all end-points measured in a single experiment need to be considered in the proper context. For high-throughput data, where the number of observations far exceeds the number of end-points measured, their utility for identifying common mechanisms across multiple agents is enhanced. These data can be used to identify mechanisms that not only seem plausible, but also have a consistent pattern of carcinogenic response across entire classes of related compounds.

(d) Susceptibility data

Individuals, populations and life-stages may have greater or lesser susceptibility to an agent, based on toxicokinetics, mechanisms of carcinogenesis and other factors. Examples of host and genetic factors that affect individual susceptibility include sex, genetic polymorphisms of genes involved in the metabolism of the agent under evaluation, differences in metabolic capacity due to life-stage or the presence of disease, differences in DNA repair capacity, competition for or alteration of metabolic capacity by medications or other chemical exposures, pre-existing hormonal imbalance that is exacerbated by a chemical exposure, a suppressed immune system, periods of higher-than-usual tissue growth or regeneration and genetic polymorphisms that lead to differences in behaviour (e.g. addiction). Such data can substantially increase the strength of the evidence from epidemiological data and enhance the linkage of in-vivo and in-vitro laboratory studies to humans.

(e) Data on other adverse effects

Data on acute, subchronic and chronic adverse effects relevant to the cancer evaluation are summarized. Adverse effects that confirm distribution and biological effects at the sites of tumour development, or alterations in physiology that could lead to tumour development, are emphasized. Effects on reproduction, embryonic and fetal survival and development are summarized briefly. The adequacy of epidemiological studies of reproductive outcome and genetic and related effects in humans is judged by the same criteria as those applied to epidemiological studies of cancer, but fewer details are given.

5. Summary

This section is a summary of data presented in the preceding sections. Summaries can be found on the *Monographs* programme web site (http://monographs.iarc.fr).

(a) Exposure data

Data are summarized, as appropriate, on the basis of elements such as production, use, occurrence and exposure levels in the workplace and environment and measurements in human tissues and body fluids. Quantitative data and time trends are given to compare exposures in different occupations and environmental settings. Exposure to biological agents is described in terms of transmission, prevalence and persistence of infection.

(b) Cancer in humans

Results of epidemiological studies pertinent to an assessment of human carcinogenicity are summarized. When relevant, case reports and correlation studies are also summarized. The target organ(s) or tissue(s) in which an increase in cancer was observed is identified. Dose–response and other quantitative data may be summarized when available.

(c) Cancer in experimental animals

Data relevant to an evaluation of carcinogenicity in animals are summarized. For each animal species, study design and route of administration, it is stated whether an increased incidence, reduced latency, or increased severity or multiplicity of neoplasms or preneoplastic lesions were observed, and the tumour sites are indicated. If the agent produced tumours after prenatal exposure or in single-dose experiments, this is also mentioned. Negative findings, inverse relationships, dose–response and other quantitative data are also summarized.

(d) Mechanistic and other relevant data

Data relevant to the toxicokinetics (absorption, distribution, metabolism, elimination) and the possible mechanism(s) of carcinogenesis (e.g. genetic toxicity, epigenetic effects) are summarized. In addition, information on susceptible individuals, populations and life-stages is summarized. This section also reports on other toxic effects, including reproductive and developmental effects, as well as additional relevant data that are considered to be important.

6. Evaluation and rationale

Evaluations of the strength of the evidence for carcinogenicity arising from human and experimental animal data are made, using standard terms. The strength of the mechanistic evidence is also characterized.

It is recognized that the criteria for these evaluations, described below, cannot encompass all of the factors that may be relevant to an evaluation of carcinogenicity. In considering all of the relevant scientific data, the Working Group may assign the agent to a higher or lower category than a strict interpretation of these criteria would indicate.

These categories refer only to the strength of the evidence that an exposure is carcinogenic and not to the extent of its carcinogenic activity (potency). A classification may change as new information becomes available.

An evaluation of the degree of evidence is limited to the materials tested, as defined physically, chemically or biologically. When the agents evaluated are considered by the Working Group to be sufficiently closely related, they may be grouped together for the purpose of a single evaluation of the degree of evidence.

(a) Carcinogenicity in humans

The evidence relevant to carcinogenicity from studies in humans is classified into one of the following categories:

Sufficient evidence of carcinogenicity: The Working Group considers that a causal relationship has been established between exposure to the agent and human cancer. That is, a positive relationship has been observed between the exposure and cancer in studies in which chance, bias and confounding could be ruled out with reasonable confidence. A statement that there is *sufficient evidence* is followed by a separate sentence that identifies the target organ(s) or tissue(s) where an increased risk of cancer was observed in humans. Identification of a specific target organ or tissue does not preclude the possibility that the agent may cause cancer at other sites.

Limited evidence of carcinogenicity: A positive association has been observed between exposure to the agent and cancer for which a causal interpretation is considered by the Working Group to be credible, but chance, bias or confounding could not be ruled out with reasonable confidence.

Inadequate evidence of carcinogenicity: The available studies are of insufficient quality, consistency or statistical power to permit a conclusion regarding the presence or absence of a causal association between exposure and cancer, or no data on cancer in humans are available.

Evidence suggesting lack of carcinogenicity: There are several adequate studies covering the full range of levels of exposure that humans are known to encounter, which are mutually consistent in not showing a positive association between exposure to the agent and any studied cancer at any observed level of exposure. The results from these studies alone or combined should have narrow confidence intervals with an upper limit close to the null value (e.g. a relative risk of 1.0). Bias and confounding should be ruled out with reasonable confidence, and the studies should have an adequate length of follow-up. A conclusion of *evidence suggesting lack of carcinogenicity* is inevitably limited to the cancer sites, conditions and levels of exposure, and length of observation covered by the available studies. In addition, the possibility of a very small risk at the levels of exposure studied can never be excluded.

In some instances, the above categories may be used to classify the degree of evidence related to carcinogenicity in specific organs or tissues.

When the available epidemiological studies pertain to a mixture, process, occupation or industry, the Working Group seeks to identify the specific agent considered most likely to be responsible for any excess risk. The evaluation is focused as narrowly as the available data on exposure and other aspects permit.

(b) Carcinogenicity in experimental animals

Carcinogenicity in experimental animals can be evaluated using conventional bioassays, bioassays that employ genetically modified animals, and other in-vivo bioassays that focus on one or more of the critical stages of carcinogenesis. In the absence of data from conventional long-term bioassays or from assays with neoplasia as the end-point, consistently positive results in several models that address several stages in the multistage process of carcinogenesis should be considered in evaluating the degree of evidence of carcinogenicity in experimental animals.

The evidence relevant to carcinogenicity in experimental animals is classified into one of the following categories:

Sufficient evidence of carcinogenicity: The Working Group considers that a causal relationship has been established between the agent and an increased incidence of malignant neoplasms or of an appropriate combination of benign and malignant neoplasms in (a) two or more species of animals or (b) two or more independent studies in one species carried out at different times or in different laboratories or under different protocols. An increased incidence of tumours in both sexes of a single species in a well conducted study, ideally conducted under Good Laboratory Practices, can also provide *sufficient evidence*.

A single study in one species and sex might be considered to provide *sufficient evidence of carcinogenicity* when malignant neoplasms occur to an unusual degree with regard to incidence, site, type of tumour or age at onset, or when there are strong findings of tumours at multiple sites.

Limited evidence of carcinogenicity: The data suggest a carcinogenic effect but are limited for making a definitive evaluation because, e.g. (a) the evidence of carcinogenicity is restricted to a single experiment; (b) there are unresolved questions regarding the adequacy of the design, conduct or interpretation of the studies; (c) the agent increases the incidence only of benign neoplasms or lesions of uncertain neoplastic potential; or (d) the evidence of carcinogenicity is restricted to studies that demonstrate only promoting activity in a narrow range of tissues or organs.

Inadequate evidence of carcinogenicity: The studies cannot be interpreted as showing either the presence or absence of a carcinogenic effect because of major qualitative or quantitative limitations, or no data on cancer in experimental animals are available.

Evidence suggesting lack of carcinogenicity: Adequate studies involving at least two species are available which show that, within the limits of the tests used, the agent is not carcinogenic. A conclusion of *evidence suggesting lack of carcinogenicity* is inevitably limited to the species, tumour sites, age at exposure, and conditions and levels of exposure studied.

(c) Mechanistic and other relevant data

Mechanistic and other evidence judged to be relevant to an evaluation of carcinogenicity and of sufficient importance to affect the overall evaluation is highlighted. This may include data on preneoplastic lesions, tumour pathology, genetic and related effects, structure–activity relationships, metabolism and toxicokinetics, physicochemical parameters and analogous biological agents.

The strength of the evidence that any carcinogenic effect observed is due to a particular mechanism is evaluated, using terms such as 'weak', 'moderate' or 'strong'. The Working Group then assesses whether that particular mechanism is likely to be operative in humans. The strongest indications that a particular mechanism operates in humans derive from data on humans or biological specimens obtained from exposed humans. The data may be considered to be especially relevant if they show that the agent in question has caused changes in exposed humans that are on the causal pathway to carcinogenesis. Such data may, however, never become available, because it is at least conceivable that certain compounds may be kept from human use solely on the basis of evidence of their toxicity and/or carcinogenicity in experimental systems.

The conclusion that a mechanism operates in experimental animals is strengthened by findings of consistent results in different experimental systems, by the demonstration of biological plausibility and by coherence of the overall database. Strong support can be obtained from studies that challenge the hypothesized mechanism experimentally, by demonstrating that the suppression of key mechanistic processes leads to the suppression of tumour development. The Working Group considers whether multiple mechanisms might contribute to tumour development, whether different mechanisms might operate in different dose ranges, whether separate mechanisms might operate in humans and experimental animals and whether a unique mechanism might operate in a susceptible group. The possible contribution of alternative mechanisms must be considered before concluding that tumours observed in experimental animals are not relevant to humans. An uneven level of experimental support for different mechanisms may reflect that disproportionate resources have been focused on investigating a favoured mechanism.

For complex exposures, including occupational and industrial exposures, the chemical composition and the potential contribution of carcinogens known to be present are considered by the Working Group in its overall evaluation of human carcinogenicity. The Working Group also determines the extent to which the materials tested in experimental systems are related to those to which humans are exposed.

(d) Overall evaluation

Finally, the body of evidence is considered as a whole, to reach an overall evaluation of the carcinogenicity of the agent to humans.

An evaluation may be made for a group of agents that have been evaluated by the Working Group. In addition, when supporting data indicate that other related agents, for which there is no direct evidence of their capacity to induce cancer in humans or in animals, may also be carcinogenic, a statement describing the rationale for this conclusion is added to the evaluation narrative; an additional evaluation may be made for this broader group of agents if the strength of the evidence warrants it.

The agent is described according to the wording of one of the following categories, and the designated group is given. The categorization of an agent is a matter of scientific judgement that reflects the strength of the evidence derived from studies in humans and in experimental animals and from mechanistic and other relevant data.

Group 1: The agent is carcinogenic to humans.

This category is used when there is *sufficient evidence of carcinogenicity* in humans. Exceptionally, an agent may be placed in this category when evidence of carcinogenicity in humans is less than *sufficient* but there is *sufficient evidence of carcinogenicity* in experimental animals and strong evidence in exposed humans that the agent acts through a relevant mechanism of carcinogenicity.

Group 2.

This category includes agents for which, at one extreme, the degree of evidence of carcinogenicity in humans is almost *sufficient*, as well as those for which, at the other extreme, there are no human data but for which there is evidence of carcinogenicity in experimental animals. Agents are assigned to either Group 2A (*probably carcinogenic to humans*) or Group 2B (*possibly carcinogenic to humans*) on the basis of epidemiological and experimental evidence of carcinogenicity and mechanistic and other relevant data. The terms *probably carcinogenic* and *possibly carcinogenic* have no quantitative significance and are used simply as descriptors of different levels of evidence of human carcinogenicity, with *probably carcinogenic* signifying a higher level of evidence than *possibly carcinogenic*.

Group 2A: The agent is probably carcinogenic to humans.

This category is used when there is *limited evidence of carcinogenicity* in humans and *sufficient evidence of carcinogenicity* in experimental animals. In some cases, an agent may be classified in this category when there is *inadequate evidence of carcinogenicity* in humans and *sufficient evidence of carcinogenicity* in experimental animals and strong evidence that the carcinogenesis is mediated by a mechanism that also operates in humans. Exceptionally, an agent may be classified in this category solely on the basis of *limited evidence of carcinogenicity* in humans. An agent may be assigned to this category if it clearly belongs, based on mechanistic considerations, to a class of agents for which one or more members have been classified in Group 1 or Group 2A.

Group 2B: The agent is possibly carcinogenic to humans.

This category is used for agents for which there is *limited evidence of carcinogenicity* in humans and less than *sufficient evidence of carcinogenicity* in experimental animals. It may also be used when there is *inadequate evidence of carcinogenicity* in humans but there is *sufficient evidence of carcinogenicity* in experimental animals. In some instances, an agent for which there is *inadequate evidence of carcinogenicity* in humans and less than *sufficient evidence of carcinogenicity* in experimental animals together with supporting evidence from mechanistic and other relevant data may be placed in this group. An agent may be classified in this category solely on the basis of strong evidence from mechanistic and other relevant data.

Group 3: The agent is not classifiable as to its carcinogenicity to humans.

This category is used most commonly for agents for which the evidence of carcinogenicity is *inadequate* in humans and *inadequate* or *limited* in experimental animals.

Exceptionally, agents for which the evidence of carcinogenicity is *inadequate* in humans but *sufficient* in experimental animals may be placed in this category when there is strong evidence that the mechanism of carcinogenicity in experimental animals does not operate in humans.

Agents that do not fall into any other group are also placed in this category.

An evaluation in Group 3 is not a determination of non-carcinogenicity or overall safety. It often means that further research is needed, especially when exposures are widespread or the cancer data are consistent with differing interpretations.

Group 4: The agent is probably not carcinogenic to humans.

This category is used for agents for which there is *evidence suggesting lack of carcinogenicity* in humans and in experimental animals. In some instances, agents for which there is *inadequate evidence of carcinogenicity* in humans but *evidence suggesting lack of carcinogenicity* in experimental animals, consistently and strongly supported by a broad range of mechanistic and other relevant data, may be classified in this group.

(e) Rationale

The reasoning that the Working Group used to reach its evaluation is presented and discussed. This section integrates the major findings from studies of cancer in humans, studies of cancer in experimental animals, and mechanistic and other relevant data. It includes concise statements of the principal line(s) of argument that emerged, the conclusions of the Working Group on the strength of the evidence for each group of studies, citations to indicate which studies were pivotal to these conclusions, and an explanation of the reasoning of the Working Group in weighing data and making evaluations. When there are significant differences of scientific interpretation among Working Group Members, a brief summary of the alternative interpretations is provided, together with their scientific rationale and an indication of the relative degree of support for each alternative.

References

Bieler GS & Williams RL (1993). Ratio estimates, the delta method, and quantal response tests for increased carcinogenicity. *Biometrics*, 49: 793–801. doi:10.2307/2532200 PMID:8241374

Breslow NE & Day NE (1980). Statistical methods in cancer research. Volume I - The analysis of case-control studies. *IARC Sci Publ*, 32: 5–338. PMID:7216345

Breslow NE & Day NE (1987). Statistical methods in cancer research. Volume II–The design and analysis of cohort studies. *IARC Sci Publ*, 82: 1–406. PMID:3329634

Buffler P, Rice J, Baan R *et al.* (2004). Workshop on Mechanisms of Carcinogenesis: Contributions of Molecular Epidemiology. Lyon, 14–17 November 2001. Workshop report. *IARC Sci Publ*, 157: 1–27. PMID:15055286

Capen CC, Dybing E, Rice JM, Wilbourn JD (1999). Species Differences in Thyroid, Kidney and Urinary Bladder Carcinogenesis. Proceedings of a consensus conference. Lyon, France, 3–7 November 1997. *IARC Sci Publ*, 147: 1–225.

Cogliano V, Baan R, Straif K *et al.* (2005). Transparency in IARC Monographs. *Lancet Oncol*, 6: 747. doi:10.1016/S1470-2045(05)70380-6

Cogliano VJ, Baan RA, Straif K *et al.* (2004). The science and practice of carcinogen identification and evaluation. *Environ Health Perspect*, 112: 1269–1274. doi:10.1289/ehp.6950 PMID:15345338

Dunson DB, Chen Z, Harry J (2003). A Bayesian approach for joint modeling of cluster size and subunit-specific outcomes. *Biometrics*, 59: 521–530. doi:10.1111/1541-0420.00062 PMID:14601753

Fung KY, Krewski D, Smythe RT (1996). A comparison of tests for trend with historical controls in carcinogen bioassay. *Can J Stat*, 24: 431–454. doi:10.2307/3315326

Gart JJ, Krewski D, Lee PN *et al.* (1986). Statistical methods in cancer research. Volume III–The design and analysis of long-term animal experiments. *IARC Sci Publ*, 79: 1–219. PMID:3301661

Greenland S (1998). Meta-analysis. In: *Modern Epidemiology*. Rothman KJ, Greenland S, editors. Philadelphia: Lippincott Williams & Wilkins, pp. 643–673

Greim H, Gelbke H-P, Reuter U *et al.* (2003). Evaluation of historical control data in carcinogenicity studies. *Hum Exp Toxicol*, 22: 541–549. doi:10.1191/0960327103ht394oa PMID:14655720

Haseman JK, Huff J, Boorman GA (1984). Use of historical control data in carcinogenicity studies in rodents. *Toxicol Pathol*, 12: 126–135. doi:10.1177/019262338401200203 PMID:11478313

Hill AB (1965). The environment and disease: Association or causation? *Proc R Soc Med*, 58: 295–300. PMID:14283879

Hoel DG, Kaplan NL, Anderson MW (1983). Implication of nonlinear kinetics on risk estimation in carcinogenesis. *Science*, 219: 1032–1037. doi:10.1126/science.6823565 PMID:6823565

Huff JE, Eustis SL, Haseman JK (1989). Occurrence and relevance of chemically induced benign neoplasms in long-term carcinogenicity studies. *Cancer Metastasis Rev*, 8: 1–22. doi:10.1007/BF00047055 PMID:2667783

IARC (1977). *IARC Monographs Programme on the Evaluation of the Carcinogenic Risk of Chemicals to Humans*. Preamble (IARC Intern Tech Rep No. 77/002)

IARC (1978). *Chemicals with Sufficient Evidence of Carcinogenicity in Experimental Animals – IARC Monographs Volumes 1–17* (IARC Intern Tech Rep No. 78/003)

IARC (1979). *Criteria to Select Chemicals for* IARC Monographs (IARC Intern Tech Rep No. 79/003)

IARC (1982). Chemicals, industrial processes and industries associated with cancer in humans (IARC Monographs, Volumes 1 to 29). *IARC Monogr Eval Carcinog Risk Chem Hum Suppl*, 4: 1-292.

IARC (1983). *Approaches to Classifying Chemical Carcinogens According to Mechanism of Action* (IARC Intern Tech Rep No. 83/001)

IARC (1987). Overall evaluations of carcinogenicity: an updating of IARC Monographs volumes 1 to 42. *IARC Monogr Eval Carcinog Risks Hum Suppl*, 7: 1–440. PMID:3482203

IARC (1988). *Report of an IARC Working Group to Review the Approaches and Processes Used to Evaluate the Carcinogenicity of Mixtures and Groups of Chemicals* (IARC Intern Tech Rep No. 88/002)

IARC (1991). *A Consensus Report of an IARC Monographs Working Group on the Use of Mechanisms of Carcinogenesis in Risk Identification* (IARC Intern Tech Rep No. 91/002)

IARC (2005). *Report of the Advisory Group to Recommend Updates to the Preamble to the* IARC Monographs (IARC Intern Rep No. 05/001)

IARC (2006). *Report of the Advisory Group to Review the Amended Preamble to the* IARC Monographs (IARC Intern Rep No. 06/001)

IARC (2004). Some drinking-water disinfectants and contaminants, including arsenic. *IARC Monogr Eval Carcinog Risks Hum*, 84: 1–477. PMID:15645577

McGregor DB, Rice JM, Venitt S, editors (1999). The use of short- and medium-term tests for carcinogens and data on genetic effects in carcinogenic hazard evaluation. Consensus report. *IARC Sci Publ*, 146: 1–536.

Montesano R, Bartsch H, Vainio H *et al.*, editors (1986). Long-term and short-term assays for carcinogenesis—a critical appraisal. *IARC Sci Publ*, 83: 1–564.

OECD (2002). *Guidance Notes for Analysis and Evaluation of Chronic Toxicity and Carcinogenicity Studies* (Series on Testing and Assessment No. 35), Paris: OECD

Peto R, Pike MC, Day NE *et al.* (1980). Guidelines for simple, sensitive significance tests for carcinogenic effects in long-term animal experiments. *IARC Monogr Eval Carcinog Risk Chem Hum Suppl*, 2: 311–426. PMID:6935185

Portier CJ & Bailer AJ (1989). Testing for increased carcinogenicity using a survival-adjusted quantal response test. *Fundam Appl Toxicol*, 12: 731–737. doi:10.1016/0272-0590(89)90004-3 PMID:2744275

Sherman CD, Portier CJ, Kopp-Schneider A (1994). Multistage models of carcinogenesis: an approximation for the size and number distribution of late-stage clones. *Risk Anal*, 14: 1039–1048. doi:10.1111/j.1539-6924.1994.tb00074.x PMID:7846311

Stewart BW, Kleihues P, editors (2003). *World Cancer Report*, Lyon: IARC

Tomatis L, Aitio A, Wilbourn J, Shuker L (1989). Human carcinogens so far identified. *Jpn J Cancer Res*, 80: 795–807. PMID:2513295

Toniolo P, Boffetta P, Shuker DEG *et al.*, editors (1997). Proceedings of the workshop on application of biomarkers to cancer epidemiology. Lyon, France, 20–23 February 1996. *IARC Sci Publ*, 142: 1–318.

Vainio H, Magee P, McGregor D, McMichael A, editors (1992). Mechanisms of carcinogenesis in risk identification. IARC Working Group Meeting. Lyon, 11–18 June 1991. *IARC Sci Publ*, 116: 1–608.

Vainio H, Wilbourn JD, Sasco AJ *et al.* (1995). [Identification of human carcinogenic risks in IARC monographs.] *Bull Cancer*, 82: 339–348. PMID:7626841

Vineis P, Malats N, Lang M *et al.*, editors (1999). Metabolic Polymorphisms and Susceptibility to Cancer. *IARC Sci Publ*, 148: 1–510. PMID:10493243

Wilbourn J, Haroun L, Heseltine E *et al.* (1986). Response of experimental animals to human carcinogens: an analysis based upon the IARC Monographs programme. *Carcinogenesis*, 7: 1853–1863. doi:10.1093/carcin/7.11.1853 PMID:3769134

GENERAL REMARKS

Part E of Volume 100 of the *IARC Monographs on the Evaluation of Carcinogenic Risks to Humans* contains updated assessments of personal habits and indoor combustions that were first classified as *carcinogenic to humans (Group 1)* in Volumes 1–99.

Volume 100 – General Information

About half of the agents classified in Group 1 were last reviewed more than 20 years ago, before mechanistic studies became prominent in evaluations of carcinogenicity. In addition, more recent epidemiological studies and animal cancer bioassays have demonstrated that many cancer hazards reported in earlier studies were later observed in other organs or through different exposure scenarios. Much can be learned by updating the assessments of agents that are known to cause cancer in humans. Accordingly, IARC has selected A Review of Human Carcinogens to be the topic for Volume 100. It is hoped that this volume, by compiling the knowledge accumulated through several decades of cancer research, will stimulate cancer prevention activities worldwide, and will be a valued resource for future research to identify other agents suspected of causing cancer in humans.

Volume 100 was developed by six separate Working Groups:

Pharmaceuticals
Biological agents
Arsenic, metals, fibres, and dusts
Radiation
Personal habits and indoor combustions
Chemical agents and related occupations

Because the scope of Volume 100 is so broad, its *Monographs* are focused on key information. Each *Monograph* presents a description of a carcinogenic agent and how people are exposed, critical overviews of the epidemiological studies and animal cancer bioassays, and a concise review of the toxicokinetic properties of the agent, plausible mechanisms of carcinogenesis, and potentially susceptible populations, and life-stages. Details of the design and results of individual epidemiological studies and animal cancer bioassays are summarized in tables. Short tables that highlight key results appear in the printed version of Volume 100, and more extensive tables that include all studies appear on the website of the *IARC Monographs* programme (http://monographs.iarc.fr). For a few well-established associations (for example, tobacco smoke and human lung cancer), it was impractical to include all studies, even in the website tables. In those instances, the rationale for inclusion or exclusion of sets of studies is given.

Each section of Volume 100 was reviewed by a subgroup of the Working Group with appropriate subject expertise; then all sections of each *Monograph* were discussed together in a plenary session of the full Working Group. As a result, the evaluation statements and other conclusions reflect the views of the Working Group as a whole.

Volume 100 compiles information on tumour sites and mechanisms of carcinogenesis. This information will be used in two scientific publications that may be considered as annexes to this volume. One publication, Tumour Site Concordance between Humans and Experimental Animals, will analyse the correspondence of tumour sites among humans and different animal species. It will discuss the predictive value of different animal tumours for cancer in humans, and perhaps identify human tumour sites for which there are no good animal models. Another publication, Mechanisms Involved in Human Carcinogenesis, will describe mechanisms known to or likely to cause cancer in humans. Joint consideration of multiple agents that act through similar mechanisms should facilitate the development of a more comprehensive discussion of these mechanisms. Because susceptibility often has its basis in a mechanism, this could also facilitate a more confident and precise description of populations that may be susceptible to agents acting through each mechanism. This publication will also suggest biomarkers that could render future research more informataive. In this way, IARC hopes that Volume 100 will serve to improve the design of future cancer studies.

Specific remarks about the agents reviewed in this volume

Billions of people around the world are exposed to one or several of these agents as part of their everyday life. A common theme is that they cause adverse health effects at levels of exposure that are commonly experienced, and collectively are responsible for a disproportionately high portion of the global burden of cancer. At the same time, some of these agents, notably tobacco in all forms and alcoholic beverages, are also mostly discretionary, although marketing and societal influences have played an important role in promoting their use. Therefore, exposure to these agents is largely preventable, through a combination of individual action and governmental intervention, the latter being especially important, for example, in promoting smoking cessation or smoke-free indoor environments.

Tobacco consumption is the single largest cause of cancer in the world. Tobacco smoking was evaluated as providing *sufficient evidence of carcinogenicity* in humans in Volumes 38 (IARC, 1986) and 83 (IARC, 2004a). Some types of smokeless tobacco were evaluated in Volume 37 (IARC, 1985) as having *sufficient evidence of carcinogenicity* in humans; two decades later, Volume 89 (IARC, 2007) classified all types of smokeless tobacco in Group 1. In this volume, the tobacco-specific nitrosamines NNK and NNN were also classified in Group 1 based on strong mechanistic evidence in exposed humans (IARC, 2007). Betel quid, a preparation that includes areca nut with betel leaf and other ingredients, and often tobacco, is chewed by over 600 million people in southern Asia and in Asian-migrant communities across the world. Betel quid with tobacco was evaluated in Volume 37 as having *sufficient evidence of carcinogenicity* in humans, and this classification was reaffirmed and extended to betel quid without tobacco in Volume 85 (IARC, 2004b). In the latter volume, areca nut, the common ingredient in all betel quid preparations, was also classified in Group 1. Alcohol consumption, another major contributor to the global burden of cancer, was classified in Group 1 in Volumes 44 (IARC, 1988) and 96 (IARC, 2010a). Ethanol and acetaldehyde associated with alcoholic beverage consumption were specifically mentioned as carcinogenic agents in the latter volume. Indoor smoke from solid fuels is yet another major contributor to the global burden of disease. The highest individual risks are seen in households that use unvented coal stoves for cooking and heating, an exposure that was classified in Group 1 in Volume 95 (IARC, 2010b). Finally, salted fish was evaluated in Volume 56 (IARC, 1993), with Chinese-style salted fish classified in Group 1.

1. Alcoholic beverages, ethanol and acetaldehyde associated with their consumption

Consumption of alcoholic beverages is one of the top-10 exposures responsible for the burden of disease worldwide. Nearly two billion adults consume alcoholic beverages regularly, with an average daily consumption of 13 g ethanol (about one drink). The Working Group that evaluated alcohol consumption recently (IARC, 2010a) concluded that it causes cancers of the oral cavity, pharynx, larynx, oesophagus, colorectum, liver and female breast. With respect to the latter cancer type, the risk increases with increasing alcohol intake by about 10% per 10 g per day. Epidemiological evidence shows little indication that the carcinogenic effects depend on the type of alcoholic beverage.

The metabolism of ethanol, the key component in alcoholic beverages, can be essentially described as a two-step dehydrogenation process. In humans, the major enzymes involved are the alcohol dehydrogenases (ADH), which oxidize ethanol to its toxic intermediate, acetaldehyde, and the aldehyde dehydrogenases (ALDH), which detoxify acetaldehyde to acetate. The two groups of dehydrogenases exhibit genetic variations that confer wide differences in enzyme kinetics and substrate specificities and that vary widely across ethnicities (figure). Studies on the carcinogenicity of alcoholic beverages consumption give a striking example of a genetic polymorphism that strongly influences the response to a carcinogen. The variant *ALDH2*2* allele, which encodes an inactive subunit of the enzyme ALDH2, is highly prevalent in certain eastern-Asian populations (28–45%), but rare in other ethnic groups. Most homozygous carriers of this allele (*ALDH2*2/*2*) are abstainers or infrequent drinkers, because the complete deficiency of enzymatic activity would cause a strong facial flushing response, physical discomfort, and severe toxic reactions when consuming alcoholic beverages. In heterozygous carriers (*ALDH2*1/*2*), who have about 10% residual ALDH2 activity, these acute adverse effects are less severe, but these persons have higher levels of acetaldehyde in their blood and saliva after alcohol drinking, and higher levels of acetaldehyde-related DNA adducts in their lymphocytes compared with those with fully active enzyme (*ALDH2*1/*1* genotype). In addition, these individuals are at high risk for several alcohol-related aerodigestive cancers. Examining the role of acetaldehyde as a cause of aerodigestive cancers is further complicated by competing risk factors such as tobacco smoking, areca nut chewing, infection by HPV; in addition, this association may be modified by microflora present in the aerodigestive tract, which have high ADH but low ALDH enzyme activity (Chang *et al.*, 2011).

The previous Working Group acknowledged the important role of acetaldehyde in the development of alcohol-related cancer, especially of the esophagus, but refrained from making a formal evaluation of this metabolite. The Working Group for this Volume considered that the available epidemiological data clearly indicates that humans who are deficient in the oxidation of acetaldehyde to acetate have a substantially increased risk for development of alcohol-related cancers, and decided to make a separate evaluation for “acetaldehyde associated with alcoholic beverage consumption”.

ADH1B*1& ADH1C*2 **(slow ethanol-oxidizing) &** ***ALDH2*2*** **(null) allele frequencies by population and incidence of head and neck cancer**

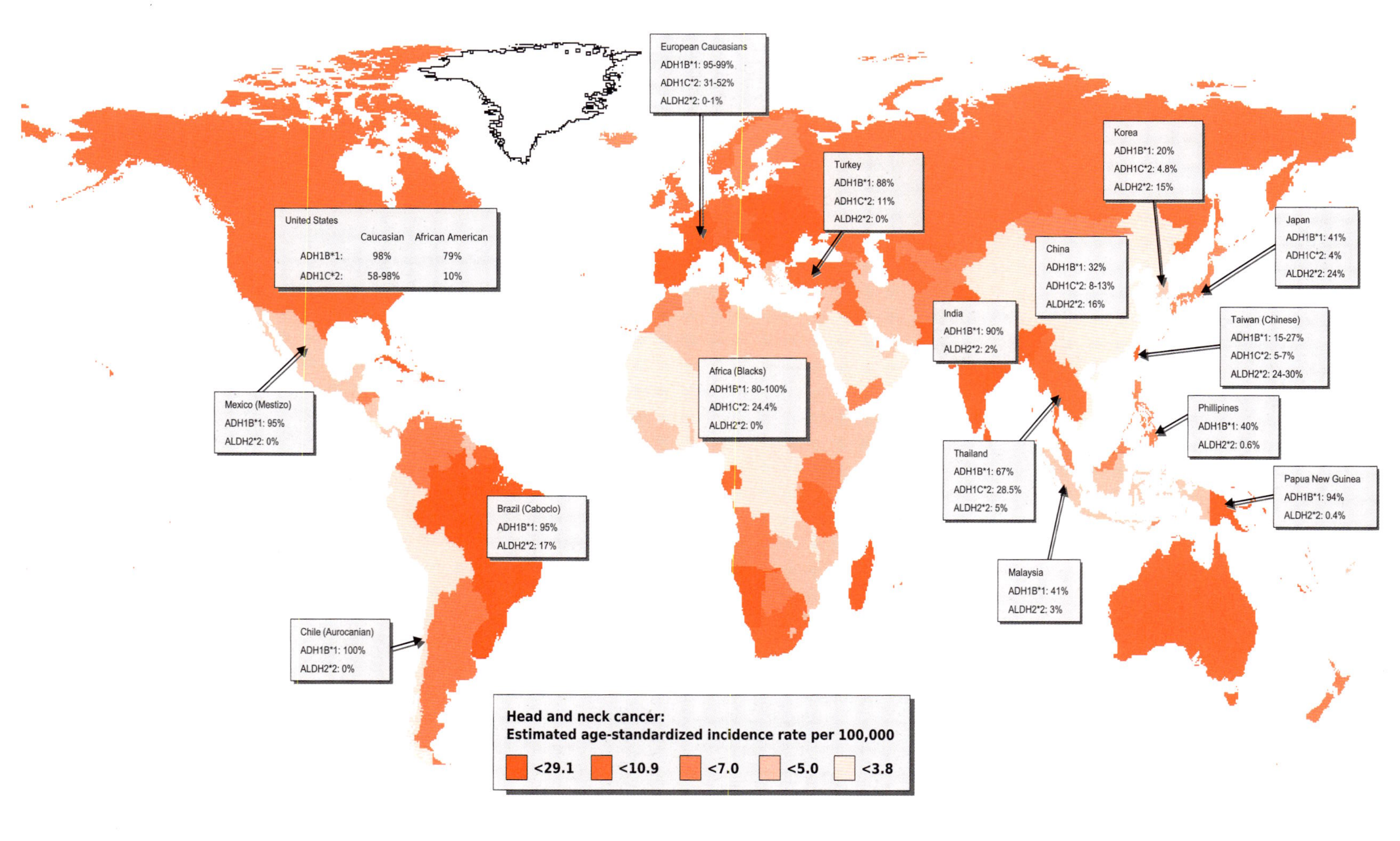

From Chang *et al.* (2011) (Supplementary figure)

2. Betel quid with and without tobacco, areca nut and smokeless tobacco

Smokeless tobacco and areca nut are consumed by millions of people across the globe and may be social practices deeply rooted in their respective cultures. In this *Monograph*, any product containing areca nut is referred to as 'betel quid', the most common name given for such products.

Smokeless tobacco and betel quid share many features. Both products are addictive (Warnakulasuriya, 2004; Chu, 2001), and most evidence suggests that users find it difficult to quit these behaviours. Both are typically used orally, being chewed and then spit out. Although generally considered as a social practice, both have other uses: for example, various forms of smokeless tobacco are used as a dentifrice in India. Both products are rarely used alone and are generally consumed with other constituents, added during manufacture or by the user. Notably, both may contain an additive that increases the pH of the product, which has the effect of unprotonating the psychoactive substance, thus making it readily bioavailable: nicotine in the case of smokeless tobacco and arecoline in the case of areca nut (for reviews, see Chu, 2001; Djordjevic *et al.*, 1995). Other additives to both smokeless tobacco and industrially manufactured betel quid may include flavourings and sweeteners.

2.1 Disentangling the effects of the various ingredients

Some populations use only areca nut and slaked lime in their betel quid. Since cancer bioassays have shown that slaked lime is not carcinogenic, studies from these populations provide evidence that areca nut is a cause of cancer in human populations. Studies of betel quids with a variety of other ingredients except tobacco provide evidence for the carcinogenicity to humans of betel quid without tobacco overall. Finally, studies that either assess specifically betel quid with tobacco, or that did not specify whether tobacco was added, or that combined individuals who may or may not include tobacco in their quid, together provide evidence for the carcinogenicity of betel quid with tobacco.

Areca nut and/or smokeless tobacco are highly prevalent in some cultures, e.g. in Sweden, up to 30% of men use smokeless tobacco. In 2002, it was estimated that 600 million people worldwide, primarily in the Indian sub-continent, used areca nut. In the successive IARC Monographs that have addressed either smokeless tobacco or areca nut, new formulations of these products and new populations with such habits have been reported.

New forms of these products are constantly being developed and introduced on the market in formulations that encourage initiation or maintenance of use of these products. For example, portion sizes and packaging render them more convenient for people to use, while flavourings may appeal to young persons.

Finally, no betel quid or tobacco product in any culture has been shown to be safe or free of risk of cancer. Despite the wide variation in added ingredients, method of preparation or manufacture of the product, mode of use and populations concerned, these products have been associated with an increased risk of cancer. Nevertheless, these products are promoted as "safe" alternatives to tobacco smoking and many people consider products such as *pan masala* to be safe. However, one study from North America found that smokers who had switched to smokeless tobacco had a higher death rate than men who quit tobacco entirely (Henley *et al.*, 2007).

2.2 Betel inflorescence

Betel inflorescence grows on Piper betel L. and is the male fruit, consumed with unripe areca nut in Taiwan, China. Betel inflorescence contains high levels of phenolic compounds including hydroxychavicol and safrole.

Of the different types of betel quid consumed in Taiwan, China, those that include betel inflorescence (*lao-hwa* quid) induced the highest risk for both oral leukoplakia and submucous fibrosis (Lee *et al.* 2003), and for oral and combined cancers of the oro- and hypopharynx (Ko *et al.* 1995; Chen *et al.* 2002).

Carcinogenic risk of betel inflorescence and mechanistic pathways should be examined in detail in the future.

2.3 Cancer burden

The magnitude of the risks associated with smokeless tobacco and betel quid vary, and can be very high. This, combined with the high prevalence of some behaviours in some parts of the world, leads to a very high cancer burden. In India for instance, the cancer burden from these habits meets or exceeds that of smoking.

3. Tobacco smoke: multiple exposures, multiple chemicals, multiple target sites

3.1 Tobacco smoke carcinogens

Tobacco smoke is the most pleiotropic carcinogen ever evaluated by the *IARC Monographs* Programme, with over 20 target sites to which it has been shown to be causally associated. The chemical compositions of mainstream smoke and sidestream smoke are qualitatively similar, although quantitatively different. Tobacco smoke contains over 60 chemicals or other agents that have been shown to be carcinogenic in rodents; for a dozen of those, there is also *sufficient evidence* of their carcinogenicity in humans.

For the agents present in tobacco smoke and that are classified as IARC Group 1 or Group 2A, the table below presents the target sites for which there is *sufficient* or *limited* evidence in humans.

3.2 Parental tobacco smoking

The prevalence of exposure to tobacco smoke from parental smoking varies by socioeconomic status and country, ranging up to 60% in some surveys. Exposure of the offspring may occur preconception, *in utero* or postnatally. Active smoking by either genitor preconception and maternal smoking during pregnancy both imply direct exposure to mainstream tobacco smoke of the germ cells (spermatozoa and ova) and of the foetus, respectively. In contrast, paternal smoking during pregnancy and parental smoking post-natally represent exposures to second-hand tobacco smoke.

How to evaluate separately the effect of the different exposures and time periods? Early studies generally only assessed the contribution of maternal exposures during pregnancy, whereas recent studies included assessments of exposure preconception, in particular from paternal smoking. Exposure may have occurred in all three periods even when a study reports on only one, or exposure may also be

Target sites associated with some carcinogenic chemical compounds and metals present in tobacco smoke

Agent	Tumour sites or types for which there is *sufficient* evidence in humans	Tumour sites or types for which there is *limited* evidence in humans
Chemicals		
1,3-Butadiene	Hematolymphatic organs	
2-Naphthylamine	Urinary bladder	
4-Aminobiphenyl	Urinary bladder	
Benzene	Acute non-lymphocytic leukaemia	Acute lymphocytic leukaemia, chronic lymphocytic leukaemia, multiple myeloma, non-Hodgkin lymphoma
Ethylene oxide		Breast, lymphoid tumours
Formaldehyde	Nasopharynx, leukaemia (particularly myeloid leukaemia)	Sinonasal cancer
o-Toluidine	Urinary bladder	
Vinyl chloride	Hepatocellular carcinoma, hepatic angiosarcoma	
Metals		
Arsenic and inorganic arsenic compounds	Lung, skin, urinary bladder	Kidney, liver, prostate
Beryllium and beryllium compounds	Lung	
Cadmium and cadmium compounds	Lung	Kidney, prostate
Chromium (VI) compounds	Lung	Nasal cavity and paranasal sinuses
Lead		Stomach
Nickel compounds	Lung, nasal cavity and paranasal sinuses	

Adapted from Cogliano *et al.* (2011)

reported as 'ever' exposed. In addition, parental smoking during each of these time periods tends to be correlated, in particular from the father, because father's smoking habits are less likely to change during pregnancy. Furthermore, paternal and maternal smoking habits are often correlated, and the risks may be increased when both parents smoke. Thus establishing a link between parental smoking and childhood cancer risk relates to several different exposures that are tightly correlated and difficult to disentangle.

The younger the child at diagnosis, the more direct prenatal exposures appear to be relevant compared to post-natal exposures. Stronger associations for cancer in offspring were observed from parental smoking preconception than from maternal smoking during pregnancy. Interestingly, the strongest and most consistent association was observed for hepatoblastoma, an embryonal tumour of presumably foetal origin, which has a median age of diagnosis of about 12 months. Cigarette smoke is a known germ-cell mutagen in mice and a likely germ-cell mutagen in humans. The effect of such mutagenicity on cancer risk in the offspring of smoking parents has now been demonstrated in human populations.

4. Coal Emissions

The use of coal in homes for cooking and heating is a major source of indoor air pollution in Asia, particularly in China. Emissions from the combustion of coal have been associated with a variety of health outcomes, especially lung cancer. The population at risk for illness from indoor air pollution numbers in the hundreds of millions in China alone, and possibly more than a billion worldwide. Women and children bear the largest share of the burden of disease from this exposure since they spend longer periods of time inside the home. Greater awareness of this exposure should be emphasized for these vulnerable groups. The development and implementation of appropriate improvement in ventilation and other strategies to reduce indoor air pollution in developing countries should be supported and encouraged from both the government and interested private parties in the commercial sector. The replacement of coal with cleaner fuels should also be a high priority. However, since many millions of people cannot afford to change the household fuels that they use, alternative efforts are necessary in the interim.

5. Salted fish

The Working Group has evaluated Chinese-style salted fish defined as salted fish consumed in Chinese populations, the majority of studies being from the Southern part of China. The evaluation of epidemiological studies has found *sufficient evidence* for an association with nasopharyngeal carcinoma, and *limited evidence* for an association with stomach cancer. The most consistent association between Chinese-style salted fish and nasopharyngeal carcinoma has been observed for ingestion during weaning or early childhood in the early studies; interestingly, the diet-related lifestyle changes that started in the second half of the 20th century in the Chinese populations, characterized by a large decrease in preserved food consumption and especially the decline in the habit of feeding young children with salted fish, coincides with the lower rate of nasopharyngeal cancer incidence observed in the most recent studies.

Defining a clear mechanism linking salted fish consumption with nasopharyngeal carcinoma has been hampered by the lack of data and by the fact that the composition of salted fish may greatly vary depending on the mode of preparation in different areas of Southern China. Possible mechanisms include the formation of *N*-nitrosamines and other *N*-nitroso compounds during the processing of the fish and/or endogenously after ingestion in the human body.

Another likely mechanism is the interaction between Chinese-style salted fish and Epstein-Baar virus (EBV). EBV involvement in the carcinogenesis of nasopharyngeal cancer in South-eastern China has been clearly demonstrated; its role is also suggested in gastric adenocarcinoma (see Volume 100B). Experimental data have shown that salted fish extracts can reactivate EBV in latently infected cells in vitro. This is an important finding, since EBV is known to be present in a latent form in almost every person unless reactivated.

Aqueous extracts of some other preserved food samples from Tunisia (e.g *harissa*, a spiced mixture) and Greenland (salted fish), two high risk areas for nasopharyngeal cancer, were also shown to activate EBV in cells in vitro. In addition, other preserved food whose consumption can potentially lead to *N*-nitroso compounds intake is consumed in many part of the world.

The Working Group recommends that IARC undertake a full review of the carcinogenic hazards of preserved food.

A summary of the findings of this volume appears in The Lancet Oncology (Secretan *et al.*, 2009).

References

Chang JS, Straif K, Guha N (2011). The role of alcohol dehydrogenase genes in head and neck cancers: a systematic review and meta-analysis of ADH1B and ADH1C. [Epub ahead of print]*Mutagenesis*, doi:10.1093/mutage/ger073 PMID:22042713

Chen PC, Kuo C, Pan CC, Chou MY (2002). Risk of oral cancer associated with human papillomavirus infection, betel quid chewing, and cigarette smoking in Taiwan–an integrated molecular and epidemiological study of 58 cases. *J Oral Pathol Med*, 31: 317–322. doi:10.1034/j.1600-0714.2002.00129.x PMID:12190813

Chu N-S (2001). Effects of Betel chewing on the central and autonomic nervous systems. *J Biomed Sci*, 8: 229–236. doi:10.1007/BF02256596 PMID:11385294

Cogliano VJ, Baan R, Straif K *et al.* (2011). Preventable exposures associated with human cancers. *J Natl Cancer Inst*, 103: 1827–1839. doi:10.1093/jnci/djr483 PMID:22158127

Djordjevic MV, Hoffmann D, Glynn T, Connolly GN (1995). US commercial brands of moist snuff, 1994. I. Assessment of nicotine, moisture, and pH. *Tob Control*, 4: 62–66. doi:10.1136/tc.4.1.62

Henley SJ, Connell CJ, Richter P *et al.* (2007). Tobacco-related disease mortality among men who switched from cigarettes to spit tobacco. *Tob Control*, 16: 22–28. doi:10.1136/tc.2006.018069 PMID:17297069

IARC (1985). Tobacco habits other than smoking; betel-quid and areca-nut chewing; and some related nitrosamines. IARC Working Group. Lyon, 23–30 October 1984. *IARC Monogr Eval Carcinog Risk Chem Hum*, 37: 1–268. PMID:3866741

IARC (1986). Tobacco smoking. *IARC Monogr Eval Carcinog Risk Chem Hum*, 38: 1–421. PMID:3866741

IARC (1988). Alcohol drinking. *IARC Monogr Eval Carcinog Risks Hum*, 44: 1–378. PMID:3236394

IARC (1993). Some naturally occurring substances: food items and constituents, heterocyclic aromatic amines and mycotoxins. *IARC Monogr Eval Carcinog Risks Hum*, 56: 1–599.

IARC (2004a). Tobacco smoke and involuntary smoking. *IARC Monogr Eval Carcinog Risks Hum*, 83: 1–1438. PMID:15285078

IARC (2004b). Betel-quid and areca-nut chewing and some areca-nut derived nitrosamines. *IARC Monogr Eval Carcinog Risks Hum*, 85: 1–334. PMID:15635762

IARC (2007). Smokeless tobacco and some tobacco-specific N-nitrosamines. *IARC Monogr Eval Carcinog Risks Hum*, 89: 1–592. PMID:18335640

IARC (2010a). Household use of solid fuels and high-temperature frying. *IARC Monogr Eval Carcinog Risks Hum*, 95: 1–430. PMID:20701241

IARC (2010b). Alcohol consumption and ethyl carbamate. *IARC Monogr Eval Carcinog Risks Hum*, 96. 1–1423.

Ko YC, Huang YL, Lee CH *et al.* (1995). Betel quid chewing, cigarette smoking and alcohol consumption related to oral cancer in Taiwan. *J Oral Pathol Med*, 24: 450–453. doi:10.1111/j.1600-0714.1995.tb01132.x PMID:8600280

Lee CH, Ko YC, Huang HL *et al.* (2003). The precancer risk of betel quid chewing, tobacco use and alcohol consumption in oral leukoplakia and oral submucous fibrosis in southern Taiwan. *Br J Cancer*, 88: 366–372. doi:10.1038/sj.bjc.6600727 PMID:12569378

Secretan B, Straif K, Baan R *et al.*WHO International Agency for Research on Cancer Monograph Working Group (2009). A review of human carcinogens–Part E: tobacco, areca nut, alcohol, coal smoke, and salted fish. *Lancet Oncol*, 10: 1033–1034. doi:10.1016/S1470-2045(09)70326-2 PMID:19891056

Warnakulasuriya S (2004). Smokeless tobacco and oral cancer. *Oral Dis*, 10: 1–4. doi:10.1046/j.1354-523X.2003.00975.x PMID:14996286

TOBACCO SMOKING

Tobacco smoking was considered by previous IARC Working Groups in 1986, 1987 and 2002 (IARC, 1986, 1987, 2004a). Since that time, new data have become available, these have been incorporated into the *Monograph*, and taken into consideration in the present evaluation.

1. Exposure Data

1.1 Smoked tobacco products

Smoked forms of tobacco include various kinds of cigarettes (manufactured, hand-rolled, filtered, un-filtered and flavoured), cigars and pipes. While cigarette smoking, particularly manufactured cigarettes, is by far the main form of tobacco smoked globally, in some countries other forms of smoked tobacco are dominant (IARC, 2004a) In India, for example, bidis (made of coarse and uncured tobacco) account for about 60% of smoked tobacco products whereas cigarettes account for 20% (Ray & Gupta, 2009; IIPS, 2010). Water pipes, another form of smoked tobacco known by other various names such as gaza, hookah, narghile, shisha, hubble-bubble, are commonly smoked in the Eastern Mediterranean region, in some parts of Asia including India, and in North Africa (Asma *et al.*, 2009).

1.2 Chemical composition of tobacco smoke

1.2.1 Smoke from cigarettes

One cubic cm of fresh, un-aged cigarette mainstream smoke [the smoke emerging from the mouth end of a cigarette during smoking] has about 4×10^9 particles with a mean diameter of about 0.2 µm (Borgerding & Klus, 2005). The size of the particles increases as the smoke ages. Temperatures in the burning cone of the cigarette are about 800 °C during the smoulder period between puffs and increase to 910–920 °C at the periphery of the cone during puffing (Borgerding & Klus, 2005). Hydrogen is generated in the glowing cone, resulting in an oxygen deficient reducing atmosphere (Borgerding & Klus, 2005). The approximate composition of mainstream smoke of a plain cigarette is summarized in Table 1.1 (Borgerding & Klus, 2005). The total particulate matter, after subtraction of the amounts of nicotine and water, is referred to as 'tar'.

Over 5300 compounds have been identified in tobacco smoke (Rodgman & Perfetti, 2009). Classes of compounds include but are not limited to neutral gases, carbon and nitrogen oxides, amides, imides, lactams, carboxylic acids, lactones, esters, aldehydes, ketones,

Table 1.1 Approximate chemical composition of mainstream smoke generated by a plain cigarette

Compound or class of components	Relative amount w/w (%)
Nitrogen	58
Oxygen	12
Carbon dioxide	13
Carbon monoxide	3.5
Hydrogen, argon	0.5
Water	1
Volatile organic substances	5
Particulate phase	8

From Borgerding & Klus (2005)

alcohols, phenols, amines, *N*-nitrosamines, *N*-heterocyclics, aliphatic hydrocarbons, monocyclic and polycyclic aromatic hydrocarbons (PAHs), nitriles, anhydrides, carbohydrates, ethers, nitro compounds and metals (Rodgman & Perfetti, 2009).

The addictive properties of tobacco smoke are attributed to nicotine, the principal tobacco alkaloid in smoke (Hukkanen *et al.*, 2005). Minor tobacco alkaloids include nornicotine, anatabine and anabasine (Hukkanen *et al.*, 2005). The tobacco alkaloids are not generally considered carcinogenic, but are accompanied by carcinogens in each puff of smoke.

There are over 70 carcinogens in tobacco smoke that have been evaluated by the *IARC Monographs* programme as having sufficient evidence for carcinogenicity in either laboratory animals or humans (IARC, 2004a). The different chemical classes of carcinogens and representatives of each are presented in Table 1.2 (IARC, 2004a). Sixteen of these – benzo[*a*]pyrene (BaP), 4-(methylnitrosamino)-1-(3-pyridyl)-1-butanone (NNK) and *N'*-nitrosonornicotine (NNN), 2-naphthylamine, 4-aminobiphenyl, formaldehyde, 1,3-butadiene, benzene, vinyl chloride, ethylene oxide, arsenic, beryllium, nickel compounds, chromium VI, cadmium, and polonium-210 – are classified as carcinogenic to humans (Group 1). Structures of some representative carcinogens in cigarette smoke are shown in Fig. 1.1. There are other likely carcinogens in cigarette smoke that have not been evaluated by the *IARC Monographs* programme. These include, for example, PAHs with incompletely characterized occurrence levels and carcinogenic activities; over 500 PAHs have been identified (Rodgman & Perfetti, 2006).

PAHs, tobacco-specific *N*-nitrosamines, aromatic amines, aldehydes and certain volatile organics likely contribute significantly to the carcinogenic activity of tobacco smoke (Hecht, 2003).

In the early part of the 20th century, PAHs were identified as carcinogenic constituents of coal tar (Phillips, 1983). They are products of incomplete combustion of all organic matter and occur, always as complex mixtures, in tars, soots, broiled foods, vehicle engine exhaust and tobacco smoke. PAHs are generally locally acting carcinogens, and some, such as the prototypic compound BaP, have strong carcinogenic activity on mouse skin and in rodent lung. Heterocyclic analogues of PAHs also occur in cigarette smoke. Concentrations of individual PAHs in mainstream cigarette smoke are generally in the range of 1–50 ng per cigarette (IARC, 2004a).

Among the carcinogenic *N*-nitrosamines in tobacco smoke are tobacco-specific *N*-nitrosamines, which are derived from, and structurally related to, the tobacco alkaloids. Two of the most important of these are NNK and NNN (Hecht & Hoffmann, 1988). Levels of NNK and NNN in cigarette smoke vary depending on tobacco type and other factors, but are frequently in the range of 50–200 ng per cigarette (IARC, 2004a).

Aromatic amines were first identified as human carcinogens from industrial exposures in the dye industry in the early part of the 20th century. They include the well known human bladder carcinogens 2-naphthylamine and 4-aminobiphenyl which, along with other

Table 1.2 Tobacco smoke carcinogens evaluated in the *IARC Monographs*

Chemical Class	Number of Carcinogens	Representative Carcinogens
Polycyclic aromatic hydrocarbons (PAHs) and their heterocyclic analogues	15	Benzo[*a*]pyrene (BaP) Dibenz[*a,h*]anthracene
N-Nitrosamines	8	4-(Methylnitrosamino)-1-(3-pyridyl)-1-butanone (NNK) *N'*-Nitrosonornicotine (NNN)
Aromatic amines	12	4-Aminobiphenyl 2-Naphthylamine
Aldehydes	2	Formaldehyde Acetaldehyde
Phenols	2	Catechol Caffeic acid
Volatile hydrocarbons	3	Benzene 1,3-Butadiene Isoprene
Other organics	12	Ethylene oxide Acrylonitrile
Inorganic compounds	8	Cadmium Polonium-210

There are many other carcinogens in cigarette smoke that have not been evaluated in an *IARC Monograph*.
From IARC (2004a)

isomers, are found in cigarette smoke, but their levels are generally quite low (1–20 ng per cigarette) (IARC, 2004a).

Aldehydes such as formaldehyde and acetaldehyde occur widely in the human environment and are also found in human blood. Concentrations of acetaldehyde and formaldehyde in cigarette smoke are far higher than those of PAHs, *N*-nitrosamines or aromatic amines but their carcinogenic activities are weak (Hecht, 2003). Cigarette mainstream smoke typically contains 10–30 μg formaldehyde/cigarette and 800–900 μg acetaldehyde/cigarette (IARC, 2004a).

Volatile hydrocarbons in cigarette smoke include 1,3-butadiene, a powerful multiorgan carcinogen in the mouse, and benzene, a known human leukaemogen. 1,3-Butadiene (20–40 μg/cigarette) and benzene (12–50 μg/cigarette) are two of the most prevalent strong carcinogens in cigarette smoke (IARC, 2004a).

In summary, cigarette smoke is an exceedingly complex mixture which contains over 5300 compounds including multiple toxicants and carcinogens.

1.2.2 Smoke from other tobacco products

Some constituents have been measured in roll-your-own cigarettes, and their levels are comparable to or higher than those in commercial brands. Carcinogen and toxicant levels expressed per unit are higher in cigars than in cigarettes because of their larger size, and in some instances are also higher per litre of smoke. Levels of nicotine and tobacco-specific nitrosamines were comparable in bidis and commercial Indian cigarettes; bidis also contain high levels of eugenol, as do kreteks. Levels of NNK and NNN in chuttas were considerably higher than in standard cigarettes (IARC, 2004a).

Fig. 1.1 Structures of some representative tobacco smoke carcinogens

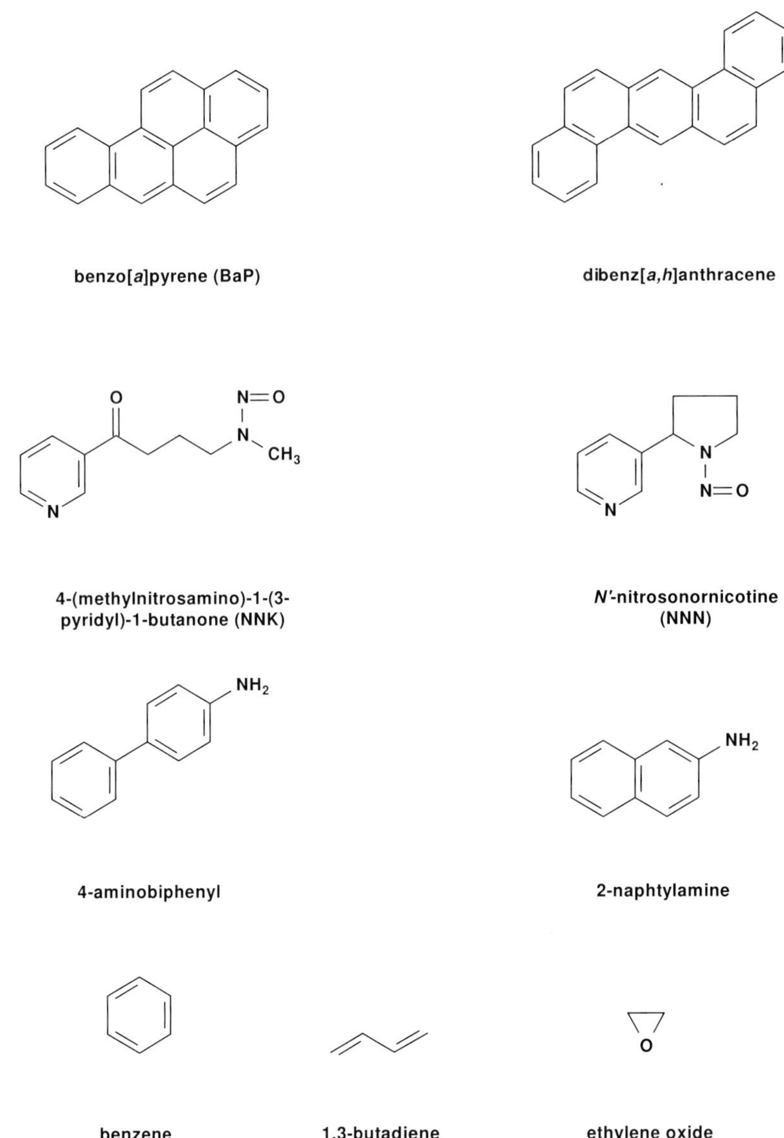

Fig. 1.2 Proportion of adult smokers by WHO region in 2009

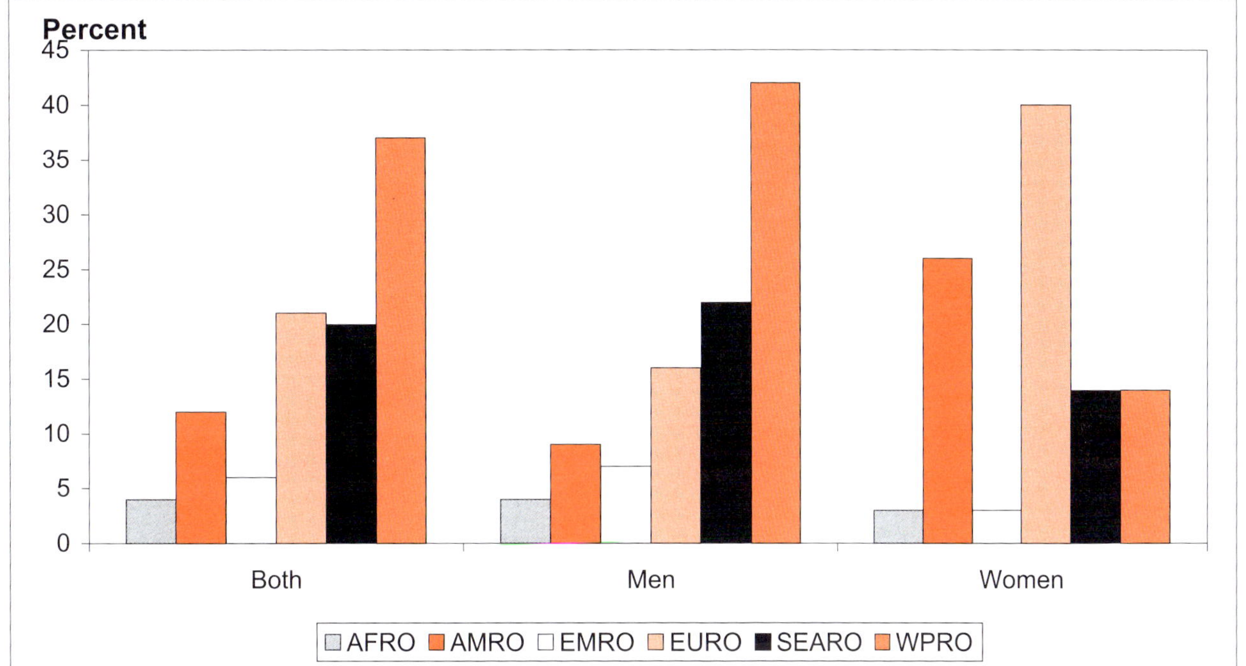

From WHO (2011)

1.3 Prevalence of tobacco smoking

1.3.1 Data collection and methods

Data on smoking tobacco are available from WHO's Global Infobase (www.who.int/infobase) and the WHO Global Health Observatory (www.who.int/gho/en) – repositories of information on tobacco use and other risk factors in young people (13–15 years old) and adults (aged 15 years and over). The data span several years and are acquired from government reports, journals and unpublished sources. WHO has in the recent past used and modelled these data to produce estimates of tobacco smoking prevalence, published in the WHO Reports on the Global Tobacco Epidemic. For a complete explanation of methods used, the reader is referred to the Technical Note on Prevalence in the 3rd WHO Report on the Global Tobacco Epidemic (WHO, 2011). The six WHO regions are: EMRO, Eastern Mediterranean Region; EURO, European Region; AFRO, African Region; WPRO, Western Pacific Region; SEARO, South East Asian Region; AMRO, Region of the Americas. A listing of the countries in each region can be viewed at http://www.who.int/about/structure/en/index.html.

1.3.2 Distribution of smokers by WHO region and country

WHO estimates that in 2009, there was about 1.1 billion adult smokers worldwide, representing nearly a quarter (22%) of the global adult population (WHO, 2011). A disaggregation by the six WHO regions (Fig. 1.2) shows that over a third of smokers worldwide live in WPRO (highly influenced by the People's Republic of China), followed by SEARO, which has around a fifth

Fig. 1.3 Proportion and cumulative percentage of smokers in high-burden countries, in men (A) and women (B) in 2009

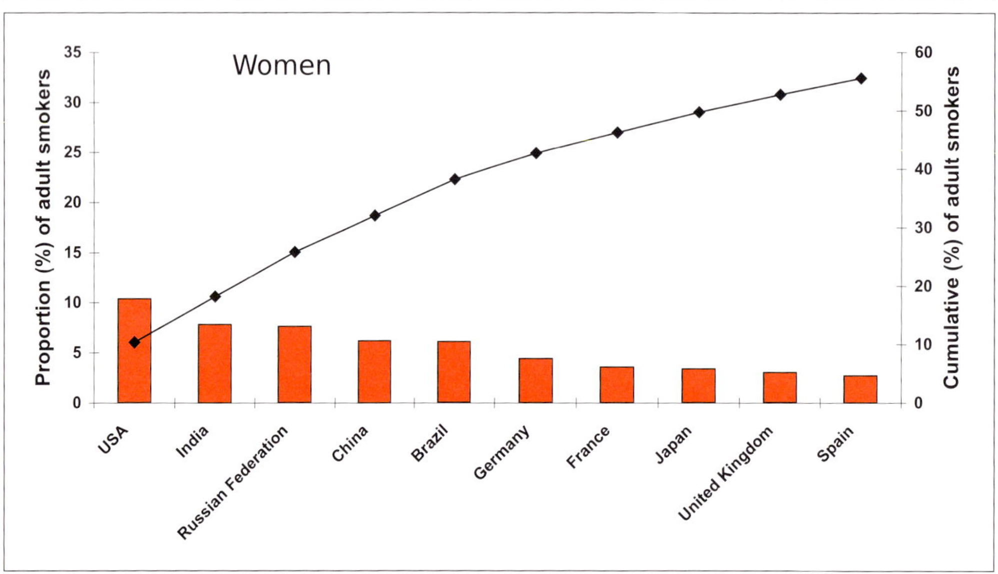

From WHO (2011)

of the world's smokers (influenced by India and Indonesia).

The number of smokers in any country is a function of both the prevalence of smoking and the size of the population. A further disaggregation of the regions by country shows that a few countries account for a large proportion of tobacco smokers. Ranked in descending order of the number of smokers, the five countries of China, India, United States of America (USA), Russian Federation and Indonesia account for about 52% of adult smokers in the world, with China and India alone accounting for 40% (Fig. 1.3). Furthermore, nearly two-thirds of the world's smokers live in only ten countries of the world.

1.3.3 Distribution of smokers by sex

With a global average smoking prevalence of 36%, men account for just over 80% of all smokers. The male adult prevalence is 4–5 times that for women, at 8%. This difference varies across WHO regions. Smoking among men, concentrated in the five countries of China, India, Indonesia, Russian Federation and USA (Fig. 1.3), accounts for about 56% of global smoking among men. Women smokers are mostly concentrated in EURO and AMRO. These two regions account for 40% and 26% of all women smokers globally, respectively. The prevalences for women in these two regions are about half of those in men, whereas the difference is substantially greater in the other regions. Just as men smoke more than women everywhere, so too among young people, boys generally smoke more than girls. There is an increasing concern, however, that the gap may diminish, not because of a reduction in boys prevalence but because of an increase in the proportion of girls who are taking up smoking (Warren *et al.*, 2006).

1.3.4 The four stage smoking model

(a) The four stages of tobacco use

Lopez *et al.* (1994) used trend data on smoking prevalence and tobacco attributable mortality to show the evolution of tobacco use in a country. Four stages of smoking and attributable mortality have been identified to represent the growth and eventual decline of smoking among men and women (Fig. 1.4).

Stage 1 is characterized by low smoking prevalence in men (less than 15%) and very low in women (less than 10%). Death and disease from smoking are not apparent in this phase, as nearly all health effects from smoking are related to past smoking habits and their cumulative effects rather than current smoking. In Stage 2, smoking prevalence in men rapidly increases while it increases more slowly in women. Towards the end of this stage, smoking prevalence in men typically peaks to lie at 50–60%, with 10% of deaths in men attributable to smoking; deaths in women are comparatively fewer. After a protracted period of high smoking prevalence, Stage 3 shows a decline in smoking prevalence in men to around 40%. Smoking prevalence in women peaks and then begins to decline; towards the end of this stage the gap between men's and women's prevalence starts to narrow. However, smoking attributable deaths in men increase from around 10% to 25–30% within a span of three decades; in women the deaths are increasing but are still quite low. In the final Stage 4, smoking prevalences in both men and women continue to decline albeit relatively slowly in comparison with Stage 3, with the gap substantially narrowing to lie at around five percentage points, and as little as one percentage point in some countries. In Stage 4, smoking mortality in men peaks to between 30–35% and then declines to below 30% at the end of this period. In women, the health effects from past smoking persist, with increasing mortality, but remain lower than in men, and recently have begun to decline in some countries.

(b) Smoking prevalence worldwide

Using prevalence data for men and women collected in 2006 for 140 countries, WHO determined at which stage of the tobacco epidemic countries are in the model of Lopez *et al.* (1994). In Fig. 1.5, countries have been ranked by smoking prevalence in men in ascending order for Stages 1 and 2, and then in descending order for Stages 3 and 4. (Smoking prevalence in men is almost always higher than in women, with a few exceptions observed in the fourth stage.) While most countries fit the classification, there are a few exceptions, most of which in the last stage. Prevalence between Stage 3 and Stage 4 is discontinuous in both sexes. This is due to the classification followed, which puts countries with a relatively narrow difference in prevalence between men and women in Stage 4 even though

Fig. 1.4 The four stages of the tobacco epidemic

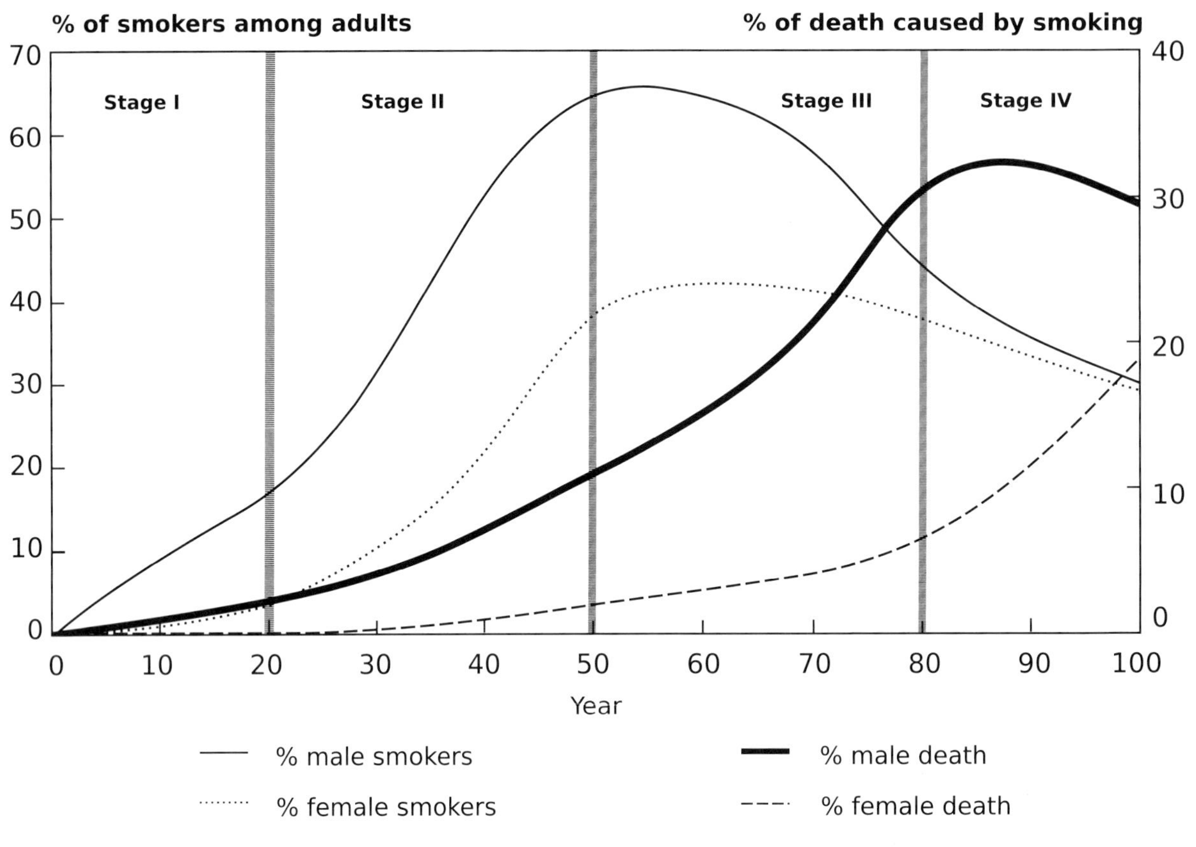

From Lopez *et al.* (1994)

their prevalence is largely comparable with those in Stage 3.

Most African countries fall in the first stage of the smoking model, characterized by low smoking prevalence in men and very low prevalence in women. Three of the five high burden countries fall in stage 2 (India, Indonesia and China), with the rest comprising a combination of countries from Africa, South East Asia, eastern Europe and the Middle East. At this stage smoking prevalences in women continue to remain very low, most countries having a prevalence in adult women of less than 10%.

Stage 3 includes the fourth high burden country (Russian Federation), along with countries in eastern Europe, South America and western Europe, which fall at the end of Stage 3. Stage 4 is populated entirely by the developed countries of western Europe, North America and Oceania. The USA, the fifth high burden country, fall in the last stage as a result of the relatively small difference in the smoking prevalence between men and women compared to the other intermediate stages. As mentioned before, Stage 4 includes countries where the smoking prevalence is higher in women than in men, with a small (< 8%) difference.

(c) Age-specific prevalence

Age-specific prevalence for men and women aged 15 years or older is presented for six representative countries for current smoking (Fig. 1.6). There are wide variations in age-specific prevalence between these countries. In men, prevalence

Fig. 1.5 Prevalence of smoking in 140 countries in 2009, staged according to the model by Lopez

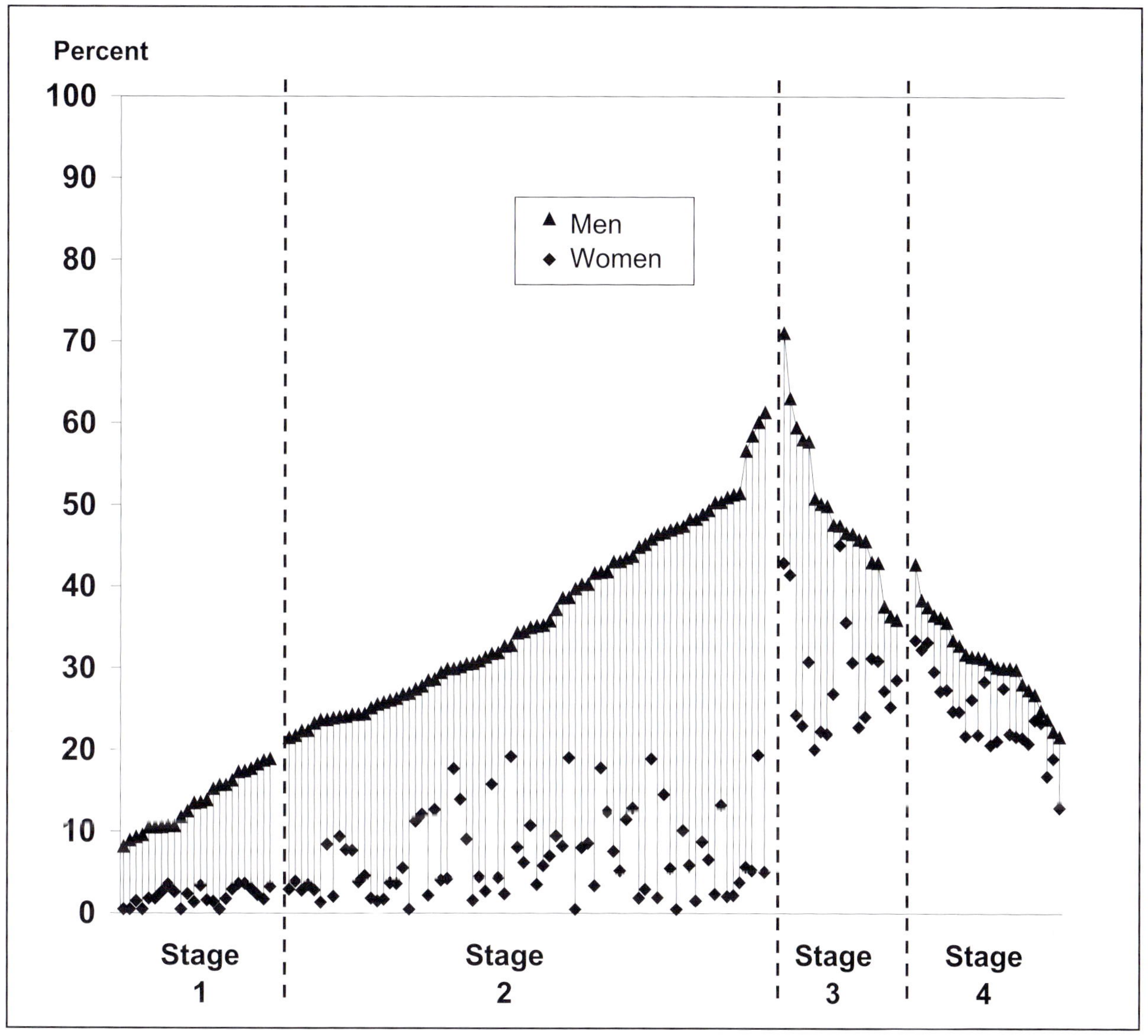

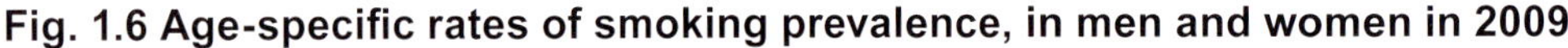

Fig. 1.6 Age-specific rates of smoking prevalence, in men and women in 2009

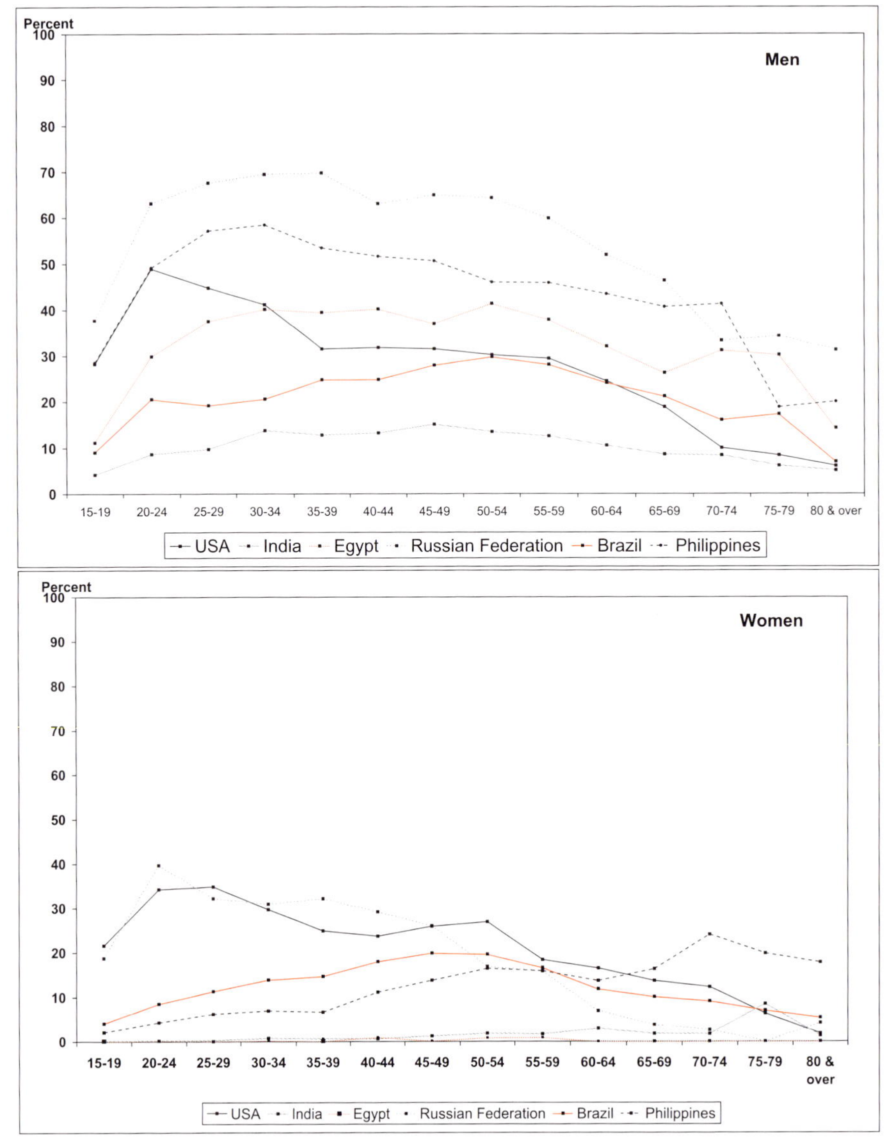

varies from less than 10% to 75% in the 15–19 years age range to lie between 10% and 55% in the oldest age range. Prevalence among women varies from less than 1% to as high as 45% in young adults (15–19 years). Unlike men, prevalence in women tends to converge after age 50, lying within 15 percentage points. Prevalence in women is almost always lower than in men in all age groups.

Initiation of smoking is shifting, and is taking place at earlier ages in both developed and developing countries. In developed countries, quitting smoking is also shifting to occur at a younger age, whereas in developing countries there is no such evidence.

(d) Smoking in youth

Information on smoking habits in youth are collected from a variety of youth surveys that include the Global Youth Tobacco Survey (GYTS), Global school-based Student Health Survey (GSHS) and Health Behaviour in School Aged Children (HBSC). Some countries have their own youth surveys, or have them as part of a general health or household survey, such as the Student Survey in Argentina, the Youth Smoking Survey in Canada, and New Zealand's Tobacco Survey.

The GYTS is a school-based survey designed to monitor tobacco use among youths aged 13 to 15 years. The GYTS uses a standard set of questions and sampling methods in over 160 countries. The survey has core questions that span seven thematic areas pertinent to tobacco. In addition to these, countries can include country-specific questions that allow assessment of tobacco use unique to the country. To assess prevalence of smoking, students are asked to report their smoking habits for both cigarettes and other tobacco products that they may have consumed over the past 30 days. Since its inception in 1999, the GYTS has covered over 2 million students. Although most GYTS are national surveys, in some countries they are limited to subnational locations. Further, countries conduct the GYTS in different years, rendering comparison for the same year difficult.

Prevalence of current tobacco use [including smokeless tobacco] in youth in 2004–09 for fourteen high burden low and middle income countries is shown in Fig. 1.7. The Russian Federation has the highest prevalence of current tobacco use among the high burden countries for which national data are available. Further, in the Americas and Europe the difference in prevalence between boys and girls is smaller than in other regions. In contrast, in Egypt, India and Thailand, prevalences in boys are significantly higher than in girls.

Fig. 1.8 shows the range of current tobacco use by WHO region for boys and for girls and for both sexes combined. There are wide variations in current tobacco use within each region. The largest variations are observed in EMRO and SEARO irrespective of sex, reflecting potentially disparate initiation rates in countries within the region. In AFRO, the range of current tobacco use between boys and girls is virtually the same. In some countries (e.g. Argentina, Peru, Sierra Leone, Bulgaria, Croatia, Cook Islands, New Zealand), tobacco use in girls exceeds that in boys; but overall boys and girls show remarkably similar propensity to take up tobacco use.

Warren *et al.* (2006) present global estimates and regional averages for current tobacco smoking in youth using GYTS data spanning 1999–2005. Their estimates show that one in five boys and one in seven girls currently smoke tobacco. Prevalence of current smoking for both boys and girls combined was highest in AMRO (22.2%) and lowest in WPRO (11.4%). AMRO have the highest average for current tobacco smoking for boys (24%) and for girls (20.4%) whereas the lowest prevalence was in WPRO among boys (15%) and in SEARO among girls (7.1%).

Fig. 1.7 Prevalence of current tobacco use in youth for selected countries, 2005–2009

Region	Group	Value (near 0)	Value (bar end)
Africa	Total	7	36
Africa	Boys	8	37
Africa	Girls	5	37
Americas	Total	8	35
Americas	Boys	10	35
Americas	Girls	7	40
Eastern Mediterranean	Total	3	60
Eastern Mediterranean	Boys	5	66
Eastern Mediterranean	Girls	2	54
Europe	Total	2	38
Europe	Boys	3	42
Europe	Girls	2	34
Southeast Asia	Total	6	57
Southeast Asia	Boys	9	60
Southeast Asia	Girls	3	53
Western Pacific	Total	4	50
Western Pacific	Boys	7	58
Western Pacific	Girls	2	42

Percent (axis 0–100)

Fig. 1.8 Range of prevalence of current tobacco use in youth, 2005–2009, by WHO region

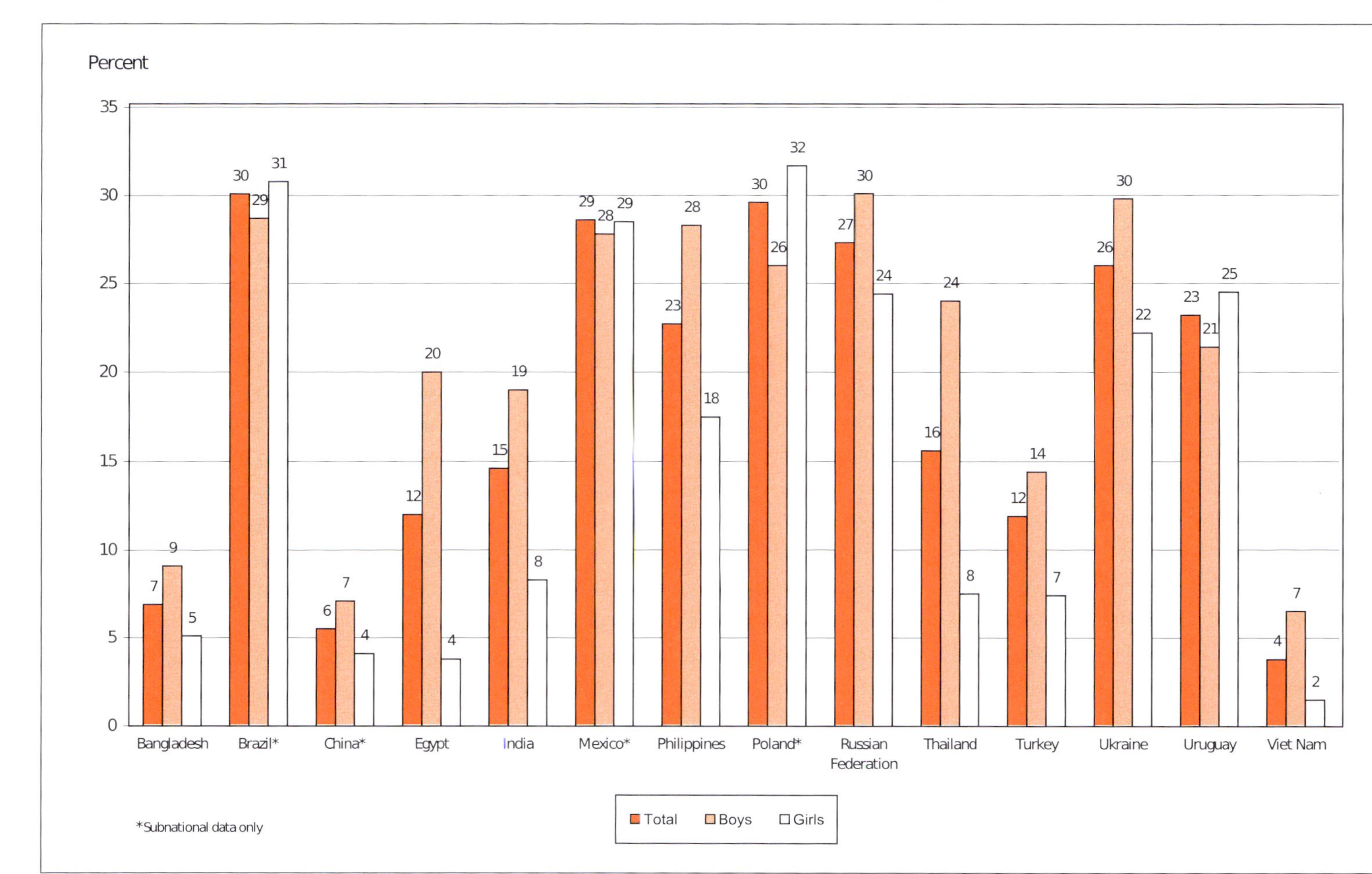

Figures have been rounded off and show prevalences in countries with national and subnational jurisdiction.

1.4 Regulations and policies: the WHO Framework Convention on Tobacco Control

The WHO Framework Convention on Tobacco Control (WHO FCTC) – the first multilateral evidence-based treaty on tobacco control – articulates tobacco control measures available to countries to counter the growing tobacco epidemic. This treaty, which entered into force in 2005, represents one of the most universal treaties in the United Nations history. In 2008, the WHO launched MPOWER, a technical assistance package comprised of six strategies that reflects one or more of the WHO FCTC measures and helps countries meet their commitments to the WHO FCTC.

2. Cancer in Humans

2.1 Introduction

The available knowledge on the relationship between tobacco smoking and a variety of human cancers is based primarily on epidemiological evidence. An immense amount of such evidence has been obtained, and only a small proportion can be referred to here. The cancers considered to be causally related to tobacco smoking in the previous *IARC Monograph* on tobacco smoking (IARC, 2004a) included lung, oral cavity, nasal cavity and paranasal sinuses, nasopharynx, oropharynx, hypopharynx, larynx, oesophagus (adenocarcinoma and squamous cell carcinoma), upper aerodigestive tract combined, stomach, pancreas, liver, kidney (body and pelvis), ureter, urinary bladder, cervix and myeloid leukaemia. In addition, it was concluded that there was evidence suggesting lack of carcinogenicity for cancers of the breast and of the endometrium.

Since 2002, there have been additional cohort and case–control studies on the relationship of tobacco smoking in different forms to these and other cancers in many countries. A large body of evidence has been obtained from cohort studies with respect to different cancer sites and types of tobacco product. These cohort studies are described briefly in Table 2.1 (available at http://monographs.iarc.fr/ENG/Monographs/vol100E/100E-01-Table2.1.pdf), listed by country. Case–control studies are described in the sections pertaining to cancer sites. More studies are now available from countries and populations that are still at an early stage of the tobacco epidemic. These studies are prone to underestimate the true strengths of the association between tobacco smoking and any specific cancer as the full effect of duration of smoking cannot be evaluated.

2.2 Cancer of the lung

2.2.1 Overview of studies

The main cause of lung cancer in humans is tobacco smoking and most information establishing this fact comes from epidemiological studies in which the assessment of exposure was based on self-reported information on personal smoking habits via self-administered questionnaire or in-person interviews. Since the previous *IARC Monograph* (IARC, 2004a), numerous studies have been published on the issues of tobacco smoking and sex and racial/ethnic susceptibility, 'tar' yields as measured by machine smoking, the relationship between histological changes and the design of cigarettes, dose–response association, genetic susceptibilities and interactions.

2.2.2 Factors affecting risk

Recent epidemiological studies incorporating measures of smoking metabolites in serum or urine are helping to refine our understanding of exposure-response relationships with tobacco smoke. Dose–response evidence has been obtained from three cohort studies (Flanders *et al.*, 2003; Boffetta *et al.*, 2006; Yuan *et al.*, 2009; Table 2.2 available at http://monographs.iarc.fr/ENG/Monographs/vol100E/100E-01-Table2.2.pdf) and four pooled analyses (Lubin & Caporaso, 2006; Lubin *et al.*, 2007a, b, 2008; Table 2.3 available at http://monographs.iarc.fr/ENG/Monographs/vol100E/100E-01-Table2.3.pdf) since the previous *IARC Monograph* (IARC, 2004a).

The US American Cancer Society Cancer Prevention Study-II (CPS-II) is the largest cohort study on smoking and lung cancer risk using questionnaire assessment of exposure (Flanders *et al.*, 2003). In this study cigarette smoking duration is a much stronger predictor of lung cancer mortality than is cigarette smoking intensity, regardless of age in both men and women. These results are qualitatively similar to those reported by Doll & Peto (1978) and are consistent with IARC (2004a).

In a questionnaire-based assessment of the association of tobacco smoking with lung cancer risk, smokers at higher smoking intensities seem to experience a "reduced potency" per pack such that for equal total exposure, the excess odds ratio per pack–year decreases with intensity (Lubin *et al.* 2008). Below 15–20 cigarettes/day, the excess odds ratio/pack–year increases with intensity (Lubin & Caporaso, 2006; Lubin *et al.*, 2007a) while above 20 cigarettes/day, there is an 'inverse-exposure-rate' effect (Lubin *et al.*, 2007a) suggesting a greater risk for total exposure delivered at lower intensity (or a longer duration) than the equivalent exposure delivered at a higher intensity. The intensity effects were also statistically homogeneous across diverse cancer types, indicating that after accounting for risk from total pack–years, intensity patterns were comparable for cancer of the lung, bladder, oral cavity, pancreas and oesophagus. These analyses suggest that the risk of lung cancer increases with increasing tobacco exposure at all dose levels, but there is some levelling-off effect at the highest intensity of tobacco smoking.

However, when serum cotinine was used as a measure of exposure to tobacco smoking, rather than questionnaire-based data, the odds ratio of lung cancer increased linearly over the full range of exposure from ≤ 5 ng/mL through ≥ 378 ng/mL, with an odds ratio of 55.1 (95% confidence interval (CI): 35.7–85.0) in the highest exposure group. These results suggest that the decreased rate of lung cancer risk at high intensity of tobacco smoke previously described is a statistical artefact. Such an effect may be due to an inaccurate assessment of total tobacco smoke exposure from questionnaire-based studies at high exposure levels (Boffetta *et al.*, 2006). Somewhat similar results were obtained when both 4-(methylnitrosamino)-1-(3-pyridyl)-1-butanol (NNAL) and total cotinine in urine were measured in subjects of two large cohort studies from Shanghai men and Singapore men and women (Yuan *et al.*, 2009). Among smokers with comparable smoking histories (as noted in questionnaire data) there is a 9-fold variation in subsequent risk of lung cancer between those with high and those with low levels of total urinary NNAL and cotinine. Thus measurements of urinary cotinine and total NNAL at a single point in time in a smoker could substantially improve the predictive power of a lung cancer assessment model based solely on self-reported smoking history (number of cigarettes/day, number of years of regular smoking). A positive NNAL-lung cancer association of comparable magnitude was observed in both Shanghai and Singapore subjects despite differences in the NNK content of tobacco smoked. The independent association between total urinary cotinine and lung cancer risk, after adjustment for total urinary NNAL and smoking history, suggests that tobacco smoke compounds other than NNK play a role in lung cancer development in smokers. Further, a single measurement of urinary NNAL may closely predict the average level of NNAL measured over a much longer period of time.

2.2.3 Types of tobacco or of cigarette

(a) Tar levels

In a previous *IARC Monograph* (IARC, 1986), it was concluded on the basis of the case–control, cohort studies and ecological evaluations available at the time that prolonged use of 'high-tar' and unfiltered cigarettes is associated with greater risks than prolonged use of filter-tipped and 'low-tar' cigarettes. More recently (IARC, 2004a), it has been recognized that the actual quantitative impact of reduced 'tar' and filter-tipped cigarettes is difficult to assess because of, respectively, the concomitant increase in tobacco-specific nitrosamines that accompanies the greater use of blend tobacco and the compensatory changes in smoking behaviour by smokers attempting to maintain their accustomed level of nicotine intake. Nevertheless, it was concluded that changes in cigarette types since the 1950s have probably tended to reduce the risk for lung cancer associated with tobacco smoking.

Additional refinement in assessing the health effects associated with smoking cigarettes of various tar content has been possible since the publication of the earlier reports. Compared with smokers of medium tar (15–21 mg) filtered cigarettes risk was higher among men and women who smoked high tar (≥ 22 mg) non-filtered brands but there was no difference in risk among men and women who smoked 'very low tar' or 'low tar' brands compared with those who smoked 'medium tar' brands (Harris *et al.*, 2004). Regardless of tar content of their cigarettes, all current smokers had a far greater risk for lung cancer than people who had stopped smoking or had never smoked (Harris *et al.*, 2004).

(b) Mentholated cigarettes

In the previous *IARC Monograph* (IARC, 2004a) the conclusion was drawn that there is no additional risk associated with smoking mentholated cigarettes when total consumption (pack–years) was controlled versus non-mentholated ones. Recent evidence supports that conclusion.

Mentholated cigarettes first appeared in the 1920s, but were not widely used until the mid-1950s (Bogen, 1929; Federal Trade Commission, 2001). Since the early 1970s, menthol varieties have accounted for 25–60% of all cigarettes sold in the USA (Federal Trade Commission, 2001). There are strong ethnic differences in the use of menthol cigarettes; more than 60% of Black smokers of both sexes use menthol brands compared to fewer than 25% of White smokers (Royce *et al.*, 1993; Hymowitz *et al.*, 1995). Studies have generally not demonstrated an increased risk of lung cancer for mentholated cigarettes versus non-mentholated cigarettes (Kabat & Hebert, 1994; Carpenter *et al.*, 1999; Brooks *et al.*, 2003; Stellman *et al.*, 2003). Recent evidence also suggests that users of mentholated cigarettes smoke fewer pack–years than those of non-mentholated cigarettes.

The higher incidence of lung cancer among Blacks is an important public health concern but the causes remain unclear. Mentholated cigarette use does not appear to explain the racial disparity observed in lung cancer risk among those having the same total tobacco consumption.

2.2.4 Histology

Compiled databases from IARC and other sources indicated that squamous cell carcinoma rates [per 100000 person-years] among men declined by 30% or more in North America and some European countries between 1980–82 and 1995–97, while changing less dramatically in other areas; small cell carcinoma rates decreased less rapidly. In contrast, the proportion of adenocarcinoma cases rose among men and women in virtually all areas, with the increases among men exceeding 50% in many areas of Europe (Devesa *et al.*, 2005).

Based on a comparison of two large cohort studies initiated by the American Cancer Society (ACS) (CPS-I and CPS-II) in 1960 and 1980, respectively, a stronger association between smoking and adenocarcinoma was observed in recent compared to earlier follow-up periods (Thun & Heath, 1997). Additionally, an association between cigarette smoking and bronchioloalveolar carcinoma was also found in several studies (Falk *et al.*, 1992; Morabia & Wynder, 1992).

A meta-analysis of 8 cohort and 14 case–control studies conducted in Japan among active smokers indicated significant excess lung cancer risks among men for both squamous cell carcinoma (relative risk (RR), 11.7) and adenocarcinoma (RR, 2.30). Among women the risks were 11.3 for squamous cell carcinoma and 1.37 for adenocarcinoma (Wakai *et al.*, 2006).

2.2.5 Population characteristics

(a) Sex

Meta-analyses on sex-specific susceptibility to lung cancer associated with tobacco smoking are presented in Table 2.4 (available at http://monographs.iarc.fr/ENG/Monographs/vol100E/100E-01-Table2.4.pdf) and cohort studies in Table 2.5 (available at http://monographs.iarc.fr/ENG/Monographs/vol100E/100E-01-Table2.5.pdf).

In the 1990s, two case–control studies indicated that relative risks for lung cancer associated with specific amounts and duration of cigarette smoking may be higher among women than among men (Risch *et al.*, 1993; Zang & Wynder, 1996).

In the large NIH-AARP [National Institutes of Health-American Association of Retired People] cohort (Freedman *et al.*, 2008), smoking was associated with lung cancer risk in both men and women. Age-standardized incidence rates for lung cancer tended to be higher in men than in women with comparable smoking histories (for current smokers and for quitters of less than 10 years), and in cases with squamous cell tumours. However, lung cancer risk was generally similar between men and women.

In a joint analysis, results from the Nurses' Health Study of women and the Health Professionals Follow-up Study in men (Bain *et al.*, 2004) suggest little difference in lung cancer susceptibility between men and women given equal smoking exposure. The hazard ratio in women ever smokers compared with men was 1.11 (95%CI: 0.95–1.31).

Serum cotinine levels were analysed in lung cancer cases and controls (Boffetta *et al.*, 2006). The lung cancer odds ratios (ORs) estimated for men and women were very similar for those with comparable serum cotinine levels. Other studies that have carefully quantified tobacco exposure via self-administered questionnaire or interview provide additional evidence of a comparable increase in lung cancer risk in the two sexes (Kreuzer *et al.*, 2000; Flanders *et al.*, 2003; Bain *et al.*, 2004).

In a meta-analysis of observational studies on cigarette smoking and cancer from 1961–2003 (conducted on 177 case–control studies, 75 cohort studies and two nested case–control studies), dose–response estimates were available in 44 studies: 19 with estimates for men only, 11 with estimates for women only and 14 with separate estimates for men and women (Gandini *et al.*, 2008). Overall, the risk of lung cancer for men and women increased by 7% for each additional cigarette smoked per day (RR, 1.07; 95%CI: 1.06–1.08). The increased risk appears to be slightly higher in women (RR, 1.08; 95%CI: 1.07–1.10) than in men (RR, 1.07; 95%CI: 1.05–1.08) ($P < 0.001$; adjusting for study type).

(b) Ethnicity

It has been postulated that susceptibility to lung cancer from tobacco smoking may differ by race and ethnicity (Schwartz & Swanson, 1997; Peto *et al.*, 1999; Stellman *et al.*, 2001; Kiyohara *et al.*, 2004, 2005, 2006; Pinsky, 2006; Wakai *et al.*, 2006; Vineis *et al.*, 2007; Takahashi *et al.*, 2008; Table 2.6 available at http://monographs.iarc.fr/ENG/Monographs/vol100E/100E-01-Table2.6.pdf). Lung cancer incidence rates vary considerable across racial/ethnic groups in the USA and elsewhere. Black men have higher rates than white men, while Hispanics, Asians and American Indians of both sexes have lower rates than whites (Stellman *et al.*, 2003; SEER, 2004). Nutritional habits, smoking patterns, type of tobacco smoked and genetic factors may play a role in such differences between racial and ethnic groups.

The association of tobacco smoking and lung cancer does not appear to be as strong among Japanese as among populations of North America or Europe (Wakai *et al.*, 2006). In a meta-analysis of 8 cohort studies and 14 case–control studies conducted in Japan, the excess lung cancer risks observed for both men (RR, 4.39; 95%CI: 3.92–4.92) and women (RR, 2.79; 95%CI: 2.44–3.20) in both case–control and cohort studies were lower than would have been expected from studies in North America and Europe. The lower lifetime consumption of cigarettes in Japanese, due in part to a later initiation of smoking and a lower consumption per day has been suggested to explain this. Other differences that may have etiological significance include tobacco ingredients, different filters on cigarettes, lifestyle factors including diet, and possibly differences in genetic susceptibility. [The Working Group noted that North American or European populations were not directly included in any of these studies.]

Data from the Asian Pacific Cohort Studies Collaboration, 31 studies involving 480125 persons, evaluated the risk of death from lung cancer associated with smoking habits in Australia, New Zealand and Asia (Huxley *et al.*, 2007b). Among Asian men the hazard ratio was 2.48 versus 9.87 in men in Australia and New Zealand. Among women, the corresponding estimates were 2.35 and 19.33, respectively. [In these studies, Asian populations smoked fewer cigarettes for a shorter period of time compared to those in Australia and New Zealand.]

Based on data from the National Cancer Institute's Surveillance, Epidemiology, and End Results program (SEER), Chinese women residing in the USA have a fourfold increased risk of lung cancer, and Filipino women a twofold increased risk, compared to that expected based on rates in non-Hispanic whites in the USA with a similar amount of cigarettes smoked (Epplein *et al.*, 2005). Among Chinese women, the increased risk was largely restricted to adenocarcinoma and large cell undifferentiated carcinoma. Chinese females residents of the western US mainland have a much higher risk of lung cancer than would be expected from their tobacco use patterns, just as they do in Asia (Peto *et al.*, 1999; Epplein *et al.*, 2005), the reason for these difference have not been identified. [Controlling for potential confounding factors was limited using aggregate data from SEER.]

Age, sex and race-specific risks of lung cancer mortality among lifetime non-smokers were compared in the two large ACS Cancer Prevention Study cohorts (CPS-I; CPS-II). The mortality rate was higher among African American women than among white women in CPS-II (hazard ratio (HR), 1.43; 95%CI: 1.11–1.36) (Thun *et al.*, 2006). This suggests an inherent susceptibility difference between white and black women but it could also be explained by access to care, diet, or exposure to environmental carcinogens.

The risk for lung cancer associated with cigarette smoking in 183813 African-American, Japanese-American, Latino, native Hawaiian and white men and women was examined in the Multiethnic Cohort Study in the USA (Haiman *et al.*, 2006). Information on demographic factors, smoking status, cigarettes/day smoked, years of smoking, years since quitting, diet, occupations, educational level and racial and ethnic group were collected for all subjects through a self-administered questionnaire at enrolment. Information about age of smoking initiation and cessation rates were collected on a subgroup of 5090 study subjects. Incident lung cancer cases were identified by linkage to the SEER cancer registries covering California and Hawaii. Among those who smoked no more than 10 cigarettes/day and those who smoked 11–20 cigarettes/day, relative risks ranged from 0.21 to 0.39 ($P < 0.001$) among Japanese Americans and Latinos and from 0.45 to 0.57 ($P < 0.001$) among whites as compared with African Americans. However, at levels exceeding 30 cigarettes/day, differences between racial/ethnic groups were no longer significant. The differences in lung cancer risk by racial group associated with smoking were observed for both men and women and for all histological types of lung cancer. These findings could not be explained by differences between populations in other known or suspected risk factors, including diet, occupation, and education level or by age at starting smoking or cessation of smoking.

Polymorphisms in glutathione-*S*-transferase (GST), GSTM1, GSTT1 and GSTP1 genes in humans are associated with reduction of enzymatic activity towards several substrates, including those found in tobacco smoke. In a population based case–control study involving early-onset lung cancer, African Americans carrying at least one G allele at the GSTP1 locus were more likely to have lung cancer compared with African Americans without a G allele after adjustment for age, sex, pack–years of smoking and a history of lung cancer in a first degree relative (OR, 2.9; 95%CI: 1.29–6.20). African Americans with either one or two risk genotypes at the GSTM1 (i.e. null genotype) and GSTP1 loci were at increased risk of having lung cancer compared with those having fully functional GSTM1 and GSTP1 genes (one risk genotype: OR, 2.8; 95%CI: 1.1–7.2 and two risk genotypes: OR, 4.0; 95%CI: 1.3–12.2). No significant single gene associations between GSTM1, GSTT1 and GSTP1 and early-onset lung cancer were observed in Caucasians, after adjusting for age, sex, pack–years and a family history of lung cancer (Cote *et al.*, 2005).

The cytochrome P450 (CYP) superfamily of enzymes catalyses one of the first steps in the metabolism of carcinogens such as polycylic aromatic hydrocarbons, nitroaromatics and arylamines. A population-based case–control study of lung cancer in the metropolitan Detroit area found that neither CYP1A1 MspI nor CYP1A1 Ile^{462}Val was associated with lung cancer susceptibility among Caucasians or African Americans. Among Caucasians, however, CYP1B1 Leu^{432} Val was significantly associated with lung cancer susceptibility (OR for at least one Val allele, 2.87; 95%CI: 1.63–5.07). Individuals with both this polymorphism and exposure to second-hand tobacco smoke were at particularly high risk for lung cancer. Combinations of particular CYP1B1 polymorphisms appeared to increase risk, although no combination differed significantly from the risk associated with CYP1B1 Leu^{432} Val alone (Cote *et al.*, 2005; Wenzlaff *et al.*, 2005).

The hypothesis that polymorphisms in TP53 may modulate the risk for lung cancer associated with tobacco smoke was evaluated in a case–control study of lung cancer in Baltimore, Maryland. African-Americans with Pro-T-A-G-G haplotype (combining the polymorphisms TP53_01 (rs1042522), TP53_65 (rs9895829), TP53_66 (re2909430), TP53_16 (rs1625895), and TP_11 (rs12951053)) had both an increased risk for lung cancer (HR, 2.32; 95%CI: 1.38–4.10) and a worsened lung cancer prognosis (HR, 2.38; 95%CI: 0.38–4.10) compared with those having the Arg-T-A-G-T haplotype. No association of TP53 polymorphisms with lung cancer was observed in Caucasians (Mechanic *et al.*, 2007). Common genetic variation in TP53 could modulate lung cancer pathways in African Americans. Differences in lung cancer susceptibility may exist based on race, tobacco exposure and selected genetic polymorphisms (Mechanic *et al.*, 2007).

2.2.6 Interactions

(a) Diet and exercise

Antioxidant vitamins, carotenoids, isothiocyanates, total dietary vegetables and fruit, and physical exercise have been associated with a decreased risk for cancer in some studies but the overall protective effect of diet and exercise account for only a small fraction of the total risk associated with tobacco smoking.

The association of fruit and vegetable with lung cancer incidence among both smokers and non-smokers was evaluated in the European Prospective Investigation into Cancer and Nutrition (EPIC). In current smokers lung cancer risk was significantly decreased with higher vegetable consumption, the hazard ratio being 0.78 (95%CI: 0.62–0.98) per 100 g increase in daily vegetable consumption, and 0.90 (95%CI: 0.81–0.99) per 100 g fruit (Linseisen *et al.*, 2007). While overall consumption of fruits and vegetables was not found to be protective of lung cancer in the NIH-AARP Diet and Health Study, higher consumption of several botanical subgroups (i.e. rosaceae, convolvulaceae, and umbelliferae) was significantly inversely associated with risk, but only in men (Wright *et al.*, 2008).

Cruciferous vegetables (i.e. broccoli, cabbage, cauliflower, Brussels sprouts, kale) are rich in isothiocyanates and have been hypothesized to have anticancer properties that may contribute to reduced risk for lung cancer. Isothiocyanates may inhibit the bioactivation of procarcinogens found in tobacco smoke such as polycyclic aromatic hydrocarbons and 4-(methylnitrosamino)-1-(3-pyridyl)-1-butanone (Hecht, 2000). Isothiocyanates may also enhance excretion of carcinogenic metabolites before they can damage DNA (Gasper *et al.*, 2005). Furthermore, sulforaphane, a major isothiocyanate found in broccoli, can induce cell cycle arrest and apoptosis (Seow *et al.*, 2005). GSTM1 and GSTT1 encode isoenzymes that play an important role in xenobiotic metabolism (Hecht, 2000). Individuals with homozygous deletion of GSTM1 and GSTT1, or both may metabolize isothiocyanates less efficiently and may be more intensely exposed to isothiocyanates after consumption of cruciferous vegetables. Epidemiological evidence from 30 studies on the association between lung cancer and either total cruciferous vegetable consumption (6 cohort and 12 case–control studies) or specific cruciferous vegetables (1 cohort and 11 case–control studies) was recently evaluated (Lam *et al.*, 2009). The risk for lung cancer among those in the highest category of total cruciferous vegetable intake was 22% lower in case–control studies (pooled OR, 0.78; 95%CI: 0.70–0.88) and 17% lower in cohort studies (pooled RR, 0.83; 95%CI: 0.62–1.08). The strongest inverse association of total cruciferous vegetable intake with lung cancer was seen among individuals with GSTM1 and GSTT1 double null genotypes (OR, 0.41; 95%CI: 0.26–0.65; p for interaction = 0.01). The inverse association was observed in both smokers and non-smokers.

The potential role of vitamin A in the development of lung cancer attracted early research interest (Bjelke, 1975). Carotenoids were thought to have anti-cancer properties and early evidence from case–control studies tended to support an inverse association of lung cancer incidence with β-carotene intake and with serum concentrations of β-carotene. However, the case–control design is not ideal for assessing the effect of serum carotenoids as a risk factor for lung cancer risk since the disease is likely to effect serum levels. In a meta-analysis of six randomized clinical trials and 25 prospective observational studies, Gallicchio *et al.* (2008) computed a pooled relative risk for studies comparing β-carotene supplements with placebo of 1.10 (95%CI: 0.89–1.36). Among observational studies, the pooled relative risk for total carotenoid dietary intake from six studies was 0.86 (95%CI: 0.75–0.99) among current smokers. For dietary intake of β-cryptoxanthin, data from six studies gave a pooled relative risk among smokers of 0.75 (95%CI: 0.58–0.96). No other carotenoids significantly reduced the risk in current, former or never smokers.

Based on a review of the literature, antioxidant vitamins show no clear protective effect on lung cancer risk in smokers or non-smokers, although there was some, albeit inconsistent, evidence pointing to a protective role for vitamin C and E. No clear protective role was observed for vitamin A (Ruano-Ravina *et al.*, 2006).

Increased physical activity has been associated with a reduction in the incidence and mortality from all-site cancer and some site-specific cancers in studies of non-smokers, but less is known about whether physical activity is associated with similar risk reduction in smokers. Several early studies suggested that physical activity is associated with decreased risk of lung cancer in men and women after adjusting for smoking, with risk reductions estimated from 18% (Peterson *et al.*, 2001) to 62% (Kubík *et al.*, 2001). The effect of physical activity on lung cancer risk was assessed in a sample drawn from participants in the Beta-Carotene and Retinol Efficacy Trial. The results suggested that physical activity may play a small role in reducing cancer risk and mortality among those with significant tobacco exposure. The incidence of lung cancer and of all cancer sites combined seemed to be more attenuated by exercise in men than in women, while the attenuation in lung cancer mortality was greater in women than in men. These effects may be more pronounced for younger people and may differ inconsistently by pack–years of smoking (Alfano *et al.*, 2004).

(b) Radon

In a pooled analysis of data from 13 case–control studies of residential radon and lung cancer from nine European countries (7148 cases of lung cancer and 14208 controls), the dose–response relation seemed to be linear with no threshold and remained significant in analyses limited to individuals from homes with measured radon < 200 Bq/m^3. The absolute risks of lung cancer by age 75 years at radon concentrations of 0, 100, and 400 Bq/m^3 would be about 0.4%, 0.5% and 0.7%, respectively, for lifelong non-smokers, and about 25 times greater (10%, 12% and 16%) for cigarette smokers. These studies show appreciable hazards from residential radon, particularly for smokers and recent ex-smokers (Darby *et al.*, 2005). Similar risks were identified in a pooling project of North American case–control studies (Krewski *et al.*, 2005).

(c) Asbestos

Exposure to asbestos and tobacco smoking are both known causes of lung cancer in humans (Doll & Peto, 1978; de Klerk *et al.*, 1996). Some studies suggest a multiplicative effect [where the effect of asbestos exposure is a multiple of the effect of smoking] (Hammond *et al.*, 1979; Doll & Peto, 1985), and meta-analyses have suggested that the additive model [where asbestos exposure and smoking are independent of each other] is unsound (Lee, 2001; Liddell, 2001). In a recent study of 2935 asbestos miners, persons exposed to asbestos and tobacco who subsequently quit smoking remained at a 90% increased risk of lung cancer up to 20 years after smoking cessation, compared to never-smoker asbestos workers (Reid *et al.*, 2006a).

(d) Genetic polymorphisms

Lung cancer is plausibly caused by the interplay between environmental factors and several low-risk alleles. Attempts in identifying specific single nucleotide polymorphisms (SNPs) responsible for modulating lung cancer risk have yielded few conclusive results. Recent studies have focused on mechanistically plausible polymorphisms in genes coding for enzymes involved in the activation, detoxification and repair of chemical damage caused by tobacco smoke. Genetic association studies indicate that several inherited genetic polymorphisms may be associated with lung cancer risk, but the data from individual studies with low statistical power are conflicting. Evidence from pooled or meta-analyses, along with some individual studies, is briefly summarized below.

(i) Metabolic genes

Most of the 70 carcinogens in tobacco smoke are procarcinogens that must be activated by phase I enzymes and may then be deactivated by phase II enzymes. Polymorphisms that alter the function of the genes involved in the activation or detoxification of tobacco smoke carcinogens can potentially influence an individual's risk of developing a tobacco-related cancer.

Meta and pooled analyses of 34 case–control, genotype-based studies were conducted to assess the effect of GSTT1 genotypes and smoking on lung cancer risk. No significant interaction was observed (Raimondi *et al.*, 2006). A pooled analysis of 21 case–control studies from the International Collaborative study of Genetic Susceptibility to Environmental Carcinogens showed no evidence of increased risk for lung cancer among carriers of the GSTM1 null genotype and there was no evidence of interaction between GSTM1 genotype and either smoking status or cumulative tobacco consumption (Benhamou *et al.*, 2002). Similarly, in another pooled analysis the summary OR indicated the slow acetylator genotype of N-acetyltransferase 2 (NAT2) detoxification enzyme was not associated with lung cancer risk among Caucasians (Borlak & Reamon-Buettner, 2006). In a pooled analysis to test the hypothesis of interaction among genetic variants in increasing the individual risk for cancer, the cumulative effect of variants in three metabolic genes, CYP1A1, GSTM1 and GSTT1 was assessed. The risk for lung cancer was increased with the combination of CYP1A1*2B or CYP1A1*4 alleles and the double deletion of both GSTM1 and GSTT1 up to an OR of 8.25 (95%CI: 2.29–29.77). The combination including CY1A1*4 among never smokers was associated with an OR of 16.19 (95%CI: 1.90–137). These estimates did not change after adjustment by the number of cigarettes smoked and duration of smoking. The results were consistent across ethnicities and were approximately the same for adenocarcinoma and squamous cell carcinoma (Vineis *et al.*, 2007).

Microsomal epoxide hydrolase 1 (EPHX1) plays an important role in both the activation and detoxification of tobacco-derived carcinogens. Polymorphisms at exons 3 and 4 of the EPHX1 gene have been reported to be associated with variations in EPHX1 activity. In a meta-analysis of 13 case–control studies the low-activity (variant) genotype of EPHX1 polymorphism at exon 3 was associated with decreased risk for lung cancer (OR, 0.65; 95%CI: 0.44–0.96) among whites. In white-populations, the high activity (variant) genotype of EPHX1 polymorphism at exon 4 was associated with a modest increased risk of lung cancer (OR, 1.22; 95%CI: 0.79–1.90) and the predicted low activity was associated with a modest decrease in risk (OR, 0.72; 95%CI: 0.43–1.22) (Kiyohara *et al.*, 2006).

(ii) DNA repair and cell cycle pathways

Data from 14 studies of lung cancer were used in a pooled analysis focusing on 18 sequence variants in 12 DNA repair genes, including APEX1, OGG1, XRCC1, XRCC2, XRCC3, ERCC1, XPD, XPF, XPG, XPA, MGMT and TP53 (Hung *et al.*, 2008a). None of the variants appeared to have a large effect on lung cancer risk. In a recent meta-analysis the X-ray repair cross-complementing protein group 3 (XRCC3) and the xeroderma pigmentosum group D (XPD)/excision repair cross-complementing group 2 (ERCC2) genes were evaluated (Manuguerra *et al.*, 2006). The authors found no association between these genes and the cancer sites investigated (skin, breast and lung). A significant association was identified for XPD/ERCC2 single nucleotide polymorphisms (codons 312 and 751) and lung cancer.

(iii) Nicotine acetylcholine receptor genes

A series of large genome-wide association studies for lung cancer have identified susceptibility loci for lung cancer in chromosome arms 5p, 6p and 15q (Landi *et al.*, 2009). In particular, the susceptibility locus at chromosome region 15q25 includes several genes, including three that encode nicotinic acetylcholine receptor subunits (CHRNA5, CHRNA3 and CHRNB4). Nicotinic acetylcholine receptor subunit genes code for proteins that form receptors present in neuronal and other tissue, in particular alveolar epithelial cells, pulmonary neuroendocrine cells, and lung cancer cell lines (Wang *et al.*, 2001; Minna, 2003) and bind to nicotine and nicotine derivatives including NNN. An association of CHRNA3 and CHRNA5 variants with nicotine dependence has been reported (Saccone *et al.*, 2007; Berrettini *et al.*, 2008). These genes may act, at least partially, upon cigarette smoking. Current smokers with one or two copies of the susceptibility variant are likely to smoke between one and two cigarettes more a day (Spitz *et al.*, 2008). Evidence for an effect of the 15q25 locus among never smokers is conflicting, with an association found in one study in Europe (Hung *et al.*, 2008b) and one in Asia (Wu *et al.*, 2009a), but not in others. Whether genes in the 15q25 locus have an effect on lung cancer beyond their propensity to increase numbers of cigarettes smoked is unclear.

Three genome-wide association studies identified genetic factors that modified disease risk. The first was a genome-wide association analysis to identify genetic polymorphisms associated with lung cancer risk in 1154 lung cancer patients of European ancestry who were current or former smokers and 1137 control subjects who were frequency matched to the lung cancer patients by age, sex, race and smoking status. Two SNPs, rs105173 and rs803419, which mapped to a region of strong linkage disequilibrium within 15q25.1, were strongly associated with risk of lung cancer, with an odds ratio for rs105173 of 1.31 ($P = 9.84 \times 10^{-6}$). This finding was replicated with an additional 711 case subjects and 632 control subjects from Texas ($P = 0.00042$) and in 2013 case subjects and 3062 control subjects in the United Kingdom ($P = 2.33 \times 10^{-10}$). The region of interest encompasses the nicotinic acetylcholine receptor subunit genes CHRNA3 and CHRNA5 (as well as CHRNB4) (Spitz *et al.*, 2008). A second genome-wide association study conducted among 1989 lung cancer cases and 2625 controls from six central European countries confirm these results (Hung *et al.*, 2008a). In a third genome-wide association study of 665 Icelandic, 269 Spanish and 90 Dutch lung cancer cases and 32244 controls a common variant in the nicotinic acetylcholine receptor gene cluster [chromosome region 15q24] was significantly associated with lung cancer risk (OR, 1.31; 95%CI: 0.1.19–1.44). The variant was observed to have a significant effect on the number of cigarettes smoked per day (Thorgeirsson *et al.*, 2008). These studies have all shown a link between this variant and lung cancer risk either through a mechanism involving nicotine dependence or a direct role in downstream signalling pathways that promote carcinogens. Together these results provide compelling evidence of a locus at 15q25 and 15q24 predisposing to lung cancer.

(iv) Alpha(1)-antitrypsin

Alpha(1)-antitrypsin deficiency (α(1)ATD) is one of the most common genetic disorders, especially among European descendents. Recent results suggest that α(1)ATD carriers are at a 70–100% increased risk of lung cancer, accounting for 11% to 12% of patients with lung cancer (Yang *et al.*, 2008). [The specific effect by smoking status was not evaluated.]

(v) Other genes

Mutations in the checkpoint CHEK2 gene have been associated with increased risk of breast, prostate and colon cancer and a decreased risk of lung cancer among those with the I157T missense variant of the CHEK2 gene. In a large Polish case–control study CHEK2 mutations were protective against lung cancer (OR, 0.3; 95%CI: 0.2–0.5) (Cybulski *et al.*, 2008).

The Swedish Family-Cancer Database was used to compare the rate of lung cancers among persons without family history of lung cancer to those with a family history (Li & Hemminki, 2004). A high risk by family history in adenocarcinoma (standardized incidence ratio (SIR), 2.03) and large cell carcinoma (SIR, 2.14) was found, a slightly lower risk among patients with squamous cell carcinoma (SIR, 1.63) and small cell carcinoma (SIR, 1.55). Among siblings, an increased risk was shown for concordant adenocarcinoma and small cell carcinoma at all ages and for all histological types when cancer was diagnosed before age 50. At young age, risks between siblings were higher than those between offspring and parents. These data suggest that a large proportion of lung cancers before age 50 are heritable and due to a high-penetrant recessive gene or genes that predispose to tobacco carcinogen susceptibility.

(e) Viral infection

Data are limited regarding lung cancer risk in human immunodeficiency virus (HIV)-infected persons with modest immune suppression, before the onset of acquired immunodeficiency syndrome (AIDS). Among 57350 HIV-infected persons registered in the USA during 1991–2002 (median CD4 counts 491 cells/mm^3), 871 cancers occurred. Risk was elevated for several non-AIDS defining malignancies, including cancer of the lung (SIR, 2.6 [n = 109]) (Engels *et al.*, 2008). [Specific evaluation with smoking status was not performed.]

2.3 Cancers of the upper aerodigestive tract

Evidence relating to cancers of the upper aerodigestive tract obtained from relevant cohort and case–control studies on specific sites is described in Sections 2.3.1 to 2.3.6; studies that looked at several subsites combined are described in Section 2.3.7. The major potential confounders for the relationship between smoking and cancers of the upper aerodigestive tract are alcohol consumption and use of any form of smokeless tobacco, and for some sites infection with human papillomavirus (HPV) (especially HPV16). In general, the studies examined by the Working Group had adjusted for these two confounders when appropriate. Some studies also adjusted for dietary intake, especially of fruits and vegetables, although few reported stratified relative risks.

2.3.1 Cancer of the oral cavity

Tobacco smoking was found to be causally related to oral cancer (IARC, 1986, 2004a). New studies on the relationship between oral cancer and cigarette smoking published since the most recent *IARC Monograph* (IARC, 2004a) include four cohort studies (Table 2.7 available at http://monographs.iarc.fr/ENG/Monographs/vol100E/100E-01-Table2.7.pdf), and eight case–control studies (Tables 2.8–2.11 online; see below).

(a) Intensity and duration of smoking

Intensity of smoking was measured in almost all cohort (Table 2.7 online) and case–control studies (IARC 2004a; Table 2.8 available at http://monographs.iarc.fr/ENG/Monographs/vol100E/100E-01-Table2.8.pdf and Table 2.9 available at http://monographs.iarc.fr/ENG/Monographs/vol100E/100E-01-Table2.9.pdf). In addition to the number of cigarettes or amount of tobacco smoked daily, cumulative exposure to cigarette smoke was also measured in terms of pack–years, tobacco-years or lifetime tobacco consumption. The link between duration of cigarette consumption and oral cancer was examined in 15 case–control studies. Seven case–control studies also considered age at starting smoking.

One cohort study (McLaughlin *et al.*, 1995) and 14 case–control studies reported a dose-dependent increase in risk with increasing number of cigarettes smoked daily or increasing daily tobacco consumption (Franceschi *et al.*, 1990, 1992, 1999; Nandakumar *et al.*, 1990; Zheng *et al.*, 1990; Choi & Kahyo, 1991; Oreggia *et al.*, 1991; Bundgaard *et al.*, 1995; Zheng *et al.*, 1997; De Stefani *et al.*, 1998; Hayes *et al.*, 1999; De Stefani *et al.*, 2007; Subapriya *et al.*, 2007; Muwonge *et al.* 2008). Whenever analysed, the trend was always statistically significant (Franceschi *et al.*, 1990, 1992; Oreggia *et al.*, 1991; Bundgaard *et al.*, 1995; McLaughlin *et al.* 1995; Hayes *et al.*, 1999; Subapriya *et al.*, 2007), except in the study of Muwonge *et al.* (2008) which also included bidi smokers.

Bundgaard *et al.* (1995) used lifetime tobacco consumption divided into four categories and reported a positive, significant trend after adjustment for life-time consumption of alcohol and other risk factors. A positive trend was also found in all studies that have analysed consumption in pack–years or tobacco-years (Zheng *et al.*, 1990; Maier *et al.*, 1992a; Macfarlane *et al.*, 1995; Hung *et al.*, 1997; Zheng *et al.*, 1997; De Stefani *et al.*, 1998, 2007; Applebaum *et al.*, 2007; Muwonge *et al.*, 2008), except Muwonge *et al.* (2008).

Ten studies (Franceschi *et al.*, 1990, 1992; Nandakumar *et al.*, 1990; Zheng *et al.*, 1990; Choi & Kahyo, 1991; Oreggia *et al.*, 1991; Zheng *et al.*, 1997; De Stefani *et al.*, 1998, 2007; Znaor *et al.*, 2003; Subapriya *et al.*, 2007; Muwonge *et al.*, 2008) classified the duration of smoking in up to four categories, and all but one (Nandakumar *et al.*, 1990) reported increased relative risks and a positive trend.

Of six studies that considered age at start of smoking (Franceschi *et al.*, 1990, 1992; Choi & Kahyo, 1991; Oreggia *et al.*, 1991; Zheng *et al.*, 1997; Balaram *et al.*, 2002) two reported a statistically significant trend of increasing risk with decreasing age at starting (Franceschi *et al.*, 1990, 1992).

(b) Cessation of smoking

Three cohort studies (McLaughlin *et al.*, 1995; Freedman *et al.*, 2007a; Friborg *et al.* 2007) and nine case–control studies (Zheng *et al.*, 1990; Choi & Kahyo, 1991; Oreggia *et al.*, 1991; Franceschi *et al.*, 1992; Ko *et al.*, 1995; Zheng *et al.*, 1997; De Stefani *et al.*, 1998, 2007; Schildt *et al.*, 1998; Balaram *et al.*, 2002; Pacella-Norman *et al.*, 2002; Muwonge *et al.* 2008) estimated risks for former smokers which were always lower than those for current smokers and in five studies almost reached unity (Zheng *et al.*, 1990; Choi & Kahyo, 1991; Zheng *et al.*, 1997; Schildt *et al.*, 1998; Muwonge *et al.*, 2008). Twelve case–control studies examined the risk by years since quitting and all reported a negative trend, with relative risks compared with those in non-smokers decreasing to near unity after 10 or more years (Franceschi *et al.*, 1990, 1992; De Stefani *et al.*, 1998, 2007; Schlecht *et al.*, 1999a; Table 2.7 online; Table 2.10 available at http://monographs.iarc.fr/ENG/Monographs/vol100E/100E-01-Table2.10.pdf).

(c) Type of cigarette

The effect of the type of cigarette smoked was examined in several case–control studies (Table 2.11 available at http://monographs.iarc.fr/ENG/Monographs/vol100E/100E-01-Table2.11.pdf). The characteristics of the cigarettes included the presence of a filter, the type of tobacco, the tar content and whether the product was manufactured or hand-rolled. Two studies reported a statistically significantly higher risk for black than for blond tobacco (Oreggia *et al.*, 1991; De Stefani *et al.*, 1998, 2007). Similarly, a much higher risk was found for hand-rolled cigarettes than for manufactured cigarettes, and plain cigarettes had a much higher risk than filter-tipped cigarettes (De Stefani *et al.*, 1998, 2007). In one study the differences between black and blond tobacco and between hand-rolled and manufactured cigarettes persisted after stratification by duration of smoking (De Stefani *et al.*, 1998). Smoking cigarettes with a high-tar content led to higher risks than smoking cigarettes with a low-tar content (Franceschi *et al.*, 1992) and the same trend was observed for cigarettes without filter compared to cigarettes with filter (De Stefani *et al.*, 2007).

(d) Sex

Sex-specific effects were examined in two case–control studies (Zheng *et al.*, 1990; Hayes *et al.*, 1999). In both studies, the relative risks for all categories of intensity, duration of smoking and pack–years were higher for women than for men. [The Working Group noted that the background risk of oral cancer is considerably lower in women than men. Thus, the higher relative risk estimates in women than men indicate a higher proportionate contribution from smoking in women than men, rather than higher absolute risk.]

2.3.2 Cancer of the pharynx

Tobacco smoking was considered to be an important cause of oropharyngeal and hypopharyngeal cancers in the previous *IARC Monographs* on tobacco smoking (IARC, 1986, 2004a). Since then, results available from three cohort (Table 2.12 available at http://monographs.iarc.fr/ENG/Monographs/vol100E/100E-01-Table2.12.pdf) and seven case–control studies (Table 2.13 available at http://monographs.iarc.fr/ENG/Monographs/vol100E/100E-01-Table2.13.pdf and Table 2.14 available at http://monographs.iarc.fr/ENG/Monographs/vol100E/100E-01-Table2.14.pdf) provide further support for the association. Many studies, however, combine cancers of the oral cavity and pharynx (see Section 2.3.7). This section summarizes the evidence from all eight cohort and 21 case–control studies that reported results specifically on oropharyngeal and hypopharyngeal cancer, or on pharyngeal cancer in general; the latter may include data on nasopharyngeal cancer.

The risk for pharyngeal cancer was significantly increased in smokers in four cohort studies (Doll *et al.*, 2005; McLaughlin *et al.*,1995; Freedman *et al.*, 2007a; Friborg *et al.*, 2007) and all but one of the case–control studies (Rao *et al.*, 1999). The trend of increasing risk associated with increasing daily or cumulative consumption of cigarettes was evident from all these studies, particularly those from Europe (Brugere *et al.*, 1986; Tuyns *et al.*, 1988; Franceschi *et al.*, 1990, 1999; Maier *et al.*, 1994; Escribano Uzcudun *et al.*, 2002; Vlajinac *et al.*, 2006), India (Znaor *et al.*, 2003; Sapkota *et al.*, 2007), Uruguay (De Stefani *et al.*, 1998, 2007) and the USA (McLaughlin *et al.*, 1995; Applebaum *et al.*, 2007), and less strongly so in studies from Canada (Elwood *et al.*, 1984) and the Republic of Korea (Choi & Kahyo, 1991). The multicentre study in Europe, North and South America of Hashibe *et al.* (2007c) showed increased risks according to frequency (cigarettes/day) and duration (years) in never drinkers. Applebaum *et al.* (2007) found a relationship between increasing risk of pharyngeal cancer and increased pack–years of smoking in subjects with negative HPV16 serology but not in those with positive HPV16 serology (p value for interaction = 0.007).

In two case–control studies the risk increased with decreasing age at starting smoking (Franceschi *et al.*, 1990; Choi & Kahyo, 1991,), but adjustment was not made for duration and intensity of smoking. In a case–control study from Spain (Escribano Uzcudun *et al.*, 2002) the risk increased with the age of starting smoking.

Former smokers had consistently lower relative risks than did current smokers in both cohort (McLaughlin *et al.*, 1995; Freedman *et al.*, 2007a) and case–control studies (Choi & Kahyo,

1991; De Stefani *et al.*, 1998; Vlajinac *et al.*, 2006). In comparison with non-smokers, the relative risks for former smokers who had quit smoking for more than 10 years were between 2 and 4 (Franceschi *et al.*, 1990; De Stefani *et al.*, 1998; La Vecchia *et al.*, 1999), whereas the relative risks for current smokers in these studies were 10–14. In one study in Brazil (Schlecht *et al.*, 1999a), relative risks for former smokers who had stopped smoking for more than 10 years approached 1, whereas that for current smokers was just below 6. Consumption of black tobacco, hand-rolled cigarettes or plain cigarettes resulted in a higher risk for pharyngeal cancer than consumption of blond tobacco, manufactured cigarettes or filter-tipped cigarettes (De Stefani *et al.*, 1998; 2007).

2.3.3 Cancer of the nasal cavity and accessory sinuses

In the Life Span Study in Japan (Akiba, 1994) the association of tobacco use with sinonasal cancer was examined. A total of 26 cases of sinonasal cancer were identified among 61505 adults during follow-up. Relative risk estimates, adjusted for sex, location, population group, atomic bomb exposure, year of birth and attained age, were 2.9 (95%CI: 0.5–) and 4.0 (95%CI: 1.2–) for former and current smokers, respectively, when compared with non-smokers [upper confidence limits were not reported]. The cohort of 34439 British doctors followed up to 50 years (Doll *et al.*, 2005) showed increased risk for current smokers and smokers of more than 25 cigarettes per day, but only six deaths from nasal cavity and sinuses cancers were observed (Table 2.15 available at http://monographs.iarc.fr/ENG/Monographs/vol100E/100E-01-Table2.15.pdf).

A total of nine case–control studies of nasal cavity and sinus cancers have been conducted. When histological types were combined, all studies found an increased risk associated with cigarette smoking, but only one was statistically significant (Caplan *et al.*, 2000). In seven studies, dose–response in terms of intensity of smoking (cigarettes/day), duration of smoking or pack-years was considered. A positive significant trend was found in five studies (Brinton *et al.*, 1984; Hayes *et al.*, 1987; Fukuda & Shibata, 1990; Zheng *et al.*, 1993; Caplan *et al.*, 2000) and suggested in the other two (Strader *et al.*, 1988; Zheng *et al.*, 1992c).

One study (Zheng *et al.*, 1993a) found a significant decrease in risk for sinonasal cancer associated with increasing number of years since cessation of smoking. In a previous study, the same authors had found a negative, non-significant association (Zheng *et al.*, 1992c).

Five studies analysed squamous-cell carcinomas and adenocarcinomas separately (Brinton *et al.*, 1984; Hayes *et al.*, 1987; Strader *et al.*, 1988; Zheng *et al.*, 1992c; 't Mannetje *et al.*, 1999). In all studies, there was a significantly increased risk for squamous-cell carcinomas, whereas the risk was generally not increased for adenocarcinomas.

2.3.4 Cancer of the nasopharynx

(a) Cohort studies

The risk for nasopharyngeal carcinoma has been examined in relation to tobacco use in six cohort studies, three of them reported since the last evaluation (IARC 2004a; Table 2.16 available at http://monographs.iarc.fr/ENG/Monographs/vol100E/100E-01-Table2.16.pdf). In one study, conducted in a low-risk area (Chow *et al.*, 1993a), a significant increase in risk among smokers and suggestive positive dose–response relationships by duration of smoking and age at starting smoking were found. In another study, conducted in Province of Taiwan, China, an area in which nasopharyngeal cancer area is endemic, a similarly increased risk was found, but it was not statistically significant (Liaw & Chen, 1998). Doll *et al.* (2005) identified a risk only for smokers of more than 25 cigarettes per day, however, this result was based on only four deaths. Friborg *et al.* (2007) in Singapore found statistically significant increased risk of nasopharyngeal cancer only for those smoking for 40 years or more. Hsu *et al.* (2009) in Taiwan, China observed increased statistically significant risks only for those smoking for 30 years or more and those with cumulative exposure of 30 pack–years or more.

(b) Case–control studies

The study designs and the results of the case–control studies on the association of nasopharyngeal carcinoma with cigarette smoking reported since the previous *IARC Monograph* (IARC, 2004a) are given in Table 2.17 (available at http://monographs.iarc.fr/ENG/Monographs/vol100E/100E-01-Table2.17.pdf) and Table 2.18 (available at http://monographs.iarc.fr/ENG/Monographs/vol100E/100E-01-Table2.18.pdf), one being a nested case–control analysis within a cohort study (Marsh *et al.*, 2007).

In total, 14 informative case–control studies were available. In almost all of these, the risk for nasopharyngeal carcinoma was higher in smokers than in non-smokers. In Taiwan, China (Cheng *et al.*, 1999) high risks were statistically significant only for duration of smoking of 20 years or more. In the five studies conducted in the USA (Mabuchi *et al.*, 1985; Nam *et al.*, 1992; Zhu *et al.*, 1995; Vaughan *et al.*, 1996; Marsh *et al.*, 2007), where the incidence of nasopharyngeal carcinoma is low, the relative risks for current smokers ranged between 2 and 4, but were not statistically significant in the two studies (Mabuchi *et al.*, 1985; Marsh *et al.*, 2007). In a study conducted in Shanghai, an area of China in which nasopharyngeal carcinoma is not endemic (Yuan *et al.*, 2000), the relative risk was just below 2. In one study from the Philippines there was a sevenfold increase in risk after more than 30 years of smoking (West *et al.*, 1993). The four studies (Lin *et al.*, 1973; Yu *et al.*, 1990; Ye *et al.*, 1995; Cao *et al.*, 2000) conducted in areas of China in which nasopharyngeal carcinoma is endemic (Taiwan, China, Guangzhou, and Sihui) found relative risks for ever smoking ranging between 2 and 5. In the study from the North of Africa (Feng *et al.*, 2009) the only statistically significant increased risk was found for differentiated nasopharyngeal cancer in those that had smoked more than 22 cigarettes/day. [The result, based only on three cases, is very unstable (RR, 313; 95%CI: 1.94–50336).]

A statistically significant dose–response relationship was detected in seven studies that evaluated the effects of daily or cumulative exposure to tobacco smoke (Yu *et al.*, 1990; Nam *et al.*, 1992; Zhu *et al.*, 1995; Vaughan *et al.*, 1996; Cao *et al.*, 2000; Yuan *et al.*, 2000; Feng *et al.*, 2009) and was suggestive in two others (Lin *et al.*, 1973; West *et al.*, 1993). In two studies the risk of nasopharyngeal carcinoma decreased with increasing time since quitting smoking (Nam *et al.*, 1992; Vaughan *et al.*, 1996).

In the remaining studies, six from areas in which nasopharyngeal carcinoma is endemic (Ng, 1986; Yu *et al.*, 1986; Sriamporn *et al.*, 1992; Zheng *et al.*, 1994; Cheng *et al.*, 1999; Feng *et al.*, 2009; Guo *et al.*, 2009) and seven from areas in which it was not endemic (Henderson *et al.*, 1976; Lanier *et al.*, 1980; Mabuchi *et al.*, 1985; Ning *et al.*, 1990; Armstrong *et al.*, 2000, Marsh *et al.*, 2007), the relative risks for nasopharyngeal carcinoma for ever smoking were not significantly increased (Lanier *et al.*, 1980; Mabuchi *et al.*, 1985; Cheng *et al.*, 1999) or were close to 1.0 (Henderson *et al.*, 1976; Ng, 1986; Yu *et al.*, 1986; Ning *et al.*, 1990; Sriamporn *et al.*, 1992; Zheng *et al.*, 1994; Guo *et al.*, 2009).

In the two studies that distinguished between different histological types, relative risks were higher for keratinized (squamous-cell) carcinoma than for unkeratinized carcinoma (Zhu *et al.*, 1995; Vaughan *et al.*, 1996).

In the three studies in which men and women were analysed separately (Lin *et al.*, 1973; Nam *et al.*, 1992; Yuan *et al.*, 2000), the relative risks were found to increase similarly in both sexes in two studies (Nam *et al.*, 1992; Yuan *et al.*, 2000) and were higher among women in the study of Lin *et al.* (1973).

2.3.5 Cancer of the oesophagus

In the previous *IARC Monograph* (IARC, 2004a), both histological subtypes of oesophageal cancer (squamous-cell carcinoma and adenocarcinoma) were considered to be causally related to cigarette smoking. Many more epidemiological studies have since been conducted, and results of these studies further support this conclusion.

(a) Squamous cell carcinoma and unspecified cancer of the oesophagus

Since the previous *IARC Monograph* (IARC, 2004a), there have been reports on 9 cohort studies (Table 2.19 available at http://monographs.iarc.fr/ENG/Monographs/vol100E/100E-01-Table2.19.pdf) and 22 case–control studies (Tables 2.20–2.23; see below), making 30 cohort and 55 case–control studies in all. All showed that the risk of oesophageal squamous cell carcinoma was associated with cigarette smoking. In one study (Li *et al.*, 1989), the elevated risk was observed only in an area with a relatively low incidence of oesophageal cancer. However, two later studies in the same area, Lin County, China, found a twofold increase in risk for oesophageal cancer among smokers (Gao *et al.*, 1994; Lu *et al.*, 2000).

In most cohort studies and in most case–control studies with relatively large sample sizes (IARC, 2004a; Table 2.19 online; Table 2.20 available at http://monographs.iarc.fr/ENG/Monographs/vol100E/100E-01-Table2.20.pdf; Table 2.21 available at http://monographs.iarc.fr/ENG/Monographs/vol100E/100E-01-Table2.21.pdf), the risk for oesophageal cancer was shown to increase with increasing duration of smoking (11 cohort and 32 case–control studies) or number of cigarettes smoked daily (18 cohort and 31 case–control studies), and to decrease with increasing age at starting smoking (12 case–control studies). In comparison with pharyngeal and laryngeal cancers, relative risks for oesophageal cancer estimated by duration and by intensity of smoking were somewhat lower (see Sections 2.3.2 and 2.3.6, respectively).

Ten cohort and 20 case–control studies (IARC, 2004a; Table 2.19 online; Table 2.22 available at http://monographs.iarc.fr/ENG/Monographs/vol100E/100E-01-Table2.22.pdf) investigated the effect of smoking cessation on risk of oesophageal cancer. Although not all studies analysed the trend, all found a decreasing relative risk with increasing number of years since quitting. In some studies, the risk first started to decrease after 10 years of cessation (Brown *et al.*, 1988; Rolón *et al.*, 1995; Gammon *et al.*, 1997; Castellsagué *et al.*, 1999; Freedman *et al.*, 2007b; Bosetti *et al.*, 2008) or after 30 years of cessation (Pandeya *et al.*, 2008).

When comparing the types of tobacco smoked (Table 2.23 available at http://monographs.iarc.fr/ENG/Monographs/vol100E/100E-01-Table2.23.pdf), consumption of black tobacco resulted in a higher risk for oesophageal cancer than did consumption of blond tobacco (De Stefani *et al.*, 1990; Rolón *et al.*, 1995; Castellsagué *et al.*, 1999; Launoy *et al.*, 2000; Vioque *et al.*, 2008). Similarly, smoking untipped cigarettes generally resulted in a higher risk than smoking filter-tipped cigarettes (Vaughan *et al.*, 1995; Gammon *et al.*, 1997; Castellsagué *et al.*, 1999).

Two studies from the USA reported risks separately for blacks and whites. After adjustment for alcohol consumption, age and income, risks were very similar for former and current smokers and for the number of cigarettes smoked per day and duration of smoking (Brown *et al.*, 1994a; Brown *et al.*, 2001).

(b) Adenocarcinoma of the oesophagus

Two decades ago it was noted that incidence rates for adenocarcinoma of the oesophagus and gastric cardia had increased steadily in the

USA, whereas the incidence rate for squamous-cell carcinoma of the oesophagus had remained relatively stable (Blot *et al.*, 1991). An increase in the incidence of adenocarcinoma of the distal oesophagus and cardia was also noted in the United Kingdom (Powell & McConkey, 1990), and in several other countries. Since 1990, several studies have focused on the risk factors for adenocarcinoma of the oesophagus. Since the last evaluation (IARC, 2004a) one cohort study (Freedman *et al.*, 2007b) and three case–control studies (Table 2.24 available at http://monographs.iarc.fr/ENG/Monographs/vol100E/100E-01-Table2.24.pdf; Table 2.25 available at http://monographs.iarc.fr/ENG/Monographs/vol100E/100E-01-Table2.25.pdf) have been reported, totaling 13 case–control studies on the association of cigarette smoking and adenocarcinoma of the oesophagus.

(i) Intensity and duration of smoking

Ten studies, three that included only cases of adenocarcinoma of the oesophagus (Menke-Pluymers *et al.*, 1993; Gammon *et al.*, 1997; Wu *et al.*, 2001), three that included cases of adenocarcinoma of the oesophagus, gastro-oesophageal junction and gastric cardia combined (Kabat *et al.*, 1993; Brown *et al.*, 1994b; Vaughan *et al.*, 1995), and four that stratified by histology (Lindblad *et al.*, 2005; Freedman *et al.*, 2007b; Hashibe *et al.*, 2007a; Pandeya *et al.*, 2008), showed a significant positive association of adenocarcinoma of the oesophagus with cigarette smoking. The relative risks were somewhat lower than those for squamous cell carcinoma of the oesophagus. Three studies, one in China (Gao *et al.*, 1994), one in Sweden (Lagergren *et al.*, 2000), and one in the USA (Zhang *et al.*, 1996), reported similarly elevated relative risks, but some of these risks were not statistically significant, probably because of relatively small numbers of cases.

Of those studies that reported risks adjusted for alcohol consumption, a positive, significant dose–response relationship was found with intensity of smoking (Kabat *et al.*, 1993; Brown *et al.*, 1994b; Gammon *et al.*, 1997; Hashibe *et al.*, 2007a), duration of smoking (Gammon *et al.*, 1997; Pandeya *et al.*, 2008) and/or pack–years (Vaughan *et al.*, 1995; Zhang *et al.*, 1996; Gammon *et al.*, 1997; Pandeya *et al.*, 2008).

(ii) Cessation of smoking

Ten studies provided point estimates for former smokers. In eight, relative risks were lower in former smokers than in current smokers, although they remained elevated (Kabat *et al.*, 1993; Gao *et al.*, 1994; Vaughan *et al.*, 1995; Gammon *et al.*, 1997; Wu *et al.*, 2001; Lindblad *et al.*, 2005; Freedman *et al.*, 2007b; Pandeya *et al.*, 2008), and were increased in the other studies (Lagergren *et al.*, 2000; Hashibe *et al.*, 2007a). The decrease in relative risk associated with years since cessation was weak, but a significant trend was found in two out of six studies (Gammon *et al.*, 1997; Wu *et al.*, 2001).

(iii) Confounding

With the exception of two studies (Levi *et al.*, 1990; Wu *et al.*, 2001), all studies adjusted for alcohol intake as a potential confounder. Three more recent studies also adjusted for fruit and vegetables intake (Freedman *et al.*, 2007b; Hashibe *et al.*, 2007a; Pandeya *et al.*, 2008). Ten of these studies were conducted in the USA (Kabat *et al.*, 1993; Brown *et al.*, 1994b; Vaughan *et al.*, 1995; Zhang *et al.*, 1996; Gammon *et al.*, 1997; Freedman *et al.*, 2007b) the Netherlands (Menke-Pluymers *et al.*, 1993), the United Kingdom (Lindblad *et al.*, 2005), central and eastern Europe (Hashibe *et al.*, 2007a) and Australia (Pandeya *et al.*, 2008), where chewing of betel quid with tobacco or use of other forms of smokeless tobacco are not likely confounders. One study conducted in Sweden was adjusted for snuff use (Lagergren *et al.*, 2000).

(iv) Sex

Kabat *et al.* (1993) examined risks for men and women separately and observed similar patterns in both sexes, although risks among current smokers and heavy smokers were somewhat higher for women than for men. Lindblad *et al.* (2005) also found higher risks in women than in men, but they were not statistically significant.

2.3.6 Cancer of the larynx

Laryngeal cancer is one of the cancers most strongly associated with cigarette smoking (IARC, 1986, 2004a). Since the previous *IARC Monograph*, more epidemiological evidence has become available to strengthen this conclusion.

(a) Potential confounders

Other causes of laryngeal cancer include alcohol consumption, some occupational exposures (e.g. sulphuric acid; IARC, 2012a) and possibly some dietary habits. In investigating associations between smoking and laryngeal cancer, potential confounding by alcohol consumption has been considered in most of the studies.

(b) Intensity and duration of smoking

Cohort and case–control studies have been carried out in Asia, Europe, North and South America, and South Africa. In all, the risk for laryngeal cancer was consistently higher in smokers, and a positive significant trend was observed with increasing duration and intensity of smoking (IARC, 2004a; Table 2.26 available at http://monographs.iarc.fr/ENG/Monographs/vol100E/100E-01-Table2.26.pdf; Table 2.27 available at http://monographs.iarc.fr/ENG/Monographs/vol100E/100E-01-Table2.27.pdf; Table 2.28 available at http://monographs.iarc.fr/ENG/Monographs/vol100E/100E-01-Table2.28.pdf).

In most case–control studies, the relative risks for laryngeal cancer were near to or greater than 10 for smokers who had smoked for longer than 40 years (Falk *et al.*, 1989; Zheng *et al.*, 1992b) or had smoked more than 20 cigarettes per day (Tuyns *et al.*, 1988; Falk *et al.*, 1989; Choi & Kahyo, 1991; Zatonski *et al.*, 1991; Muscat & Wynder, 1992; Zheng *et al.*, 1992b; Hedberg *et al.*, 1994; Sokić *et al.*, 1994; Talamini *et al.*, 2002). Cancer of the larynx in non-smokers is so rare that several studies used as the reference category light smokers (Herity *et al.*, 1982; Olsen *et al.*, 1985a; De Stefani *et al.*, 1987; Zatonski *et al.*, 1991; López-Abente *et al.*, 1992; Maier & Tisch, 1997), or former smokers (Hashibe *et al.*, 2007b). Consequently, relative risks were lower in these studies, although the increases were still statistically significant.

Three case–control studies reported odds ratios for cancer of the larynx that increased with decreasing age of starting smoking (Franceschi *et al.*, 1990; Zatonski *et al.*, 1991; Talamini *et al.*, 2002).

(c) Cessation of smoking

The risk for cancer of the larynx declines rather rapidly after cessation of smoking (IARC, 2004a; Table 2.29 available at http://monographs.iarc.fr/ENG/Monographs/vol100E/100E-01-Table2.29.pdf). No detectable higher risk compared with never-smokers was seen among subjects who had quit smoking for at least 10 years (Franceschi *et al.*, 1990; Ahrens *et al.*, 1991; Schlecht *et al.*, 1999a, b; Bosetti *et al.*, 2006; Hashibe *et al.*, 2007b).

(d) Types of tobacco or of cigarette

Some investigators considered the role of type of tobacco (IARC, 2004a; Table 2.30 available at http://monographs.iarc.fr/ENG/Monographs/vol100E/100E-01-Table2.30.pdf). An average 2.5-fold higher risk was observed in smokers of black tobacco compared to smokers of blond tobacco (De Stefani *et al.*, 1987; Tuyns *et al.*, 1988; López-Abente *et al.*, 1992). Smoking untipped cigarettes also led to a higher risk than smoking filter-tipped cigarettes (Wynder & Stellman, 1979; Tuyns *et al.*, 1988; Falk *et al.*, 1989). Those that smoke cigarettes only had higher risks of larynx cancer than those that smoke cigars only (Hashibe *et al.*, 2007b).

(e) Subsites

Six studies investigated the risk for glottic and supraglottic cancer separately (Olsen *et al.*, 1985a; Tuyns *et al.*, 1988; López-Abente *et al.*, 1992; Maier *et al.*, 1992b; Muscat & Wynder, 1992; Sapkota *et al.*, 2007). The cancer risk increased with increasing amount smoked per day and with cumulative exposure for both subsites (IARC, 2004a; Table 2.28 online). In addition, the observed relative risks were higher for supraglottic cancer than for glottic cancer (Maier *et al.*, 1992b; Sapkota *et al.*, 2007).

(f) Sex

Few studies investigated sex-specific effects. In one cohort study (Raitiola & Pukander, 1997) similar risks were found for men and women, whereas in two case–control studies (Zheng *et al.*, 1992b; Tavani *et al.*, 1994), the relative risks for women were up to 10-fold higher than for the corresponding categories in men, though a small number of cases were involved. However, Freedman *et al.* (2007a) observed higher relative risks in men than women (Table 2.26 online). One study looked at women only and found higher risks of laryngeal cancer in former and current smokers relative to non-smokers, and also according to the number of cigarettes per day with a clear dose–response effect ($P < 0.001$) (Gallus *et al.*, 2003b).

2.3.7 Cancer of the upper aerodigestive tract combined

In epidemiological studies, especially in cohort studies in which there are few cases at some sites, investigators often combine cancers of the oral cavity, pharynx, larynx and oesophagus and term these 'cancer of the upper aerodigestive tract'. This section summarizes the data from 19 cohort studies (IARC, 2004a; Table 2.31 available at http://monographs.iarc.fr/ENG/Monographs/vol100E/100E-01-Table2.31.pdf), and 40 case–control studies (IARC, 2004a; Tables 2.32–2.35; see below).

(a) Intensity and duration of smoking

In all but two cohort studies from Japan (Kono *et al.*, 1987; Akiba, 1994), the risk for cancer of the upper aerodigestive tract was strongly associated with cigarette smoking. Relative risks increased with increasing daily cigarette consumption (Hammond & Horn, 1958; Doll *et al.*, 1980, 1994; Akiba & Hirayama, 1990; Kuller *et al.*, 1991; Chyou *et al.*, 1995; Engeland *et al.*, 1996; Murata *et al.*, 1996; Yuan *et al.*, 1996; Kjaerheim *et al.*, 1998; Liaw & Chen, 1998; Yun *et al.*, 2005; Freedman *et al.*, 2007a), duration of smoking (Chyou *et al.*, 1995; Yun *et al.* 2005; Friborg *et al.*, 2007) or pack–years (Liaw & Chen, 1998; Freedman *et al.*, 2007a).

The main characteristics and results of the case–control studies are presented in IARC (2004a), and in Table 2.32 (available at http://monographs.iarc.fr/ENG/Monographs/vol100E/100E-01-Table2.32.pdf) and Table 2.33 (available at http://monographs.iarc.fr/ENG/Monographs/vol100E/100E-01-Table2.33.pdf), respectively. Intensity of smoking was measured in most of these studies. The link between duration of smoking and cancer of the upper aerodigestive tract was examined in 20 case–control studies (Blot *et al.*, 1988; Merletti *et al.*, 1989; Barra *et al.*, 1991; De Stefani *et al.*, 1992, 2007; Franceschi *et al.*, 1992; Day *et al.*, 1993; Mashberg *et al.*, 1993; Kabat *et al.*, 1994; Lewin *et al.*, 1998; Bosetti *et al.*, 2000a; Garrote *et al.*, 2001; Gallus *et al.*, 2003a; Lissowska *et al.*, 2003; Znaor *et al.*, 2003; Castellsagué *et al.*, 2004; Menvielle *et al.*, 2004a, b; Rodriguez *et al.*, 2004; Hashibe *et al.*, 2007c; Sapkota *et al.*, 2007). Nine also considered age at starting smoking (Blot *et al.*, 1988; Merletti *et al.*, 1989; Barra *et al.*, 1991; Franceschi *et al.*, 1992; Day *et al.*, 1993; Lewin *et al.*, 1998; Garrote *et al.* 2001; Lissowska *et al.* 2003; Menvielle *et al.* 2004a).

In all but one study (Rao *et al.*, 1999) there was an increased risk for cancer of the upper aerodigestive tract associated with cigarette smoking. A clear dose–response relationship was seen with increasing daily tobacco consumption and duration of smoking as well as with decreasing age at starting smoking in most of the studies examined.

(b) Cessation of smoking

Twelve cohort studies (Doll *et al.*, 1980, 1994; Tomita *et al.*, 1991; Akiba, 1994; Chyou *et al.*, 1995; Engeland *et al.*, 1996; Nordlund *et al.*, 1997; Kjaerheim *et al.*, 1998; Yun *et al.*, 2005; Freedman *et al.*, 2007a; Friborg *et al.*, 2007; Ide *et al.*, 2008) provided point estimates for former smokers (IARC 2004a; Table 2.31 online). The relative risks for former smokers were always lower than those for current smokers.

In 16 case–control studies the relative risk by years since quitting was examined and generally a statistically significant negative trend was found (Table 2.34 available at http://monographs.iarc.fr/ENG/Monographs/vol100E/100E-01-Table2.34.pdf).

(c) Types of cigarette

The characteristics studied in several case–control studies included the use of a filter, the type of tobacco, the tar content and whether the product was manufactured or hand-rolled (IARC, 2004a; Table 2.35 available at http://monographs.iarc.fr/ENG/Monographs/vol100E/100E-01-Table2.35.pdf). Consumption of black tobacco, cigars, untipped cigarettes, hand-rolled cigarettes, or cigarettes with a high-tar yield generally resulted in a higher risk than consumption of blond tobacco (Merletti *et al.*, 1989; Castellsagué *et al.*, 2004; De Stefani *et al.*, 2007), filter-tipped cigarettes (Merletti *et al.*, 1989; Mashberg *et al.*, 1993; Kabat *et al.*, 1994; Lissowska *et al.*, 2003; De Stefani *et al.*, 2007), manufactured cigarettes (De Stefani *et al.*, 1992, 2007) or low-tar cigarettes (Franceschi *et al.*, 1992). Two studies from India (Znaor *et al.*, 2003; Sapkota *et al.* 2007) revealed higher risks of *bidi* smoking related to cigarettes smoking.

(d) Sex

Sex-specific effects were analysed in four cohort studies (IARC 2004a; Table 2.31 online). In three cohort studies (Hammond & Seidman, 1980; Akiba & Hirayama, 1990; Freedman *et al.*, 2007a) a higher relative risk was found for male smokers than for female smokers; however, Ide *et al.* (2008) detected a higher risk among women in a study with a small number of cases.

In three case–control studies (Blot *et al.*, 1988; Kabat *et al.*, 1994; Muscat *et al.*, 1996) the relative risks were higher for women than for men in all categories of intensity of smoking (number of cigarettes per day), cumulative exposure (cumulative tar consumption, pack–years, duration of smoking) and age at starting smoking, as well as for former smokers. However, the trends in men were always in the same direction and of the same order of magnitude. An exception to the pattern was that in one study (Merletti *et al.*, 1989) the relative risk for smoking filter-tipped cigarettes was higher than that for smoking untipped cigarettes for women.

Overall, the strength of association by sex was generally similar, especially when taking into account the fact that women generally underreport levels of smoking and that most studies included many fewer women than men.

(e) Ethnicity

Relative risks were reported separately for blacks and whites in a large case–control study from the USA (Day *et al.*, 1993). Relative risks adjusted for alcohol consumption, sex and other relevant variables were very similar for the number of cigarettes smoked per day, years of cigarette smoking, age at starting smoking and number of years since stopping smoking.

2.4 Cancer of the stomach

2.4.1 Overview of studies

In the previous *IARC Monograph* (IARC, 2004a) it was concluded that there was *sufficient evidence* that tobacco smoking causes cancer of the stomach. Three meta-analyses have since examined the evidence for gastric cancer in 42 independent cohort studies published between 1958 and July 2007 (Ladeiras-Lopes *et al.*, 2008), in 46 case–control studies published between 1997 and June 2006 (La Torre *et al.*, 2009), and in 10 cohort and 16 case–control studies conducted in Japanese populations published between 1966 and March 2005 (Nishino *et al.*, 2006; Table 2.36 available at http://monographs.iarc.fr/ENG/Monographs/vol100E/100E-01-Table2.36.pdf). For current smokers compared to never smokers, the risk for stomach cancer was found to be statistically significantly increased by 53% (Ladeiras-Lopes *et al.*, 2008), 56% (Nishino *et al.*, 2006), and 57% when considering high quality case–control studies (La Torre *et al.*, 2009), with moderate to high heterogeneity.

Since the previous *IARC Monograph* (IARC, 2004a), the association between cigarette smoking and stomach cancer risk (15 studies) and mortality (4 studies) has been examined in 19 cohort studies (Table 2.37 available at http://monographs.iarc.fr/ENG/Monographs/vol100E/100E-01-Table2.37.pdf). Eleven of these were conducted in Asia (Sasazuki *et al.*, 2002; Jee *et al.*, 2004; Koizumi *et al.*, 2004; Wen *et al.*, 2004; Fujino *et al.*, 2005; Sauvaget *et al.*, 2005; Tran *et al.*, 2005; Kurosawa *et al.*, 2006; Kim *et al.*, 2007; Sung *et al.*, 2007; Shikata *et al.*, 2008), seven in Europe (Simán *et al.*, 2001; González *et al.*, 2003; Doll *et al.*, 2005; Lindblad *et al.*, 2005; Sjödahl *et al.*, 2007; Batty *et al.*, 2008; Zendehdel *et al.*, 2008) and one in the USA (Freedman *et al.*, 2007a). Only the updated British Doctors' study (Doll *et al.*, 2005) and the most recent studies (Shikata *et al.*, 2008; Zendehdel *et al.*, 2008) were not included in the meta-analysis of cohort studies (Ladeiras-Lopes *et al.*, 2008). Elevated risks in current smokers were found in all studies. The reported association of current smoking with mortality in the four cohort studies conducted in Taiwan, China (Wen *et al.*, 2004), Japan (Kurosawa *et al.*, 2006) and the United Kingdom (Doll *et al.*, 2005; Batty *et al.*, 2008) was comparable to that with incidence.

In addition, the association between smoking and stomach cancer risk has been reported in 37 case–control studies since the previous *IARC Monograph*, of which 22 are hospital-based and 15 population-based. With the exception of three studies (Campos *et al.*, 2006; García-González *et al.*, 2007; Suwanrungruang *et al.*, 2008; Table 2.38 available at http://monographs.iarc.fr/ENG/Monographs/vol100E/100E-01-Table2.38.pdf), all these studies were included in the meta-analysis conducted by (La Torre *et al.*, 2009).

2.4.2 Factors affecting risk

(a) Intensity and duration

Clear evidence has been provided by the meta-analyses as well as by the additional cohort studies that the risk for stomach cancer increases significantly with increasing daily cigarette consumption, duration or pack–years of smoking, although individual studies did not always find statistically significant dose–response relationships. In one meta-analysis based on 21 cohort studies, the risk for stomach cancer increased statistically significantly by 53% with consumption of approximately 20 cigarettes per day (Ladeiras-Lopes *et al.*, 2008). Using trend estimation analysis as proposed by Greenland & Longnecker (1992), the authors found an increase in relative risk from 1.3 for the lowest consumption to 1.7 for smoking 30 cigarettes per day.

(b) Cessation of smoking

Risk for stomach cancer has been generally found to be lower in former smokers than in current smokers. In six of the cohort studies decreasing risk with increasing years since stopping smoking was found although none found statistically significant dose–response relationships (González *et al.*, 2003; Koizumi *et al.*, 2004; Sauvaget *et al.*, 2005; Freedman *et al.*, 2007a; Kim *et al.*, 2007; Zendehdel *et al.*, 2008). Risk in former smokers was comparable to never smokers after quitting for 5 years (Kim *et al.*, 2007), 10 years (González *et al.*, 2003; Sauvaget *et al.*, 2005; Freedman *et al.*, 2007a) or 15 years (Koizumi *et al.*, 2004).

2.4.3 Subsites

The effect of current smoking on the risk for stomach cancer by subsite was assessed in ten cohort studies. Elevated risks were found for both cardia and non-cardia cancers. In six studies higher risks were found for cancer of the gastric cardia than for cancer of the distal stomach (Simán *et al.* 2001; González *et al.*, 2003; Freedman *et al.*, 2007a; Sung *et al.*, 2007; Shikata *et al.*, 2008; Zendehdel *et al.*, 2008), three studies found no difference (Sasazuki *et al.*, 2002; Lindblad *et al.*, 2005; Tran *et al.*, 2005), and in one study higher risk for cancer in the antrum rather than the body or the cardia was found (Koizumi *et al.*, 2004). A meta-analysis yielded statistically significant summary relative risks of 1.87 for cardia cancers and 1.60 for non-cardia cancers based on nine cohort studies (Ladeiras-Lopes *et al.*, 2008). However, there was substantial heterogeneity across studies for cardia cancers. For case–controls studies, the corresponding odds ratios were 2.05 (95%CI: 1.50–2.81) and 2.04 (95%CI: 1.66–2.50), respectively, with greater heterogeneity for non-cardia cancers. Criteria for the classification by subsite were not always described (Simán *et al.*, 2001; Koizumi *et al.*, 2004; Lindblad *et al.*, 2005; Tran *et al.*, 2005) and some studies included tumours located in the upper third of the stomach in the group of cardia cancer (Sasazuki *et al.*, 2002; Sung *et al.*, 2007; Shikata *et al.* 2008).

In three studies risk estimates for smoking associated stomach cancer were estimated by histological type (Sasazuki *et al.*, 2002; Koizumi *et al.*, 2004; Shikata *et al.*, 2008). The relative risks were 2.1 (95%CI: 1.2–3.6), 1.6 (95%CI: 1.1–2.3) and 2.3 (95%CI: 1.3–4.1) for the differentiated type, respectively, and 0.6 (95%CI: 0.3–1.1), 2.1 (95%CI: 1.1–4.1), and 1.3 (95%CI: 0.5–3.5) for the non-differentiated type, respectively.

2.4.4 Population characteristics

In four of the additional cohort studies risk was reported separately for men and women (González *et al.*, 2003; Jee *et al.*, 2004; Fujino *et al.*, 2005; Kim *et al.*, 2007), in three studies only for men (Koizumi *et al.*, 2004; Tran *et al.*, 2005; Sung *et al.*, 2007) and in one mortality study for men as well as for women (Wen *et al.*, 2004). Generally, the relative risks were smaller in women than in men. For all stomach cancers, risk in current smokers compared to never smokers was found to be significantly increased by 62% in men (based on 18 studies) and by 20% in women (based on nine studies) in the meta-analysis of cohort studies (Ladeiras-Lopes *et al.*, 2008). The men–women differences were independent of exposure level but could be explained by the sex difference in the distribution by histological type and other factors associated with socioeconomic status.

Ethnicity does not appear to modify the effect of smoking on stomach cancer risk. In the meta-analysis of case–control studies risk in current smokers was increased by 78% in Caucasians and by 48% in Asians (La Torre *et al.*, 2009). The summary risk based on the cohort studies increased by 46% and 47% in Caucasian and Asian studies, respectively. In a meta-regression analysis including the variables sex, population, and fruit and vegetable consumption, sex but not origin of the population showed significant differences in risk estimates (Ladeiras-Lopes *et al.*, 2008).

2.4.5 Bias and confounding

Generally, most cohort studies have relied on baseline information and did not update the exposure information, possibly leading to misclassification of smoking status. Most of the recent cohort studies have accounted for confounding by alcohol consumption (Fujino *et al.*, 2005; Lindblad *et al.*, 2005; Sjödahl *et al.*, 2007; Sung *et al.*, 2007) as well as fruit and vegetable consumption (González *et al.*, 2003; Koizumi *et al.*, 2004; Freedman *et al.* 2007a) and still observed significantly increased risk of stomach cancer in current smokers.

2.4.6 Helicobacter pylori infection

The association between tobacco smoking and stomach cancer could be confounded or modified by the effect of *H. pylori* infection, an established risk factor for stomach cancer. In three case–control studies (Zaridze *et al.*, 2000; Brenner *et al.*, 2002; Wu *et al.* 2003), and two cohort studies (Simán *et al.*, 2001; Shikata *et al.*, 2008) the joint effects and possible interaction between *H. pylori* status and smoking in relation to risk for stomach cancer was investigated. Among subjects who had *H. pylori* infection, the risk for stomach cancer was higher in current smokers than in non-smokers by 1.6 to 2.7 fold, providing evidence for a causal effect of tobacco smoking independently of *H. pylori* infection. Smoking was associated with risk elevations of the same order of magnitude among subjects without *H. pylori* infection. Smoking and *H. pylori* therefore may act synergistically, leading to very high risks in current smokers with *H. pylori* infection compared to non-smokers without *H. pylori* infection. In one study that examined risk by subsite an effect of smoking independent of *H. pylori* infection for gastric cardia as well as distal gastric cancer was found (Wu *et al.*, 2003). In none of the studies was there statistically significant evidence for interaction.

2.5 Cancer of the pancreas

2.5.1 Overview of studies

Previous *IARC Monographs* (IARC, 1986, 2004a) concluded that exposure to tobacco smoke caused cancer of the pancreas. Additional evidence has come from a pooled analysis of eight cohort studies with almost 1500 incident cases of pancreatic cancer and an equal number of controls (Lynch *et al.*, 2009) as well as a meta-analysis of 82 independent studies (42 case–control studies, 40 cohort studies) published between 1950 and 2007 (Iodice *et al.*, 2008; Table 2.39 available at http://monographs.iarc.fr/ENG/Monographs/vol100E/100E-01-Table2.39.pdf). In the meta-analysis 74% and 20% significant increased risks for current and former smokers, respectively, were found with significant heterogeneity of effect regarding current smoking across studies. Adjustment for confounders explained some of the heterogeneity (Iodice *et al.*, 2008). A similar significant risk elevation of 77% for current smokers was found in the pooled analysis, without study heterogeneity (Lynch *et al.*, 2009). For former smokers, risk was increased non-significantly by 9%.

Since the previous *IARC Monograph* (IARC, 2004a), a total of 15 cohort studies have reported on the association between cigarette smoking and pancreatic cancer incidence (8 studies) and mortality (5 studies) or both (one study) (Table 2.40 available at http://monographs.iarc.fr/ENG/Monographs/vol100E/100E-01-Table2.40.pdf), two of which were included in the pooled analysis (Coughlin *et al.*, 2000; Vrieling *et al.*, 2009). Excluding case–control studies that did not report odds ratios for current smokers, there were three additional case–control studies (Duell *et al.*, 2002; Inoue *et al.*, 2003; Alguacil & Silverman, 2004; Table 2.41 available at http://monographs.iarc.fr/ENG/Monographs/vol100E/100E-01-Table2.41.pdf). The effect of cigar and pipe smoking on pancreatic cancer was also examined in the ACS Cancer Prevention Study II regarding mortality (Shapiro *et al.*, 2000; Henley *et al.*, 2004) and in the Kaiser Permanente Medical Care Program regarding incidence (Iribarren *et al.*, 1999). All the additional studies showed an increased risk for pancreatic cancer associated with tobacco smoking, generally higher in current than in former smokers. The reported risk estimates were not always statistically significant, predominantly due to the small size of some studies and therefore lack of statistical precision.

2.5.2 Factors affecting risks

(a) Intensity and duration

Clear evidence has been provided by the meta-analysis, the pooled analysis as well as the additional studies that the risk for cancer of the pancreas increases significantly with increasing daily cigarette consumption, duration and pack–years of smoking (Coughlin *et al.*, 2000; Gapstur *et al.*, 2000; Nilsen & Vatten, 2000; Nilsson *et al.*, 2001; Isaksson *et al.*, 2002; Doll *et al.*, 2005; Yun *et al.*, 2005; Ansary-Moghaddam *et al.*, 2006; Gallicchio *et al.*, 2006; Vrieling *et al.*, 2009). In the meta-analysis risk of pancreatic cancer increased significantly by 62% with an increase of 20 cigarettes per day (based on 45 studies) and by 16% with a 10-year increase in smoking duration (based on 16 studies), but with significant study heterogeneity. In the pooled analysis, the excess odds ratio per pack–years generally declined with increasing smoking intensity (Lynch *et al.*, 2009).

(b) Cessation of smoking

A reduction in risk in former smokers who had stopped smoking for at least 10 years was found in the meta-analysis (Iodice *et al.*, 2008) and the pooled study (Lynch *et al.*, 2009). In some cohort studies risk was already comparable to never smokers five years after quitting (Boyle *et al.*, 1996; Fuchs *et al.*, 1996; Nilsen & Vatten, 2000; Vrieling *et al.*, 2009).

(c) Types of tobacco

In non-cigarette smokers, mortality from pancreatic cancer was increased although not statistically significantly so in cigar smokers in the CPS-II cohort study (Shapiro *et al.*, 2000) as well as a large case–control study (Alguacil & Silverman, 2004) but was less clearly elevated in the smaller Kaiser Permanente cohort study (Iribarren *et al.*, 1999). There was a significantly increased mortality for current cigar smokers who reported inhaling cigar smoke (Shapiro *et al.*, 2000). Pipe smoking was also found to be associated with an increased risk of cancer of the pancreas, which was stronger in those who reported that they inhaled the smoke (Henley *et al.*, 2004). A limitation of the cohort studies is that smoking habits were reported only at baseline, misclassification of smoking exposure is likely to underestimate the associated risks. In the meta-analysis there was a significant increase in risk of 47% associated with current cigar and/or pipe smoking (18 studies) and a non-significant risk elevation of 29% with former cigar and/or pipe smoking (5 studies) (Iodice *et al.*, 2008).

2.5.3 Population characteristics

The effect of sex on pancreatic cancer risk was investigated in two cohort studies (Nilsen & Vatten, 2000; Larsson *et al.*, 2005) and on pancreatic cancer mortality in four cohort studies (Coughlin *et al.*, 2000; Gapstur *et al.*, 2000; Nilsson *et al.*, 2001; Lin *et al.*, 2002a). The relative risks were comparable between men and women and no consistent evidence for an effect modification by sex was observed.

Ethnicity does not appear to modify the association of smoking with pancreatic cancer risk. The roughly twofold elevated risk in current smokers compared to never smokers was observed both in studies of Caucasians (Lynch *et al.*, 2009) and of Asians (Lin *et al.*, 2002a; Jee *et al.*, 2004; Yun *et al.*, 2005; Li *et al.*, 2006). In populations of the Asia-Pacific Region, there was also no difference in the strength of association between Asia and Australia/New Zealand (Ansary-Moghaddam *et al.*, 2006).

2.5.4 Confounding factors

In two large cohort studies the risk estimates for pancreatic cancer associated with cigarette smoking were not substantially influenced by adjustment for further potential confounding factors, including diabetes, body mass index (BMI), alcohol and dietary intake (Coughlin *et al.*, 2000; Vrieling *et al.*, 2009).

2.6 Cancer of the colorectum

2.6.1 Overview of studies

In the previous *IARC Monograph* (IARC, 2004a) it was not possible to conclude that the association between tobacco smoking and colorectal cancer is casual, principally because of concern about confounding by other risk factors. That evaluation was based on a total of 60 epidemiologic studies, although only few were specifically designed to study the effects of smoking. Studies have however shown consistently that cigarette smoking is a risk factor for colorectal adenomatous polyps, which are recognized precursor lesions of colorectal cancer (Hill, 1978). To explain this discrepancy, Giovannucci *et al.* (1994) hypothesized that a long induction period is required for tobacco to play a role in colorectal carcinogenesis, which would not be captured by studies with shorter follow-up time.

Four recent meta-analyses consistently showed a strong association between cigarette smoking and colorectal cancer (Botteri *et al.*, 2008a; Liang *et al.*, 2009; Huxley *et al.*, 2009; Tsoi *et al.*, 2009).

2.6.2 Cohort studies

Since the previous *IARC Monograph* (IARC, 2004a), 22 additional cohort studies have investigated the association between tobacco smoke and colorectal cancer (Table 2.42 available at http://monographs.iarc.fr/ENG/Monographs/vol100E/100E-01-Table2.42.pdf). [Studies that did not provide point estimates of risk (Andersen *et al.*, 2009; Hansen *et al.*, 2009; Murphy *et al.*, 2009) and included prevalent colorectal cancer in patients with other diagnosis (Chan *et al.*, 2007) are excluded from this review]. Seven of the studies were conducted in Europe, nine in Asia and five in the USA. In eleven studies, risk estimates were reported solely for colorectal cancer (Tiemersma *et al.*, 2002a; Limburg *et al.*, 2003; Otani *et al.*, 2003; Colangelo *et al.*, 2004; Sanjoaquin *et al.*, 2004; Lüchtenborg *et al.*, 2005a; Kim *et al.*, 2006; Akhter *et al.*, 2007; Huxley, 2007a; Kenfield *et al.*, 2008; Hannan *et al.*, 2009), five studies separately for colon cancer and rectal cancer (Shimizu *et al.*, 2003; Wakai *et al.*, 2003; Jee *et al.*, 2004; Yun *et al.*, 2005; Batty *et al.*, 2008) and five studies both for colorectal cancer as well as for colon and rectal cancers (Terry *et al.*, 2002a; van der Hel *et al.*, 2003a; Doll *et al.*, 2005; Paskett *et al.*, 2007; Tsong *et al.*, 2007; Gram *et al.*, 2009). Six studies were restricted to women (Terry *et al.*, 2002a; Limburg *et al.*, 2003; van der Hel *et al.*, 2003a; Paskett *et al.*, 2007; Kenfield *et al.*, 2008; Gram *et al.*, 2009), and two studies to men (Doll *et al.*, 2005; Yun *et al.*, 2005; Akhter *et al.*, 2007). One study reported both colorectal incidence and mortality (Limburg *et al.*, 2003) and three studies only reported colorectal cancer mortality (Doll *et al.*, 2005; Huxley, 2007a; Batty *et al.*, 2008; Kenfield *et al.*, 2008).

(a) Smoking status

Virtually all studies reported elevated risk associated with smoking, although results were not always statistically significant. The largest meta-analysis based on 36 prospective studies with data from a total of 3007002 subjects found that compared to never smokers, current smokers had a 15% significantly higher risk of developing colorectal cancer and 27% significantly higher risk of colorectal cancer mortality (Liang *et al.*, 2009; Table 2.43 available at http://monographs.iarc.fr/ENG/Monographs/vol100E/100E-01-Table2.43.pdf). In former smokers, colorectal cancer risk was also significantly elevated by 20% whereas colorectal cancer mortality was non-significantly increased by 20%. The risk estimates were not significantly different between colon and rectal cancer for current smokers (RR, 1.10 versus 1.19) and for former smokers (RR, 1.10 versus 1.20). There was no heterogeneity among colorectal cancer studies and no evidence for publication bias. Comparable risk elevations in current and former smokers were found in the other meta-analyses. For current smokers, the risk for colorectal cancer increased significantly by 16% when using data from 22 cohort studies (Huxley *et al.*, 2009), by 20% based on 28 cohort studies (Tsoi *et al.*, 2009), and by 7% based on data from 45 cohort and case–control studies (Botteri *et al.*, 2008a). In the latter meta-analysis a 17% significantly higher risk of colorectal cancer in former smokers was found.

(b) Intensity of smoking

All but three of the recent 21 cohort studies (van der Hel *et al.*, 2003a; Jee *et al.*, 2004; Sanjoaquin *et al.*, 2004) investigated dose–response relationships, using at least one of number of cigarettes smoked, duration of smoking, pack–years of smoking, age at smoking initiation, time since smoking cessation. In two further studies (Tiemersma *et al.*, 2002a; Batty *et al.*, 2008) these parameters were examined separately in current and former smokers, as by Chao *et al.* (2000). Statistically significant dose–response trends with amount smoked daily were reported for colorectal cancer (Lüchtenborg *et al.*, 2005a; Akhter *et al.*, 2007; Paskett *et al.*, 2007; Kenfield *et al.*, 2008), for colon cancer (Paskett *et al.*, 2007), and for rectal cancer (Paskett *et al.*, 2007; Tsong *et al.*, 2007). The dose–response of daily cigarette consumption and colorectal cancer was assessed in two meta-analyses (Liang *et al.*, 2009; Tsoi *et al.*, 2009) and both found statistically significant relationships. Based on eleven studies, Liang *et al.* (2009) found that risk for colorectal cancer increased significantly by 17% with an increase of 20 cigarettes/day and by 38% with an increase of 40 cigarettes/day, while colorectal cancer mortality increased by 41% and 98%, respectively (Table 2.43 online). The risk elevation associated with an increase of 20 cigarettes/day was greater for rectal than for colon cancer (13% versus 3%) but this difference was not statistically significant.

(c) Duration of smoking

In addition to two previously reported studies (Hsing *et al.*, 1998; Chao *et al.*, 2000), thirteen studies have examined duration of smoking and colorectal cancer risk. A statistically significant trend of increasing risk with increasing duration was found for colorectal (Limburg *et al.*, 2003; Kim *et al.*, 2006; Paskett *et al.*, 2007; Gram *et al.*, 2009), for colon cancer (Paskett *et al.*, 2007) and for rectal cancer (Terry *et al.*, 2002a; Paskett *et al.*, 2007; Tsong *et al.*, 2007). In one study, increasing duration of smoking was significantly associated with risk for colorectal cancer solely in former smokers (Tiemersma *et al.*, 2002a). Based on eight studies (Terry *et al.*, 2002a; Tiemersma *et al.*, 2002a; Limburg *et al.*, 2003; Lüchtenborg *et al.*, 2005a; Kim *et al.*, 2006; Akhter *et al.*, 2007; Paskett *et al.*, 2007; Tsong *et al.*, 2007), a meta-analysis for duration of smoking and colorectal cancer incidence yielded highly significant results (Liang *et al.*, 2009). Risk was increased by 9.4% with a 20-year increase in smoking duration and 19.7% with a 40-year increase. Smoking duration was also significantly associated with risk for rectal cancer but not for colon cancer. In another meta-analysis where dose–response relationship was modelled, a nonlinear increase in risk with increasing duration was observed (Botteri *et al.*, 2008a). The risk started to increase after approximately 10 years of smoking and reached statistical significance after 30 years.

(d) Pack–years

Since the previous *IARC Monograph*, the association of colorectal cancer with pack–years of cigarette smoking has been evaluated in six studies (Limburg *et al.*, 2003; Otani *et al.*, 2003; Shimizu *et al.*, 2003; Wakai *et al.*, 2003; Kim *et al.*, 2006; Gram *et al.*, 2009). In addition to the previously reported significant results (Giovannucci *et al.*, 1994; Heineman *et al.*, 1994; Chao *et al.*, 2000; Stürmer *et al.*, 2000), a statistically significant trend of increasing risk with increasing pack–years was found for colorectal cancer in two studies (Limburg *et al.*, 2003; Gram *et al.*, 2009), and for colon cancer in one study (Gram *et al.*, 2009). In their dose–response analysis of pack–years and colorectal incidence, Liang *et al.* (2009) included five studies (Giovannucci *et al.*, 1994; Stürmer *et al.*, 2000; Limburg *et al.*, 2003; Otani *et al.*, 2003; Kim *et al.*, 2006) and found a statistically significant trend of increasing risk with increasing pack–years of smoking for colorectal cancer but not specifically for colon or rectal cancer. Risk for colorectal cancer increased by 27% for an increase of 35 pack–years and by 50% for an increase of 60 pack–years.

(e) Age at initiation

In nine of the cohort studies the age at smoking initiation in relation to colorectal cancer (eight studies) or colon and rectal cancer (four studies) was investigated. In four studies a statistically significant trend of increasing risk with decreasing age at initiation of smoking for colorectal cancer was found (Limburg *et al.*, 2003; Kim *et al.*, 2006; Akhter *et al.*, 2007; Gram *et al.*, 2009) and for colon cancer (Gram *et al.*, 2009) and rectal cancer (Tsong *et al.*, 2007). In one meta-analysis (Liang *et al.*, 2009), a highly significant association was found for age at smoking initiation and colorectal cancer incidence based on six studies (Limburg *et al.*, 2003; Kim *et al.*, 2006; Akhter *et al.*, 2007; Paskett *et al.*, 2007; Tsong *et al.*, 2007; Gram *et al.*, 2009). Risk for colorectal cancer was reduced by 2.2% for a 5-year delay in smoking initiation and by 4.4% for a 10-year delay.

(f) Smoking cessation

The effect of smoking cessation by years since stopping was assessed in seven studies, six for colorectal cancer (Tiemersma *et al.*, 2002a; Lüchtenborg *et al.*, 2005a, 2007; Paskett *et al.*, 2007; Kenfield *et al.*, 2008; Gram *et al.*, 2009; Hannan *et al.*, 2009) and three for colon and/or rectal cancer (Wakai *et al.*, 2003; Paskett *et al.*, 2007; Gram *et al.*, 2009). In one study a statistically significant trend in risk reduction with years since quitting was found both overall as well as separately for men and for women (Hannan *et al.*, 2009).

(g) Population characteristics

It has been suggested that the association between smoking and colorectal cancer may be stronger in men than in women. In the three recent cohort studies reporting sex-specific results (Shimizu *et al.*, 2003; Wakai *et al.*, 2003; Colangelo *et al.*, 2004), this was only observed in studies in Japan (Shimizu *et al.*, 2003; Wakai *et al.*, 2003), but could be attributed to the very low prevalence of smoking in women. The studies restricted to women have generally shown associations with cigarette smoking that were of comparable magnitude to those observed in men (Terry *et al.*, 2002a; Limburg *et al.*, 2003; van der

Hel *et al.*, 2003a; Paskett *et al.*, 2007; Kenfield *et al.*, 2008; Gram *et al.*, 2009).

Recent studies have been carried out either in Europe and in USA, with predominantly Caucasian study subjects, or in Asia, mostly in Japan and in the Republic of Korea. The results from these studies suggest no differences in the association between tobacco smoking and colorectal cancer between different ethnic groups.

(h) Subsites

Smoking and risks for colon cancer and for rectal cancer were investigated in eleven of the 21 additional studies. Risk patterns are generally consistent between colon and rectal cancer (Otani *et al.*, 2003; van der Hel *et al.*, 2003a; Wakai *et al.*, 2003; Jee *et al.*, 2004; Yun *et al.*, 2005; Batty *et al.*, 2008). In some studies, dose–response relationships were stronger for rectal cancer than for colon cancer (Terry *et al.*, 2002a; Paskett *et al.*, 2007) or were statistically significant only for rectal cancer (Shimizu *et al.*, 2003; Doll *et al.*, 2005; Tsong *et al.*, 2007). In a meta-analysis (Liang *et al.*, 2009) the association was stronger for rectal cancer than for colon cancer in the subset of cohort studies that differentiated cancer by site. Most dose–response variables were not associated with colon cancer incidence whereas associations were stronger for rectal cancer incidence and statistically significant with longer duration of smoking, albeit based only on a small number of studies. In one cohort study the increased risk associated with smoking was more apparent for proximal than for distal colon cancer (Lüchtenborg *et al.*, 2005a), which was not found in an earlier study (Heineman *et al.*, 1994).

(i) Confounding and effect modification

Smokers have been shown to be more likely than non-smokers to be physically inactive, to use alcohol, to have lower consumption of fruits and vegetables and higher consumption of fat and meat, and they are less likely to be screened for colorectal cancer (Le Marchand *et al.*, 1997; Ghadirian *et al.*, 1998; Nkondjock & Ghadirian, 2004; Reid *et al.*, 2006b; Mutch *et al.*, 2009).

Few potential confounders were considered in the cohort studies evaluated in the previous *IARC Monograph* (IARC, 2004a). Of the cohort studies published since, all except three (van der Hel *et al.*, 2003a; Jee *et al.*, 2004; Doll *et al.*, 2005) considered two or more potential confounders. In eleven of the recent studies adjustments were made for physical activity, alcohol consumption, overweight/obesity (Terry *et al.*, 2002a; Limburg *et al.*, 2003; Otani *et al.*, 2003; Wakai *et al.*, 2003; Yun *et al.*, 2005; Akhter *et al.*, 2007; Ashktorab *et al.*, 2007; Paskett *et al.*, 2007; Tsong *et al.*, 2007; Kenfield *et al.*, 2008; Hannan *et al.*, 2009), and seven also adjusted for dietary habits (e.g. intake of fruits and vegetables, dietary fibres, fat, red meat). Among the studies with the latter adjustments, eight (Giovannucci *et al.*, 1994; Chao *et al.*, 2000; Stürmer *et al.*, 2000; Limburg *et al.*, 2003; Yun *et al.*, 2005; Akhter *et al.*, 2007; Paskett *et al.*, 2007; Hannan *et al.*, 2009) found significant dose–response relationships with at least one of the smoking variables. In two studies a significant association of smoking with colorectal cancer risk was observed after accounting for history of colonoscopy (Paskett *et al.*, 2007; Hannan *et al.*, 2009). Risk factors in multivariable analyses in several studies were level of education, use of menopausal hormone therapy, family history and regular aspirin use. The association between smoking and colorectal cancer was not modified by these other characteristics, or by alcohol consumption in two studies (Otani *et al.*, 2003; Tsong *et al.*, 2007). Therefore, confounding factors do not seem to affect the observed significant increase in risk for colorectal cancer associated with tobacco smoking and the dose–response relationships with smoking variables.

When considering other types of smoking, it is generally found that cigar and pipe smoking are less associated with socioeconomic class and other life-style habits than cigarette smoking. Therefore, it is logical to assume that, for these types of smoking, risk associations derived from epidemiologic studies may be less prone to potential confounding. In all the cohort studies reviewed in the previous *IARC Monograph* (IARC, 2004a) an elevated, though not always statistically significant, risk was consistently reported for cancers of the colon and the rectum associated with exclusive pipe and/or cigar smoking.

Infection with JC virus has been proposed as a potential risk factor for colon cancer (Rollison *et al.*, 2009) but results still need further validation.

Three cohort studies assessed possible modifying effects by genetic susceptibility. Rapid acetylator phenotype (as determined by polymorphisms of the *NAT2* gene involved in metabolism of heterocyclic aromatic amines) was found to increase the risk for colorectal cancer in smokers, in one (van der Hel *et al.*, 2003a) but not in another study (Tiemersma *et al.*, 2002a). For genes involved in the metabolism of polycyclic aromatic hydrocarbons such as *GSTM1* or *GSTT1*, no statistical contribution to the risk of colorectal cancer associated with smoking was observed (Tiemersma *et al.*, 2002a; Lüchtenborg *et al.*, 2005a).

2.6.3 Case–control studies

Thirty-one case–control studies were included in the previous *IARC Monograph* (IARC, 2004a). Although results were inconsistent with respect to risk association in ever versus former and current smokers, a dose–response relationship with smoking variables was found in some studies. Since then, seventeen case–control studies investigating the association between tobacco smoke and colorectal cancer risk have been published, seven carried out in Asia, four in Europe, five in North America and one in Hawaii (Table 2.44 available at http://monographs.iarc.fr/ENG/Monographs/vol100E/100E-01-Table2.44.pdf). Six studies reported solely for colorectal cancer (Ateş *et al.*, 2005; Chia *et al.*, 2006; Verla-Tebit *et al.*, 2006; Lüchtenborg *et al.*, 2007; Steinmetz *et al.*, 2007; Wu *et al.*, 2009b), four separately for colon and rectal cancer (Ji *et al.*, 2002; Sharpe *et al.*, 2002; Minami & Tateno, 2003; Goy *et al.*, 2008), two for colorectal cancer as well as for colon and rectal cancer (Ho *et al.*, 2004; Gao *et al.*, 2007; Wei *et al.*, 2009), three for colon cancer only (Diergaarde *et al.*, 2003; Kim *et al.*, 2003; Hu *et al.*, 2007) and one for rectal cancer only (Slattery *et al.*, 2003). Nine of the studies reported risk estimates separately for men and for women.

(a) Smoking status

Most case–control studies considered the effects of current and former smoking separately. A positive association between smoking and colorectal cancer was found in virtually all the studies, although the results were generally not statistically significant. Statistically significant increased risk was reported in current smokers for colorectal cancer (Chia *et al.*, 2006; Wu *et al.*, 2009b), for rectal cancer (Slattery *et al.*, 2003; Ho *et al.*, 2004), and in former smokers for colorectal cancer both in men and women combined (Chia *et al.*, 2006) and in women only (Lüchtenborg *et al.*, 2007). Five studies, which did not focus on the main effects of smoking, only evaluated risks for ever smoking (Diergaarde *et al.*, 2003; Kim *et al.*, 2003; Ateş *et al.*, 2005; Gao *et al.*, 2007; Hu *et al.*, 2007); none of these reported significant risk estimates.

(b) Intensity of smoking

Nine case–control studies investigated dose–response relationships considering at least one smoking variable. Number of cigarettes smoked daily was evaluated in seven studies, three for colorectal cancer (Verla-Tebit *et al.*, 2006; Lüchtenborg *et al.*, 2007; Wu *et al.*, 2009b), two for colon and rectal cancer (Ji *et al.*, 2002; Minami & Tateno, 2003), one for rectal cancer (Slattery *et al.*, 2003) and one for colorectal cancer and both subsites (Ho *et al.*, 2004). Statistically significant positive trends of increasing risk with increasing number of cigarettes smoked daily were found for colorectal cancer in only one study (Wu *et al.*, 2009b).

(c) Duration of smoking, pack–years, age at initiation, smoking cessation

Duration of smoking was examined in several studies in relation to colorectal cancer (Ho *et al.*, 2004; Chia *et al.*, 2006; Verla-Tebit *et al.*, 2006; Lüchtenborg *et al.*, 2007; Wu *et al.*, 2009b) and/or to colorectal cancer by subsite (Ji *et al.*, 2002; Minami & Tateno, 2003; Ho *et al.*, 2004). A statistically significant trend with increasing number of years smoked was found in two of the five studies of colorectal cancer (Chia *et al.*, 2006; Wu *et al.*, 2009b). In one study, increasing duration of smoking was significantly associated with risk for rectal cancer in ever smokers but not in current smokers (Ho *et al.*, 2004). In only one earlier case–control study was a significant association in ever smokers with increasing number of years of smoking for colon as well as rectal cancer found (Newcomb *et al.*, 1995).

Duration of smoking exposure was assessed by pack–years of smoking in seven studies (Ji *et al.*, 2002; Slattery *et al.*, 2003; Chia *et al.*, 2006; Verla-Tebit *et al.*, 2006; Lüchtenborg *et al.*, 2007; Goy *et al.*, 2008; Wu *et al.*, 2009b) and by age at smoking initiation in three studies (Ji *et al.*, 2002; Slattery *et al.*, 2003; Wu *et al.*, 2009b). All four studies that evaluated pack–years of smoking with respect to colorectal cancer risk found statistically significant associations. Two studies found a significant association with increasing pack–years in men and women combined; when investigated separately, the increasing trend was statistically significant only in women (Verla-Tebit *et al.*, 2006) or only in men (Wu *et al.*, 2009b). In one study a statistically significant trend with pack–years of smoking in both men and women was found only with non-filtered cigarettes (Lüchtenborg *et al.*, 2007); the relative risk was significant for colon as well as rectal cancer and was greater for rectal cancer.

In two studies a non-significant trend of decreasing risk with increasing time since stopped smoking was found (Verla-Tebit *et al.*, 2006; Lüchtenborg *et al.*, 2007).

(d) Subsites and molecular subtypes

A stronger association between tobacco smoking and rectal cancer compared with colon cancer has generally been observed in the studies that reported risk estimates by cancer site. In a recent meta-analysis including both cohort and case–control studies, higher smoking-related risk estimates for rectal cancer were found than for proximal and distal colon cancer (Botteri *et al.*, 2008a). Stronger relative risk in ever smokers, but not in current smokers, was found for proximal compared to distal tumours in one recent study (Hu *et al.*, 2007).

Colorectal cancer is a multipathway disease. A molecular approach to its classification utilizes: (1) the type of genetic instability, specifically microsatellite instability, and (2) the presence of DNA methylation or the CpG island methylator phenotype (CIMP) (Jass, 2007). Smoking has been associated with microsatellite instability in sporadic colon cancer. Higher risk for microsatellite-unstable than for microsatellite-stable tumours was found in four studies (Slattery *et al.*, 2000; Yang *et al.*, 2000; Chia *et al.*, 2006; Campbell *et al.*, 2009). The observed twofold risk elevation for colorectal cancer showing microsatellite instability is similar in order of magnitude to that found for colorectal polyps. In only one small study similar risk estimates for stable and unstable tumours were found (Diergaarde *et al.*, 2003). Microsatellite instability is characteristic of hereditary nonpolyposis colorectal cancer syndrome and smoking has been associated with colorectal cancer in patients with this syndrome (Watson *et al.*, 2004; Diergaarde *et al.*, 2007). Among sporadic colorectal tumours with microsatellite instability, about 11–28% carry somatic genetic mutations. In addition, the association of colon cancer with smoking was increased two to threefold when widespread CIMP and/or *BRAF* mutation, irrespective of microsatellite instability status, was present (Samowitz *et al.*, 2006). These data indicate that the association with MSI-high tumours may be attributed to the association of smoking with CIMP and *BRAF* mutation.

(e) Effect modification

Effect modification by genetic polymorphisms in enzymes metabolizing tobacco smoke constituents could provide further evidence for a causal association between smoking and colorectal cancer. Most studies that have investigated modification of colorectal cancer risk associated with smoking by genetic polymorphisms of xenobiotic enzymes were too small to be informative (Inoue *et al.*, 2000; Smits *et al.*, 2003; Jin *et al.*, 2005; Tranah *et al.*, 2005; van den Donk *et al.*, 2005; Tijhuis *et al.*, 2008). Studies on the possible differential effect by acetylation status have reported stronger association of tobacco smoking (in terms of pack–years) with colorectal cancer risk in slow acetylators phenotypes (Lilla *et al.*, 2006), and with rectal cancer in rapid acetylators phenotypes (Curtin *et al.*, 2009). Furthermore, *CYP1A1* and *GSTM1* variant alleles were found to greatly affect colon cancer or rectal cancer risk in smokers (Slattery *et al.*, 2004).

2.6.4 Colorectal polyps

Colorectal adenomas and possibly some hyperplastic polyps are considered precursors of colorectal cancer. The epidemiologic evidence on the relationship between cigarette smoking and colorectal polyps has been generally consistent. Since the previous *IARC Monograph* (IARC, 2004a), twelve further independent studies have investigated this association (Table 2.45 available at http://monographs.iarc.fr/ENG/Monographs/vol100E/100E-01-Table2.45.pdf). All studies found a significantly increased risk for polyps in association with one or more smoking variables. A recent meta-analysis including 42 studies reported a statistically significant positive association between smoking and colorectal adenomas (Botteri *et al.*, 2008b). The meta-analysis, which included several studies that did not explicitly report relative risks for tobacco smoking (Cardoso *et al.*, 2002; Voskuil *et al.*, 2002; Sparks *et al.*, 2004; Gong *et al.*, 2005; Jiang *et al.*, 2005; Kim *et al.*, 2005; Mitrou *et al.*, 2006; Otani *et al.*, 2006; Skjelbred *et al.*, 2006), found a twofold risk elevation for colorectal adenomas in current smokers and a 50% increase in former smokers. The association had been previously found to be equally strong in men and women. In one of two recent studies, there was no difference in the results for men and women separately (Tranah *et al.*, 2004) but significantly greater effects in women were found in the other (Hermann *et al.*, 2009).

Significant positive trends with number of cigarettes per day were found in four (Ji *et al.*, 2006; Larsen *et al.*, 2006; Stern *et al.*, 2006; Shrubsole *et al.*, 2008) of five studies (Tiemersma *et al.*, 2004). Dose–response with duration of smoking was assessed in four studies (Ji *et al.*, 2002; Tiemersma *et al.*, 2004; Stern *et al.*, 2006; Shrubsole *et al.*, 2008) and with pack–years of smoking in five studies (Hoshiyama *et al.*, 2000; Ulrich *et al.*, 2001; Tranah *et al.*, 2004; Ji *et al.*, 2006; Shrubsole *et al.*, 2008; Omata *et al.*, 2009). All nine studies found statistically significant trends, which were consistent with those for adenomas and hyperplastic polyps when reported separately (Ulrich *et al.*, 2001; Ji *et al.*, 2006; Shrubsole *et al.*, 2008). Ever smokers were estimated to have a 13% (95%CI: 9–18%) increasing risk of presenting with adenomatous polyps for every additional 10 pack–years smoked in comparison to never smokers, based on data from 19 studies (Botteri *et al.*, 2008b).

Decreasing risks with years since quitting smoking were found in four studies (Ulrich *et al.*, 2001; Tiemersma *et al.*, 2004; Ji *et al.*, 2006;

Shrubsole *et al.*, 2008), statistically significant so in the latter three studies. In comparison to never smokers, former smokers retained moderately elevated risk for colorectal polyps even 20 years after quitting smoking. One study examined both dose metrics (cigarettes per day, duration, and pack–years) and recency of tobacco use: in subjects who had quit smoking for at least 20 years, only the heaviest users of tobacco still had modest excess risks (Ji *et al.*, 2006).

It has been proposed that the association between cigarette smoking and polyps may be stronger with non-progressing adenomas, such as those that are smaller and less villous but the hypothesis is not supported in most studies (Anderson *et al.*, 2003; Toyomura *et al.*, 2004; Ji *et al.*, 2006; Skjelbred *et al.*, 2006). In one study a clearly higher risk for large and multiple adenomas in every anatomic site of the colon was found in a dose–response manner (Toyomura *et al.*, 2004). A meta-analysis found that the combined risk estimate for high-risk adenomas associated with smoking was greater than that for low-risk adenomas and that the difference was statistically significant for current smokers but not former smokers (Botteri *et al.*, 2008b). In addition, a stronger association of smoking with hyperplastic polyps than with adenomas was found in some studies (Ulrich *et al.*, 2001; Ji *et al.*, 2006; Shrubsole *et al.*, 2008) but not in another (Erhardt *et al.*, 2002). The risk associated with smoking may be even higher in subjects presenting with concurrent benign hyperplastic and adenomatous polyps (Ji *et al.*, 2006; Shrubsole *et al.*, 2008).

Relative risk estimates for tobacco smoking and polyps generally range between 2 and 3 whereas those for colorectal cancer range between 1.2 and 1.4. One possible explanation is the effect dilution due to the inclusion of a high proportion of individuals with precursor lesions in the unscreened control groups in most colorectal cancer studies (Terry & Neugut, 1998). Some indirect evidence for this hypothesis is provided by the meta-analysis of colorectal adenomas, which showed that the smoking-associated risk for adenomas was significantly higher in studies including subjects who had undergone complete colonoscopy in comparison to those in which some or all controls had undergone incomplete examination (i.e. only sigmoidoscopy) (Abrams *et al.*, 2008; Botteri *et al.*, 2008b).

It is also possible that smoking is associated with a subset of colorectal cancers so that relative risk estimates for colorectal cancer as a whole are diluted. The pattern of risk observed for colorectal cancer by microsatellite instability status and for type of colorectal polyps suggests that the traditional (non-serrated) adenoma-carcinoma sequence may proceed through a hyperplastic polyps-mixed polyps-serrated adenoma progression and that smoking may be more strongly related to the development of these subtypes (Jass *et al.*, 2000; Hawkins & Ward, 2001). More recently, a *BRAF* mutation was shown to be a specific marker for the serrated polyp neoplasia pathway originating from a hyperplastic polyp, in which the CIMP-high develops early and the microsatellite instability carcinoma develops late (O'Brien *et al.*, 2006). The findings of strong associations between smoking and colon cancer with CIMP and/or BRAF mutation, irrespective of microsatellite status, are compatible with this observation (Samowitz *et al.*, 2006).

2.7 Hepatocellular carcinoma

2.7.1 Overview of studies

In the previous *IARC Monograph* (IARC, 2004a), a causal relationship between liver cancer (hepatocellular carcinoma) and smoking was established. Two case–control and one cohort studies have been published since (Table 2.46 available at http://monographs.iarc.fr/ENG/Monographs/vol100E/100E-01-Table2.46.pdf). Overall, most cohort studies and the largest case–control studies, most notably those that included community controls, showed a moderate association between tobacco smoking and risk for hepatocellular carcinoma.

Confounding from alcohol has been addressed in the best studies. The association between alcohol drinking and hepatocellular carcinoma is strong, and alcohol intake is frequently misclassified, leading to potential residual confounding. However an association with smoking has been demonstrated also among non-drinkers.

A meta-analysis was based on 38 cohort studies and 58 case–control studies (Lee *et al.*, 2009). Compared to never smokers, the meta-relative risks adjusted for appropriate confounders were 1.51 (95%CI: 1.37–1.67) for current smokers and 1.12 (0.78–1.60) for former smokers. The increased liver cancer risk among current smokers appeared to be consistent in strata of different regions, study designs, study sample sizes, and publication periods. The association with smoking was observed in non-alcohol-drinkers (RR, 1.34; 95%CI: 0.92–1.94 in men and 1.31; 95%CI: 0.70–2.44 in women). Further supportive evidence is provided by the association between smoking and liver cancer observed among Chinese women and Japanese women, in whom alcohol drinking is extremely rare (Li *et al.*, 2011). One difficulty is that sometimes studies do not specify the histology of liver cancer (hepatocellular versus intra-hepatic biliary tract).

In the update of the Whitehall study (Batty *et al.*, 2008) (a cohort of 17363 government employees in London, followed-up for 38 years), the hazard ratio for death from liver cancer was 1.03 (0.49–2.16) in former smokers and 1.43 (0.69–2.95) in current smokers (based on 57 deaths). In the 50-year follow-up of the British doctors cohort (Doll *et al.*, 2005), there were 74 deaths from liver cancer. Death rates per 100000 per year were 4.4 in never smokers, 10.7 in smokers of 1–14 cigarettes/day, 2.6 in smokers of 15–24 cigarettes/day, and 31.3 in smokers of ≥ 25 cigarettes/day.

2.7.2 Factors affecting risks

(a) Dose–response relationship

Most studies, including the recent ones (Table 2.46 online), show a dose–response relationship with the number of cigarettes smoked and with smoking duration, with exceptions such as Franceschi *et al.* (2006) and some older studies from Asia. Relative risk estimates increased to 2.0 after 20 years of smoking.

(b) Cessation

Though former smokers tend to have lower relative risks than current smokers, there were no consistent patterns of risks after cessation, including in the recent studies (Table 2.46 online).

2.7.3 Interaction with hepatitis B or C

Infection with hepatitis B virus (HBV) is one of the major causes of liver cancer worldwide, whereas hepatis C virus (HCV) infection causes a large fraction of liver cancer in Japan, Northern Africa and southern Europe. While many studies, most notably from Asia, have found no attenuation of the association between smoking and liver cancer after adjustment/stratification for markers of HBV or HCV infection, an apparent interaction between smoking and HBV or HCV infection has been reported. The increase in risk for liver cancer associated with cigarette smoking appears to be greater among HBV carriers than among uninfected persons in some studies (Tu *et al.*, 1985), but not in others (Kuper *et al.*, 2000a). Two recent reports (Franceschi *et al.*, 2006; Hassan *et al.*, 2008a) studied possible interactions between smoking and hepatitis virus infection and both reported an apparent interaction between smoking and hepatitis C infection. Interactions between smoking and hepatitis B infection were not found among men in one study (Hassan *et al.*, 2008a) and the rarity of HBsAg prevented the evaluation of HBV and smoking in the other (Franceschi *et al.*, 2006;

Table 2.46 online). In the meta-analysis by Lee *et al.* (2009) adjustment for HBV reduced the relative risks in both men and women, while adjustment for HCV did not change the risk in women and increased it in men.

2.8 Renal cell carcinoma

2.8.1 Overview of studies

The previous *IARC Monograph* (IARC, 2004a) concluded that renal-cell carcinoma is associated with tobacco smoking in both men and women. Four case–control studies and no cohort studies have become available since then (Table 2.47 available at http://monographs.iarc.fr/ENG/Monographs/vol100E/100E-01-Table2.47.pdf). Overall these confirm the previous evidence, though with some conflicting results. In particular, both the study by Hu *et al.* (2005) in Canada and the multicentre European study by Brennan *et al.* (2008) do not show a clear effect of smoking. In contrast, the study by Theis *et al.* (2008) shows an increased risk with smoking duration (irregular, levelling-off after 40 years) and a statistically significant dose–response relationship with pack–years.

In the update of the Whitehall study (Batty *et al.*, 2008) (a cohort of 17363 government employees in London, followed for 38 years), the hazard ratio for deaths from kidney cancer was 0.64 (0.32–1.26) for former smokers, and 1.29 (0.69–2.41) for current smokers (based on 68 deaths). In the 50-year follow-up of the British doctor cohort (Doll *et al.*, 2005) there were 140 deaths from kidney cancer. Mortality rates per 100000 per year were 9.3 in never smokers, 16.4 in smokers of 1–14 cigarettes/day, 16.6 in smokers of 15–24 cigarettes/day, and 15.5 in smokers of ≥ 25 cigarettes/day (age-adjusted).

Hunt *et al.* (2005) performed a meta-analysis based on 19 case–control studies and 5 cohort studies (total 8032 cases in case–control and 1326 in cohort studies). The relative risk for smoking men was 1.54 (1.42–1.68), and for smoking women was 1.22 (1.09–1.36). A dose–response relationship was found in both men and women. The association observed was more convincing in population-based compared to hospital-based studies.

2.8.2 Confounding

Hypertension is a well established risk factor for kidney cancer but the association with smoking is only indirect. Potential confounding from hypertension was considered only by Brennan *et al.* (2008).

Other potential confounders such as BMI have been appropriately addressed in most studies.

2.8.3 Cessation

Most studies reviewed in the previous *Monograph* showed a lower risk for former smokers compared to current smokers, with a significant negative trend with increasing number of years since quitting (IARC, 2004a). In case–control study on smoking cessation and renal-cell carcinoma, the decrease in risk became significant only after 30 years of quitting (Parker *et al.*, 2003). In the meta-analysis (Hunt *et al.*, 2005), former smokers were at reduced risk after 10 years or more of quitting. A clear decline in risk after cessation was also reported by Theis *et al.* (2008). [The Working Group noted the poor quality of the study, considering the low response rate among controls.]

2.9 Cancer of the lower urinary tract (including cancer of the bladder, ureter, and renal pelvis)

2.9.1 Overview of studies

The previous *IARC Monograph* (IARC, 2004a) clearly identified a causal relationship of smoking with transitional-cell carcinomas and squamous-cell carcinomas of the bladder, ureter and renal pelvis both in men and women. Two new case–control studies (Cao *et al.*, 2005; Samanic *et al.*, 2006; Table 2.48 available at http://monographs.iarc.fr/ENG/Monographs/vol100E/100E-01-Table2.48.pdf) and two cohort studies (Bjerregaard *et al.*, 2006; Alberg *et al.*, 2007; Table 2.49 available at http://monographs.iarc.fr/ENG/Monographs/vol100E/100E-01-Table2.49.pdf) have been reported since then in addition to updates of cohort studies with longer follow-up.

In the update of the Whitehall study (Batty *et al.*, 2008) (a cohort of 17363 government employees in London, followed-up for 38 years), the hazard ratio for death from bladder cancer was 0.98 (0.62–1.54) in former smokers and 1.66 (1.06–2.59) in current smokers (based on 164 deaths). In the 50-year follow-up of the British doctors cohort (Doll *et al.*, 2005), there were 220 deaths from bladder cancer. Death rates per 100000 per year were 13.7 in never smokers, 37.7 in smokers of 1–14 cigarettes/day, 31.8 in smokers of 15–24 cigarettes/day, and 51.4 in smokers of ≥ 25 cigarettes/day. All the new studies confirm the existence of a dose–response relationship with the number of cigarettes smoked and with duration, and a decline in relative risk with time since quitting smoking, compared to non-quitters.

2.9.2 Types of tobacco

The risk of lower urinary tract cancer was more strongly associated with smoking air-cured (black) tobacco than smoking flue-cured (blond) tobacco in several studies (IARC, 2004a). The stronger association with air-cured (black) than blond tobacco among current smokers has not been clearly confirmed in a re-analysis of the Spanish multicentre case–control study (Samanic *et al.*, 2006). Relative risks in current smokers were 7.3 (4.9–10.9) in black tobacco smokers and 5.8 (3.4–10.0) in blond tobacco smokers; in former smokers, 4.2 (2.9–6.0) for black tobacco and 1.8 (1.0–3.2) for blond tobacco (Table 2.48 online). The effect of cessation was more pronounced in blond tobacco smokers than in black tobacco smokers, suggesting potentially different mechanisms of action of the two types of tobacco. Air-cured (black) tobacco is richer in arylamines.

2.9.3 Gene–environment interactions

A large number of studies have considered gene–environment interactions between tobacco smoking and genetic polymorphisms, including DNA repair genes (Vineis *et al.*, 2009) and genes involved in carcinogen metabolism (Malats, 2008; Dong *et al.*, 2008). Overall, there is evidence that the slow acetylator variant of the *NAT2* gene is involved in bladder carcinogenesis and may interact with smoking. The meta-relative risk for *NAT2* slow acetylator and bladder cancer was 1.46 (95%CI: 1.26–1.68; $P = 2.5 \times 10^{-7}$), based on 36 studies and 5747 cases (Dong *et al.*, 2008). Similar but weaker evidence has been provided for *GSTM1* (Malats, 2008).

The extent of interaction between *NAT2* variants and smoking is still unclear. In one study the *NAT2* acetylation status was found to modulate the association of bladder cancer and cigarette smoking through smoking intensity and not smoking duration (Lubin *et al.*, 2007). Studies are not consistent concerning the three-way association between smoking intensity, *NAT2* and bladder cancer. Some studies found greater effects at a lower level of exposure and others the opposite (Malats, 2008). Genome-wide association studies have indicated 8q24 as a region that may confer high risk for bladder cancer (Kiemeney *et al.*, 2008).

2.10 Myeloid leukaemia (acute and chronic)

Myeloid leukaemia in adults was observed to be causally related to cigarette smoking in the previous *IARC Monograph* (IARC, 2004a). Risk increased with amount of tobacco smoked in a substantial number of adequate studies, with evidence of a dose–response relationship. Biological plausibility for a causal relationship of smoking with myeloid leukaemia is provided by the finding of known leukaemogens in tobacco smoke, one of which (benzene) is present in relatively large amounts. No evidence was found for an association with acute lymphocytic leukaemia.

One recently published cohort study included information on acute and chronic myeloid leukaemias (Fernberg *et al.*., 2007), based on 372 incident cases. A weak association was found between acute myeloid leukaemia and intensity of smoking, and a statistically significant association with current smoking (RR, 1.5; 95%CI: 1.06–2.11). No association was found with chronic myeloid leukaemia.

In the update of the Whitehall study (Batty *et al.*., 2008) (a cohort of 17363 government employees in London, followed-up for 38 years), the hazard ratio for mortality from myeloid leukaemias (acute plus chronic) was 5.08 (95%CI: 1.78–14.5) for current smokers, and 3.84 (95%CI: 1.35–11.0) for former smokers (based on 66 deaths). In the 50-year follow-up of the British doctors cohort (Doll *et al.*., 2005), there were 100 deaths from myeloid leukaemias. The mortality rates per 100000 per year were 6.3 in never smokers, 2.8 in smokers of 1–14 cigarettes/day, 14.0 in smokers of 15–24, and 18.3 in smokers of ≥ 25 cigarettes/day (age-adjusted).

2.11 Other leukaemias and lymphomas

2.11.1 Non-Hodgkin lymphoma

Six cohort studies have been published on the association between non-Hodgkin lymphoma and smoking, all reviewed in the previous *IARC Monograph* (IARC, 2004a). In five of these, no increased risk among smokers was evident (Doll *et al.*, 1994; McLaughlin *et al.*, 1995; Adami *et al.*, 1998; Herrinton & Friedman, 1998; Parker *et al.*, 2000). However, in one study, men who had ever smoked cigarettes had a twofold increase in risk for non-Hodgkin lymphoma, and the risk was still higher among the heaviest smokers (Linet *et al.*, 1992). Data from case–control studies generally also fail to support an effect of smoking on the incidence of non-Hodgkin lymphoma (Peach & Barnett, 2001; Stagnaro *et al.*, 2001; Schöllkopf *et al.*, 2005; Bracci & Holly, 2005; Table 2.50 available at http://monographs.iarc.fr/ENG/Monographs/vol100E/100E-01-Table2.50.pdf). Reanalysis of data of an Italian study (Stagnaro *et al.*, 2004) found a statistically significant association (OR, 1.4; 95%CI: 1.1–1.7) for blond tobacco exposure and non-Hodgkin lymphoma risk.

Three studies and a pooled analysis have examined histological subtypes of non-Hodgkin lymphoma. In one cohort study in women, smoking was associated with increased risk for follicular non-Hodgkin lymphoma (Parker *et al.*, 2000). Similarly, two other studies reported a weak positive association between smoking and risk for follicular lymphoma, but no effect for other histological types (Herrinton & Friedman, 1998; Stagnaro *et al.*, 2001). A large pooled analysis based on nine North-American and European case–control studies found an overall odds ratio of 1.07 (95%CI: 1.0–1.15) for smokers; the association was particularly strong for follicular lymphoma (OR, 1.31; 95%CI: 1.12–1.52) (Morton *et al.*, 2005).

2.11.2 Hodgkin lymphoma

In the previous *IARC Monograph* (IARC, 2004a) seven studies on the association between Hodgkin lymphoma and smoking were examined and null or weakly positive associations were noted. Among studies published since, a positive association was observed in two case–control (Willett *et al.*, 2007; Kanda *et al.*, 2009) and three cohort studies (Nieters *et al.*, 2006; Lim *et al.*, 2007; Nieters *et al.*, 2008), while one study found no clear association (Monnereau *et al.*, 2008). Several other recent studies also reported a positive association, but with some internal inconsistencies. In a European multicentre case–control study, no association was observed between tobacco and Hodgkin lymphoma for subjects below age 35 years, whereas for older subjects, ever-smokers experienced a doubled risk of Hodgkin lymphoma as compared to never smokers (Besson *et al.*, 2006). In contrast, a positive association was observed in young adults participating in the International Twin Study (Cozen *et al.*, 2009). A positive association was observed in a Scandinavian case–control study, but without a clear dose–response (Hjalgrim *et al.*, 2007). In a case-control study addressing infectious precursors, particularly Epstein-Barr virus (EBV), an increased risk for EBV-positive Hodgkin lymphoma was found among current smokers (Glaser *et al.*, 2004; Table 2.50 online).

Several of the above studies found positive associations for Hodgkin lymphoma while also demonstrating null or inverse associations with non-Hodgkin lymphoma (Nieters *et al.*, 2006; Lim *et al.*, 2007; Nieters *et al.*, 2008; Kanda *et al.*, 2009).

2.11.3 Multiple myeloma

In the previous *IARC Monograph* (IARC, 2004a), the large majority of studies on tobacco smoking and risk for multiple myeloma evaluated showed no clear association. More recently, two case–control studies found a positive association (Vlajinac *et al.*, 2003; Nieters *et al.*, 2006), whereas no clear association was observed in another case–control study (Monnereau *et al.*, 2008) or in a cohort study in Sweden (Fernberg *et al.*, 2007; Table 2.51 available at http://monographs.iarc.fr/ENG/Monographs/vol100E/100E-01-Table2.51.pdf).

2.12 Cancer of the breast

Approximately 150 epidemiological studies have been published on the relationship between breast cancer and active and passive smoking. The results from these studies have been comprehensively examined in peer-reviewed literature (Palmer & Rosenberg, 1993; Terry *et al.*, 2002a; Johnson *et al.*, 2002; Johnson, 2005; Terry & Goodman, 2006; Miller *et al.*, 2007). The previous *IARC Monograph* (IARC, 2004a) considered studies conducted through June 2002 and concluded that there is evidence suggesting lack of carcinogenicity of tobacco smoking in humans for cancers of the female breast.

Other consensus reviews have drawn different conclusions, based partly on the availability of new data, and partly on differences in interpretation:

- The 2001 US Surgeon General Report on Women and Smoking (Department of Health & Human Services, 2001) concluded that tobacco smoking does not appear to appreciably affect breast cancer risk overall. However, several issues were not entirely resolved, including whether starting to smoke at an early age increases risk, whether certain subgroups defined by genetic polymorphisms are differentially affected by smoking, and whether exposure to second-hand smoke affects risk.
- The 2004 US Surgeon General report on "The Health Consequences of Smoking" (Department of Health & Human

Services, 2004) concluded the evidence is suggestive of no causal relationship between tobacco smoking and breast cancer.
- The 2009 Canadian Expert Panel on Tobacco Smoke and Breast Cancer Risk (Collishaw *et al.*, 2009) concludes that based on the weight of evidence from epidemiological and toxicological studies and understanding of biological mechanisms, the associations between tobacco smoking and both pre- and post-menopausal breast cancer are consistent with causality.

The lack of agreement in the conclusions from these groups is not surprising, given that the observed associations are weaker and less consistent for breast cancer than for other tobacco-related cancers. Furthermore, several methodological considerations could either obscure a small increase in risk caused by tobacco smoking, or alternatively introduce a spurious association where no causal relationship exists.

2.12.1 *Methodological and related issues*

The principal concerns about studies of tobacco smoking and breast cancer are the following: timing of exposure, the relevant disease endpoint, the potential for confounding by factors associated with both smoking and the occurrence/detection of breast cancer, the hypothesis that tobacco smoking may have opposing effects on breast cancer risk (protective and detrimental), and the hypothesis that some women may be genetically more susceptible to develop breast cancer from smoking, and that increased risk in these subgroups may be obscured in analyses of average risk in the population.

(a) Misclassification of exposure

Self-reported information on tobacco smoking is generally considered more reliable than questionnaire information on exposure to second-hand tobacco smoke. However, studies of tobacco smoking have not uniformly considered the duration of smoking (years), the average amount smoked (cigarettes/day), or the timing of initiation in relation to first full-term pregnancy. Only one (Al-Delaimy *et al.*, 2004) of the seven available cohort studies updated the information on smoking behaviour during follow-up. Whereas some exposure variables, such as age at initiation and age at first full-term pregnancy remain constant over time, others, such as smoking status, duration and age at cessation do not. Furthermore, the average age at initiation and duration of smoking are highly correlated with birth cohort and attained age. While the number of years of smoking before first full term pregnancy has been proposed as a potentially relevant measure of exposure, the range of this variable is constrained except among women whose first pregnancy occurs at an older age, which is itself an independent risk factor for breast cancer.

(b) Specificity of disease endpoints

Breast cancer is not a single disease. Accordingly, some researchers have postulated that exposure to tobacco smoke (from tobacco smoking or second-hand tobacco smoke) could differentially affect certain clinical subtypes of breast such as pre- or post-menopausal cancers or tumours with or without hormonal receptors. It is also possible that smoking might affect the survival of women with breast cancer, whether or not it affects incidence rates. Most published studies have measured incidence rates as the endpoint, although some have measured mortality rates or effects on survival.

(c) Confounding

Alcohol consumption is positively correlated with tobacco smoking (Marshall *et al.*, 1999) and is an established cause of breast cancer (IARC, 2010a; *Monograph* on Consumption of Alcoholic Beverages in this Volume). Most epidemiologic studies attempt to control for alcohol consumption using questionnaire information on usual drinking patterns. This approach is vulnerable to residual confounding, because self-reported data on lifetime alcohol consumption leave room for misclassification. Potential confounding by alcohol consumption is of greater concern for current than for former smokers, since, on average, current smokers drink more than former smokers (Reynolds *et al.*, 2004a, b). One study by the Collaborative Group on Hormonal Factors and Breast Cancer (Hamajima *et al.*, 2002) controlled rigorously for alcohol consumption by restricting the analysis of smoking and breast cancer to women who reported drinking no alcohol.

Conversely, mammography screening can be a negative confounder in studies of tobacco smoking and breast cancer incidence. Few studies of tobacco smoking in relation to breast cancer have controlled for mammography screening. Current smokers report a lower frequency of mammographic screening than never-smokers, whereas health conscious former smokers report higher screening rates (Gross *et al.*, 2006). Mammography screening affects the detection rather than the occurrence of breast cancer; it detects some tumours that might otherwise never have been recognized and allows earlier diagnosis of others, thereby increasing breast cancer incidence in the short-term. The consequence of uncontrolled confounding by mammography screening would be to underestimate an association between current smoking and breast cancer incidence, and to overestimate the association in former smokers. Confounding by screening would be expected to have the opposite effect in studies of breast cancer mortality.

Other correlates of tobacco smoking might also confound a potential association between tobacco smoking and breast cancer, although their net effect is likely to be smaller and harder to predict than confounding by alcohol and mammography screening. Women who smoke undergo menopause about two to three years earlier than never-smokers (Baron *et al.*, 1990). The effect of this may be partly or wholly offset by the greater likelihood of girls who experience early menarche to initiate smoking in early adolescence (Jean *et al.*, 2011). There is no documentation that smokers and never-smokers differ with respect to average years of ovulation. Tobacco smoking also has a complex relationship to body mass index. Post-menopausal women who smoke are less likely to be overweight or obese than former or never smokers, but overweight adolescent girls are more likely to begin smoking for weight control (Fine *et al.*, 2004). Similarly complex relationships exist between smoking and physical activity. Current smokers report less physical activity than either former or never smokers (Kaczynski *et al.*, 2008; Trost *et al.*, 2002), but only a small proportion of the population engages in the vigorous physical activity that is needed to protect against breast cancer. The socioeconomic correlates of smoking have changed over time. Women who attended college during the 1960s and 1970s were more likely to initiate smoking than less educated women, but subsequently college-educated women have been more likely to quit. Thus, the potential for confounding by reproductive patterns and use of post-menopausal hormone treatment varies by birth cohort and differs for current and former smokers.

Most epidemiological studies have attempted to control for factors that might confound the relationship between breast cancer and tobacco smoking using questionnaire information collected on these factors. None of the published studies have been able to control for all of the potential confounders, however. Most studies lack data on screening behaviour and have limited information on alcohol consumption, use of post-menopausal hormones, and physical activity.

(d) Potential anti-estrogenic effects of tobacco smoking

Indirect evidence suggests that tobacco smoking may have anti-estrogenic effects that might offset the adverse effects of tobacco smoke carcinogens on breast cancer risk. Baron *et al.* (1990) pointed to observations suggesting lower estrogen activity levels in women who smoke compared to those who do not. Smokers have lower risk of endometrial cancer (Department of Health & Human Services, 2004), higher risk of osteoporosis (Jensen *et al.*, 1985; Jensen & Christiansen, 1988), earlier age at natural menopause (Baron *et al.*, 1990) and lower mammography density (Roubidoux *et al.*, 2003) than women who do not smoke. Smoking also attenuates the effects of hormone replacement therapy (HRT) on lipid profiles (Jensen & Christiansen, 1988) and serum estrone (McDivit *et al.*, 2008). No difference in serum concentrations of estradiol and estrone between post-menopausal smokers and non-smokers have been reported in several studies (Cassidenti *et al.*, 1992; Khaw *et al.*, 1988; Berta *et al.*, 1991; Longcope *et al.*, 1986; Berta *et al.*, 1992; Cauley *et al.*, 1989; Friedman *et al.*, 1987; Key *et al.*, 1991). However, smokers have been observed to have higher levels of androgens (Cassidenti *et al.*, 1992) (specifically androstenedione) (Khaw *et al.*, 1988; Cauley *et al.*, 1989; Friedman *et al.*, 1987; Key *et al.*, 1991), prolactin (Berta *et al.*, 1991), and unbound serum estradiol (Cassidenti *et al.*, 1992).

(e) Genetically susceptible subgroups

Certain subgroups of women may have greater risk of breast cancer when exposed to tobacco smoke because of genetic or other factors affecting cancer susceptibility. Potential interactions between inherited polymorphisms and tobacco smoking have been studied for selected candidate genes that affect carcinogen metabolism, modulation of oxidative damage, immune responses, and DNA repair (see Sections 2.12.4b and 4.2).

2.12.2 Analytical studies

Over 130 epidemiological studies on tobacco smoking and breast cancer were reviewed.

(a) Incidence in current and former smokers

Since the previous *IARC Monograph* (IARC, 2004a), seven reports on cohort studies (Al-Delaimy *et al.*, 2004; Reynolds *et al.*, 2004a; Gram *et al.*, 2005; Hanaoka *et al.*, 2005; Olson *et al.*, 2005; Cui *et al.*, 2006; Ha *et al.*, 2007) have been published on breast cancer incidence in relation to tobacco smoking (Table 2.52 available at http://monographs.iarc.fr/ENG/Monographs/vol100E/100E-01-Table2.52.pdf). Breast cancer incidence was significantly associated with current tobacco smoking in three studies (Reynolds *et al.*, 2004a; Olson *et al.*, 2005; Cui *et al.*, 2006), with relative risk estimates among the larger studies ranging from 1.12 (95%CI: 0.92–1.37) (Al-Delaimy *et al.*, 2004) to 1.32 (95%CI:1.10–1.57) (Reynolds *et al.*, 2004a). Former smoking was significantly associated with risk in only one cohort (Al-Delaimy *et al.*, 2004), with relative risk estimates across all of the cohorts ranging from 1.00 (95%CI: 0.93–1.08) (Cui *et al.*, 2006) to 1.18 (95%CI: 1.02–1.36) (Al-Delaimy *et al.*, 2004). The association with breast cancer is stronger in current than in former smokers in four of the seven cohort studies (Reynolds *et al.*, 2004a; Hanaoka *et al.*, 2005; Olson *et al.*, 2005; Cui *et al.*, 2006), although the confidence intervals overlap widely in all but one (Cui *et al.*, 2006). [The Working group noted that three cohort studies (Gram *et al.*, 2005; Hanaoka *et al.*, 2005; Olson *et al.*, 2005) provided data on both the age-adjusted and the multivariate-adjusted risk estimates for current and former smoking. None of these showed attenuation of the estimate associated with current smoking, and two (Hanaoka *et al.*, 2005; Olson *et al.*, 2005) reported somewhat stronger estimates when adjusted for established risk factors besides age. None of the studies adjusted for the frequency of mammography screening. Residual confounding by screening and incomplete control for other risk factors would be expected to cause underestimation of the association with current smoking, and overestimation of the association with former smoking.]

Since the previous *IARC Monograph* (IARC, 2004a), a total of 12 case–control studies on tobacco smoking and breast cancer incidence have been published (Table 2.53 available at http://monographs.iarc.fr/ENG/Monographs/vol100E/100E-01-Table2.53.pdf). Results from the case–control studies are less consistent than those from the cohort studies. Six studies (Li *et al.*, 2004; Mechanic *et al.*, 2006; Magnusson *et al.*, 2007; Prescott *et al.*, 2007; Roddam *et al.*, 2007; Slattery *et al.*, 2008) differentiated between current and former smokers, while the six other reports (Band *et al.*, 2002; Lash & Aschengrau, 2002; Gammon *et al.*, 2004; Rollison *et al.*, 2008; Ahern *et al.*, 2009; Young *et al.*, 2009) specify only ever or never smokers. Only one study (Li *et al.*, 2004) reported a borderline significant increase in risk associated with current smoking, and two studies (Band *et al.*, 2002; Rollison *et al.*, 2008) with ever smoking.

None of the six case–control studies that presented data on breast cancer incidence separately for current and former smokers found a significant difference in risk between the two smoking categories; the relative risk estimates were higher for former than for current smokers in four of the studies (Mechanic *et al.*, 2006; Prescott *et al.*, 2007; Roddam *et al.*, 2007; Slattery *et al.*, 2008) and identical in the fifth (Magnusson *et al.*, 2007).

(b) Years of cessation

When the relative risk for breast cancer incidence in former smokers is examined by years since cessation in cohort studies (Table 2.54 available at http://monographs.iarc.fr/ENG/Monographs/vol100E/100E-01-Table2.54.pdf), the point estimates do not consistently decrease with longer time since cessation. In none of the four cohort studies (London *et al.*, 1989b; Egan *et al.*, 2002; Reynolds *et al.*, 2004a; Cui *et al.*, 2006) and in only one (Li *et al.*, 2005) of the five case–control studies (Chu *et al.*, 1990; Gammon *et al.*, 1998; Johnson *et al.*, 2000; Kropp & Chang-Claude, 2002; Li *et al.*, 2005) that formally tested for trend (Table 2.55 available at http://monographs.iarc.fr/ENG/Monographs/vol100E/100E-01-Table2.55.pdf) was there a statistically significant decrease in relative risk observed with longer time since cessation. Only one study has reported data on breast cancer mortality in relation to years since quitting or age at cessation (Calle *et al.*, 1994). A statistically significant inverse trend in the relative risk estimates was reported with both years since quitting (p trend = 0.04) and younger age at cessation (p trend = 0.02). [The Working Group noted that the inverse trends in the relative risk of dying from breast cancer observed in this study are weaker than those observed with most other cancers designated as causally associated with smoking.]

(c) Duration of smoking and age at initiation

Tables 2.56–2.61 (see below for links) list the published epidemiologic studies that relate breast cancer incidence to duration of tobacco smoking, age at initiation and/or timing relative to first full term pregnancy.

Longer duration of smoking is associated with higher breast cancer incidence in five of seven cohort studies (Table 2.56 available at http://monographs.iarc.fr/ENG/Monographs/vol100E/100E-01-Table2.56.pdf). A similar trend is seen inconsistently among the 33 case–control studies that report relative risk estimates by duration of smoking (Table 2.57 available at http://monographs.iarc.fr/ENG/Monographs/vol100E/100E-01-Table2.57.pdf). Among the 18 studies that reported a formal test of trend, eight studies (Gammon *et al.*, 1998; Johnson *et al.*, 2000; Reynolds *et al.*, 2004a; Gram *et al.*, 2005; Li *et al.*, 2005; van der Hel *et al.*, 2005; Cui *et al.*, 2006; Mechanic *et al.*, 2006) reported a statistically significant or borderline increase in the relative risk of incident breast cancer with the duration of smoking; seven studies (Ewertz, 1990; Palmer *et al.*, 1991; Egan *et al.*, 2002; Al-Delaimy *et al.*, 2004; Lissowska *et al.*, 2006; Magnusson *et al.*, 2007; Prescott *et al.*, 2007) reported no trend, and one study (Brinton *et al.*, 1986) reported an inverse relationship.

Thirty studies, including cohort (Tables 2.58 available at http://monographs.iarc.fr/ENG/Monographs/vol100E/100E-01-Table2.58.pdf) and case–control studies (Table 2.59 available at http://monographs.iarc.fr/ENG/Monographs/vol100E/100E-01-Table2.59.pdf) related breast cancer incidence to age at smoking initiation. Fifteen of these (Chu *et al.*, 1990; Ewertz, 1990; Palmer *et al.*, 1991; Nordlund *et al.*, 1997; Gammon *et al.*, 1998; Johnson *et al.*, 2000; Egan *et al.*, 2002; Kropp & Chang-Claude, 2002; Gram *et al.*, 2005; Cui *et al.*, 2006; Lissowska *et al.*, 2006; Ha *et al.*, 2007; Lissowska *et al.*, 2007; Magnusson *et al.*, 2007; Prescott *et al.*, 2007; Slattery *et al.*, 2008) reported a formal test of trend. Among these, only two (Gram *et al.*, 2005; Ha *et al.*, 2007) found a statistically significant or borderline significantly higher risk in women who began smoking at a younger ages; twelve studies (Chu *et al.*, 1990; Ewertz, 1990; Palmer *et al.*, 1991; Nordlund *et al.*, 1997; Gammon *et al.*, 1998; Johnson *et al.*, 2000; Egan *et al.*, 2002; Cui *et al.*, 2006; Lissowska *et al.*, 2006; Magnusson *et al.*, 2007; Prescott *et al.*, 2007; Slattery *et al.*, 2008) found no relationship with age at initiation, and one (Kropp & Chang-Claude, 2002) reported higher risk among women who began smoking later. [The Working Group noted that at least two studies (Cui *et al.*, 2006; Slattery *et al.*, 2008) appear to have included never-smokers in the tests of trend and that the categories that define age at initiation differ across studies.]

The relative risk of incident breast cancer according to the timing of smoking initiation relative to first full-term pregnancy was reported in 21 studies, of cohort (Table 2.60 available at http://monographs.iarc.fr/ENG/Monographs/vol100E/100E-01-Table2.60.pdf) and case–control (Table 2.61 available at http://monographs.iarc.fr/ENG/Monographs/vol100E/100E-01-Table2.61.pdf) design. For nine studies (Hunter *et al.*, 1997; Egan *et al.*, 2002; Al-Delaimy *et al.*, 2004; Reynolds *et al.*, 2004a; Li *et al.*, 2005; Cui *et al.*, 2006; Prescott *et al.*, 2007; Rollison *et al.*, 2008; Young *et al.*, 2009) categorical data on years of smoking before first pregnancy are presented, whereas for 12 (Lash & Aschengrau, 1999; Innes & Byers, 2001; Band *et al.*, 2002; Kropp & Chang-Claude, 2002; Lash & Aschengrau, 2002; Fink & Lash, 2003; Lawlor *et al.*, 2004; Gram *et al.*, 2005; Olson *et al.*, 2005; Lissowska *et al.*, 2006; Magnusson *et al.*, 2007; Slattery *et al.*, 2008) whether smoking was initiated before or after the initial pregnancy was considered. Breast cancer incidence is consistently higher when smoking began before or during first pregnancy in most (Hunter *et al.*, 1997; Lash & Aschengrau, 1999; Innes & Byers, 2001; Band *et al.*, 2002; Egan *et al.*, 2002; Al-Delaimy *et al.*, 2004; Reynolds *et al.*, 2004a; Gram *et al.*, 2005; Li *et al.*, 2005; Olson *et al.*, 2005; Cui *et al.*, 2006; Slattery *et al.*, 2008; Young *et al.*, 2009) but not all (Kropp & Chang-Claude, 2002; Lash & Aschengrau, 2002; Fink & Lash, 2003; Prescott *et al.*, 2007) studies that tested this. [The Working Group noted that the number of years of smoking before first pregnancy is highly correlated with age at first full-term pregnancy, which is itself an independent risk factor for breast cancer.]

It has been argued that some studies, and especially cohort studies, may underestimate the true association between tobacco smoking and breast cancer risk by ignoring or underestimating lifetime exposure to second-hand tobacco smoke of those in the referent group (California Environmental Protection Agency, 2005; Johnson, 2005; Collishaw *et al.*, 2009). This criticism is based on the hypothesis that exposure to second-hand smoke may confer almost the same degree of breast cancer risk as tobacco smoking. Under this hypothesis, the inclusion of women exposed to second-hand smoke in the referent group dilutes the contrast between exposed and unexposed women in studies of tobacco smoking, and causes underestimation of the association between tobacco smoking and breast cancer. In several case–control studies the association between breast cancer and tobacco smoking strengthened when the referent group was defined as women with "never active, never-passive" exposure to tobacco smoke (Morabia *et al.*, 1996; Lash & Aschengrau, 1999; Johnson *et al.*, 2000; Kropp & Chang-Claude, 2002). In contrast, a stronger association between tobacco smoking and breast cancer risk, when women exposed only to second-hand smoke are excluded from the referent group, has not been observed in cohort studies (Egan *et al.*, 2002; Reynolds *et al.*, 2004a). Debate continues over whether the case–control studies should be considered "of highest quality" because they provide "lifetime exposure assessment" (Collishaw *et al.*, 2009) or whether the cohort studies are more credible, because prospectively-collected exposure data are not susceptible to the recall bias that can affect retrospective studies.

(d) Survival and mortality from breast cancer

The relationship between smoking and the natural history of breast cancer has been examined in several studies (Daniell, 1988; Ewertz *et al.*, 1991; Daniell *et al.*, 1993; Scanlon *et al.*, 1995; Yu *et al.*, 1997; Manjer *et al.*, 2000; Murin & Inciardi, 2001; Holmes *et al.*, 2007). In cross-sectional analyses, Daniell *et al.* (1993) found that smokers with breast cancer had more and larger lymph node metastases than non-smokers, after controlling for primary tumour size and other variables. Further, a case–control study (Murin & Inciardi, 2001) and a retrospective cohort study (Scanlon *et al.*, 1995) found smoking to be associated with an increased risk of developing pulmonary metastases from breast cancer. However, these studies could not definitively distinguish lung metastases from primary lung cancers.

Five cohort studies have focused specifically upon the association of tobacco smoking with either breast cancer survival (Ewertz *et al.*, 1991; Yu *et al.*, 1997; Manjer *et al.*, 2000; Holmes *et al.*, 2007) or breast cancer death rates (Calle *et al.*, 1994). A study of 1774 Danish women showed no association between smoking and breast cancer survival (Ewertz *et al.*, 1991), as did a study of 5056 women with breast cancer in the Nurse's Health Study (Holmes *et al.*, 2007). In contrast, follow-up of 792 women with in situ or invasive breast cancer detected in a screening study in Malmø, Sweden found a crude relative risk for smokers and ex-smokers, compared to never smokers, of 1.44 (95%CI: 1.01–2.06) and of 1.13 (95%CI: 0.66–1.94), respectively (Manjer *et al.*, 2000). The relative risk associated with smoking remained significant after adjustment for age and stage at diagnosis (RR, 2.14; 95%CI: 1.47–3.10). A study based on the ACS Cancer Prevention Study II reported an association between current smoking and increased breast cancer death rates after six years of follow-up (Table 2.56 online; Calle *et al.*, 1994). Risk of death attributed to breast cancer was positively and significantly related to the duration of current smoking reported at the time of enrolment. However, the authors acknowledge that mortality studies cannot exclude biases arising from the effect of smoking on overall death rates, which could increase the potential for prevalent breast cancer to be coded as the underlying cause of death on the death certificate (Calle *et al.*, 1994).

2.12.3 Subtypes

(a) Pre- versus post-menopausal

Since the previous *IARC Monograph* (IARC, 2004a), 19 case–control studies have published data on tobacco smoking in relation to pre- and post-menopausal breast cancer (Table 2.62 available at http://monographs.iarc.fr/ENG/Monographs/vol100E/100E-01-Table2.62.pdf). The results are inconsistent. Of the 12 studies that provide information separately for current smokers (Schechter *et al.*, 1985; Brinton *et al.*, 1986; Rohan & Baron, 1989; Ewertz, 1990; Baron *et al.*, 1996; Gammon *et al.*, 1998; Millikan *et al.*, 1998; Johnson *et al.*, 2000; Zheng *et al.*, 2002; Magnusson *et al.*, 2007; Slattery *et al.*, 2008), only five (Schechter *et al.*, 1985; Johnson *et al.*, 2000; Magnusson *et al.*, 2007; Slattery *et al.*, 2008) found a stronger association with pre- than with post-menopausal breast cancer. The other analyses show either similar associations (Brinton *et al.*, 1986; Ewertz, 1990; Baron *et al.*, 1996; Gammon *et al.*, 1998; Millikan *et al.*, 1998; Zheng *et al.*, 2002) or a stronger association with post-menopausal breast cancer (Rohan & Baron, 1989; Millikan *et al.*, 1998; Johnson *et al.*, 2000; Zheng *et al.*, 2002).

(b) Hormone receptor status

Two cohort studies (London *et al.*, 1989a; Manjer *et al.*, 2001), one case–control study (Morabia *et al.*, 1998) and a case series (Yoo *et al.*, 1997) have examined the association between quantitative measures of cigarette smoking and breast cancer risk according to estrogen receptor (ER) status. In one of the cohort studies (Manjer *et al.*, 2001), a statistically significant increased risk (RR, 1.6) of ER negative tumours associated with current smoking was found but no clear association between smoking and ER positive tumours, and no difference in the association with progestogen receptor (PR)-positive and PR-negative tumours. In the other three studies there was no clear difference in the association related to ER or PR receptor status.

2.12.4 Susceptible populations

More than 30 studies and meta-analyses (Alberg *et al.*, 2004; Terry & Goodman, 2006; Ambrosone *et al.*, 2008; Collishaw *et al.*, 2009) have evaluated whether a family history of breast cancer and/or inherited polymorphisms in various genes may confer greater susceptibility to develop breast cancer from exposure to tobacco smoke. These are described below in relation to the measure indicating potential susceptibility.

(a) Family history

In two studies, whether a family history of breast cancer modifies susceptibility to develop breast cancer from tobacco smoking has been examined. Couch *et al.* (2001) measured breast cancer incidence among female family members in a cohort of breast cancer cases diagnosed between 1944 and 1952 at the University of Minnesota. Sisters and daughters in families with at least three breast and/or ovarian cancers were at 2.4 fold higher risk for breast cancer (95%CI: 1.2–5.1) if they smoked compared to never-smokers. No dose–response was observed in relation to pack–years of smoking.

Suzuki *et al.* (2007) reported a statistically significant interaction between family history of breast cancer and smoking history in a hospital-based case–control study of 3861 breast cancer cases treated at a large cancer centre in Japan between 1988 and 2000. A family history of breast cancer in the absence of smoking was associated with a relative risk of 1.44 (95%CI: 1.21–1.71); the relative risk estimate was 1.95 (95%CI: 1.36–2.81) in women who reported < 30 pack–years of tobacco smoking, and 4.33 (95%CI: 1.65–11.40) in women who reported > 30 pack–years of smoking.

[The Working group noted that Japanese women who smoked during this time period may have differed from never-smokers in other characteristics related to breast cancer. Besides its strong correlation with female smoking, "Westernization" might be associated with delayed childbearing, smaller families, higher body mass index, and greater use of post-menopausal hormones.]

(b) Genetic polymorphisms

Studies of breast cancer, smoking and low penetrance genetic polymorphisms are summarized in Table 2.63 (available at http://monographs.iarc.fr/ENG/Monographs/vol100E/100E-01-Table2.63.pdf). The candidate genes in these studies are involved in carcinogen metabolism [*N*-acetyltransferases (*NAT1, NAT2*), cytochrome P450s (*CYP1A1, CYP1B1, CYP2E2*), GSTs], host responses to oxidative stress (superoxide dismutase) or to infectious organisms (myeloperoxidase and immunoglobulin binding protein) and DNA repair (O^6-methylguanine DNA methyltransferase, nucleotide excision repair).

The most consistent associations with breast cancer risk have been observed among long-term smokers with the *NAT2* slow acetylation genotype (Terry & Goodman, 2006). *NAT2* slow acetylation genotype is thought to confer less capability to detoxify tobacco smoke carcinogens and is associated with an increase in breast cancer risk (Ambrosone *et al.*, 1996, 2008). Approximately 50–60% of Caucasian women are reported to be slow acetylators.

Table 2.63 (online) lists 15 studies of polymorphisms in *NAT2*, of which 9 were included in a pooled analysis and 13 in a meta-analysis (Ambrosone *et al.*, 2008). [The study by Delfino *et al.* (2000) was excluded from these analyses because cases included women with benign breast disease; the study by Lilla *et al.* (2005) was not considered because it is based on the same population as that by Chang-Claude *et al.* (2002).] The meta-analysis found a statistically significant association between ever tobacco smoking and breast cancer risk among women with the *NAT2* slow acetylator genotype (meta-RR, 1.27; 95%CI: 1.16–1.40) but not in those with rapid acetylator genotype (meta-RR, 1.05; 95%CI: 0.95–1.17). Pack–years of tobacco smoking was significantly associated with increasing breast cancer risk among women with *NAT2* slow acetylator genotype (meta-RR for ever smokers, 1.44; 95%CI: 1.23–1.68, for > 20 pack–years versus never smokers), but not among rapid acetylators (Ambrosone *et al.*, 2008). No main effect was seen between *NAT2* status and breast cancer risk (meta-RR, 1.0; 95%CI: 0.93–1.07). In contrast to an earlier meta-analysis (Alberg *et al.*, 2004), this study observed no difference in risk for pre- or post-menopausal breast cancer. The pooled analysis of nine studies (Ambrosone *et al.*, 2008) reported pooled risk estimates for pre- and post-menopausal women of 1.49 (95%CI: 1.08–2.04) and 1.42 (95%CI: 1.16–1.74), respectively, among women with slow *NAT2* genotype and at least 20 pack–years of smoking compared to never-smokers. The corresponding values for women with rapid acetylator genotype were 1.29 (95%CI: 0.89–1.86) and 0.88 (95%CI: 0.69–1.13). A statistically significant interaction was observed between pack–years of smoking as a continuous variable and *NAT2* genotype (p interaction = 0.03).

A population-based case–control study published after the meta-analysis by Ambrosone *et al.* compared the prevalence of the *NAT2* genotypes and their joint effect with smoking on breast cancer risk in Hispanic and non-Hispanic white women (Baumgartner *et al.*, 2009). Non-Hispanic white women were more likely ($P < 0.001$) than Hispanics to have a slow (41.7% versus 33.5%) or very slow (19.0% versus 11.1%) *NAT2* acetylator status. Breast cancer risk was significantly increased in non-Hispanic smoking white women with a very slow acetylator genotype (RR, 2.46; 95%CI: 1.07–5.65 for current versus never).

[The Working Group noted that publication bias remains a concern in the studies of *NAT2* published to date. All of the studies included in the meta-analysis by Ambrosone *et al.* were published between 1996 and 2006; some among them (Morabia *et al.*, 2000; Sillanpää *et al.*, 2007) reported very strong associations that seem inconsistent with the rest of the data. Because genetic studies often examine multiple genes, it is plausible that studies that find no main effect with *NAT2* have not examined this association or that null results for smoking have not been published.]

Fewer studies with less consistent findings have been published on polymorphisms in other genes such as *NAT1*, *CYP1A1*, *GST*, *NOS3*, *MPO*, *MnSOD2* and various DNA repair genes (Table 2.63 online).

2.12.5 High penetrance genes & prognosis

At least seven studies have examined the hypothesis that tobacco smoking may modify breast cancer risk among women who carry *BRCA1* and *BRCA2* mutations (Brunet *et al.*, 1998; Ghadirian *et al.*, 2004; Colilla *et al.*, 2006; Gronwald *et al.*, 2006; Nkondjock *et al.*, 2006; Breast Cancer Family Registry, 2008; Ginsburg *et al.*, 2009). The results have been inconsistent. A recent case–control study of women under age 50 years who were carriers of mutations in *BRCA1* or *BRCA2* reported increased risk for breast cancer associated with as little as five pack–years of smoking. Compared to non-smokers, the risk associated with five or more pack–years of smoking was 2.3 (95%CI: 1.6–3.5) for *BRCA1* mutation carriers and 2.6 (95%CI: 1.8–3.9) for *BRCA2* mutation carriers (Breast Cancer Family Registry, 2008). In contrast, six other studies reported no increased risk among *BRCA1* or *BRCA2* carriers who smoke. The Canadian Panel review (Collishaw *et al.*, 2009) postulated that the five previous studies (Brunet *et al.*, 1998; Ghadirian *et al.*, 2004; Colilla *et al.*, 2006; Gronwald *et al.*, 2006; Nkondjock *et al.*, 2006) may have failed to observe a relationship because they included prevalent cases. However, a sixth study published since the Canadian panel review is also negative (Ginsburg *et al.*, 2009).

2.13 Cancer of the cervix

The association between smoking and cervical cancer has been examined in many epidemiological studies over the past few decades.

Since the previous *IARC Monograph* (IARC, 2004a), additional epidemiological studies have been published. Study design and results of the case–control studies restricted to HPV positive women or that adjusted for HPV status are presented in Table 2.64 (available at http://monographs.iarc.fr/ENG/Monographs/vol100E/100E-01-Table2.64.pdf) and Table 2.65 (available at http://monographs.iarc.fr/ENG/Monographs/vol100E/100E-01-Table2.65.pdf). Cohort studies and pooled analyses are presented in Table 2.66 (available at http://monographs.iarc.fr/ENG/Monographs/vol100E/100E-01-Table2.66.pdf) and Table 2.67 (available at http://monographs.iarc.fr/ENG/Monographs/vol100E/100E-01-Table2.67.pdf), respectively. Table 2.68 (available at http://monographs.iarc.fr/ENG/Monographs/vol100E/100E-01-Table2.68.pdf) and Table 2.69 (available at http://monographs.iarc.fr/ENG/Monographs/vol100E/100E-01-Table2.69.pdf) present additional cohort studies and pooled analyses on tobacco smoking and cervical, cervical intraepithelia neoplasia and carcinoma in situ, with our without controlling for HPV status, respectively.

2.13.1 Dose–response relationship

A positive association between smoking and incidence of cervical squamous-cell carcinoma, which account for approximately 90% of all cervical cancers, has been shown consistently over several decades in many epidemiological studies of various designs conducted across different geographic regions. Dose–response associations with smoking intensity and duration were noted in many of the studies where such associations were examined (Berrington de González *et al.*, 2004; Appleby *et al.*, 2006). Conversely, no clear association was found among former smokers. For adenocarcinoma of the cervix, which usually account for less than 10% of the total of all types of cervical cancer, there appears to be no clear association with smoking (Berrington de González *et al.*, 2004).

2.13.2 Interaction with HPV positivity

Epidemiological studies of smoking and cervical cancer increasingly have considered the effects of HPV infection, which is recognized as the main etiological factor for invasive and pre-invasive cervical neoplasia worldwide (IARC, 1995, 2012b). HPV infection has been considered not only with respect to possible effect modification (Hellberg & Stendahl, 2005; Gunnell *et al.*, 2006), but also to confounding, as both HPV infection and smoking habits are directly associated with number of sexual partners and other indications of high-risk sexual behaviours (Sikström *et al.*, 1995; Wang *et al.* 2004; Hellberg & Stendahl, 2005; McIntyre-Seltman *et al.*, 2005; Syrjänen *et al.*, 2007). Although there have been exceptions (Syrjänen *et al.*, 2007), recent studies have generally continued to show that statistical adjustment for the potential confounding effects of HPV infection, or restricting studies to women with high risk HPV infection (Plummer *et al.*, 2003), does not appreciably alter the finding of a positive association or its magnitude (McIntyre-Seltman *et al.*, 2005; Appleby *et al.*, 2006; Tolstrup *et al.*, 2006; Tsai *et al.*, 2007; Nishino *et al.*, 2008; Kapeu *et al.*, 2009).

Statistical adjustment for the potentially confounding effect of HPV infection was usually based on the measured presence of HPV DNA in cervical cells or anti-HPV serum antibodies in multivariate analytical models; as noted above, studies have also restricted their analyses to HPV-positive cases and controls. As there is currently no reliable marker of persistent HPV infection, case–control studies based on a cross-sectional measurement of HPV cannot distinguish between transient and persistent infections (Franco *et al.*, 1999). Tobacco smoking is suspected to facilitate acquisition or persistence of an HPV infection through a reduced number of Langerhans cells and CD4 lymphocytes, which are markers of local immune response in the cervix (Vaccarella *et al.*, 2008). In addition, smoking may affect innate immunity (Ferson *et al.*, 1979). Current smokers have been shown to have a slightly higher HPV prevalence than non-smokers in a broad range of world populations after adjustment for life-time number of sexual partners (OR, 1.18; 95%CI: 1.01–1.39) (Vaccarella *et al.*, 2008). Studies have evaluated the effect of smoking on HPV persistence. One study shows lower probability of HPV clearance among ever smokers (Giuliano *et al.*, 2002) but a few others found no relationship (Molano *et al.*, 2003; Richardson *et al.*, 2005).

2.14 Cancer of the endometrium

2.14.1 Overview of studies

To date, at least 42 epidemiological studies have examined the association between smoking and endometrial cancer, 25 reviewed in the previous *IARC Monograph* (IARC, 2004a) and 17 published since then (Petridou *et al.*, 2002; Folsom *et al.*, 2003; Furberg & Thune, 2003; Newcomb & Trentham-Dietz, 2003; Beral *et al.*, 2005; Matthews *et al.*, 2005; Viswanathan *et al.*, 2005; Okamura *et al.*, 2006; Strom *et al.*, 2006; Trentham-Dietz *et al.*, 2006; Weiss *et al.*, 2006a; Al-Zoughool *et al.*, 2007; Bjørge *et al.*, 2007; Lacey *et al.*, 2007; Loerbroks *et al.*, 2007; Setiawan *et al.*, 2007; Lindemann *et al.*, 2008). Study design and results of the additional studies are presented separately for the case–control studies (Table 2.70 available at http://monographs.iarc.fr/ENG/Monographs/vol100E/100E-01-Table2.70.pdf and Table 2.71 available at http://monographs.iarc.fr/ENG/Monographs/vol100E/100E-01-Table2.71.pdf, respectively) and for the cohort studies (Table 2.72 available at http://monographs.iarc.fr/ENG/Monographs/vol100E/100E-01-Table2.72.pdf and Table 2.73 available at http://monographs.iarc.fr/ENG/Monographs/vol100E/100E-01-Table2.73.pdf, respectively).

(a) Cohort studies

The majority of the 13 cohort studies (Engeland *et al.*, 1996; Terry *et al.*, 1999, 2002b; Folsom *et al.*, 2003; Furberg & Thune 2003; Beral *et al.*, 2005; Viswanathan *et al.*, 2005; Al-Zoughool *et al.*, 2007; Bjørge *et al.*, 2007; Lacey *et al.*, 2007; Loerbroks *et al.*, 2007; Setiawan *et al.*, 2007; Lindemann *et al.*, 2008) suggest a decreased risk among current smokers, including the largest study with over 9000 cases (Bjørge *et al.*, 2007). In five of these studies quantitative smoking measures have been examined in relation to endometrial cancer risk (Terry *et al.*, 1999, 2002b; Viswanathan *et al.*, 2005; Al-Zoughool *et al.*, 2007; Loerbroks *et al.*, 2007). Of these, one (Terry *et al.*, 1999) found a 50% reduced risk among current smokers in the highest level of intensity (11 cigarettes per day or more) compared with non-smokers, but the number of cases was low and the confidence intervals correspondingly wide. A more recent and larger cohort study (Terry *et al.*, 2002b) found a statistically significant 40% reduced risk among current smokers of more than 20 cigarettes per day, but showed somewhat weaker and statistically non-significant reductions in risk with smoking of long duration or high cumulative consumption (i.e. pack–years). In contrast, the risk among former smokers was similar to that among never smokers. The largest of these studies generally showed decreasing risk of endometrial cancer with increasing smoking intensity, duration, and pack–years of consumption (Viswanathan *et al.*, 2005). Three studies examined the association between time since smoking cessation and endometrial cancer risk. Two of these studies suggested a positive association with time since quitting (compared with non-smokers) (Viswanathan *et al.*, 2005; Loerbroks *et al.*, 2007), whereas one found no association (Terry *et al.*, 2002b).

(b) Case–control studies

The results of 17 population-based case–control studies (Smith *et al.*, 1984; Tyler *et al.*, 1985; Franks *et al.*, 1987; Elliott *et al.*, 1990; Rubin *et al.*, 1990; Brinton *et al.*, 1993; Goodman *et al.*, 1997; Shields *et al.*, 1999; Jain *et al.*, 2000; McCann *et al.*, 2000; Newcomer *et al.*, 2001; Weiderpass & Baron, 2001; Newcomb & Trentham-Dietz, 2003; Matthews *et al.*, 2005; Strom *et al.*, 2006; Trentham-Dietz *et al.*, 2006; Weiss *et al.*, 2006a), that have included between 46 and 1304 endometrial cancer cases, generally have shown reductions in risk among current smokers compared with never smokers (although the magnitude of the reduction in risk has varied somewhat); results among former smokers compared with never smokers were equally variable, albeit somewhat weaker overall. The results of eight hospital-based case–control studies (Kelsey *et al.*, 1982; Lesko *et al.*, 1985; Levi *et al.*, 1987; Stockwell & Lyman, 1987; Koumantaki *et al.*, 1989; Austin *et al.*, 1993; Petridou *et al.*, 2002; Okamura *et al.*, 2006), which included between 83 and 1374 endometrial cancer cases, are somewhat consistent with those of population-based studies. They showed moderate (e.g. 30–40%) reduction in risks among current compared with never smokers, and unaltered risks (or perhaps a small 10–20% reduction in risk) in former compared with never smokers. The largest of the hospital-based studies (Stockwell & Lyman, 1987), with 1374 cases and 3921 controls, found both former and current smokers to be at moderately (approximately 30%) reduced risk of endometrial cancer. To date, six population-based case–control studies (Tyler *et al.*, 1985; Lawrence *et al.*, 1987, 1989; Brinton *et al.*, 1993; Newcomer *et al.*, 2001; Weiderpass & Baron, 2001) have examined quantitative measures of smoking in relation to endometrial cancer risk, generally showing inverse associations to be strongest among current smokers of high intensity or long duration.

2.14.2 Confounders

Whereas the majority of these studies adjusted their relative risk estimates for potentially confounding variables, such as BMI, HRT, parity, diabetes, and age at menopause, studies that did not adjust for these variables tended to show similar inverse associations. Within individual studies, statistical adjustment for the effects of BMI and other covariates often made little difference, although some attenuation of relative risk estimates has been noted (Weiderpass & Baron, 2001; Terry *et al.*, 2002c).

2.14.3 Effect modification

The association between smoking and endometrial cancer risk according to factors that are known determinants of endogenous hormone concentrations, and which may counteract or augment possible tobacco-related hormonal changes, have been examined in several studies. These factors include menopausal status, HRT and BMI. Effect modification can reflect true underlying differences in the association across strata (for example, if cigarette smoking acts to reduce or modify estrogen concentrations differently in one group compared with another), but can also reflect methodological factors, such as differences that occur by chance or through the varying prevalence of confounding variables.

(a) Menopausal status

Although endometrial cancer is rare among pre-menopausal women, several studies have examined the association between cigarette smoking and endometrial cancer risk according to menopausal status, because the effect of smoking (if any) might vary according to the underlying hormonal milieu. The studies have included two cohort studies (Terry *et al.*, 2002b; Al-Zoughool *et al.*, 2007), five population-based case–control studies (Smith *et al.*, 1984; Franks *et al.*, 1987; Lawrence *et al.*, 1987; Brinton *et al.*, 1993; Weiderpass & Baron, 2001), and four hospital-based case–control studies (Lesko *et al.*, 1985; Levi *et al.*, 1987; Stockwell & Lyman, 1987; Koumantaki *et al.*, 1989). In all but one of these studies, a study of early stage endometrial cancer (Lawrence *et al.*, 1987), the inverse association was (to varying degrees) stronger among post-menopausal than pre-menopausal women. Among pre-menopausal women, the relative risk estimates for cigarette smoking have been inconsistent, sometimes showing increased risks with certain measures of cigarette smoking (Smith *et al.*, 1984; Stockwell & Lyman, 1987; Koumantaki *et al.*, 1989; Brinton *et al.*, 1993; Al-Zoughool *et al.*, 2007), sometimes showing decreased risks (Lawrence *et al.*, 1987; Levi *et al.*, 1987; Brinton *et al.*, 1993; Terry *et al.*, 2002b), and sometimes showing practically no association (Lesko *et al.*, 1985; Weiderpass & Baron, 2001; Al-Zoughool *et al.*, 2007). In analyses limited to post-menopausal women, on the other hand, all showed between 10% and 80% reduced risks of endometrial cancer with the various smoking measures.

(b) Hormone replacement therapy

Given the possibility that cigarette smoking affects hormone concentrations mostly among women who are taking HRT (Jensen *et al.*, 1985; Jensen & Christiansen, 1988; Cassidenti *et al.*, 1990), the inverse association between tobacco smoking and endometrial cancer risk might be stronger among HRT users than among non-users. However, the results of studies that have examined the association between smoking and endometrial cancer risk according to HRT use have been equivocal (Weiss *et al.*, 1980; Franks *et al.*, 1987; Lawrence *et al.*, 1987; Levi *et al.*, 1987; Terry *et al.*, 2002b; Beral *et al.*, 2005). Whereas in two studies (Franks *et al.*, 1987; Levi *et al.*, 1987) a larger reduction in risk among smokers taking HRT than among smokers not taking HRT was observed, in two other studies (Lawrence *et al.*, 1987; Terry *et al.*, 2002b) there was no difference in the association according to HRT status. A cohort study that examined associations only among women using HRT showed no clear association among users of continuous combined HRT and cyclic combined HRT, but some suggestion of increased risk among smokers who used tibolone (perhaps more clearly among former smokers) (Beral *et al.*, 2005). Thus, although effect modification by HRT status is biologically plausible, the available epidemiological evidence is equivocal.

(c) Relative body weight

Obesity is an established risk factor for endometrial cancer (IARC, 2002). Smokers tend to have a lower BMI than non-smokers, although former smokers tend to have a higher BMI than current or never smokers (Baron *et al.*, 1990). Two case–control studies have examined the association between cigarette smoking and endometrial cancer risk according to BMI, one population-based (Elliott *et al.*, 1990) and one hospital-based (Levi *et al.*, 1987). Neither of these studies found clear differences in the association between smoking and endometrial cancer risk according to BMI. In a population-based case–control study of early stage endometrial cancer (Lawrence *et al.*, 1987), the inverse association with cigarette smoking tended to become stronger with increasing absolute rather than relative body weight.

2.14.4 Gene polymorphisms

Cigarette smoking and estrogen are both thought to influence cancer risk through pathways that are under the control of specific genes, such as those involved in the formation of bulky DNA adducts by estrogen metabolites (Cavalieri *et al.*, 2000) and both bulky and non-bulky adducts formed by carcinogens in tobacco smoke (Terry & Rohan, 2002). Therefore, studies have been conducted to examine the association between smoking and endometrial cancer risk according to genes that repair these types of DNA damage. In a moderately-sized population-based case–control study no clear effect modification according to certain polymorphisms in the *XPA* and *XPC* genes, both of which are involved in the nucleotide excision repair of bulky DNA adducts and may influence endometrial cancer risk, were found (Weiss *et al.*, 2005, 2006b). A nested case–control study also showed no clear effect modification according to three polymorphisms in *CYP1A1* (McGrath *et al.*, 2007), a gene that encodes microsomal CYP1A1, which contributes to aryl hydrocarbon hydroxylase activity, catalysing the metabolism of PAHs and other carcinogens found in tobacco smoke (Masson *et al.*, 2005). In another nested case–control study some evidence was found that the association between smoking and endometrial cancer may vary according to a polymorphism (Ile^{143}Val) in O^6-methylguanine DNA methyltransferase (*MGMT*). Overall, studies that address the association between smoking and endometrial cancer risk according to genotype are scarce.

2.15 Cancer of the prostate

Many epidemiological studies have examined the association between cigarette smoking and prostate cancer risk, and most have shown no consistent association (Hickey *et al.*, 2001; Levi & La Vecchia, 2001; Batty *et al.*, 2008; Butler *et al.*, 2009; Huncharek *et al.*, 2010; Table 2.74 available at http://monographs.iarc.fr/ENG/Monographs/vol100E/100E-01-Table2.74.pdf; Table 2.75 available at http://monographs.iarc.fr/ENG/Monographs/vol100E/100E-01-Table2.75.pdf). However, questions remain regarding whether smoking may alter risk in various population subgroups, for example, those defined by certain genotypes, and whether any association with smoking may be stronger for, or limited to, advanced tumours or prostate cancer mortality. Regarding this latter issue, the majority of epidemiological studies, including several large, long-term cohort studies, have reported a positive association between smoking and prostate cancer mortality (Rohrmann *et al.*, 2007; Zu & Giovannucci, 2009). Several studies that examined smoking in relation to both prostate cancer incidence and mortality tend to show positive results only for the latter (Rohrmann *et al.*, 2007; Zu & Giovannucci, 2009). Given the largely null results with respect to prostate cancer incidence, the latter findings suggest that smoking is less likely to be a causal agent in prostate cancer initiation than an agent that acts on existing tumours to promote their progression (Zu & Giovannucci, 2009).

A recent review of smoking and prostate cancer that focused specifically on aggressive and fatal tumours, considered the findings from 14 cohort studies (Zu & Giovannucci, 2009). Nine of these studies showed statistically significant increased risk with at least one smoking measure, and five showed increased risks that were not statistically significant for any measure. Only one study showed no association with any measure of tobacco consumption. Seven studies of various designs examined smoking with respect to indicators of cancer aggressive behaviour at the time of diagnosis. In these studies smoking was associated positively with tumour grade, risk of regional, distant, extraprostatic or metastatic disease, Gleason score, and biochemical outcome (failure) after prostate brachytherapy and in several dose–response associations with the respective endpoint were demonstrated. In one study smoking cessation was associated with a decline in risk compared with that among current smokers.

The association between smoking and prostate cancer risk according to genotype and other potentially effect-modifying factors have been examined in several studies. For example, in a population-based case–control study tobacco use was a risk factor for prostate cancer primarily among men with high BMI (Sharpe & Siemiatycki, 2001). The results of a cohort study in Switzerland suggest that risk of prostate cancer mortality is increased in smokers, particularly those with low plasma vitamin E levels (Eichholzer *et al.*, 1999). These latter associations, as well as those regarding several genotypes that may modify the association (Mao *et al.*, 2004; Nock *et al.*, 2006; Quiñones *et al.*, 2006; Yang *et al.*, 2006; Iguchi *et al.*, 2009; Kesarwani *et al.*, 2009), have yet to be fully clarified.

[The Working Group noted that several of the studies of smoking and prostate cancer mortality did not demonstrate clear dose–response associations with risk, and noted the possibility of bias due to confounding by screening behaviour. However, in the Health Professionals Follow-up Study, screening behaviour was not found to differ appreciably between smokers and non-smokers. In an analysis limited to men with a negative digital rectal examination in the prior two years, stronger associations were found between smoking and metastatic prostate cancer risk among high intensity smokers (RR, 4.2; 95%CI: 1.6–10.9) (Zu & Giovannucci, 2009). This finding was evidence against bias from screening behaviour.]

2.16 Cancer of the ovary

2.16.1 Overview of studies

A total of over 30 epidemiological studies have investigated the association between tobacco smoking and ovarian cancer risk. Of these, 24 were case–control studies (IARC, 2004a; Table 2.76 available at http://monographs.iarc.fr/ENG/Monographs/vol100E/100E-01-Table2.76.pdf; Table 2.77 available at http://monographs.iarc.fr/ENG/Monographs/vol100E/100E-01-Table2.77.pdf) and six were cohort studies (IARC, 2004a; Table 2.78 available at http://monographs.iarc.fr/ENG/Monographs/vol100E/100E-01-Table2.78.pdf; Table 2.79 available at http://monographs.iarc.fr/ENG/Monographs/vol100E/100E-01-Table2.79.pdf). Most studies showed no statistically significant association between a measure of smoking and risk for ovarian cancer overall (Newhouse *et al.*, 1977; Smith *et al.*, 1984; Tzonou *et al.*, 1984; Baron *et al.*, 1986; Stockwell & Lyman, 1987; Whittemore *et al.*, 1988; Hartge *et al.*, 1989; Polychronopoulou *et al.*, 1993; Engeland *et al.*, 1996; Goodman *et al.*, 2001; Goodman & Tung, 2003; Pan *et al.*, 2004; Zhang *et al.*, 2004; Kurian *et al.*, 2005; Niwa *et al.*, 2005; Baker *et al.*, 2006; Huusom *et al.*, 2006; Fujita *et al.*, 2008; Lurie *et al.*, 2008; Nagle *et al.*, 2008; Tworoger *et al.*, 2008); some showed positive associations (Doll *et al.*, 1980; Tverdal *et al.*, 1993; Kuper *et al.*, 2000b; Marchbanks *et al.*, 2000; Green *et al.*, 2001; Modugno *et al.*, 2002; Gram *et al.*, 2008; Rossing *et al.*, 2008) and one (Riman *et al.*, 2004) showed an inverse association.

2.16.2 Histological subtypes

Differences in ovarian cancer risk factor profiles have been observed according to histological type, on the basis of which it has been suggested that mucinous and non-mucinous tumours are etiologically distinct diseases (Risch *et al.*, 1996). Epidemiological studies that have considered histological type tend to support a positive association primarily between cigarette smoking and mucinous ovarian tumours (Kuper *et al.*, 2000b; Marchbanks *et al.*, 2000; Green *et al.*, 2001; Modugno *et al.*, 2002; Pan *et al.*, 2004; Zhang *et al.*, 2004; Kurian *et al.*, 2005; Tworoger *et al.*, 2008). In contrast, two studies showed no clear association between smoking and risk of mucinous or non-mucinous ovarian tumours (Riman *et al.*, 2004; Baker *et al.*, 2006). In addition, one early case–control study (Newhouse *et al.*, 1977), with 300 ovarian cancer cases and with both population and hospital controls, found no clear association with "ever" compared with "never" smoking, and reported no differences according to histological type.

A pooled analysis of 10 case–control studies (Kurian *et al.*, 2005) with 254 cases of mucinous and 1580 non-mucinous tumours found an increased risk of mucinous tumours among current smokers (RR, 2.4; 95%CI: 1.5–3.8), a positive association that was not observed with other histological types. Former smokers in that analysis did not have an increased risk of any histological type of ovarian cancer. This type of dose–response, whereby current smokers have a higher risk than former smokers, was observed in most, but not all, studies of mucinous ovarian cancer (Tables 2.77 and 2.79 online). Overall, the positive association between cigarette smoking and risk of mucinous ovarian tumours is generally consistent across both case–control and cohort studies conducted among various populations. In contrast, associations with smoking have been mostly null with respect to non-mucinous ovarian tumours, suggesting that recall bias is unlikely to explain the association with mucinous tumours.

[The Working Group considered the possibility that women who smoke may come to medical attention more frequently. This raises the possibility of detection bias, because mucinous tumours, benign or malignant, tend to be quite large and could be more easily detected on routine physical exam or testing. However, the

Working Group felt that detection bias would not account for the association entirely.

2.17 Cancer of the thyroid

The previous *IARC Monograph* (IARC, 2004a) noted inconsistent associations between smoking and thyroid cancer risk. In 2003, a pooled analysis of 14 case–control studies showed that smoking was inversely associated with thyroid cancer risk (Mack *et al.*, 2003; Table 2.80 available at http://monographs.iarc.fr/ENG/Monographs/vol100E/100E-01-Table2.80.pdf; Table 2.81 available at http://monographs.iarc.fr/ENG/Monographs/vol100E/100E-01-Table2.81.pdf). The sample consisted of 2725 thyroid cancer cases (2247 women, 478 men) and 4776 controls (3699 women, 1077 men). The inverse association was stronger among current smokers (RR, 0.6; 9% CI: 0.6–0.7) than former smokers (RR, 0.9; 9% CI: 0.8–1.1) and were similar in both men and women, for both papillary and follicular thyroid cancers, as well as by age and region. An inverse association between smoking and thyroid cancer risk was also found in a subsequent case–control study (Nagano *et al.*, 2007). In contrast, two case–control studies (Zivaljevic *et al.*, 2004; Bufalo *et al.*, 2006) reported no clear association between smoking and thyroid cancer risk (no risk ratio estimates were reported; hence, data are not shown in the tables) and a cohort study with 169 incident cases of thyroid cancer, also found no clear association with any qualitative or quantitative smoking measure (Navarro Silvera *et al.*, 2005; Table 2.82 available at http://monographs.iarc.fr/ENG/Monographs/vol100E/100E-01-Table2.82.pdf; Table 2.83 available at http://monographs.iarc.fr/ENG/Monographs/vol100E/100E-01-Table2.83.pdf).

2.18 Other cancers

The cancers reviewed in this section generally have low incidence and mortality rates and are not considered to be strongly associated with cigarette smoking. This raises the possibility of preferential reporting of positive associations in epidemiological studies.

2.18.1 Cancer of the salivary gland

Studies of smoking and cancers of the salivary gland reviewed in the previous *IARC Monograph* (IARC, 2004a) were sparse and their results were inconsistent (Spitz *et al.*, 1990; Swanson & Burns, 1997; Hayes *et al.*, 1999). A few additional studies also show inconsistent results (Kotwall, 1992; Pinkston & Cole, 1996; Horn-Ross *et al.*, 1997; Vories & Ramirez, 1997; Muscat & Wynder, 1998). Studies that focused specifically on Warthin's tumour [papillary cystadenoma lymphomatosum or adenolymphoma, a benign tumour of the parotid gland] tend to show strong positive associations with smoking (Kotwall, 1992; Pinkston & Cole, 1996; Vories & Ramirez, 1997). One study (Pinkston & Cole, 1996) compared the risk for Warthin's tumour with that for other salivary gland tumours and found that smoking increased risk significantly only for Warthin's tumour.

2.18.2 Cancer of the small intestine

Epidemiological studies (all of case–control design) reviewd in the previous *IARC Monograph* (IARC, 2004a) have been inconsistent in showing a positive association between smoking and cancers of the small intestine (Chow *et al.*, 1993b; Chen *et al.*, 1994; Wu *et al.*, 1997; Negri *et al.*, 1999; Kaerlev *et al.*, 2002). A more recent study showed no clear association (Hassan *et al.*, 2008b).

2.18.3 Cancers of the gallbladder and extra-hepatic bile ducts

Epidemiological studies of smoking and risk of cancers of the gallbladder and extra-hepatic bile ducts reviewed in the previous *IARC Monograph* (IARC, 2004a) tended to show null, weak, or moderately strong positive associations. More recent studies also tend to show either no clear association with biliary tract carcinoma/extra-hepatic cholangiocarcinoma (Shaib *et al.*, 2007; Welzel *et al.*, 2007) or suggest positive associations with gallbladder/biliary cancers (Pandey & Shukla, 2003; Yagyu *et al.*, 2008; Grainge *et al.*, 2009). Attention should be paid to potential confounders, especially BMI, when considering the results of epidemiological studies of risk of cancers of the gallbladder and extra-hepatic bile ducts. Recent studies that statistically adjusted for BMI, on gallbladder disease risk (Grainge *et al.*, 2009) or on extrahepatic biliary tract carcinoma risk (Ahrens *et al.*, 2007), showed a positive and null association with smoking, respectively. To date, there are too few studies with adequate control for potentially confounding factors to determine any clear pattern.

2.18.4 Soft-tissue sarcoma

As reported in the previous *IARC Monograph* (IARC, 2004a), one cohort study found an association between cigarette smoking and mortality from soft-tissue sarcoma after 26 years of follow-up but no dose–response relationship with the number of cigarettes/day, duration of smoking or pack–years (Zahm *et al.*, 1992). No effect of cigarette smoking was detected in an Italian hospital-based case–control study (Franceschi & Serraino, 1992).

2.18.5 Cancer of the skin

(a) Melanoma

Several case–control studies found no difference in the prevalence of tobacco smoking between patients with malignant melanoma and controls, and one study found an inverse association (IARC, 2004a). An inverse association with smoking was also found in the US Radiologic Technologists cohort Study (Freedman *et al.*, 2003a). In that study, smoking for at least 30 years compared with never smoking was inversely related to melanoma risk (RR, 0.6; 95%CI: 0.3–1.3), though risk was not associated with number of cigarettes/day. An inverse association was also observed in a cohort of Swedish construction workers (Odenbro *et al.*, 2007). In this study, the risk for malignant melanoma was reduced in a dose-dependant manner for both cigarette and pipe smokers. The possibility that smoking may reduce the risk for melanoma should, therefore, be considered.

(b) Non-melanoma skin cancer

Four studies showed a positive association between smoking and non-melanoma skin cancer risk (De Stefani *et al.*, 1995; Wojno, 1999; Smith & Randle, 2001; Boyd *et al.*, 2002), and two found no clear association (van Dam *et al.*, 1999; Corona *et al.*, 2001). When distinguishing between histological subtypes, tobacco smoking was linked to the incidence of squamous-cell carcinoma of the skin in most studies, whereas the results for basal cell carcinoma remain inconsistent (Zak-Prelich *et al.*, 2004). No clear association between smoking and risk for basal cell carcinoma was found in a cohort study (Freedman *et al.*, 2003b).

2.18.6 Cancer of the penis

Case–control studies of smoking and penile cancer (Hellberg *et al.*, 1987; Daling *et al.*, 1992, 2005; Maden *et al.*, 1993; Harish & Ravi, 1995;

Table 2.84 available at http://monographs.iarc.fr/ENG/Monographs/vol100E/100E-01-Table2.84.pdf; Table 2.85 available at http://monographs.iarc.fr/ENG/Monographs/vol100E/100E-01-Table2.85.pdf) and reviews of studies of smoking and penile cancer and population surveys (Dillner *et al.*, 2000; Favorito *et al.*, 2008; Bleeker *et al.*, 2009; Table 2.86 available at http://monographs.iarc.fr/ENG/Monographs/vol100E/100E-01-Table2.86.pdf; Table 2.87 available at http://monographs.iarc.fr/ENG/Monographs/vol100E/100E-01-Table2.87.pdf) consistently showed a positive association. In most studies there was a dose–response relationship, with higher risks among those with increased smoking intensity and/or duration. A study in Brazil showed a positive correlation with penile tumour grade (Favorito *et al.*, 2008). Based on the two reviews (Dillner *et al.*, 2000; Bleeker *et al.*, 2009), relative risks were generally increased twofold to fivefold among smokers.

Most studies did not adjust for HPV infection. In one case–control study (Daling *et al.*, 2005), current smoking was associated with a 160% increased risk of HPV-positive penile cancer (n = 75), and a 180% increased risk of HPV-negative penile cancer (n = 19), suggesting no important effect modification.

2.18.7 Cancer of the testis

Studies reviewed in the previous *IARC Monograph* (IARC, 2004a) showed no association between cigarette smoking and risk for testicular cancer. More recently, two case–control studies showed positive associations with smoking, one in Canada (Srivastava & Kreiger, 2004) and one in the Czech Republic (Dusek *et al.*, 2008).

2.18.8 Cancer of the central nervous system

A recent meta-analysis was conducted on smoking in relation to glioma risk (Mandelzweig *et al.*, 2009), which included 17 epidemiological studies (6 cohort and 11 case–control). It was concluded that smoking is not associated with risk of glioma, despite a small significant increased risk seen in cohort studies. A recent cohort study found no association between smoking and carcinoma of the brain (Batty *et al.*, 2008). There have been no consistent associations of smoking with other CNS tumours (IARC, 2004a). In a population-based case–control study in the USA, smoking was associated with increased risk of intracranial meningioma in men (OR, 2.1; 95%CI: 1.1–4.2) but not in women (Phillips *et al.*, 2005).

2.18.9 Cancer of the adrenal gland

Data on risk factors for adrenal carcinoma are sparse. In the US Veterans' Study there was a fivefold increase in risk among current cigarette smokers during 26 years of follow-up, with risk being particularly high among those who smoked most intensely (Chow *et al.*, 1996). Other forms of tobacco use were associated with a statistically non-significant increase in risk. A case–control study in the USA found a twofold increase in risk for adrenal cancer among heavy smokers in men, but not in women (Hsing *et al.*, 1996).

2.19 Bidi smoking

2.19.1 Cancer of the oral cavity

(a) Overview of studies

The association between cancers of oral cavity and bidi smoking has been examined in 10 case–control studies conducted in India (Sankaranarayanan *et al.*, 1989a, b, 1990a; Rao *et al.*, 1994; Rao & Desai, 1998; Dikshit & Kanhere, 2000; Balaram *et al.*, 2002; Znaor *et al.*, 2003; Subapriya *et al.*, 2007; Muwonge *et al.*, 2008; Table 2.88 available at http://monographs.iarc.fr/ENG/Monographs/vol100E/100E-01-Table2.88.pdf). In these studies both cases and controls were interviewed and analyses were restricted to men, except for the studies by Balaram *et al.* (2002) and Subapriya *et al.* (2007), because very few women smoked among study subjects.

Three hospital-based case–control studies considered cancers of subsites of the oral cavity (gingiva, tongue and floor of the mouth, buccal and labial mucosa) (Sankaranarayanan *et al.*, 1989a, b, 1990a). All three studies showed a higher oral cancer risk for bidi smoking. In one early study an unadjusted relative risk of 1.6 (95%CI: 1.3–2.0) for oral cancer in bidi smokers was reported (Rao *et al.*, 1994). [The Working Group noted that the study had several deficiencies, particularly in the selection of controls that resulted in cigarette smoking apparently being protective for oral cancer.] In another early study (Rao & Desai, 1998) relative risks were estimated after stratification by age and place of residence. Bidi smoking was a significant risk factor for cancer of the base of the tongue (RR, 5.9; 95%CI: 4.2–8.2) but not significant for cancer of the anterior tongue. Relative risk for bidi smoking adjusted for alcohol drinking, illiteracy, non-vegetarian diet and tobacco chewing showed significant risk for cancer of the base of the tongue (RR, 4.7; 95%CI: 3.5–6.3) but not for cancer of the anterior tongue. In a population-based case–control study a relative risk of 1.5 (95%CI: 0.9–2.4), adjusted for age and tobacco quid chewing for smokers (bidis and/or cigarettes), was found (Dikshit & Kanhere, 2000).

Two hospital-based multi centre case–control studies on cancer of the oral cavity were conducted in southern India. One included 309 cases and 292 controls (Balaram *et al.*, 2002). The risk for oral cavity cancer among those who smoked < 20 bidis per day was 2.0 (95%CI: 1.1–3.8) and 2.5 (95%CI: 1.4–4.4) for ≥ 20 per day. The second study included 1563 cases and 3638 controls and found a risk for bidi smoking only of 2.2 (95%CI: 1.75–2.63) compared to never smokers, adjusted for age, centre, level of education, alcohol consumption and chewing (Znaor *et al.*, 2003).

In a hospital-based case–control study with 388 oral squamous cell carcinoma cases (202 men and 186 women) and an equal number of age and sex-matched controls the effect of lifestyle factors (tobacco chewing, smoking and alcohol drinking, diet and dental care) on the risk of oral cancer was evaluated (Subapriya *et al.*, 2007). Both cases and controls were interviewed using a structured questionnaire. The risk estimate for bidi smoking based on 22 cases (84 cases included in the model) and 22 controls was 4.6 (95%CI not given).

Data from a randomized control trial conducted between 1996 and 2004 in Trivandrum, southern India were used in a nested case–control analysis with 282 (163 men and 119 women) incident oral cancer cases and 1410 matched population controls aged 35 years and over (Muwonge *et al.*, 2008). Oral cancer risk among men, adjusted for education and religion, was 1.9 (95%CI: 1.1–3.2) for bidi smokers only compared to never smokers. No association was found between mixed smoking of bidi and cigarette and risk of oral cancer.

Rahman *et al.* (2003) performed a meta-analysis to investigate the relationship between bidi smoking and oral cancer. They identified 12 case–control studies published in English during 1996–2002 with quantitative information on bidi smoking and oral cancer. Of these, ten studies were conducted in India, one in Sri Lanka and one in Pakistan. All cases were confirmed histologically and exposure data were collected by direct interview. In these studies ORs were not adjusted for tobacco chewing or alcohol drinking. The OR for bidi smokers compared to never smokers based on random effects model was 3.1 (95%CI: 2.0 –5.0). The ORs ranged from 2.0 to 3.6 in different regions of India: studies conducted in Mumbai had an OR of 3.6 (95%CI: 1.6 –7.9), in central India 2.7 (95%CI: 1.6–4.6), in Kerala 2.0 (95%CI: 1.5–2.9) and in Bangalore 2.0 (95%CI: 1.1–3.7).

(b) Dose–response evidence

The trends in relative risks by intensity and duration of bidi smoking were both statistically significant in two studies (Rao *et al.*, 1994; Rao & Desai, 1998). A meta-analysis based on three studies on duration of bidi smoking and on five studies on number of bidi sticks per day, showed a dose–response relationship for duration of bidi smoking but not for number of sticks used per day (Rahman *et al.*, 2003).

In a nested case–control analysis (Muwonge *et al.*, 2008) a dose–response relationship was observed for duration of bidi smoking ($P = 0.045$). [It is not clear if the analysis was restricted to bidi smokers only (n = 40 men) and if smokers with combined smoking habits (bidi and cigarette) were excluded. Moreover, ORs for the dose–response analysis were not reported.]

2.19.2 Cancer of the pharynx

Five case–control studies, two hospital-based (Wasnik *et al.*, 1998; Rao *et al.*, 1999), one population-based (Dikshit & Kanhere, 2000) and two multicentric studies (Znaor *et al.*, 2003; Sapkota *et al.*, 2007) were conducted on cancers of oropharynx and hypopharynx in India (Table 2.88 online). In all these studies, analyses were restricted to men because very few women smoked among study subjects.

Wasnik *et al.* (1998) conducted a case–control study on oropharyngeal cancers with cases and controls were matched on age and sex. Odds ratios for tobacco smoking, predominantly in the form of bidi and/or chillum, were 2.3 (95%CI: 1.2–3.7) after adjustment for tobacco chewing and outdoor occupation. [The Working Group noted some problems with the data analysis.]

Rao *et al.* (1999) reported a relative risk for bidi smoking adjusted for alcohol, illiteracy, diet and tobacco chewing of 4.7 (3.6–6.3) for oropharyngeal cancer and of 2.8 (2.1–3.7) for cancer of the hypopharynx. Dikshit & Kanhere (2000) found an odds ratio for oropharyngeal cancer among bidi smokers only of 7.9 (95%CI: 5.1–12.4).

Znaor *et al.* (2003) reported a risk for bidi smoking only for pharyngeal cancer of 4.7 (95%CI: 3.5–6.3) and for combined bidi and cigarette smoking of 3.6 (95%CI: 2.55–4.98). Sapkota *et al.* (2007) reported an odds ratio for hypopharyngeal cancer of 6.8 (95%CI: 4.6–10.0) for bidi smokers compared to never smokers.

A dose–response relationship was observed for intensity and duration of bidi smoking for both cancers of oropharynx and hypopharynx (Rao *et al.*, 1999; Dikshit & Kanhere, 2000; Sapkota *et al.*, 2007).

2.19.3 Cancer of the lung

One cohort study (Jayalekshmy *et al.*, 2008), one population-based case–control study (Dikshit & Kanhere, 2000) and two hospital-based case–control studies (Gupta *et al.*, 2001; Gajalakshmi *et al.*, 2003) in India (Table 2.88 online) have investigated the relationship between bidi smoking and lung cancer. In all these studies both cases and controls were interviewed and analyses were restricted to men because very few women smoked among study subjects. One hospital-based case–control study in Chiang Mai, Thailand, looked at the association between lung cancer and *khii yoo,* hand-rolled cigars. The risk for lung cancer for *khii yoo* smoking was 1.2 in men and 1.5 in women, $P > 0.05$ (Simarak *et al.*, 1977).

In the population based case–control study by Dikshit & Kanhere (2000) the age-adjusted relative risk for lung cancer among bidi smokers only was 11.6 (95%CI: 6.4–21.3).

Gupta *et al.* (2001) reported an odds ratio for bidi smoking of 5.8 (95%CI: 3.4–9.7) from a hospital-based case–control study of lung cancer conducted in Chandigarh. Gajalakshmi *et al.* (2003) conducted a case–control study in two centres in which all subjects were interviewed by trained social investigators with standard questionnaires. Odds ratios were adjusted for age, educational level, centre, chewing and alcohol habit. The odds ratios of lung cancer for former and current bidi smokers were 3.4 (95%CI: 2.1–5.4) and 5.3 (95%CI: 3.8–7.3), respectively. Odds ratios for former and current smokers of cigarette and bidi combined were 4.0 (95%CI: 2.5–6.6) and 9.1 (95%CI: 6.2–13.2), respectively.

Baseline data of a cohort of 359 619 residents in Kerala, India was collected by direct interview using standardized questionnaires during 1990–97 (Jayalekshmy *et al.*, 2008). After excluding rare earth workers, those who died, were diagnosed with cancer before 1997 or died within three years of interview, there were 65 829 bidi-smoking men aged 30–84 years old. Two hundred and twelve lung cancer cases were identified by the Karunagappally Cancer Registry between 1997 and 2004. The relative risk for lung cancer for current compared to never bidi smokers calculated by Poisson regression analysis and adjusted for age, religion and education was 3.9 (95%CI: 2.6–6.0; $P < 0.001$). The risk was lower among former than among current smokers.

(a) Dose–response evidence

Lung cancer risks increased with increasing bidi smoking intensities. The highest odds ratio was found for 9 pack–years (3.9; 95%CI: 2.1–7.1) (Gupta *et al.*, 2001). In a cohort study Jayalekshmy *et al.* (2008) found increased lung cancer incidence with increasing number of bidi sticks smoked per day ($P < 0.001$) and with increasing duration of bidi smoking ($P < 0.001$). [The number of lung cancer cases was small in each category, resulting in wide confidence intervals.] Gajalakshmi *et al.* (2003) also reported increased risk with duration and intensity of bidi smoking.

(b) Cessation of smoking

In two case–control studies (Gupta *et al.*, 2001; Gajalakshmi *et al.*, 2003) there was a clear decreasing trend in risk for years since quitting. Gajalakshmi *et al.* (2003) reported that lung cancer risk of former bidi smokers fell to 0.4 (0.1–1.2) after quitting for more than 15 years. The cohort study conducted in Kerala did not have the power to assess the risk associated with stopping bidi smoking (Jayalekshmy *et al.*, 2008).

2.19.4 Cancer of the larynx

Two hospital based case–control studies (Sankaranarayanan *et al.*, 1990b; Rao *et al.*, 1999) showed a higher risk for bidi smokers (Table 2.88 online). The relative risk was adjusted for age and religion in Sankaranarayanan *et al.* (1990b) study and for alcohol use, illiteracy, vegetarian/non-vegetarian diet and tobacco chewing in Rao *et al.* (1999) study. A multicentre case–control study on laryngeal cancer was conducted in four Indian centres using standardized questionnaires adjusting risks for centre, age, socio-economic status, alcohol consumption, tobacco snuffing and tobacco chewing (Sapkota *et al.*, 2007). Compared to never smokers bidi smokers had a higher risk for cancers of the supraglottis (OR, 7.5; 95%CI: 3.8–14.7), glottis (OR, 5.3; 95%CI: 3.2–8.9) and rest of larynx (OR, 9.6; 95%CI: 5.6–16.4).

All levels of intensity and duration of bidi smoking were associated with significant relative risk estimates and dose–response for laryngeal cancer (Sankaranarayanan *et al.*, 1990b; Rao *et al.*, 1999). A strong dose–response relationship was observed for duration and frequency of bidi smoking for cancers of supraglottis, glottis and rest of larynx (Sapkota *et al.*, 2007).

2.19.5 Cancer of the oesophagus

Three hospital-based case–control studies and one multicentre study (Sankaranarayanan *et al.*, 1991; Nandakumar *et al.*, 1996; Nayar *et al.*, 2000; Znaor *et al.* 2003) showed increased risk for oesophageal cancer among bidi smokers in India (Table 2.88 online). A significantly elevated risk for all three segments of the oesophagus was reported (Nandakumar *et al.*, 1996). One study (Nayar *et al.*, 2000) adjusted for chewing of betel leaf with tobacco and low consumption of vegetables other than leafy vegetables. The multicentre case–control study conducted in two centres in South India found an increased risk for oesophageal cancer for bidi smoking only (OR, 3.3; 95%CI: 2.45–4.39) (Znaor *et al.*, 2003). Odds ratios were adjusted for age, centre, level of education, alcohol consumption and chewing. Only men were analysed in all the above studies.

Significant effects were noted in men for all levels of intensity and for duration of more than 20 years of bidi smoking (Sankaranarayanan *et al.*, 1991).

2.19.6 Cancer of the stomach

In a hospital-based case–control study the association between stomach cancer and bidi smoking was analysed as part of a multicentre study (Gajalakshmi & Shanta, 1996). Cases and controls were matched on age, sex, religion and mother tongue. The odds ratio for stomach cancer for current bidi smokers only was 3.2 (95%CI: 1.8–5.7) and for current smokers of any type of tobacco was 2.7 (95%CI: 1.8–4.1).

Table 2.88 (online) summarizes the studies published since the last *IARC Monograph* (IARC, 2004a). A hospital-based case–control study of stomach cancer included 170 stomach cancer cases (121 men and 49 women) and 2184 controls (1309 men and 875 women) aged 30–75 years (Rao *et al.*, 2002). The association between bidi smoking and stomach cancer was not significant (RR, 0.8; 95%CI: 0.5–1.2) in a univariate analysis. The risk increased with increase in lifetime exposure to bidi smoking and was highly significant ($P < 0.001$).

One study investigated stomach cancer risk in association with smoking of *meiziol*, a local cigarette in Mizoram, India (Phukan *et al.*, 2005). Statistically significant higher risks were seen for smokers of combined users of tobacco (cigarette and *meiziol*), with an odds ratio of 3.1 (95%CI: 2.0–11.1). Among users of a single type of tobacco, higher risks were seen for *meiziol* smokers (OR, 2.2; 95%CI: 1.3–9.3) in the multivariate model in comparison to cigarette smokers. Overall, the excess risk was limited to smokers of > 10 *meiziols* per day.

2.20 Synergistic effects of tobacco smoking and alcohol drinking

This section addresses the combined effects of smoking and alcohol consumption on cancers of oral cavity, pharynx, larynx and oesophagus, which have been examined extensively. For the purposes of this report interdependence of effects is termed *effect modification*, and *synergism* and *antagonism* are used to describe the consequences of the interdependence of disease risk when both risk factors are present (Rothman & Greenland, 1998). The studies varied in their methods and in the approaches used to assess effect modification, which ranged from descriptive to formal estimation of interaction terms in multivariate models. Study designs of the case–control and cohort studies are presented in Table 2.89 (available at http://monographs.iarc.fr/ENG/Monographs/vol100E/100E-01-Table2.89.pdf) and Table 2.90 (available at http://monographs.iarc.fr/ENG/Monographs/vol100E/100E-01-Table2.90.pdf), respectively; and the results for both study designs are presented in Table 2.91 (available at http://monographs.iarc.fr/ENG/Monographs/vol100E/100E-01-Table2.91.pdf).

2.20.1 Cancers of the upper aerodigestive tract

It was noted in the previous *IARC Monograph* (IARC, 2004a) with relatively large numbers of cases and controls that the pattern of increasing cancer risk with increasing alcohol consumption is strong (Mashberg *et al.*, 1993; Kabat *et al.*, 1994).

For cancers of the oral cavity, recent evidence comes from seven case–control studies and one cohort study. The pattern of odds ratios for smoking, across categories of alcohol consumption, is consistent with synergism. In four case–control studies with relatively large numbers of cases and controls (more than 200 cases and equivalent number of controls), the pattern of increasing cancer risks with increasing alcohol consumption was strong (Schlecht *et al.*, 1999b; Znaor *et al.*, 2003; Castellsagué *et al.*, 2004; Hashibe *et al.*, 2009). In the cohort study from Taiwan, China (Yen *et al.*, 2008) similar strong risks were also observed. In all four case–control studies in which the estimate of formal statistical interaction was examined, the tests were statistically significant (Schlecht *et al.*, 1999b; Znaor *et al.*, 2003; Castellsagué *et al.*, 2004; Hashibe *et al.*, 2009). In two case–control studies from India (Znaor *et al.*, 2003; Muwonge *et al.*, 2008) and in the cohort study from Taiwan, China (Yen *et al.*, 2008) the interaction of tobacco smoking, alcohol and betel quid chewing was examined. In general, the results suggested increasing risks when betel quid chewing was included in the model.

Five case–control studies and one cohort study examined the effect of interaction between tobacco and alcohol in pharyngeal cancer. The results from case–control studies were similar to those observed for oral cancer (Olsen *et al.*, 1985b; Choi & Kahyo, 1991; Schlecht *et al.*, 1999b; Znaor *et al.*, 2003; Hashibe *et al.*, 2009). In a Singapore cohort study (Friborg *et al.*, 2007) the pattern of odds ratios for smoking across categories of alcohol consumption was consistent with synergism for oropharyngeal but not for nasopharyngeal cancer.

Two cohort and fourteen case–control studies reported on joint effects of tobacco smoking and alcohol drinking on the risk for oesophageal cancer. Since multiple logistic regression models were used for analysing most of these studies, some of them tested likelihood ratio test for departure from multiplicativity of the individual effects of tobacco and alcohol. Generally, the positive results were stronger for squamous cell carcinoma. However, these tests for interaction are inadequate to assess synergy. Four studies from India and Taiwan, China, included betel quid chewing to the joint effect analysis of tobacco smoking and alcohol consumption and the results suggested increasing risks of oesophageal cancer.

Most of the twenty case–control studies of laryngeal cancer provided strong evidence for synergism of tobacco smoking and alcohol consumption. Only Zheng *et al.* (1992) did not find consistent evidence with synergism. In several studies, tests for interaction were carried out and reported to be 'non significant.' These were tests for departure from the multiplicative models, typically multiple logistic regression models, used to analyse the case–control data, and not tests for departure from additive model.

Several studies (14 case–control, 3 cohort) reported on cancer of the 'mixed upper aerodigestive tract', comprising studies on squamous cell carcinomas, regardless of specific sites. These studies also provided strong evidence for synergism.

The Working Group considers that there is strong evidence of tobacco smoking and alcohol consumption interaction on the incidence of upper aerodigestive tract cancers, as well as with regard to cancer of specific subsites of this anatomical region.

2.21 Synthesis

2.21.1 Lung

Tobacco smoking is the major cause of lung cancer, primarily from cigarettes. Duration of smoking is the strongest determinant of lung cancer in smokers. Risk also increases in proportion to the number of cigarettes smoked. The strong dose– and duration–response relationships between lung cancer and tobacco smoking have been confirmed more recently in both questionnaire-based and biomarker-based studies. Tobacco smoking increases the risk of all histological types of lung cancer.

Differences in the intensity and/or duration of tobacco smoking may explain, in part, the lower lung cancer risks in Asian populations relative to whites. However, several studies of genetic polymorphisms among African-American and Caucasian populations provide some preliminary evidence supporting the hypothesis of a racial/ethnic disparity in susceptibility.

The results from observational studies do not provide strong support that a higher intake or a greater circulating concentration of carotenoids reduce lung cancer risk, particular in light of the elevated risk of lung cancer observed in the randomized trials of β-carotene supplementation. Residual confounding from smoking and the possibility that carotenoid measurements are serving as markers for a diet rich in total fruit and vegetables mitigate the likelihood of any protective role for total carotenoids or β-cryptoxanthins.

The specific genes that are responsible for enhanced lung cancer risk remain poorly understood, in spite of hundreds of candidate gene studies. Single-gene studies conducted to date have several limitations which contribute to inconclusive results, including small sample size and associated low power to detect moderate risks when allele frequencies are low.

2.21.2 Upper areodigestive tract

(a) Oral cavity

Tobacco smoking is causally associated with cancer of the oral cavity in both men and women. Since the previous *Monograph*, additional evidence has accumulated that further confirms the association. Risk increases with duration and intensity of smoking, and decreases after quitting.

(b) Pharynx

Tobacco smoking is an important cause of oropharyngeal and hypopharyngeal cancers. The risk increases with increasing duration and intensity of smoking and decreases with increasing time since quitting.

(c) Nasal cavity and accessory sinuses

The evidence of an association between tobacco smoking and sinonasal cancer is based on the results from case–control studies, each of which may be subject to different sources of bias. However, presence of a dose–response relationship in most studies, the decrease in risk associated with time since quitting, the consistently higher risks for squamous-cell carcinoma than for adenocarcinoma and the lack of potential confounders support the existence of a causal association.

(d) Nasopharynx

Although the interpretation of the results is complicated by small sample sizes in several studies, by different criteria used for the selection of controls and by the control groups in some studies including smoking-related diseases, the combined evidence shows an association between tobacco smoking and nasopharyngeal carcinoma in both endemic and non-endemic areas. Most studies that adjusted for known and suspected causes of nasopharyngeal carcinoma such as intake of Chinese-style salted fish, other dietary factors, alcohol drinking and family history of nasopharyngeal carcinoma, suggested only a limited confounding effect of these factors. Adjustment for infection with Epstein–Barr virus (human herpes virus 4), a major cause of nasopharyngeal carcinoma worldwide, was possible in just one of the available studies. However, it is unlikely that confounding by infection with Epstein–Barr virus would explain the observed association between tobacco smoking and risk for nasopharyngeal carcinoma.

(e) Oesophagus

Several well conducted case–control studies found a statistically significant higher risk for adenocarcinoma of the oesophagus in smokers than in nonsmokers. Positive dose–response relationships obtained using various indicators of amount smoked support a causal association, which is further corroborated by the findings of decreasing risks after smoking cessation. Several of these studies reported relative risks adjusted for alcohol consumption and other potential confounders. Further risk factors, such as chewing betel quid with tobacco or use of other forms of smokeless tobacco, have not been considered in these populations, but are not likely to be strong confounders. Studies from Australia, China and Europe also found increased risks for smokers.

(f) Larynx

Laryngeal cancer is one of the cancers most strongly associated with cigarette smoking. Recent epidemiological evidence strengthens this conclusion.

2.21.3 Stomach

The additional epidemiologic data showing a consistent association of stomach cancer with tobacco smoking in both men and women greatly strengthens the previous conclusion of a causal association. There was insufficient evidence for differential risks between cardia and non-cardia stomach cancer. Confounding and effect modification by H. pylori has not been found.

2.21.4 Pancreas

The additional data supports the previous evaluation that cancer of the pancreas is causally associated with tobacco smoking. The risk increases with increasing daily consumption levels and duration of smoking and decreases with increasing time since cessation of smoking. The risk remains elevated after accounting for potential confounding factors.

2.21.5 Colorectum

At the previous evaluation, there was already some evidence from prospective cohort and case–control studies that the risk of colorectal cancer is increased among tobacco smokers. However, inadequate adjustment for various potential confounders was considered to possibly account for some of the small increase in risk that appears to be associated with smoking. Since then, an appreciable amount of data has accumulated to support a causal association with smoking. In virtually all the cohort studies published since elevated risk associated with smoking was found, although not always statistically significant. More than half of the cohort studies that assessed dose–response relationships found statistically significant increasing risks with increasing daily cigarette consumption, duration of smoking and/or pack–years of smoking. Risk of colorectal cancer decreased with increasing delay in smoking initiation and years since cessation of smoking. A meta-analysis based on 36 cohort studies with data from a total of 3 million subjects found a significantly 15% increased risk of colorectal cancer and 27% higher risk of colorectal cancer mortality in current smokers compared to never smokers. A stronger association with smoking for rectal cancer than for colon cancer was found in the meta-analysis of the subset of cohort studies that differentiated colorectal cancer by site. Risk for colorectal cancer increased significantly by 17% and by 38% with 20 cigarettes and 40 cigarettes/day, respectively, and was elevated by 9.4% and by 19.7% with a 20-year and a 40-year duration of smoking, respectively. While these results are persuasive, this meta-analysis could not correct for the potential confounders in the individual studies. Convincing evidence has been provided by three large cohort studies that adjusted for at least four important potential confounders (i.e. physical activity, alcohol consumption, body mass index and dietary intake of fruits and vegetables and/or meat); two studies also adjusted for history of colonoscopy. Significant dose–response relationships were found with one or more of the smoking variables, for risk of colorectal cancer and/or colon cancer and/or rectal cancer. Earlier cohort studies may not have been able to establish the association because of insufficient follow-up time and a limited number of cases. Updated results of several large cohort studies, which now show clearly significant increased risk of colorectal cancer associated with smoking, provide support for the lag-time hypothesis for smoking and colorectal risk.

Recent evidence suggests that smoking may be associated with the subtype of colorectal cancer characterized by microsatellite instability, and by CIMP status and BRAF mutation. For this subtype, the magnitude of risk associated with smoking reaches the twofold risk elevation consistently observed for colorectal adenomas and supported by a recent meta-analysis. Smoking has been associated with a stronger risk for hyperplastic polyps than for adenomas. Also, CIMP positivity and BRAF mutations have been associated with hyperplastic polyps, particularly serrated polyps. These data suggest that smoking may be associated primarily with a subtype of colorectal cancer that develops through a hyperplastic (serrated) polyp progression. The association with smoking may therefore be diluted when considering colon cancers overall.

2.21.6 Liver

Recent studies on smoking and hepatocellular carcinoma supports the established causal relationship. Supporting evidence comes from the consistency of the findings across regions (with the best evidence coming from Asian studies), and the observations of an association among non-drinkers and after controlling for hepatitis B or C virus infection.

2.21.7 Kidney

Recent evidence supports a causal association between kidney cancer and smoking. After adjustment for body mass index and hypertension, current and former smokers still had a greater risk for renal-cell cancer. A dose–response relationship with the number of cigarettes smoked has been noted in most studies, and a few also noted a reduction in risk after cessation.

2.21.8 Urinary bladder

Tobacco smoking is causally associated to bladder cancer, based on a large number of case–control and cohort studies that showed statistically significant associations not explained by confounding or bias. Risk increased with the duration of smoking and the number of cigarettes smoked. Also, stopping smoking at any age avoids the further increase in risk incurred by continued smoking. The evidence supporting a modulating role by *NAT2* polymorphisms is convincing.

2.21.9 Myeloid leukaemia

There is evidence for a causal association of tobacco smoking with myeloid leukaemia.

2.21.10 Breast

New evidence from cohort and case–control studies and from meta-analyses of genetic polymorphisms has become available since the previous *IARC Monograph* (IARC, 2004a). Results from seven new cohort studies consistently show a small overall association between current smoking and breast cancer incidence, with relative risk estimates ranging from 1.1–1.3 in studies with at least 100 exposed cases. The overall association is weaker than that observed with other cancers that have been designated as causally related to smoking, and the dose–response relationships (with years of smoking, cigarettes smoked per day, age at initiation) are correspondingly small.

Emerging evidence from case–control studies suggests that inherited polymorphisms in the *NAT2* gene, which encode the slow acetylator phenotype, may modify (increase) the association between smoking and breast cancer. The p-value for interaction with pack–years of smoking as a continuous variable is statistically significant ($P = 0.03$) and another small study published since this meta-analysis supports the conclusion. The potential for publication bias remains of concern.

It is biologically plausible that tobacco smoke could be causally related to breast cancer risk. There are multiple chemicals in tobacco smoke that are known to cause mammary cancer in rodents. These substances reach the breast in humans; some are stored in adipose tissue, and some can be detected in nipple aspirate and DNA adducts.

Hypotheses have been proposed to explain why numerous well conducted epidemiological studies have generally not observed strong or consistent associations between tobacco smoking and breast cancer. Underlying all of these is the theory that tobacco smoking may have both protective and detrimental effects on breast cancer risk, which cancel each other out and which could explain the atypical dose–response relationship that has been reported between tobacco smoke and breast cancer from some studies.

2.21.11 Cervix

The largely positive findings observed in studies of cohort design, the relatively high consistency of positive associations found for squamous-cell carcinoma of the cervix (but not adenocarcinomas) across all epidemiological studies, including those with adjustment for a wide range of potentially confounding variables, and the positive associations observed in studies restricted to HPV-positive individuals, all argue against the observed positive association being due to recall or selection bias or confounding.

2.21.12 Endometrium

The results of epidemiological studies to date, including recent studies, largely show inverse associations of smoking with risk of postmenopausal endometrial cancer. However, the Working Group noted the few studies of premenopausal cancer that were less consistent, as well as indications of an increased risk among smokers in a recent multicentre European study.

2.21.13 Prostate

Many epidemiological studies have examined the association between cigarette smoking and prostate cancer risk, and most have shown no consistent association. The question remains whether smoking may alter risk in various population subgroups.

2.21.14 Ovary

A causal association between cigarette smoking and risk for mucinous ovarian tumours is indicated by 1) the consistency of the positive association across the large majority of ten pooled case–control studies and ten additional independent epidemiological studies of both case–control and cohort design, 2) the relatively strong magnitude of the association (typically greater than a doubling of risk among current smokers), 3) the tendency to show dose–response associations with risk, such that current smokers generally have higher risk than former smokers and the dose–response observed with measures of smoking intensity in some (but not all) studies, and 4) the specificity of the positive association with the mucinous histological type, which argues against recall bias as an explanation of the findings.

2.21.15 Thyroid

A pooled analysis of 14 case–control studies showed that smoking was inversely associated with thyroid cancer risk. Similar inverse associations were also observed in two subsequent case–control studies.

2.21.16 Other sites

There is inconsistent or sparse evidence for an association between tobacco smoking and other cancer sites that were considered by the Working Group.

2.21.17 Bidi smoking

Overall, bidi smoking increases the risk for cancers of the oral cavity, oropharynx, hypopharynx, larynx, lung, oesophagus and stomach.

3. Cancer in Experimental Animals

3.1 Mainstream tobacco smoke

3.1.1 Mouse

There have been multiple studies of the carcinogenic potential of tobacco smoke in mice (Table 3.1). Lifetime exposure of several mouse strains to cigarette smoke failed to result in the production of lung tumours (Harris & Negroni, 1967; Otto & Elmenhorst, 1967; Henry & Kouri, 1986). However, studies involving lifetime exposure of C57BL mice to a mixture of flue-cured or air-cured cigarette smoke or to the gas phase of flue-cured cigarette smoke led to significant increases in the number of lung tumours (adenomas) (Harris *et al.*, 1974). Similarly, lifetime exposure of Snell's mice to the gas phase of cigarette smoke led to an increased incidence of lung adenocarcinomas (Leuchtenberger & Leuchtenberger, 1970). Exposure of $B6C3F_1$ female mice to smoke for lifetime led to increased incidence of lung adenomas, bronchiolar papillomas and lung adenocarcinomas in smoke-exposed mice. In addition, the occurrence of squamous cell carcinomas of the nasal cavity in smoke-exposed mice was increased (Hutt *et al.*, 2005). In a recent study, Swiss mice were exposed whole-body to cigarette smoke for 120 days, starting within 12 hours of the birth. Smoke-exposed mice developed microscopic lung tumours beginning only 75 days after birth and reaching an overall incidence of 78.3% after 181–230 days. The mean lung tumour multiplicity was 6.1 and 13.6 tumours per mouse in males and females, respectively. In addition, malignant tumours, some of which may have had a metastatic origin, were detected in the urinary tract of smoke-exposed mice (Balansky *et al.*, 2007).

3.1.2 Rat

Several studies have evaluated the carcinogenic potential of mainstream tobacco smoke in rats (Table 3.1). Exposure of Wistar rats to cigarette smoke for lifetime did not increase the lung tumour incidence (Davis *et al.*, 1975). In contrast, exposure of Fischer 344 rats to a mixture of non-filter cigarette smoke for 128 weeks resulted in an increased incidence of nasal and lung tumours. There was also an increase in subcutaneous sarcomas at forelimb ulceration sites (Dalbey *et al.*, 1980). CDF rats were exposed to low-dose cigarette smoke (LCS) or high-dose cigarette smoke (HCS) for 126 weeks. The incidence of lung tumours was significantly higher only in female rats that received HCS (Finch *et al.*, 1995). In a recent study, Fischer 344 rats received whole body exposure to smoke containing either 100 mg (LCS) or 250 mg (HCS) total particulate matter/m^3 for 30 months. This led to significant increases in the incidence of lung and nasal cavity tumours in male rats treated with HCS but not with LCS. In female rats, there were significant increases in the incidence of lung adenomas in animals treated with HCS and of all lung tumours in animals treated with both LCS and HCS. There was also a significant increase in the occurrence of nasal cavity tumours in female rats treated with HCS (Mauderly *et al.*, 2004).

3.1.3 Hamster

Four studies have evaluated the ability of mainstream tobacco smoke to induce tumours in hamsters (Table 3.1). Syrian golden hamsters were exposed to either a mixture of German reference cigarette smoke or of dark air-cured cigarette smoke for lifetime. There were increases in the incidence of laryngeal carcinomas in hamsters exposed to both smoke preparations (Dontenwill *et al.*, 1973). In a subsequent study, hamsters were exposed to a mixture of German reference cigarette smoke containing 1.5 mg nicotine, 0.173 mg phenol and 12.7 mL carbon monoxide/cigarette for lifetime. The incidence of laryngeal tumours in smoke-exposed hamsters was higher than in controls (Dontenwill *et al.*, 1977). BIO male hamsters exposed to a mixture of US reference smoke for 100 weeks developed laryngeal and nasopharyngeal tumours (Bernfeld *et al.*, 1974) In a subsequent study, male BIO hamsters exposed to smoke from commercial British filter cigarettes developed higher incidence of laryngeal tumours than controls (Bernfeld *et al.*, 1979).

3.2 Co-administration of tobacco smoke with known carcinogens and other agents

Study design and results of the studies on co-administration of tobacco smoke with known carcinogens and other agents are summarized in Table 3.2.

3.2.1 Rat

(a) Benzo[a]pyrene

Wistar rats received a single intratracheal instillation of 2 mg benzo[*a*]pyrene followed by lifetime exposure to cigarette smoke. This treatment led to a low incidence of lung tumours that was not significantly higher than in controls (Davis *et al.*, 1975). In another study Wistar rats were given intratracheal instillations of benzo[*a*]pyrene mixed with ferric oxide and exposed to cigarette smoke either during initiation and post-initiation or only after treatment with benzo[*a*]pyrene/ferric oxide (post-initiation). Inhalation of cigarette smoke during the initiation and post-initiation phases of carcinogenesis resulted in a higher lung tumour (squamous-cell carcinoma) multiplicity than that seen in rats exposed during the post-initiation phase only (Gupta *et al.*, 1990).

(b) Radon progeny

Sprague-Dawley rats were exposed to radon progeny at cumulative doses of 4000, 500 or 100 work-level-months (WLM), with or without concurrent exposure to cigarette smoke by inhalation for one year. Rats exposed to 4000 WLM radon progeny, without exposure to smoke, developed lung carcinomas (17/50). Thirty four carcinomas were seen in 50 rats exposed to radon and cigarette smoke. The 500 WLM radon progeny group exposed to radon only had 2/28 lung carcinomas as compared with 8/30 rats exposed to radon and cigarette smoke. No tumours were observed in rats treated with 100 WLM radon and one carcinoma was seen among 30 rats exposed to 100 WLM radon and cigarette smoke. Seventy five percent of the lung tumours were squamous-cell carcinomas, 20% were adenocarcinomas, and the remainder were undifferentiated carcinomas (Chameaud *et al.*, 1982).

Table 3.1 Carcinogenicity in response to mainstream tobacco smoke in animals

Species, strain (sex) Reference	Animals/group at start Dosing regimen Duration	Lung burden	Results Target organ Incidence and/or multiplicity of tumours (%)	Significance	Comments
Mice, C57BL (M, F) Harris & Negroni (1967)	100 animals/sex/group Nose-only, mixture of fresh non-filter cigarette smoke/air (1/39, v/v), nicotine, 0.1 mg/mL; CO, 0.064% (v/v), 12 min/every other d; lifetime	Nicotine, 14–17 µg	Alveologenic adenocarcinomas:		
			M–4/100 (alveologenic AdC) Controls–0/100	*P* = 0.06	
			F–4/100 (alveologenic AdC) Controls–0/100	*P* = 0.06	
Mice, C57BL and BLH (sex, NR) Otto & Elmenhorst (1967)	126 animals/group Whole-body, gas phase of 12 cigarettes puffed 2 sec/min, concentration (NR), 90 min/d; lifetime (~27 mo)	NR	Lung (adenomas):		
			C57BL–7/126 (5.5%) Controls–3/90 (3%)	NS	
			BLH–40/126 (32%) Controls–19/60 (32%)	NS	
Mice, (C57BL/Cum × C3H/Anf Cum)F_1 (F) Henry & Kouri (1986)	2053, 1 014 sham Nose-only, 10% smoke from US reference cigarettes, concentration (NR), smoke 20 sec/min, 6–8 min/d, 5 d/wk for 110 wk; 116 wk	Particulate deposition, 125–200 µg	Alveolar adenocarcinomas: 19/978 (2%) Sham-exposed controls–7/651 (1%)	*P* = 0.10	Shorter latency of tumour occurrence in smoke-exposed group suggested
Mice, C57BL (M, F) Harris *et al.* (1974)	100 animals/sex/group Nose-only, mixture of fresh flue-cured or air-cured cigarette smoke/air (1/39, v/v), concentration (NR), 12 min/d on alternate d; lifetime	NR	M: 9/162[a] (5%, flue-cured), 7/189[a] (4%, air-cured) Controls–3/160[a] (2%)	*P* = 0.07, flue-cured *P* > 0.05, air-cured	
			F: 7/164[a] (4%, flue-cured), 0/173 (air-cured) Controls–1/159[a] (1%)	*P* = 0.04, flue-cured	
	Nose-only, gas phase of flue-cured cigarette smoke, concentration (NR), 12 min/d on alternate d; lifetime	NR	M: 3/8[a] (37%) Controls–3/160[a] (2%)	*P* > 0.05	
			F: 2/88[a] (2%) Controls–1/159[a] (1%)	*P* > 0.05	

Table 3.1 (continued)

Species, strain (sex) Reference	Animals/group at start Dosing regimen Duration	Lung burden	Results Target organ Incidence and/or multiplicity of tumours (%)	Significance	Comments
Mice, Snell (M, F) Leuchtenberger & Leuchtenberger (1970)	160 M, 118 F Whole-body, whole fresh cigarette smoke, concentration (NR), 2 puffs, 1 × /d, lifetime (26 mo)	Nicotine, 5 µg	M:		
			Lung A–7/107 (6.5%) Controls–8/106 (7.5%)	NS	
			Lung AdC–11/107 (10%) Controls–5/106 (4.7%)	$P = 0.15$	
			F: Lung A–2/65 (3%) Controls–1/78 (1.2%)	$P = 0.475$	
			Lung AdC–5/65 (7.7%) Controls–3/78 (3.8%)	$P = 0.035$	
	100 M, 89 F Whole-body, gas phase of fresh cigarette smoke, concentration (NR), 2 puffs, 1 × /d, lifetime (26 mo)	NR	M: Lung A–1/44 (2%) Controls–8/106 (7%)	NS	
			Lung AdC–10/44 (23%) Controls–5/106 (5%)	$P = 0.005$	
			F: Lung A–3/44 (7%) Controls–1/78 (1%)	$P = 0.15$	
			Lung AdC–5/44 (11%) Controls–3/78 (4%)	$P = 0.15$	
Mice, B6C3F1 (F) Hutt *et al.* (2005)	330, 326 controls Whole-body, smoke from Kentucky 2R1 unfiltered reference cigarettes, 250 mg total particulate matter/m³, 6 h/d, 5 d/wk for 30 mo; 30 mo or lifetime	NR	Lung A: 93/330 (28%) Sham-exposed controls–22/326 (7%)	$P < 0.001$ $P < 0.007$	
			Bronchiolar papillomas: 15/330 (4%) Controls–0/326	$P < 0.001$	
			Lung AdC: 67/330 (20%) Controls–9/326	$P < 0.001$	
			All lung tumours: 148/330 (45%) Controls–31/326	$P < 0.001$[b]	
			Nasal cavity tumours: 20/330 (6%) Controls–0/326	$P = 0.002$, one-tailed Fisher	
			Squamous-cell carcinomas: 9/330 (3%) Controls–0/326		

Table 3.1 (continued)

Species, strain (sex) Reference	Animals/group at start Dosing regimen Duration	Lung burden	Results Target organ Incidence and/or multiplicity of tumours (%)	Significance	Comments
Mice, Swiss (M, F) Balansky *et al.* (2007)	38, 36 controls (neonatal mice, 21 h of age) Whole-body, cigarette smoke/air, 818 mg total particulate matter/m³, 65 min/d for 120 d	NR	Lung A: 15/38(19%) Sham-exposed controls–0/36	$P < 0.001$	
			Lung AdC: 7/38 (18%) Controls–0/38	$P < 0.01$	
			Kidney A: 6/16 (16%) (F only) Controls–0/21	$P < 0.01$	
			Liver carcinomas: 2/16 (5%) (F only) Controls–0/21		
Rats, Wistar (F) Davis *et al.* (1975)	408, 102 untreated, 102 sham Nose-only, mixture of cigarette smoke/air (1/5), concentration (NR), 15 sec/min, 2 × 11 min/d, 5 d/wk, lifetime	NR	4/408 (1%) (1 lung C and 3 lung neoplasms of uncertain malignancy) Controls–0/102 Sham treated controls–0/102	NS	
Rats, F344 (F) Dalbey *et al.* (1980)	80, 63 untreated, 30 sham Nose-only, mixture of non-filter cigarette smoke/air (1/10), 18.4 mg smoke particulate and 0.89 mg nicotine/cigarette, 1 cigarette/h, 7 cigarettes/d, 5 d/wk for 128 wk; 160 wk	Particulate deposition, 1.75 mg/d	10/80 (12%) (1 nasal AdC, 1 nasal C, 5 pulmonary A, 1 pulmonary C, 2 alveologenic C) Controls–3/93 (3%)	$P < 0.05$	
			Subcutaneous sarcomas at forelimb ulceration sites: 21/80 (26%) Controls–0/93	$P < 0.05$	
Rats, CDF* (F344)/CrlBR (M, F) Finch *et al.* (1995)	2165 animals Whole-body, cigarette smoke/air, 100 mg (LCS) or 250 mg (HCS) total particulate matter/m³, 6 h/d, 5 d/wk for 30 mo; lifetime	NR	Lung tumours: M: LCS 3/173 (2%) HCS 7/78 (9%) Filtered air 3/119 (2%)	$P < 0.05$	
			F: LCS–4/145 (3%) HCS–6/83 (7%) Filtered air–0/113	$P < 0.05$	

Table 3.1 (continued)

Species, strain (sex) Reference	Animals/group at start Dosing regimen Duration	Lung burden	Results Target organ Incidence and/or multiplicity of tumours (%)	Significance	Comments
Rats, F344 (M, F) Mauderly *et al.* (2004)	M: 178 LCS, 82 HCS F: 175 LCS, 81 HCS Whole-body, smoke from Kentucky 1R3 unfiltered reference cigarettes, 100 mg (LCS) or 250 mg (HCS) total particulate matter/m^3, 6 h/d, 5 d/wk for 30 mo; lifetime	NR	M: Lung A– LCS 4/178 (2%) HCS 2/82 (2%) Sham-exposed controls 1/118 (1%)	NS	
			Lung AdC– LCS 1/178 (1%) HCS 5/82 (6%) Controls 3/118 (3%)	NS	
			All lung tumours– LCS 4/178 (2%) HCS 7/82 (8%) Controls 4/118	NS; trend, $P = 0.055$	
			Nasal cavity (all tumour types)– LCS 1/178 (1%) HCS 5/82 (6%) Controls 1/118 (1%)	$P = 0.032$ (HCS); trend, $P = 0.010$	
			F: Lung A– LCS 7/175 (6%) HCS 7/81 (9%) Sham-exposed controls 0/119	NS (LCS); $P < 0.001$ (HCS)	
			AdC– LCS 4/175 (2%) HCS 4/81 (5%) Controls 0/119	NS	
			All lung tumours– LCS 10/175 (6%) HCS 11/81 (13%) Controls 0/119	$P = 0.023$ (LCS); $P = 0.001$ (HCS)	
			Nasal cavity (all tumour types)– LCS 0/175 HCS 3/81 Controls 0/119	$P = 0.020$ (HCS); trend, $P = 0.003$	

Table 3.1 (continued)

Species, strain (sex) Reference	Animals/group at start Dosing regimen Duration	Lung burden	Results Target organ Incidence and/or multiplicity of tumours (%)	Significance	Comments
Hamsters, Syrian golden (M, F) Dontenwill *et al.* (1973)	80 animals/sex/group Whole-body, mixture of German reference cigarette smoke/air (1/15), concentration (NR), smoke of 30 cigarettes for 7–10 min; 1, 2 or 3 × /d, 5 d/wk, lifetime	NR	Laryngeal carcinomas: 1/160 (1%), 17/160 (11%) and 11/160 (7%) Controls–0/80		
	Whole-body, mixture of dark air-cured cigarette smoke/air (1/15), concentration (NR), Smoke of 30 cigarettes for 7–10 min: twice/d, 5 d/wk, lifetime	NR	Laryngeal carcinomas: 2/160 (1%) Controls–0/80		
Hamsters, Syrian golden (M, F) Dontenwill *et al.* (1977)	80 animals/group Whole-body, mixture of German reference cigarette smoke/air (1/15), 1.5 mg nicotine, 0.173 mg phenol and 12.7 mL CO/cigarette, smoke of 30 cigarettes for 7–10 min; 1, 2 or 3 × /d, 5 d/wk, lifetime	NR	M: Laryngeal C–0, 4, 6 and 11%, Controls–0% F: Laryngeal C–0, 1, 2 and 7% Controls–0%		
Rats, Inbred BIO 15.16 & Inbred BIO 87.20 (M) Bernfeld *et al.* (1974)	102 animals/group Whole-body, mixture of US reference cigarette smoke/air (1/5), concentration (NR), duration (NR)		Inbred BIO 15.16: Laryngeal tumours–9/84 (10%) Nasopharyngeal tumours–2/84 (2%) Sham-exposed controls 0/42 Controls 0/40 Inbred BIO 87.20: Laryngeal tumours–2/87 (2%) Sham-exposed controls 0/44 Controls 0/48		
Rats, Inbred BIO 15.16 (M) Bernfeld *et al.* (1979)	Number at start (NR) Whole-body, 11 or 22% smoke from commercial British filter cigarettes, concentration (NR), 2 × 12 min/d, 7 d/wk for 35–42 wk; up to 74–80 wk	NR	Laryngeal carcinomas: 11% smoke–3/44 (7%) 22% smoke–27/57 (47%) Sham-exposed controls 0/36; Controls 0/50		

[a] Most of these lung tumours are adenomas

[b] Nasal cavity tumours included 14 squamous cell carcinomas (5 in situ), 5 hemangiomas, and 1 respiratory papilloma

A, adenoma; AdC, adenocarcinoma; C, carcinoma; CO, carbon monoxide; d, day or days; F, female; h, hour or hours; HCS, high cigarette smoke; LCS, low cigarette smoke; M, male; min, minute or minutes; mo, month or months; NR, not reported; NS, not significant; sec, second or seconds; wk, week or weeks; yr, year or years

Table 3.2 Carcinogenicity in response to exposure to mainstream tobacco smoke in conjunction with exposure to known carcinogens or other agents in animals

Species, strain (sex) Reference	Animals/group at start Dosing regimen Duration	Results Target organ Incidence and/or multiplicity of tumours (%)	Significance
Rats, Wistar (F) Davis *et al.* (1975)	84 or 408 animals/group A single intratracheal instillation of benzo[*a*] pyrene (2 mg) + infusine + carbon black followed by British reference cigarette smoke/air (1/5); 1 cigarette, twice/d, 5 d/wk, lifetime	3/84 (4%, lung C), 1/84 (1%, lung C; benzo[*a*]pyrene alone), 4/408 (1%, 3 A + 1 malignant neoplasm; cigarette smoke only), 0/204 (controls + sham-exposed controls)	NS
Rats, Wistar (M) Gupta *et al.* (1990)	35 animals/group Cigarette smoke; 5 cigarettes/8.2 L air; 1 h/d during 2nd–24th wk or 10th–24th wk of the study Benzo[*a*]pyrene (20 mg) + Fe_2O_3; intratracheally (3 weekly doses) during 6th–8th wk of the study; 24 wk	Conventional diet: 2nd–24th wk, 2.14 lung C/animal; 10th–24th wk, 1.33 lung C/animal; benzo[*a*]pyrene control, 1.22 lung C/animal. Vitamin A-deficient diet: 2nd–24th wk, 2.86 lung C/animal; 10th–24th wk, 1.67 lung C/animal; benzo[*a*] pyrene control, 1.83 lung C/animal	
Rats, Sprague-Dawley, sex NR) Chameaud *et al.* (1982)	28–50 animals/group French reference cigarette smoke (9 cigarettes/ 500 L air); 10–15 min session, 4 d/wk for 1 yr Radon progeny (4 000, 500 or 100 WLM) Lifetime	4000 WLM: 34/50 (68%, lung C); 17/50 (34%, lung C; radon progeny alone) 500 WLM: 8/30 (27%, lung C); 2/28 (7%, lung C; radon progeny alone) 100 WLM: 1/30 (3%, lung C); 0/50 (radon progeny alone)	$P = 0.0015$
CDF*(F344)/CrlBR (M, F) Finch *et al.* (1995)	Number at start (NR) Cigarette smoke/air, 100 mg (LCS) or 250 mg (HCS) total particulate matter/m^3; 6 h/d, 5 d/wk for 126 wk $^{239}PuO_2$ aerosol, 1 wk (6th wk of the study); > 52 wk	49–61% (lung tumours, LCS + $^{239}PuO_2$) 72–74% (HCS + $^{239}PuO_2$) 20–33% ($^{239}PuO_2$) 2–3% (LCS) 7–8% (HCS)	
Syrian golden (M, F) Dontenwill *et al.* (1973)	80 animals/sex/group German reference cigarette smoke/air (1/15); Smoke of 30 cigarettes for 7–10 min; twice/d, 5 d/wk, lifetime DMBA (0.5 mg); intratracheally 10 d before the beginning of smoke exposure	32/160 (20%, laryngeal C), 17/160 (11%, laryngeal C; smoke only), 0/160 (DMBA alone)	

Table 3.2 (continued)

Species, strain (sex) Reference	Animals/group at start Dosing regimen Duration	Results Target organ Incidence and/or multiplicity of tumours (%)	Significance
Syrian golden, (sex NR) Hoffmann *et al.* (1979)	20 or 40 animals/group Cigarette smoke/air (1/7); Cigarette smoke 2 × 10 min/d, 5 d/wk, 48 wk DMBA (0.24 mg); intralaryngeally	3/40 (7%, laryngeal C), 0/20 (smoke only), 0/20 (DMBA alone)	
Syrian golden (M) Takahashi *et al.* (1992)	10 or 30 animals/group Cigarette smoke/air (1/7); Smoke of 30 cigarettes for 9 min; twice/d, 5 d/wk, 12 wk NDEA (100 mg/kg bw); subcutaneously	Non-filter cigarettes (2.10 ± 1.74 P+H/animal) and filter cigarettes (1.93 ± 1.55 P + H/animal) versus sham-exposed (0.97 ± 1.03 P + H/animal)	*P* < 0.01 *P* < 0.01
Syrian golden (M) Harada *et al.* (1985)	30 animals/group Non-filter cigarette smoke/air (1/7); Smoke of 30 cigarettes for 6 min: twice/d, 5 d/wk, 58 wk NDEA (10 mg/hamster); subcutaneously (12 weekly doses)	Nasal cavity tumours 14/30 (47%, smoke + NDEA), 5/30 (17%, NDEA alone)	*P* < 0.05

A, adenoma; bw, body weight; C, carcinoma; d, day or days; DMBA, 7,12-dimethylbenz[*a*]anthracene; F, female; h, hour or hours; HCS, high cigarette smoke; LCS, low cigarette smoke; M, male; min, minute or minutes; mo, month or months; NDEA, *N*-nitrosodiethylamine; NR, not reported; NS, not significant; P + H, epithelial hyperplasias and papillomas; sec, second or seconds; wk, week or weeks; WLM, work-level-months; yr, year or years

(c) Plutonium oxide

CDF®/CrlBR rats were exposed to either filtered air or mainstream cigarette smoke at concentrations of either 100 or 250 mg total particulate matter/m^3 (LCS and HCS groups, respectively). At 12 weeks, rats were removed from smoke chambers and exposed nose-only to plutonium oxide ($^{239}PuO_2$) then returned to the smoke chambers one week later for 30 months of continuous exposure to either filtered air or cigarette smoke. The incidence and multiplicity of lung tumours (adenocarcinomas, squamous-cell carcinomas, adenosquamous carcinomas) in animals exposed to both concentrations of cigarette smoke and $^{239}PuO_2$ were higher than those in animals exposed to $^{239}PuO_2$, LCS or HCS alone (Finch *et al.*, 1995).

3.2.2 Hamster

(a) 7,12-Dimethylbenz[a]anthracene

Groups of 160 Syrian golden hamsters received 7,12-dimethylbenz[*a*]anthracene (DMBA) intratracheally, followed by cigarette smoke for life, or treated with cigarette smoke or DMBA only. A total of 32 squamous-cell carcinomas of the larynx were observed in animals treated with both DMBA and cigarette smoke, in comparison with 17 in hamsters exposed to cigarette smoke only and none in hamsters treated with DMBA alone (Dontenwill *et al.*, 1973). Similar results were reported from other experiments in which Syrian golden hamsters were exposed to DMBA and cigarette smoke (Hoffmann *et al.*, 1979).

(b) N-Nitrosodiethylamine

Groups of hamsters received a single subcutaneous injection of *N*-nitrosodiethylamine (NDEA) and then were exposed to smoke from unfiltered cigarettes, filtered cigarettes and sham smoke. Controls were exposed to either unfiltered cigarette smoke, filtered cigarette smoke or sham smoke. In the NDEA-smoke-treated groups, epithelial hyperplasias and/or papillomas of the larynx were induced at higher frequency than in controls (Takahashi *et al.*, 1992). Hamsters exposed to cigarette smoke in air also received 12 weekly subcutaneous injections of NDEA (total dose, 10 mg/hamster). Treatment with NDEA only resulted in both benign and malignant tumours of the respiratory tract, and co-exposure to cigarette smoke potentiated the development of tumours in the nasal cavity (Harada *et al.*, 1985).

3.3 Smoke condensates

Study design and results of the studies on administration of tobacco smoke condensates are summarized in Table 3.3.

3.3.1 Skin application

(a) Mouse

Cigarette-smoke condensate produces both benign and malignant tumours on mouse skin. The carcinogenic potency of the cigarette-smoke condensate depends upon tobacco variety, composition of cigarette paper and the presence of additives (Wynder *et al.*, 1957; Gargus *et al.*, 1976; Gori, 1976).

(b) Rabbit

Cigarette-smoke condensate induced skin papillomas and carcinomas when applied to the ears of rabbits for lifetime (Graham *et al.*, 1957).

3.3.2 Intrapulmonary administration

Injection of 24 mg cigarette-smoke condensate into the lungs of female Osborne Mendel rats led to the development of squamous cell carcinomas (Stanton *et al.*, 1972). These observations were confirmed by Dagle *et al.* (1978) who observed a dose-dependent incidence of lung carcinomas when cigarette-smoke condensate prepared from two types of cigarettes were given.

Table 3.3 Carcinogenicity in response to exposure to cigarette-smoke condensate in animals

Species, strain (sex) Reference	Animals/group at start Dosing regimen Duration	Results Target organ Incidence and/or multiplicity of tumours (%)	Significance
Mice CAF1 (M, F) Wynder *et al.* (1953)	112, 44 controls Skin painting (dorsal) of CSC, CSC/acetone solution (40 mg CSC/ application), 3 × /wk, lifetime	36/81 (44%, skin epidermoid C), 0/30 (acetone controls)	
Mice ICR Swiss (F) Gargus *et al.* (1976)	5200 Skin painting (dorsal) of CSC, CSC/acetone solution (150 mg or 300 mg CSC/wk), 6 × /wk, 78 wk	482/5200 (9%, skin C), 3/800 (0.4%, acetone controls)[a]	
Mice ICR Swiss (F) Gori (1976)	4900 Skin painting (dorsal) of CSC, CSC/acetone solution (25 mg or 50 mg CSC/application), 6 × /wk, 78 wk	1157/4900 (24%, skin C), 0/800 (acetone controls)	
Mice, ICR/Ha Swiss (F) Hoffmann & Wynder (1971)	30 animals/group Skin painting (dorsal) with CSC active fraction with or without subsequent painting of the skin with croton oil, CSC active fraction/acetone (2.5 mg of 0.6% CSC/application), 10 times on alternate d Croton oil (2.5%), 3 × /wk, up to 12 mo, 10 d after last CSC active fraction application; 15 mo	After 12 and 15 mo: 4/30 (13%, skin C), 0/65 (croton oil controls)	
Mice, Swiss (F) Wynder & Hoffmann (1961)	30–50 animals/group Skin painting (dorsal) of CSC with or without initiation by DMBA application; DMBA (75 µg); CSC/acetone (75 mg CSC/application, start: 1 wk after DMBA application), 2–3 × /wk, 12 mo; 15 mo	DMBA: 2/30 (7%, skin C) 2 × CSC: 1/40 (3%, skin C) DMBA + 2 × CSC: 8/30 (27%, skin C) 3 × CSC: 11/50 (22%, skin C) DMBA + 3 × CSC: 11/30 (37%, skin C)	
Mice, SENCAR (F) Meckley *et al.* (2004a)	40 animals/group Skin painting (dorsal) of CSC from Kentucky 1R4F reference cigarettes, with or without initiation by DMBA application; DMBA (75 µg) or acetone, 1x. Then starting 1 wk after DMBA or acetone: CSC in acetone, 0, 10, 20 or 40 mg/application, 3 × /wk, 29 wk; 31 wk	Mean mice with tumours/mice per group at 31 wk[c]: No DMBA: 0/40 acetone-acetone, 9/40 (22%) acetone-CSC 40 mg/treatment DMBA/CSC: 0/40, 3/40 (1.0), 16/40 (75 tumours/16 mice = 4.7), 32/40 (200 tumours/32 mice = 6.3)	
Mice, SENCAR (F) Meckley *et al.* (2004b)	40 animals/group Skin painting (dorsal) of CSC from Kentucky 1R4F reference cigarettes or ECLIPSE (non-burned) cigarettes, with or without initiation by DMBA application; DMBA (75 µg) or acetone, 1 × . Then starting 1 wk after DMBA or acetone: CSC in acetone, 0, 10, 20 or 40 mg/application, 3 × /wk, 29 wk; 31 wk	No DMBA: acetone/acetone 0/40 (0); acetone/1R4F CSC 40 mg, 9/40 (1.8); acetone/ECLIPSE CSC 40 mg, 0/40 (0) DMBA/CSC: acetone, 0/40 (0); 1R4F CSC 10 mg, 6/40 (1.8); 1R4F CSC 12 mg, 28/40 (6.6); 1R4F CSC 40 mg, 36/40 (6.8); ECLIPSE CSC, 0/40 (0); ECLIPSE CSC 10 mg, 1/40 (1); ECLIPSE CSC 20 mg, 2/40 (5.5); ECLIPSE CSC 40 mg, 12/40 (2.6)	

Table 3.3 (continued)

Species, strain (sex) Reference	Animals/group at start Dosing regimen Duration	Results Target organ Incidence and/or multiplicity of tumours (%)	Significance
Mice, SENCAR (F) Hayes *et al.* (2007)	40 or 50 animals/group Skin painting (dorsal) of CSC from heat-exchanged flue cured tobacco (HE; low TSNA) or direct-fire (DF) cured tobacco, with or without initiation by DMBA application; DMBA (75 µg) or acetone, 1 ×. Then starting 1 wk after DMBA or acetone: CSC/acetone, 0, 9, 18, or 36 mg/application, 3 × /wk, 29 wk; 31 wk	No DMBA: acetone/acetone 0/40; acetone/DF CSC 36 mg, 5/50 (1.4); acetone/HE CSC 36 mg, 8/50 (1.3) DMBA/CSC: DF CSC, 0/40, DF CSC 9 mg, 15/40 (5.5); DF CSC 18 mg, 30/40 (10.0); DF CSC 36 mg, 43/50 (8.2); HE CSC, 0/40, HE CSC 9 mg, 17/40 (4.8); HE CSC 18 mg, 32/40 (7.3); HE CSC 36 mg, 42/50 (8.5)	 $P < 0.05$ $P < 0.05$ $P < 0.05$
Mice, Swiss albino (M) Pakhale *et al.* (1988)	20 animals/group Oral gavage of Indian bidi smoke condensate; 1 mg bidi smoke condensate/0.1 mg DMSO, 5 d/wk, 55 wk; 90 wk	4/15 (27%, hepatic haemangiomas); 1/15 (7%, stomach papilloma); 1/15 (7%, stomach carcinoma); 1/15 (7%, oesophageal carcinoma); 0/15 (untreated or DMSO-treated controls)	
Rats, Osborne Mendel (F) Stanton *et al.* (1972)	Number/group at start (NR) Intrapulmonary administration of CSC pellet; CSC/beeswax:tricaprylin (24 mg CSC/injection), up to 107 wk after implantation	14/40[c] (35%, lung squamous-cell C), 0/63[c] (beeswax:tricaprylin controls)	
Rats, OM/NCR (F) Dagle *et al.* (1978)	120[d] Intrapulmonary administration of CSC pellet; CSC/beeswax:tricaprylin (5, 10, 20 or 67 mg CSC/injection), 120 wk after implantation	4, 10, 20 and 42% pulmonary C prevalence; 0% C prevalence for 3 control groups of about 190 rats each	
Rabbits, Albino New Zealand (M, F) Graham *et al.* (1957)	38, 7 controls Skin painting of CSC (both ears); CSC/acetone solution (100 mg CSC/application/ear), 5 × /wk, lifetime (4–6 yr)	4/38 (11%, 2 skin C + 1 skin liposarcoma + 1 skin fibrosarcoma), 0/7 (acetone controls)	

[a] Skin papillomas
[b] Mostly adenomas
[c] Incidence in animals that died 43–107 weeks after injection
[d] 4 × 10 rats/group terminated before 120 weeks
[e] Total visually identified and histologically confirmed skin tumours included mostly squamous papillomas and carcinomas [Tumour incidences and multiplicities estimated from graphs]
C, carcinoma; CSC, cigarette-smoke condensate; d, day or days; DMBA, 7,12-dimethylbenz[*a*]anthracene; DMSO, dimethyl sulfoxide; F, female; M, male; NR, not reported; TSNA, tobacco-specific *N*-nitrosamines; wk, week or weeks

3.3.3 Initiation-promotion skin painting studies

Cigarette-smoke condensate and its fractions can act as skin co-carcinogens in Swiss and SENCAR mice when tested in conjunction with croton oil (Hoffmann & Wynder, 1971) or DMBA (Wynder & Hoffmann, 1961; Meckley *et al.*, 2004a, b; Hayes *et al.*, 2007).

3.3.4 Bidi smoke

Swiss albino mice administered 1 mg bidi smoke condensate in dimethyl sulfoxide (DMSO) by oral gavage developed haemangiomas (4/15), stomach carcinoma (1/15), and esophageal carcinoma (1/15), whereas no tumours were observed in controls (Pakhale *et al.*, 1988).

3.4 Synthesis

Mainstream tobacco smoke induced lung tumours in mice, lung and nasal cavity tumours in rats and laryngeal carcinomas in hamsters.

Co-administration of tobacco smoke with benzo[*a*]pyrene, radon progeny and plutonium resulted in higher lung tumour responses in rats than administration of either agent alone. Hamsters exposed to cigarette smoke and either DMBA or NDEA had higher lung tumour responses compared to cigarette smoke, DMBA or NDEA alone.

Topical application of cigarette-smoke condensate led to the development of skin tumours in mice and rabbits; intrapulmonary administration of cigarette-smoke condensate induced squamous cell carcinomas in rat lung.

4. Other Relevant Data

4.1 Overview of the mechanistic evidence for the carcinogenicity of tobacco

4.1.1 Conceptual model of the carcinogenesis of tobacco and tobacco smoke

A conceptual model for understanding mechanisms by which tobacco smoke causes cancer is shown in Fig. 4.1 (Hecht, 1999, 2003). This model also applies to smokeless tobacco and other forms of smoked tobacco and, in theory, to second-hand tobacco smoke since it contains all of the same carcinogens and toxicants as mainstream cigarette smoke, although at lower doses.

The major accepted mechanistic pathway is summarized in the central track of Fig. 4.1. Smokers inhale carcinogens which, either directly or after metabolism, covalently bind to DNA, forming DNA adducts. DNA adducts are central to chemical carcinogenesis because they can cause miscoding and permanent mutations. If these mutations occur in critical regions of oncogenes and tumour suppressor genes, which are essential in growth control, the result can be loss of normal cellular proliferation mechanisms, genomic instability, and cancer. A study that sequenced 623 cancer-related genes in 188 human lung adenocarcinomas validated this premise by finding multiple somatic mutations in critical growth control genes, consistent with the chronic bombardment of cellular DNA by tobacco smoke carcinogens and their metabolically activated forms (Ding *et al.*, 2008).

Each step of this conceptual model is considered in detail below.

Most people begin smoking cigarettes when they are teenagers, and become addicted to nicotine. Nicotine is not generally considered to be a carcinogen (Schuller, 2009), but it is accompanied in each puff of each cigarette by a complex

Fig. 4.1 Conceptual model for understanding mechanisms of tobacco carcinogenesis

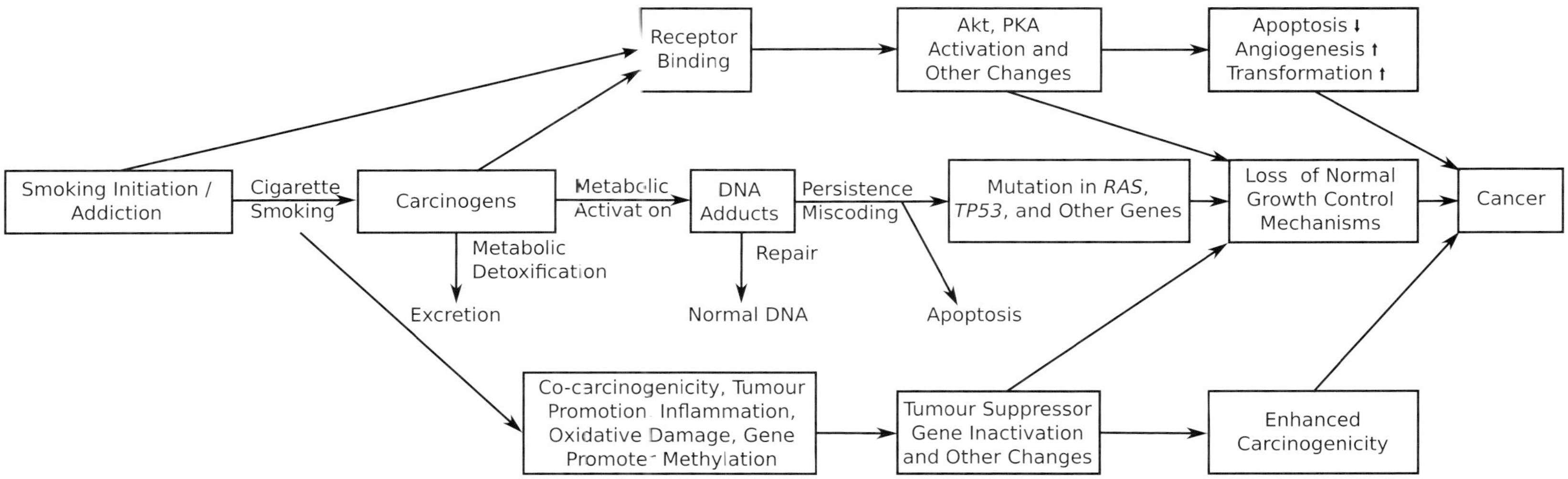

Smoking Initiation / Addiction
Cigarette Smoking
Carcinogens
Receptor Binding
Akt, PKA Activation and Other Changes
Apoptosis ↓ Angiogenesis ↑ Transformation ↑
Metabolic Activation
Metabolic Detoxification
Excretion
DNA Adducts
Repair
Normal DNA
Persistence Miscoding
Apoptosis
Mutation in *RAS*, *TP53*, and Other Genes
Loss of Normal Growth Control Mechanisms
Cancer
Co-carcinogenicity, Tumour Promotion, Inflammation, Oxidative Damage, Gene Promoter Methylation
Tumour Suppressor Gene Inactivation and Other Changes
Enhanced Carcinogenicity

There may be overlap between these three tracks: e.g. mutation in *TP53* leading to tumour suppressor gene inactivation.

mixture of carcinogens and toxicants. There are over 60 carcinogens in cigarette smoke that have been evaluated in the previous *IARC Monograph* as having *sufficient evidence* for carcinogenicity in laboratory animals (IARC, 2004a), sixteen of which are considered to be *carcinogenic to humans (Group 1)*. There are also many other carcinogens and potential carcinogens in cigarette smoke that have not been evaluated (Rodgman & Perfetti, 2006; see Section 1.1). Structures of tobacco smoke constituents and biomarkers discussed here are presented in Fig. 4.2.

Numerous studies demonstrate the uptake of tobacco smoke carcinogens and toxicants by smokers, and showed higher levels of their metabolites in urine and blood of smokers than non-smokers (Sections 4.1.1 and 4.1.2). There are substantial differences in carcinogen exposure among people because of the number and types of cigarettes they smoke and the ways in which they smoke them. These differences can be monitored in part by biomarkers of exposure such as urinary metabolites or haemoglobin adducts (Section 4.1.2). Haemoglobin adducts of multiple aromatic amines and volatile carcinogens have been demonstrably related to tobacco (Hatsukami *et al.*, 2006a). There may also be differences in carcinogen exposure due to genetic variations (Section 4.2).

The body's response to cigarette smoke constituents is similar to its response to pharmaceutical agents and other foreign compounds. Drug metabolizing enzymes, most frequently CYPs, convert these compounds to more water soluble forms, facilitating excretion. During this natural protective attempt, some reactive intermediates are formed. These intermediates are frequently electrophilic (electron seeking, or bearing a partial or full positive charge). Electrophilic intermediates may react with water, generally resulting in detoxification, or may covalently bind to nucleophilic (electron rich) sites in DNA, forming DNA adducts (Guengerich, 2001; Jalas *et al.*, 2005), which are critical in the carcinogenic process (see Section 4.1.3c). CYP1A1 and CYP1B1, repeatedly shown to be inducible by cigarette smoke via interactions of smoke compounds with the aryl hydrocarbon receptor (AhR), are particularly important in the metabolic activation of PAHs, while CYP2A13 is critical for the metabolism of NNK (Nebert *et al.*, 2004; Jalas *et al.*, 2005). The inducibility of certain CYPs may be a critical aspect of cancer susceptibility in smokers (Nebert *et al.*, 2004). CYP1A2, CYP2A6, CYP2E1 and CYP3A4 are also important in the metabolism of cigarette smoke carcinogens to DNA binding intermediates (Jalas *et al.*, 2005), and aldo-keto reductase enzymes, also induced by tobacco smoke (Quinn *et al.*, 2008), are involved in the metabolism of NNK, BaP and other tobacco smoke carcinogens. Competing with this process of "metabolic activation" resulting in DNA binding is the intended metabolic detoxification, which leads to harmless excretion of carcinogen metabolites, and is also catalysed by CYPs and a variety of other enzymes including GSTs, uridine diphosphate-glucuronosyl transferases (UGTs), and arylsulfatases. The relative amounts of carcinogen metabolic activation and detoxification differ among individuals. It is widely hypothesized that this balance will affect cancer risk with those having higher activation and lower detoxification capacity being the most susceptible. This premise is supported in part by molecular epidemiologic studies of polymorphisms, or variants in more than 1% of the population, in certain genes coding for these enzymes (Vineis *et al.*, 2003; Carlsten *et al.*, 2008).

DNA adducts are thought to be a critical lesion in carcinogenesis. Many investigations demonstrate the presence of DNA adducts in human tissues, and some of these are summarized in Section 4.1.2c. There is massive evidence, particularly from studies which use relatively non-specific DNA adduct measurement methods, that DNA adduct levels in the lung and other tissues of smokers are higher than in non-smokers, and some epidemiologic data link

Fig. 4.2 Structures of compounds discussed in the text

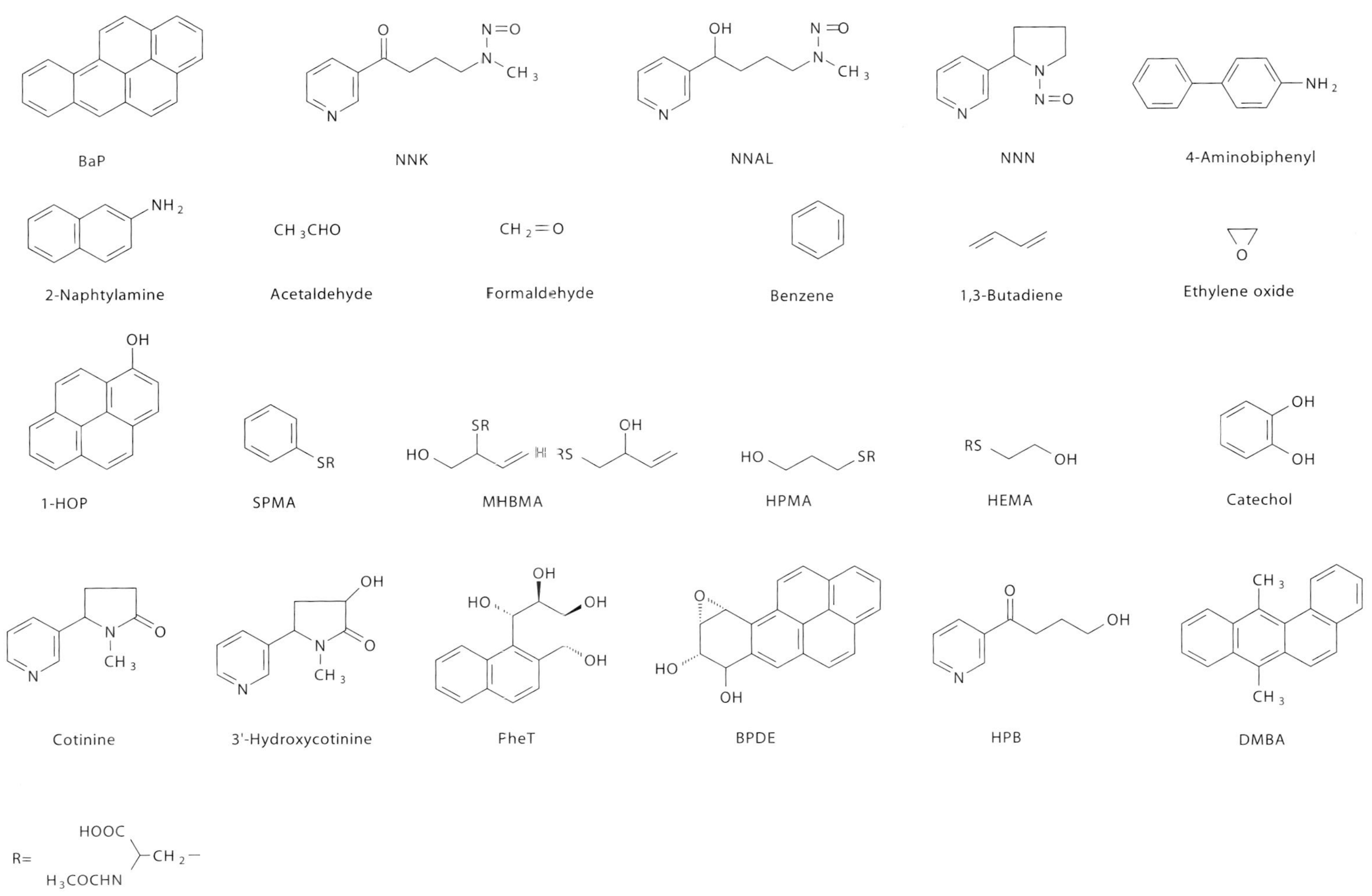

BaP
NNK
NNAL
NNN
4-Aminobiphenyl

2-Naphtylamine
CH_3CHO Acetaldehyde
$CH_2=O$ Formaldehyde
Benzene
1,3-Butadiene
Ethylene oxide

1-HOP
SPMA
MHBMA
HPMA
HEMA
Catechol

Cotinine
3'-Hydroxycotinine
PheT
BPDE
HPB
DMBA

R= $HOOC(H_3COCHN)CH-CH_2-$

BaP, Benzo[*a*]pyrene; BPDE, Benzo[*a*]pyrene diol epoxyde; DMBA, dimethylbenz[*a*]anthracene; 1-HOP, 1-hydroxypyrene; HEMA, 2-hydroxyethyl-mercapturic acid; HPMA, 3-hydroxypropyl-mercapturic acid; HPB, 4-hydroxy-1-(3-pyridyl)-1-butanone; HPMA, 3-hydroxypropyl-mercapturic acid; MHBMA, monohydroxybutyl-mercapturic acid; NNAL, 4-(methylnitrosamino)-1-(3-pyridyl)-1-butanol; NNK, 4-(methylnitrosamino)-1-(3-pyridyl)-1-butanone; NNN, *N'*-nitrosonornicotine; PheT, phenanthrenetetrol; SPMA, S-phenyl-mercapturic acid these higher adduct levels to increased cancer risk (IARC, 2004b; Veglia *et al.*, 2008). However, there is much more limited evidence from studies using specific carcinogen-derived DNA adducts as biomarkers (Pfeifer *et al.*, 2002). Oxidative DNA damage has also been observed, and this may result partially from exposure to metals in cigarette smoke (Stavrides, 2006).

Cellular DNA repair systems can excise DNA adducts and restore normal DNA structure (Christmann *et al.*, 2003). These complex multiple systems include direct base repair by alkyltransferases, removal of DNA damage by base and nucleotide excision repair, mismatch repair, and double strand repair. If these DNA repair systems are unsuccessful in fixing the damage, then the DNA adducts can persist, increasing the probability of a permanent mutation. There are polymorphisms in genes coding for some DNA repair enzymes. If these variants lead to deficient DNA repair, the probability of cancer development can increase (Vineis *et al.*, 2009).

DNA adducts can cause miscoding during replication when DNA polymerase enzymes misread the DNA adduct and consequently insert the wrong base opposite to it. There is some specificity in the relationship between specific DNA adducts formed from cigarette smoke carcinogens and the types of mutations which they cause. G to T and G to A mutations have often been observed (Section 4.1.3) (Hecht, 1999). Extensive studies have characterized the mutations which occur because of specific carcinogen-DNA adducts (Delaney & Essigmann, 2008). Mutations have been reported in the *KRAS* oncogene in lung cancer and in the *TP53* tumour suppressor gene in a variety of cigarette smoke-induced cancers (Ahrendt *et al.*, 2001; Pfeifer *et al.*, 2002; Ding *et al.*, 2008). The cancer causing role of these genes has been firmly established in animal studies (Lubet *et al.*, 2000; Johnson *et al.*, 2001). A selection and promotion process may also play a role in the final mutation spectrum seen in genes in smoking-associated tumours (Rodin & Rodin, 2005; Sudo *et al.*, 2008).

Urinary mutagenicity, sister chromatid exchanges, micronuclei in buccal cells, and other genetic effects have been consistently observed in smokers at higher levels than in non-smokers (IARC, 2004a; Proia *et al.*, 2006). In addition to mutations, numerous cytogenetic changes are observed in lung cancer, and chromosome damage throughout the field of the aerodigestive tract is strongly associated with cigarette smoke exposure. Mutations resulting from DNA adducts can cause loss of normal cellular growth control functions, via a complex process of signal transduction pathways, ultimately resulting in genomic instability, cellular proliferation and cancer (Ding *et al.*, 2008). Apoptosis, or programmed cell death, is a protective process, and can remove cells which have DNA damage, thus serving as a counterbalance to these mutational events. The balance between apoptotic mechanisms and those suppressing apoptosis will have a major impact on tumour growth.

While the central track of Fig. 4.1 is the major pathway by which tobacco smoke carcinogens cause cancer, other mechanisms also contribute, as indicated in the top and bottom tracks (Hecht, 2003). Nicotine, NNK, and NNN bind to nicotinic and other cellular receptors, resulting in activation of serine/threonine kinase Akt (also known as protein kinase B), protein kinase A, and other changes. Nicotine and NNK increase expression of survivin, an inhibitor of apoptosis in normal human bronchial epithelial cells, and survivin mRNA is detected in bronchial brush samples from heavy smokers (Jin *et al.*, 2008). This can cause decreased apoptosis, increased angiogenesis, and increased transformation (Heeschen *et al.*, 2001; West *et al.*, 2003). Thus, although nicotine is not carcinogenic, it may enhance carcinogenicity in various ways (Schuller, 2009). Cigarette smoke also contains well established oxidants, co-carcinogens, tumour promoting fractions, and inflammatory agents, as well as cilia-toxic compounds such as acrolein, which impede clearance. Many studies demonstrate the co-carcinogenic and cytotoxic effects of catechol, an important constituent of cigarette smoke. An epigenetic pathway frequently observed in tobacco-induced cancers is enzymatic methylation of promoter regions of genes such as *p16* and *FHIT* [fragile histidine triad gene, a gene coding for a dinucleoside 5′, 5‴- P[1], P[3]-triphosphate hydrolase, a putative tumour suppressor protein] resulting in gene silencing, which are also strongly implicated in tobacco-induced lung cancer (D'Agostini *et al.*, 2006; Bhutani *et al.*, 2008). When this occurs in tumour suppressor genes, the result can be unregulated proliferation (Belinsky, 2005). Inflammation due to smoking is associated with tumour promotion and activation of factors such as NFκB. Inflammation also plays a role in chronic obstructive pulmonary disease (COPD), which in turn is an independent risk factor for lung cancer (Smith *et al.*, 2006; Turner *et al.*, 2007; Lee *et al.*, 2008a).

This conceptual model can be applied to smokeless tobacco products. Smokeless tobacco products have much lower levels of carcinogens and toxicants that result from combustion, so the effects of these agents are not seen to a significant extent. The most prevalent strong carcinogens in smokeless tobacco are the tobacco-specific nitrosamines; other nitrosamines, PAHs, aldehydes and metals are also present, and there are large amounts of some inorganic salts that may contribute to inflammation (IARC, 2007a; Stepanov *et al.*, 2008). An additional factor in carcinogenesis by betel quid with tobacco is the basic pH resulting from addition of slaked lime to the quid, leading to oxidative damage and inflammation (IARC, 2004b).

Multiple studies demonstrate that tobacco-specific nitrosamines are absorbed and metabolised in smokeless tobacco users (IARC, 2007a).

There is evidence for DNA adduct formation in oral tissues of smokeless tobacco users, and sister chromatid exchanges, chromosomal aberrations, and micronuclei – consequences of DNA adduct formation – have been reported (Proia *et al.*, 2006; Warnakulasuriya & Ralhan, 2007). Many studies have demonstrated *RAS* and *TP53* mutations in smokeless tobacco users (Warnakulasuriya & Ralhan, 2007) consistent with the conceptual framework.

Oxidative stress and reactive oxygen species could play a significant role in cancer induction in smokeless tobacco users, particularly at high pH (Boffetta *et al.*, 2008). Chronic local inflammation and irritation induced by smokeless tobacco and its constituents could have a tumour promoting or co-carcinogenic effect (Boffetta *et al.*, 2008). Upregulation of cyclooxygenase-2, involved in prostaglandin synthesis and inflammation, has been observed in animal studies upon exposure to smokeless tobacco (Boffetta *et al.*, 2008). Smokeless tobacco products have relatively high levels of sodium chloride (NaCl), which could contribute to inflammation, tumour promotion, and co-carcinogenesis. Cancer of the oral cavity is strongly associated with tobacco smoking (IARC, 2004a) or chewing (IARC, 2007a) and alcoholic beverage drinking (IARC, 2010a) However only a fraction of exposed subjects develop tumours, which suggests that other exposures such as HPV may be independently involved or act as cofactors. HPV is known to infect the oral cavity of healthy individuals and several HPV-related lesions have been characterized (IARC, 2007b). Herpes simplex virus has also been shown to enhance the carcinogenicity of smokeless tobacco products in animal studies (Park *et al.*, 1986). These factors may contribute significantly to the local carcinogenic effects characteristic of smokeless tobacco use.

4.1.2 Absorption, distribution, metabolism and excretion

There are examples of toxicant and carcinogen metabolism and excretion for representatives of virtually every major class of compounds;

some of these are summarized in Table 4.1. Nicotine and five of its urinary metabolites – cotinine, 3′-hydroxycotinine and their glucuronides, and nicotine glucuronide – comprise about 73–96% of the nicotine dose (Hukkanen *et al.*, 2005), and are found in blood, sweat, hair and toenails (Al Delaimy, 2002; Hukkanen *et al.*, 2005; Stepanov *et al.*, 2007; Al Delaimy & Willett, 2008). Metabolites of various polycyclic aromatic hydrocarbons including pyrene, phenanthrene, fluorene, and benzo[*a*]pyrene have been quantified in human urine and are higher in smokers than in non-smokers (Hecht, 2002; Hecht *et al.*, 2005a; Jacob *et al.*, 2007; Hansen *et al.*, 2008). Metabolites of tobacco-specific nitrosamines – NNAL and its glucuronides (total NNAL) from NNK; and NNN and its glucuronides (total NNN) from NNN – are present in human urine (Hecht, 2002; Stepanov & Hecht, 2005; Hecht *et al.*, 2008a; Stepanov *et al.*, 2008). Total NNAL has also been quantified in blood and toenails (Hecht *et al.*, 2002; Stepanov *et al.*, 2007). Aromatic amine-haemoglobin adducts have been frequently measured in human blood, and their levels increase with smoking (Hecht, 2002; Hatsukami *et al.*, 2006a). Mercapturic acids of several tobacco smoke compounds such as benzene, 1,3-butadiene, acrolein, and ethylene oxide are present in human urine and are related to smoking (Carmella *et al.*, 2009). Haemoglobin adducts of acrylonitrile and related compounds are elevated in smokers' blood, and levels of metals such as Cd are increased in smokers' urine (Carmella *et al.*, 2002; IARC, 2004b).

All of the metabolites listed in Table 4.1 are elevated in cigarette smokers; in studies of second-hand smoke exposure, only nicotine metabolites and urinary total NNAL are consistently increased in exposed versus non-exposed subjects, although one very large study also observed an increase in PAH metabolites (Pirkle *et al.*, 2006; Hecht, 2008; Suwan-ampai *et al.*, 2009). Smokeless tobacco users have significantly raised levels of nicotine metabolites and tobacco-specific nitrosamine metabolites compared to non-tobacco users (Hecht *et al.*, 2007).

4.1.3 Biomarkers

Tobacco carcinogen biomarkers are quantifiable entities that can be *specifically* related to tobacco carcinogens. Specificity to a given carcinogen is critical because tobacco carcinogens vary widely in their potency and target organs.

Considering the mechanistic framework outlined in Fig. 4.1, one could visualize various types of biomarkers. Currently, biomarkers of carcinogen/toxicant dose, reflecting the second box of the central track of Fig. 4.1, are by far the most extensively used and validated. The second most common are measurements of DNA adducts (or protein adducts as their surrogates), but fewer of these have both practical utility and validation with respect to tobacco carcinogen specificity.

The use of tobacco carcinogen biomarkers bypasses many uncertainties in estimation of dose. The most commonly used estimation of dose is self-reported number of cigarettes/day, but this is not a very good marker. It may not be reported accurately and it provides no information on the way in which the cigarettes were smoked, which is critical when one considers the common phenomenon of smoker's compensation. Brand information together with machine smoking measurements of specific components is another way of obtaining a measure of dose. However, machine smoking measurements are known to have limitations and the application of a given machine smoking protocol to a given smoker requires smoking topography measurements for that smoker. A disadvantage of tobacco carcinogen biomarkers is that they are affected to some extent by individual differences in metabolism, which may complicate interpretation of dose.

Table 4.1 Examples of toxicant or carcinogen metabolites in tobacco users

Toxicant or carcinogen	Examples of metabolites in tobacco users	References
Nicotine	Cotinine, 3′-hydroxycotinine and their glucuronides in urine, blood or saliva; nicotine and cotinine in toenails	Al Delaimy (2002), Hukkanen *et al.* (2005), Al Delaimy & Willett (2008), Stepanov *et al.* (2007)
Polycyclic Aromatic Hydrocarbons (PAHs)	1-hydroxypyrene, phenanthrols, phenanthrene tetraols, fluorenols, benzo[*a*]pyrenols, benzo[*a*]pyrene tetraols in urine	Hecht (2002), Hecht *et al.* (2005a), Hansen *et al.* (2008), Jacob *et al.* (2007)
Tobacco-specific nitrosamines	NNAL and its glucuronides (total NNAL) in urine or blood, total NNN in urine; NNAL and NNN in toenails	Hecht (2002), Hecht *et al.* (2002, 2008a), Stepanov & Hecht (2005), Stepanov *et al.*, (2007, 2008)
Aromatic amines	Parent amines in urine and haemoglobin adducts in blood	Hecht (2002), Hatsukami *et al.* (2006a)
Volatile hydrocarbons		
Benzene 1,3-Butadiene	Muconic acid and S-phenyl-mercapturic acid (SPMA) in urine; Monohydroxybutyl-mercapturic acid (MHBMA) in urine	Hecht (2002), Carmella *et al.* (2009)
Acrolein	3-hydroxypropyl-mercapturic acid (HPMA) in urine	Carmella *et al.* (2009)
Ethylene oxide	2-hydroxyethyl-mercapturic acid (HEMA) in urine, haemoglobin adducts in blood	Bono *et al.* (2002), Carmella *et al.* (2009)
Acrylonitrile	Haemoglobin adducts in blood	Carmella *et al.* (2002)
Metals	Cadmium in urine	IARC (2004a)

(a) Urinary biomarkers

Probably the most practical and, to date, the most extensively applied tobacco carcinogen biomarkers are urinary metabolites of tobacco carcinogens, and these have been comprehensively reviewed (Hecht, 2002; IARC, 2004a). Advantages include the ready availability of samples, and concentrations in urine that are easily quantifiable using modern analytical chemistry methods, most frequently liquid chromatography-tandem mass spectrometry (LC-MS/MS). The urinary metabolites listed in Table 4.1 have all been used as biomarkers and all are validated with respect to exposure in cigarette smokers (Carmella *et al.*, 2009). Total nicotine equivalents (the sum of nicotine and the five metabolites in Table 4.1) is a particularly effective way of estimating nicotine dose from tobacco products.

Total NNAL, the sum of NNAL and its glucuronides, is a highly useful biomarker of NNK exposure (Hecht, 2002, 2003; Hatsukami *et al.*, 2006a). The tobacco-specificity of NNK, and therefore total NNAL, is a key feature of this biomarker because studies in which it is applied are not confounded by other environmental or dietary exposures. It also has a considerably longer half-life than cotinine and several other urinary biomarkers. Total NNAL has been used in numerous studies that estimated uptake of NNK in smokers under varying circumstances. In one example, smokers reduced their number of cigarettes smoked per day, but there was not a corresponding decrease in NNK uptake due to compensation (Hecht *et al.*, 2004). In another study, NNK and PAH uptake, estimated by total NNAL and 1-hydroxypyrene, respectively, were compared in smokers of regular, light, and ultra-light cigarettes, and found to be similar, consistent with epidemiologic studies that demonstrate no protection against lung cancer in smokers of light compared to regular cigarettes (Hecht *et al.*, 2005b). Other studies evaluated NNK uptake in smokers who switched from their current cigarette brand to products advertised as being less hazardous, but the results generally did not support these claims (Hatsukami *et al.*, 2004). One of the most useful applications of total NNAL has been in studies of non-smokers exposed to second-hand tobacco smoke (Hecht, 2003). The sensitivity and specificity of this biomarker are ideal for such studies, and it is the most commonly elevated tobacco carcinogen biomarker in non-smokers exposed to second-hand smoke. Total NNAL has also found utility in establishing NNK uptake in smokeless tobacco users (Hecht *et al.*, 2002, 2007, 2008a, b; Hecht, 2008)

The relationship of urinary total NNAL to lung cancer was demonstrated in a study of stored urine samples collected years before diagnosis of lung cancer from smokers in Shanghai, China and Singapore (Yuan *et al.*, 2009). There was a significant relationship between total NNAL and lung cancer incidence, after correction for numbers of cigarettes smoked per day and duration of smoking. An 8.5 fold increased risk for lung cancer was observed for those smokers in the highest tertile of total NNAL and cotinine, relative to smokers with the same smoking history but in the lowest tertiles of total NNAL and cotinine. Urinary biomarkers were also used to demonstrate higher uptake of nicotine and NNK per cigarette in smokers with polymorphisms in the nicotinic acetylcholine genes associated with lung cancer in genome-wide association studies (see Section 4.2; Le Marchand *et al.*, 2008). Collectively, these results indicate that urinary total NNAL is not only a biomarker of exposure, but also a biomarker of risk for lung cancer.

(b) Serum and saliva metabolites

Serum and saliva metabolites have been used as biomarkers much less often than urine metabolites. The most frequently measured tobacco smoke toxicant in serum and saliva is cotinine, documented as a useful biomarker of cigarette smoking in many studies (Lee, 1999; Hukkanen *et al.*, 2005). Total NNAL can be readily quantified in serum and its levels remain relatively constant in a given smoker sampled at bimonthly intervals over a one year period. Consistent with the results described above, one study showed a significant relationship between total NNAL in prospectively collected serum samples from smokers and lung cancer risk (Church *et al.*, 2009). Other biomarkers that have been measured in serum include cadmium, benzene, styrene and *r*-1,*t*-2,3,*c*-4-tetrahydroxy-1,2,3,4-tetrahydrophenanthrene (PheT) (IARC, 2004a; Church *et al.*, 2009).

(c) DNA adducts

Fig. 4.3 presents an overview of metabolism and DNA adduct formation from eight tobacco smoke compounds (clockwise from top left): BaP, NNK, *N*-nitrosodimethylamine (NDMA), NNN, acrolein, ethylene oxide, acetaldehyde and 4-aminobiphenyl. Evidence exists for DNA adduct formation from each of these carcinogens in smokers, based on studies carried out with tissues or blood cells. DNA adduct biomarkers have been applied mainly in studies of smokers, and there is far less evidence from studies of second-hand tobacco smoke or smokeless tobacco use.

The structures of DNA adducts of tobacco smoke carcinogens have been characterized in detail, but a complete description of these structures is beyond the scope of this section. Selected DNA adduct structures are shown in Fig. 4.4. A major DNA adduct of BaP results from *trans*- addition of the benzo[*a*]pyrene diol epoxide (BPDE) to the N^2-position of dG (Szeliga

Fig. 4.3 Overview of metabolism and DNA adduct formation from eight tobacco smoke constituents

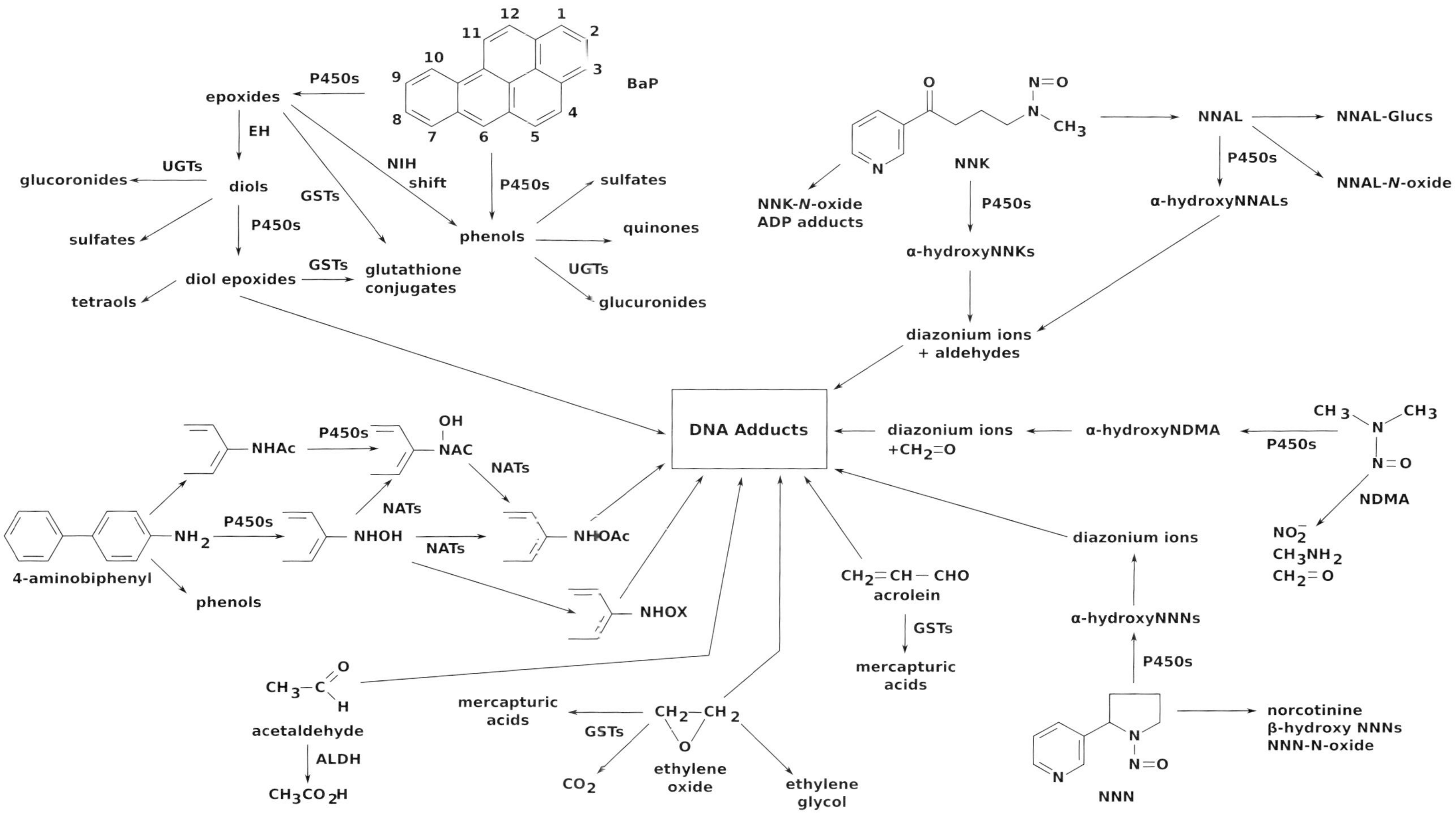

4-ABP, 4-aminobiphenyl; AC, acetyl; ADP, adenosine diphosphate; ALDH, aldehyde dehydrogenase; AKR, aldo-ketoreductase; B[*a*]P, benzo[*a*]pyrene; EH, epoxide hydrolase; Gluc, glucuronide; GSTs, glutathione *S*-transferases; NATs, *N*-acetyltransferases; NDMA, *N*-nitrosodimethylamine; NIH shift, phenomenon of hydroxylation-induced intramolecular migration; NNAL, 4-(methylnitrosamino)-1-(3-pyridyl)-1-butanol; NNK, 4-(methylnitrosamino)-1-(3-pyridyl)-1-butanone; NNN, *N'*-nitrosonornicotine; P450s, cytochrome P450 enzymes; UGTs, uridine-5'-diphosphate-glucuronosyl transferases

Adapted from Cooper *et al.* (1983), Preussmann & Stewart (1984), Kadlubar & Beland (1985), Hecht (1998, 1999), Penning & Drury (2007), IARC (2008, 2010b).

Fig. 4.4 Structures of some DNA adducts of tobacco smoke constituents

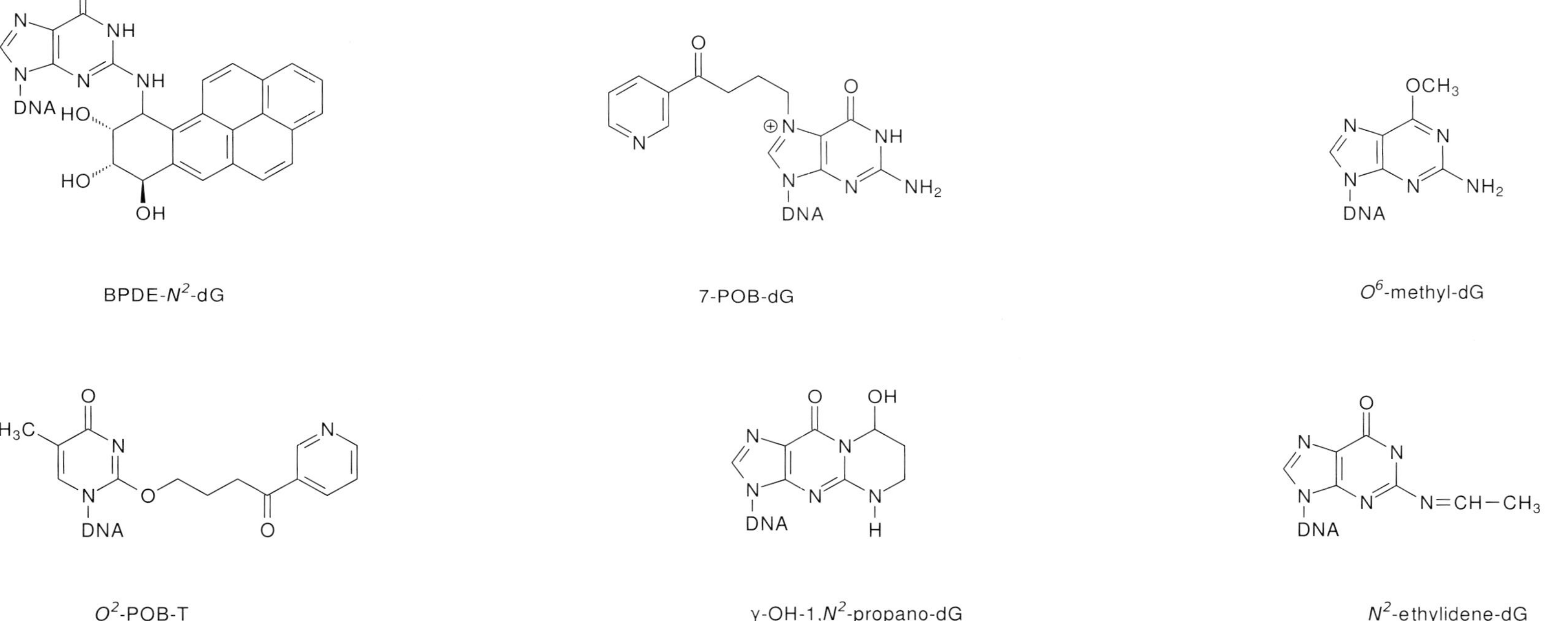

BPDE-N^2-dG, benzo[*a*]pyrene diol epoxide-N^2-deoxyguanosine; 7-POB-dG, pyridyloxobutyl-deoxyguanosine; O^2-POB-T, O^2-pyridyloxobutyl-thymidine

& Dipple, 1998). Pyridyloxobutyl (POB)-DNA adducts of NNK and NNN are formed at the 7- and O^6-positions of deoxyguanosine dG, the O^2-position of thymidine, and the O^2-position of deoxycytidine (Hecht, 2008). They can be measured in part as 4-hydroxy-1-(3-pyridyl)-1-butanone (HPB) released upon hydrolysis. Metabolic activation of NNK also leads to 7-methyl-dG and O^6-methyl-dG, identical to the DNA adducts formed from NDMA and other DNA methylating agents (Hecht, 2008). Ethylating agents and ethylene oxide in cigarette smoke also alkylate dG (Zhao *et al.*, 1999; Singh *et al.*, 2005). Acrolein and crotonaldehyde react with DNA to produce exocyclic 1,N^2-dG adducts, while acetaldehyde forms a Schiff base adduct with the exocyclic N^2 amino group of dG. There is evidence for the presence of all these DNA adducts in tissues or blood cells of smokers, but there are also many studies in which these specific adducts have been sought but not found (Boysen & Hecht, 2003).

Measurement of these DNA adducts as biomarkers potentially can provide the most direct link between cellular exposure and cancer, because DNA adducts are so critical in carcinogenesis. However, it is challenging because their levels are extremely low, frequently ranging from 1 per 10^6 to 1 per 10^8 normal bases, and the tissue or blood samples containing them are usually available in only small quantities. Fortunately, the routine detection of amol levels [attomole, equivalent to 10 moles] of DNA adducts by conventional LC-MS/MS techniques is now feasible (Singh & Farmer, 2006). There are still relatively few examples of quantitation of *specific* DNA adducts of tobacco carcinogens in tissues of smokers using mass spectrometry, high pressure liquid chromatography (HPLC)-fluorescence, HPLC with electrochemical detection, or postlabelling techniques (Pfeifer *et al.*, 2002). A much larger body of work has used the highly sensitive, but relatively non-specific ^{32}P-postlabelling and immunoassay methods of DNA adduct detection. Although the adducts detected using ^{32}P-postlabelling are often referred to as "aromatic DNA adducts," there is strong evidence that they are not related to PAHs (Arif *et al.*, 2006). Adduct levels are generally higher in lung tissues of smokers than non-smokers while studies using blood DNA have produced varied results. Adducts have also been detected in the larynx, oral and nasal mucosa, bladder, cervix, breast, pancreas, stomach, placenta, foetal tissue, cardiovascular tissues, sputum, and sperm of smokers (IARC, 2004a). A meta-analysis of the relationship of DNA adduct levels in smokers to cancer, as determined by ^{32}P-postlabelling in the majority of studies or enzyme linked immunosorbent assay (ELISA), demonstrated a positive relationship in current smokers (Veglia *et al.*, 2003; 2008).

(d) Protein adducts

Carcinogen-haemoglobin (Hb) and serum albumin adducts are regarded as surrogates for DNA adduct measurements. Although these proteins are not targets for carcinogenesis, virtually all carcinogens that react with DNA will also react with protein. Advantages of haemoglobin adducts include the ready availability of haemoglobin from blood and the relatively long lifetime of the erythrocyte in humans – 120 days –,which provides an opportunity for adducts to accumulate. Studies on protein adducts in smokers have been comprehensively reviewed (IARC, 2004a).

Haemoglobin adducts of aromatic amines are a highly informative type of carcinogen biomarker, with levels that are consistently higher in smokers than non-smokers, particularly for 3-aminobiphenyl and 4-aminobiphenyl-Hb adducts. Haemoglobin binds aromatic amines efficiently because heme accelerates the rate of nitrosoarene formation from the hydroxylamine, which is produced metabolically from the aromatic amine by CYP1A2 (Fig. 4.3; Skipper & Tannenbaum, 1990). Binding of the nitrosoarene occurs at the β-93 cysteine residue of human haemoglobin; the adduct is hydrolysed releasing the free amine, which is quantified by GC-MS (Skipper & Tannenbaum, 1990). Adduct levels are clearly related to cigarette smoking (Skipper & Tannenbaum, 1990). Adducts that form at the terminal valine of haemoglobin are also useful biomarkers: examples include those derived from ethylene oxide, acrylonitrile and acrylamide (Bergmark, 1997; Fennell *et al.*, 2000). Ethylated N-terminal valine of haemoglobin is also higher in smokers than in non-smokers (Carmella *et al.*, 2002).

HPB-releasing Hb adducts of NNK and NNN have been quantified in studies of smokers and smokeless tobacco users (IARC, 2004a, 2007a). These adducts are thought to be tobacco-specific, but some studies report their presence in non-smokers (Falter *et al.*, 1994; Schlöbe *et al.*, 2008).

4.1.4 Genetic and related effects

(a) Mutagenicity and cytogenetic effects

Tobacco smoke and its condensates are mutagenic in a wide variety of test systems from bacteria to mammalian cells in culture to rodents and humans (DeMarini, 2004; IARC, 2004a; Husgafvel-Pursiainen, 2004). In bacterial systems, the heterocyclic amines and aromatic amines in condensates account for much of the frameshift mutagenicity, whereas the PAHs and nitrosamines may account for some of the base-substitution mutagenicity (DeMarini *et al.*, 1995). G to T is the predominant class of base-substitution mutation induced by condensates in experimental systems and found in oncogenes and tumour-suppressor genes in smoking-associated lung tumours (IARC, 2004a). The genotoxic potencies of a variety of condensates in several genotoxicity assays likely have only qualitative value with regard to health risk assessment (DeMarini *et al.*, 2008). This is consistent with findings that smokers of low- or high-tar cigarettes have similar urinary levels of lung carcinogens (Hecht *et al.*, 2005b; Hatsukami *et al.*, 2006b) and similar risks for lung cancer (Harris *et al.*, 2004).

In rodents, cigarette smoke induces sister chromatid exchange and micronuclei in bone marrow and lung cells. Human newborns of smoking mothers have increased frequencies of *HPRT* mutations, chromosomal translocations, and DNA strand breaks. Sperm of smokers has increased frequencies of aneuploidy, DNA adducts, strand breaks, and oxidative damage. Cigarette smoke also causes germ-cell mutations in mice (Yauk *et al.*, 2007). Collectively, these data suggest that smoking is likely a germ-cell mutagen in humans. Smoking produces mutagenic urine and somatic-cell mutations in humans, including *HPRT* mutations, sister chromatid exchange, microsatellite instability and DNA damage in a variety of tissues. Genotoxic effects have been found in eight organ sites at which tobacco smoke causes cancer in humans (DeMarini, 2004; IARC, 2004a).

(b) Mutations in TP53, KRAS and related genes

Gene mutation data from a variety of databases, including the IARC Cancer *TP53* Mutation Database (http://www-p53.iarc.fr/), have been collated in the Genetic Alterations in Cancer (GAC) database (http://dir-apps.niehs.nih.gov/gac/) so that mutations in a variety of genes in various cancerous tissues can be compared. An assessment of the Gene Alterations in Cancer database showed that at least three genes were mutated more frequently in lung tumours from smokers than non-smokers (Lea *et al.*, 2007): *TP53* (39 versus 26%), *K-RAS* (20 versus 3%), and loss of heterozygosity at *FHIT* (57 versus 27%). Thus, genes in the cell cycle (*TP53*), cell signalling (*KRAS*) and apoptotic (*FHIT*) pathways are mutated more frequently in smoking- rather than in nonsmoking-associated lung tumours. Genomic sequencing of lung tumours has identified other mutated genes that are associated with smoking; ten times more genes are mutated in lung tumours from smokers compared to non-smokers (Ding *et al.*, 2008).

GC to TA transversions were the predominant class of base-substitution mutation found in *TP53* and *KRAS* genes in lung tumours from smokers, with the frequency of this mutation in *TP53* being 30% in smokers versus 22% in non-smokers. In smoking-associated oral cancers, the percentage of GC to TA mutations in *TP53* was 15% versus 2%, respectively. This mutation spectrum is consistent with that produced by a variety of known carcinogens present in tobacco smoke (IARC, 2004a). At the codon level, the most frequently mutated codons in *TP53* in lung tumours of smokers were 157, 175, 245, 248, and 273, all of which occur in the DNA-binding domain of the protein; among these codons, only 273 was mutated in lung tumours from non-smokers. Only three of these codons (157, 245 and 273) were mutated in smoking-associated larynx tumours, and only codon 157 was mutated in smoking-associated oral tumours. Thus, the mutational specificity at *TP53* is different among smoking- and nonsmoking-associated tumours and among smoking-associated tumours at various organs (Lea *et al.*, 2007). Thus, different pathways are involved in the development of different types of tumours (Le Calvez *et al.*, 2005; Mounawar *et al.*, 2007; Subramanian & Govindan, 2008).

4.1.5 Effects on gene expression profile

As indicated in a review by Sen *et al.* (2007) involving microarray analysis of 18 studies in human smokers, 7 in smoke-exposed rodents, and 3 in condensate-exposed mammalian cells, smoking generally upregulated a wide variety of genes, especially those involved in the stress response, phase I metabolism, and immune response. Genes that were consistently expressed differentially in smokers (as assessed in alveolar macrophages, lung cells or peripheral lymphocytes) included metallothioneins, heat-shock proteins, superoxide dismutase, glutathione transferase, heme oxygenase, *CYP* genes (*1A2, 1A1* and *1B1*), interleukins and chemokines.

Spira *et al.* (2004) analysed global gene expression in bronchial epithelial cells and found that the expression levels of metabolizing and antioxidant genes had reverted to control levels after two years of smoking cessation. However, expression of potential oncogenes and tumour-suppressor genes never reverted to never-smoker levels even after years of smoking cessation. Consistently, expression of microRNAs is generally downregulated by cigarette smoke (Izzotti *et al.*, 2009). As discussed below, smoking also altered methylation patterns and gene expression in smoking-associated tumours.

4.1.6 Other effects associated with carcinogenesis

(a) Proliferation, differentiation, apoptosis, and inflammation

As noted above, the signal-transduction pathways in lung tumours from smokers are distinctly different from those of non-smokers (Mountzios *et al.*, 2008). Fig 4.5 shows details of signalling pathways that are deregulated by tobacco smoke. The involvement of high frequencies of mutated *K-RAS* and *TP53* genes in smoking-associated lung tumours results in altered regulation of cell proliferation, differentiation, cytoskeletal organization and protein trafficking. Cigarette smoking activates *NF-κB*, which induces pro-inflammatory cytokine expression and induces growth factors and proliferative signals (Mountzios *et al.*, 2008). This gene also influences the expression of the anti-apoptotic gene *BCL2* and pro-apoptotic gene *BAX*. Smoking produces chronic inflammation, which promotes cancer (Walser *et al.*, 2008). Smoking results in high levels of reactive oxygen species, which damage epithelial and endothelial cells and impair their function. In smoking-associated lung cancer, elevated levels of cyclooxygenase-2 (COX-2) and

Fig. 4.5 General scheme of some cell-signalling pathways that are deregulated by tobacco smoke in lung carcinogenesis

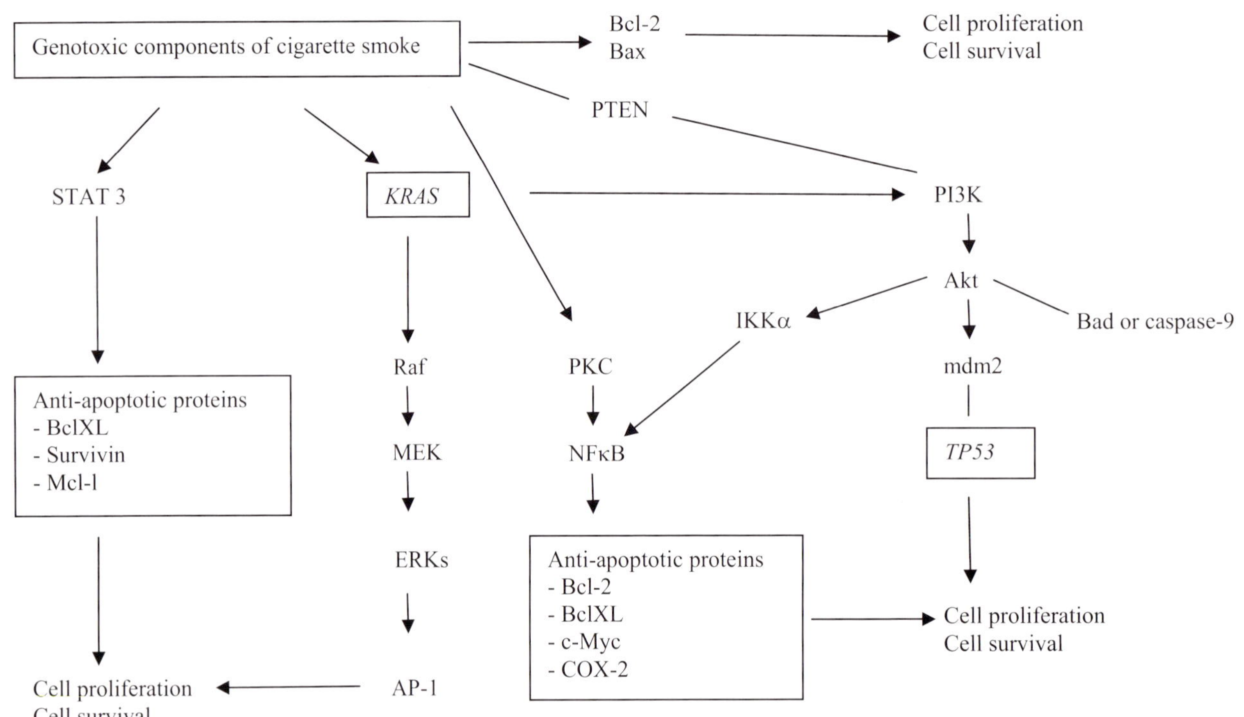

Akt, serine/threonine protein kinase; ERKs, extracellular regulated kinases; MEK, mitogen-activated protein kinase; Bad, Bcl2-associated agonist of cell death; PI3K, phosphatidylinositol 3-kinase; PKC, protein kinase C; NF-κB, nuclear factor κB; IKKα, inhibitor of nuclear factor κ-B kinase; PTEN, phosphatase and tensin homologue; STAT3, signal transducer and activator of transcription; COX-2, cyclooxygenase-2

prostaglandin (PGE_2) indicate apoptosis resistance, proliferation, immunosuppression, angiogenesis, invasion, and epithelial-mesenchymal transition (Walser *et al.*, 2008).

(b) Endogenous nitrosation

Intragastric formation of *N*-nitroso compounds, measured using urinary nitrosamino acids excreted in urine, was increased in smokers compared to non-smokers (Hoffmann & Brunnemann, 1983). Two recent studies demonstrated that NNN forms endogenously in some users of nicotine replacement therapy products (Stepanov *et al.*, 2009a, b).

(c) Hormonal changes

These are described in Section 4.3.2a.

4.2 Polymorphisms in carcinogen-metabolizing genes

4.2.1 Introduction

It has been long proposed that the known variation among individuals in their capacity to activate and detoxify carcinogens may be associated with increased susceptibility to cancer, and that polymorphisms of carcinogen-metabolising genes may play a significant role. The most intensively studied genes involved in the metabolism of carcinogens include the various *CYP* genes, the *GST* genes and the *NAT* genes. Other relevant xenobiotic-metabolising genes, such as *EPHX*, sulfotransferase (*SULT*), *UGT*, myeloperoxidase (*MPO*), and NAD(P)H quinone oxidoreductase-1 (*NQO1*) genes, have also been studied. Recently, extensive pooled studies and reviews have been published on polymorphisms of carcinogen-metabolising genes and their role in cancer susceptibility, especially in tobacco-related lung cancer and cancers at other sites. Similarly, various biomarkers of exposure and genotoxicity that are presumed to provide a mechanistic basis for such associations have been comprehensively investigated in relation to these polymorphisms. A brief overview based largely on reviews and the meta- and pooled analyses is presented here.

4.2.2 Genetic polymorphisms of carcinogen metabolism: some central genes

(a) CYP genes

CYPs comprise the principal enzyme system catalysing various phase I oxidation reactions, including metabolic activation and detoxification of many carcinogenic substances in tobacco smoke such as PAHs. Of the various CYP enzymes expressed in humans, many of those belonging to CYP1 to CYP3 families play a role in carcinogen metabolism, producing highly reactive DNA-damaging metabolites as well as detoxified metabolites (Guengerich & Shimada, 1998; Lang & Pelkonen, 1999; Ingelman-Sundberg, 2004). CYPs have evolved into a wide superfamily with close to 60 different active genes currently identified; most of these genes exhibit polymorphism (www.cypalleles.ki.se).

(i) CYP1A1

Several allelic variants of the human *CYP1A1* gene are currently known (www.cypalleles.ki.se). The major variant forms of the *CYP1A1* gene (wildtype allele *CYP1A1*1*) mostly frequently studied for association to cancer susceptibility include the following two alleles: (i) *CYP1A1*2A* allele (m1 allele; *Msp* I) and (ii) *CYP1A1*2B* (Cascorbi *et al.*, 1996) or *CYP1A1*2C* (www.cypalleles.ki.se) allele (m2 allele; Ile^{462}Val). Importantly, the *CYP1A1* m1 allele and m2 allele are in complete linkage disequilibrium in Caucasians (Kawajiri, 1999; Bartsch *et al.*, 2000). In addition, *CYP1A1*4* allele (m4; Thr^{461}Asn) (Cascorbi *et al.*, 1996), and *CYP1A1*3* (m3) allele found in African-Americans but not in Caucasians or Asians (Crofts *et al.*, 1993) are included in some studies (Bartsch *et al.*, 2000).

In smoking-related lung cancer, the various *CYP1A1* polymorphisms as well as the differences in the frequencies of the rare variant alleles between ethnicities contribute to the differences in findings. There are collective analyses of data predominantly indicating an overall mild to moderate effect of *CYP1A1* polymorphisms on lung cancer risk (Kawajiri, 1999; Bartsch *et al.*, 2000; Houlston, 2000; Le Marchand *et al.*, 2003; Vineis *et al.*, 2003; Vineis *et al.*, 2004; Lee *et al.*, 2008a; Shi *et al.*, 2008). In many reviews and meta- or pooled analyses the increased risk associated with *CYP1A1* polymorphism has most clearly been seen in Asian populations (Kawajiri, 1999; Le Marchand *et al.*, 2003; Vineis *et al.*, 2003; Lee *et al.*, 2008a; Shi *et al.*, 2008).

Multiple studies have also analysed the gene-gene interactions between *CYP1A1*, *GSTM1* and *GSTT1* polymorphisms and lung cancer (d'Errico *et al.*, 1999; Houlston, 1999; Benhamou *et al.*, 2002; Bolt & Thier, 2006; Raimondi *et al.*, 2006; Ye *et al.*, 2006; Carlsten *et al.*, 2008). Some of the analyses have indicated that the elevated risk for lung cancer may be more pronounced for some *CYP1A1/GSTM1* null genotype combinations (Le Marchand *et al.*, 1998; Bartsch *et al.*, 2000; Vineis *et al.*, 2004, 2007; Lee *et al.*, 2008a; Shi *et al.*, 2008).

(ii) CYP1A2

CYP1A2 is highly inducible and metabolises, including deacetylation reactions, many tobacco smoke carcinogens such as aromatic and heterocyclic amines and nitro-aromatic compounds, and tobacco-specific nitrosamines such as NNK (Nebert *et al.*, 2004; Jalas *et al.*, 2005; IARC, 2007a). A few major variant alleles have been described (www.cypalleles.ki.se), some of which may have been reported to influence inducibility (Nakajima *et al.*, 1999; Ingelman-Sundberg *et al.*, 2007). Overall, the phenotype-genotype relations have not been well established for *CYP1A2*, although current evidence points towards contribution of genetic variation (Murayama *et al.*, 2004; Ingelman-Sundberg *et al.*, 2007); data on possible associations with tobacco related cancer are sparse (Agundez, 2004; Nebert & Dalton, 2006).

(iii) CYP2A6

Several aspects of smoking behaviour are likely to be influenced by *CYP2A6* genetic variation, which influences nicotine metabolism (Malaiyandi *et al.*, 2005; Mwenifumbo & Tyndale, 2007). The most important functionally altered allele is *CYP2A6*4* (gene deletion), which confers a poor-metabolizer phenotype in homozygous individuals (Malaiyandi *et al.*, 2005; Ingelman-Sundberg *et al.*, 2007; Mwenifumbo & Tyndale, 2007). In some studies, polymorphic variants of *CYP2A6* gene have been implicated in susceptibility to smoking-related cancers (Gambier *et al.*, 2005; Malaiyandi *et al.*, 2005; Nakajima, 2007). In line with this, the accumulated data have suggested that *CYP2A6* polymorphism may affect cancer risk in smokers but not in non-smokers (Tan *et al.*, 2001; Kamataki *et al.*, 2005; Malaiyandi *et al.*, 2005; Canova *et al.*, 2009).

(iv) CYP2A13

From human CYPs, CYP2A13 is the primary form involved in the metabolic activation of the tobacco-specific nitrosamines NNK and NNN (Jalas *et al.*, 2005; IARC, 2007a). The *CYP2A13* gene exhibits polymorphism in humans (Zhang *et al.*, 2002; Jalas *et al.*, 2005), and experimental studies suggest that some of the polymorphisms may affect the hydroxylation of NNN and NNK (Jalas *et al.*, 2005; Schlicht *et al.*, 2007). However, the data on possible effects of these polymoprhisms on the risk of tobacco-related cancers in humans are still limited (Wang *et al.*, 2003; Song *et al.*, 2009; Timofeeva *et al.*, 2009).

(v) CYP2D6

The *CYP2D6* gene shows high variability in expression. The enzyme is not inducible, and therefore genetic variation largely contributes to the interindividual variation in enzyme activity. Currently, more than 100 different functional CYP2D6 gene variants have been described, and these are divided into alleles causing abolished, decreased, normal, and ultrarapid enzyme activity (Ingelman-Sundberg, 2005; Ingelman-Sundberg *et al.*, 2007). The most important null alleles leading to poor-metabolizer phenotype are *CYP2D6*4* (splice defect) and *CYP2D6*5* (gene deletion) (Ingelman-Sundberg, 2005; Ingelman-Sundberg *et al.*, 2007).

A large series of studies have been carried out over the past 20 years on the association between *CYP2D6* polymorphism and susceptibility to lung cancer and to some other tobacco-related cancers (Wolf & Smith, 1999). Despite some indication of an association between CYP2D6 poor-metabolizer and decreased risk for lung cancer, no major role for CYP2D6 in carcinogen metabolism or a molecular basis for such an association have been discovered (Wolf & Smith, 1999; Ingelman-Sundberg, 2005).

(vi) Other CYP genes

CYP1B1 allelic variants that affect the catalytic activity have been described but they have been studied to a lesser extent for the association with susceptibility to smoking-related cancers (Thier *et al.*, 2003). Some positive findings have been reported on head and neck cancer (Ko *et al.*, 2001), and lung cancer (Zienolddiny *et al.*, 2008).

Several polymorphisms have been characterized in the *CYP2E1* gene and several positive associations with the risk of different cancers have been reported, in particular for cancers of the upper aerodigestive tract, lung and gastrointestinal tract (Section 2.19). *CYP2E1* may also play an important role in the interaction of the carcinogenic effects of alcohol and tobacco (Section 4.4).

From the human *CYP3A* locus (*CYP3A4*, *CYP3A5* and *CYP3A7*), the *CYP3A4*1B* allele has been associated with lung cancer and prostate cancer in some studies but not in all (Dally *et al.*, 2003; Rodriguez-Antona & Ingelman-Sundberg, 2006). However, the role of these variants in relation to tobacco smoking is unknown.

(b) GSTM1 and other GST genes

Polymorphic *GST* genes have long been proposed to modify susceptibility to lung cancer (Seidegård *et al.*, 1986; Ketterer *et al.*, 1992). The polymorphic genes encoding the various classes of cytosolic GST enzymes include the *GSTM1* and *GSTM3* genes (mu class), the *GSTP1* gene (pi class), and the *GSTT1* gene (theta class). The gene deletion (null) allele of the *GSTM1* gene (*GSTM1*0*) and of the *GSTT1* gene (*GSTT1*0*) have been the most intensively studied polymorphisms in relation to increased susceptibility to cancer (Strange *et al.*, 2001; Bolt & Thier, 2006; McIlwain *et al.*, 2006). For the *GSTP1* gene, the form most abundantly present in lung tissue, genetic variation in exon 5 (*GSTP1*2*; $Ile^{105}Val$), in exon 6 ($Ala^{114}Val$), as well as a combination of these, are the variations most frequently studied for cancer susceptibility (Watson *et al.*, 1998; Cote *et al.*, 2009).

Numerous reviews, meta- and pooled analyses have been published over the past 15 years or so for the *GST* genes with systematic assessments covering altogether tens of thousands of cases and controls. For the *GSTM1* null genotype, such analyses have largely provided negative, suggestive or at most moderately positive results for an association with an increased risk for lung cancer (d'Errico *et al.*, 1999; Houlston, 1999; Benhamou *et al.*, 2002; Ye *et al.*, 2006; Carlsten *et al.*, 2008). The larger the studies, the less significant the estimates for the role of *GSTM1* emerge in systematic analysis (Ye *et al.*, 2006; Carlsten *et al.*, 2008). Also the varying allele frequencies related to ethnic background affect the findings for *GSTM1* as well as for many other genes (Garte *et al.*, 2001; Ye *et al.*, 2006; Carlsten *et al.*, 2008; Lee *et al.*, 2008a).

In a meta-analysis of the association between the *GSTT1* gene polymorphism and lung cancer no association between *GSTT1* null genotype and risk for lung cancer in Caucasians was observed, but a positive association was found for Asians (Raimondi *et al.*, 2006). A significant association for either Caucasians or Asians was also not found in a pooled analysis (Raimondi *et al.*, 2006). A meta-analysis found no significant association between lung cancer risk and the *GSTP1* $Ile^{105}Val$ polymorphism; but the pooled analysis suggested an overall statistically significant mild association between lung cancer and homozygosity or heterozygosity for the Val^{105} allele (Cote *et al.*, 2009).

A recent body of epidemiologic data suggests an inverse association between cruciferous vegetables/isothiocyanates intake and cancers of the colorectum, lung and breast; the studies also provide evidence that this protective effect is greater among individuals who possess the *GSTM1* or *T1* null genotype, who would be expected to accumulate higher levels of isothiocyanates at the target tissue level, a pre-requisite for their enzyme-inducing effects (Seow *et al.*, 2005). The association between isothiocyanates and cancer, and its modification by *GSTM1* and *GSTT1* status, is most consistent for lung cancer and appears to be strongest among current smokers who possess the combined *GSTM1* and *GSTT1* null genotypes (London *et al.*, 2000a; Spitz *et al.*, 2000; Zhao *et al.*, 2001; Brennan *et al.*, 2005; Seow *et al.*, 2005).

(c) NAT1 and NAT2 genes

The pooled and meta-analyses carried out on *NAT1* and *NAT2* polymorphisms and bladder cancer risk have consistently reported significantly increased risk for *NAT2* slow acetylators

(Dong *et al.*, 2008; Malats, 2008; see also Section 2.9). Data on *NAT1* fast acetylators are inconsistent, as are the studies suggesting an increased risk for *NAT2* rapid acetylator status. Additionally, genotypes for other genes, specially *GSTM1*, have also been implicated (Vineis *et al.* 2001; García-Closas *et al.*, 2005; Hein, 2006; Sanderson *et al.*, 2007; Dong *et al.*, 2008; Malats, 2008).

In a recent large study on tobacco-related lung cancer and upper aerodigestive cancers, the *NAT* genes, in particular *NAT*10* haplotype, emerged from a set of 16 genes as involved in the risk (McKay *et al.*, 2008). When more than one hundred single nucleotide polymorphisms for 31 genes involved in phase I or phase II metabolism or in antioxidant defence were investigated, only four of the previously reported polymorphisms of the *GSTP1*, *EPHX1* and superoxide dismutase *SOD2* genes and the *NAT1* fast acetylator phenotype remained significantly associated with risk of non-small cell lung cancer after correction for multiple testing (Zienolddiny *et al.*, 2008).

In breast cancer, several recent meta-analyses of epidemiological studies have suggested increased risk among smokers with the *NAT2* slow acetylator genotype; such an association has been observed especially among long-term smokers and post-menopausal women (Terry & Goodman, 2006; Ambrosone *et al.*, 2008; Ochs-Balcom *et al.*, 2007; Baumgartner *et al.*, 2009).

In all, the role of the *NAT* gene polymorphisms in tobacco-related cancers, with the exceptions of increased risk of bladder cancer and possibly breast cancer in *NAT2* slow acetylators, remains largely open due to the incomplete understanding of phenotype-genotype relationships, and the interplay between these two genes and their polymorphisms (Hein, 2002, 2006).

(d) Others

Genes coding for EPHX, UGT and SULT enzymes, mainly but not exclusively involved in detoxification reactions, exhibit polymorphisms with numerous gene variants discovered (Mackenzie *et al.*, 1997; London *et al.*, 2000b; Glatt *et al.*, 2001; Burchell, 2003). Additional polymorphic genes studied for their significance in cancer susceptibility are the *NQO1* and *MPO* genes, with NQO1 playing a dual role in the detoxification and activation of procarcinogens, and MPO converting lipophilic carcinogens into hydrophilic forms (Nebert *et al.*, 2002). All these genes have been studied for their possible association with tobacco-related cancer risk to a varying extent and with variable outcomes (London *et al.*, 2000b; Bamber *et al.*, 2001; Garte, 2001; To-Figueras *et al.*, 2001; Tiemersma *et al.*, 2002b; Guillemette, 2003; Wells *et al.*, 2004; Kiyohara *et al.*, 2005; Moreno *et al.*, 2005; Nagar & Remmel, 2006; Gallagher *et al.*, 2007).

4.2.3 Biomarkers of tobacco carcinogenesis and polymorphic genes of carcinogen metabolism

A myriad of studies have investigated association between various biomarkers of tobacco-related carcinogenesis and genetic variation of genes involved in carcinogen metabolism. For involvement in increased cancer susceptibility, a large variety of intermediate biomarker have been studied, including PAH metabolites in urine, urinary mutagenicity, DNA and protein adducts, cytogenetic alterations, *HPRT* mutant lymphocytes, as well as somatic mutations of the tumour suppressor gene *TP53* and *KRAS* oncogene occurring in cancer tissue.

(a) PAH metabolites and mutagenicity in urine

(i) PAH metabolites in urine

Increased excretion of 1-hydroxypyrene in urine in association with the *GSTM1* null genotype has been reported in many studies on individuals with occupational or environmental exposure to PAHs (Yang *et al.*, 1999; Alexandrie *et al.*, 2000; Lee *et al.*, 2001; Kuljukka-Rabb *et al.*, 2002; Kato *et al.*, 2004). The associations seen between *GSTT1* polymorphism and the

PAH metabolites are somewhat more variable. Similarly, the joint effect of *GSTM1* and *GSTT1* null genotypes, as well as the effects of some other genes of xenobiotic metabolism, such as *EPHX*, *CYP1A1*, *CYP1A2* and the aryl hydrocarbon receptor (*AhR*) gene have been either positive or negative (Yang *et al.*, 1999; Alexandrie *et al.*, 2000; Lee *et al.*, 2001; Zhang *et al.*, 2001; Kuljukka-Rabb *et al.*, 2002; Yang *et al.*, 2003; Chen *et al.*, 2007; Cocco *et al.*, 2007; Bin *et al.*, 2008).

Another PAH metabolite studied in this context is phenanthrene, the simplest PAHs with a bay region, a feature closely associated with carcinogenicity. A study quantified ratios of urinary products of metabolic activation (such as PheT) and detoxification (such as phenanthrols, HOPhe) of phenanthrene in 346 smokers, who were also genotyped for 11 polymorphisms in genes involved in PAHs metabolism, including the *CYP1A1* and *GSTM1* genes. A significant association between the presence of the *CYP1A1* Ile^{462}Val polymorphism and high PheT/3-HOPhe ratios was found, particularly in combination with the *GSTM1* null polymorphism (Hecht *et al.*, 2006).

Overall, the data on the influence of genetic variation in PAHs metabolism on the levels of the urinary metabolite biomarkers are variable, and currently inconclusive.

(ii) Urinary mutagenicity

One relatively early line of research investigated the relationship between urinary mutagenicity and genetic variation in activation or detoxification genes. These studies, however, have seldom been focused on smokers only but rather on other sources of exposure (Pavanello & Clonfero, 2000).

In some studies, *NAT2* slow acetylator genotype either alone or in combination with *GSTM1* null genotype has been associated with increased urinary mutagenicity in the *Salmonella* test in individuals with occupational, environmental or medicinal PAH-related exposure, or in smokers (Vineis & Malats, 1999; Pavanello & Clonfero, 2000). In another study, CYP1A2 activity, but not *NAT2*, *GSTM1* or *GSTT1* genotypes influenced urinary mutagen excretion in smokers (Pavanello *et al.*, 2002). A further study also suggested contribution of the *CYP1A2* gene variation to increased urinary mutagenicity in heavy smokers (Pavanello *et al.*, 2005). Associations with variants of other xenobiotic-metabolising genes (such as *EPHX1*) have also been reported, with somewhat complex results (Kuljukka-Rabb *et al.*, 2002).

(b) DNA adducts

The relationship between the variants of polymorphic genes of carcinogen metabolism and tobacco smoke-related DNA adduct formation has been addressed in an abundant number of studies among smokers, occupationally exposed groups, and patients with smoking-related cancer. In addition, multiple *in vitro* studies on this relationship have been carried out (Bartsch *et al.*, 2000; Pavanello & Clonfero, 2000; Alexandrov *et al.*, 2002; Wiencke, 2002).

The intensive efforts to study the relationship between *CYP1A1* and *GSTM1* gene polymorphism and the level of aromatic-hydrophobic/bulky PAH-DNA adducts in human lungs have so far provided little evidence for a role of a single metabolic genotype or their combinations on DNA adduct formation, with largely weak, non-significant or contradictory results. However, a trend of increasing adduct levels in subjects with the *CYP1A1*2-GSTM1*0* genotype combination has been observed, which was reinforced when BPDE-DNA adducts were specifically assessed. These results suggest a gene-gene interaction, supported by biological data from other studies (Bartsch *et al.*, 2000; Alexandrov *et al.*, 2002; Wiencke, 2002). Such gene-gene interaction lends support to the increased risk for lung cancer found in carriers of these genotypes in Japanese, among whom the frequency of the variant *CYP1A1* allele is much higher (Bartsch *et al.*, 2000; Alexandrov *et al.*, 2002).

A wide selection of genes and genotypes included in the various studies have made it difficult to assess the overall role of the polymorphisms of *GSTM1* and other genes alone or in combination. Differences between the studies in the types of adducts determined, the various tissues, cell types and cancers studied, detection methods, variation in sources and types of exposure, sample size, gender differences, and sometimes poor knowledge regarding the alleles, genotypes and haplotypes under study also contribute to the large variability seen in these studies (d'Errico *et al.*, 1999; Hemminki *et al.*, 2001; Alexandrov *et al.*, 2002; Wiencke, 2002).

(c) Cytogenetic biomarkers of genotoxicity

(i) Chromosome aberrations and sister chromatid exchanges

Early studies investigating whether homozygosity for the *GSTM1* null allele affects prevalence of cytogenetic changes in lymphocytes of smokers reported positive results (Seidegård *et al.*, 1990; van Poppel *et al.*, 1992; Cheng *et al.*, 1995). Since then, studies have investigated the association between genetic polymorphisms of xenobiotic-metabolising genes and cytogenetic biomarkers in smokers and in some occupational groups (Rebbeck, 1997; Autrup, 2000; Pavanello & Clonfero, 2000; Norppa, 2003, 2004).

Collectively, the reported findings are in support of increased susceptibility of smokers to chromosomal effects in association with *GSTM1* and *GSTT1* null variants deficient in detoxification of tobacco smoke carcinogens. Exposure to genotoxicants generated from other environmental sources (e.g. polluted air, diet, endogenous sources such as reactive oxygen species) may contribute to the observed associations, and it is likely that other polymorphic metabolic genes such as *NAT2* may be involved (Pavanello & Clonfero, 2000; Norppa, 2001, 2003).

(ii) Micronucleus induction

The relationship between formation of micronuclei and genetic polymorphisms of carcinogen metabolism has been addressed in a wide range of human population studies (Norppa, 2003, 2004). Induction of micronuclei in smokers may be little, if at all, affected by *GSTM1*, *GSTT1* or *NAT2* genotypes. In contrast, the *NAT1* rapid genotype appears to show an association with increased susceptibility to smoking-related micronuclei (Norppa, 2004).

A recent review evaluated more than seventy human studies on genetic polymorphisms and micronucleus frequency detected either in peripheral blood lymphocytes or exfoliated cells in populations exposed to various genotoxic agents. There were no significant genotype effects involved in micronucleus induction in smokers (Iarmarcovai *et al.*, 2008). The relationship between genetic polymorphisms and micronucleus formation is complex, and is influenced to a variable extent by several genes of xenobiotic metabolism and DNA repair, as well as the variety of chromosomal alterations known to contribute to micronucleus formation (Iarmarcovai *et al.*, 2008).

(iii) Chromosomal damage induced in vitro

The effects of genotypes or genotype combinations *in vitro* on the induction of various cytogenetic endpoints by tobacco-smoke carcinogens and their metabolites have been studied, initially focused on the *GSTM1* and *GSTT1* null genotypes (Norppa, 2001, 2004). In a study investigating NNK *in vitro*, lymphocytes from *GSTM1* null donors were more sensitive to induction of chromosomal aberrations and sister chromatid exchanges by NNK than lymphocytes from *GSTM1* positive donors (Salama *et al.*, 1999).

(d) Gene mutations

(i) HPRT mutant lymphocytes

Associations between the frequencies of *HPRT* mutant T-lymphocytes in populations exposed to genotoxic agents, such as smokers, and the polymorphism of xenobiotic-metabolising genes have been studied. In the early studies, positive, weak, or negative associations were reported for *GSTM1* null genotype, and negative findings were published for *NAT2* slow acetylator genotype in occupationally exposed or non-exposed subjects (Rebbeck, 1997; Vineis & Malats, 1999). When healthy, non-smoking and occupationally non-exposed young adults were studied for HPRT mutant frequency and polymorphisms in *CYP1A1*, *GSTM1* and *NAT2* genes, none of these polymorphisms, analysed individually, were found to influence the *HPRT* mutant frequency (Davies *et al.*, 1999). A significant interaction between the *GSTM1* null genotype and *NAT2* slow acetylator was associated with higher mutant frequency, but no other genotype combinations (Davies *et al.*, 1999). Some later studies have reported variable associations between *HPRT* mutant frequency and polymorphisms for either individual genes (*GSTM1*, *GSTT1* or *EPHX1*) or some of the genotypes in combination among exposed (Viezzer *et al.*, 1999; Abdel-Rahman *et al.*, 2001, 2003).

(ii) Mutations of the TP53 gene and other cancer-related genes

Whether the frequency of somatic mutations detected in tumour tissue in cancer-related genes, primarily the *TP53* tumour suppressor gene and *KRAS* oncogene, may be modified by polymorphisms in carcinogen metabolizing genes was first investigated assessing the effects of the *GSTM1* genotype, alone or in combination with other genetic polymorphisms. Several, but not all, such studies showed significant association between *GSTM1* null genotype and either the frequency or type of *TP53* mutations in smoking-induced lung cancer or other cancer type (Rebbeck, 1997; Vineis & Malats, 1999; Autrup, 2000). Fewer studies examined the association between *TP53* mutations and *GSTT1* polymorphism, and some results suggested the involvement of both null genotypes (Vineis & Malats, 1999; Autrup, 2000).

In smokers with non-small cell lung cancer, the risk of mutation was found to be the highest among the homozygous carriers of the *CYP1A1* rare allele *CYP1A1 MspI* (*Ile*^{462}*Val*) who also exhibited the *GSTM1* null genotype (Kawajiri *et al.*, 1996). Similarly, positive associations between *K-RAS* mutations and homozygosity for the *CYP1A1* rare allele were observed; the risk of mutation was enhanced when the *CYP1A1* susceptible genotype was combined with *GSTM1* null genotype (Kawajiri *et al.*, 1996). In another study, also carried out in a Japanese study population, *K-RAS* mutations occurred with greater frequency in lung adenocarcinoma smoking patients and of the *GSTM1* null genotype as compared with the *GSTM1* positive genotype (Noda *et al.*, 2004).

Many of the studies that assessed *NAT2* acetylator genotypes have found non-significant associations with the frequency or type of *TP53* mutation in bladder, lung, or other cancers (Vineis & Malats, 1999; Autrup, 2000). A study on bladder cancer did not find an overall association between *TP53* mutation frequency and *GSTM1*, *GSTT1*, *GSTP1* or *NAT2* genotypes. However, among patients with *TP53* mutations, transversion mutations were more frequent in those with *GSTM1* null genotype as compared to those with GSTM1 positive genotype; no significant associations were found for the *NAT2* gene (Ryk *et al.*, 2005).

In rectal cancer, overall negative results for an association between *TP53* or *KRAS* mutations and *GSTM1* and *NAT2* polymorphisms among smokers and non-smokers exposed to tobacco smoke were found (Curtin *et al.*, 2009). An interaction of second-hand tobacco smoke and *NAT2* was found in *TP53* mutation positive tumours but not in smokers (Curtin *et al.*, 2009). Earlier, an increased risk of *TP53* transversion mutations among *GSTM1* positive individuals who smoked cigarettes was found in colon cancer (Slattery *et al.*, 2002).

A statistically significant association was observed between the *GSTT1* null genotype and *TP53* mutation status of breast tumour in one study (Gudmundsdottir *et al.*, 2001), while in another larger study none of the genotypes for *CYP1B1*, *GSTM1*, *GSTT1* and *GSTP1* genes alone were associated with somatic *TP53* mutations (Van Emburgh *et al.*, 2008).

In summary, data from various cancer types on the association between genetic polymorphisms of carcinogen-metabolizing genes and somatic mutations of the *TP53* and *K-RAS* genes vary widely and do not permit to conclude (Rebbeck, 1997; Vineis & Malats, 1999; Autrup, 2000).

4.3 Site-specific mechanisms of carcinogenicity of tobacco smoke

4.3.1 Sites with sufficient evidence of carcinogenicity of tobacco smoking

(a) Lung

The conceptual model presented in Section 4.1 (Fig. 4.1) depicts the main mechanistic steps by which cigarette smoke causes cancer. Smokers inhale into their lungs carcinogens which, either directly or after metabolism, covalently bind to DNA, forming DNA adducts (see Section 4.1, Fig. 4.3). Tobacco smoke contains multiple strong lung carcinogens such as NNN, NNK, PAHs, 1,3-butadiene and cadmium. Levels of tobacco smoke-related DNA adducts, mainly ^{32}P-postlabelled aromatic-hydrophobic/PAH-related bulky DNA adducts, in the lung are higher in smokers than in non-smokers (Phillips, 2002; IARC, 2004a; Hecht, 2008). Higher levels of DNA adducts have further been linked to increased risk for cancer in pooled and meta-analyses (IARC, 2004a; Veglia *et al.*, 2008).

Mutations in *TP53* and *K-RAS* genes, two central genes of human carcinogenesis, are more frequently mutated in smokers' lung cancer as compared to lung cancer from non-smokers (DeMarini, 2004; IARC, 2004a; Lea *et al.*, 2007; Ding *et al.*, 2008; see Section 4.1.3). In particular, *TP53* but also to some extent *K-RAS* mutations found in smoking-associated lung tumours exhibit mutational specificity that is consistent with the pattern produced by PAH diol epoxides in experimental studies and different from that observed in non-smokers' lung cancer (Pfeifer *et al.*, 2002; DeMarini, 2004; IARC, 2004a; Le Calvez *et al.*, 2005; Section 4.1.3). Keeping with such exposure-specific mutation profile, lung cancer in non-smokers exposed to second-hand tobacco smoke shows mutational similarity to smokers' lung cancer, although less data are available (Husgafvel-Pursiainen, 2004; IARC, 2004a; Le Calvez *et al.*, 2005; Subramanian & Govindan, 2008). The different pathways of lung carcinogenesis for smokers and non-smokers are likely to involve somatic mutations and other genetic alterations in a larger set of genes that are critical in controlling normal cellular growth via signal transduction (Bode & Dong, 2005; Lea *et al.*, 2007; Ding *et al.*, 2008).

Smoking-related lung carcinogenesis also involves a multitude of other alterations influencing the complex pathogenic pathways involved in lung cancer development, such as increased inflammation, aberrant apoptosis, increased angiogenesis, tumour progression and tumour metastasis (Wolff *et al.*, 1998; Heeschen *et al.*, 2001; Schuller, 2002; West *et al.*, 2003; Smith *et al.*, 2006; Lee *et al.*, 2008b; Section 4.1.5). Continued exposure to toxicants, genotoxicants, carcinogens, co-carcinogens and tumour promoters present in tobacco smoke has major effects on biological processes at all steps of multistep tumourigenesis of human lung (Hecht,

2003, 2008; Section 4.1). For example, nicotine in tobacco smoke is currently not described as a full carcinogen, but it exerts its biological effects via binding to nicotinic and other cellular receptors and likely enhances cell transformation and carcinogenicity through mechanisms not yet defined (Heeschen *et al.*, 2001; West *et al.*, 2003).

Numerous studies have provided evidence that the human genome may contain one or several loci that confer susceptibility to lung cancer. There are low-penetrance genes involved in the metabolism of tobacco smoke carcinogens, DNA repair and cell cycle control that may influence individual susceptibility to lung cancer (Spitz *et al.*, 2006). The role of the polymorphisms of these various classes of genes in lung carcinogenesis requires a systematic evaluation of the genetic evidence with stringent criteria (Ioannidis, 2008; Risch & Plass, 2008; Vineis *et al.*, 2009; Sections 4.1 and 4.2). Recently, genome-wide association studies have identified a susceptibility locus at chromosome 15q25.1 (Amos *et al.*, 2008; Hung *et al.*, 2008; Thorgeirsson *et al.*, 2008). The identity or function of the gene is not yet known, nor is the mechanism through which it may predispose to lung cancer. It is however likely that lung cancer susceptibility is related to the nicotine receptor gene residing at 15q25.1, and there is some evidence suggesting that it may be related to increased uptake of nicotine and NNK per cigarette (Le Marchand *et al.*, 2008).

In addition to genetic alterations, a growing body of evidence shows that epigenetic mechanisms, such as aberrant DNA methylation, histone modifications and RNA-mediated gene silencing are involved in cancer development (Jones & Baylin, 2007; Cortez & Jones, 2008). In lung carcinogenesis, gene promoter-associated (CpG island-specific) hypermethylation is an early and frequent event causing transcriptional inactivation of genes involved in regulation of cellular growth and differentiation (Belinsky, 2004). For example, several studies have indicated that the tumour suppressor gene *p16* ($p16^{INK4a/CDKN2A}$), a cell cycle regulator, is among the genes most frequently inactivated by aberrant methylation in lung cancer from smokers (Belinsky, 2004), with differences seen between smokers and never-smokers (Toyooka *et al.*, 2006). Significant associations have been established between smoking and promoter hypermethylation of tumour suppressor genes in lung tumours from smokers, and in plasma, serum or sputum DNA from cancer-free smokers (Belinsky, 2004; Belinsky *et al.*, 2005, 2006; Toyooka *et al.*, 2006).

(b) Oral cavity

PAHs can be carcinogenic at the site of application, which could include the human oral cavity. DMBA, a highly carcinogenic PAH not present in tobacco or tobacco smoke, is a standard model compound for induction of oral tumours in the hamster cheek pouch; less is known about the effects on the oral cavity of PAHs that do occur in tobacco products (Shklar, 1972; Rao, 1984; Vairaktaris *et al.*, 2008). A mixture of NNN and NNK induced oral tumours in rats when applied locally (Hecht *et al.*, 1986), and DNA adduct formation from NNN, NNK and NNAL has been observed in the rat oral cavity (Zhang *et al.*, 2009a, b). HPB-releasing DNA adducts from NNK and/or NNN have been reported in exfoliated oral cells from smokers and smokeless tobacco users (Heling *et al.*, 2008) and HPB-releasing heamoglobin adducts are elevated in smokeless tobacco users (IARC, 2007a). Unidentified DNA adduct levels are consistently elevated in oral cells and tissues from smokers compared to non-smokers (IARC, 2004a). Mutations in the *TP53* gene have been observed in oral tumours from smokers and smokeless tobacco users (IARC, 2006b, 2007a; Warnakulasuriya & Ralhan, 2007). Tobacco-associated genetic mutations including micronuclei, gene mutations, DNA polymorphisms, and chromosomal abnormalities have been reported in studies of buccal cells from smokers and smokeless tobacco users (Proia *et al.*, 2006). The use of lime by betel quid chewers is associated with enhanced oxidative damage that could play a role in inflammation or tumour promotion (IARC, 2004b).

(c) Larynx and nasopharynx

Hamsters exposed to cigarette smoke by inhalation consistently developed benign and malignant tumours of the larynx; tumours were produced by inhalation of the particulate phase, but not the gas phase of cigarette smoke (IARC, 1986). In related studies in which hamsters were treated with DMBA by intratracheal instillation followed by exposure to cigarette smoke, a significantly higher incidence of laryngeal tumours was observed than in hamsters exposed only to cigarette smoke or to DMBA (IARC, 1986). Collectively, these results indicate an initiation-promotion mechanism for the production of laryngeal tumours, and are consistent with the results of experiments in which tobacco smoke condensate is applied to mouse skin (IARC, 1986). The combined data implicate PAHs and tumour promoters in tobacco smoke as potential etiologic agents for cancer of the larynx in hamsters. Levels of DNA adducts measured by non-specific methods were higher in larynx tissue from smokers than from non-smokers (IARC, 2004a). Analyses of mutations in the *TP53* gene from tumours of the larynx in smokers show a pattern similar to that observed in lung tumours, and both are consistent with the pattern produced by PAH diol epoxides (IARC, 2006b). The available data are consistent with the conceptual framework illustrated in Fig. 4.1 (Szyfter *et al.*, 1999).

Formaldehyde, a constituent of cigarette smoke, causes nasopharyngeal cancer in humans (IARC, 2006a). A recent study demonstrates a 10-fold higher level of the formaldehyde-DNA adduct N^6-hydroxymethyldeoxyadenosine in leukocytes of smokers compared to non-smokers, suggesting its possible involvement in nasopharyngeal cancer in smokers (Wang *et al.*, 2009). Acetaldehyde, another carcinogenic constituent of tobacco smoke, which also forms genotoxic adducts (Section 4.1), may also contribute to the development of these forms of head and neck cancer.

(d) Oesophagus

Nitrosamines are probably the most effective oesophageal carcinogens known, with particularly strong activity in the rat (Lijinsky, 1992). NNN and NDEA are both present in cigarette smoke, and levels of NNN greatly exceed those of NDEA (IARC, 2004a). NNN is also present in considerable quantities in smokeless tobacco and betel quid containing tobacco (IARC, 2004a, 2007a). Thus, NNN is a likely candidate as a causative agent for esophageal cancer in smokers, smokeless tobacco users, and chewers of betel-quid with tobacco. While considerable mechanistic data are available from studies of NNN in laboratory animals (Hecht, 1998; Wong *et al.*, 2005; Lao *et al.*, 2007; Zhang *et al.*, 2009a), there are little comparable data in humans.

Increased acetaldehyde production derived both from tobacco smoke and from microbial alcohol oxidation may play a role in the synergistic carcinogenic action of alcohol and smoking on oesophagus, as well as on other upper aerodigestive locations (Homann *et al.*, 2000; Salaspuro & Salaspuro, 2004; Lee *et al.*, 2007a).

(e) Stomach

Hypermethylation of the E-cadherin 1 gene (*CDH1*) was observed preferentially in gastric tumours from smokers rather than non-smokers (Poplawski *et al.*, 2008). *CDH1* can act as a tumour-suppressor gene, preventing cells from growing and dividing in an uncontrolled way to form a cancerous tumour. Because the protein encoded by this gene helps cells stick together, altered regulation may lead to metastasis.

Boccia *et al.* (2007) found an increased risk for stomach cancer among smokers who had the *SULT1A1 His* genotype, and Lee *et al.* (2006) found an increased risk for those who had the *m2* allelic variant of *CYP1A1*. A nested case–control study found that smokers had an increased risk of gastric cancer if they carried at least one variant allele A in Ex7+129 C > A (*Thr*[461]*Asn, m4*) of *CYP1A1* (Agudo *et al.*, 2006). Stomach cancer tissue from smokers had higher levels of stable DNA adducts than did those from non-smokers; however, the number of non-smokers was quite small (Dyke *et al.*, 1992).

(f) Pancreas

NNK and its metabolite NNAL are the only pancreatic carcinogens known to be present in tobacco and tobacco smoke. NNK was detected in the pancreatic juice of 15 of 18 samples from smokers, at levels significantly higher than in non-smokers; NNAL and NNN were also detected in some samples (Prokopczyk *et al.*, 2002). DNA adducts of NNK and NNAL were present in pancreatic tissue of rats treated with these nitrosamines (Zhang *et al.*, 2009b), but were not detected in most human pancreatic tissue samples (Prokopczyk *et al.*, 2005).

(g) Colorectum

Tobacco smoke contains heterocyclic amines, such as 2-amino-1-methyl-6-phenylimidazo[4,5,6]pyridine (PhIP), which are intestinal carcinogens in rats and mutate the adenomatous polyposis coli (*Apc*) gene in mice (Møllersen *et al.*, 2004). The *APC* gene is frequently mutated and has altered expression in human colon cancer (Samowitz *et al.*, 2007; Samowitz, 2008). A recent model of colon cancer by Sweeney *et al.* (2009) suggests that this disease can develop via at least three independent mechanistic pathways. One pathway is initiated by methylation of *MINT* (methylation in tumour) markers that proceeds down a pathway predisposing to microsatellite instability, followed by methylation of the mismatch repair gene mutL homologue 1 (*MHL1*) and the tumour-suppressor gene *TP16*, followed by mutation in *BRAF* (a homologue of a viral raf oncogen). A second independent pathway is initiated with a mutation in the *APC* gene, followed by a mutation in the *TP53* gene. A third independent pathway involves only *KRAS2* mutations. One study found BPDE-DNA adducts at a higher frequency in colon DNA from smokers than from non-smokers (Alexandrov *et al.*, 1996). Mutations or epigenetic changes in some or all of these genes have been found in smoking-associated colon or colorectal tumours.

Microsatellite instability, which is the expansion or contraction of short nucleotide repeats, occurs in approximately 10–15% of sporadic colorectal cancer, and is usually associated with smoking and hypermethylation of the promoter of the mismatch repair gene *MLH1* (Samowitz, 2008). Smoking-associated colorectal tumours also have high frequencies of methylation at CpG islands (Samowitz, 2008).

In a case–control study of colorectal cancer, Kasahara *et al.* (2008) found that the genetic polymorphism *APEX1/APE1* (apurinic/apyrimidinic endonuclease-1) Asp[148]Glu, which is a gene involved in DNA repair, was associated with risk for colorectal cancer among smokers but not non-smokers. Other studies have also found associations between polymorphisms in the DNA repair genes *XRCC1* and smoking and risk for colorectal cancer (Stern *et al.*, 2007; Campbell *et al.*, 2009).

(h) Liver

Tobacco smoke contains liver carcinogens such as furan and certain nitrosamines. Liver tumours exhibit increased expression of *C-MYC*, *P16*^{INK4A}, epidermal growth factor receptor (*EGFR*), telomerase, transforming growth factor-α (*TGF-*α), insulin-like growth factor-2 (*IGF-2*) and *RAF* oncogene (Abou-Alfa, 2006). Smokers show altered expression of some of these genes or of genes in the same or similar pathways (Sen *et al.*, 2007). A genome-wide association study found that SNP rs1447295 in the 8q24 chromosome was positively associated with liver cancer among ever-smokers (Park *et al.*, 2008). Thus, tobacco smoke appears to have epigenetic effects on the liver that may contribute to hepatocellular carcinoma.

(i) Urinary bladder

Tobacco smoke contains aromatic amines such as 4-aminobiphenyl and 2-naphthylamine, which are human bladder carcinogens (see IARC, 2012a). In bladder tumours, smoking was associated with a more than twofold increase risk of methylation of the promoter region of the *P16*^{INK4A} gene and of the soluble Frizzled receptor protein (*SFRP*) gene (Marsit *et al.*, 2006). In addition, Tang *et al.* (2009) suggested that epigenetic silencing of *Wnt* antagonists through hypermethylation may play a role in smoking-related invasive bladder cancer (Tang *et al.*, 2009). SNP rs6983267 of the 8q24 chromosome was inversely associated with bladder cancer among ever-smokers (Park *et al.*, 2008). Smokers generally have mutagenic urine and smoking is associated with specific cytogenetic changes and DNA breaks in bladder tumours (DeMarini, 2004). Smoking-associated stable DNA adducts have been found in bladder tissue or exfoliated urothelial cells, supporting a role for DNA damage in smoking-associated bladder cancer (Phillips, 2002).

(j) Cervix

The cervical mucus of smokers is more mutagenic than that of non-smokers, and cervical epithelia of smokers have higher frequencies of micronuclei than those of non-smokers (DeMarini, 2004). Several studies have found increased levels of DNA adducts in cervical tissue from smokers relative to non-smokers, suggesting a role for smoking-associated DNA damage in cervical cancer (Phillips, 2002).

(k) Ovary

It has been observed that the inverse associations reported for serous and endometrioid tumours with respect to parity and oral contraceptives did not hold for the mucinous tumours. Based on these observations, Risch *et al.* (1996) suggested that mucinous ovarian tumours may be etiologically unrelated to the other types of epithelial tumours. Whereas mucinous elements such as gastric or intestinal type glands may be seen in mature teratomas, a form of germ cell neoplasia, overall mucinous tumours are classified as surface epithelial tumours because transitions among the subtypes may be observed. The major difference between mucinous and serous tumours is their biologic behaviour. Mucinous carcinomas of the ovary are slow growing tumours that appear to develop from their benign counterparts. The fact that the transitions between the benign, borderline, and malignant form of the disease can be seen in the same tumour suggests that over time, there is a progression from benign to malignant (Riopel *et al.*, 1999). *K-ras* mutational analysis, for example, demonstrates a heterogeneous distribution of the mutation within different parts of the same neoplasm, suggesting that acquisition of the *K-ras* mutation occurs in malignant transformation (Mandai *et al.*, 1998). Serous carcinomas seem to develop de novo rather than from a benign pre-existing lesion; alternatively, the rate of progression is rapid and the precursor lesion is obliterated before the detection of the tumour. In some data, current smoking is associated with a shorter interval to detection of mucinous than non-mucinous tumours. Because the mucinous tumour is slow growing, smoking could contribute to the malignant progression of the adenoma-carcinoma sequence, as the benign form of the tumour may have been present for some time.

(l) Leukaemia

Tobacco smoke contains known leukaemogens such as benzene, 1,3-butadiene and formaldehyde (IARC, 2012a). The mechanisms of leukaemogenesis are currently not well understood. Data indicate that leukaemogenic agents, such as benzene, cause toxicity to the haemotopoietic system, as well as genotoxicity at low levels, and that genetic polymorphisms may be involved in these processes (Aksoy, 1989; Lan *et al.*, 2004; Garte *et al.*, 2008; Hosgood *et al.*, 2009; Lau *et al.*, 2009; Rappaport *et al.*, 2009). Recent studies suggest the importance in carcinogen-related leukaemogenesis of damage to haematopoietic stem/progenitor cells circulating in the peripheral blood, or, alternatively, damage to primitive pluripotent progenitor cells present in other tissues (Zhang *et al.*, 2009c). In these two models, damaged stem/progenitor cells would then travel to the bone marrow and become initiated leukaemic stem cells. Mechanisms considered central in these models are: disruption of bone marrow DNA, through e.g. formation of DNA adducts, DNA–protein crosslinks, the action of free radicals or active states of oxygen; intercalation of metals within the DNA structure; or inhibition of enzymes involved in cell division (Zhang *et al.*, 2007, 2009c).

4.3.2 Sites with limited evidence of carcinogenicity or evidence suggesting lack of carcinogenicity

(a) Breast

(i) Carcinogenic pathway

Carcinogens found in tobacco smoke pass through the alveolar membrane and into the blood stream, by means of which they can be transported to the breast via plasma lipoproteins (Yamasaki & Ames, 1977; Shu & Bymun, 1983; Plant *et al.*, 1985). Tobacco smoke contains known rodent mammary carcinogens, including PAHs and aromatic amines (IARC, 1986, 2004a; el-Bayoumy, 1992; Ambrosone & Shields, 1999; Ambrosone, 2001; Hoffmann *et al.*, 2001) which, due to their lipophilicity, can be stored in breast adipose tissue (Obana *et al.*, 1981; Morris & Seifter, 1992) and then metabolized and activated by human mammary epithelial cells (MacNicoll *et al.*, 1980). Tobacco smoke constituents reach the breast as demonstrated by the detection of cotinine in breast fluid (Petrakis *et al.*, 1978). There is evidence suggesting the presence of mutagenic arylamines (Thompson *et al.*, 2002) and PAHs (Zanieri *et al.*, 2007) in human breast milk. Cigarette smoke condensate has been shown to transform normal human breast epithelial cells *in vitro* (Narayan *et al.*, 2004), perhaps by blocking long-patch base excision repair (Kundu *et al.*, 2007). Transformation and cytogenetic effects have been observed in human mammary epithelial cells after exposure to chemical carcinogens such as PAHs or arylamine (Mane *et al.*, 1990; Eldridge *et al.*, 1992; Calaf & Russo, 1993).

The formation of specific adducts from PAHs and aromatic amines has been observed in human breast epithelial cells *in vitro*, and unspecified-DNA adducts have been found in exfoliated ductal epithelial cells in human breast milk (Gorlewska-Roberts *et al.*, 2002; Thompson *et al.*, 2002).

Mutations in the *TP53* tumour suppressor gene have been found in 15–30% of breast cancers (Goldman & Shields, 1998; Olivier & Hainaut, 2001). An increased prevalence and altered spectrum of *TP53* mutations in breast tumours have been observed among current smokers compared with never smokers (Conway *et al.*, 2002). The breast tumours with the most pronounced smoking-related mutational pattern (for example, a greater number of G:C→T:A transversions) were from women who had smoked for more than 20 years, although total *TP53* mutations were not associated with smoking duration (Conway *et al.*, 2002). This increased frequency of G to T transversions in smokers versus non-smokers is also observed in the IARC TP53 database (IARC, 2006b; Van Emburgh *et al.*, 2008).

Recent meta-analyses of epidemiological studies tend to show positive associations of breast cancer with long-term smoking among *NAT2* slow acetylators, especially among post-menopausal women (who are more likely than pre-menopausal women to be very long-term smokers). Firozi *et al.* (2002) showed that breast tissue from *NAT2* slow acetylators had significantly higher levels of the diagonal radioactive zone (smoking-related) DNA adduct pattern than that from fast acetylators.

High rates of breast cancer in women exposed to ionizing radiation during adolescence (aged 10–19 years at exposure) (Tokunaga *et al.*, 1987) suggested that the adolescent breast may also be sensitive to the DNA-damaging effects of other exposures. This might also be true for the genotoxic compounds contained in tobacco smoke. Although some studies have supported such association, the results have been sparse and mixed. In addition, it is difficult to separate the effects of early life exposure to tobacco and smoking duration (Terry & Rohan, 2002).

Early age at first full-term pregnancy has been associated with reduced breast cancer risk (Kelsey *et al.*, 1993), hypothetically due to terminal differentiation of the breast epithelium that occurs late in the first trimester. It has been suggested that in the early stages of pregnancy, when growth-promoting hormone levels are high, but before terminal differentiation (Montelongo *et al.*, 1992), the breast may be particularly susceptible to the cancer-promoting chemicals in tobacco smoke. Several epidemiological studies compared measures of smoking before and after a first full-term pregnancy. Although suggestive, the data did not consistently show an increased risk for breast cancer among women who smoked before a first full-term pregnancy (Adami *et al.*, 1988; Hunter *et al.*, 1997; Band *et al.*, 2002; Egan *et al.*, 2003; Gram *et al.*, 2005; Li *et al.*, 2005; Olson *et al.*, 2005; Cui *et al.*, 2006). Smoking was associated with a 50% increased risk among women with slow *NAT2* acetylation genotype (Egan *et al.*, 2003). Overall, studies of risk in association with the timing of smoking relative to a first pregnancy are inconclusive; nevertheless, the breast tissue appears to have a greater susceptibility to the carcinogenic chemicals in tobacco smoke before compared to after terminal differentiation of breast epithelium.

(ii) Estrogenic pathway

The "anti-estrogenic" mechanism through which tobacco smoking may inhibit breast cancer progression is unclear. Estrogen is a known risk factor for breast cancer and several hypotheses have been proposed: earlier age at menopause among smokers, a reduction in the gastrointestinal absorption or distribution of estrogen, enhanced metabolism of estradiol to inactive catechol estrogens, increased binding of estrogens by serum sex hormone-binding globulin, lowered levels of estrogen derived from adipose tissue (Baron, 1984; Baron *et al.*, 1990; Terry & Rohan, 2002). Several studies of cigarette smoking and mammographically-defined breast density showed lower measures of breast density in current smokers than in non-smokers (Sala *et al.*, 2000; Vachon *et al.*, 2000; Warwick *et al.*, 2003; Jeffreys *et al.*, 2004; Modugno *et al.*, 2006; Bremnes *et al.*, 2007; Butler *et al.*, 2008). Since exposure to estrogen has been associated positively with breast density, a strong risk factor for breast cancer (McCormack & dos Santos Silva, 2006), the results of these studies are consistent with an anti-estrogenic effect of cigarette smoking. Although smokers and non-smokers may have the same concentrations of estrogens overall, it may be the type rather than the absolute levels of circulating estrogens that is important. Smokers might have a lower concentration of more biologically active estrogens, primarily 16-α-hydroxyestrone (16α-OHE1) (Michnovicz *et al.*, 1986, 1988; Berta *et al.*, 1992; Berstein *et al.*, 2000; Terry *et al.*, 2002b). Estrogen can be metabolized along three pathways, to 16α-OHE1 or to 2-OHE1 or to 4-OHE1. 16α-OHE1 and 4-OHE1 have been observed to increase mammary epithelial cell proliferation rates in experimental studies (Schütze *et al.*, 1993, 1994; IARC, 2007c). In contrast, 2-OHE1 might decrease epithelial cell proliferation rates (Bradlow *et al.*, 1996;

Muti *et al.*, 2000). If cigarette smoking increases estradiol 2-hydroxylation, as has been suggested (Michnovicz *et al.*, 1986), thereby increasing the ratio of 2-OHE1:16-α-OHE1, an inverse association between smoking and breast cancer risk might be observed. However, only one study has directly examined 2-hydroxylation in relation to cigarette smoking (Michnovicz *et al.*, 1986). Using injected radiolabelled estradiol, a 50% increased estradiol 2-hydroxylation was found in premenopausal women who smoked at least 15 cigarettes/day compared with non-smokers. Two studies of urinary estrogens found increased excretion of 2-OHE1 and decreased excretion of estriol among smokers (Michnovicz *et al.*, 1988; Berstein *et al.*, 2000), which may also support the hypothesis that smoking decreases the formation of active estrogen metabolites along the 16α-hydroxylation pathway. However, the ratio of urinary 2-OHE1:16α-OHE1 was not related to breast cancer risk in the one case–control study that examined the association (Ursin *et al.*, 1999). The 4-hydroxylation of estrogens is catalysed by CYP1B1, which is induced by tobacco smoke (Nebert *et al.*, 2004). This has been postulated as an additional pathway that could lead to formation of DNA adducts via catechol estrogen-quinones (Gaikwad *et al.*, 2008) and oxidative/DNA damage via redox-cycling (Zhu & Conney, 1998). The ratio of 2-OHE1:4-OHE1 has been studied in relation to breast cancer risk and smoking in one study (Berstein *et al.*, 2000). Smokers carrying the *CYP1B1 Val* allele [associated with high hydroxylation activity] had a significantly higher risk for breast cancer compared to never smokers with the *Leu/Leu* [wildtype] genotype (Saintot *et al.*, 2003).

(b) Endometrium

Exogenous estrogens unopposed by progesterone have been shown to increase the risk for endometrial cancer through increased mitotic activity of endometrial cells, increased number of DNA replication errors, and somatic mutations resulting in the malignant phenotype (IARC, 2007c, 2012c). Hence, factors associated with estrogen absorption or metabolism may alter the risk of this malignancy. Several investigators have hypothesized that cigarette smoking might be have anti-estrogenic effects, and through this mechanism reduce the risk of endometrial cancer (Baron, 1984; Baron *et al.*, 1990; Terry *et al.*, 2002b, 2004a).

Whether mediated through changes in the amount of adipose tissue, altered age at menopause, or anti-estrogenic effects, blood hormone concentrations might be an important link between smoking and the reduced risk of endometrial cancer observed in most epidemiological studies. The estrogens that have typically been studied in relation to cigarette smoking include estrone, sex hormone binding globulin (SHBG)-bound estradiol, and estriol. Blood concentrations of androgens, typically androstenedione and dehydroepiandrosterone sulfate (DHEAS), have also been studied, because these are biological precursors of estrone. Studies that have examined blood concentrations of SHBG are less common, and studies of unbound (free) estradiol are scarce.

Studies of cigarette smoking and blood hormone concentrations have been conducted mostly among post-menopausal women who were not taking HRT. Of these studies, nine examined serum (Friedman *et al.*, 1987; Cauley *et al.*, 1989; Slemenda *et al.*, 1989; Schlemmer *et al.*, 1990; Cassidenti *et al.*, 1992; Austin *et al.*, 1993; Law *et al.*, 1997) or plasma (Khaw *et al.*, 1988; Longcope & Johnston, 1988) estrone, ten examined serum (Friedman *et al.*, 1987; Cauley *et al.*, 1989; Slemenda *et al.*, 1989; Schlemmer *et al.*, 1990; Key *et al.*, 1991; Cassidenti *et al.*, 1992; Austin *et al.*, 1993; Law *et al.*, 1997) or plasma (Khaw *et al.*, 1988; Longcope & Johnston, 1988) estradiol, and two examined serum (Cassidenti *et al.*, 1992) or plasma (Longcope & Johnston, 1988) free estradiol. These studies consistently showed little or no association between smoking and blood estrogen concentrations among post-menopausal women who were not taking hormone replacement therapy. Among pre-menopausal women, three studies (Longcope & Johnston, 1988; Key *et al.*, 1991; Berta *et al.*, 1992) found no clear association between cigarette smoking and estrogen concentrations. Studies that adjusted hormone measurements for the effects of BMI (and other covariates) showed similar results to those that did not, suggesting that BMI is not a strong confounder of this association.

In two studies the association between cigarette smoking and blood estrogen concentrations after randomization of women to groups receiving either estradiol or placebo were examined (Jensen & Christiansen, 1988; Cassidenti *et al.*, 1990). In a small study of 25 post-menopausal women, unbound estradiol was significantly lower among smokers than non-smokers both at baseline and shortly after taking micronized estradiol orally (Cassidenti *et al.*, 1990). No important differences were observed between smokers and non-smokers in serum concentrations of either estrone or bound estradiol. In contrast, in a study in which 110 post-menopausal women were randomized to take hormones (either orally or percutaneously) or a placebo (Jensen & Christiansen, 1988), smokers had lower concentrations of both estrone and bound estradiol than non-smokers after oral (but not percutaneous) hormone treatment for at least one year (concentrations of free estrogens were not examined). These results indicate that smoking might affect the absorption or metabolism of hormones used in replacement therapy.

Of the five studies that have examined the association between cigarette smoking and serum (Lapidus *et al.*, 1986; Cassidenti *et al.*, 1992; Law *et al.*, 1997) or plasma (Khaw *et al.*, 1988; Longcope & Johnston, 1988) SHBG, none found any clear association. However, one of these studies (Khaw *et al.*, 1988) found an inverse association between smoking and the ratio of bound estradiol to SHBG, a measure of estrogen activity. In this context, Cassidenti *et al.* (1990) found unbound (but not SHBG-bound) estradiol was significantly lower among smokers than non-smokers both at baseline and after taking oral estradiol, suggesting an increased SHBG-binding capacity in the women who smoked.

In post-menopausal women, androgens are the major source of estrone, converted through aromatization in fat deposits. Thus, adiposity is positively correlated with estrogen concentrations in post-menopausal women. Of the nine studies in which blood concentrations of androstenedione were examined in smokers (Friedman *et al.*, 1987; Khaw *et al.*, 1988; Longcope & Johnston, 1988; Cauley *et al.*, 1989; Slemenda *et al.*, 1989; Schlemmer *et al.*, 1990; Cassidenti *et al.*, 1992; Austin *et al.*, 1993; Law *et al.*, 1997), higher circulating concentrations were found among current than among never or former smokers in all studies. However, there was no clear variation in blood estrone concentrations by smoking status, suggesting a reduced conversion of androstenedione to estrone among smokers. Of the five studies where cigarette smoking and DHEAS concentrations were examined, three (Khaw *et al.*, 1988; Cassidenti *et al.*, 1992; Law *et al.*, 1997) found increased blood concentrations among current smokers, one (Friedman *et al.*, 1987) found also an increase that was not statistically significant, whereas another (Key *et al.*, 1991) found no clear differences according to smoking status.

Cigarette smoking and urinary estrogen concentrations have been examined in seven studies (MacMahon *et al.*, 1982; Michnovicz *et al.*, 1986; Trichopoulos *et al.*, 1987; Michnovicz *et al.*, 1988; Berta *et al.*, 1992; Key *et al.*, 1996; Berstein *et al.*, 2000). Of these, three found no major differences according to smoking status (Trichopoulos *et al.*, 1987; Michnovicz *et al.*, 1988; Berta *et al.*, 1992). The remaining four studies all showed lower urinary estriol concentrations among smokers than among non-smokers, but mixed results for urinary estrone and estradiol.

Two of these studies (Michnovicz *et al.*, 1988; Berstein *et al.*, 2000) showed higher concentrations of 2-hydroxyestrone among smokers, than non-smokers but only after estrogen treatment in Berstein *et al.* (2000).

Age at natural menopause varies substantially under the influence of genetic and environmental factors (McKinlay, 1996). A relatively early age at menopause has been associated with reduced risk of endometrial cancer (Kelsey *et al.*, 1982; Baron, 1984; Baron *et al.*, 1990; Akhmedkhanov *et al.*, 2001). A one year decrease in age at menopause has been associated approximately with a 7% decrease in risk (Kelsey *et al.*, 1982). It has been proposed that cigarette smoking decreases the age at natural menopause (Baron *et al.*, 1990), more clearly with qualitative than quantitative smoking measures (Parente *et al.*, 2008), and thus might reduce endometrial cancer risk through reduced exposure to endogenous estrogens. On average, smokers have menopause approximately 1 to 1.5 years earlier than non-smokers (Terry *et al.*, 2002b, 2004a). Adjustment for obesity and other covariates did not alter the results (Terry *et al.*, 2002b).

4.4 Mechanistic considerations of the interaction of ethanol and tobacco carcinogens

The combined effects of alcoholic beverages and tobacco on the risk for cancer incidence and mortality have been widely studied in human populations. When tested for multiplicative and additive interactions, synergistic effects of alcoholic beverages and tobacco have been found, especially for oropharyngeal and oesophageal cancers (Homann *et al.*, 2000; Castellsagué *et al.*, 2004; Salaspuro & Salaspuro, 2004; Lee *et al.*, 2005a; Lee *et al.*, 2007b).

Data support at least four possible mechanisms for the modifying effects of alcoholic beverages on cancer risk due to tobacco.

1. Alcohol may have a local permeabilizing effect on penetration of the oral mucosa by tobacco carcinogens (Du *et al.*, 2000), particularly important in the case of oropharyngeal and oesophageal cancer.
2. CYP2E1 and other CYPs may both activate and detoxify carcinogens present in tobacco smoke, including NDMA, NDEA, NNK, benzene and other tobacco-derived carcinogens in two ways: CYP induction increases metabolic activation of tobacco carcinogens leading to enhanced formation of proximate reactive chemical species at target sites; and alteration of phase II conjugation/detoxification enzymes by ethanol may also occur, changing the effective dose at the target site.
3. Competitive inhibition of CYP metabolism leads to reduced central hepatic and gastrointestinal clearance thus increasing dose delivery of carcinogens to peripheral target tissues (reviewed in Meskar *et al.*, 2001).
4. Effects of acetaldehyde derived by microbial alcohol oxidation and from the tobacco smoke (Homann *et al.*, 2000; Salaspuro & Salaspuro, 2004).

Supportive evidence for ii) and iii) is briefly presented below.

4.4.1 Effects of induction of CYPs by ethanol

(a) CYP2E1

Ethanol induces CYP2E1 in the human liver and in all species tested. Over 70 substrates of CYP2E1 have been compiled (Raucy & Carpenter, 1993; Guengerich *et al.*, 1994; Djordjević *et al.*, 1998; Klotz & Ammon, 1998; Cederbaum, 2006). Among those are tobacco carcinogens such as benzene, vinyl chloride, NDMA, NDEA and *N*-nitrosopyrrolidine, as well as many low-molecular-weight compounds. Induction of CYP2E1 by ethanol generated increased levels of toxic metabolites from the metabolism of many of these chemicals (Novak & Woodcroft, 2000). Pyridine, a constituent of tobacco smoke and substrate of CYP2E1, generates DNA damaging products by redox-cycling (Kim & Novak, 1990).

In humans, in addition to the prominent CYP2E1 expression in the centrilobular regions of the liver, the enzyme is also detectable in the kidney cortex and, at lower levels, in organs such as the oropharynx, nasal mucosa, ovary, testis, small intestine, colon and pancreas (Ingelman-Sundberg *et al.*, 1994; Lieber, 1999, 2004).

In rats, ethanol induced CYP2E1 in epithelia of the cheek, tongue and oesophagus (Shimizu *et al.*, 1990). As a result of CYP2E1 induction by ethanol in the upper respiratory tract and possibly of inhibition of carcinogen clearance, hamsters had a significant increase of nasal cavity and tracheal tumours after intraperitoneal injection of *N*-nitrosopyrrolidine (McCoy *et al.*, 1981). Thus, induction of CYP2E1 by ethanol may participate in the genesis of cancers at several sites via metabolic activation of tobacco carcinogens into reactive species in target tissues.

(b) Other xenobiotic-activating CYPs

In addition to CYP2E1, several CYPs, including CYP3A4 and probably CYP1A2 in humans, and CYP1A1, 2B1 and 3A in rat liver, may be induced by ethanol. Of particular interest are members of the CYP3A family, which have wide substrate specificity and have been implicated in the activation of several known or suspected human carcinogens, including those derived from tobacco (Wojnowski & Kamdem, 2006). Both CYP3A4 and CYP1A2 metabolize NNK (Jalas *et al.*, 2005). Based on the Michaelis constant (Km) data (IARC, 2007a), the relative efficiencies in NNK metabolism by human CYP are (from greatest catalyst to least): 2A13 > 2B6 > 2A6 > 1A2 ~1A1 > 2D6 ~2E1 ~3A4. As the amount of CYP enzymes with overlapping substrate specificity that participate in nitrosamine metabolism varies according to organ and species, it is difficult to determine their individual contribution at target sites.

4.4.2 Effects of inhibition of CYPs by ethanol

Ethanol is a competitive inhibitor of CYP2E1 (reviewed in Anderson, 1992). It also inhibits the activities of CYP1A1, 2B6 and 2C19 but not those of CYP1A2.

Direct inhibition of CYPs by ethanol in target tissues may reduce metabolic activation of xenobiotics and hence local toxic and tumorigenic effects. Thus CYP inhibition in the liver could increase extrahepatic exposure to genotoxic metabolites from tobacco carcinogens that are substrates for these CYP enzymes. This mechanism is supported by several studies.

Ethanol caused a fivefold increase in oesophageal DNA adducts in rats induced by NDEA (Swann, 1984). In monkeys, O^6-methylguanine-DNA adducts after an oral dose of NDMA with or without ethanol were increased by co-exposure to ethanol in all tissues except the liver (Anderson *et al.*, 1996). Effects were seen in the oesophagus (17-fold increase), colonic mucosa (12-fold), pancreas (sixfold), urinary bladder (11-fold), ovary (ninefold), uterus (eightfold), brain (ninefold), spleen (13-fold) and nasal mucosa (fivefold). In these studies, ethanol treatment was acute, so that enzyme induction was improbable, and the oesophagus was not directly exposed to either ethanol or carcinogen. This indicates that a systemic interaction, most likely inhibition of hepatic carcinogen clearance, was responsible for the observed effects in the oesophagus and other extrahepatic tissues. The 17-fold increase in DNA adducts in the monkey oesophagus is similar to the 18-fold increased risk for human oesophageal cancers in tobacco smokers combined with heavy alcohol drinking (Tuyns *et al.*, 1977).

The relevance of increased genotoxic effects in extrahepatic target sites by ethanol is confirmed by many rodent experiments. Oral dosing of mice with NDMA in ethanol resulted in nasal cavity tumours (olfactory neuroblastoma) that were not seen with NDMA or ethanol alone (Griciute *et al.*, 1981). Ethanol in the drinking-water led to a ninefold increase in oesophageal tumours in rats induced by NDEA (Aze *et al.*, 1993). Ethanol given by gavage to nursing dams together with NDMA or NNK (Chhabra *et al.*, 2000) increased O^6-methylguanine-DNA adducts in maternal mammary glands, by 10-fold with NDMA and to a lesser extent with NNK. In the suckling infants, DNA adducts were detected in the lungs and kidneys after maternal exposure to NDMA and increased about fourfold after maternal co-treatment with ethanol. In mice, ethanol given with NDMA in the drinking-water resulted in a fourfold increase in lung tumours, but had no significant effect when NDMA was given intragastrically, intraperitoneally, subcutaneously or intravenously (Anderson, 1992). These negative findings support that direct inhibition of hepatic carcinogen clearance by ethanol is the main operative mechanism.

There is indirect evidence that ethanol can inhibit the *in vivo* clearance of the carcinogen NDMA in humans: individuals with chronic renal failure showed detectable blood and urine levels of NDMA, which were increased by consumption of ethanol (Dunn *et al.*, 1990). Other studies that involved sources of NDMA from tobacco smoke, diet or pharmaceuticals are consistent with ethanol reducing its clearance rate in humans (Anderson, 1992).

Other possible modifying effects of ethanol in tobacco-related tumorigenesis are presented in Section 4 of the *Monograph* on Consumption of Alcoholic Beverages in this Volume.

4.5 Synthesis

4.5.1 Mechanisms of tobacco-related carcinogenesis

The pathways by which tobacco products cause cancer essentially recapitulate established mechanisms of carcinogenesis by individual compounds, which were elaborated by landmark studies during the second half of the 20th century. These studies demonstrate that most carcinogens, either directly or after metabolism catalyzed by multiple cytochrome P450 enzymes, react with nucleophilic sites in DNA to form covalent binding products called adducts (a contraction for "addition products"). These DNA adducts, if left unrepaired by cellular DNA repair enzymes, persist and cause mistakes during DNA replication leading to incorporation of the wrong base in a DNA strand and consequent permanent mutations. If these permanent mutations occur in important regions of critical growth control genes such as the oncogene *KRAS* or the tumor suppressor gene *p53*, cellular growth processes can become severely unregulated and cancer can result. Multiple studies of mutations in *KRAS*, *p53*, and other growth control genes in lung tumours from smokers, some of which report thousands of mutations, are fully consistent with this overall concept.

It is the complexity of tobacco carcinogenesis which challenges investigators to identify specific mechanisms that fully explain the ways in which tobacco products cause each type of cancer. There are over 70 established carcinogens in cigarette smoke, and analyses of smokers' urine and blood clearly demonstrate higher uptake of these compounds in smokers than in non-smokers. The urine of smokers is consistently mutagenic. Similar considerations apply to smokeless tobacco users, although there are fewer identified carcinogens. Multiple DNA adducts are present in the lungs and other tissues of smokers, and sister chromatid exchanges as well as other genetic effects are consistently observed. But much less is known about the specifics of the process. Only relatively few DNA adducts in smokers' lungs have been structurally characterized and the relationship between specific adducts and the consequent mutations in critical genes is still somewhat unsettled.

There are other processes which contribute to cancer induction by tobacco products, based on multiple studies in both laboratory animals and humans. These include inflammation, tumor promotion, oxidative damage, co-carcinogenesis, and direct activation of cellular growth pathways by constituents of smoke. Many studies demonstrate the involvement of these processes in tobacco carcinogenesis but the details by which they interact with the DNA damage pathways and their roles in specific cancers caused by tobacco products are still not fully understood.

4.5.2 Genetic polymorphisms

Multiple studies have been carried out on the role of genetic polymorphisms of xenobiotic metabolism in smoking-related carcinogenesis in humans. These studies have covered various cancer types, with lung cancer representing one of the most intensively studied. The polymorphic genes, their variant forms, and the genotype combinations investigated in these studies have similarly been numerous. In addition to the associations with increased risk of cancer, much data have accumulated on relationships between the polymorphisms and the various biomarkers of tobacco carcinogenesis in non-cancer control populations, whether smokers or non-smokers, in subjects with work-related exposure or in patients with other cancers.

Despite the massive body of research, many observations remain ambiguous. Some associations between genetic polymorphism and increased risk for cancer, such as for the *GSTM1* null genotype, alone or in combination with *CYP1A1* polymorphism, in lung cancer, or the *NAT2* slow acetylator genotype in bladder cancer and breast cancer appear stronger and more consistent, but not without controversies. Similarly, the data on the various biomarkers of tobacco-related carcinogenesis exhibit inconsistencies.

The variability in the data is at least partially likely due to differences between the studies in the genes and gene variants included (many of which are still of unknown functional or regulatory consequence), in the types of cancer studied, in levels and sources of exposure, in ethnic backgrounds, in sex, in histological types and in the features of the genome such as haplotype blocks and copy number variation resulting in linkage disequilibrium. In addition, gene-gene interactions and gene-environment interactions are likely to contribute to the discrepancies in current data. Mechanisms of tobacco-related carcinogenesis also involve genes from numerous other classes, such as those encoding for DNA repair proteins and many other regulators of cell cycle and growth. In addition; there are well described mechanistic pathways of carcinogenesis mediated via epigenetic alterations and genetic instability, to mention a few.

4.5.3 Site-specific mechanisms

The Working Group reviewed the mechanistic evidence relative to specific target sites for which there is sufficient evidence of carcinogenicity in humans, i.e. lung, oral cavity, oesophagus, larynx and nasopharynx, pancreas, stomach, liver, urinary bladder, leukaemia, cervix and ovary. Genotoxic effects have been found in eight organ sites at which tobacco smoke causes cancer in humans (DeMarini, 2004).

Sites with limited evidence of carcinogenicity or evidence suggesting lack of carcinogenicity in humans include the breast and the endothelium and relevant mechanisms are presented below.

Breast — There are several plausible mechanisms by which smoking may increase breast cancer risk, and some data support such an effect, including the increased risk among long-term smokers with *NAT2* slow genotype. Despite the overall lack of clear association in epidemiological studies, and the potential anti-estrogenic effects of smoking, the possibility that smoking increases breast cancer risk is biologically plausible.

Endothelium — The mechanisms by which cigarette smoking reduces the risk for endometrial cancer among current smokers, mainly among postmenopausal, remain unclear.

4.5.4 Interaction of ethanol and tobacco carcinogens

Data in rodents and non-human primates on the relationships between a) inhibition of hepatic clearance of nitrosamines by ethanol, b) the formation of promutagenic DNA adducts and c) tumours in extra-hepatic targets, likely also pertain in humans.

5. Evaluation

There is *sufficient evidence* in humans for the carcinogenicity of tobacco smoking.

Tobacco smoking causes cancers of the lung, oral cavity, naso-, oro- and hypopharynx, nasal cavity and accesory sinuses, larynx, oesophagus, stomach, pancreas, colorectum, liver, kidney (body and pelvis), ureter, urinary bladder, uterine cervix and ovary (mucinous), and myeloid leukaemia. Also, a positive association has been observed between tobacco smoking and cancer of the female breast. For cancers of the endometrium (post-menopausal) and of the thyroid, there is *evidence suggesting lack of carcinogenicity*.

There is *sufficient evidence* in humans for the carcinogenicity of parental smoking. Parental smoking causes hepatoblastoma in children. Also, a positive association has been observed between parental smoking and childhood leukaemia (particularly acute lymphocytic leukaemia).

There is *sufficient evidence* in experimental animals for the carcinogenicity of tobacco smoke and of tobacco smoke condensates.

Tobacco smoking is *carcinogenic to humans (Group 1)*.

References

Abdel-Rahman SZ, Ammenheuser MM, Ward JB Jr (2001). Human sensitivity to 1,3-butadiene: role of microsomal epoxide hydrolase polymorphisms. *Carcinogenesis*, 22: 415–423. doi:10.1093/carcin/22.3.415 PMID:11238181

Abdel-Rahman SZ, El-Zein RA, Ammenheuser MM *et al.* (2003). Variability in human sensitivity to 1,3-butadiene: Influence of the allelic variants of the microsomal epoxide hydrolase gene. *Environ Mol Mutagen*, 41: 140–146. doi:10.1002/em.10142 PMID:12605384

Abou-Alfa GK (2006). Hepatocellular carcinoma: molecular biology and therapy. *Semin Oncol*, 33: Suppl 11S79–S83. doi:10.1053/j.seminoncol.2006.10.015 PMID:17178294

Abrams JA, Terry MB, Neugut AI (2008). Cigarette smoking and the colorectal adenoma-carcinoma sequence. *Gastroenterology*, 134: 617–619. doi:10.1053/j.gastro.2007.12.015 PMID:18242224

Adami HO, Lund E, Bergström R, Meirik O (1988). Cigarette smoking, alcohol consumption and risk of breast cancer in young women. *Br J Cancer*, 58: 832–837. PMID:3224085

Adami J, Nyrén O, Bergström R *et al.* (1998). Smoking and the risk of leukemia, lymphoma, and multiple myeloma (Sweden). *Cancer Causes Control*, 9: 49–56. doi:10.1023/A:1008897203337 PMID:9486463

Agudo A, Sala N, Pera G *et al.* (2006). Polymorphisms in metabolic genes related to tobacco smoke and the risk of gastric cancer in the European prospective investigation into cancer and nutrition. *Cancer Epidemiol Biomarkers Prev*, 15: 2427–2434. doi:10.1158/1055-9965.EPI-06-0072 PMID:17164366

Agundez JA (2004). Cytochrome P450 gene polymorphism and cancer. *Curr Drug Metab*, 5: 211–224. doi:10.2174/1389200043335621 PMID:15180491

Ahern TP, Lash TL, Egan KM, Baron JA (2009). Lifetime tobacco smoke exposure and breast cancer incidence. *Cancer Causes Control*, 20: 1837–1844. doi:10.1007/s10552-009-9376-1 PMID:19533391

Ahrendt SA, Decker PA, Alawi EA *et al.* (2001). Cigarette smoking is strongly associated with mutation of the *K-ras* gene in patients with primary adenocarcinoma of the lung. *Cancer*, 92: 1525–1530. doi:10.1002/1097-0142(20010915)92:6<1525::AID-CNCR1478>3.0.CO;2-H PMID:11745231

Ahrens W, Jöckel KH, Patzak W, Elsner G (1991). Alcohol, smoking, and occupational factors in cancer of the larynx: a case-control study. *Am J Ind Med*, 20: 477–493. doi:10.1002/ajim.4700200404 PMID:1785612

Ahrens W, Timmer A, Vyberg M *et al.* (2007). Risk factors for extrahepatic biliary tract carcinoma in men: medical conditions and lifestyle: results from a European multicentre case-control study. *Eur J Gastroenterol Hepatol*,

19: 623–630. doi:10.1097/01.meg.0000243876.79325.a1 PMID:17625430

Akhmedkhanov A, Zeleniuch-Jacquotte A, Toniolo P (2001). Role of exogenous and endogenous hormones in endometrial cancer: review of the evidence and research perspectives. *Ann N Y Acad Sci*, 943: 296–315. PMID:11594550

Akhter M, Nishino Y, Nakaya N *et al.* (2007). Cigarette smoking and the risk of colorectal cancer among men: a prospective study in Japan. *Eur J Cancer Prev*, 16: 102–107. doi:10.1097/01.cej.0000228412.98847.bc PMID:17297385

Akiba S (1994). Analysis of cancer risk related to longitudinal information on smoking habits. *Environ Health Perspect*, 102: Suppl 815–19. PMID:7851325

Akiba S & Hirayama T (1990). Cigarette smoking and cancer mortality risk in Japanese men and women–results from reanalysis of the six-prefecture cohort study data. *Environ Health Perspect*, 87: 19–26. doi:10.2307/3431001 PMID:2269225

Aksoy M (1989). Hematotoxicity and carcinogenicity of benzene. *Environ Health Perspect*, 82: 193–197. doi:10.2307/3430775 PMID:2676498

Al-Delaimy WK (2002). Hair as a biomarker for exposure to tobacco smoke. *Tob Control*, 11: 176–182. doi:10.1136/tc.11.3.176 PMID:12198265

Al-Delaimy WK, Cho E, Chen WY *et al.* (2004). A prospective study of smoking and risk of breast cancer in young adult women. *Cancer Epidemiol Biomarkers Prev*, 13: 398–404. PMID:15006915

Al-Delaimy WK & Willett WC (2008). Measurement of tobacco smoke exposure: comparison of toenail nicotine biomarkers and self-reports. *Cancer Epidemiol Biomarkers Prev*, 17: 1255–1261. doi:10.1158/1055-9965.EPI-07-2695 PMID:18483348

Al-Zoughool M, Dossus L, Kaaks R *et al.* (2007). Risk of endometrial cancer in relationship to cigarette smoking: results from the EPIC study. *Int J Cancer*, 121: 2741–2747. doi:10.1002/ijc.22990 PMID:17657712

Alberg AJ, Daudt A, Huang HY *et al.* (2004). N-acetyltransferase 2 (*NAT2*) genotypes, cigarette smoking, and the risk of breast cancer. *Cancer Detect Prev*, 28: 187–193. doi:10.1016/j.cdp.2004.04.001 PMID:15225898

Alberg AJ, Kouzis A, Genkinger JM *et al.* (2007). A prospective cohort study of bladder cancer risk in relation to active cigarette smoking and household exposure to secondhand cigarette smoke. *Am J Epidemiol*, 165: 660–666. doi:10.1093/aje/kwk047 PMID:17204516

Alexandrie AK, Warholm M, Carstensen U *et al.* (2000). CYP1A1 and GSTM1 polymorphisms affect urinary 1-hydroxypyrene levels after PAH exposure. *Carcinogenesis*, 21: 669–676. doi:10.1093/carcin/21.4.669 PMID:10753202

Alexandrov K, Cascorbi I, Rojas M *et al.* (2002). CYP1A1 and GSTM1 genotypes affect benzo[a]pyrene DNA adducts in smokers' lung: comparison with aromatic/hydrophobic adduct formation. *Carcinogenesis*, 23: 1969–1977. doi:10.1093/carcin/23.12.1969 PMID:12507920

Alexandrov K, Rojas M, Kadlubar FF *et al.* (1996). Evidence of *anti*-benzo[*a*]pyrene diolepoxide-DNA adduct formation in human colon mucosa. *Carcinogenesis*, 17: 2081–2083. doi:10.1093/carcin/17.9.2081 PMID:8824539

Alfano CM, Klesges RC, Murray DM *et al.* (2004). Physical activity in relation to all-site and lung cancer incidence and mortality in current and former smokers. *Cancer Epidemiology, Biomarkers & Prevention*, 13: 2233–2241.

Alguacil J & Silverman DT (2004). Smokeless and other noncigarette tobacco use and pancreatic cancer: a case-control study based on direct interviews. *Cancer Epidemiol Biomarkers Prev*, 13: 55–58. doi:10.1158/1055-9965.EPI-03-0033 PMID:14744733

Ambrosone CB (2001). Impact of genetics on the relationship between smoking and breast cancer risk. *Journal of Women's Cancer*, 3: 17–22.

Ambrosone CB, Freudenheim JL, Graham S *et al.* (1996). Cigarette smoking, N-acetyltransferase 2 genetic polymorphisms, and breast cancer risk. *JAMA*, 276: 1494–1501. doi:10.1001/jama.276.18.1494 PMID:8903261

Ambrosone CB, Kropp S, Yang J *et al.* (2008). Cigarette smoking, *N-acetyltransferase 2* genotypes, and breast cancer risk: pooled analysis and meta-analysis. *Cancer Epidemiol Biomarkers Prev*, 17: 15–26. doi:10.1158/1055-9965.EPI-07-0598 PMID:18187392

Ambrosone CB, Shields PG (1999). *Smoking as a risk factor for breast cancer.* In: *Breast cancer: molecular genetics, pathogenesis, and therapeutics.* Bowcock AM, editor. Tetowa, NJ: Humana Press, pp. 519–536,.

Amos CI, Wu X, Broderick P *et al.* (2008). Genome-wide association scan of tag SNPs identifies a susceptibility locus for lung cancer at 15q25.1. *Nat Genet*, 40: 616–622. doi:10.1038/ng.109 PMID:18385676

Andersen V, Agerstjerne L, Jensen D *et al.* (2009). The multidrug resistance 1 (MDR1) gene polymorphism G-rs3789243-A is not associated with disease susceptibility in Norwegian patients with colorectal adenoma and colorectal cancer; a case control study. *BMC Med Genet*, 10: 18 doi:10.1186/1471-2350-10-18 PMID:19250544

Anderson JC, Attam R, Alpern Z *et al.* (2003). Prevalence of colorectal neoplasia in smokers. *Am J Gastroenterol*, 98: 2777–2783. doi:10.1111/j.1572-0241.2003.08671.x PMID:14687832

Anderson LM (1992). *Modulation of nitrosamine metabolism by ethanol: implications for cancer risk.* In: *Alcohol and Cancer.* Watson RR, editor. Boca Raton, FL: CRC Press, pp. 17–54.

Anderson LM, Souliotis VL, Chhabra SK *et al.* (1996). *N*-nitrosodimethylamine-derived O[6]-methylguanine in DNA of monkey gastrointestinal and urogenital organs and enhancement by ethanol. *Int J Cancer*, 66: 130–134. doi:10.1002/(SICI)1097-0215(19960328)66:1<130::AID-IJC22>3.0.CO;2-G PMID:8608956

Ansary-Moghaddam A, Huxley R, Barzi F *et al.*Asia Pacific Cohort Studies Collaboration (2006). The effect of modifiable risk factors on pancreatic cancer mortality in populations of the Asia-Pacific region. *Cancer Epidemiol Biomarkers Prev*, 15: 2435–2440. doi:10.1158/1055-9965.EPI-06-0368 PMID:17164367

Applebaum KM, Furniss CS, Zeka A *et al.* (2007). Lack of association of alcohol and tobacco with HPV16-associated head and neck cancer. *J Natl Cancer Inst*, 99: 1801–1810. doi:10.1093/jnci/djm233 PMID:18042931

Appleby P, Beral V, Berrington de González A *et al.* International Collaboration of Epidemiological Studies of Cervical Cancer (2006). Carcinoma of the cervix and tobacco smoking: collaborative reanalysis of individual data on 13,541 women with carcinoma of the cervix and 23,017 women without carcinoma of the cervix from 23 epidemiological studies. *Int J Cancer*, 118: 1481–1495. doi:10.1002/ijc.21493 PMID:16206285

Arif JM, Dresler C, Clapper ML *et al.* (2006). Lung DNA adducts detected in human smokers are unrelated to typical polyaromatic carcinogens. *Chem Res Toxicol*, 19: 295–299. doi:10.1021/tx0502443 PMID:16485906

Armstrong RW, Imrey PB, Lye MS *et al.* (2000). Nasopharyngeal carcinoma in Malaysian Chinese: occupational exposures to particles, formaldehyde and heat. *Int J Epidemiol*, 29: 991–998. doi:10.1093/ije/29.6.991 PMID:11101539

Ashktorab H, Begum R, Akhgar A *et al.* (2007). Folate status and risk of colorectal polyps in African Americans. *Dig Dis Sci*, 52: 1462–1470. doi:10.1007/s10620-006-9236-8 PMID:17372834

Asma S, Bettcher DW, Samet J *et al.* (2009). *Tobacco*. In: *Oxford Textbook Of Public Health*. Detels R, editor. Oxford: Oxford University Press.

Ateş NA, Tamer L, Ateş C *et al.* (2005). Glutathione S-transferase M1, T1, P1 genotypes and risk for development of colorectal cancer. *Biochem Genet*, 43: 149–163. doi:10.1007/s10528-005-1508-z PMID:15932063

Austin H, Drews C, Partridge EE (1993). A case-control study of endometrial cancer in relation to cigarette smoking, serum estrogen levels, and alcohol use. *Am J Obstet Gynecol*, 169: 1086–1091. PMID:8238164

Autrup H (2000). Genetic polymorphisms in human xenobiotica metabolizing enzymes as susceptibility factors in toxic response. *Mutat Res*, 464: 65–76. PMID:10633178

Aze Y, Toyoda K, Furukawa F *et al.* (1993). Enhancing effect of ethanol on esophageal tumor development in rats by initiation of diethylnitrosamine. *Carcinogenesis*, 14: 37–40. doi:10.1093/carcin/14.1.37 PMID:8425269

Bain C, Feskanich D, Speizer FE *et al.* (2004). Lung cancer rates in men and women with comparable histories of smoking. *J Natl Cancer Inst*, 96: 826–834. PMID:15173266

Baker JA, Odunuga OO, Rodabaugh KJ *et al.* (2006). Active and passive smoking and risk of ovarian cancer. *Int J Gynecol Cancer*, 16: Suppl 1211–218. doi:10.1111/j.1525-1438.2006.00473.x PMID:16515593

Balansky R, Ganchev G, Iltcheva M *et al.* (2007). Potent carcinogenicity of cigarette smoke in mice exposed early in life. *Carcinogenesis*, 28: 2236–2243. doi:10.1093/carcin/bgm122 PMID:17522065

Balaram P, Sridhar H, Rajkumar T *et al.* (2002). Oral cancer in southern India: the influence of smoking, drinking, paan-chewing and oral hygiene. *Int J Cancer*, 98: 440–445. doi:10.1002/ijc.10200 PMID:11920597

Bamber DE, Fryer AA, Strange RC *et al.* (2001). Phenol sulphotransferase *SULT1A1*1* genotype is associated with reduced risk of colorectal cancer. *Pharmacogenetics*, 11: 679–685. doi:10.1097/00008571-200111000-00006 PMID:11692076

Band PR, Le ND, Fang R, Deschamps M (2002). Carcinogenic and endocrine disrupting effects of cigarette smoke and risk of breast cancer. *Lancet*, 360: 1044–1049. doi:10.1016/S0140-6736(02)11140-8 PMID:12383984

Baron JA (1984). Smoking and estrogen-related disease. *Am J Epidemiol*, 119: 9–22. PMID:6362403

Baron JA, Byers T, Greenberg ER *et al.* (1986). Cigarette smoking in women with cancers of the breast and reproductive organs. *J Natl Cancer Inst*, 77: 677–680. PMID:3462409

Baron JA, La Vecchia C, Levi F (1990). The antiestrogenic effect of cigarette smoking in women. *Am J Obstet Gynecol*, 162: 502–514. PMID:2178432

Baron JA, Newcomb PA, Longnecker MP *et al.* (1996). Cigarette smoking and breast cancer. *Cancer Epidemiol Biomarkers Prev*, 5: 399–403. PMID:9162307

Barra S, Barón AE, Franceschi S *et al.* (1991). Cancer and non-cancer controls in studies on the effect of tobacco and alcohol consumption. *Int J Epidemiol*, 20: 845–851. doi:10.1093/ije/20.4.845 PMID:1800421

Bartsch H, Nair U, Risch A *et al.* (2000). Genetic polymorphism of *CYP* genes, alone or in combination, as a risk modifier of tobacco-related cancers. *Cancer Epidemiol Biomarkers Prev*, 9: 3–28. PMID:10667460

Batty GD, Kivimaki M, Gray L *et al.* (2008). Cigarette smoking and site-specific cancer mortality: testing uncertain associations using extended follow-up of the original Whitehall study. *Ann Oncol*, 19: 996–1002. doi:10.1093/annonc/mdm578 PMID:18212091

Baumgartner KB, Schlierf TJ, Yang D *et al.* (2009). N-acetyltransferase 2 genotype modification of active cigarette smoking on breast cancer risk among hispanic and non-hispanic white women. *Toxicol Sci*, 112: 211–220. PMID:19692670

Belinsky SA (2004). Gene-promoter hypermethylation as a biomarker in lung cancer. *Nat Rev Cancer*, 4: 707–717. PMID:15343277

Belinsky SA (2005). Silencing of genes by promoter hypermethylation: key event in rodent and human lung cancer. *Carcinogenesis*, 26: 1481–1487. doi:10.1093/carcin/bgi020 PMID:15661809

Belinsky SA, Klinge DM, Dekker JD *et al.* (2005). Gene promoter methylation in plasma and sputum increases with lung cancer risk. *Clin Cancer Res*, 11: 6505–6511. PMID:16166426

Belinsky SA, Liechty KC, Gentry FD *et al.* (2006). Promoter hypermethylation of multiple genes in sputum precedes lung cancer incidence in a high-risk cohort. *Cancer Res*, 66: 3338–3344. PMID:16540689

Benhamou S, Lee WJ, Alexandrie AK *et al.* (2002). Meta- and pooled analyses of the effects of glutathione *S*-transferase M1 polymorphisms and smoking on lung cancer risk. *Carcinogenesis*, 23: 1343–1350. doi:10.1093/carcin/23.8.1343 PMID:12151353

Beral V, Bull D, Reeves GMillion Women Study Collaborators (2005). Endometrial cancer and hormone-replacement therapy in the Million Women Study. *Lancet*, 365: 1543–1551. doi:10.1016/S0140-6736(05)66455-0 PMID:15866308

Bergmark E (1997). Hemoglobin adducts of acrylamide and acrylonitrile in laboratory workers, smokers and nonsmokers. *Chem Res Toxicol*, 10: 78–84. doi:10.1021/tx960113p PMID:9074806

Bernfeld P, Homburger F, Russfield AB (1974). Strain differences in the response of inbred Syrian hamsters to cigarette smoke inhalation. *J Natl Cancer Inst*, 53: 1141–1157. PMID:4279301

Bernfeld P, Homburger F, Soto E, Pai KJ (1979). Cigarette smoke inhalation studies in inbred Syrian golden hamsters. *J Natl Cancer Inst*, 63: 675–689. PMID:288930

Berrettini W, Yuan X, Tozzi F *et al.* (2008). Alpha-5/alpha-3 nicotinic receptor subunit alleles increase risk for heavy smoking. *Mol Psychiatry*, 13: 368–373. doi:10.1038/sj.mp.4002154 PMID:18227835

Berrington de González A, Sweetland S, Green J (2004). Comparison of risk factors for squamous cell and adenocarcinomas of the cervix: a meta-analysis. *Br J Cancer*, 90: 1787–1791. PMID:15150591

Berstein LM, Tsyrlina EV, Kolesnik OS *et al.* (2000). Catecholestrogens excretion in smoking and non-smoking postmenopausal women receiving estrogen replacement therapy. *J Steroid Biochem Mol Biol*, 72: 143–147. doi:10.1016/S0960-0760(00)00038-8 PMID:10775805

Berta L, Fortunati N, Gennari P *et al.* (1991). Influence of cigarette smoking on pituitary and sex hormone balance in healthy premenopausal women. *Fertil Steril*, 56: 788–789. PMID:1915961

Berta L, Frairia R, Fortunati N *et al.* (1992). Smoking effects on the hormonal balance of fertile women. *Horm Res*, 37: 45–48. doi:10.1159/000182280 PMID:1398476

Besson H, Brennan P, Becker N *et al.* (2006). Tobacco smoking, alcohol drinking and Hodgkin's lymphoma: A European multicenter case-control study (Epilymph). *Br J Cancer*, 95: 378–384.

Bhutani M, Pathak AK, Fan YH *et al.* (2008). Oral epithelium as a surrogate tissue for assessing smoking-induced molecular alterations in the lungs. *Cancer Prev Res (Phila)*, 1: 39–44. PMID:19138934

Bin P, Leng S, Cheng J *et al.* (2008). Association of aryl hydrocarbon receptor gene polymorphisms and urinary 1-hydroxypyrene in polycyclic aromatic hydrocarbon-exposed workers. *Cancer Epidemiol Biomarkers Prev*, 17: 1702–1708. doi:10.1158/1055-9965.EPI-07-2812 PMID:18628420

Bjelke E (1975). Dietary vitamin A and human lung cancer. *Int J Cancer*, 15: 561–565. doi:10.1002/ijc.2910150405 PMID:1140863

Bjerregaard BK, Raaschou-Nielsen O, Sørensen M *et al.* (2006). Tobacco smoke and bladder cancer–in the European Prospective Investigation into Cancer and Nutrition. *Int J Cancer*, 119: 2412–2416. doi:10.1002/ijc.22169 PMID:16894557

Bjørge T, Engeland A, Tretli S, Weiderpass E (2007). Body size in relation to cancer of the uterine corpus in 1 million Norwegian women. *Int J Cancer*, 120: 378–383. doi:10.1002/ijc.22260 PMID:17066451

Bleeker MC, Heideman DA, Snijders PJ *et al.* (2009). Penile cancer: epidemiology, pathogenesis and prevention. *World J Urol*, 27: 141–150. doi:10.1007/s00345-008-0302-z PMID:18607597

Blot WJ, Devesa SS, Kneller RW, Fraumeni JF Jr (1991). Rising incidence of adenocarcinoma of the esophagus and gastric cardia. *JAMA*, 265: 1287–1289. doi:10.1001/jama.265.10.1287 PMID:1995976

Blot WJ, McLaughlin JK, Winn DM *et al.* (1988). Smoking and drinking in relation to oral and pharyngeal cancer. *Cancer Res*, 48: 3282–3287. PMID:3365707

Boccia S, Sayed-Tabatabaei FA, Persiani R *et al.* (2007). Polymorphisms in metabolic genes, their combination and interaction with tobacco smoke and alcohol consumption and risk of gastric cancer: a case-control study in an Italian population. *BMC Cancer*, 7: 206 PMID:17996038

Bode AM & Dong Z (2005). Signal transduction pathways in cancer development and as targets for cancer prevention. *Prog Nucleic Acid Res Mol Biol*, 79: 237–297. PMID:16096030

Boffetta P, Clark S, Shen M *et al.* (2006). Serum cotinine level as predictor of lung cancer risk. *Cancer Epidemiol Biomarkers Prev*, 15: 1184–1188. doi:10.1158/1055-9965.EPI-06-0032 PMID:16775179

Boffetta P, Hecht SS, Gray N *et al.* (2008). Smokeless tobacco and cancer. *Lancet Oncol*, 9: 667–675. doi:10.1016/S1470-2045(08)70173-6 PMID:18598931

Bogen E (1929). The composition of cigarets and cigaret smoke. *Journal of the American Medical Association*, 93: 1110–1114.

Bolt HM & Thier R (2006). Relevance of the deletion polymorphisms of the glutathione *S*-transferases *GSTT1* and *GSTM1* in pharmacology and toxicology. *Curr Drug Metab*, 7: 613–628. doi:10.2174/138920006778017786 PMID:16918316

Bono R, Vincenti M, Saglia U *et al.* (2002). Tobacco smoke and formation of *N*-(2-hydroxyethyl)valine in human hemoglobin. *Arch Environ Health*, 57: 416–421. doi:10.1080/00039890209601430 PMID:12641182

Borgerding M & Klus H (2005). Analysis of complex mixtures–cigarette smoke. *Exp Toxicol Pathol*, 57: Suppl 143–73. doi:10.1016/j.etp.2005.05.010 PMID:16092717

Borlak J & Reamon-Buettner SM (2006). N-acetyltransferase 2 (NAT2) gene polymorphisms in colon and lung cancer patients. *BMC Med Genet*, 7: 58 doi:10.1186/1471-2350-7-58 PMID:16827944

Bosetti C, Gallus S, Peto R *et al.* (2008). Tobacco smoking, smoking cessation, and cumulative risk of upper aerodigestive tract cancers. *Am J Epidemiol*, 167: 468–473. doi:10.1093/aje/kwm318 PMID:18056925

Bosetti C, Garavello W, Gallus S, La Vecchia C (2006). Effects of smoking cessation on the risk of laryngeal cancer: an overview of published studies. *Oral Oncol*, 42: 866–872. doi:10.1016/j.oraloncology.2006.02.008 PMID:16931120

Bosetti C, Negri E, Franceschi S *et al.* (2000a). Risk factors for oral and pharyngeal cancer in women: a study from Italy and Switzerland. *Br J Cancer*, 82: 204–207. PMID:10638990

Botteri E, Iodice S, Bagnardi V *et al.* (2008a). Smoking and colorectal cancer: a meta-analysis. *JAMA*, 300: 2765–2778. doi:10.1001/jama.2008.839 PMID:19088354

Botteri E, Iodice S, Raimondi S *et al.* (2008b). Cigarette smoking and adenomatous polyps: a meta-analysis. *Gastroenterology*, 134: 388–395. doi:10.1053/j.gastro.2007.11.007 PMID:18242207

Boyd AS, Shyr Y, King LE Jr (2002). Basal cell carcinoma in young women: an evaluation of the association of tanning bed use and smoking. *J Am Acad Dermatol*, 46: 706–709. doi:10.1067/mjd.2002.120467 PMID:12004311

Boyle P, Maisonneuve P, Bueno de Mesquita B *et al.* (1996). Cigarette smoking and pancreas cancer: a case control study of the search programme of the IARC. *Int J Cancer*, 67: 63–71. doi:10.1002/(SICI)1097-0215(19960703)67:1<63::AID-IJC12>3.0.CO;2-D PMID:8690527

Boysen G & Hecht SS (2003). Analysis of DNA and protein adducts of benzo[a]pyrene in human tissues using structure-specific methods. *Mutat Res*, 543: 17–30. doi:10.1016/S1383-5742(02)00068-6 PMID:12510015

Bracci PM & Holly EA (2005). Tobacco use and non-Hodgkin lymphoma: results from a population-based case-control study in the San Francisco Bay Area, California. *Cancer Causes Control*, 16: 333–346.

Bradlow HL, Telang NT, Sepkovic DW, Osborne MP (1996). 2-hydroxyestrone: the 'good' estrogen. *J Endocrinol*, 150: SupplS259–S265. PMID:8943806

Breast Cancer Family Registry; Kathleen Cuningham Consortium for Research into Familial Breast Cancer (Australasia) Ontario Cancer Genetics Network (Canada) (2008). Smoking and risk of breast cancer in carriers of mutations in BRCA1 or BRCA2 aged less than 50 years. *Breast Cancer Res Treat*, 109: 67–75. doi:10.1007/s10549-007-9621-9 PMID:17972172

Bremnes Y, Ursin G, Bjurstam N, Gram IT (2007). Different measures of smoking exposure and mammographic density in postmenopausal Norwegian women: a cross-sectional study. *Breast Cancer Res*, 9: R73 doi:10.1186/bcr1782 PMID:17963507

Brennan P, Hsu CC, Moullan N *et al.* (2005). Effect of cruciferous vegetables on lung cancer in patients stratified by genetic status: a mendelian randomisation approach. *Lancet*, 366: 1558–1560. PMID:16257343

Brennan P, van der Hel O, Moore LE *et al.* (2008). Tobacco smoking, body mass index, hypertension, and kidney cancer risk in central and eastern Europe. *Br J Cancer*, 99: 1912–1915. doi:10.1038/sj.bjc.6604761 PMID:19034282

Brenner H, Arndt V, Bode G *et al.* (2002). Risk of gastric cancer among smokers infected with Helicobacter pylori. *Int J Cancer*, 98: 446–449. doi:10.1002/ijc.10201 PMID:11920598

Brinton LA, Barrett RJ, Berman ML *et al.* (1993). Cigarette smoking and the risk of endometrial cancer. *Am J Epidemiol*, 137: 281–291. PMID:8452136

Brinton LA, Blot WJ, Becker JA *et al.* (1984). A case-control study of cancers of the nasal cavity and paranasal sinuses. *Am J Epidemiol*, 119: 896–906. PMID:6731431

Brinton LA, Schairer C, Stanford JL, Hoover RN (1986). Cigarette smoking and breast cancer. *Am J Epidemiol*, 123: 614–622. PMID:3953540

Brooks DR, Palmer JR, Strom BL, Rosenberg L (2003). Menthol cigarettes and risk of lung cancer. *Am J Epidemiol*, 158: 609–616, discussion 617–620. doi:10.1093/aje/kwg182 PMID:14507595

Brown LM, Blot WJ, Schuman SH *et al.* (1988). Environmental factors and high risk of esophageal cancer among men in coastal South Carolina. *J Natl Cancer Inst*, 80: 1620–1625. doi:10.1093/jnci/80.20.1620 PMID:3193480

Brown LM, Hoover R, Silverman D *et al.* (2001). Excess incidence of squamous cell esophageal cancer among US Black men: role of social class and other risk factors.

Am J Epidemiol, 153: 114–122. doi:10.1093/aje/153.2.114 PMID:11159155

Brown LM, Hoover RN, Greenberg RS *et al.* (1994a). Are racial differences in squamous cell esophageal cancer explained by alcohol and tobacco use? *J Natl Cancer Inst*, 86: 1340–1345. doi:10.1093/jnci/86.17.1340 PMID:8064893

Brown LM, Silverman DT, Pottern LM *et al.* (1994b). Adenocarcinoma of the esophagus and esophagogastric junction in white men in the United States: alcohol, tobacco, and socioeconomic factors. *Cancer Causes Control*, 5: 333–340. doi:10.1007/BF01804984 PMID:8080945

Brugere J, Guenel P, Leclerc A, Rodriguez J (1986). Differential effects of tobacco and alcohol in cancer of the larynx, pharynx, and mouth. *Cancer*, 57: 391–395. doi:10.1002/1097-0142(19860115)57:2<391::AID-CNCR2820570235>3.0.CO;2-Q PMID:3942973

Brunet JS, Ghadirian P, Rebbeck TR *et al.* (1998). Effect of smoking on breast cancer in carriers of mutant BRCA1 or BRCA2 genes. *J Natl Cancer Inst*, 90: 761–766. doi:10.1093/jnci/90.10.761 PMID:9605646

Bufalo NE, Leite JL, Guilhen ACT *et al.* (2006). Smoking and susceptibility to thyroid cancer: an inverse association with CYP1A1 allelic variants. *Endocr Relat Cancer*, 13: 1185–1193. doi:10.1677/ERC-06-0002 PMID:17158763

Bundgaard T, Wildt J, Frydenberg M *et al.* (1995). Case-control study of squamous cell cancer of the oral cavity in Denmark. *Cancer Causes Control*, 6: 57–67. doi:10.1007/BF00051681 PMID:7718736

Burchell B (2003). Genetic variation of human UDP-glucuronosyltransferase: implications in disease and drug glucuronidation. *Am J Pharmacogenomics*, 3: 37–52. PMID:12562215

Butler LM, Gold EB, Greendale GA *et al.* (2008). Menstrual and reproductive factors in relation to mammographic density: the Study of Women's Health Across the Nation (SWAN). *Breast Cancer Res Treat*, 112: 165–174. doi:10.1007/s10549-007-9840-0 PMID:18066689

Butler LM, Wang R, Wong AS *et al.* (2009). Cigarette smoking and risk of prostate cancer among Singapore Chinese. *Cancer Causes Control*, 20: 1967–1974.

Calaf G & Russo J (1993). Transformation of human breast epithelial cells by chemical carcinogens. *Carcinogenesis*, 14: 483–492. doi:10.1093/carcin/14.3.483 PMID:8453725

California Environmental Protection Agency (2005). *Health effects assessment for ETS: final.* Sacramento, CA: California Environmental Protection Agency, Office of Environmental Health Hazard Assesment.

Calle EE, Miracle-McMahill HL, Thun MJ, Heath CW Jr (1994). Cigarette smoking and risk of fatal breast cancer. *Am J Epidemiol*, 139: 1001–1007. PMID:8178779

Campbell PT, Curtin K, Ulrich CM *et al.* (2009). Mismatch repair polymorphisms and risk of colon cancer, tumour microsatellite instability and interactions with lifestyle factors. *Gut*, 58: 661–667. doi:10.1136/gut.2007.144220 PMID:18523027

Campos F, Carrasquilla G, Koriyama C *et al.* (2006). Risk factors of gastric cancer specific for tumor location and histology in Cali, Colombia. *World J Gastroenterol*, 12: 5772–5779. PMID:17007041

Canova C, Hashibe M, Simonato L *et al.* (2009). Genetic associations of 115 polymorphisms with cancers of the upper aerodigestive tract across 10 European countries: the ARCAGE project. *Cancer Res*, 69: 2956–2965. doi:10.1158/0008-5472.CAN-08-2604 PMID:19339270

Cao SM, Liu Q, Huang TB (2000). Analysis for risk factors of nasopharyngeal carcinoma in Sihui city. [chinese] *Cancer*, 19: 987–989.

Cao W, Cai L, Rao JY *et al.* (2005). Tobacco smoking, GSTP1 polymorphism, and bladder carcinoma. *Cancer*, 104: 2400–2408. doi:10.1002/cncr.21446 PMID:16240451

Caplan LS, Hall HI, Levine RS, Zhu K (2000). Preventable risk factors for nasal cancer. *Ann Epidemiol*, 10: 186–191. doi:10.1016/S1047-2797(99)00049-6 PMID:10813512

Cardoso MA, Maruta LM, Kida AA *et al.* (2002). Micronutrients and the risk of colorectal adenomas: a case-control study in São Paulo, Brazil. *IARC Sci Publ*, 156: 361–363. PMID:12484206

Carlsten C, Sagoo GS, Frodsham AJ *et al.* (2008). Glutathione *S*-transferase M1 (*GSTM1*) polymorphisms and lung cancer: a literature-based systematic HuGE review and meta-analysis. *Am J Epidemiol*, 167: 759–774. doi:10.1093/aje/kwm383 PMID:18270371

Carmella SG, Chen M, Han S *et al.* (2009). Effects of smoking cessation on eight urinary tobacco carcinogen and toxicant biomarkers. *Chem Res Toxicol*, 22: 734–741. doi:10.1021/tx800479s PMID:19317515

Carmella SG, Chen M, Villalta PW *et al.* (2002). Ethylation and methylation of hemoglobin in smokers and non-smokers. *Carcinogenesis*, 23: 1903–1910. doi:10.1093/carcin/23.11.1903 PMID:12419839

Carpenter CL, Jarvik ME, Morgenstern H *et al.* (1999). Mentholated cigarette smoking and lung-cancer risk. *Ann Epidemiol*, 9: 114–120. doi:10.1016/S1047-2797(98)00042-8 PMID:10037555

Cascorbi I, Brockmöller J, Roots I (1996). A C4887A polymorphism in exon 7 of human *CYP1A1*: population frequency, mutation linkages, and impact on lung cancer susceptibility. *Cancer Res*, 56: 4965–4969. PMID:8895751

Cassidenti DL, Pike MC, Vijod AG *et al.* (1992). A reevaluation of estrogen status in postmenopausal women who smoke. *Am J Obstet Gynecol*, 166: 1444–1448. PMID:1534446

Cassidenti DL, Vijod AG, Vijod MA *et al.* (1990). Short-term effects of smoking on the pharmacokinetic profiles of micronized estradiol in postmenopausal women. *Am J Obstet Gynecol*, 163: 1953–1960. PMID:2256508

Castellsagué X, Muñoz N, De Stefani E *et al.* (1999). Independent and joint effects of tobacco smoking and alcohol drinking on the risk of esophageal cancer in men and women. *Int J Cancer*, 82: 657–664. doi:10.1002/(SICI)1097-0215(19990827)82:5<657::AID-IJC7>3.0.CO;2-C PMID:10417762

Castellsagué X, Quintana MJ, Martínez MC *et al.* (2004). The role of type of tobacco and type of alcoholic beverage in oral carcinogenesis. *Int J Cancer*, 108: 741–749. doi:10.1002/ijc.11627 PMID:14696101

Cauley JA, Gutai JP, Kuller LH *et al.* (1989). The epidemiology of serum sex hormones in postmenopausal women. *Am J Epidemiol*, 129: 1120–1131. PMID:2729251

Cavalieri E, Frenkel K, Liehr JG *et al.* (2000). Estrogens as endogenous genotoxic agents–DNA adducts and mutations. *J Natl Cancer Inst Monogr*, 2775–93. PMID:10963621

Cederbaum AI (2006). CYP2E1–biochemical and toxicological aspects and role in alcohol-induced liver injury. *Mt Sinai J Med*, 73: 657–672. PMID:16878272

Chameaud J, Perraud R, Chrétien J *et al.* (1982). Lung carcinogenesis during in vivo cigarette smoking and radon daughter exposure in rats. *Recent Results Cancer Res*, 82: 11–20. PMID:7111833

Chan AO, Jim MH, Lam KF *et al.* (2007). Prevalence of colorectal neoplasm among patients with newly diagnosed coronary artery disease. *JAMA*, 298: 1412–1419. PMID:17895457

Chang-Claude J, Kropp S, Jäger B *et al.* (2002). Differential effect of NAT2 on the association between active and passive smoke exposure and breast cancer risk. *Cancer Epidemiol Biomarkers Prev*, 11: 698–704. PMID:12163321

Chao A, Thun MJ, Jacobs EJ *et al.* (2000). Cigarette smoking and colorectal cancer mortality in the cancer prevention study II. *J Natl Cancer Inst*, 92: 1888–1896. doi:10.1093/jnci/92.23.1888 PMID:11106680

Chen B, Hu Y, Jin T *et al.* (2007). The influence of metabolic gene polymorphisms on urinary 1-hydroxypyrene concentrations in Chinese coke oven workers. *Sci Total Environ*, 381: 38–46. doi:10.1016/j.scitotenv.2007.02.021 PMID:17498780

Chen CC, Neugut AI, Rotterdam H (1994). Risk factors for adenocarcinomas and malignant carcinoids of the small intestine: preliminary findings. *Cancer Epidemiol Biomarkers Prev*, 3: 205–207. PMID:8019367

Cheng TJ, Christiani DC, Xu X *et al.* (1995). Glutathione S-transferase *mu* genotype, diet, and smoking as determinants of sister chromatid exchange frequency in lymphocytes. *Cancer Epidemiol Biomarkers Prev*, 4: 535–542. PMID:7549811

Cheng YJ, Hildesheim A, Hsu MM *et al.* (1999). Cigarette smoking, alcohol consumption and risk of nasopharyngeal carcinoma in Taiwan. *Cancer Causes Control*, 10: 201–207. doi:10.1023/A:1008893109257 PMID:10454065

Chhabra SK, Anderson LM, Perella C *et al.* (2000). Coexposure to ethanol with N-nitrosodimethylamine or 4-(Methylnitrosamino)-1-(3-pyridyl)-1-butanone during lactation of rats: marked increase in O^6-methylguanine-DNA adducts in maternal mammary gland and in suckling lung and kidney. *Toxicol Appl Pharmacol*, 169: 191–200. doi:10.1006/taap.2000.9068 PMID:11097872

Chia VM, Newcomb PA, Bigler J *et al.* (2006). Risk of microsatellite-unstable colorectal cancer is associated jointly with smoking and nonsteroidal anti-inflammatory drug use. *Cancer Res*, 66: 6877–6883. doi:10.1158/0008-5472.CAN-06-1535 PMID:16818666

Choi SY & Kahyo H (1991). Effect of cigarette smoking and alcohol consumption in the aetiology of cancer of the oral cavity, pharynx and larynx. *Int J Epidemiol*, 20: 878–885. doi:10.1093/ije/20.4.878 PMID:1800426

Chow WH, Hsing AW, McLaughlin JK, Fraumeni JF Jr (1996). Smoking and adrenal cancer mortality among United States veterans. *Cancer Epidemiol Biomarkers Prev*, 5: 79–80. PMID:8850265

Chow WH, Linet MS, McLaughlin JK *et al.* (1993b). Risk factors for small intestine cancer. *Cancer Causes Control*, 4: 163–169. doi:10.1007/BF00053158 PMID:8481495

Chow WH, McLaughlin JK, Hrubec Z *et al.* (1993a). Tobacco use and nasopharyngeal carcinoma in a cohort of US veterans. *Int J Cancer*, 55: 538–540. doi:10.1002/ijc.2910550403 PMID:8406978

Christmann M, Tomicic MT, Roos WP, Kaina B (2003). Mechanisms of human DNA repair: an update. *Toxicology*, 193: 3–34. doi:10.1016/S0300-483X(03)00287-7 PMID:14599765

Chu SY, Stroup NE, Wingo PA *et al.* (1990). Cigarette smoking and the risk of breast cancer. *Am J Epidemiol*, 131: 244–253. PMID:2404408

Church TR, Anderson KE, Caporaso NE *et al.* (2009). A prospectively measured serum biomarker for a tobacco-specific carcinogen and lung cancer in smokers. *Cancer Epidemiol Biomarkers Prev*, 18: 260–266. doi:10.1158/1055-9965.EPI-08-0718 PMID:19124507

Chyou PH, Nomura AM, Stemmermann GN (1995). Diet, alcohol, smoking and cancer of the upper aerodigestive tract: a prospective study among Hawaii Japanese men. *Int J Cancer*, 60: 616–621. doi:10.1002/ijc.2910600508 PMID:7860134

Cocco P, Moore PS, Ennas MG *et al.* (2007). Effect of urban traffic, individual habits, and genetic polymorphisms on background urinary 1-hydroxypyrene excretion. *Ann Epidemiol*, 17: 1–8. doi:10.1016/j.annepidem.2005.11.001 PMID:16406813

Colangelo LA, Gapstur SM, Gann PH, Dyer AR (2004). Cigarette smoking and colorectal carcinoma mortality in a cohort with long-term follow-up. *Cancer*, 100: 288–293. doi:10.1002/cncr.11923 PMID:14716762

Colilla S, Kantoff PW, Neuhausen SL *et al.* (2006). The joint effect of smoking and AIB1 on breast cancer risk in BRCA1 mutation carriers. *Carcinogenesis*, 27: 599–605. doi:10.1093/carcin/bgi246 PMID:16244359

Collishaw NE, Boyd NF, Cantor KP *et al.* (2009). *Canadian expert panel on tobacco smoke and breast cancer risk.* Toronto: Ontario Tobacco Research Unit.

Conway K, Edmiston SN, Cui L *et al.* (2002). Prevalence and spectrum of p53 mutations associated with smoking in breast cancer. *Cancer Res*, 62: 1987–1995. PMID:11929815

Cooper CS, Grover PL, Sims P (1983). *The metabolism and activation of benzo[a]pyrene.* In: *Progress in Drug Metabolism*, Vol. 7. Bridges JW, Chasseaud LF, editors. London: Wiley & Sons, pp. 295–396

Corona R, Dogliotti E, D'Errico M *et al.* (2001). Risk factors for basal cell carcinoma in a Mediterranean population: role of recreational sun exposure early in life. *Arch Dermatol*, 137: 1162–1168. PMID:11559211

Cortez CC & Jones PA (2008). Chromatin, cancer and drug therapies. *Mutat Res*, 647: 44–51. PMID:18691602

Cote ML, Chen W, Smith DW *et al.* (2009). Meta- and pooled analysis of *GSTP1* polymorphism and lung cancer: a HuGE-GSEC review. *Am J Epidemiol*, 169: 802–814. doi:10.1093/aje/kwn417 PMID:19240225

Cote ML, Kardia SL, Wenzlaff AS *et al.* (2005). Combinations of glutathione S-transferase genotypes and risk of early-onset lung cancer in Caucasians and African Americans: a population-based study. *Carcinogenesis*, 26: 811–819. doi:10.1093/carcin/bgi023 PMID:15661806

Couch FJ, Cerhan JR, Vierkant RA *et al.* (2001). Cigarette smoking increases risk for breast cancer in high-risk breast cancer families. *Cancer Epidemiol Biomarkers Prev*, 10: 327–332. PMID:11319172

Coughlin SS, Calle EE, Patel AV, Thun MJ (2000). Predictors of pancreatic cancer mortality among a large cohort of United States adults. *Cancer Causes Control*, 11: 915–923. doi:10.1023/A:1026580131793 PMID:11142526

Cozen W, Hamilton AS, Zhao P *et al.* (2009). A protective role for early oral exposures in the etiology of young adult Hodgkin lymphoma. *Blood*, 114: 4014–4020.

Crofts F, Cosma GN, Currie D *et al.* (1993). A novel CYP1A1 gene polymorphism in African-Americans. *Carcinogenesis*, 14: 1729–1731. doi:10.1093/carcin/14.9.1729 PMID:8104732

Cui Y, Miller AB, Rohan TE (2006). Cigarette smoking and breast cancer risk: update of a prospective cohort study. *Breast Cancer Res Treat*, 100: 293–299. doi:10.1007/s10549-006-9255-3 PMID:16773435

Curtin K, Samowitz WS, Wolff RK *et al.* (2009). Somatic alterations, metabolizing genes and smoking in rectal cancer. *Int J Cancer*, 125: 158–164. doi:10.1002/ijc.24338 PMID:19358278

Cybulski C, Masojc B, Oszutowska D *et al.* (2008). Constitutional CHEK2 mutations are associated with a decreased risk of lung and laryngeal cancers. *Carcinogenesis*, 29: 762–765. doi:10.1093/carcin/bgn044 PMID:18281249

D'Agostini F, Izzotti A, Balansky R *et al.* (2006). Early loss of Fhit in the respiratory tract of rodents exposed to environmental cigarette smoke. *Cancer Res*, 66: 3936–3941. doi:10.1158/0008-5472.CAN-05-3666 PMID:16585223

d'Errico A, Malats N, Vineis P, Boffetta P (1999). Review of studies of selected metabolic polymorphisms and cancer. *IARC Sci Publ*, 148: 323–393. PMID:10493265

Dagle GE, McDonald KE, Smith LG, Stevens DL Jr (1978). Pulmonary carcinogenesis in rats given implants of cigarette smoke condensate in beeswax pellets. *J Natl Cancer Inst*, 61: 905–910. PMID:278868

Dalbey WE, Nettesheim P, Griesemer R *et al.* (1980). Chronic inhalation of cigarette smoke by F344 rats. *J Natl Cancer Inst*, 64: 383–390. PMID:6928229

Daling JR, Madeleine MM, Johnson LG *et al.* (2005). Penile cancer: importance of circumcision, human papillomavirus and smoking in in situ and invasive disease. *Int J Cancer*, 116: 606–616. doi:10.1002/ijc.21009 PMID:15825185

Daling JR, Sherman KJ, Hislop TG *et al.* (1992). Cigarette smoking and the risk of anogenital cancer. *Am J Epidemiol*, 135: 180–189. PMID:1311142

Dally H, Edler L, Jäger B *et al.* (2003). The *CYP3A4*1B* allele increases risk for small cell lung cancer: effect of gender and smoking dose. *Pharmacogenetics*, 13: 607–618. doi:10.1097/00008571-200310000-00004 PMID:14515059

Daniell HW (1988). Increased lymph node metastases at mastectomy for breast cancer associated with host obesity, cigarette smoking, age, and large tumor size. *Cancer*, 62: 429–435. doi:10.1002/1097-0142(19880715)62:2<429::AID-CNCR2820620230>3.0.CO;2-4 PMID:3383142

Daniell HW, Tam E, Filice A (1993). Larger axillary metastases in obese women and smokers with breast cancer–an influence by host factors on early tumor behavior. *Breast Cancer Res Treat*, 25: 193–201. doi:10.1007/BF00689833 PMID:8369520

Darby S, Hill D, Auvinen A *et al.* (2005). Radon in homes and risk of lung cancer: collaborative analysis of individual data from 13 European case-control studies. *BMJ*, 330: 223 doi:10.1136/bmj.38308.477650.63 PMID:15613366

Davies MJ, Turner JG, Vives-Bauza C, Rumsby PC (1999). Investigation of mutant frequency at the *HPRT* locus and changes in microsatellite sequences in healthy young adults. *Mutat Res*, 431: 317–323. PMID:10635997

Davis BR, Whitehead JK, Gill ME *et al.* (1975). Response of rat lung to inhaled tobacco smoke with or without prior exposure to 3,4-benzpyrene (BP) given by intratracheal instillation. *Br J Cancer*, 31: 469–484. PMID:1156528

Day GL, Blot WJ, Austin DF *et al.* (1993). Racial differences in risk of oral and pharyngeal cancer: alcohol, tobacco, and other determinants. *J Natl Cancer Inst*, 85: 465–473. doi:10.1093/jnci/85.6.465 PMID:8445674 de Klerk NH, Musk AW, Eccles JL *et al.* (1996). Exposure to crocidolite and the incidence of different histological types of lung cancer. *Occup Environ Med*, 53: 157–159. doi:10.1136/oem.53.3.157 PMID:8704855

De Stefani E, Boffetta P, Deneo-Pellegrini H *et al.* (2007). The effect of smoking and drinking in oral and pharyngeal cancers: a case-control study in Uruguay. *Cancer Lett*, 246: 282–289. doi:10.1016/j.canlet.2006.03.008 PMID:16624486

De Stefani E, Boffetta P, Oreggia F *et al.* (1998). Smoking patterns and cancer of the oral cavity and pharynx: a case-control study in Uruguay. *Oral Oncol*, 34: 340–346. doi:10.1016/S1368-8375(98)00014-1 PMID:9861338

De Stefani E, Correa P, Oreggia F *et al.* (1987). Risk factors for laryngeal cancer. *Cancer*, 60: 3087–3091. doi:10.1002/1097-0142(19871215)60:12<3087::AID-CNCR2820601238>3.0.CO;2-6 PMID:3677031

De Stefani E, Espasandin J, Ronco A *et al.* (1995). Tobacco smoking and the risk of non-melanoma skin cancer. *Tob Control*, 4(2): 175–179. PMCID: PMC1759430 doi:10.1136/tc.4.2.175

De Stefani E, Muñoz N, Estève J *et al.* (1990). Mate drinking, alcohol, tobacco, diet, and esophageal cancer in Uruguay. *Cancer Res*, 50: 426–431. PMID:2295081

De Stefani E, Oreggia F, Rivero S, Fierro L (1992). Hand-rolled cigarette smoking and risk of cancer of the mouth, pharynx, and larynx. *Cancer*, 70: 679–682. doi:10.1002/1097-0142(19920801)70:3<679::AID-CNCR2820700323>3.0.CO;2-Z PMID:1623483

Delaney JC & Essigmann JM (2008). Biological properties of single chemical-DNA adducts: a twenty year perspective. *Chem Res Toxicol*, 21: 232–252. doi:10.1021/tx700292a PMID:18072751

Delfino RJ, Smith C, West JG *et al.* (2000). Breast cancer, passive and active cigarette smoking and N-acetyltransferase 2 genotype. *Pharmacogenetics*, 10: 461–469. doi:10.1097/00008571-200007000-00009 PMID:10898115

DeMarini DM (2004). Genotoxicity of tobacco smoke and tobacco smoke condensate: a review. *Mutat Res*, 567: 447–474. doi:10.1016/j.mrrev.2004.02.001 PMID:15572290

DeMarini DM, Gudi R, Szkudlinska A *et al.* (2008). Genotoxicity of 10 cigarette smoke condensates in four test systems: comparisons between assays and condensates. *Mutat Res*, 650: 15–29. PMID:18006367

DeMarini DM, Shelton ML, Levine JG (1995). Mutation spectrum of cigarette smoke condensate in Salmonella: comparison to mutations in smoking-associated tumors. *Carcinogenesis*, 16: 2535–2542. doi:10.1093/carcin/16.10.2535 PMID:7586163

Department of Health and Human Services (2001). *Women and Smoking: A Report of the Surgeon General.* Washington: Centers for Disease Control and Prevention, National Center for Chronic Disease Prevention and Health Promotion, Office on Smoking and Health.

Department of Health and Human Services (2004). *The Health Consequences of Smoking: A Report of the Surgeon General.* Atlanta, Georgia: U.S. Department of Health and Human Services, Centers for Disease Control and Prevention, National Center for Chronic Disease Prevention and Health Promotion, Office on Smoking and Health.

Devesa SS, Bray F, Vizcaino AP, Parkin DM (2005). International lung cancer trends by histologic type: male:female differences diminishing and adenocarcinoma rates rising. *Int J Cancer*, 117: 294–299. doi:10.1002/ijc.21183 PMID:15900604

Diergaarde B, Braam H, Vasen HF *et al.* (2007). Environmental factors and colorectal tumor risk in individuals with hereditary nonpolyposis colorectal cancer. *Clin Gastroenterol Hepatol*, 5: 736–742. PMID:17544999

Diergaarde B, Vrieling A, van Kraats AA *et al.* (2003). Cigarette smoking and genetic alterations in sporadic colon carcinomas. *Carcinogenesis*, 24: 565–571. doi:10.1093/carcin/24.3.565 PMID:12663519

Dikshit RP & Kanhere S (2000). Tobacco habits and risk of lung, oropharyngeal and oral cavity cancer: a population-based case-control study in Bhopal, India. *Int J Epidemiol*, 29: 609–614. doi:10.1093/ije/29.4.609 PMID:10922335

Dillner J, von Krogh G, Horenblas S, Meijer CJLM (2000). Etiology of squamous cell carcinoma of the penis. *Scand J Urol Nephrol Suppl*, 34: 189–193. doi:10.1080/00365590050509913 PMID:11144896

Ding L, Getz G, Wheeler DA *et al.* (2008). Somatic mutations affect key pathways in lung adenocarcinoma. *Nature*, 455: 1069–1075. doi:10.1038/nature07423 PMID:18948947

Djordjević D, Nikolić J, Stefanović V (1998). Ethanol interactions with other cytochrome P450 substrates including drugs, xenobiotics, and carcinogens. *Pathol Biol (Paris)*, 46: 760–770. PMID:9922992

Doll R, Gray R, Hafner B, Peto R (1980). Mortality in relation to smoking: 22 years' observations on female British doctors. *Br Med J*, 280: 967–971. doi:10.1136/bmj.280.6219.967 PMID:7417764

Doll R & Peto R (1978). Cigarette smoking and bronchial carcinoma: dose and time relationships among regular smokers and lifelong non-smokers. *J Epidemiol Community Health*, 32: 303–313. doi:10.1136/jech.32.4.303 PMID:744822

Doll R, Peto R (1985). *Effects on health of exposure to asbestos.* London: Health and Safety Commission.

Doll R, Peto R, Boreham J, Sutherland I (2005). Mortality from cancer in relation to smoking: 50 years observations on British doctors. *Br J Cancer*, 92: 426–429. PMID:15668706

Doll R, Peto R, Wheatley K *et al.* (1994). Mortality in relation to smoking: 40 years' observations on male British doctors. *BMJ*, 309: 901–911. PMID:7755693

Dong LM, Potter JD, White E *et al.* (2008). Genetic susceptibility to cancer: the role of polymorphisms in candidate genes. *JAMA*, 299: 2423–2436. doi:10.1001/jama.299.20.2423 PMID:18505952

Dontenwill W, Chevalier HJ, Harke HP *et al.* (1973). Investigations on the effects of chronic cigarette-smoke inhalation in Syrian golden hamsters. *J Natl Cancer Inst*, 51: 1781–1832. PMID:4765388

Dontenwill W, Chevalier HJ, Harke HP *et al.* (1977). Untersuchungen über den Effekt der chronischen Zigarettenrauchinhalation beim syrischen Goldhamster und über die Bedeutung des Vitamin A auf die bei Berauchung gefundenen Organveründerungen *Z Krebsforsch Klin Onkol Cancer Res Clin Oncol*, 89: 153–180. doi:10.1007/BF00308516 PMID:143143

Du X, Squier CA, Kremer MJ, Wertz PW (2000). Penetration of N-nitrosonornicotine (NNN) across oral mucosa in the presence of ethanol and nicotine. *J Oral Pathol Med*, 29: 80–85. doi:10.1034/j.1600-0714.2000.290205.x PMID:10718403

Duell EJ, Holly EA, Bracci PM *et al.* (2002). A population-based, case-control study of polymorphisms in carcinogen-metabolizing genes, smoking, and pancreatic adenocarcinoma risk. *J Natl Cancer Inst*, 94: 297–306. PMID:11854392

Dunn SR, Simenhoff ML, Lele PS *et al.* (1990). *N*-nitrosodimethylamine blood levels in patients with chronic renal failure: modulation of levels by ethanol and ascorbic acid. *J Natl Cancer Inst*, 82: 783–787. doi:10.1093/jnci/82.9.783 PMID:2325149

Dusek L, Abrahamova J, Lakomy R *et al.* (2008). Multivariate analysis of risk factors for testicular cancer: a hospital-based case-control study in the Czech Republic. *Neoplasma*, 55: 356–368. PMID:18505349

Dyke GW, Craven JL, Hall R, Garner RC (1992). Smoking-related DNA adducts in human gastric cancers. *Int J Cancer*, 52: 847–850. doi:10.1002/ijc.2910520602 PMID:1459723

Egan KM, Newcomb PA, Titus-Ernstoff L *et al.* (2003). Association of NAT2 and smoking in relation to breast cancer incidence in a population-based case-control study (United States). *Cancer Causes Control*, 14: 43–51. doi:10.1023/A:1022517506689 PMID:12708724

Egan KM, Stampfer MJ, Hunter D *et al.*Nurses' Health Study (2002). Active and passive smoking in breast cancer: prospective results from the Nurses' Health Study. *Epidemiology*, 13: 138–145. doi:10.1097/00001648-200203000-00007 PMID:11880753

Eichholzer M, Stähelin HB, Lüdin E, Bernasconi F (1999). Smoking, plasma vitamins C, E, retinol, and carotene, and fatal prostate cancer: seventeen-year follow-up of the prospective basel study. *Prostate*, 38: 189–198. doi:10.1002/(SICI)1097-0045(19990215)38:3<189::AID-PROS3>3.0.CO;2-N PMID:10068343

el-Bayoumy K (1992). Environmental carcinogens that may be involved in human breast cancer etiology. *Chem Res Toxicol*, 5: 585–590. doi:10.1021/tx00029a001 PMID:1445997

Eldridge SR, Gould MN, Butterworth BE (1992). Genotoxicity of environmental agents in human mammary epithelial cells. *Cancer Res*, 52: 5617–5621. PMID:1394185

Elliott EA, Matanoski GM, Rosenshein NB *et al.* (1990). Body fat patterning in women with endometrial cancer. *Gynecol Oncol*, 39: 253–258. doi:10.1016/0090-8258(90)90247-I PMID:2258066

Elwood JM, Pearson JC, Skippen DH, Jackson SM (1984). Alcohol, smoking, social and occupational factors in the aetiology of cancer of the oral cavity, pharynx and larynx. *Int J Cancer*, 34: 603–612. doi:10.1002/ijc.2910340504 PMID:6500740

Engeland A, Andersen A, Haldorsen T, Tretli S (1996). Smoking habits and risk of cancers other than lung cancer: 28 years' follow-up of 26,000 Norwegian men and women. *Cancer Causes Control*, 7: 497–506. doi:10.1007/BF00051881 PMID:8877046

Engels EA, Biggar RJ, Hall HI *et al.* (2008). Cancer risk in people infected with human immunodeficiency virus in the United States. *International Journal of Cancer*, 123: 187–194. doi:10.1002/ijc.23487

Epplein M, Schwartz SM, Potter JD, Weiss NS (2005). Smoking-adjusted lung cancer incidence among Asian-Americans (United States). *Cancer Causes Control*, 16: 1085–1090. doi:10.1007/s10552-005-0330-6 PMID:16184474

Erhardt JG, Kreichgauer HP, Meisner C *et al.* (2002). Alcohol, cigarette smoking, dietary factors and the risk of colorectal adenomas and hyperplastic polyps–a case control study. *Eur J Nutr*, 41: 35–43. doi:10.1007/s003940200004 PMID:11990006

Escribano Uzcudun A, Rabanal Retolaza I, García Grande A *et al.* (2002). Pharyngeal cancer prevention: evidence from a case–control study involving 232 consecutive patients. *J Laryngol Otol*, 116: 523–531. PMID:12238672

Ewertz M (1990). Smoking and breast cancer risk in Denmark. *Cancer Causes Control*, 1: 31–37. doi:10.1007/BF00053181 PMID:2102274

Ewertz M, Gillanders S, Meyer L, Zedeler K (1991). Survival of breast cancer patients in relation to factors which affect the risk of developing breast cancer. *Int J Cancer*, 49: 526–530. doi:10.1002/ijc.2910490409 PMID:1917153

Falk RT, Pickle LW, Brown LM *et al.* (1989). Effect of smoking and alcohol consumption on laryngeal cancer risk in coastal Texas. *Cancer Res*, 49: 4024–4029. PMID:2736543

Falk RT, Pickle LW, Fontham ET *et al.* (1992). Epidemiology of bronchioloalveolar carcinoma. *Cancer Epidemiology, Biomarkers & Prevention*, 1: 339–344.

Falter B, Kutzer C, Richter E (1994). Biomonitoring of hemoglobin adducts: aromatic amines and tobacco-specific nitrosamines. *Clin Investig*, 72: 364–371. doi:10.1007/BF00252829 PMID:8086771

Favorito LA, Nardi AC, Ronalsa M *et al.* (2008). Epidemiologic study on penile cancer in Brazil. *Int Braz J Urol*, 34: 587–591, discussion 591–593. doi:10.1590/S1677-55382008000500007 PMID:18986562

Federal Trade Commission (2001). *Cigarette report for 1999*. C. Department. Washington D.C.

Feng BJ, Khyatti M, Ben-Ayoub W *et al.* (2009). Cannabis, tobacco and domestic fumes intake are associated with nasopharyngeal carcinoma in North Africa. *Br J Cancer*, 101: 1207–1212. doi:10.1038/sj.bjc.6605281 PMID:19724280

Fennell TR, MacNeela JP, Morris RW *et al.* (2000). Hemoglobin adducts from acrylonitrile and ethylene oxide in cigarette smokers: effects of *glutathione S-transferase T1*-null and *M1*-null genotypes. *Cancer Epidemiol Biomarkers Prev*, 9: 705–712. PMID:10919741

Fernberg P, Odenbro A, Bellocco R *et al.* (2007). Tobacco use, body mass index, and the risk of leukemia and multiple myeloma: a nationwide cohort study in Sweden. *Cancer Res*, 67: 5983–5986. doi:10.1158/0008-5472.CAN-07-0274 PMID:17575169

Ferson M, Edwards A, Lind A *et al.* (1979). Low natural killer-cell activity and immunoglobulin levels associated with smoking in human subjects. *Int J Cancer*, 23: 603–609. doi:10.1002/ijc.2910230504 PMID:457307

Finch GL, Nikula KJ, Barr EB *et al.* (1995). *Effects of combined exposure of F344 rats to radiation and chronically inhaled cigarette smoke*. In: *Annual Report of the Inhalation Toxicology Research Institute. ITRI-149*. Bice DE, Hahn FF, Hoover R *et al.*,editors

Fine LJ, Philogene GS, Gramling R *et al.* (2004). Prevalence of multiple chronic disease risk factors. 2001 National Health Interview Survey. *Am J Prev Med*, 27: Suppl18–24. doi:10.1016/j.amepre.2004.04.017 PMID:15275670

Fink AK & Lash TL (2003). A null association between smoking during pregnancy and breast cancer using Massachusetts registry data (United States). *Cancer Causes Control*, 14: 497–503. doi:10.1023/A:1024922824237 PMID:12946045

Firozi PF, Bondy ML, Sahin AA *et al.* (2002). Aromatic DNA adducts and polymorphisms of *CYP1A1*, *NAT2*, and *GSTM1* in breast cancer. *Carcinogenesis*, 23: 301–306. doi:10.1093/carcin/23.2.301 PMID:11872636

Flanders WD, Lally CA, Zhu BP *et al.* (2003). Lung cancer mortality in relation to age, duration of smoking, and daily cigarette consumption: results from Cancer Prevention Study II. *Cancer Res*, 63: 6556–6562. PMID:14559851

Folsom AR, Demissie Z, Harnack LIowa Women's Health Study (2003). Glycemic index, glycemic load, and incidence of endometrial cancer: the Iowa women's health study. *Nutr Cancer*, 46: 119–124. doi:10.1207/S15327914NC4602_03 PMID:14690786

Franceschi S, Barra S, La Vecchia C *et al.* (1992). Risk factors for cancer of the tongue and the mouth. A case-control study from northern Italy. *Cancer*, 70: 2227–2233. doi:10.1002/1097-0142(19921101)70:9<2227::AID-CNCR2820700902>3.0.CO;2-Z PMID:1394055

Franceschi S, Levi F, La Vecchia C *et al.* (1999). Comparison of the effect of smoking and alcohol drinking between oral and pharyngeal cancer. *Int J Cancer*, 83: 1–4. doi:10.1002/(SICI)1097-0215(19990924)83:1<1::AID-IJC1>3.0.CO;2-8 PMID:10449598

Franceschi S, Montella M, Polesel J *et al.* (2006). Hepatitis viruses, alcohol, and tobacco in the etiology of hepatocellular carcinoma in Italy. *Cancer Epidemiol Biomarkers Prev*, 15: 683–689. doi:10.1158/1055-9965.EPI-05-0702 PMID:16614109

Franceschi S & Serraino D (1992). Risk factors for adult soft tissue sarcoma in northern Italy. *Ann Oncol*, 3: Suppl 2S85–S88. PMID:1622876

Franceschi S, Talamini R, Barra S *et al.* (1990). Smoking and drinking in relation to cancers of the oral cavity, pharynx, larynx, and esophagus in northern Italy. *Cancer Res*, 50: 6502–6507. PMID:2208109

Franco EL, Villa LL, Sobrinho JP *et al.* (1999). Epidemiology of acquisition and clearance of cervical human papillomavirus infection in women from a high-risk area for cervical cancer. *J Infect Dis*, 180: 1415–1423. doi:10.1086/315086 PMID:10515798

Franks AL, Kendrick JS, Tyler CW Jr (1987) Postmenopausal smoking, estrogen replacement therapy, and the risk of endometrial cancer. *Am J Obstet Gynecol*, 156: 20–23. PMID:3799753

Freedman DM, Sigurdson A, Doody MM *et al.* (2003a). Risk of melanoma in relation to smoking, alcohol intake, and other factors in a large occupational cohort. *Cancer Causes Control*, 14: 847–857. doi:10.1023/B:CACO.0000003839.56954.73 PMID:14682442

Freedman DM, Sigurdson A, Doody MM *et al.* (2003b). Risk of basal cell carcinoma in relation to alcohol intake and smoking. *Cancer Epidemiol Biomarkers Prev*, 12: 1540–1543. PMID:14693751

Freedman ND, Abnet CC, Leitzmann MF *et al.* (2007a). Prospective investigation of the cigarette smoking-head and neck cancer association by sex. *Cancer*, 110: 1593–1601. doi:10.1002/cncr.22957 PMID:17724671

Freedman ND, Abnet CC, Leitzmann MF *et al.* (2007b). A prospective study of tobacco, alcohol, and the risk of esophageal and gastric cancer subtypes. *Am J Epidemiol*, 165: 1424–1433. doi:10.1093/aje/kwm051 PMID:17420181

Freedman ND, Leitzmann MF, Hollenbeck AR *et al.* (2008). Cigarette smoking and subsequent risk of lung cancer in men and women: analysis of a prospective cohort study. *Lancet Oncol*, 9: 649–656. doi:10.1016/S1470-2045(08)70154-2 PMID:18556244

Friborg JT, Yuan JM, Wang R *et al.* (2007). A prospective study of tobacco and alcohol use as risk factors for pharyngeal carcinomas in Singapore Chinese. *Cancer*, 109: 1183–1191.

Friedman AJ, Ravnikar VA, Barbieri RL (1987). Serum steroid hormone profiles in postmenopausal smokers and nonsmokers. *Fertil Steril*, 47: 398–401. PMID:2951278

Fuchs CS, Colditz GA, Stampfer MJ *et al.* (1996). A prospective study of cigarette smoking and the risk of pancreatic cancer. *Arch Intern Med*, 156: 2255–2260. doi:10.1001/archinte.156.19.2255 PMID:8885826

Fujino Y, Mizoue T, Tokui N *et al.*JACC Study Group (2005). Cigarette smoking and mortality due to stomach cancer: findings from the JACC Study. *J Epidemiol*, 15: Suppl 2S113–S119. doi:10.2188/jea.15.S113 PMID:16127222

Fujita M, Tase T, Kakugawa Y *et al.* (2008). Smoking, earlier menarche and low parity as independent risk factors for gynecologic cancers in Japanese: a case-control study. *Tohoku J Exp Med*, 216: 297–307. doi:10.1620/tjem.216.297 PMID:19060444

Fukuda K & Shibata A (1990). Exposure-response relationships between woodworking, smoking or passive smoking, and squamous cell neoplasms of the maxillary sinus. *Cancer Causes Control*, 1: 165–168. doi:10.1007/BF00053168 PMID:2102286

Furberg AS & Thune I (2003). Metabolic abnormalities (hypertension, hyperglycemia and overweight), lifestyle (high energy intake and physical inactivity) and endometrial cancer risk in a Norwegian cohort. *Int J Cancer*, 104: 669–676. doi:10.1002/ijc.10974 PMID:12640672

Gaikwad NW, Yang L, Muti P *et al.* (2008). The molecular etiology of breast cancer: evidence from biomarkers of risk. *Int J Cancer*, 122: 1949–1957. PMID:18098283

Gajalakshmi CK & Shanta V (1996). Lifestyle and risk of stomach cancer: a hospital-based case-control study. *Int J Epidemiol*, 25: 1146–1153. doi:10.1093/ije/25.6.1146 PMID:9027518

Gajalakshmi V, Hung RJ, Mathew A *et al.* (2003). Tobacco smoking and chewing, alcohol drinking and lung cancer risk among men in southern India. *Int J Cancer*, 107: 441–447. doi:10.1002/ijc.11377 PMID:14506745

Gallagher CJ, Muscat JE, Hicks AN *et al.* (2007). The UDP-glucuronosyltransferase 2B17 gene deletion polymorphism: sex-specific association with urinary 4-(methylnitrosamino)-1-(3-pyridyl)-1-butanol glucuronidation phenotype and risk for lung cancer. *Cancer Epidemiol Biomarkers Prev*, 16: 823–828. doi:10.1158/1055-9965.EPI-06-0823 PMID:17416778

Gallicchio L, Boyd K, Matanoski G *et al.* (2008). Carotenoids and the risk of developing lung cancer: a systematic review. *Am J Clin Nutr*, 88: 372–383. PMID:18689373

Gallicchio L, Kouzis A, Genkinger JM *et al.* (2006). Active cigarette smoking, household passive smoke exposure, and the risk of developing pancreatic cancer. *Prev Med*, 42: 200–205. doi:10.1016/j.ypmed.2005.12.014 PMID:16458957

Gallus S, Altieri A, Bosetti C *et al.* (2003a). Cigarette tar yield and risk of upper digestive tract cancers: case-control studies from Italy and Switzerland. *Ann Oncol*, 14: 209–213. doi:10.1093/annonc/mdg074 PMID:12562646

Gallus S, Bosetti C, Franceschi S *et al.* (2003b). Laryngeal cancer in women: tobacco, alcohol, nutritional, and hormonal factors. *Cancer Epidemiol Biomarkers Prev*, 12: 514–517. PMID:12814996

Gambier N, Batt AM, Marie B *et al.* (2005). Association of *CYP2A6*1B* genetic variant with the amount of smoking in French adults from the Stanislas cohort. *Pharmacogenomics J*, 5: 271–275. doi:10.1038/sj.tpj.6500314 PMID:15940289

Gammon MD, Eng SM, Teitelbaum SL *et al.* (2004). Environmental tobacco smoke and breast cancer incidence. *Environ Res*, 96: 176–185. doi:10.1016/j.envres.2003.08.009 PMID:15325878

Gammon MD, Schoenberg JB, Ahsan H *et al.* (1997). Tobacco, alcohol, and socioeconomic status and adenocarcinomas of the esophagus and gastric cardia. *J Natl Cancer Inst*, 89: 1277–1284. doi:10.1093/jnci/89.17.1277 PMID:9293918

Gammon MD, Schoenberg JB, Teitelbaum SL *et al.* (1998). Cigarette smoking and breast cancer risk among young women (United States). *Cancer Causes Control*, 9: 583–590. doi:10.1023/A:1008868922799 PMID:10189043

Gandini S, Botteri E, Iodice S *et al.* (2008). Tobacco smoking and cancer: a meta-analysis. *International Journal of Cancer*, 122: 155–164. doi:10.1002/ijc.23033

Gao CM, Takezaki T, Wu JZ *et al.* (2007). CYP2E1 Rsa I polymorphism impacts on risk of colorectal cancer association with smoking and alcohol drinking. *World J Gastroenterol*, 13: 5725–5730. PMID:17963298

Gao YT, McLaughlin JK, Blot WJ *et al.* (1994). Risk factors for esophageal cancer in Shanghai, China. I. Role of cigarette smoking and alcohol drinking. *Int J Cancer*, 58: 192–196. doi:10.1002/ijc.2910580208 PMID:8026880

Gapstur SM, Gann PH, Lowe W *et al.* (2000). Abnormal glucose metabolism and pancreatic cancer mortality. *JAMA*, 283: 2552–2558. doi:10.1001/jama.283.19.2552 PMID:10815119

García-Closas M, Malats N, Silverman D *et al.* (2005). NAT2 slow acetylation, GSTM1 null genotype, and risk of bladder cancer: results from the Spanish Bladder Cancer Study and meta-analyses. *Lancet*, 366: 649–659. doi:10.1016/S0140-6736(05)67137-1 PMID:16112301

García-González MA, Lanas A, Quintero E *et al.*Spanish Gastroenterological Association AEG (2007). Gastric cancer susceptibility is not linked to pro-and anti-inflammatory cytokine gene polymorphisms in whites: a Nationwide Multicenter Study in Spain. *Am J Gastroenterol*, 102: 1878–1892. doi:10.1111/j.1572-0241.2007.01423.x PMID:17640324

Gargus JL, Powers MB, Habermann RT *et al.* (1976). *Mouse dermal bioassays of cigarette smoke condensates.* In: *Report No. 1. Toward Less Hazardous Cigarettes. The First Set of Experimental Cigarettes (DHEW Publ. No. (NIH)76-905).* Washington DC: Public Health Service, National Institutes of Health, National Cancer Institute, pp. 85–94.

Garrote LF, Herrero R, Reyes RM *et al.* (2001). Risk factors for cancer of the oral cavity and oro-pharynx in Cuba. *Br J Cancer*, 85: 46–54. doi:10.1054/bjoc.2000.1825 PMID:11437401

Garte S (2001). Metabolic susceptibility genes as cancer risk factors: time for a reassessment? *Cancer Epidemiol Biomarkers Prev*, 10: 1233–1237. PMID:11751439

Garte S, Gaspari L, Alexandrie AK *et al.* (2001). Metabolic gene polymorphism frequencies in control populations. *Cancer Epidemiol Biomarkers Prev*, 10: 1239–1248. PMID:11751440

Garte S, Taioli E, Popov T *et al.* (2008). Genetic susceptibility to benzene toxicity in humans. *J Toxicol Environ Health A*, 71: 1482–1489. PMID:18836923

Gasper AV, Al-Janobi A, Smith JA *et al.* (2005). Glutathione S-transferase M1 polymorphism and metabolism of sulforaphane from standard and high-glucosinolate broccoli. *Am J Clin Nutr*, 82: 1283–1291. PMID:16332662

Ghadirian P, Lubinski J, Lynch H *et al.* (2004). Smoking and the risk of breast cancer among carriers of BRCA mutations. *Int J Cancer*, 110: 413–416. doi:10.1002/ijc.20106 PMID:15095307

Ghadirian P, Maisonneuve P, Perret C *et al.* (1998). Epidemiology of sociodemographic characteristics, lifestyle, medical history, and colon cancer: a case-control study among French Canadians in Montreal. *Cancer Detect Prev*, 22: 396–404. doi:10.1046/j.1525-1500.1998.00058.x PMID:9727620

Ginsburg O, Ghadirian P, Lubinski J *et al.*Hereditary Breast Cancer Clinical Study Group (2009). Smoking and the risk of breast cancer in BRCA1 and BRCA2 carriers: an update. *Breast Cancer Res Treat*, 114: 127–135. doi:10.1007/s10549-008-9977-5 PMID:18483851

Giovannucci E, Rimm EB, Stampfer MJ *et al.* (1994). A prospective study of cigarette smoking and risk of colorectal adenoma and colorectal cancer in U.S. men. *J Natl Cancer Inst*, 86: 183–191. PMID:8283490

Giuliano AR, Sedjo RL, Roe DJ *et al.* (2002). Clearance of oncogenic human papillomavirus (HPV) infection: effect of smoking (United States). *Cancer Causes Control*, 13: 839–846. doi:10.1023/A:1020668232219 PMID:12462549

Glaser SL, Keegan TH, Clarke CA *et al.* (2004). Smoking and Hodgkin lymphoma risk in women United States. *Cancer Causes Control*, 15: 387–397.

Glatt H, Boeing H, Engelke CE *et al.* (2001). Human cytosolic sulphotransferases: genetics, characteristics, toxicological aspects. *Mutat Res*, 482: 27–40. PMID:11535246

Goldman R & Shields PG (1998). Molecular epidemiology of breast cancer. *In Vivo*, 12: 43–48. PMID:9575425

Gong Z, Xie D, Deng Z *et al.* (2005). The PPARgamma Pro12Ala polymorphism and risk for incident sporadic colorectal adenomas. *Carcinogenesis*, 26: 579–585. doi:10.1093/carcin/bgh343 PMID:15564289

González CA, Pera G, Agudo A *et al.* (2003). Smoking and the risk of gastric cancer in the European Prospective Investigation Into Cancer and Nutrition (EPIC). *Int J Cancer*, 107: 629–634. doi:10.1002/ijc.11426 PMID:14520702

Goodman MT, Hankin JH, Wilkens LR *et al.* (1997). Diet, body size, physical activity, and the risk of endometrial cancer. *Cancer Res*, 57: 5077–5085. PMID:9371506

Goodman MT, McDuffie K, Kolonel LN *et al.* (2001). Case-control study of ovarian cancer and polymorphisms in genes involved in catecholestrogen formation and metabolism. *Cancer Epidemiol Biomarkers Prev*, 10: 209–216. PMID:11303589

Goodman MT & Tung KH (2003). Active and passive tobacco smoking and the risk of borderline and invasive ovarian cancer (United States). *Cancer Causes Control*, 14: 569–577. doi:10.1023/A:1024828309874 PMID:12948288

Gori GB (1976). *Report on the second set of experimental cigarettes.* In: *Report No. 2. Toward Less Hazardous Cigarettes. The Second Set of Experimental Cigarettes (DHEW Publ. No. (NIH) 76-1111).* Washington DC: Public Health Service, National Institutes of Health, National Cancer Institute.

Gorlewska-Roberts K, Green B, Fares M *et al.* (2002). Carcinogen-DNA adducts in human breast epithelial cells. *Environ Mol Mutagen*, 39: 184–192. doi:10.1002/em.10060 PMID:11921188

Goy J, Rosenberg MW, King WD (2008). Health risk behaviors: examining social inequalities in bladder and colorectal cancers. *Ann Epidemiol*, 18: 156–162. PMID:18191762

Graham EA, Croninger AB, Wynder EL (1957). Experimental production of carcinoma with cigarette tar. IV. Successful experiments with rabbits. *Cancer Res*, 17: 1058–1066. PMID:13489709

Grainge MJ, West J, Solaymani-Dodaran M *et al.* (2009). The antecedents of biliary cancer: a primary care case-control study in the United Kingdom. *Br J Cancer*, 100: 178–180. doi:10.1038/sj.bjc.6604765 PMID:19018260

Gram IT, Braaten T, Adami HO *et al.* (2008). Cigarette smoking and risk of borderline and invasive epithelial ovarian cancer. *Int J Cancer*, 122: 647–652.

Gram IT, Braaten T, Lund E *et al.* (2009). Cigarette smoking and risk of colorectal cancer among Norwegian women. *Cancer Causes Control*, 20: 895–903. doi:10.1007/s10552-009-9327-x PMID:19274482

Gram IT, Braaten T, Terry PD *et al.* (2005). Breast cancer risk among women who start smoking as teenagers. *Cancer Epidemiol Biomarkers Prev*, 14: 61–66. PMID:15668477

Green A, Purdie D, Bain C *et al.* (2001). Cigarette smoking and risk of epithelial ovarian cancer (Australia). *Cancer Causes Control*, 12: 713–719. doi:10.1023/A:1011297403819 PMID:11562111

Greenland S & Longnecker MP (1992). Methods for trend estimation from summarized dose-response data, with applications to meta-analysis. *Am J Epidemiol*, 135: 1301–1309. PMID:1626547

Griciute L, Castegnaro M, Bereziat JC (1981). Influence of ethyl alcohol on carcinogenesis with *N*-nitrosodimethylamine. *Cancer Lett*, 13: 345–352. doi:10.1016/0304-3835(81)90063-X PMID:7306961

Gronwald J, Byrski T, Huzarski T *et al.* (2006). Influence of selected lifestyle factors on breast and ovarian cancer risk in BRCA1 mutation carriers from Poland. *Breast Cancer Res Treat*, 95: 105–109. doi:10.1007/s10549-005-9051-5 PMID:16261399

Gross CP, Filardo G, Singh HS *et al.* (2006). The relation between projected breast cancer risk, perceived cancer risk, and mammography use. Results from the National Health Interview Survey. *J Gen Intern Med*, 21: 158–164. PMID:16390511

Gudmundsdottir K, Tryggvadottir L, Eyfjord JE (2001). *GSTM1*, *GSTT1*, and *GSTP1* genotypes in relation to breast cancer risk and frequency of mutations in the *p53* gene. *Cancer Epidemiol Biomarkers Prev*, 10: 1169–1173. PMID:11700265

Guengerich FP (2001). Common and uncommon cytochrome P450 reactions related to metabolism and chemical toxicity. *Chem Res Toxicol*, 14: 611–650. doi:10.1021/tx0002583 PMID:11409933

Guengerich FP & Shimada T (1998). Activation of procarcinogens by human cytochrome P450 enzymes. *Mutat Res*, 400: 201–213. PMID:9685642

Guengerich FP, Shimada T, Yun CH *et al.* (1994). Interactions of ingested food, beverage, and tobacco components involving human cytochrome P4501A2, 2A6, 2E1, and 3A4 enzymes. *Environ Health Perspect*, 102: Suppl 949–53. PMID:7698084

Guillemette C (2003). Pharmacogenomics of human UDP-glucuronosyltransferase enzymes. *Pharmacogenomics J*, 3: 136–158. doi:10.1038/sj.tpj.6500171 PMID:12815363

Gunnell AS, Tran TN, Torrång A *et al.* (2006). Synergy between cigarette smoking and human papillomavirus type 16 in cervical cancer in situ development. *Cancer Epidemiol Biomarkers Prev*, 15: 2141–2147. doi:10.1158/1055-9965.EPI-06-0399 PMID:17057029

Guo X, Johnson RC, Deng H *et al.* (2009). Evaluation of nonviral risk factors for nasopharyngeal carcinoma in a high-risk population of Southern China. *Int J Cancer*, 124: 2942–2947. doi:10.1002/ijc.24293 PMID:19296536

Gupta D, Boffetta P, Gaborieau V, Jindal SK (2001). Risk factors of lung cancer in Chandigarh, India. *Indian J Med Res*, 113: 142–150. PMID:11558323

Gupta MP, Khanduja KL, Koul IB, Sharma RR (1990). Effect of cigarette smoke inhalation on benzo[a]pyrene-induced lung carcinogenesis in vitamin A deficiency in the rat. *Cancer Lett*, 55: 83–88. doi:10.1016/0304-3835(90)90015-P PMID:2265418

Ha M, Mabuchi K, Sigurdson AJ *et al.* (2007). Smoking cigarettes before first childbirth and risk of breast cancer. *Am J Epidemiol*, 166: 55–61. doi:10.1093/aje/kwm045 PMID:17426039

Haiman CA, Stram DO, Wilkens LR *et al.* (2006). Ethnic and racial differences in the smoking-related risk of lung cancer. *N Engl J Med*, 354: 333–342.

Hamajima N, Hirose K, Tajima K *et al.*Collaborative Group on Hormonal Factors in Breast Cancer (2002). Alcohol, tobacco and breast cancer–collaborative reanalysis of individual data from 53 epidemiological studies, including 58,515 women with breast cancer and 95,067 women without the disease. *Br J Cancer*, 87: 1234–1245. doi:10.1038/sj.bjc.6600596 PMID:12439712

Hammond EC & Horn D (1958). Smoking and death rates: report on forty-four months of follow-up of 187,783 men. 2. Death rates by cause. *J Am Med Assoc*, 166: 1294–1308. PMID:12308037

Hammond EC & Seidman H (1980). Smoking and cancer in the United States. *Prev Med*, 9: 169–174. doi:10.1016/0091-7435(80)90071-7 PMID:7383981

Hammond EC, Selikoff IJ, Seidman H (1979). Asbestos exposure, cigarette smoking and death rates. *Ann N Y Acad Sci*, 330: 1 Health Hazard473–490. doi:10.1111/j.1749-6632.1979.tb18749.x PMID:294198

Hanaoka T, Yamamoto S, Sobue T *et al.*Japan Public Health Center-Based Prospective Study on Cancer and Cardiovascular Disease Study Group (2005). Active and passive smoking and breast cancer risk in middle-aged Japanese women. *Int J Cancer*, 114: 317–322. doi:10.1002/ijc.20709 PMID:15540214

Hannan LM, Jacobs EJ, Thun MJ (2009). The association between cigarette smoking and risk of colorectal cancer in a large prospective cohort from the United States. *Cancer Epidemiol Biomarkers Prev*, 18: 3362–3367. doi:10.1158/1055-9965.EPI-09-0661 PMID:19959683

Hansen AM, Mathiesen L, Pedersen M, Knudsen LE (2008). Urinary 1-hydroxypyrene (1-HP) in environmental and occupational studies–a review. *Int J Hyg Environ Health*, 211: 471–503. doi:10.1016/j.ijheh.2007.09.012 PMID:18222724

Hansen RD, Krath BN, Frederiksen K *et al.* (2009). GPX1 Pro(198)Leu polymorphism, erythrocyte GPX activity, interaction with alcohol consumption and smoking, and risk of colorectal cancer. *Mutat Res*, 664: 13–19. PMID:19428376

Harada T, Kitazawa T, Maita K, Shirasu Y (1985). Effects of vitamin C on tumor induction by diethylnitrosamine in the respiratory tract of hamsters exposed to cigarette smoke. *Cancer Lett*, 26: 163–169. doi:10.1016/0304-3835(85)90022-9 PMID:3978606

Harish K & Ravi R (1995). The role of tobacco in penile carcinoma. *Br J Urol*, 75: 375–377.

Harris JE, Thun MJ, Mondul AM, Calle EE (2004). Cigarette tar yields in relation to mortality from lung cancer in the cancer prevention study II prospective cohort, 1982–1998. *BMJ (Clinical Research Ed.)*, 328: 72–78. doi:10.1136/bmj.37936.585382.44

Harris RJ & Negroni G (1967). Production of lung carcinomas in C57BL mice exposed to a cigarette smoke and air mixture. *Br Med J*, 4: 637–641. doi:10.1136/bmj.4.5580.637 PMID:4293822

Harris RJ, Negroni G, Ludgate S *et al.* (1974). The incidence of lung tumours in c57bl mice exposed to cigarette smoke: air mixtures for prolonged periods. *Int J Cancer*, 14: 130–136. doi:10.1002/ijc.2910140116 PMID:4617705

Hartge P, Schiffman MH, Hoover R *et al.* (1989). A case-control study of epithelial ovarian cancer. *Am J Obstet Gynecol*, 161: 10–16. PMID:2750791

Hashibe M, Boffetta P, Janout V *et al.* (2007a). Esophageal cancer in Central and Eastern Europe: tobacco and alcohol. *Int J Cancer*, 120: 1518–1522. doi:10.1002/ijc.22507 PMID:17205526

Hashibe M, Boffetta P, Zaridze D *et al.* (2007b). Contribution of tobacco and alcohol to the high rates of squamous cell carcinoma of the supraglottis and glottis in Central Europe. *Am J Epidemiol*, 165: 814–820. doi:10.1093/aje/kwk066 PMID:17244634

Hashibe M, Brennan P, Benhamou S *et al.* (2007c). Alcohol drinking in never users of tobacco, cigarette smoking in never drinkers, and the risk of head and neck cancer: pooled analysis in the International Head and Neck Cancer Epidemiology Consortium. *J Natl Cancer Inst*, 99: 777–789. doi:10.1093/jnci/djk179 PMID:17505073

Hashibe M, Brennan P, Chuang SC *et al.* (2009). Interaction between tobacco and alcohol use and the risk of head and neck cancer: pooled analysis in the International Head and Neck Cancer Epidemiology Consortium. *Cancer Epidemiol Biomarkers Prev*, 18: 541–550. doi:10.1158/1055-9965.EPI-08-0347 PMID:19190158

Hassan MM, Phan A, Li D *et al.* (2008b). Risk factors associated with neuroendocrine tumors: A U.S.-based case-control study. *Int J Cancer*, 123: 867–873. doi:10.1002/ijc.23529 PMID:18491401

Hassan MM, Spitz MR, Thomas MB *et al.* (2008a). Effect of different types of smoking and synergism with hepatitis C virus on risk of hepatocellular carcinoma in American men and women: case-control study. *Int J Cancer*, 123: 1883–1891. doi:10.1002/ijc.23730 PMID:18688864

Hatsukami DK, Benowitz NL, Rennard SI *et al.* (2006a). Biomarkers to assess the utility of potential reduced exposure tobacco products. *Nicotine Tob Res*, 8: 600–622. PMID:16920658

Hatsukami DK, Le CT, Zhang Y *et al.* (2006b). Toxicant exposure in cigarette reducers versus light smokers. *Cancer Epidemiol Biomarkers Prev*, 15: 2355–2358. doi:10.1158/1055-9965.EPI-06-0240 PMID:17164356

Hatsukami DK, Lemmonds C, Zhang Y *et al.* (2004). Evaluation of carcinogen exposure in people who used "reduced exposure" tobacco products. *J Natl Cancer Inst*, 96: 844–852. PMID:15173268

Hawkins NJ & Ward RL (2001). Sporadic colorectal cancers with microsatellite instability and their possible origin in hyperplastic polyps and serrated adenomas. *J Natl Cancer Inst*, 93: 1307–1313. PMID:11535705

Hayes JR, Meckley DR, Stavanja MS *et al.* (2007). Effect of a flue-curing process that reduces tobacco specific nitrosamines on the tumor promotion in SENCAR mice by cigarette smoke condensate. *Food Chem Toxicol*, 45: 419–430. doi:10.1016/j.fct.2006.08.024 PMID:17070977

Hayes RB, Bravo-Otero E, Kleinman DV *et al.* (1999). Tobacco and alcohol use and oral cancer in Puerto Rico. *Cancer Causes Control*, 10: 27–33. doi:10.1023/A:1008876115797 PMID:10334639

Hayes RB, Kardaun JW, de Bruyn A (1987). Tobacco use and sinonasal cancer: a case-control study. *Br J Cancer*, 56: 843–846. PMID:3435710

Hecht SS (1998). Biochemistry, biology, and carcinogenicity of tobacco-specific *N*-nitrosamines. *Chem Res Toxicol*, 11: 559–603. doi:10.1021/tx980005y PMID:9625726

Hecht SS (1999). Tobacco smoke carcinogens and lung cancer. *J Natl Cancer Inst*, 91: 1194–1210. doi:10.1093/jnci/91.14.1194 PMID:10413421

Hecht SS (2000). Inhibition of carcinogenesis by isothiocyanates. *Drug Metab Rev*, 32: 395–411. doi:10.1081/DMR-100102342 PMID:11139137

Hecht SS (2002). Human urinary carcinogen metabolites: biomarkers for investigating tobacco and cancer. *Carcinogenesis*, 23: 907–922. doi:10.1093/carcin/23.6.907 PMID:12082012

Hecht SS (2003). Tobacco carcinogens, their biomarkers and tobacco-induced cancer. *Nat Rev Cancer*, 3: 733–744. doi:10.1038/nrc1190 PMID:14570033

Hecht SS (2008). Progress and challenges in selected areas of tobacco carcinogenesis. *Chem Res Toxicol*, 21: 160–171. doi:10.1021/tx7002068 PMID:18052103

Hecht SS, Carmella SG, Edmonds A *et al.* (2008b). Exposure to nicotine and a tobacco-specific carcinogen increase with duration of use of smokeless tobacco. *Tob Control*, 17: 128–131. doi:10.1136/tc.2007.023242 PMID:18375734

Hecht SS, Carmella SG, Murphy SE *et al.* (2007). Similar exposure to a tobacco-specific carcinogen in smokeless tobacco users and cigarette smokers. *Cancer Epidemiol*

Biomarkers Prev, 16: 1567–1572. doi:10.1158/1055-9965.EPI-07-0227 PMID:17684130

Hecht SS, Carmella SG, Stepanov I *et al.* (2008a). Metabolism of the tobacco-specific carcinogen 4-(methylnitrosamino)-1-(3-pyridyl)-1-butanone to its biomarker total NNAL in smokeless tobacco users. *Cancer Epidemiol Biomarkers Prev*, 17: 732–735. doi:10.1158/1055-9965.EPI-07-2843 PMID:18349296

Hecht SS, Carmella SG, Ye M *et al.* (2002). Quantitation of metabolites of 4-(methylnitrosamino)-1-(3-pyridyl)-1-butanone after cessation of smokeless tobacco use. *Cancer Res*, 62: 129–134. PMID:11782369

Hecht SS, Carmella SG, Yoder A *et al.* (2006). Comparison of polymorphisms in genes involved in polycyclic aromatic hydrocarbon metabolism with urinary phenanthrene metabolite ratios in smokers. *Cancer Epidemiol Biomarkers Prev*, 15: 1805–1811. doi:10.1158/1055-9965.EPI-06-0173 PMID:17035385

Hecht SS, Chen M, Yoder A *et al.* (2005a). Longitudinal study of urinary phenanthrene metabolite ratios: effect of smoking on the diol epoxide pathway. *Cancer Epidemiol Biomarkers Prev*, 14: 2969–2974. doi:10.1158/1055-9965.EPI-05-0396 PMID:16365018

Hecht SS & Hoffmann D (1988). Tobacco-specific nitrosamines, an important group of carcinogens in tobacco and tobacco smoke. *Carcinogenesis*, 9: 875–884. doi:10.1093/carcin/9.6.875 PMID:3286030

Hecht SS, Murphy SE, Carmella SG *et al.* (2004). Effects of reduced cigarette smoking on the uptake of a tobacco-specific lung carcinogen. *J Natl Cancer Inst*, 96: 107–115. PMID:14734700

Hecht SS, Murphy SE, Carmella SG *et al.* (2005b). Similar uptake of lung carcinogens by smokers of regular, light, and ultralight cigarettes. *Cancer Epidemiol Biomarkers Prev*, 14: 693–698. doi:10.1158/1055-9965.EPI-04-0542 PMID:15767351

Hecht SS, Rivenson A, Braley J *et al.* (1986). Induction of oral cavity tumors in F344 rats by tobacco-specific nitrosamines and snuff. *Cancer Res*, 46: 4162–4166. PMID:3731083

Hedberg K, Vaughan TL, White E *et al.* (1994). Alcoholism and cancer of the larynx: a case-control study in western Washington (United States). *Cancer Causes Control*, 5: 3–8. doi:10.1007/BF01830720 PMID:8123776

Heeschen C, Jang JJ, Weis M *et al.* (2001). Nicotine stimulates angiogenesis and promotes tumor growth and atherosclerosis. *Nat Med*, 7: 833–839. doi:10.1038/89961 PMID:11433349

Hein DW (2002). Molecular genetics and function of NAT1 and NAT2: role in aromatic amine metabolism and carcinogenesis. *Mutat Res*, 506–507: 65–77. PMID:12351146

Hein DW (2006). *N*-acetyltransferase 2 genetic polymorphism: effects of carcinogen and haplotype on urinary bladder cancer risk. *Oncogene*, 25: 1649–1658. doi:10.1038/sj.onc.1209374 PMID:16550165

Heineman EF, Zahm SH, McLaughlin JK, Vaught JB (1994). Increased risk of colorectal cancer among smokers: results of a 26-year follow-up of US veterans and a review. *Int J Cancer*, 59: 728–738. doi:10.1002/ijc.2910590603 PMID:7989109

Heling A-K, Schutte-Borkovec K, Heppel C *et al.* (2008). *Pyridyloxobutylated DNA adducts in oral mucosa of nonsmokers, smokers and snuff dippers in relation to other biomarkers of exposure.* AACR Meeting Abstracts, April 2008, Abstract 1883

Hellberg D & Stendahl U (2005). The biological role of smoking, oral contraceptive use and endogenous sexual steroid hormones in invasive squamous epithelial cervical cancer. *Anticancer Res*, 25: 3041–3046. PMID:16080563

Hellberg D, Valentin J, Eklund T, Nilsson S (1987). Penile cancer: is there an epidemiological role for smoking and sexual behaviour? *Br Med J (Clin Res Ed)*, 295: 1306–1308. doi:10.1136/bmj.295.6609.1306 PMID:3120988

Hemminki K, Koskinen M, Zhao C (2001). DNA adducts as a marker for cancer risk? *Int J Cancer*, 92: 923–925. doi:10.1002/ijc.1273 PMID:11351318

Henderson BE, Louie E, SooHoo Jing J *et al.* (1976). Risk factors associated with nasopharyngeal carcinoma. *N Engl J Med*, 295: 1101–1106. PMID:980005

Henley SJ, Thun MJ, Chao A, Calle EE (2004). Association between exclusive pipe smoking and mortality from cancer and other diseases. *J Natl Cancer Inst*, 96: 853–861. doi:10.1093/jnci/djh144 PMID:15173269

Henry CJ & Kouri RE (1986). Chronic inhalation studies in mice. II. Effects of long-term exposure to 2R1 cigarette smoke on (C57BL/Cum x C3H/AnfCum)F1 mice. *J Natl Cancer Inst*, 77: 203–212. PMID:3459913

Herity B, Moriarty M, Daly L *et al.* (1982). The role of tobacco and alcohol in the aetiology of lung and larynx cancer. *Br J Cancer*, 46: 961–964. PMID:7150489

Hermann S, Rohrmann S, Linseisen J (2009). *Lifestyle factors, obesity and the risk of colorectal adenomas in EPIC-Heidelberg.* Cancer Causes Control.

Herrinton LJ & Friedman GD (1998). Cigarette smoking and risk of non-Hodgkin's lymphoma subtypes. *Cancer Epidemiol Biomarkers Prev*, 7: 25–28. PMID:9456239

Hickey K, Do KA, Green A (2001). Smoking and prostate cancer. *Epidemiol Rev*, 23: 115–125. PMID:11588835

Hill M (1978). Etiology of the adenoma-carcinoma sequence. *Major Probl Pathol*, 10: 153–162. PMID:616868

Hjalgrim H, Ekström-Smedby K, Rostgaard K *et al.* (2007). Cigarette smoking and risk of Hodgkin lymphoma: a population-based case-control study. *Cancer Epidemiol Biomarkers Prev*, 16: 1561–1566.

Ho JW, Lam TH, Tse CW *et al.* (2004). Smoking, drinking and colorectal cancer in Hong Kong Chinese: a case-control study. *Int J Cancer*, 109: 587–597. doi:10.1002/ijc.20018 PMID:14991582

Hoffmann D & Brunnemann KD (1983). Endogenous formation of *N*-nitrosoproline in cigarette smokers. *Cancer Res*, 43: 5570–5574. PMID:6616484

Hoffmann D, Hoffmann I, El-Bayoumy K (2001). The less harmful cigarette: a controversial issue. a tribute to Ernst L. Wynder. *Chem Res Toxicol*, 14: 767–790. doi:10.1021/tx000260u PMID:11453723

Hoffmann D, Rivenson A, Hecht SS *et al.* (1979). Model studies in tobacco carcinogenesis with the Syrian golden hamster. *Prog Exp Tumor Res*, 24: 370–390. PMID:395571

Hoffmann D & Wynder EL (1971). A study of tobacco carcinogenesis. XI. Tumor initiators, tumor accelerators, and tumor promoting activity of condensate fractions. *Cancer*, 27: 848–864. doi:10.1002/1097-0142(197104)27:4<848::AID-CNCR2820270415>3.0.CO;2-4 PMID:5574075

Holmes MD, Murin S, Chen WY *et al.* (2007). Smoking and survival after breast cancer diagnosis. *Int J Cancer*, 120: 2672–2677. doi:10.1002/ijc.22575 PMID:17278091

Homann N, Tillonen J, Meurman JH *et al.* (2000). Increased salivary acetaldehyde levels in heavy drinkers and smokers: a microbiological approach to oral cavity cancer. *Carcinogenesis*, 21: 663–668. doi:10.1093/carcin/21.4.663 PMID:10753201

Horn-Ross PL, Ljung BM, Morrow M (1997). Environmental factors and the risk of salivary gland cancer. *Epidemiology*, 8: 414–419. doi:10.1097/00001648-199707000-00011 PMID:9209856

Hosgood HD 3rd, Zhang L, Shen M *et al.* (2009). Association between genetic variants in *VEGF*, *ERCC3* and occupational benzene haematotoxicity. *Occup Environ Med*, 66: 848–853. PMID:19773279

Hoshiyama Y, Kono S, Sasaba T *et al.* (2000). Relation of Cigarette Smoking, Alcohol Use, and Dietary Habits to Colon Adenomas: A Case-Control Study in Saitama, Japan. *Asian Pac J Cancer Prev*, 1: 139–146. PMID:12718681

Houlston RS (1999). Glutathione *S*-transferase M1 status and lung cancer risk: a meta-analysis. *Cancer Epidemiol Biomarkers Prev*, 8: 675–682. PMID:10744127

Houlston RS (2000). *CYP1A1* polymorphisms and lung cancer risk: a meta-analysis. *Pharmacogenetics*, 10: 105–114. doi:10.1097/00008571-200003000-00002 PMID:10761998

Hsing AW, McLaughlin JK, Chow WH *et al.* (1998). Risk factors for colorectal cancer in a prospective study among U.S. white men. *Int J Cancer*, 77: 549–553. doi:10.1002/(SICI)1097-0215(19980812)77:4<549::AID-IJC13>3.0.CO;2-1 PMID:9679757

Hsing AW, Nam JM, Co Chien HT *et al.* (1996). Risk factors for adrenal cancer: an exploratory study. *Int J Cancer*, 65: 432–436. doi:10.1002/(SICI)1097-0215(19960208)65:4<432::AID-IJC6>3.0.CO;2-Y PMID:8621222

Hsu WL, Chen JY, Chien YC *et al.* (2009). Independent effect of EBV and cigarette smoking on nasopharyngeal carcinoma: a 20-year follow-up study on 9,622 males without family history in Taiwan. *Cancer Epidemiol Biomarkers Prev*, 18: 1218–1226. doi:10.1158/1055-9965.EPI-08-1175 PMID:19336547

Hu J, Morrison H, Mery L *et al.*Canadian Cancer Registries Epidemiology Research Group (2007). Diet and vitamin or mineral supplementation and risk of colon cancer by subsite in Canada. *Eur J Cancer Prev*, 16: 275–291. doi:10.1097/01.cej.0000228411.21719.25 PMID:17554200

Hu J & Ugnat AMCanadian Cancer Registries Epidemiology Research Group (2005). Active and passive smoking and risk of renal cell carcinoma in Canada. *Eur J Cancer*, 41: 770–778. doi:10.1016/j.ejca.2005.01.003 PMID:15763654

Hukkanen J, Jacob P 3rd, Benowitz NL (2005). Metabolism and disposition kinetics of nicotine. *Pharmacol Rev*, 57: 79–115. doi:10.1124/pr.57.1.3 PMID:15734728

Huncharek M, Haddock KS, Reid R, Kupelnick B (2010). Smoking as a risk factor for prostate cancer: a meta-analysis of 24 prospective cohort studies. *Am J Public Health*, 100: 693–701. doi:10.2105/AJPH.2008.150508 PMID:19608952

Hung HC, Chuang J, Chien YC *et al.* (1997). Genetic polymorphisms of CYP2E1, GSTM1, and GSTT1; environmental factors and risk of oral cancer. *Cancer Epidemiol Biomarkers Prev*, 6: 901–905.

Hung RJ, Christiani DC, Risch A *et al.* (2008a). International lung cancer consortium: pooled analysis of sequence variants in DNA repair and cell cycle pathways. *Cancer Epidemiology, Biomarkers & Prevention*, 17: 3081–3089. doi:10.1158/1055-9965.EPI-08-0411

Hung RJ, McKay JD, Gaborieau V *et al.* (2008). A susceptibility locus for lung cancer maps to nicotinic acetylcholine receptor subunit genes on 15q25. *Nature*, 452: 633–637. doi:10.1038/nature06885 PMID:18385738

Hung RJ, McKay JD, Gaborieau V *et al.* (2008b). A susceptibility locus for lung cancer maps to nicotinic acetylcholine receptor subunit genes on 15q25. *Nature*, 452: 633–637. doi:10.1038/nature06885 PMID:18385738

Hunt JD, van der Hel OL, McMillan GP *et al.* (2005). Renal cell carcinoma in relation to cigarette smoking: meta-analysis of 24 studies. *Int J Cancer*, 114: 101–108. doi:10.1002/ijc.20618 PMID:15523697

Hunter DJ, Hankinson SE, Hough H *et al.* (1997). A prospective study of *NAT2* acetylation genotype, cigarette smoking, and risk of breast cancer. *Carcinogenesis*, 18: 2127–2132. doi:10.1093/carcin/18.11.2127 PMID:9395212

Husgafvel-Pursiainen K (2004). Genotoxicity of environmental tobacco smoke: a review. *Mutat Res*, 567: 427–445. doi:10.1016/j.mrrev.2004.06.004 PMID:15572289

Hutt JA, Vuillemenot BR, Barr EB *et al.* (2005). Life-span inhalation exposure to mainstream cigarette smoke induces lung cancer in B6C3F1 mice through genetic and epigenetic pathways. *Carcinogenesis*, 26: 1999–2009. doi:10.1093/carcin/bgi150 PMID:15944214

Huusom LD, Frederiksen K, Høgdall EV *et al.* (2006). Association of reproductive factors, oral contraceptive use and selected lifestyle factors with the risk of ovarian borderline tumors: a Danish case-control study. *Cancer Causes Control*, 17: 821–829. doi:10.1007/s10552-006-0022-x PMID:16783610

Huxley R; Asia Pacific Cohort Studies Collaboration (2007a). The role of lifestyle risk factors on mortality from colorectal cancer in populations of the Asia-Pacific region. *Asian Pac J Cancer Prev*, 8: 191–198. PMID:17696730

Huxley R, Jamrozik K, Lam TH *et al.*Asia Pacific Cohort Studies Collaboration (2007b). Impact of smoking and smoking cessation on lung cancer mortality in the Asia-Pacific region. *Am J Epidemiol*, 165: 1280–1286. doi:10.1093/aje/kwm002 PMID:17369610

Huxley RR, Ansary-Moghaddam A, Clifton P *et al.* (2009). The impact of dietary and lifestyle risk factors on risk of colorectal cancer: a quantitative overview of the epidemiological evidence. *Int J Cancer*, 125: 171–180. doi:10.1002/ijc.24343 PMID:19350627

Hymowitz N, Corle D, Royce J *et al.* (1995). Smokers' baseline characteristics in the COMMIT trial. *Prev Med*, 24: 503–508. doi:10.1006/pmed.1995.1080 PMID:8524726

IARC (1986). Tobacco smoking. *IARC Monogr Eval Carcinog Risk Chem Hum*, 38: 1–421.

IARC (1987). Overall evaluations of carcinogenicity: an updating of IARC Monographs volumes 1 to 42. *IARC Monogr Eval Carcinog Risks Hum Suppl*, 7: 1–440. PMID:3482203

IARC (1995). Human papillomaviruses. *IARC Monogr Eval Carcinog Risks Hum*, 64: 1–378. PMID:16755705

IARC (2002). *IARC handbook of cancer prevention, vol. 6. Weight control and physical activity.* IARC Press, Lyon: International Agency for Research on Cancer

IARC (2004a). Tobacco smoke and involuntary smoking. *IARC Monogr Eval Carcinog Risks Hum*, 83: 1–1438. PMID:15285078

IARC (2004b). Betel-quid and areca-nut chewing and some areca-nut derived nitrosamines. *IARC Monogr Eval Carcinog Risks Hum*, 85: 1–334. PMID:15635762

IARC (2006a). Formaldehyde, 2-butoxyethanol and 1-tert-butoxypropan-2-ol. *IARC Monogr Eval Carcinog Risks Hum*, 88: 1–478. PMID:17366697

IARC (2006b). *TP53 mutation database.* http://www.p53.iarc.fr/index.htlm.

IARC (2007a). Smokeless tobacco and some tobacco-specific N-nitrosamines. *IARC Monogr Eval Carcinog Risks Hum*, 89: 1–592. PMID:18335640

IARC (2007b). Human papillomaviruses. *IARC Monogr Eval Carcinog Risks Hum*, 90: 1–636. PMID:18354839

IARC (2007c). Combined estrogen-progestogen contraceptives and combined estrogen-progestogen menopausal therapy. *IARC Monogr Eval Carcinog Risks Hum*, 91: 1–528. PMID:18756632

IARC (2008). 1,3-Butadiene, ethylene oxide and vinyl halides (vinyl fluoride, vinyl chloride and vinyl bromide). *IARC Monogr Eval Carcinog Risks Hum*, 97: 1–510.

IARC (2010a). Alcohol consumption and ethyl carbamate. *IARC Monogr Eval Carcinog Risks Hum*, 96: 1–1428.

IARC (2010b). Some Aromatic Amines, Organic Dyes, and Related Exposures *IARC Monogr Eval Carcinog Risks Hum*, 99: 1–692.

IARC (2012c). Pharmaceuticals. *IARC Monogr Eval Carcinog Risks Hum*, 100A: 1–437. PMID:18335640

IARC (2012b). Biological agents. *IARC Monogr Eval Carcinog Risks Hum*, 100B: 1–475. PMID:18335640

IARC (2012a). Chemical agents and related occupations. *IARC Monogr Eval Carcinog Risks Hum*, 100F: PMID:18335640

Iarmarcovai G, Bonassi S, Botta A *et al.* (2008). Genetic polymorphisms and micronucleus formation: a review of the literature. *Mutat Res*, 658: 215–233. doi:10.1016/j.mrrev.2007.10.001 PMID:18037339

Ide R, Mizoue T, Fujino Y *et al.*JACC Study Group (2008). Cigarette smoking, alcohol drinking, and oral and pharyngeal cancer mortality in Japan. *Oral Dis*, 14: 314–319. doi:10.1111/j.1601-0825.2007.01378.x PMID:18449960

Iguchi T, Sugita S, Wang CY *et al.* (2009). MnSOD genotype and prostate cancer risk as a function of NAT genotype and smoking status. *In Vivo*, 23: 7–12. PMID:19368118

IIPS; International Institute for Population Sciences (2010).* *Mumbai and Ministry of Health and Family Welfare, Government of India. Global Adult Tobacco Survey India (GATS India).* New Delhi, India: Ministry of Health and Family Welfare, Government of India

Ingelman-Sundberg M (2004). Human drug metabolising cytochrome P450 enzymes: properties and polymorphisms. *Naunyn Schmiedebergs Arch Pharmacol*, 369: 89–104. doi:10.1007/s00210-003-0819-z PMID:14574440

Ingelman-Sundberg M (2005). Genetic polymorphisms of cytochrome P450 2D6 (CYP2D6): clinical consequences, evolutionary aspects and functional diversity. *Pharmacogenomics J*, 5: 6–13. doi:10.1038/sj.tpj.6500285 PMID:15492763

Ingelman-Sundberg M, Ronis MJ, Lindros KO *et al.* (1994). Ethanol-inducible cytochrome P4502E1: regulation, enzymology and molecular biology. *Alcohol Alcohol Suppl*, 2: 131–139. PMID:8974327

Ingelman-Sundberg M, Sim SC, Gomez A, Rodriguez-Antona C (2007). Influence of cytochrome P450 polymorphisms on drug therapies: pharmacogenetic, pharmacoepigenetic and clinical aspects. *Pharmacol Ther*, 116: 496–526. doi:10.1016/j.pharmthera.2007.09.004 PMID:18001838

Innes KE & Byers TE (2001). Smoking during pregnancy and breast cancer risk in very young women (United States). *Cancer Causes Control*, 12: 179–185. doi:10.1023/A:1008961512841 PMID:11246847

Inoue H, Kiyohara C, Marugame T *et al.* (2000). Cigarette smoking, CYP1A1 MspI and GSTM1 genotypes, and colorectal adenomas. *Cancer Res*, 60: 3749–3752. PMID:10919645

Inoue M, Tajima K, Takezaki T *et al.* (2003). Epidemiology of pancreatic cancer in Japan: a nested case-control study from the Hospital-based Epidemiologic Research Program at Aichi Cancer Center (HERPACC). *Int J Epidemiol*, 32: 257–262. doi:10.1093/ije/dyg062 PMID:12714546

Ioannidis JP (2008). Calibration of credibility of agnostic genome-wide associations. *Am J Med Genet B Neuropsychiatr Genet*, 147B: 964–972. PMID:18361430

Iodice S, Gandini S, Maisonneuve P, Lowenfels AB (2008). Tobacco and the risk of pancreatic cancer: a review and meta-analysis. *Langenbecks Arch Surg*, 393: 535–545. doi:10.1007/s00423-007-0266-2 PMID:18193270

Iribarren C, Tekawa IS, Sidney S, Friedman GD (1999). Effect of cigar smoking on the risk of cardiovascular disease, chronic obstructive pulmonary disease, and cancer in men. *N Engl J Med*, 340: 1773–1780. doi:10.1056/NEJM199906103402301 PMID:10362820

Isaksson B, Jonsson F, Pedersen NL *et al.* (2002). Lifestyle factors and pancreatic cancer risk: a cohort study from the Swedish Twin Registry. *Int J Cancer*, 98: 480–482. doi:10.1002/ijc.10256 PMID:11920604

Izzotti A, Calin GA, Arrigo P *et al.* (2009). Downregulation of microRNA expression in the lungs of rats exposed to cigarette smoke. *FASEB J*, 23: 806–812. doi:10.1096/fj.08-121384 PMID:18952709

Jacob P 3rd, Wilson M, Benowitz NL (2007). Determination of phenolic metabolites of polycyclic aromatic hydrocarbons in human urine as their pentafluorobenzyl ether derivatives using liquid chromatography-tandem mass spectrometry. *Anal Chem*, 79: 587–598. doi:10.1021/ac060920l PMID:17222024

Jain MG, Howe GR, Rohan TE (2000). Nutritional factors and endometrial cancer in Ontario, Canada. *Cancer Control*, 7: 288–296. PMID:10832115

Jalas JR, Hecht SS, Murphy SE (2005). Cytochrome P450 enzymes as catalysts of metabolism of 4-(methylnitrosamino)-1-(3-pyridyl)-1-butanone, a tobacco specific carcinogen. *Chem Res Toxicol*, 18: 95–110. doi:10.1021/tx049847p PMID:15720112

Jass JR (2007). Molecular heterogeneity of colorectal cancer: Implications for cancer control. *Surg Oncol*, 16: Suppl 1S7–S9. doi:10.1016/j.suronc.2007.10.039 PMID:18023574

Jass JR, Young J, Leggett BA (2000). Hyperplastic polyps and DNA microsatellite unstable cancers of the colorectum. *Histopathology*, 37: 295–301. PMID:11012735

Jayalekshmy PA, Akiba S, Nair MK *et al.* (2008). Bidi smoking and lung cancer incidence among males in Karunagappally cohort in Kerala, India. *Int J Cancer*, 123: 1390–1397. doi:10.1002/ijc.23618 PMID:18623085

Jean RT, Wilkinson AV, Spitz MR *et al.* (2011). Psychosocial risk and correlates of early menarche in Mexican-American girls. *Am J Epidemiol*, 173: 1203–1210. Epub 2011 Mar 31.

Jee SH, Samet JM, Ohrr H *et al.* (2004). Smoking and cancer risk in Korean men and women. *Cancer Causes Control*, 15: 341–348. doi:10.1023/B:CACO.0000027481.48153.97 PMID:15141135

Jeffreys M, Warren R, Gunnell D *et al.* (2004). Life course breast cancer risk factors and adult breast density (United Kingdom). *Cancer Causes Control*, 15: 947–955. PMID:15577297

Jensen J & Christiansen C (1988). Effects of smoking on serum lipoproteins and bone mineral content during postmenopausal hormone replacement therapy. *Am J Obstet Gynecol*, 159: 820–825. PMID:2972209

Jensen J, Christiansen C, Rødbro P (1985). Cigarette smoking, serum estrogens, and bone loss during hormone-replacement therapy early after menopause. *N Engl J Med*, 313: 973–975. doi:10.1056/NEJM198510173131602 PMID:4047104

Ji BT, Dai Q, Gao YT *et al.* (2002). Cigarette and alcohol consumption and the risk of colorectal cancer in Shanghai, China. *Eur J Cancer Prev*, 11: 237–244. doi:10.1097/00008469-200206000-00007 PMID:12131657

Ji BT, Weissfeld JL, Chow WH *et al.* (2006). Tobacco smoking and colorectal hyperplastic and adenomatous polyps. *Cancer Epidemiol Biomarkers Prev*, 15: 897–901. doi:10.1158/1055-9965.EPI-05-0883 PMID:16702367

Jiang J, Suzuki S, Xiang J *et al.* (2005). Plasma carotenoid, alpha-tocopherol and retinol concentrations and risk of colorectal adenomas: A case-control study in Japan. *Cancer Lett*, 226: 133–141. doi:10.1016/j.canlet.2005.03.040 PMID:15885891

Jin MJ, Chen K, Song L *et al.* (2005). The association of the DNA repair gene XRCC3 Thr241Met polymorphism with susceptibility to colorectal cancer in a Chinese population. *Cancer Genet Cytogenet*, 163: 38–43. doi:10.1016/j.cancergencyto.2005.05.001 PMID:16271954

Jin Q, Menter DG, Mao L *et al.* (2008). Survivin expression in normal human bronchial epithelial cells: an early and critical step in tumorigenesis induced by tobacco exposure. *Carcinogenesis*, 29: 1614–1622. doi:10.1093/carcin/bgm234 PMID:18635526

Johnson KC (2005). Accumulating evidence on passive and active smoking and breast cancer risk. *Int J Cancer*, 117: 619–628. doi:10.1002/ijc.21150 PMID:15929073

Johnson KC, Goodman M, Kelsh M *et al.* (2002). Passive and active smoking as possible confounders in studies of breast cancer risk. *Epidemiology*, 13: 610–611, author reply 610–611. doi:10.1097/00001648-200209000-00029 PMID:12192238

Johnson KC, Hu J, Mao YCanadian Cancer Registries Epidemiology Research Group (2000). Passive and active smoking and breast cancer risk in Canada, 1994–97. *Cancer Causes Control*, 11: 211–221. doi:10.1023/A:1008906105790 PMID:10782655

Johnson L, Mercer K, Greenbaum D *et al.* (2001). Somatic activation of the K-ras oncogene causes early onset lung cancer in mice. *Nature*, 410: 1111–1116. doi:10.1038/35074129 PMID:11323676

Jones PA & Baylin SB (2007). The epigenomics of cancer. *Cell*, 128: 683–692. doi:10.1016/j.cell.2007.01.029 PMID:17320506

Kabat GC, Chang CJ, Wynder EL (1994). The role of tobacco, alcohol use, and body mass index in oral and pharyngeal cancer. *Int J Epidemiol*, 23: 1137–1144. doi:10.1093/ije/23.6.1137 PMID:7721514

Kabat GC & Hebert JR (1994). Use of mentholated cigarettes and oropharyngeal cancer. *Epidemiology*, 5: 183–188. PMID:8172993

Kabat GC, Ng SKC, Wynder EL (1993). Tobacco, alcohol intake, and diet in relation to adenocarcinoma of the esophagus and gastric cardia. *Cancer Causes Control*, 4: 123–132.

Kaczynski AT, Manske SR, Mannell RC, Grewal K (2008). Smoking and physical activity: a systematic review. *Am J Health Behav*, 32: 93–110. PMID:18021037

Kadlubar FF, Beland FA (1985). *Chemical properties of ultimate carcinogenic metabolites of arylamines and arylamides.* In: *Polycyclic Hydrocarbons and Carcinogenesis.* Harvey RG, editor. Washington, D.C.: American Chemical Society.

Kaerlev L, Teglbjaerg PS, Sabroe S *et al.* (2002). The importance of smoking and medical history for development of small bowel carcinoid tumor: a European population-based case-control study. *Cancer Causes Control*, 13: 27–34.

Kamataki T, Fujieda M, Kiyotani K *et al.* (2005). Genetic polymorphism of CYP2A6 as one of the potential determinants of tobacco-related cancer risk. *Biochem Biophys Res Commun*, 338: 306–310. doi:10.1016/j.bbrc.2005.08.268 PMID:16176798

Kanda J, Matsuo K, Kawase T *et al.* (2009). Association of alcohol intake and smoking with malignant lymphoma risk in Japanese: a hospital-based case-control study at Aichi Cancer Center. *Cancer Epidemiol Biomarkers Prev*, 18: 2436–2441. Epub 2009 Sep 1.

Kapeu AS, Luostarinen T, Jellum E *et al.* (2009). Is smoking an independent risk factor for invasive cervical cancer? A nested case-control study within Nordic biobanks. *Am J Epidemiol*, 169: 480–488. doi:10.1093/aje/kwn354 PMID:19074773

Kasahara M, Osawa K, Yoshida K *et al.* (2008). Association of *MUTYH Gln324His* and *APEX1 Asp148Glu* with colorectal cancer and smoking in a Japanese population. *J Exp Clin Cancer Res*, 27: 49 doi:10.1186/1756-9966-27-49 PMID:18823566

Kato M, Loomis D, Brooks LM *et al.* (2004). Urinary biomarkers in charcoal workers exposed to wood smoke in Bahia State, Brazil. *Cancer Epidemiol Biomarkers Prev*, 13: 1005–1012. PMID:15184257

Kawajiri K (1999). CYP1A1. *IARC Sci Publ*, 148: 159–172. PMID:10493257

Kawajiri K, Eguchi H, Nakachi K *et al.* (1996). Association of *CYP1A1* germ line polymorphisms with mutations of the *p53* gene in lung cancer. *Cancer Res*, 56: 72–76. PMID:8548778

Kelsey JL, Gammon MD, John EM (1993). Reproductive factors and breast cancer. *Epidemiol Rev*, 15: 36–47. PMID:8405211

Kelsey JL, LiVolsi VA, Holford TR *et al.* (1982). A case-control study of cancer of the endometrium. *Am J Epidemiol*, 116: 333–342. PMID:7114042

Kenfield SA, Stampfer MJ, Rosner BA, Colditz GA (2008). Smoking and smoking cessation in relation to mortality in women. *JAMA*, 299: 2037–2047. doi:10.1001/jama.299.17.2037 PMID:18460664

Kesarwani P, Singh R, Mittal RD (2009). Association of GSTM3 intron 6 variant with cigarette smoking, tobacco chewing and alcohol as modifier factors for prostate cancer risk. *Arch Toxicol*, 83: 351–356. doi:10.1007/s00204-008-0343-5 PMID:18668224

Ketterer B, Harris JM, Talaska G *et al.* (1992). The human glutathione *S*-transferase supergene family, its polymorphism, and its effects on susceptibility to lung cancer. *Environ Health Perspect*, 98: 87–94. doi:10.2307/3431252 PMID:1486868

Key TJ, Pike MC, Baron JA *et al.* (1991). Cigarette smoking and steroid hormones in women. *J Steroid Biochem Mol Biol*, 39: 4A529–534. doi:10.1016/0960-0760(91)90247-3 PMID:1832941

Key TJ, Pike MC, Brown JB *et al.* (1996). Cigarette smoking and urinary oestrogen excretion in premenopausal and post-menopausal women. *Br J Cancer*, 74: 1313–1316. PMID:8883424

Khaw KT, Tazuke S, Barrett-Connor E (1988). Cigarette smoking and levels of adrenal androgens in post-menopausal women. *N Engl J Med*, 318: 1705–1709. doi:10.1056/NEJM198806303182601 PMID:2967432

Kiemeney LA, Thorlacius S, Sulem P *et al.* (2008). Sequence variant on 8q24 confers susceptibility to urinary bladder cancer. *Nat Genet*, 40: 1307–1312. doi:10.1038/ng.229 PMID:18794855

Kim CS, Kim MC, Cheong HK *et al.* (2005[The association of obesity and left colonic adenomatous polyps in Korean adult men]). *J Prev Med Pub Health*, 38: 415–419. PMID:16358826.

Kim HJ, Lee SM, Choi NK *et al.* (2006). [Smoking and colorectal cancer risk in the Korean elderly][Article in Korean]*J Prev Med Pub Health*, 39: 123–129.

Kim JI, Park YJ, Kim KH *et al.* (2003). hOGG1 Ser326Cys polymorphism modifies the significance of the environmental risk factor for colon cancer. *World J Gastroenterol*, 9: 956–960. PMID:12717837

Kim SG & Novak RF (1990). Role of P450IIE1 in the metabolism of 3-hydroxypyridine, a constituent of tobacco smoke: redox cycling and DNA strand scission by the metabolite 2,5-dihydroxypyridine. *Cancer Res*, 50: 5333–5339. PMID:2167153

Kim Y, Shin A, Gwack J *et al.* (2007). Cigarette smoking and gastric cancer risk in a community-based cohort study in Korea *J Prev Med Public Health*, 40: 467–474. doi:10.3961/jpmph.2007.40.6.467 PMID:18063902

Kiyohara C, Yoshimasu K, Shirakawa T, Hopkin JM (2004). Genetic polymorphisms and environmental risk of lung cancer: a review. *Rev Environ Health*, 19: 15–38. PMID:15186038

Kiyohara C, Yoshimasu K, Takayama K, Nakanishi Y (2005). NQO1, MPO, and the risk of lung cancer: a HuGE review. *Genet Med*, 7: 463–478. doi:10.1097/01.gim.0000177530.55043.c1 PMID:16170238

Kiyohara C, Yoshimasu K, Takayama K, Nakanishi Y (2006). EPHX1 polymorphisms and the risk of lung cancer: a HuGE review. *Epidemiology*, 17: 89–99. PMID:16357600

Kjaerheim K, Gaard M, Andersen A (1998). The role of alcohol, tobacco, and dietary factors in upper aerogastric tract cancers: a prospective study of 10,900 Norwegian men. *Cancer Causes Control*, 9: 99–108. doi:10.1023/A:1008809706062 PMID:9486469

Klotz U & Ammon E (1998). Clinical and toxicological consequences of the inductive potential of ethanol. *Eur J Clin Pharmacol*, 54: 7–12. doi:10.1007/s002280050412 PMID:9591923

Ko Y, Abel J, Harth V *et al.* (2001). Association of CYP1B1 codon 432 mutant allele in head and neck squamous cell cancer is reflected by somatic mutations of p53 in tumor tissue. *Cancer Res*, 61: 4398–4404. PMID:11389067

Ko YC, Huang YL, Lee CH *et al.* (1995). Betel quid chewing, cigarette smoking and alcohol consumption related to oral cancer in Taiwan. *J Oral Pathol Med*, 24: 450–453. doi:10.1111/j.1600-0714.1995.tb01132.x PMID:8600280

Koizumi Y, Tsubono Y, Nakaya N *et al.* (2004). Cigarette smoking and the risk of gastric cancer: a pooled analysis of two prospective studies in Japan. *Int J Cancer*, 112: 1049–1055. doi:10.1002/ijc.20518 PMID:15386347

Kono S, Ikeda M, Tokudome S *et al.* (1987). Cigarette smoking, alcohol and cancer mortality: a cohort study of male Japanese physicians. *Jpn J Cancer Res*, 78: 1323–1328. PMID:3123436

Kotwall CA (1992). Smoking as an etiologic factor in the development of Warthin's tumor of the parotid gland. *Am J Surg*, 164: 646–647. doi:10.1016/S0002-9610(05)80725-1 PMID:1334381

Koumantaki Y, Tzonou A, Koumantakis E *et al.* (1989). A case-control study of cancer of endometrium in Athens. *Int J Cancer*, 43: 795–799. doi:10.1002/ijc.2910430509 PMID:2714884

Kreuzer M, Boffetta P, Whitley E *et al.* (2000). Gender differences in lung cancer risk by smoking: a multicentre case-control study in Germany and Italy. *Br J Cancer*, 82: 227–233. PMID:10638994

Krewski D, Lubin JH, Zielinski JM *et al.* (2005). Residential radon and risk of lung cancer: a combined analysis of 7 North American case-control studies. *Epidemiology*, 16: 137–145. PMID:15703527

Kropp S & Chang-Claude J (2002). Active and passive smoking and risk of breast cancer by age 50 years among German women. *Am J Epidemiol*, 156: 616–626. doi:10.1093/aje/kwf093 PMID:12244030

Kubík A, Zatloukal P, Boyle P *et al.* (2001). A case-control study of lung cancer among Czech women. *Lung Cancer*, 31: 111–122. PMID:11165390

Kuljukka-Rabb T, Nylund L, Vaaranrinta R *et al.* (2002). The effect of relevant genotypes on PAH exposure-related biomarkers. *J Expo Anal Environ Epidemiol*, 12: 81–91. doi:10.1038/sj.jea.7500204 PMID:11859435

Kuller LH, Ockene JK, Meilahn E *et al.*MRFIT Research Group (1991). Cigarette smoking and mortality. *Prev Med*, 20: 638–654. doi:10.1016/0091-7435(91)90060-H PMID:1758843

Kundu CN, Balusu R, Jaiswal AS *et al.* (2007). Cigarette smoke condensate-induced level of adenomatous polyposis coli blocks long-patch base excision repair in breast epithelial cells. *Oncogene*, 26: 1428–1438. doi:10.1038/sj.onc.1209925 PMID:16924228

Kuper H, Titus-Ernstoff L, Harlow BL, Cramer DW (2000b). Population based study of coffee, alcohol and tobacco use and risk of ovarian cancer. *Int J Cancer*, 88: 313–318. doi:10.1002/1097-0215(20001015)88:2<313::AID-IJC26>3.0.CO;2-5 PMID:11004686

Kuper H, Tzonou A, Kaklamani E *et al.* (2000a). Tobacco smoking, alcohol consumption and their interaction in the causation of hepatocellular carcinoma. *Int J Cancer*, 85: 498–502. doi:10.1002/(SICI)1097-0215(20000215)85:4<498::AID-IJC9>3.0.CO;2-F PMID:10699921

Kurian AW, Balise RR, McGuire V, Whittemore AS (2005). Histologic types of epithelial ovarian cancer: have they different risk factors? *Gynecol Oncol*, 96: 520–530. doi:10.1016/j.ygyno.2004.10.037 PMID:15661246

Kurosawa M, Kikuchi S, Xu J, Inaba Y (2006). Highly salted food and mountain herbs elevate the risk for stomach cancer death in a rural area of Japan. *J Gastroenterol Hepatol*, 21: 1681–1686. doi:10.1111/j.1440-1746.2006.04290.x PMID:16984589

La Torre G, Chiaradia G, Gianfagna F *et al.* (2009). Smoking status and gastric cancer risk: an updated meta-analysis of case-control studies published in the past ten years. *Tumori*, 95: 13–22. PMID:19366050

La Vecchia C, Franceschi S, Bosetti C *et al.* (1999). Time since stopping smoking and the risk of oral and pharyngeal cancers. *J Natl Cancer Inst*, 91: 726–728. doi:10.1093/jnci/91.8.726a PMID:10218516

Lacey JV Jr, Leitzmann MF, Chang SC *et al.* (2007). Endometrial cancer and menopausal hormone therapy in the National Institutes of Health-AARP Diet and Health Study cohort. *Cancer*, 109: 1303–1311. doi:10.1002/cncr.22525 PMID:17315161

Ladeiras-Lopes R, Pereira AK, Nogueira A *et al.* (2008). Smoking and gastric cancer: systematic review and meta-analysis of cohort studies. *Cancer Causes Control*, 19: 689–701. doi:10.1007/s10552-008-9132-y PMID:18293090

Lagergren J, Bergström R, Lindgren A, Nyrén O (2000). The role of tobacco, snuff and alcohol use in the aetiology of cancer of the oesophagus and gastric cardia. *Int J Cancer*, 85: 340–346. doi:10.1002/(SICI)1097-0215(20000201)85:3<340::AID-IJC8>3.0.CO;2-N PMID:10652424

Lam TK, Gallicchio L, Lindsley K *et al.* (2009). Cruciferous vegetable consumption and lung cancer risk: a systematic review. *Cancer Epidemiol Biomarkers Prev*, 18: 184–195. doi:10.1158/1055-9965.EPI-08-0710 PMID:19124497

Lan Q, Zhang L, Li G *et al.* (2004). Hematotoxicity in workers exposed to low levels of benzene. *Science*, 306: 1774–1776. doi:10.1126/science.1102443 PMID:15576619

Landi MT, Chatterjee N, Yu K *et al.* (2009). A genome-wide association study of lung cancer identifies a region of chromosome 5p15 associated with risk for adenocarcinoma. *Am J Hum Genet*, 85: 679–691. doi:10.1016/j.ajhg.2009.09.012 PMID:19836008

Lang M & Pelkonen O (1999). Metabolism of xenobiotics and chemical carcinogenesis. *IARC Sci Publ*, 14813–22. PMID:10493245

Lanier A, Bender T, Talbot M *et al.* (1980). Nasopharyngeal carcinoma in Alaskan Eskimos Indians, and Aleuts: a review of cases and study of Epstein-Barr virus, HLA, and environmental risk factors. *Cancer*, 46: 2100–2106. doi:10.1002/1097-0142(19801101)46:9<2100::AID-CNCR2820460932>3.0.CO;2-G PMID:6253051

Lao Y, Yu N, Kassie F *et al.* (2007). Analysis of pyridyloxobutyl DNA adducts in F344 rats chronically treated with (*R*)- and (*S*)-*N*′-nitrosonornicotine. *Chem Res Toxicol*, 20: 246–256. doi:10.1021/tx060208j PMID:17305408

Lapidus L, Lindstedt G, Lundberg PA *et al.* (1986). Concentrations of sex-hormone binding globulin and corticosteroid binding globulin in serum in relation to cardiovascular risk factors and to 12-year incidence of cardiovascular disease and overall mortality in postmenopausal women. *Clin Chem*, 32: 146–152. PMID:3940696

Larsen IK, Grotmol T, Almendingen K, Hoff G (2006). Lifestyle as a predictor for colonic neoplasia in asymptomatic individuals. *BMC Gastroenterol*, 6: 5 doi:10.1186/1471-230X-6-5 PMID:16412216

Larsson SC, Permert J, Håkansson N *et al.* (2005). Overall obesity, abdominal adiposity, diabetes and cigarette smoking in relation to the risk of pancreatic cancer in two Swedish population-based cohorts. *Br J Cancer*, 93: 1310–1315. doi:10.1038/sj.bjc.6602868 PMID:16288300

Lash TL & Aschengrau A (1999). Active and passive cigarette smoking and the occurrence of breast cancer. *Am J Epidemiol*, 149: 5–12. PMID:9883788

Lash TL & Aschengrau A (2002). A null association between active or passive cigarette smoking and breast cancer risk. *Breast Cancer Res Treat*, 75: 181–184. doi:10.1023/A:1019625102365 PMID:12243511

Lau A, Belanger CL, Winn LM (2009). *In utero* and acute exposure to benzene: investigation of DNA double-strand breaks and DNA recombination in mice. *Mutat Res*, 676: 74–82. PMID:19486867

Launoy G, Milan C, Faivre J *et al.* (2000). Tobacco type and risk of squamous cell cancer of the oesophagus in males: a French multicentre case-control study. *Int J Epidemiol*, 29: 36–42. doi:10.1093/ije/29.1.36 PMID:10750601

Law MR, Cheng R, Hackshaw AK *et al.* (1997). Cigarette smoking, sex hormones and bone density in women. *Eur J Epidemiol*, 13: 553–558. doi:10.1023/A:1007389712487 PMID:9258568

Lawlor DA, Ebrahim S, Smith GD (2004). Smoking before the birth of a first child is not associated with increased risk of breast cancer: findings from the British Women's Heart and Health Cohort Study and a meta-analysis. *Br J Cancer*, 91: 512–518. doi:10.1038/sj.bjc.6601916 PMID:15226777

Lawrence C, Tessaro I, Durgerian S *et al.* (1987). Smoking, body weight, and early-stage endometrial cancer. *Cancer*, 59: 1665–1669. doi:10.1002/1097-0142(19870501)59:9<1665::AID-CNCR2820590924>3.0.CO;2-2 PMID:3828966

Lawrence C, Tessaro I, Durgerian S *et al.* (1989). Advanced-stage endometrial cancer: contributions of estrogen use, smoking, and other risk factors. *Gynecol Oncol*, 32: 41–45. doi:10.1016/0090-8258(89)90847-0 PMID:2909447

Le Calvez F, Mukeria A, Hunt JD *et al.* (2005). *TP53* and *KRAS* mutation load and types in lung cancers in relation to tobacco smoke: distinct patterns in never, former, and current smokers. *Cancer Res*, 65: 5076–5083. doi:10.1158/0008-5472.CAN-05-0551 PMID:15958551

Le Marchand L, Derby KS, Murphy SE *et al.* (2008). Smokers with the *CHRNA* lung cancer-associated variants are exposed to higher levels of nicotine equivalents and a carcinogenic tobacco-specific nitrosamine. *Cancer Res*, 68: 9137–9140. doi:10.1158/0008-5472.CAN-08-2271 PMID:19010884

Le Marchand L, Guo C, Benhamou S *et al.* (2003). Pooled analysis of the *CYP1A1* exon 7 polymorphism and lung cancer (United States). *Cancer Causes Control*, 14: 339–346. doi:10.1023/A:1023956201228 PMID:12846365

Le Marchand L, Sivaraman L, Pierce L *et al.* (1998). Associations of *CYP1A1*, GSTM1, and *CYP2E1* polymorphisms with lung cancer suggest cell type specificities to tobacco carcinogens. *Cancer Res*, 58: 4858–4863. PMID:9809991

Le Marchand L, Wilkens LR, Kolonel LN *et al.* (1997). Associations of sedentary lifestyle, obesity, smoking, alcohol use, and diabetes with the risk of colorectal cancer. *Cancer Res*, 57: 4787–4794. PMID:9354440

Lea IA, Jackson MA, Li X *et al.* (2007). Genetic pathways and mutation profiles of human cancers: site- and exposure-specific patterns. *Carcinogenesis*, 28: 1851–1858. doi:10.1093/carcin/bgm176 PMID:17693665

Lee CH, Wu DC, Lee JM *et al.* (2007a). Carcinogenetic impact of alcohol intake on squamous cell carcinoma risk of the oesophagus in relation to tobacco smoking. *Eur J Cancer*, 43: 1188–1199. doi:10.1016/j.ejca.2007.01.039 PMID:17383866

Lee CH, Wu DC, Lee JM *et al.* (2007b). Anatomical subsite discrepancy in relation to the impact of the consumption of alcohol, tobacco and betel quid on esophageal cancer. *Int J Cancer*, 120: 1755–1762. doi:10.1002/ijc.22324 PMID:17230518

Lee CY, Lee JY, Kang JW, Kim H (2001). Effects of genetic polymorphisms of CYP1A1, CYP2E1, GSTM1, and GSTT1 on the urinary levels of 1-hydroxypyrene and 2-naphthol in aircraft maintenance workers. *Toxicol Lett*, 123: 115–124. doi:10.1016/S0378-4274(01)00374-5 PMID:11641039

Lee JM, Yanagawa J, Peebles KA *et al.* (2008b). Inflammation in lung carcinogenesis: new targets for lung cancer chemoprevention and treatment. *Crit Rev Oncol Hematol*, 66: 208–217. doi:10.1016/j.critrevonc.2008.01.004 PMID:18304833

Lee K, Cáceres D, Varela N *et al.* (2006). Allelic variants of cytochrome P4501A1 (CYP1A1), glutathione S transferase M1 (GSTM1) polymorphisms and their association with smoking and alcohol consumption as gastric cancer susceptibility biomarkers *Rev Med Chil*, 134: 1107–1115. PMID:17171211

Lee KM, Kang D, Clapper ML *et al.* (2008a). *CYP1A1*, *GSTM1*, and *GSTT1* polymorphisms, smoking, and lung cancer risk in a pooled analysis among Asian populations. *Cancer Epidemiol Biomarkers Prev*, 17: 1120–1126. doi:10.1158/1055-9965.EPI-07-2786 PMID:18463401

Lee KW, Kuo WR, Tsai SM *et al.* (2005a). Different impact from betel quid, alcohol and cigarette: risk factors for pharyngeal and laryngeal cancer. *Int J Cancer*, 117: 831–836. doi:10.1002/ijc.21237 PMID:15957167

Lee PN (1999). *Uses and abuses of cotinine as a marker of tobacco smoke exposure*. In: *Analytical Determination of Nicotine and Related Compounds and Their Metabolites*. Gorrod JW, Jacob P III, editors. Amsterdam: Elsevier, pp. 669–719

Lee PN (2001). Relation between exposure to asbestos and smoking jointly and the risk of lung cancer. *Occup Environ Med*, 58: 145–153. doi:10.1136/oem.58.3.145 PMID:11171926

Lee YCA, Cohet C, Yang YC *et al.* (2009). Meta-analysis of epidemiologic studies on cigarette smoking and liver cancer. *Int J Epidemiol*, 38: 1497–1511. doi:10.1093/ije/dyp280 PMID:19720726

Lesko SM, Rosenberg L, Kaufman DW *et al.* (1985). Cigarette smoking and the risk of endometrial cancer. *N Engl J Med*, 313: 593–596. doi:10.1056/NEJM198509053131001 PMID:4022045

Leuchtenberger C, Leuchtenberger R (1970). *Effects of chronic inhalation of whole fresh cigarette smoke and of its gas phase on pulmonary tumorigenesis in Snell's mice.* In: *Morphology of Experimental Respiratory Carcinogenesis. Proceedings of a Biology Division.* Nettesheim P, Hanna MGJ, Deathevage JWJ, editors. Oak Ridge National Laboratory Conference, US Atomic Energy Commission, pp. 329–346.

Levi F & La Vecchia C (2001). Tobacco smoking and prostate cancer: time for an appraisal. *Ann Oncol*, 12: 733–738. doi:10.1023/A:1011124523984 PMID:11484946

Levi F, la Vecchia C, Decarli A (1987). Cigarette smoking and the risk of endometrial cancer. *Eur J Cancer Clin Oncol*, 23: 1025–1029. doi:10.1016/0277-5379(87)90353-1 PMID:3665988

Levi F, Ollyo JB, La Vecchia C *et al.* (1990). The consumption of tobacco, alcohol and the risk of adenocarcinoma in Barrett's oesophagus. *Int J Cancer*, 45: 852–854. doi:10.1002/ijc.2910450511 PMID:2335388

Lewin F, Norell SE, Johansson H *et al.* (1998). Smoking tobacco, oral snuff, and alcohol in the etiology of squamous cell carcinoma of the head and neck: a population-based case-referent study in Sweden. *Cancer*, 82: 1367–1375.

Li CI, Malone KE, Daling JR (2005). The relationship between various measures of cigarette smoking and risk of breast cancer among older women 65–79 years of age (United States). *Cancer Causes Control*, 16: 975–985. doi:10.1007/s10552-005-2906-6 PMID:16132806

Li JY, Ershow AG, Chen ZJ *et al.* (1989). A case-control study of cancer of the esophagus and gastric cardia in Linxian. *Int J Cancer*, 43: 755–761. doi:10.1002/ijc.2910430502 PMID:2714880

Li W, Ray RM, Gao DL *et al.* (2006). Occupational risk factors for pancreatic cancer among female textile workers in Shanghai, China. *Occup Environ Med*, 63: 788–793. doi:10.1136/oem.2005.026229 PMID:16847032

Li X & Hemminki K (2004). Inherited predisposition to early onset lung cancer according to histological type. *International Journal of Cancer*, 112: 451–457. doi:10.1002/ijc.20436

Li Y, Jiang Y, Zhang M *et al.* (2011). Drinking behaviour among men and women in China: the 2007 China Chronic Disease and Risk Factor Surveillance. *Addiction*, 106: 1946–1956.

Li Y, Millikan RC, Bell DA *et al.* (2004). Cigarette smoking, cytochrome P4501A1 polymorphisms, and breast cancer among African-American and white women. *Breast Cancer Res*, 6: R460–R473. doi:10.1186/bcr814 PMID:15217514

Liang PS, Chen TY, Giovannucci E (2009). Cigarette smoking and colorectal cancer incidence and mortality: systematic review and meta-analysis. *Int J Cancer*, 124: 2406–2415. doi:10.1002/ijc.24191 PMID:19142968

Liaw KM & Chen CJ (1998). Mortality attributable to cigarette smoking in Taiwan: a 12-year follow-up study. *Tob Control*, 7: 141–148. doi:10.1136/tc.7.2.141 PMID:9789932

Liddell FD (2001). The interaction of asbestos and smoking in lung cancer. *Ann Occup Hyg*, 45: 341–356. PMID:11418084

Lieber CS (1999). Microsomal ethanol-oxidizing system (MEOS): the first 30 years (1968–1998)–a review. *Alcohol Clin Exp Res*, 23: 991–1007. doi:10.1111/j.1530-0277.1999.tb04217.x PMID:10397283

Lieber CS (2004). The discovery of the microsomal ethanol oxidizing system and its physiologic and pathologic role. *Drug Metab Rev*, 36: 511–529. doi:10.1081/DMR-200033441 PMID:15554233

Lijinsky W (1992). *Chemistry and biology of N-Nitroso compounds.* Monographs on Cancer Research. Cambridge University Press

Lilla C, Risch A, Kropp S, Chang-Claude J (2005). SULT1A1 genotype, active and passive smoking, and breast cancer risk by age 50 years in a German case-control study. *Breast Cancer Res*, 7: R229–R237. doi:10.1186/bcr976 PMID:15743503

Lilla C, Verla-Tebit E, Risch A *et al.* (2006). Effect of NAT1 and NAT2 genetic polymorphisms on colorectal cancer risk associated with exposure to tobacco smoke and meat consumption. *Cancer Epidemiol Biomarkers Prev*, 15: 99–107. PMID:16434594

Lim U, Morton LM, Subar AF *et al.* (2007). Alcohol, smoking, and body size in relation to incident Hodgkin's and non-Hodgkin's lymphoma risk. *Am J Epidemiol*, 166: 697–708.

Limburg PJ, Vierkant RA, Cerhan JR *et al.* (2003). Cigarette smoking and colorectal cancer: long-term, subsite-specific risks in a cohort study of postmenopausal women. *Clin Gastroenterol Hepatol*, 1: 202–210. PMID:15017492

Lin TM, Chen KP, Lin CC *et al.* (1973). Retrospective study on nasopharyngeal carcinoma. *J Natl Cancer Inst*, 51: 1403–1408. PMID:4762926

Lin Y, Tamakoshi A, Kawamura T *et al.*JACC Study Group. Japan Collaborative Cohort (2002a). A prospective cohort study of cigarette smoking and pancreatic cancer in Japan. *Cancer Causes Control*, 13: 249–254. doi:10.1023/A:1015052710213 PMID:12020106

Lindblad M, Rodríguez LA, Lagergren J (2005). Body mass, tobacco and alcohol and risk of esophageal, gastric cardia, and gastric non-cardia adenocarcinoma among men and women in a nested case-control study. *Cancer Causes Control*, 16: 285–294. doi:10.1007/s10552-004-3485-7 PMID:15947880

Lindemann K, Vatten LJ, Ellstrøm-Engh M, Eskild A (2008). Body mass, diabetes and smoking, and endometrial cancer risk: a follow-up study. *Br J Cancer*, 98: 1582–1585. doi:10.1038/sj.bjc.6604313 PMID:18362938

Linet MS, McLaughlin JK, Hsing AW *et al.* (1992). Is cigarette smoking a risk factor for non-Hodgkin's lymphoma or multiple myeloma? Results from the Lutheran Brotherhood Cohort Study. *Leuk Res*, 16: 621–624. doi:10.1016/0145-2126(92)90011-U PMID:1635380

Linseisen J, Rohrmann S, Miller AB *et al.* (2007). Fruit and vegetable consumption and lung cancer risk: updated information from the European Prospective Investigation into Cancer and Nutrition (EPIC). *International Journal of Cancer*, 121: 1103–1114. doi:10.1002/ijc.22807

Lissowska J, Brinton LA, Garcia-Closas M (2007). Re: more data regarding the effects of passive smoking on breast cancer risk among younger women. *Int J Cancer*, 120: 2517–2518. doi:10.1002/ijc.22610 PMID:17290385

Lissowska J, Brinton LA, Zatonski W *et al.* (2006). Tobacco smoking, NAT2 acetylation genotype and breast cancer risk. *Int J Cancer*, 119: 1961–1969. doi:10.1002/ijc.22044 PMID:16721725

Lissowska J, Pilarska A, Pilarski P *et al.* (2003). Smoking, alcohol, diet, dentition and sexual practices in the epidemiology of oral cancer in Poland. *Eur J Cancer Prev*, 12: 25–33. doi:10.1097/00008469-200302000-00005 PMID:12548107

Loerbroks A, Schouten LJ, Goldbohm RA, van den Brandt PA (2007). Alcohol consumption, cigarette smoking, and endometrial cancer risk: results from the Netherlands Cohort Study. *Cancer Causes Control*, 18: 551–560. doi:10.1007/s10552-007-0127-x PMID:17437180

London SJ, Colditz GA, Stampfer MJ *et al.* (1989a). Prospective study of relative weight, height, and risk of breast cancer. *JAMA*, 262: 2853–2858. doi:10.1001/jama.262.20.2853 PMID:2810620

London SJ, Colditz GA, Stampfer MJ *et al.* (1989b). Prospective study of smoking and the risk of breast cancer. *J Natl Cancer Inst*, 81: 1625–1631. doi:10.1093/jnci/81.21.1625 PMID:2795691

London SJ, Smart J, Daly AK (2000b). Lung cancer risk in relation to genetic polymorphisms of microsomal epoxide hydrolase among African-Americans and Caucasians in Los Angeles County. *Lung Cancer*, 28: 147–155. doi:10.1016/S0169-5002(99)00130-0 PMID:10717332

London SJ, Yuan JM, Chung FL *et al.* (2000a). Isothiocyanates, glutathione S-transferase M1 and T1 polymorphisms, and lung-cancer risk: a prospective study of men in Shanghai, China. *Lancet*, 356: 724–729. doi:10.1016/S0140-6736(00)02631-3 PMID:11085692

Longcope C, Baker R, Johnston CC Jr (1986). Androgen and estrogen metabolism: relationship to obesity. *Metabolism*, 35: 235–237. doi:10.1016/0026-0495(86)90206-4 PMID:3456482

Longcope C & Johnston CC Jr (1988). Androgen and estrogen dynamics in pre- and postmenopausal women: a comparison between smokers and nonsmokers. *J Clin Endocrinol Metab*, 67: 379–383. doi:10.1210/jcem-67-2-379 PMID:3392163

Lopez AD, Collishaw N, Piha T (1994). A descriptive model of the cigarette epidemic in developed countries. *Tobacco Control*, 3: 242–247. doi:10.1136/tc.3.3.242

López-Abente G, Pollán M, Monge V, Martínez-Vidal A (1992). Tobacco smoking, alcohol consumption, and laryngeal cancer in Madrid. *Cancer Detect Prev*, 16: 265–271. PMID:1473116

Lu J, Lian S, Sun X *et al.* (2000). A case-control study on the risk factors of esophageal cancer in Linzhou *Zhonghua Liu Xing Bing Xue Za Zhi*, 21: 434–436. PMID:11860829

Lubet RA, Zhang Z, Wiseman RW, You M (2000). Use of p53 transgenic mice in the development of cancer models for multiple purposes. *Exp Lung Res*, 26: 581–593. doi:10.1080/01902140150216684 PMID:11195457

Lubin JH, Alavanja MC, Caporaso N *et al.* (2007a). Cigarette smoking and cancer risk: modeling total exposure and intensity. *Am J Epidemiol*, 166: 479–489. doi:10.1093/aje/kwm089 PMID:17548786

Lubin JH, Caporaso N, Hatsukami DK *et al.* (2007b). The association of a tobacco-specific biomarker and cigarette consumption and its dependence on host characteristics. *Cancer Epidemiology, Biomarkers & Prevention*, 16: 1852–1857. doi:10.1158/1055-9965.EPI-07-0018

Lubin JH & Caporaso NE (2006). Cigarette smoking and lung cancer: modeling total exposure and intensity. *Cancer Epidemiology, Biomarkers & Prevention*, 15: 517–523. doi:10.1158/1055-9965.EPI-05-0863

Lubin JH, Kogevinas M, Silverman D *et al.* (2007). Evidence for an intensity-dependent interaction of NAT2 acetylation genotype and cigarette smoking in the Spanish Bladder Cancer Study. *Int J Epidemiol*, 36: 236–241. doi:10.1093/ije/dym043 PMID:17510079

Lubin JH, Virtamo J, Weinstein SJ, Albanes D (2008). Cigarette smoking and cancer: intensity patterns in the alpha-tocopherol, beta-carotene cancer prevention study in Finnish men. *Am J Epidemiol*, 167: 970–975. doi:10.1093/aje/kwm392 PMID:18250081

Lüchtenborg M, Weijenberg MP, Kampman E *et al.* (2005a). Cigarette smoking and colorectal cancer: APC mutations, hMLH1 expression, and GSTM1 and GSTT1 polymorphisms. *Am J Epidemiol*, 161: 806–815. doi:10.1093/aje/kwi114 PMID:15840612

Lüchtenborg M, White KK, Wilkens L *et al.* (2007). Smoking and colorectal cancer: different effects by type of cigarettes? *Cancer Epidemiol Biomarkers Prev*, 16: 1341–1347. doi:10.1158/1055-9965.EPI-06-0519 PMID:17626999

Lurie G, Wilkens LR, Thompson PJ *et al.* (2008). Genetic polymorphisms in the Paraoxonase 1 gene and risk of ovarian epithelial carcinoma. *Cancer Epidemiol Biomarkers Prev*, 17: 2070–2077. doi:10.1158/1055-9965.EPI-08-0145 PMID:18708400

Lynch SM, Vrieling A, Lubin JH *et al.* (2009). Cigarette smoking and pancreatic cancer: a pooled analysis from the pancreatic cancer cohort consortium. *Am J Epidemiol*, 170: 403–413. doi:10.1093/aje/kwp134 PMID:19561064

Mabuchi K, Bross DS, Kessler II (1985). Cigarette smoking and nasopharyngeal carcinoma. *Cancer*, 55: 2874–2876. doi:10.1002/1097-0142(19850615)55:12<2874::AID-CNCR2820551228>3.0.CO;2-4 PMID:3995493

Macfarlane GJ, Zheng T, Marshall JR *et al.* (1995). Alcohol, tobacco, diet and the risk of oral cancer: a pooled analysis of three case-control studies. *Eur J Cancer B Oral Oncol*, 31B: 181–187. doi:10.1016/0964-1955(95)00005-3 PMID:7549758

Mack WJ, Preston-Martin S, Dal Maso L *et al.* (2003). A pooled analysis of case-control studies of thyroid cancer: cigarette smoking and consumption of alcohol, coffee, and tea. *Cancer Causes Control*, 14: 773–785. doi:10.1023/A:1026349702909 PMID:14674742

Mackenzie PI, Owens IS, Burchell B *et al.* (1997). The UDP glycosyltransferase gene superfamily: recommended nomenclature update based on evolutionary divergence. *Pharmacogenetics*, 7: 255–269. PMID:9295054

MacMahon B, Trichopoulos D, Cole P, Brown J (1982). Cigarette smoking and urinary estrogens. *N Engl J Med*, 307: 1062–1065. PMID:7121516

MacNicoll AD, Easty GC, Neville AM *et al.* (1980). Metabolism and activation of carcinogenic polycyclic hydrocarbons by human mammary cells. *Biochem Biophys Res Commun*, 95: 1599–1606. doi:10.1016/S0006-291X(80)80081-7 PMID:6774726

Maden C, Sherman KJ, Beckmann AM *et al.* (1993). History of circumcision, medical conditions, and sexual activity and risk of penile cancer. *J Natl Cancer Inst*, 85: 19–24. doi:10.1093/jnci/85.1.19 PMID:8380060

Magnusson C, Wedrén S, Rosenberg LU (2007). Cigarette smoking and breast cancer risk: a population-based study in Sweden. *Br J Cancer*, 97: 1287–1290. doi:10.1038/sj.bjc.6604007 PMID:17912245

Maier H, Dietz A, Gewelke U *et al.* (1992a). Tobacco and alcohol and the risk of head and neck cancer. *Clin Investig*, 70: 320–327. doi:10.1007/BF00184668 PMID:1521046

Maier H, Gewelke U, Dietz A *et al.* (1992b[). Laryngeal cancer and occupation — results of the Heidelberg laryngeal cancer study]*HNO*, 40: 44–51.

Maier H, Sennewald E, Heller GF, Weidauer H (1994). Chronic alcohol consumption–the key risk factor for pharyngeal cancer. *Otolaryngol Head Neck Surg*, 110: 168–173. PMID:7906410

Maier H & Tisch M (1997). Epidemiology of laryngeal cancer: results of the Heidelberg case-control study. *Acta Otolaryngol Suppl*, 527: 160–164. doi:10.3109/00016489709124063 PMID:9197510

Malaiyandi V, Sellers EM, Tyndale RF (2005). Implications of *CYP2A6* genetic variation for smoking behaviors and nicotine dependence. *Clin Pharmacol Ther*, 77: 145–158. doi:10.1016/j.clpt.2004.10.011 PMID:15735609

Malats N (2008). Genetic epidemiology of bladder cancer: scaling up in the identification of low-penetrance genetic markers of bladder cancer risk and progression. *Scand J Urol Nephrol Suppl*, 42: 131–140. doi:10.1080/03008880802285172 PMID:18815927

Mandai M, Konishi I, Kuroda H *et al.* (1998). Heterogeneous distribution of K-ras-mutated epithelia in mucinous ovarian tumors with special reference to histopathology. *Hum Pathol*, 29: 34–40. doi:10.1016/S0046-8177(98)90387-2 PMID:9445131

Mandelzweig L, Novikov I, Sadetzki S (2009). *Smoking and risk of glioma: a meta-analysis.* Cancer Causes Control.

Mane SS, Purnell DM, Hsu IC (1990). Genotoxic effects of five polycyclic aromatic hydrocarbons in human and rat mammary epithelial cells. *Environ Mol Mutagen*, 15: 78–82. doi:10.1002/em.2850150204 PMID:2307152

Manjer J, Andersson I, Berglund G *et al.* (2000). Survival of women with breast cancer in relation to smoking. *Eur J Surg*, 166: 852–858. doi:10.1080/110241500447227 PMID:11097150

Manjer J, Malina J, Berglund G *et al.* (2001). Smoking associated with hormone receptor negative breast cancer. *Int J Cancer*, 91: 580–584. doi:10.1002/1097-0215(200002)9999:9999<::AID-IJC1091>3.0.CO;2-V PMID:11251985

Manuguerra M, Saletta F, Karagas MR *et al.* (2006). XRCC3 and XPD/ERCC2 single nucleotide polymorphisms and the risk of cancer: a HuGE review. *Am J Epidemiol*, 164: 297–302. doi:10.1093/aje/kwj189 PMID:16707649

Mao GE, Morris G, Lu QY *et al.* (2004). Glutathione S-transferase P1 Ile105Val polymorphism, cigarette smoking and prostate cancer. *Cancer Detect Prev*, 28: 368–374. doi:10.1016/j.cdp.2004.07.003 PMID:15542263

Marchbanks PA, Wilson H, Bastos E *et al.* (2000). Cigarette smoking and epithelial ovarian cancer by histologic type. *Obstet Gynecol*, 95: 255–260. doi:10.1016/S0029-7844(99)00531-1 PMID:10674590

Marsh GM, Youk AO, Buchanich JM *et al.* (2007). Work in the metal industry and nasopharyngeal cancer mortality among formaldehyde-exposed workers. *Regul Toxicol Pharmacol*, 48: 308–319. doi:10.1016/j.yrtph.2007.04.006 PMID:17544557

Marshall JR, Hastrup JL, Ross JS (1999). Mismeasurement and the resonance of strong confounders: correlated errors. *Am J Epidemiol*, 150: 88–96. PMID:10400558

Marsit CJ, Karagas MR, Schned A, Kelsey KT (2006). Carcinogen exposure and epigenetic silencing in bladder cancer. *Ann N Y Acad Sci*, 1076: 810–821. doi:10.1196/annals.1371.031 PMID:17119258

Mashberg A, Boffetta P, Winkelman R, Garfinkel L (1993). Tobacco smoking, alcohol drinking, and cancer of the oral cavity and oropharynx among U.S. veterans. *Cancer*, 72: 1369–1375. doi:10.1002/1097-0142(19930815)72:4<1369::AID-CNCR2820720436>3.0.CO;2-L PMID:8339227

Masson LF, Sharp L, Cotton SC, Little J (2005). Cytochrome P-450 1A1 gene polymorphisms and risk of breast cancer: a HuGE review. *Am J Epidemiol*, 161: 901–915. doi:10.1093/aje/kwi121 PMID:15870154

Matthews CE, Xu WH, Zheng W *et al.* (2005). Physical activity and risk of endometrial cancer: a report from the Shanghai endometrial cancer study. *Cancer Epidemiol Biomarkers Prev*, 14: 779–785. doi:10.1158/1055-9965.EPI-04-0665 PMID:15824143

Mauderly JL, Gigliotti AP, Barr EB *et al.* (2004). Chronic inhalation exposure to mainstream cigarette smoke increases lung and nasal tumor incidence in rats. *Toxicol Sci*, 81: 280–292. doi:10.1093/toxsci/kfh203 PMID:15213336

McCann SE, Freudenheim JL, Marshall JR *et al.* (2000). Diet in the epidemiology of endometrial cancer in western New York (United States). *Cancer Causes Control*, 11: 965–974. doi:10.1023/A:1026551309873 PMID:11142531

McCormack VA & dos Santos Silva I (2006). Breast density and parenchymal patterns as markers of breast cancer risk: a meta-analysis. *Cancer Epidemiol Biomarkers Prev*, 15: 1159–1169. doi:10.1158/1055-9965.EPI-06-0034 PMID:16775176

McCoy GD, Hecht SS, Katayama S, Wynder EL (1981). Differential effect of chronic ethanol consumption on the carcinogenicity of *N*-nitrosopyrrolidine and *N'*-nitrosonornicotine in male Syrian golden hamsters. *Cancer Res*, 41: 2849–2854. PMID:7248945

McDivit AM, Greendale GA, Stanczyk FZ, Huang M-H (2008). Effects of alcohol and cigarette smoking on change in serum estrone levels in postmenopausal women randomly assigned to fixed doses of conjugated equine estrogens with or without a progestin. *Menopause*, 15: 382–385. doi:10.1097/gme.0b013e3181407cb2 PMID:18000469

McGrath M, Hankinson SE, De Vivo I (2007). Cytochrome P450 1A1, cigarette smoking, and risk of endometrial cancer (United States). *Cancer Causes Control*, 18: 1123–1130. doi:10.1007/s10552-007-9051-3 PMID:17717632

McIlwain CC, Townsend DM, Tew KD (2006). Glutathione *S*-transferase polymorphisms: cancer incidence and therapy. *Oncogene*, 25: 1639–1648. doi:10.1038/sj.onc.1209373 PMID:16550164

McIntyre-Seltman K, Castle PE, Guido R *et al.* ALTS Group (2005). Smoking is a risk factor for cervical intraepithelial neoplasia grade 3 among oncogenic human papillomavirus DNA-positive women with equivocal or mildly abnormal cytology. *Cancer Epidemiol Biomarkers Prev*, 14: 1165–1170. doi:10.1158/1055-9965.EPI-04-0918 PMID:15894667

McKay JD, Hashibe M, Hung RJ *et al.* (2008). Sequence variants of *NAT1* and *NAT2* and other xenometabolic genes and risk of lung and aerodigestive tract cancers in Central Europe. *Cancer Epidemiol Biomarkers Prev*, 17: 141–147. doi:10.1158/1055-9965.EPI-07-0553 PMID:18199719

McKinlay SM (1996). The normal menopause transition: an overview. *Maturitas*, 23: 137–145. doi:10.1016/0378-5122(95)00985-X PMID:8735352

McLaughlin JK, Hrubec Z, Blot WJ, Fraumeni JF Jr (1995). Smoking and cancer mortality among U.S. veterans: a 26-year follow-up. *Int J Cancer*, 60: 190–193. doi:10.1002/ijc.2910600210 PMID:7829214

Mechanic LE, Bowman ED, Welsh JA *et al.* (2007). Common genetic variation in TP53 is associated with lung cancer risk and prognosis in African Americans and somatic mutations in lung tumors. *Cancer Epidemiology, Biomarkers & Prevention*, 16: 214–222. doi:10.1158/1055-9965.EPI-06-0790

Mechanic LE, Millikan RC, Player J *et al.* (2006). Polymorphisms in nucleotide excision repair genes, smoking and breast cancer in African Americans and whites: a population-based case-control study. *Carcinogenesis*, 27: 1377–1385. doi:10.1093/carcin/bgi330 PMID:16399771

Meckley D, Hayes JR, Van Kampen KR *et al.* (2004a). A responsive, sensitive, and reproducible dermal tumor promotion assay for the comparative evaluation of cigarette smoke condensates. *Regul Toxicol Pharmacol*, 39: 135–149. doi:10.1016/j.yrtph.2003.12.003 PMID:15041145

Meckley DR, Hayes JR, Van Kampen KR *et al.* (2004b). Comparative study of smoke condensates from 1R4F cigarettes that burn tobacco versus ECLIPSE cigarettes that primarily heat tobacco in the SENCAR mouse dermal tumor promotion assay. *Food Chem Toxicol*, 42: 851–863. doi:10.1016/j.fct.2004.01.009 PMID:15046832

Menke-Pluymers MB, Hop WC, Dees J *et al.* The Rotterdam Esophageal Tumor Study Group (1993). Risk factors for the development of an adenocarcinoma in columnar-lined (Barrett) esophagus. *Cancer*, 72: 1155–1158. doi:10.1002/1097-0142(19930815)72:4<1155::AID-CNCR2820720404>3.0.CO;2-C PMID:8339208

Menvielle G, Luce D, Goldberg P *et al.* (2004a). Smoking, alcohol drinking and cancer risk for various sites of the larynx and hypopharynx. A case-control study in France. *Eur J Cancer Prev*, 13: 165–172. doi:10.1097/01.cej.0000130017.93310.76 PMID:15167214

Menvielle G, Luce D, Goldberg P, Leclerc A (2004b). Smoking, alcohol drinking, occupational exposures and social inequalities in hypopharyngeal and laryngeal cancer. *Int J Epidemiol*, 33: 799–806. doi:10.1093/ije/dyh090 PMID:15155704

Merletti F, Boffetta P, Ciccone G *et al.* (1989). Role of tobacco and alcoholic beverages in the etiology of cancer of the oral cavity/oropharynx in Torino, Italy. *Cancer Res*, 49: 4919–4924. PMID:2758421

Meskar A, Plee-Gautier E, Amet Y *et al.* (2001). Alcohol-xenobiotic interactions. Role of cytochrome P450 2E1 *Pathol Biol (Paris)*, 49: 696–702. doi:10.1016/S0369-8114(01)00235-8 PMID:11762131

Michnovicz JJ, Hershcopf RJ, Naganuma H *et al.* (1986). Increased 2-hydroxylation of estradiol as a possible mechanism for the anti-estrogenic effect of cigarette smoking. *N Engl J Med*, 315: 1305–1309. PMID:3773953

Michnovicz JJ, Naganuma H, Hershcopf RJ *et al.* (1988). Increased urinary catechol estrogen excretion in female smokers. *Steroids*, 52: 69–83. doi:10.1016/0039-128X(88)90218-8 PMID:2854668

Miller MD, Marty MA, Broadwin R *et al.* California Environmental Protection Agency (2007). The association between exposure to environmental tobacco smoke and breast cancer: a review by the California Environmental Protection Agency. *Prev Med*, 44: 93–106. doi:10.1016/j.ypmed.2006.08.015 PMID:17027075

Millikan RC, Pittman GS, Newman B *et al.* (1998). Cigarette smoking, N-acetyltransferases 1 and 2, and breast cancer risk. *Cancer Epidemiol Biomarkers Prev*, 7: 371–378. PMID:9610785

Minami Y & Tateno H (2003). Associations between cigarette smoking and the risk of four leading cancers in Miyagi Prefecture, Japan: a multi-site case-control study. *Cancer Sci*, 94: 540–547. doi:10.1111/j.1349-7006.2003.tb01480.x PMID:14529588

Minna JD (2003). Nicotine exposure and bronchial epithelial cell nicotinic acetylcholine receptor expression in the pathogenesis of lung cancer. *J Clin Invest*, 111: 31–33. PMID:12511585

Mitrou PN, Watson MA, Loktionov AS *et al.* (2006). MTHFR (C677T and A1298C) polymorphisms and risk of sporadic distal colorectal adenoma in the UK Flexible Sigmoidoscopy Screening Trial (United Kingdom). *Cancer Causes Control*, 17: 793–801. doi:10.1007/s10552-006-0016-8 PMID:16783607

Modugno F, Ness RB, Cottreau CM (2002). Cigarette smoking and the risk of mucinous and nonmucinous epithelial ovarian cancer. *Epidemiology*, 13: 467–471. doi:10.1097/00001648-200207000-00016 PMID:12094103

Modugno F, Ngo DL, Allen GO *et al.* (2006). Breast cancer risk factors and mammographic breast density in women over age 70. *Breast Cancer Res Treat*, 97: 157–166. doi:10.1007/s10549-005-9105-8 PMID:16362132

Molano M, Van den Brule A, Plummer M *et al.* (2003). Determinants of clearance of human papillomavirus infections in Colombian women with normal cytology: a population-based, 5-year follow-up study. *Am J Epidemiol*, 158: 486–494.

Møllersen L, Vikse R, Andreassen A *et al.* (2004). Adenomatous polyposis coli truncation mutations in 2-amino-1-methyl-6-phenylimidazo[4,5-b]pyridine (PhIP)-induced intestinal tumours of multiple intestinal neoplasia mice. *Mutat Res*, 557: 29–40. PMID:14706516

Monnereau A, Orsi L, Troussard X *et al.* (2008). Cigarette smoking, alcohol drinking, and risk of lymphoid neoplasms: results of a French case-control study. *Cancer Causes Control*, 19: 1147–1160.

Montelongo A, Lasunción MA, Pallardo LF, Herrera E (1992). Longitudinal study of plasma lipoproteins and hormones during pregnancy in normal and diabetic women. *Diabetes*, 41: 1651–1659. doi:10.2337/diabetes.41.12.1651 PMID:1446807

Morabia A, Bernstein M, Héritier S, Khatchatrian N (1996). Relation of breast cancer with passive and active exposure to tobacco smoke. *Am J Epidemiol*, 143: 918–928. PMID:8610705

Morabia A, Bernstein M, Ruiz J *et al.* (1998). Relation of smoking to breast cancer by estrogen receptor status. *Int J Cancer*, 75: 339–342. doi:10.1002/(SICI)1097-0215(19980130)75:3<339::AID-IJC2>3.0.CO;2-3 PMID:9455790

Morabia A, Bernstein MS, Bouchardy I *et al.* (2000). Breast cancer and active and passive smoking: the role of the N-acetyltransferase 2 genotype. *Am J Epidemiol*, 152: 226–232. doi:10.1093/aje/152.3.226 PMID:10933269

Morabia A & Wynder EL (1992). Relation of bronchioloalveolar carcinoma to tobacco. *BMJ*, 304: 541–543. doi:10.1136/bmj.304.6826.541 PMID:1313719

Moreno V, Glatt H, Guino E *et al.*Bellvitge Colorectal Cancer Study Group (2005). Polymorphisms in sulfotransferases *SULT1A1* and *SULT1A2* are not related to colorectal cancer. *Int J Cancer*, 113: 683–686. doi:10.1002/ijc.20613 PMID:15455379

Morris JJ & Seifter E (1992). The role of aromatic hydrocarbons in the genesis of breast cancer. *Med Hypotheses*, 38: 177–184. doi:10.1016/0306-9877(92)90090-Y PMID:1513270

Morton LM, Hartge P, Holford TR *et al.* (2005). Cigarette smoking and risk of non-Hodgkin lymphoma: a pooled analysis from the International Lymphoma Epidemiology Consortium (interlymph). *Cancer Epidemiol Biomarkers Prev*, 14: 925–933.

Mounawar M, Mukeria A, Le Calvez F *et al.* (2007). Patterns of *EGFR*, *HER2*, *TP53*, and *KRAS* mutations of *p14[arf]* expression in non-small cell lung cancers in relation to smoking history. *Cancer Res*, 67: 5667–5672. doi:10.1158/0008-5472.CAN-06-4229 PMID:17575133

Mountzios G, Fouret P, Soria J-C (2008). Mechanisms of Disease: signal transduction in lung carcinogenesis – a comparison of smokers and never-smokers. *Nat Clin Pract Oncol*, 5: 610–618. doi:10.1038/ncponc1181 PMID:18628738

Murata M, Takayama K, Choi BCK, Pak AWP (1996). A nested case-control study on alcohol drinking, tobacco smoking, and cancer. *Cancer Detect Prev*, 20: 557–565. PMID:8939341

Murayama N, Soyama A, Saito Y *et al.* (2004). Six novel nonsynonymous *CYP1A2* gene polymorphisms: catalytic activities of the naturally occurring variant enzymes. *J Pharmacol Exp Ther*, 308: 300–306. doi:10.1124/jpet.103.055798 PMID:14563787

Murin S & Inciardi J (2001). Cigarette smoking and the risk of pulmonary metastasis from breast cancer. *Chest*, 119: 1635–1640. doi:10.1378/chest.119.6.1635 PMID:11399684

Murphy G, Shu XO, Gao YT *et al.* (2009). *Family cancer history affecting risk of colorectal cancer in a prospective cohort of Chinese women*. Cancer Causes Control.

Muscat JE, Richie JP Jr, Thompson S, Wynder EL (1996). Gender differences in smoking and risk for oral cancer. *Cancer Res*, 56: 5192–5197. PMID:8912856

Muscat JE & Wynder EL (1992). Tobacco, alcohol, asbestos, and occupational risk factors for laryngeal cancer. *Cancer*, 69: 2244–2251. doi:10.1002/1097-0142(19920501)69:9<2244::AID-CNCR2820690906>3.0.CO;2-O PMID:1562970

Muscat JE & Wynder EL (1998). A case/control study of risk factors for major salivary gland cancer. *Otolaryngol Head Neck Surg*, 118: 195–198. doi:10.1016/S0194-5998(98)80013-2 PMID:9482552

Mutch MG, Schoen RE, Fleshman JW *et al.* (2009). A multicenter study of prevalence and risk factors for aberrant crypt foci. *Clin Gastroenterol Hepatol*, 7: 568–574. doi:10.1016/j.cgh.2009.01.016 PMID:19418605

Muti P, Bradlow HL, Micheli A *et al.* (2000). Estrogen metabolism and risk of breast cancer: a prospective study of the 2:16alpha-hydroxyestrone ratio in premenopausal and postmenopausal women. *Epidemiology*, 11: 635–640. doi:10.1097/00001648-200011000-00004 PMID:11055622

Muwonge R, Ramadas K, Sankila R *et al.* (2008). Role of tobacco smoking, chewing and alcohol drinking in the risk of oral cancer in Trivandrum, India: a nested case-control design using incident cancer cases. *Oral Oncol*, 44: 446–454. doi:10.1016/j.oraloncology.2007.06.002 PMID:17933578

Mwenifumbo JC & Tyndale RF (2007). Genetic variability in CYP2A6 and the pharmacokinetics of nicotine. *Pharmacogenomics*, 8: 1385–1402. doi:10.2217/14622416.8.10.1385 PMID:17979512

Nagano J, Mabuchi K, Yoshimoto Y *et al.* (2007). A case-control study in Hiroshima and Nagasaki examining non-radiation risk factors for thyroid cancer. *J Epidemiol*, 17: 76–85. doi:10.2188/jea.17.76 PMID:17545694

Nagar S & Remmel RP (2006). Uridine diphosphoglucuronosyltransferase pharmacogenetics and cancer. *Oncogene*, 25: 1659–1672. doi:10.1038/sj.onc.1209375 PMID:16550166

Nagle CM, Olsen CM, Webb PM *et al.*Australian Cancer Study Group; Australian Ovarian Cancer Study Group (2008). Endometrioid and clear cell ovarian cancers: a comparative analysis of risk factors. *Eur J Cancer*, 44: 2477–2484. doi:10.1016/j.ejca.2008.07.009 PMID:18707869

Nakajima M (2007). Smoking behavior and related cancers: the role of *CYP2A6* polymorphisms. *Curr Opin Mol Ther*, 9: 538–544. PMID:18041664

Nakajima M, Yokoi T, Mizutani M *et al.* (1999). Genetic polymorphism in the 5⊠-flanking region of human *CYP1A2* gene: effect on the CYP1A2 inducibility in humans. *J Biochem*, 125: 803–808. PMID:10101295

Nam JM, McLaughlin JK, Blot WJ (1992). Cigarette smoking, alcohol, and nasopharyngeal carcinoma: a case-control study among U.S. whites. *J Natl Cancer Inst*, 84: 619–622. doi:10.1093/jnci/84.8.619 PMID:1556772

Nandakumar A, Anantha N, Pattabhiraman V *et al.* (1996). Importance of anatomical subsite in correlating risk factors in cancer of the oesophagus–report of a case–control study. *Br J Cancer*, 73: 1306–1311. PMID:8630297

Nandakumar A, Thimmasetty KT, Sreeramareddy NM *et al.* (1990). A population-based case-control investigation on cancers of the oral cavity in Bangalore, India. *Br J Cancer*, 62: 847–851. PMID:2245179

Narayan S, Jaiswal AS, Kang D *et al.* (2004). Cigarette smoke condensate-induced transformation of normal human breast epithelial cells in vitro. *Oncogene*, 23: 5880–5889. doi:10.1038/sj.onc.1207792 PMID:15208684

Navarro Silvera SA, Miller AB, Rohan TE (2005). Risk factors for thyroid cancer: a prospective cohort study. *Int J Cancer*, 116: 433–438. doi:10.1002/ijc.21079 PMID:15818623

Nayar D, Kapil U, Joshi YK *et al.* (2000). Nutritional risk factors in esophageal cancer. *J Assoc Physicians India*, 48: 781–787. PMID:11273469

Nebert DW & Dalton TP (2006). The role of cytochrome P450 enzymes in endogenous signalling pathways and environmental carcinogenesis. *Nat Rev Cancer*, 6: 947–960. doi:10.1038/nrc2015 PMID:17128211

Nebert DW, Dalton TP, Okey AB, Gonzalez FJ (2004). Role of aryl hydrocarbon receptor-mediated induction of the CYP1 enzymes in environmental toxicity and cancer. *J Biol Chem*, 279: 23847–23850. doi:10.1074/jbc.R400004200 PMID:15028720

Nebert DW, Roe AL, Vandale SE *et al.* (2002). NAD(P)H:quinone oxidoreductase (*NQO1*) polymorphism, exposure to benzene, and predisposition to disease: a HuGE review. *Genet Med*, 4: 62–70. doi:10.1097/00125817-200203000-00003 PMID:11882782

Negri E, Bosetti C, La Vecchia C *et al.* (1999). Risk factors for adenocarcinoma of the small intestine. *Int J Cancer*, 82: 171–174. doi:10.1002/(SICI)1097-0215(19990719)82:2<171::AID-IJC3>3.0.CO;2-T PMID:10389747

Newcomb PA, Storer BE, Marcus PM (1995). Cigarette smoking in relation to risk of large bowel cancer in women. *Cancer Res*, 55: 4906–4909. PMID:7585528

Newcomb PA & Trentham-Dietz A (2003). Patterns of postmenopausal progestin use with estrogen in relation to endometrial cancer (United States). *Cancer Causes Control*, 14: 195–201. doi:10.1023/A:1023066304473 PMID:12749724

Newcomer LM, Newcomb PA, Trentham-Dietz A, Storer BE (2001). Hormonal risk factors for endometrial cancer: modification by cigarette smoking (United States). *Cancer Causes Control*, 12: 829–835. doi:10.1023/A:1012297905601 PMID:11714111

Newhouse ML, Pearson RM, Fullerton JM *et al.* (1977). A case control study of carcinoma of the ovary. *Br J Prev Soc Med*, 31: 148–153. PMID:588853

Ng TP (1986). A case-referent study of cancer of the nasal cavity and sinuses in Hong Kong. *Int J Epidemiol*, 15: 171–175. doi:10.1093/ije/15.2.171 PMID:3721678

Nieters A, Deeg E, Becker N (2006). Tobacco and alcohol consumption and risk of lymphoma: results of a population-based case-control study in Germany. *Int J Cancer*, 118: 422–430.

Nieters A, Rohrmann S, Becker N *et al.* (2008). Smoking and lymphoma risk in the European prospective investigation into cancer and nutrition. *Am J Epidemiol*, 167: 1081–1089.

Nilsen TI & Vatten LJ (2000). A prospective study of lifestyle factors and the risk of pancreatic cancer in Nord-Trøndelag, Norway. *Cancer Causes Control*, 11: 645–652. doi:10.1023/A:1008916123357 PMID:10977109

Nilsson S, Carstensen JM, Pershagen G (2001). Mortality among male and female smokers in Sweden: a 33 year follow up. *J Epidemiol Community Health*, 55: 825–830. doi:10.1136/jech.55.11.825 PMID:11604439

Ning JP, Yu MC, Wang QS, Henderson BE (1990). Consumption of salted fish and other risk factors for nasopharyngeal carcinoma (NPC) in Tianjin, a low-risk region for NPC in the People's Republic of China. *J Natl Cancer Inst*, 82: 291–296. doi:10.1093/jnci/82.4.291 PMID:2299678

Nishino K, Sekine M, Kodama S *et al.* (2008). Cigarette smoking and glutathione S-transferase M1 polymorphism associated with risk for uterine cervical cancer. *J Obstet Gynaecol Res*, 34: 994–1001.

Nishino Y, Inoue M, Tsuji I *et al.*Research Group for the Development and Evaluation of Cancer Prevention Strategies in Japan (2006). Tobacco smoking and gastric cancer risk: an evaluation based on a systematic review of epidemiologic evidence among the Japanese population. *Jpn J Clin Oncol*, 36: 800–807. doi:10.1093/jjco/hyl112 PMID:17210611

Niwa Y, Wakai K, Suzuki S *et al.*JACC Study Group (2005). Cigarette smoking and the risk of ovarian cancer in the Japanese population: findings from the Japanese Collaborate Cohort study. *J Obstet Gynaecol Res*, 31: 144–151. doi:10.1111/j.1447-0756.2005.00261.x PMID:15771641

Nkondjock A & Ghadirian P (2004). Dietary carotenoids and risk of colon cancer: case-control study. *Int J Cancer*, 110: 110–116. doi:10.1002/ijc.20066 PMID:15054875

Nkondjock A, Robidoux A, Paredes Y *et al.* (2006). Diet, lifestyle and BRCA-related breast cancer risk among French-Canadians. *Breast Cancer Res Treat*, 98: 285–294. doi:10.1007/s10549-006-9161-8 PMID:16541324

Nock NL, Liu X, Cicek MS *et al.* (2006). Polymorphisms in polycyclic aromatic hydrocarbon metabolism and conjugation genes, interactions with smoking and prostate cancer risk. *Cancer Epidemiol Biomarkers Prev*, 15: 756–761. doi:10.1158/1055-9965.EPI-05-0826 PMID:16614120

Noda N, Matsuzoe D, Konno T *et al.* (2004). Risk for K-ras gene mutations in smoking-induced lung cancer is associated with cytochrome P4501A1 and glutathione S-transferase micro1 polymorphisms. *Oncol Rep*, 12: 773–779. PMID:15375499

Nordlund LA, Carstensen JM, Pershagen G (1997). Cancer incidence in female smokers: a 26-year follow-up. *Int J Cancer*, 73: 625–628. doi:10.1002/(SICI)1097-0215(19971127)73:5<625::AID-IJC2>3.0.CO;2-Z PMID:9398036

Norppa H (2001). Genetic polymorphisms and chromosome damage. *Int J Hyg Environ Health*, 204: 31–38. doi:10.1078/1438-4639-00069 PMID:11725342

Norppa H (2003). Genetic susceptibility, biomarker respones, and cancer. *Mutat Res*, 544: 339–348. doi:10.1016/j.mrrev.2003.09.006 PMID:14644336

Norppa H (2004). Cytogenetic biomarkers and genetic polymorphisms. *Toxicol Lett*, 149: 309–334. doi:10.1016/j.toxlet.2003.12.042 PMID:15093278

Novak RF & Woodcroft KJ (2000). The alcohol-inducible form of cytochrome P450 (CYP 2E1): role in toxicology and regulation of expression. *Arch Pharm Res*, 23: 267–282. doi:10.1007/BF02975435 PMID:10976571

O'Brien MJ, Yang S, Mack C *et al.* (2006). Comparison of microsatellite instability, CpG island methylation phenotype, BRAF and KRAS status in serrated polyps and traditional adenomas indicates separate pathways to distinct colorectal carcinoma end points. *Am J Surg Pathol*, 30: 1491–1501.

Obana H, Hori S, Kashimoto T, Kunita N (1981). Polycyclic aromatic hydrocarbons in human fat and liver. *Bull Environ Contam Toxicol*, 27: 23–27. doi:10.1007/BF01610981 PMID:7296033

Ochs-Balcom HM, Wiesner G, Elston RC (2007). A meta-analysis of the association of *N*-acetyltransferase 2 gene (*NAT2*) variants with breast cancer. *Am J Epidemiol*, 166: 246–254. PMID:17535831

Odenbro A, Gillgren P, Bellocco R *et al.* (2007). The risk for cutaneous malignant melanoma, melanoma in situ and intraocular malignant melanoma in relation to tobacco use and body mass index. *Br J Dermatol*, 156: 99–105. doi:10.1111/j.1365-2133.2006.07537.x PMID:17199574

Okamura C, Tsubono Y, Ito K *et al.* (2006). Lactation and risk of endometrial cancer in Japan: a case-control study. *Tohoku J Exp Med*, 208: 109–115. doi:10.1620/tjem.208.109 PMID:16434833

Olivier M & Hainaut P (2001). TP53 mutation patterns in breast cancers: searching for clues of environmental carcinogenesis. *Semin Cancer Biol*, 11: 353–360. doi:10.1006/scbi.2001.0390 PMID:11562177

Olsen J, Sabreo S, Fasting U (1985a). Interaction of alcohol and tobacco as risk factors in cancer of the laryngeal region. *J Epidemiol Community Health*, 39: 165–168. doi:10.1136/jech.39.2.165 PMID:4009100

Olsen J, Sabroe S, Ipsen J (1985b). Effect of combined alcohol and tobacco exposure on risk of cancer of the hypopharynx. *J Epidemiol Community Health*, 39: 304–307. doi:10.1136/jech.39.4.304 PMID:4086960

Olson JE, Vachon CM, Vierkant RA *et al.* (2005). Prepregnancy exposure to cigarette smoking and subsequent risk of postmenopausal breast cancer. *Mayo Clin Proc*, 80: 1423–1428. doi:10.4065/80.11.1423 PMID:16295021

Omata F, Brown WR, Tokuda Y *et al.* (2009). Modifiable risk factors for colorectal neoplasms and hyperplastic polyps. *Intern Med*, 48: 123–128. doi:10.2169/internalmedicine.48.1562 PMID:19182421

Oreggia F, De Stefani E, Correa P, Fierro L (1991). Risk factors for cancer of the tongue in Uruguay. *Cancer*, 67: 180–183. doi:10.1002/1097-0142(19910101)67:1<180::AID-CNCR2820670130>3.0.CO;2-R PMID:1985715

Otani T, Iwasaki M, Ikeda S *et al.* (2006). Serum triglycerides and colorectal adenoma in a case-control study among cancer screening examinees (Japan). *Cancer Causes Control*, 17: 1245–1252. doi:10.1007/s10552-006-0065-z PMID:17111255

Otani T, Iwasaki M, Yamamoto S *et al.*Japan Public Health Center-based Prospective Study Group (2003). Alcohol consumption, smoking, and subsequent risk of colorectal cancer in middle-aged and elderly Japanese men and women: Japan Public Health Center-based prospective study. *Cancer Epidemiol Biomarkers Prev*, 12: 1492–1500. PMID:14693743

Otto H & Elmenhorst H (1967). Experimental studies on tumour induction with the gas phase of cigarette smoke.] *Z Krebsforsch*, 70: 45–47. doi:10.1007/BF00524450

Pacella-Norman R, Urban MI, Sitas F *et al.* (2002). Risk factors for oesophageal, lung, oral and laryngeal cancers in black South Africans. *Br J Cancer*, 86: 1751–1756. doi:10.1038/sj.bjc.6600338 PMID:12087462

Pakhale SS, Sarkar S, Jayant K, Bhide SV (1988). Carcinogenicity of Indian bidi and cigarette smoke condensate in Swiss albino mice. *J Cancer Res Clin Oncol*, 114: 647–649. doi:10.1007/BF00398193 PMID:3204112

Palmer JR & Rosenberg L (1993). Cigarette smoking and the risk of breast cancer. *Epidemiol Rev*, 15: 145–156. PMID:8405197

Palmer JR, Rosenberg L, Clarke EA *et al.* (1991). Breast cancer and cigarette smoking: a hypothesis. *Am J Epidemiol*, 134: 1–13. PMID:1853854

Pan SY, Ugnat AM, Mao Y *et al.*Canadian Cancer Registries Epidemiology Research Group (2004). Association of cigarette smoking with the risk of ovarian cancer. *Int J Cancer*, 111: 124–130. doi:10.1002/ijc.20242 PMID:15185353

Pandey M & Shukla VK (2003). Lifestyle, parity, menstrual and reproductive factors and risk of gallbladder cancer. *Eur J Cancer Prev*, 12: 269–272. doi:10.1097/00008469-200308000-00005 PMID:12883378

Pandeya N, Williams GM, Sadhegi S *et al.* (2008). Associations of duration, intensity, and quantity of smoking with adenocarcinoma and squamous cell carcinoma of the esophagus. *Am J Epidemiol*, 168: 105–114. doi:10.1093/aje/kwn091 PMID:18483122

Parente RC, Faerstein E, Celeste RK, Werneck GL (2008). The relationship between smoking and age at the menopause: A systematic review. *Maturitas*, 61: 287–298. doi:10.1016/j.maturitas.2008.09.021 PMID:19019585

Park NH, Sapp JP, Herbosa EG (1986). Oral cancer induced in hamsters with herpes simplex infection and simulated snuff dipping. *Oral Surg Oral Med Oral Pathol*, 62: 164–168. doi:10.1016/0030-4220(86)90039-3 PMID:3462612

Park SL, Chang S-C, Cai L *et al.* (2008). Associations between variants of the 8q24 chromosome and nine smoking-related cancer sites. *Cancer Epidemiol Biomarkers Prev*, 17: 3193–3202. doi:10.1158/1055-9965.EPI-08-0523 PMID:18990762

Parker AS, Cerhan JR, Dick F *et al.* (2000). Smoking and risk of non-Hodgkin lymphoma subtypes in a cohort of older women. *Leuk Lymphoma*, 37: 341–349. PMID:10752985

Parker AS, Cerhan JR, Janney CA *et al.* (2003). Smoking cessation and renal cell carcinoma. *Ann Epidemiol*, 13: 245–251. doi:10.1016/S1047-2797(02)00271-5 PMID:12684190

Paskett ED, Reeves KW, Rohan TE *et al.* (2007). Association between cigarette smoking and colorectal cancer in the Women's Health Initiative. *J Natl Cancer Inst*, 99: 1729–1735. doi:10.1093/jnci/djm176 PMID:18000222

Pavanello S & Clonfero E (2000). Biological indicators of genotoxic risk and metabolic polymorphisms. *Mutat Res*, 463: 285–308. doi:10.1016/S1383-5742(00)00051-X PMID:11018745

Pavanello S, Pulliero A, Lupi S *et al.* (2005). Influence of the genetic polymorphism in the 5⊠-noncoding region of the *CYP1A2* gene on *CYP1A2* phenotype and urinary mutagenicity in smokers. *Mutat Res*, 587: 59–66. PMID:16188490

Pavanello S, Simioli P, Lupi S *et al.* (2002). Exposure levels and cytochrome P450 1A2 activity, but not *N*-acetyltransferase, glutathione *S*-transferase (GST) *M1* and *T1*, influence urinary mutagen excretion in smokers. *Cancer Epidemiol Biomarkers Prev*, 11: 998–1003. PMID:12376499

Peach HG & Barnett NE (2001). Critical review of epidemiological studies of the association between smoking and non-Hodgkin's lymphoma. *Hematol Oncol*, 19: 67–80. doi:10.1002/hon.677 PMID:11438976

Penning TM & Drury JE (2007). Human aldo-keto reductases: Function, gene regulation, and single nucleotide polymorphisms. *Arch Biochem Biophys*, 464: 241–250. doi:10.1016/j.abb.2007.04.024 PMID:17537398

Peterson GM, Schmitz K *et al.* (2001). *Physical activity among smokers is inversely associated with lung cancer incidence in Iowa Women's Health Study*. 25th Annual Meeting of the American Society of Preventive Oncology

Peto R, Chen ZM, Boreham J (1999). Tobacco the growing epidemic. *Nat Med*, 5: 15–17. doi:10.1038/4691 PMID:9883828

Petrakis NL, Gruenke LD, Beelen TC *et al.* (1978). Nicotine in breast fluid of nonlactating women. *Science*, 199: 303–305. doi:10.1126/science.619458 PMID:619458

Petridou E, Koukoulomatis P, Dessypris N *et al.* (2002). Why is endometrial cancer less common in Greece than in other European Union countries? *Eur J Cancer Prev*, 11: 427–432. doi:10.1097/00008469-200210000-00004 PMID:12394239

Pfeifer GP, Denissenko MF, Olivier M *et al.* (2002). Tobacco smoke carcinogens, DNA damage and p53 mutations in smoking-associated cancers. *Oncogene*, 21: 7435–7451. doi:10.1038/sj.onc.1205803 PMID:12379884

Phillips DH (1983). Fifty years of benzo(a)pyrene. *Nature*, 303: 468–472. doi:10.1038/303468a0 PMID:6304528

Phillips DH (2002). Smoking-related DNA and protein adducts in human tissues. *Carcinogenesis*, 23: 1979–2004. doi:10.1093/carcin/23.12.1979 PMID:12507921

Phillips LE, Longstreth WT Jr, Koepsell T *et al.* (2005). Active and passive cigarette smoking and risk of intracranial meningioma. *Neuroepidemiology*, 24: 117–122. Epub 2004 Dec 30.

Phukan RK, Zomawia E, Narain K *et al.* (2005). Tobacco use and stomach cancer in Mizoram, India. *Cancer Epidemiol Biomarkers Prev*, 14: 1892–1896.

Pinkston JA & Cole P (1996). Cigarette smoking and Warthin's tumor. *Am J Epidemiol*, 144: 183–187. PMID:8678050

Pinsky PF (2006). Racial and ethnic differences in lung cancer incidence: how much is explained by differences in smoking patterns? (United States). *Cancer Causes Control*, 17: 1017–1024. doi:10.1007/s10552-006-0038-2 PMID:16933052

Pirkle JL, Bernert JT, Caudill SP *et al.* (2006). Trends in the exposure of nonsmokers in the U.S. population to secondhand smoke: 1988–2002. *Environ Health Perspect*, 114: 853–858. PMID:16759984

Plant AL, Benson DM, Smith LC (1985). Cellular uptake and intracellular localization of benzo(a)pyrene by digital fluorescence imaging microscopy. *J Cell Biol*, 100: 1295–1308. doi:10.1083/jcb.100.4.1295 PMID:3980583

Plummer M, Herrero R, Franceschi S *et al.*IARC Multi-centre Cervical Cancer Study Group (2003). Smoking and cervical cancer: pooled analysis of the IARC multi-centric case–control study. *Cancer Causes Control*, 14: 805–814. doi:10.1023/B:CACO.0000003811.98261.3e PMID:14682438

Polychronopoulou A, Tzonou A, Hsieh CC *et al.* (1993). Reproductive variables, tobacco, ethanol, coffee and somatometry as risk factors for ovarian cancer. *Int J Cancer*, 55: 402–407. doi:10.1002/ijc.2910550312 PMID:8375923

Poplawski T, Tomaszewska K, Galicki M *et al.* (2008). Promoter methylation of cancer-related genes in gastric carcinoma. *Exp Oncol*, 30: 112–116. PMID:18566573

Powell J & McConkey CC (1990). Increasing incidence of adenocarcinoma of the gastric cardia and adjacent sites. *Br J Cancer*, 62: 440–443. PMID:2206952

Prescott J, Ma H, Bernstein L, Ursin G (2007). Cigarette smoking is not associated with breast cancer risk in young women. *Cancer Epidemiol Biomarkers Prev*, 16: 620–622. doi:10.1158/1055-9965.EPI-06-0873 PMID:17372262

Preussmann R, Stewart BW (1984). *N-Nitroso Carcinogens.* In: *Chemical Carcinogens, Second Edition, ACS Monograph 182.* Searle CE, editor. Washington, DC: American Chemical Society.

Proia NK, Paszkiewicz GM, Nasca MA *et al.* (2006). Smoking and smokeless tobacco-associated human buccal cell mutations and their association with oral cancer–a review. *Cancer Epidemiol Biomarkers Prev*, 15: 1061–1077. doi:10.1158/1055-9965.EPI-05-0983 PMID:16775162

Prokopczyk B, Hoffmann D, Bologna M *et al.* (2002). Identification of tobacco-derived compounds in human pancreatic juice. *Chem Res Toxicol*, 15: 677–685. doi:10.1021/tx0101088 PMID:12018989

Prokopczyk B, Leder G, Trushin N *et al.* (2005). 4-Hydroxy-1-(3-pyridyl)-1-butanone, an indicator for 4-(methylnitrosamino)-1-(3-pyridyl)-1-butanone-induced DNA damage, is not detected in human pancreatic tissue. *Cancer Epidemiol Biomarkers Prev*, 14: 540–541. doi:10.1158/1055-9965.EPI-04-0626 PMID:15734986

Quinn AM, Harvey RG, Penning TM (2008). Oxidation of PAH *trans*-dihydrodiols by human aldo-keto reductase AKR1B10. *Chem Res Toxicol*, 21: 2207–2215. doi:10.1021/tx8002005 PMID:18788756

Quiñones LA, Irarrázabal CE, Rojas CR *et al.* (2006). Joint effect among p53, CYP1A1, GSTM1 polymorphism combinations and smoking on prostate cancer risk: an exploratory genotype-environment interaction study. *Asian J Androl*, 8: 349–355. doi:10.1111/j.1745-7262.2006.00135.x PMID:16625286

Rahman M, Sakamoto J, Fukui T (2003). Bidi smoking and oral cancer: a meta-analysis. *Int J Cancer*, 106: 600–604. doi:10.1002/ijc.11265 PMID:12845659

Raimondi S, Paracchini V, Autrup H *et al.* (2006). Meta- and pooled analysis of GSTT1 and lung cancer: a HuGE-GSEC review. *Am J Epidemiol*, 164: 1027–1042. doi:10.1093/aje/kwj321 PMID:17000715

Raitiola HS & Pukander JS (1997). Etiological factors of laryngeal cancer. *Acta Otolaryngol Suppl*, 529: 215–217. doi:10.3109/00016489709124126 PMID:9288314

Rao AR (1984). Modifying influences of betel quid ingredients on B(a)P-induced carcinogenesis in the buccal pouch of hamster. *Int J Cancer*, 33: 581–586. doi:10.1002/ijc.2910330506 PMID:6327538

Rao DN & Desai PB (1998). Risk assessment of tobacco, alcohol and diet in cancers of base tongue and oral tongue–a case control study. *Indian J Cancer*, 35: 65–72. PMID:9849026

Rao DN, Desai PB, Ganesh B (1999). Alcohol as an additional risk factor in laryngopharyngeal cancer in Mumbai–a case-control study. *Cancer Detect Prev*, 23: 37–44. doi:10.1046/j.1525-1500.1999.09906.x PMID:9892989

Rao DN, Ganesh B, Dinshaw KA, Mohandas KM (2002). A case-control study of stomach cancer in Mumbai, India. *Int J Cancer*, 99: 727–731. doi:10.1002/ijc.10339 PMID:12115507

Rao DN, Ganesh B, Rao RS, Desai PB (1994). Risk assessment of tobacco, alcohol and diet in oral cancer–a case-control study. *Int J Cancer*, 58: 469–473. doi:10.1002/ijc.2910580402 PMID:8056441

Rappaport SM, Kim S, Lan Q *et al.* (2009). Evidence that humans metabolize benzene via two pathways. *Environ Health Perspect*, 117: 946–952. PMID:19590688

Raucy JL & Carpenter SJ (1993). The expression of xenobiotic-metabolizing cytochromes P450 in fetal tissues. *J Pharmacol Toxicol Methods*, 29: 121–128. doi:10.1016/1056-8719(93)90062-J PMID:8364226

Ray CS & Gupta P (2009). Bidis and Smokeless Tobacco. *Current Science*, 96: 1324–1334.

Rebbeck TR (1997). Molecular epidemiology of the human glutathione *S*-transferase genotypes *GSTM1* and *GSTT1* in cancer susceptibility. *Cancer Epidemiol Biomarkers Prev*, 6: 733–743. PMID:9298582

Reid A, de Klerk NH, Ambrosini GL *et al.* (2006a). The risk of lung cancer with increasing time since ceasing exposure to asbestos and quitting smoking. *Occup Environ Med*, 63: 509–512. doi:10.1136/oem.2005.025379 PMID:16849527

Reid ME, Duffield-Lillico AJ, Sunga A *et al.* (2006b). Selenium supplementation and colorectal adenomas: an analysis of the nutritional prevention of cancer trial. *Int J Cancer*, 118: 1777–1781. doi:10.1002/ijc.21529 PMID:16217756

Reynolds P, Hurley S, Goldberg DE *et al.* (2004a). Active smoking, household passive smoking, and breast cancer: evidence from the California Teachers Study. *J Natl Cancer Inst*, 96: 29–37. doi:10.1093/jnci/djh002 PMID:14709736

Reynolds P, Hurley SE, Hoggatt K *et al.* (2004b). Correlates of active and passive smoking in the California Teachers Study cohort. *J Womens Health (Larchmt)*, 13: 778–790. doi:10.1089/jwh.2004.13.778 PMID:15385072

Richardson H, Abrahamowicz M, Tellier PP *et al.* (2005). Modifiable risk factors associated with clearance of type-specific cervical human papillomavirus infections in a cohort of university students. *Cancer Epidemiol Biomarkers Prev*, 14: 1149–1156. doi:10.1158/1055-9965.EPI-04-0230 PMID:15894665

Riman T, Dickman PW, Nilsson S *et al.* (2004). Some life-style factors and the risk of invasive epithelial ovarian cancer in Swedish women. *Eur J Epidemiol*, 19: 1011–1019. doi:10.1007/s10654-004-1633-8 PMID:15648594

Riopel MA, Ronnett BM, Kurman RJ (1999). Evaluation of diagnostic criteria and behavior of ovarian intestinal-type mucinous tumors: atypical proliferative (borderline) tumors and intraepithelial, microinvasive, invasive, and metastatic carcinomas. *Am J Surg Pathol*, 23: 617–635. doi:10.1097/00000478-199906000-00001 PMID:10366144

Risch A & Plass C (2008). Lung cancer epigenetics and genetics. *Int J Cancer*, 123: 1–7. PMID:18425819

Risch HA, Howe GR, Jain M *et al.* (1993). Are female smokers at higher risk for lung cancer than male smokers? A case-control analysis by histologic type. *Am J Epidemiol*, 138: 281–293. PMID:8395141

Risch HA, Marrett LD, Jain M, Howe GR (1996). Differences in risk factors for epithelial ovarian cancer by histologic type. Results of a case-control study. *Am J Epidemiol*, 144: 363–372. PMID:8712193

Roddam AW, Pirie K, Pike MC *et al.* (2007). Active and passive smoking and the risk of breast cancer in women aged 36–45 years: a population based case-control study in the UK. *Br J Cancer*, 97: 434–439. doi:10.1038/sj.bjc.6603859 PMID:17579618

Rodgman A & Perfetti TA (2006). The composition of cigarette smoke: a catalogue of the polycyclic aromatic hydrocarbons. *Beitr. Tabakforschung Inti.*, 22: 13–69.

Rodgman A, Perfetti TA (2009). *Alphabetical Component Index*. In: *The Chemical Components of Tobacco and Tobacco Smoke*. Rodgman A, Perfetti TA, editors. Boca Raton, FL: CRC Press, pp. 1483–1784.

Rodin SN & Rodin AS (2005). Origins and selection of p53 mutations in lung carcinogenesis. *Semin Cancer Biol*, 15: 103–112. doi:10.1016/j.semcancer.2004.08.005 PMID:15652455

Rodriguez T, Altieri A, Chatenoud L *et al.* (2004). Risk factors for oral and pharyngeal cancer in young adults. *Oral Oncol*, 40: 207–213. doi:10.1016/j.oraloncology.2003.08.014 PMID:14693246

Rodriguez-Antona C & Ingelman-Sundberg M (2006). Cytochrome *P450* pharmacogenetics and cancer. *Oncogene*, 25: 1679–1691. doi:10.1038/sj.onc.1209377 PMID:16550168

Rohan TE & Baron JA (1989). Cigarette smoking and breast cancer. *Am J Epidemiol*, 129: 36–42. PMID:2910070

Rohrmann S, Genkinger JM, Burke A *et al.* (2007). Smoking and risk of fatal prostate cancer in a prospective U.S. study. *Urology*, 69: 721–725. doi:10.1016/j.urology.2006.12.020 PMID:17445658

Rollison DE, Brownson RC, Hathcock HL, Newschaffer CJ (2008). Case-control study of tobacco smoke exposure and breast cancer risk in Delaware. *BMC Cancer*, 8: 157 doi:10.1186/1471-2407-8-157 PMID:18518960

Rollison DE, Helzlsouer KJ, Lee JH *et al.* (2009). Prospective study of JC virus seroreactivity and the development of colorectal cancers and adenomas. *Cancer Epidemiol Biomarkers Prev*, 18: 1515–1523. doi:10.1158/1055-9965.EPI-08-1119 PMID:19383887

Rolón PA, Castellsagué X, Benz M, Muñoz N (1995). Hot and cold mate drinking and esophageal cancer in Paraguay. *Cancer Epidemiol Biomarkers Prev*, 4: 595–605. PMID:8547825

Rossing MA, Cushing-Haugen KL, Wicklund KG, Weiss NS (2008). Cigarette smoking and risk of epithelial ovarian cancer. *Cancer Causes Control*, 19: 413–420. doi:10.1007/s10552-007-9103-8 PMID:18080774

Rothman KJ, Greenland S (1998). *Modern Epidemiology*, 2nd ed. Philadelphia, USA: Lippincott-Raven Publishers.

Roubidoux MA, Kaur JS, Griffith KA *et al.* (2003). Relationship of mammographic parenchymal patterns to breast cancer risk factors and smoking in Alaska Native women. *Cancer Epidemiol Biomarkers Prev*, 12: 1081–1086. PMID:14578146

Royce JM, Hymowitz N, Corbett K *et al.*COMMIT Research Group (1993). Smoking cessation factors among African Americans and whites. *Am J Public Health*, 83: 220–226. doi:10.2105/AJPH.83.2.220 PMID:8427327

Ruano-Ravina A, Figueiras A, Freire-Garabal M, Barros-Dios JM (2006). Antioxidant vitamins and risk of lung cancer. *Curr Pharm Des*, 12: 599–613. doi:10.2174/138161206775474396 PMID:16472151

Rubin GL, Peterson HB, Lee NC *et al.* (1990). Estrogen replacement therapy and the risk of endometrial cancer: remaining controversies. *Am J Obstet Gynecol*, 162: 148–154. PMID:2301483

Ryk C, Berggren P, Kumar R *et al.* (2005). Influence of *GSTM1*, *GSTT1*, *GSTP1* and *NAT2* genotypes on the *p53* mutational spectrum in bladder tumours. *Int J Cancer*, 113: 761–768. doi:10.1002/ijc.20650 PMID:15499621

Saccone SF, Hinrichs AL, Saccone NL *et al.* (2007). Cholinergic nicotinic receptor genes implicated in a nicotine dependence association study targeting 348 candidate genes with 3713 SNPs. *Hum Mol Genet*, 16: 36–49. doi:10.1093/hmg/ddl438 PMID:17135278

Saintot M, Malaveille C, Hautefeuille A, Gerber M (2003). Interactions between genetic polymorphism of cytochrome P450–1B1, sulfotransferase 1A1, catechol-o-methyltransferase and tobacco exposure in breast cancer risk. *Int J Cancer*, 107: 652–657. doi:10.1002/ijc.11432 PMID:14520706

Sala E, Warren R, McCann J *et al.* (2000). Smoking and high-risk mammographic parenchymal patterns: a case-control study. *Breast Cancer Res*, 2: 59–63. doi:10.1186/bcr29 PMID:11056684

Salama SA, Abdel-Rahman SZ, Sierra-Torres CH *et al.* (1999). Role of polymorphic *GSTM1* and *GSTT1* genotypes on NNK-induced genotoxicity. *Pharmacogenetics*, 9: 735–743. doi:10.1097/00008571-199912000-00008 PMID:10634136

Salaspuro V & Salaspuro M (2004). Synergistic effect of alcohol drinking and smoking on *in vivo* acetaldehyde concentration in saliva. *Int J Cancer*, 111: 480–483. doi:10.1002/ijc.20293 PMID:15239123

Samanic C, Kogevinas M, Dosemeci M *et al.* (2006). Smoking and bladder cancer in Spain: effects of tobacco type, timing, environmental tobacco smoke, and gender. *Cancer Epidemiol Biomarkers Prev*, 15: 1348–1354. doi:10.1158/1055-9965.EPI-06-0021 PMID:16835335

Samowitz WS (2008). Genetic and epigenetic changes in colon cancer. *Exp Mol Pathol*, 85: 64–67. doi:10.1016/j.yexmp.2008.03.008 PMID:18482722

Samowitz WS, Albertsen H, Sweeney C *et al.* (2006). Association of smoking, CpG island methylator phenotype, and V600E BRAF mutations in colon cancer. *J Natl Cancer Inst*, 98: 1731–1738. doi:10.1093/jnci/djj468 PMID:17148775

Samowitz WS, Slattery ML, Sweeney C *et al.* (2007). *APC* mutations and other genetic and epigenetic changes in colon cancer. *Mol Cancer Res*, 5: 165–170. doi:10.1158/1541-7786.MCR-06-0398 PMID:17293392

Sanderson S, Salanti G, Higgins J (2007). Joint effects of the *N*-acetyltransferase 1 and 2 (*NAT1* and *NAT2*) genes and smoking on bladder carcinogenesis: a literature-based systematic HuGE review and evidence synthesis. *Am J Epidemiol*, 166: 741–751. doi:10.1093/aje/kwm167 PMID:17675654

Sanjoaquin MA, Appleby PN, Thorogood M *et al.* (2004). Nutrition, lifestyle and colorectal cancer incidence: a prospective investigation of 10998 vegetarians and non-vegetarians in the United Kingdom. *Br J Cancer*, 90: 118–121. doi:10.1038/sj.bjc.6601441 PMID:14710217

Sankaranarayanan R, Duffy SW, Day NE *et al.* (1989b). A case-control investigation of cancer of the oral tongue and the floor of the mouth in southern India. *Int J Cancer*, 44: 617–621. doi:10.1002/ijc.2910440410 PMID:2793234

Sankaranarayanan R, Duffy SW, Nair MK *et al.* (1990b). Tobacco and alcohol as risk factors in cancer of the larynx in Kerala, India. *Int J Cancer*, 45: 879–882. doi:10.1002/ijc.2910450517 PMID:2335391

Sankaranarayanan R, Duffy SW, Padmakumary G *et al.* (1989a). Tobacco chewing, alcohol and nasal snuff in cancer of the gingiva in Kerala, India. *Br J Cancer*, 60: 638–643. PMID:2803939

Sankaranarayanan R, Duffy SW, Padmakumary G *et al.* (1990a). Risk factors for cancer of the buccal and labial mucosa in Kerala, southern India. *J Epidemiol Community Health*, 44: 286–292. doi:10.1136/jech.44.4.286 PMID:2277249

Sankaranarayanan R, Duffy SW, Padmakumary G *et al.* (1991). Risk factors for cancer of the oesophagus in Kerala, India. *Int J Cancer*, 49: 485–489. doi:10.1002/ijc.2910490402 PMID:1917146

Sapkota A, Gajalakshmi V, Jetly DH *et al.* (2007). Smokeless tobacco and increased risk of hypopharyngeal and laryngeal cancers: a multicentric case-control study from India. *Int J Cancer*, 121: 1793–1798. doi:10.1002/ijc.22832 PMID:17583577

Sasazuki S, Sasaki S, Tsugane SJapan Public Health Center Study Group (2002). Cigarette smoking, alcohol consumption and subsequent gastric cancer risk by subsite and histologic type. *Int J Cancer*, 101: 560–566. doi:10.1002/ijc.10649 PMID:12237898

Sauvaget C, Lagarde F, Nagano J *et al.* (2005). Lifestyle factors, radiation and gastric cancer in atomic-bomb survivors (Japan). *Cancer Causes Control*, 16: 773–780. doi:10.1007/s10552-005-5385-x PMID:16132787

Scanlon EF, Suh O, Murthy SM *et al.* (1995). Influence of smoking on the development of lung metastases from breast cancer. *Cancer*, 75: 2693–2699. doi:10.1002/1097-0142(19950601)75:11<2693::AID-CNCR2820751109>3.0.CO;2-E PMID:7743472

Schechter MT, Miller AB, Howe GR (1985). Cigarette smoking and breast cancer: a case-control study of screening program participants. *Am J Epidemiol*, 121: 479–487. PMID:4014139

Schildt EB, Eriksson M, Hardell L, Magnuson A (1998). Oral snuff, smoking habits and alcohol consumption in relation to oral cancer in a Swedish case-control study. *Int J Cancer*, 77: 341–346. doi:10.1002/(SICI)1097-0215(19980729)77:3<341::AID-IJC6>3.0.CO;2-O PMID:9663593

Schlecht NF, Franco EL, Pintos J *et al.* (1999b). Interaction between tobacco and alcohol consumption and the risk of cancers of the upper aero-digestive tract in Brazil. *Am J Epidemiol*, 150: 1129–1137. PMID:10588073

Schlecht NF, Franco EL, Pintos J, Kowalski LP (1999a). Effect of smoking cessation and tobacco type on the risk of cancers of the upper aero-digestive tract in Brazil. *Epidemiology*, 10: 412–418. doi:10.1097/00001648-199907000-00012 PMID:10401876

Schlemmer A, Jensen J, Riis BJ, Christiansen C (1990). Smoking induces increased androgen levels in early post-menopausal women. *Maturitas*, 12: 99–104. doi:10.1016/0378-5122(90)90087-M PMID:2123959

Schlicht KE, Michno N, Smith BD *et al.* (2007). Functional characterization of CYP2A13 polymorphisms. *Xenobiotica*, 37: 1439–1449. PMID:17922361

Schlöbe D, Hölzle D, Hatz D *et al.* (2008). 4-Hydroxy-1-(3-pyridyl)-1-butanone-releasing DNA adducts in lung, lower esophagus and cardia of sudden death victims. *Toxicology*, 245: 154–161. doi:10.1016/j.tox.2007.12.021 PMID:18243467

Schöllkopf C, Smedby KE, Hjalgrim H *et al.* (2005). Cigarette smoking and risk of non-Hodgkin's lymphoma — a population-based case-control study. *Cancer Epidemiol Biomarkers Prev*, 14: 1791–1796.

Schuller HM (2002). Mechanisms of smoking-related lung and pancreatic adenocarcinoma development. *Nat Rev Cancer*, 2: 455–463. PMID:12189387

Schuller HM (2009). Is cancer triggered by altered signalling of nicotinic acetylcholine receptors? *Nat Rev Cancer*, 9: 195–205. doi:10.1038/nrc2590 PMID:19194381

Schütze N, Vollmer G, Knuppen R (1994). Catecholestrogens are agonists of estrogen receptor dependent gene expression in MCF-7 cells. *J Steroid Biochem Mol Biol*, 48: 453–461. doi:10.1016/0960-0760(94)90193-7 PMID:8180106

Schütze N, Vollmer G, Tiemann I *et al.* (1993). Catecholestrogens are MCF-7 cell estrogen receptor agonists. *J Steroid Biochem Mol Biol*, 46: 781–789. doi:10.1016/0960-0760(93)90319-R PMID:8274412

Schwartz AG & Swanson GM (1997). Lung carcinoma in African Americans and whites. A population-based study in metropolitan Detroit, Michigan. *Cancer*, 79: 45–52. doi:10.1002/(SICI)1097-0142(19970101)79:1<45::AID-CNCR7>3.0.CO;2-L PMID:8988725

SEER (2004). *Surveillance research Program, Cancer Statistics Branch.* http://www.seer.cancer.gov/publications/csr.html

Seidegård J, Pero RW, Markowitz MM *et al.* (1990). Isoenzyme(s) of glutathione transferase (class Mu) as a marker for the susceptibility to lung cancer: a follow up study. *Carcinogenesis*, 11: 33–36. doi:10.1093/carcin/11.1.33 PMID:2295125

Seidegård J, Pero RW, Miller DG, Beattie EJ (1986). A glutathione transferase in human leukocytes as a marker for the susceptibility to lung cancer. *Carcinogenesis*, 7: 751–753. doi:10.1093/carcin/7.5.751 PMID:3698203

Sen B, Mahadevan B, DeMarini DM (2007). Transcriptional responses to complex mixtures: a review. *Mutat Res*, 636: 144–177. doi:10.1016/j.mrrev.2007.08.002 PMID:17888717

Seow A, Vainio H, Yu MC (2005). Effect of glutathione-S-transferase polymorphisms on the cancer preventive potential of isothiocyanates: an epidemiological perspective. *Mutat Res*, 592: 58–67. doi:10.1016/j.mrfmmm.2005.06.004 PMID:16019037

Setiawan VW, Pike MC, Kolonel LN *et al.* (2007). Racial/ethnic differences in endometrial cancer risk: the multiethnic cohort study. *Am J Epidemiol*, 165: 262–270. doi:10.1093/aje/kwk010 PMID:17090617

Shaib YH, El-Serag HB, Nooka AK *et al.* (2007). Risk factors for intrahepatic and extrahepatic cholangiocarcinoma: a hospital-based case-control study. *Am J Gastroenterol*, 102: 1016–1021. doi:10.1111/j.1572-0241.2007.01104.x PMID:17324130

Shapiro JA, Jacobs EJ, Thun MJ (2000). Cigar smoking in men and risk of death from tobacco-related cancers. *J Natl Cancer Inst*, 92: 333–337. doi:10.1093/jnci/92.4.333 PMID:10675383

Sharpe CR & Siemiatycki J (2001). Joint effects of smoking and body mass index on prostate cancer risk. *Epidemiology*, 12: 546–551. doi:10.1097/00001648-200109000-00014 PMID:11505174

Sharpe CR, Siemiatycki JA, Rachet BP (2002). The effects of smoking on the risk of colorectal cancer. *Dis Colon Rectum*, 45: 1041–1050. PMID:12195188

Shi X, Zhou S, Wang Z *et al.* (2008). *CYP1A1* and *GSTM1* polymorphisms and lung cancer risk in Chinese populations: a meta-analysis. *Lung Cancer*, 59: 155–163. doi:10.1016/j.lungcan.2007.08.004 PMID:17900751

Shields TS, Weiss NS, Voigt LF, Beresford SA (1999). The additional risk of endometrial cancer associated with unopposed estrogen use in women with other risk factors. *Epidemiology*, 10: 733–738. doi:10.1097/00001648-199911000-00014 PMID:10535788

Shikata K, Doi Y, Yonemoto K *et al.* (2008). Population-based prospective study of the combined influence of cigarette smoking and Helicobacter pylori infection on gastric cancer incidence: the Hisayama Study. *Am J Epidemiol*, 168: 1409–1415. doi:10.1093/aje/kwn276 PMID:18945691

Shimizu M, Lasker JM, Tsutsumi M, Lieber CS (1990). Immunohistochemical localization of ethanol-inducible P450IIE1 in the rat alimentary tract. *Gastroenterology*, 99: 1044–1053. PMID:2203661

Shimizu N, Nagata C, Shimizu H *et al.* (2003). Height, weight, and alcohol consumption in relation to the risk of colorectal cancer in Japan: a prospective study. *Br J Cancer*, 88: 1038–1043. doi:10.1038/sj.bjc.6600845 PMID:12671701

Shklar G (1972). Experimental oral pathology in the Syrian hamster. *Prog Exp Tumor Res*, 16: 518–538. PMID:4557243

Shrubsole MJ, Wu H, Ness RM *et al.* (2008). Alcohol drinking, cigarette smoking, and risk of colorectal adenomatous and hyperplastic polyps. *Am J Epidemiol*, 167: 1050–1058. doi:10.1093/aje/kwm400 PMID:18304959

Shu HP & Bymun EN (1983). Systemic excretion of benzo(a)pyrene in the control and microsomally induced rat: the influence of plasma lipoproteins and albumin as carrier molecules. *Cancer Res*, 43: 485–490. PMID:6293698

Sikström B, Hellberg D, Nilsson S, Mårdh PA (1995). Smoking, alcohol, sexual behaviour and drug use in women with cervical human papillomavirus infection. *Arch Gynecol Obstet*, 256: 131–137. doi:10.1007/BF01314641 PMID:7574905

Sillanpää P, Heikinheimo L, Kataja V *et al.* (2007). CYP1A1 and CYP1B1 genetic polymorphisms, smoking and breast cancer risk in a Finnish Caucasian population. *Breast Cancer Res Treat*, 104: 287–297. doi:10.1007/s10549-006-9414-6 PMID:17063266

Simán JH, Forsgren A, Berglund G, Florén C-H (2001). Tobacco smoking increases the risk for gastric adenocarcinoma among Helicobacter pylori-infected individuals. *Scand J Gastroenterol*, 36: 208–213. doi:10.1080/003655201750065988 PMID:11252415

Simarak S, de Jong UW, Breslow N *et al.* (1977). Cancer of the oral cavity, pharynx/larynx and lung in North Thailand: case-control study and analysis of cigar smoke. *Br J Cancer*, 36: 130–140. PMID:19028

Singh R & Farmer PB (2006). Liquid chromatography-electrospray ionization-mass spectrometry: the future of DNA adduct detection. *Carcinogenesis*, 27: 178–196. doi:10.1093/carcin/bgi260 PMID:16272169

Singh R, Kaur B, Farmer PB (2005). Detection of DNA damage derived from a direct acting ethylating agent present in cigarette smoke by use of liquid chromatography-tandem mass spectrometry. *Chem Res Toxicol*, 18: 249–256. doi:10.1021/tx049793j PMID:15720129

Sjödahl K, Lu Y, Nilsen TI *et al.* (2007). Smoking and alcohol drinking in relation to risk of gastric cancer: a population-based, prospective cohort study. *Int J Cancer*, 120: 128–132. doi:10.1002/ijc.22157 PMID:17036324

Skipper PL & Tannenbaum SR (1990). Protein adducts in the molecular dosimetry of chemical carcinogens. *Carcinogenesis*, 11: 507–518. doi:10.1093/carcin/11.4.507 PMID:2182215

Skjelbred CF, Saebø M, Wallin H *et al.* (2006). Polymorphisms of the XRCC1, XRCC3 and XPD genes and risk of colorectal adenoma and carcinoma, in a Norwegian cohort: a case control study. *BMC Cancer*, 6: 67 doi:10.1186/1471-2407-6-67 PMID:16542436

Slattery ML, Curtin K, Anderson K *et al.* (2000). Associations between cigarette smoking, lifestyle factors, and microsatellite instability in colon tumors. *J Natl Cancer Inst*, 92: 1831–1836. doi:10.1093/jnci/92.22.1831 PMID:11078760

Slattery ML, Curtin K, Giuliano AR *et al.* (2008). Active and passive smoking, IL6, ESR1, and breast cancer risk. *Breast Cancer Res Treat*, 109: 101–111. doi:10.1007/s10549-007-9629-1 PMID:17594514

Slattery ML, Curtin K, Ma K *et al.* (2002). *GSTM*-1 and *NAT2* and genetic alterations in colon tumors. *Cancer Causes Control*, 13: 527–534. doi:10.1023/A:1016376016716 PMID:12195642

Slattery ML, Edwards S, Curtin K *et al.* (2003). Associations between smoking, passive smoking, GSTM-1, NAT2, and rectal cancer. *Cancer Epidemiol Biomarkers Prev*, 12: 882–889. PMID:14504199

Slattery ML, Samowtiz W, Ma K *et al.* (2004). CYP1A1, cigarette smoking, and colon and rectal cancer. *Am J Epidemiol*, 160: 842–852. doi:10.1093/aje/kwh298 PMID:15496536

Slemenda CW, Hui SL, Longcope C, Johnston CC Jr (1989). Cigarette smoking, obesity, and bone mass. *J Bone Miner Res*, 4: 737–741. PMID:2816518

Smith CJ, Perfetti TA, King JA (2006). Perspectives on pulmonary inflammation and lung cancer risk in cigarette smokers. *Inhal Toxicol*, 18: 667–677. doi:10.1080/08958370600742821 PMID:16864557

Smith EM, Sowers MF, Burns TL (1984). Effects of smoking on the development of female reproductive cancers. *J Natl Cancer Inst*, 73: 371–376. PMID:6589429

Smith JB & Randle HW (2001). Giant basal cell carcinoma and cigarette smoking. *Cutis*, 67: 73–76. PMID:11204609

Smits KM, Gaspari L, Weijenberg MP *et al.* (2003). Interaction between smoking, GSTM1 deletion and colorectal cancer: results from the GSEC study. *Biomarkers*, 8: 299–310. doi:10.1080/1354750031000121467 PMID:12944179

Sokić SI, Adanja BJ, Marinković JP, Vlajinac HD (1994). Case-control study of risk factors in laryngeal cancer. *Neoplasma*, 41: 43–47. PMID:8202195

Song DK, Xing DL, Zhang LR *et al.* (2009). Association of *NAT2*, *GSTM1*, *GSTT1*, *CYP2A6*, and *CYP2A13* gene polymorphisms with susceptibility and clinicopathologic characteristics of bladder cancer in Central China. *Cancer Detect Prev*, 32: 416–423. PMID:19303722

Sparks R, Bigler J, Sibert JG *et al.* (2004). TGFbeta1 polymorphism (L10P) and risk of colorectal adenomatous and hyperplastic polyps. *Int J Epidemiol*, 33: 955–961. doi:10.1093/ije/dyh102 PMID:15020570

Spira A, Beane J, Shah V *et al.* (2004). Effects of cigarette smoke on the human airway epithelial cell transcriptome. *Proc Natl Acad Sci U S A*, 101: 10143–10148. doi:10.1073/pnas.0401422101 PMID:15210990

Spitz MR, Amos CI, Dong Q *et al.* (2008). The CHRNA5–A3 region on chromosome 15q24–25.1 is a risk factor both for nicotine dependence and for lung cancer. *J Natl Cancer Inst*, 100: 1552–1556. doi:10.1093/jnci/djn363 PMID:18957677

Spitz MR, Duphorne CM, Detry MA *et al.* (2000). Dietary intake of isothiocyanates: evidence of a joint effect with glutathione *S*-transferase polymorphisms in lung cancer risk. *Cancer Epidemiol Biomarkers Prev*, 9: 1017–1020. PMID:11045782

Spitz MR, Fueger JJ, Goepfert H, Newell GR (1990). Salivary gland cancer. A case-control investigation of risk factors. *Arch Otolaryngol Head Neck Surg*, 116: 1163–1166. PMID:2206501

Spitz MR, Wu X, Wilkinson A, Wei D (2006). *Cancer of the Lung*. In: *Cancer Epidemiology and Prevention*. Schottenfeld D, Fraumeni JF, editors. New York: Oxford University Press, Chap 33, pp. 638–658.

Sriamporn S, Vatanasapt V, Pisani P *et al.* (1992). Environmental risk factors for nasopharyngeal carcinoma: a case-control study in northeastern Thailand. *Cancer Epidemiol Biomarkers Prev*, 1: 345–348. PMID:1305465

Srivastava A & Kreiger N (2004). Cigarette smoking and testicular cancer. *Cancer Epidemiol Biomarkers Prev*, 13: 49–54. doi:10.1158/1055-9965.EPI-03-0133 PMID:14744732

Stagnaro E, Ramazzotti V, Crosignani P *et al.* (2001). Smoking and hematolymphopoietic malignancies. *Cancer Causes Control*, 12: 325–334. doi:10.1023/A:1011216102871 PMID:11456228

Stagnaro E, Tumino R, Parodi S *et al.* (2004). Non-Hodgkin's lymphoma and type of tobacco smoke. *Cancer Epidemiol Biomarkers Prev*, 13: 431–437.

Stanton MF, Miller E, Wrench C, Blackwell R (1972). Experimental induction of epidermoid carcinoma in the lungs of rats by cigarette smoke condensate. *J Natl Cancer Inst*, 49: 867–877. PMID:4647499

Stavrides JC (2006). Lung carcinogenesis: pivotal role of metals in tobacco smoke. *Free Radic Biol Med*, 41: 1017–1030. doi:10.1016/j.freeradbiomed.2006.06.024 PMID:16962926

Steinmetz J, Spyckerelle Y, Guéguen R, Dupré C (2007). Alcohol, tobacco and colorectal adenomas and cancer. Case-control study in a population with positive fecal occult blood tests *Presse Med*, 36: 1174–1182. PMID:17350789

Stellman SD, Chen Y, Muscat JE *et al.* (2003). Lung cancer risk in white and black Americans. *Ann Epidemiol*, 13: 294–302. doi:10.1016/S1047-2797(02)00420-9 PMID:12684197

Stellman SD, Takezaki T, Wang L *et al.* (2001). Smoking and lung cancer risk in American and Japanese men: an international case-control study. *Cancer Epidemiol Biomarkers Prev*, 10: 1193–1199. PMID:11700268

Stepanov I, Carmella SG, Briggs A *et al.* (2009a). Presence of the carcinogen *N'*-nitrosonornicotine in the urine of some users of oral nicotine replacement therapy products. *Cancer Res*, 69: 8236–8240. PMID:19843845

Stepanov I, Carmella SG, Han S *et al.* (2009b). Evidence for endogenous formation of *N'*-nitrosonornicotine in some long-term nicotine patch users. *Nicotine Tob Res*, 11: 99–105. PMID:19246447

Stepanov I & Hecht SS (2005). Tobacco-specific nitrosamines and their pyridine-*N*-glucuronides in the urine of smokers and smokeless tobacco users. *Cancer Epidemiol Biomarkers Prev*, 14: 885–891. doi:10.1158/1055-9965.EPI-04-0753 PMID:15824160

Stepanov I, Hecht SS, Lindgren B *et al.* (2007). Relationship of human toenail nicotine, cotinine, and 4-(methylnitrosamino)-1-(3-pyridyl)-1-butanol to levels of these biomarkers in plasma and urine. *Cancer Epidemiol Biomarkers Prev*, 16: 1382–1386. doi:10.1158/1055-9965.EPI-07-0145 PMID:17627002

Stepanov I, Upadhyaya P, Carmella SG *et al.* (2008). Extensive metabolic activation of the tobacco-specific carcinogen 4-(methylnitrosamino)-1-(3-pyridyl)-1-butanone in smokers. *Cancer Epidemiol Biomarkers Prev*, 17: 1764–1773. doi:10.1158/1055-9965.EPI-07-2844 PMID:18628430

Stern MC, Conti DV, Siegmund KD *et al.* (2007). DNA repair single-nucleotide polymorphisms in colorectal cancer and their role as modifiers of the effect of cigarette smoking and alcohol in the Singapore Chinese Health Study. *Cancer Epidemiol Biomarkers Prev*, 16: 2363–2372. doi:10.1158/1055-9965.EPI-07-0268 PMID:18006925

Stern MC, Siegmund KD, Conti DV *et al.* (2006). XRCC1, XRCC3, and XPD polymorphisms as modifiers of the effect of smoking and alcohol on colorectal adenoma risk. *Cancer Epidemiol Biomarkers Prev*, 15: 2384–2390. doi:10.1158/1055-9965.EPI-06-0381 PMID:17164360

Stockwell HG & Lyman GH (1987). Cigarette smoking and the risk of female reproductive cancer. *Am J Obstet Gynecol*, 157: 35–40. PMID:3605266

Strader CH, Vaughan TL, Stergachis A (1988). Use of nasal preparations and the incidence of sinonasal cancer. *J Epidemiol Community Health*, 42: 243–248. doi:10.1136/jech.42.3.243 PMID:2471766

Strange RC, Spiteri MA, Ramachandran S, Fryer AA (2001). Glutathione-*S*-transferase family of enzymes. *Mutat Res*, 482: 21–26. PMID:11535245

Strom BL, Schinnar R, Weber AL *et al.* (2006). Case-control study of postmenopausal hormone replacement therapy and endometrial cancer. *Am J Epidemiol*, 164: 775–786. doi:10.1093/aje/kwj316 PMID:16997897

Stürmer T, Glynn RJ, Lee IM *et al.* (2000). Lifetime cigarette smoking and colorectal cancer incidence in the Physicians' Health Study I. *J Natl Cancer Inst*, 92: 1178–1181. doi:10.1093/jnci/92.14.1178 PMID:10904092

Subapriya R, Thangavelu A, Mathavan B *et al.* (2007). Assessment of risk factors for oral squamous cell carcinoma in Chidambaram, Southern India: a case-control study. *Eur J Cancer Prev*, 16: 251–256. doi:10.1097/01.cej.0000228402.53106.9e PMID:17415096

Subramanian J & Govindan R (2008). Molecular genetics of lung cancer in people who have never smoked. *Lancet Oncol*, 9: 676–682. doi:10.1016/S1470-2045(08)70174-8 PMID:18598932

Sudo H, Li-Sucholeiki X-C, Marcelino LA *et al.* (2008). Fetal-juvenile origins of point mutations in the adult human tracheal-bronchial epithelium: absence of detectable effects of age, gender or smoking status. *Mutat Res*, 646: 25–40. PMID:18824180

Sung NY, Choi KS, Park EC *et al.* (2007). Smoking, alcohol and gastric cancer risk in Korean men: the National Health Insurance Corporation Study. *Br J Cancer*, 97: 700–704. doi:10.1038/sj.bjc.6603893 PMID:17637680

Suwan-ampai P, Navas-Acien A, Strickland PT, Agnew J (2009). Involuntary tobacco smoke exposure and urinary levels of polycyclic aromatic hydrocarbons in the United States, 1999 to 2002. *Cancer Epidemiol Biomarkers Prev*, 18: 884–893. doi:10.1158/1055-9965.EPI-08-0939 PMID:19258471

Suwanrungruang K, Sriamporn S, Wiangnon S *et al.* (2008). Lifestyle-related risk factors for stomach cancer in northeast Thailand. *Asian Pac J Cancer Prev*, 9: 71–75. PMID:18439078

Suzuki T, Matsuo K, Wakai K *et al.* (2007). Effect of familial history and smoking on common cancer risks in Japan. *Cancer*, 109: 2116–2123. doi:10.1002/cncr.22685 PMID:17410537

Swann PF (1984). Effect of ethanol on nitrosamine metabolism and distribution. Implications for the role of nitrosamines in human cancer and for the influence of alcohol consumption on cancer incidence. *IARC Sci Publ*, 57501–512. PMID:6533040

Swanson GM & Burns PB (1997). Cancers of the salivary gland: workplace risks among women and men. *Ann Epidemiol*, 7: 369–374. doi:10.1016/S1047-2797(97)00041-0 PMID:9279445

Sweeney C, Boucher KM, Samowitz WS *et al.* (2009). Oncogenetic tree model of somatic mutations and DNA methylation in colon tumors. *Genes Chromosomes Cancer*, 48: 1–9. doi:10.1002/gcc.20614 PMID:18767147

Syrjänen K, Shabalova I, Petrovichev N *et al.* (2007). Smoking is an independent risk factor for oncogenic human papillomavirus (HPV) infections but not for high-grade CIN. *Eur J Epidemiol*, 22: 723–735. doi:10.1007/s10654-007-9180-8 PMID:17828436

Szeliga J & Dipple A (1998). DNA adduct formation by polycyclic aromatic hydrocarbon dihydrodiol epoxides. *Chem Res Toxicol*, 11: 1–11. doi:10.1021/tx970142f PMID:9477220

Szyfter K, Szmeja Z, Szyfter W *et al.* (1999). Molecular and cellular alterations in tobacco smoke-associated larynx cancer. *Mutat Res*, 445: 259–274. PMID:10575435

't Mannetje A, Kogevinas M, Luce D *et al.* (1999). Sinonasal cancer, occupation, and tobacco smoking in European women and men. *Am J Ind Med*, 36: 101–107. doi:10.1002/(SICI)1097-0274(199907)36:1<101::AID-AJIM14>3.0.CO;2-A PMID:10361593

Takahashi I, Matsuzaka M, Umeda T *et al.* (2008). Differences in the influence of tobacco smoking on lung cancer between Japan and the USA: possible explanations for the 'smoking paradox' in Japan. *Public Health*, 122: 891–896. doi:10.1016/j.puhe.2007.10.004 PMID:18420238

Takahashi M, Imaida K, Mitsumori K *et al.* (1992). Promoting effects of cigarette smoke on the respiratory tract carcinogenesis of Syrian golden hamsters treated with diethylnitrosamine. *Carcinogenesis*, 13: 569–572. doi:10.1093/carcin/13.4.569 PMID:1576708

Talamini R, Bosetti C, La Vecchia C *et al.* (2002). Combined effect of tobacco and alcohol on laryngeal cancer risk: a case-control study. *Cancer Causes Control*, 13: 957–964. doi:10.1023/A:1021944123914 PMID:12588092

Tan W, Chen GF, Xing DY *et al.* (2001). Frequency of *CYP2A6* gene deletion and its relation to risk of lung and esophageal cancer in the Chinese population. *Int J Cancer*, 95: 96–101. doi:10.1002/1097-0215(20010320)95:2<96::AID-IJC1017>3.0.CO;2-2 PMID:11241319

Tang Y, Simoneau AR, Liao WX *et al.* (2009). WIF1, a Wnt pathway inhibitor, regulates SKP2 and c-myc expression leading to G1 arrest and growth inhibition of human invasive urinary bladder cancer cells. *Mol Cancer Ther*, 8: 458–468. doi:10.1158/1535-7163.MCT-08-0885 PMID:19174556

Tavani A, Negri E, Franceschi S *et al.* (1994). Attributable risk for laryngeal cancer in northern Italy. *Cancer Epidemiol Biomarkers Prev*, 3: 121–125. PMID:8049633

Terry MB & Neugut AI (1998). Cigarette smoking and the colorectal adenoma-carcinoma sequence: a hypothesis to explain the paradox. *Am J Epidemiol*, 147: 903–910. PMID:9596467

Terry P, Baron JA, Weiderpass E *et al.* (1999). Lifestyle and endometrial cancer risk: a cohort study from the Swedish Twin Registry. *Int J Cancer*, 82: 38–42. doi:10.1002/(SICI)1097-0215(19990702)82:1<38::AID-IJC8>3.0.CO;2-Q PMID:10360818

Terry P, Rohan TE, Franceschi S *et al.* (2004a). *Endometrial cancer*. In: *Tobacco: Science, Policy and Public Health*. Boyle P, Gray N, Henningfield J *et al.*, editors. Oxford University Press.

Terry PD & Goodman M (2006). Is the association between cigarette smoking and breast cancer modified by genotype? A review of epidemiologic studies and meta-analysis. *Cancer Epidemiol Biomarkers*

Prev, 15: 602–611. doi:10.1158/1055-9965.EPI-05-0853 PMID:16614098

Terry PD, Miller AB, Rohan TE (2002a). Prospective cohort study of cigarette smoking and colorectal cancer risk in women. *Int J Cancer*, 99: 480–483. doi:10.1002/ijc.10364 PMID:11992421

Terry PD, Miller AB, Rohan TE (2002b). A prospective cohort study of cigarette smoking and the risk of endometrial cancer. *Br J Cancer*, 86: 1430–1435. PMID:11986776

Terry PD & Rohan TE (2002). Cigarette smoking and the risk of breast cancer in women: a review of the literature. *Cancer Epidemiol Biomarkers Prev*, 11: 953–971. PMID:12376493

Terry PD, Rohan TE, Franceschi S, Weiderpass E (2002c). Cigarette smoking and the risk of endometrial cancer. *Lancet Oncol*, 3: 470–480. doi:10.1016/S1470-2045(02)00816-1 PMID:12147433

Theis RP, Dolwick Grieb SM, Burr D *et al.* (2008). Smoking, environmental tobacco smoke, and risk of renal cell cancer: a population-based case-control study. *BMC Cancer*, 8: 387 doi:10.1186/1471-2407-8-387 PMID:19108730

Thier R, Brüning T, Roos PH *et al.* (2003). Markers of genetic susceptibility in human environmental hygiene and toxicology: the role of selected CYP, NAT and GST genes. *Int J Hyg Environ Health*, 206: 149–171. doi:10.1078/1438-4639-00209 PMID:12872524

Thompson PA, DeMarini DM, Kadlubar FF *et al.* (2002). Evidence for the presence of mutagenic arylamines in human breast milk and DNA adducts in exfoliated breast ductal epithelial cells. *Environ Mol Mutagen*, 39: 134–142. doi:10.1002/em.10067 PMID:11921181

Thorgeirsson TE, Geller F, Sulem P *et al.* (2008). A variant associated with nicotine dependence, lung cancer and peripheral arterial disease. *Nature*, 452: 638 642. doi:10.1038/nature06846 PMID:18385739

Thun MJ & Heath CW Jr (1997). Changes in mortality from smoking in two American Cancer Society prospective studies since 1959. *Prev Med*, 26: 422–426. doi:10.1006/pmed.1997.0182 PMID:9245660

Thun MJ, Henley SJ, Burns D *et al.* (2006). Lung cancer death rates in lifelong nonsmokers. *J Natl Cancer Inst*, 98: 691–699. PMID:16705123

Tiemersma EW, Bunschoten A, Kok FJ *et al.* (2004). Effect of SULT1A1 and NAT2 genetic polymorphism on the association between cigarette smoking and colorectal adenomas. *Int J Cancer*, 108: 97–103. doi:10.1002/ijc.11533 PMID:14618622

Tiemersma EW, Kampman E, Bueno de Mesquita HB *et al.* (2002a). Meat consumption, cigarette smoking, and genetic susceptibility in the etiology of colorectal cancer: results from a Dutch prospective study. *Cancer Causes Control*, 13: 383–393. doi:10.1023/A:1015236701054 PMID:12074508

Tiemersma EW, Kloosterman J, Bunschoten A *et al.* (2002b). Role of EPHX genotype in the associations of smoking and diet with colorectal adenomas. *IARC Sci Publ*, 156: 491–493. PMID:12484240

Tijhuis MJ, Visker MH, Aarts JM *et al.* (2008). NQO1 and NFE2L2 polymorphisms, fruit and vegetable intake and smoking and the risk of colorectal adenomas in an endoscopy-based population. *Int J Cancer*, 122: 1842–1848. doi:10.1002/ijc.23246 PMID:18074351

Timofeeva MN, Kropp S, Sauter W *et al.*LUCY-Consortium (2009). CYP450 polymorphisms as risk factors for early-onset lung cancer: gender-specific differences. *Carcinogenesis*, 30: 1161–1169. doi:10.1093/carcin/bgp102 PMID:19414505

To-Figueras J, Gené M, Gómez-Catalán J *et al.* (2001). Lung cancer susceptibility in relation to combined polymorphisms of microsomal epoxide hydrolase and glutathione S-transferase P1. *Cancer Lett*, 173: 155–162. doi:10.1016/S0304-3835(01)00626-7 PMID:11597790

Tokunaga M, Land CE, Yamamoto T *et al.* (1987). Incidence of female breast cancer among atomic bomb survivors, Hiroshima and Nagasaki, 1950–1980. *Radiat Res*, 112: 243–272. doi:10.2307/3577254 PMID:3685255

Tolstrup J, Munk C, Thomsen BL *et al.* (2006). The role of smoking and alcohol intake in the development of high-grade squamous intraepithelial lesions among high-risk HPV-positive women. *Acta Obstet Gynecol Scand*, 85: 1114–1119. doi:10.1080/00016340600677027 PMID:16929418

Tomita M, Odaka M, Matsumoto M *et al.* (1991). Cigarette smoking and mortality among Japanese males in a prospective cohort study *Nippon Koshu Eisei Zasshi*, 38: 492–497. PMID:1747539

Toyomura K, Yamaguchi K, Kawamoto H *et al.* (2004). Relation of cigarette smoking and alcohol use to colorectal adenomas by subsite: the self-defense forces health study. *Cancer Sci*, 95: 72–76. doi:10.1111/j.1349-7006.2004.tb03173.x PMID:14720330

Toyooka S, Tokumo M, Shigematsu H *et al.* (2006). Mutational and epigenetic evidence for independent pathways for lung adenocarcinomas arising in smokers and never smokers. *Cancer Res*, 66: 1371–1375. PMID:16452191

Tran GD, Sun XD, Abnet CC *et al.* (2005). Prospective study of risk factors for esophageal and gastric cancers in the Linxian general population trial cohort in China. *Int J Cancer*, 113: 456–463. doi:10.1002/ijc.20616 PMID:15455378

Tranah GJ, Giovannucci E, Ma J *et al.* (2004). Epoxide hydrolase polymorphisms, cigarette smoking and risk of colorectal adenoma in the Nurses' Health Study and the Health Professionals Follow-up Study. *Carcinogenesis*, 25: 1211–1218. doi:10.1093/carcin/bgh126 PMID:14988221

Tranah GJ, Giovannucci E, Ma J *et al.* (2005). APC Asp1822Val and Gly2502Ser polymorphisms and risk of colorectal cancer and adenoma. *Cancer Epidemiol Biomarkers Prev*, 14: 863–870. doi:10.1158/1055-9965.EPI-04-0687 PMID:15824157

Trentham-Dietz A, Nichols HB, Hampton JM, Newcomb PA (2006). Weight change and risk of endometrial cancer. *Int J Epidemiol*, 35: 151–158. doi:10.1093/ije/dyi226 PMID:16278243

Trichopoulos D, Brown J, MacMahon B (1987). Urine estrogens and breast cancer risk factors among post-menopausal women. *Int J Cancer*, 40: 721–725. doi:10.1002/ijc.2910400602 PMID:3692620

Trost SG, Owen N, Bauman AE *et al.* (2002). Correlates of adults' participation in physical activity: review and update. *Med Sci Sports Exerc*, 34: 1996–2001. doi:10.1097/00005768-200212000-00020 PMID:12471307

Tsai HT, Tsai YM, Yang SF *et al.* (2007). Lifetime cigarette smoke and second-hand smoke and cervical intraepithelial neoplasm — a community-based case-control study. *Gynecol Oncol*, 105: 181–188. Epub 2007 Jan 3.

Tsoi KK, Pau CY, Wu WK *et al.* (2009). Cigarette smoking and the risk of colorectal cancer: a meta-analysis of prospective cohort studies. *Clin Gastroenterol Hepatol*, 7: 682–688, e1–e5. PMID:19245853

Tsong WH, Koh WP, Yuan JM *et al.* (2007). Cigarettes and alcohol in relation to colorectal cancer: the Singapore Chinese Health Study. *Br J Cancer*, 96: 821–827. PMID:17311023

Tu JT, Gao RN, Zhang DH, Gu BC (1985). Hepatitis B virus and primary liver cancer on Chongming Island, People's Republic of China. *Natl Cancer Inst Monogr*, 69: 213–215. PMID:3834335

Turner MC, Chen Y, Krewski D *et al.* (2007). Chronic obstructive pulmonary disease is associated with lung cancer mortality in a prospective study of never smokers. *Am J Respir Crit Care Med*, 176: 285–290. doi:10.1164/rccm.200612-1792OC PMID:17478615

Tuyns AJ, Estève J, Raymond L *et al.* (1988). Cancer of the larynx/hypopharynx, tobacco and alcohol: IARC international case-control study in Turin and Varese (Italy), Zaragoza and Navarra (Spain), Geneva (Switzerland) and Calvados (France). *Int J Cancer*, 41: 483–491. doi:10.1002/ijc.2910410403 PMID:3356483

Tuyns AJ, Péquignot G, Jensen OM (1977). [Esophageal cancer in Ille-et-Vilaine in relation to levels of alcohol and tobacco consumption. Risks are multiplying] *Bull Cancer*, 64: 45–60. PMID:861389

Tverdal A, Thelle D, Stensvold I *et al.* (1993). Mortality in relation to smoking history: 13 years' follow-up of 68,000 Norwegian men and women 35–49 years. *J Clin Epidemiol*, 46: 475–487. doi:10.1016/0895-4356(93)90025-V PMID:8501474

Tworoger SS, Gertig DM, Gates MA *et al.* (2008). Caffeine, alcohol, smoking, and the risk of incident epithelial ovarian cancer. *Cancer*, 112: 1169–1177. doi:10.1002/cncr.23275 PMID:18213613

Tyler CW Jr, Webster LA, Ory HW, Rubin GL (1985). Endometrial cancer: how does cigarette smoking influence the risk of women under age 55 years having this tumor? *Am J Obstet Gynecol*, 151: 899–905. PMID:3985056

Tzonou A, Day NE, Trichopoulos D *et al.* (1984). The epidemiology of ovarian cancer in Greece: a case-control study. *Eur J Cancer Clin Oncol*, 20: 1045–1052. doi:10.1016/0277-5379(84)90107-X PMID:6540687

Ulrich CM, Bigler J, Whitton JA *et al.* (2001). Epoxide hydrolase Tyr113His polymorphism is associated with elevated risk of colorectal polyps in the presence of smoking and high meat intake. *Cancer Epidemiol Biomarkers Prev*, 10: 875–882. PMID:11489754

Ursin G, London S, Stanczyk FZ *et al.* (1999). Urinary 2-hydroxyestrone/16alpha-hydroxyestrone ratio and risk of breast cancer in postmenopausal women. *J Natl Cancer Inst*, 91: 1067–1072. doi:10.1093/jnci/91.12.1067 PMID:10379970

Vaccarella S, Herrero R, Snijders PJ *et al.*IARC HPV Prevalence Surveys (IHPS) Study Group (2008). Smoking and human papillomavirus infection: pooled analysis of the International Agency for Research on Cancer HPV Prevalence Surveys. *Int J Epidemiol*, 37: 536–546. doi:10.1093/ije/dyn033 PMID:18316350

Vachon CM, Kuni CC, Anderson K *et al.* (2000). Association of mammographically defined percent breast density with epidemiologic risk factors for breast cancer (United States). *Cancer Causes Control*, 11: 653–662. doi:10.1023/A:1008926607428 PMID:10977110

Vairaktaris E, Spyridonidou S, Papakosta V *et al.* (2008). The hamster model of sequential oral oncogenesis. *Oral Oncol*, 44: 315–324. doi:10.1016/j.oraloncology.2007.08.015 PMID:18061531

van Dam RM, Huang Z, Rimm EB *et al.* (1999). Risk factors for basal cell carcinoma of the skin in men: results from the health professionals follow-up study. *Am J Epidemiol*, 150: 459–468. PMID:10472945

van den Donk M, Buijsse B, van den Berg SW *et al.* (2005). Dietary intake of folate and riboflavin, MTHFR C677T genotype, and colorectal adenoma risk: a Dutch case-control study. *Cancer Epidemiol Biomarkers Prev*, 14: 1562–1566. doi:10.1158/1055-9965.EPI-04-0419 PMID:15941973

van der Hel OL, Bueno de Mesquita HB, Sandkuijl L *et al.* (2003a). Rapid N-acetyltransferase 2 imputed phenotype and smoking may increase risk of colorectal cancer in women (Netherlands). *Cancer Causes Control*, 14: 293–298. doi:10.1023/A:1023601922106 PMID:12814209

van der Hel OL, Bueno-de-Mesquita HB, van Gils CH *et al.* (2005). Cumulative genetic defects in carcinogen metabolism may increase breast cancer risk (The Netherlands). *Cancer Causes Control*, 16: 675–681. doi:10.1007/s10552-005-1227-0 PMID:16049806

Van Emburgh BO, Hu JJ, Levine EA *et al.* (2008). Polymorphisms in drug metabolism genes, smoking, and *p53* mutations in breast cancer. *Mol Carcinog*, 47: 88–99. doi:10.1002/mc.20365 PMID:17683074

van Poppel G, de Vogel N, van Balderen PJ, Kok FJ (1992). Increased cytogenetic damage in smokers deficient in glutathione S-transferase isozyme *mu*. *Carcinogenesis*, 13:303–305.doi:10.1093/carcin/13.2.303PMID:1740022

Vaughan TL, Davis S, Kristal A, Thomas DB (1995). Obesity, alcohol, and tobacco as risk factors for cancers of the esophagus and gastric cardia: adenocarcinoma versus squamous cell carcinoma. *Cancer Epidemiol Biomarkers Prev*, 4: 85–92. PMID:7742727

Vaughan TL, Shapiro JA, Burt RD *et al.* (1996). Nasopharyngeal cancer in a low-risk population: defining risk factors by histological type. *Cancer Epidemiol Biomarkers Prev*, 5: 587–593. PMID:8824359

Veglia F, Loft S, Matullo G *et al.*Genair-EPIC Investigators (2008). DNA adducts and cancer risk in prospective studies: a pooled analysis and a meta-analysis. *Carcinogenesis*, 29: 932–936. doi:10.1093/carcin/bgm286 PMID:18343884

Veglia F, Matullo G, Vineis P (2003). Bulky DNA adducts and risk of cancer: a meta-analysis. *Cancer Epidemiol Biomarkers Prev*, 12: 157–160. PMID:12582026

Verla-Tebit E, Lilla C, Hoffmeister M *et al.* (2006). Cigarette smoking and colorectal cancer risk in Germany: a population-based case-control study. *Int J Cancer*, 119: 630–635. doi:10.1002/ijc.21875 PMID:16496385

Viezzer C, Norppa H, Clonfero E *et al.* (1999). Influence of *GSTM1*, *GSTT1*, *GSTP1*, and *EPHX* gene polymorphisms on DNA adduct level and *HPRT* mutant frequency in coke-oven workers. *Mutat Res*, 431: 259–269. PMID:10635992

Vineis P, Anttila S, Benhamou S *et al.* (2007). Evidence of gene gene interactions in lung carcinogenesis in a large pooled analysis. *Carcinogenesis*, 28: 1902–1905. doi:10.1093/carcin/bgm039 PMID:17307802

Vineis P & Malats N (1999). Strategic issues in the design and interpretation of studies on metabolic polymorphisms and cancer. *IARC Sci Publ*, 148: 51–61. PMID:10493248

Vineis P, Manuguerra M, Kavvoura FK *et al.* (2009). A field synopsis on low-penetrance variants in DNA repair genes and cancer susceptibility. *J Natl Cancer Inst*, 101: 24–36. PMID:19116388

Vineis P, Marinelli D, Autrup H *et al.* (2001). Current smoking, occupation, *N*-acetyltransferase-2 and bladder cancer: a pooled analysis of genotype-based studies. *Cancer Epidemiol Biomarkers Prev*, 10: 1249–1252. PMID:11751441

Vineis P, Veglia F, Anttila S *et al.* (2004). CYP1A1, GSTM1 and GSTT1 polymorphisms and lung cancer: a pooled analysis of gene-gene interactions. *Biomarkers*, 9: 298–305. doi:10.1080/13547500400011070 PMID:15764294

Vineis P, Veglia F, Benhamou S *et al.* (2003). CYP1A1 $T^{3801}C$ polymorphism and lung cancer: a pooled analysis of 2451 cases and 3358 controls. *Int J Cancer*, 104: 650–657. doi:10.1002/ijc.10995 PMID:12594823

Vioque J, Barber X, Bolumar F *et al.*PANESOES Study Group (2008). Esophageal cancer risk by type of alcohol drinking and smoking: a case-control study in Spain. *BMC Cancer*, 8: 221 doi:10.1186/1471-2407-8-221 PMID:18673563

Viswanathan AN, Feskanich D, De Vivo I *et al.* (2005). Smoking and the risk of endometrial cancer: results from the Nurses' Health Study. *Int J Cancer*, 114: 996–1001. doi:10.1002/ijc.20821 PMID:15645490

Vlajinac HD, Marinkovic JM, Sipetic SB *et al.* (2006). Case-control study of oropharyngeal cancer. *Cancer Detect Prev*, 30: 152–157. doi:10.1016/j.cdp.2006.02.001 PMID:16647226

Vlajinac HD, Pekmezović TD, Adanja BJ *et al.* (2003). Case-control study of multiple myeloma with special reference to diet as risk factor. *Neoplasma*, 50: 79–83.

Vories AA & Ramirez SG (1997). Warthin's tumor and cigarette smoking. *South Med J*, 90: 416–418. PMID:9114834

Voskuil DW, Kampman E, Grubben MJ *et al.* (2002). Meat consumption and meat preparation in relation to colorectal adenomas among sporadic and HNPCC family patients in The Netherlands. *Eur J Cancer*, 38: 2300–2308. doi:10.1016/S0959-8049(02)00455-0 PMID:12441267

Vrieling A, Bueno-De-Mesquita B, Boshuizen HC *et al.* (2009). Fruit and vegetable consumption and pancreatic cancer risk in the European Prospective Investigation into Cancer and Nutrition. *Int J Cancer*, 124: 1926–1934. PMID:19107929

Wakai K, Hayakawa N, Kojima M *et al.*JACC Study Group (2003). Smoking and colorectal cancer in a non-Western population: a prospective cohort study in Japan. *J Epidemiol*, 13: 323–332. PMID:14674660

Wakai K, Inoue M, Mizoue T *et al.*Research Group for the Development and Evaluation of Cancer Prevention Strategies in Japan (2006). Tobacco smoking and lung cancer risk: an evaluation based on a systematic review of epidemiological evidence among the Japanese population. *Jpn J Clin Oncol*, 36: 309–324. doi:10.1093/jjco/hyl025 PMID:16735374

Walser T, Cui X, Yanagawa J *et al.* (2008). Smoking and lung cancer: the role of inflammation. *Proc Am Thorac Soc*, 5: 811–815. doi:10.1513/pats.200809-100TH PMID:19017734

Wang H, Tan W, Hao B *et al.* (2003). Substantial reduction in risk of lung adenocarcinoma associated with genetic polymorphism in CYP2A13, the most active cytochrome P450 for the metabolic activation of tobacco-specific carcinogen NNK. *Cancer Res*, 63: 8057–8061. PMID:14633739

Wang M, Cheng G, Balbo S *et al.* (2009). Clear differences in levels of a formaldehyde-DNA adduct in leukocytes of smokers and non-smokers. *Cancer Research*, 69:7170–7174.

Wang SS, Schiffman M, Herrero R *et al.* (2004). Determinants of human papillomavirus 16 serological conversion and persistence in a population-based cohort of 10 000 women in Costa Rica. *Br J Cancer*, 91: 1269–1274. doi:10.1038/sj.bjc.6602088 PMID:15292929

Wang Y, Pereira EF, Maus AD *et al.* (2001). Human bronchial epithelial and endothelial cells express alpha7 nicotinic acetylcholine receptors. *Mol Pharmacol*, 60: 1201–1209. PMID:11723227

Warnakulasuriya KA & Ralhan R (2007). Clinical, pathological, cellular and molecular lesions caused by oral smokeless tobacco–a review. *J Oral Pathol Med*, 36: 63–77. PMID:17238967

Warren CW, Jones NR, Eriksen MP, Asma SGlobal Tobacco Surveillance System (GTSS) collaborative group (2006). Patterns of global tobacco use in young people and implications for future chronic disease burden in adults. *Lancet*, 367: 749–753. doi:10.1016/S0140-6736(06)68192-0 PMID:16517275

Warwick J, Pinney E, Warren RM *et al.* (2003). Breast density and breast cancer risk factors in a high-risk population. *Breast*, 12: 10–16. doi:10.1016/S0960-9776(02)00212-6 PMID:14659350

Wasnik KS, Ughade SN, Zodpey SP, Ingole DL (1998). Tobacco consumption practices and risk of oro-pharyngeal cancer: a case-control study in Central India. *Southeast Asian J Trop Med Public Health*, 29: 827–834. PMID:10772572

Watson MA, Stewart RK, Smith GB *et al.* (1998). Human glutathione *S*-transferase P1 polymorphisms: relationship to lung tissue enzyme activity and population frequency distribution. *Carcinogenesis*, 19: 275–280. doi:10.1093/carcin/19.2.275 PMID:9498276

Watson P, Ashwathnarayan R, Lynch HT, Roy HK (2004). Tobacco use and increased colorectal cancer risk in patients with hereditary nonpolyposis colorectal cancer (Lynch syndrome). *Arch Intern Med*, 164: 2429–2431. PMID:15596632

Wei YS, Lu JC, Wang L *et al.* (2009). Risk factors for sporadic colorectal cancer in southern Chinese. *World J Gastroenterol*, 15: 2526–2530. PMID:19469004

Weiderpass E & Baron JA (2001). Cigarette smoking, alcohol consumption, and endometrial cancer risk: a population-based study in Sweden. *Cancer Causes Control*, 12: 239–247. doi:10.1023/A:1011201911664 PMID:11405329

Weiss JM, Saltzman BS, Doherty JA *et al.* (2006a). Risk factors for the incidence of endometrial cancer according to the aggressiveness of disease. *Am J Epidemiol*, 164: 56–62. doi:10.1093/aje/kwj152 PMID:16675538

Weiss JM, Weiss NS, Ulrich CM *et al.* (2005). Interindividual variation in nucleotide excision repair genes and risk of endometrial cancer. *Cancer Epidemiol Biomarkers Prev*, 14: 2524–2530. doi:10.1158/1055-9965.EPI-05-0414 PMID:16284373

Weiss JM, Weiss NS, Ulrich CM *et al.* (2006b). Nucleotide excision repair genotype and the incidence of endometrial cancer: effect of other risk factors on the association. *Gynecol Oncol*, 103: 891–896. doi:10.1016/j.ygyno.2006.05.020 PMID:16806437

Weiss NS, Farewall VT, Szekely DR *et al.* (1980). Oestrogens and endometrial cancer: effect of other risk factors on the association. *Maturitas*, 2: 185–190. doi:10.1016/0378-5122(80)90003-1 PMID:7442552

Wells PG, Mackenzie PI, Chowdhury JR *et al.* (2004). Glucuronidation and the UDP-glucuronosyltransferases in health and disease. *Drug Metab Dispos*, 32: 281–290. doi:10.1124/dmd.32.3.281 PMID:14977861

Welzel TM, Graubard BI, El-Serag HB *et al.* (2007). Risk factors for intrahepatic and extrahepatic cholangiocarcinoma in the United States: a population-based case-control study. *Clin Gastroenterol Hepatol*, 5: 1221–1228. doi:10.1016/j.cgh.2007.05.020 PMID:17689296

Wen CP, Tsai SP, Chen CJ, Cheng TY (2004). The mortality risks of smokers in Taiwan: Part I: cause-specific mortality. *Prev Med*, 39: 528–535. doi:10.1016/j.ypmed.2004.02.010 PMID:15313092

Wenzlaff AS, Cote ML, Bock CH *et al.* (2005). CYP1A1 and CYP1B1 polymorphisms and risk of lung cancer among never smokers: a population-based study. *Carcinogenesis*, 26: 2207–2212. doi:10.1093/carcin/bgi191 PMID:16051642

West KA, Brognard J, Clark AS *et al.* (2003). Rapid Akt activation by nicotine and a tobacco carcinogen modulates the phenotype of normal human airway epithelial cells. *J Clin Invest*, 111: 81–90. PMID:12511591

West S, Hildesheim A, Dosemeci M (1993). Non-viral risk factors for nasopharyngeal carcinoma in the Philippines: results from a case-control study. *Int J Cancer*, 55: 722–727. doi:10.1002/ijc.2910550504 PMID:7503957

Whittemore AS, Wu ML, Paffenbarger RS Jr *et al.* (1988). Personal and environmental characteristics related to epithelial ovarian cancer. II. Exposures to talcum powder, tobacco, alcohol, and coffee. *Am J Epidemiol*, 128: 1228–1240. PMID:3195564

WHO (2011).* *Third WHO Report on the Global Tobacco Epidemic*. World Health Organization. http://www.who.int/tobacco/global_report/2011/en/index.html

Wiencke JK (2002). DNA adduct burden and tobacco carcinogenesis. *Oncogene*, 21: 7376–7391. doi:10.1038/sj.onc.1205799 PMID:12379880

Willett EV, O'Connor S, Smith AG, Roman E (2007). Does smoking and alcohol modify the risk of Epstein-Barr virus-positive or -negative Hodgkin lymphoma. *Epidemiology*, 18: 130–136.

Wojno TH (1999). The association between cigarette smoking and basal cell carcinoma of the eyelids in women. *Ophthal Plast Reconstr Surg*, 15: 390–392. doi:10.1097/00002341-199911000-00004 PMID:10588245

Wojnowski L & Kamdem LK (2006). Clinical implications of *CYP3A* polymorphisms. *Expert Opin Drug Metab Toxicol*, 2: 171–182. doi:10.1517/17425255.2.2.171 PMID:16866606

Wolf CR & Smith G (1999). Cytochrome P450 CYP2D6. *IARC Sci Publ*, 148: 209–229. PMID:10493260

Wolff H, Saukkonen K, Anttila S *et al.* (1998). Expression of cyclooxygenase-2 in human lung carcinoma. *Cancer Res*, 58: 4997–5001. PMID:9823297

Wong HL, Murphy SE, Hecht SS (2005). Cytochrome P450 2A-catalyzed metabolic activation of structurally similar carcinogenic nitrosamines: *N'*-nitrosonornicotine enantiomers, *N*-nitrosopiperidine, and *N*-nitrosopyrrolidine. *Chem Res Toxicol*, 18: 61–69. doi:10.1021/tx0497696 PMID:15651850

Wright ME, Park Y, Subar AF *et al.* (2008). Intakes of fruit, vegetables, and specific botanical groups in relation to lung cancer risk in the NIH-AARP Diet and Health Study. *Am J Epidemiol*, 168: 1024–1034. doi:10.1093/aje/kwn212 PMID:18791192

Wu AH, Crabtree JE, Bernstein L *et al.* (2003). Role of Helicobacter pylori CagA+ strains and risk of adenocarcinoma of the stomach and esophagus. *Int J Cancer*, 103: 815–821. doi:10.1002/ijc.10887 PMID:12516104

Wu AH, Wan P, Bernstein L (2001). A multiethnic population-based study of smoking, alcohol and body size and risk of adenocarcinomas of the stomach and esophagus (United States). *Cancer Causes Control*, 12: 721–732. doi:10.1023/A:1011290704728 PMID:11562112

Wu AH, Yu MC, Mack TM (1997). Smoking, alcohol use, dietary factors and risk of small intestinal adenocarcinoma. *Int J Cancer*, 70: 512–517. doi:10.1002/(SICI)1097-0215(19970304)70:5<512::AID-IJC4>3.0.CO;2-0 PMID:9052748

Wu C, Hu Z, Yu D *et al.* (2009a). Genetic variants on chromosome 15q25 associated with lung cancer risk in Chinese populations. *Cancer Res*, 69: 5065–5072. doi:10.1158/0008-5472.CAN-09-0081 PMID:19491260

Wu IC, Lee CH, Kuo CH *et al.* (2009b). Consumption of cigarettes but not betel quid or alcohol increases colorectal cancer risk. *J Formos Med Assoc*, 108: 155–163. doi:10.1016/S0929-6646(09)60046-2 PMID:19251551

Wynder EL, Gottlieb S, Wright G (1957). A study of tobacco carcinogenesis. IV. Different tobacco types. *Cancer*, 10: 1206–1209. doi:10.1002/1097-0142(195711/12)10:6<1206::AID-CNCR2820100618>3.0.CO;2-P PMID:13489672

Wynder EL, Graham EA, Croninger AB (1953). Experimental production of carcinoma with cigarette tar. *Cancer Res*, 13: 855–864. PMID:13116124

Wynder EL & Hoffmann D (1961). A study of tobacco carcinogenesis. VIII. The role of the acidic fractions as promoters. *Cancer*, 14: 1306–1315. doi:10.1002/1097-0142(196111/12)14:6<1306::AID-CNCR2820140621>3.0.CO;2-T PMID:14008628

Wynder EL & Stellman SD (1979). Impact of long-term filter cigarette usage on lung and larynx cancer risk: a case-control study. *J Natl Cancer Inst*, 62: 471–477. PMID:283277

Yagyu K, Kikuchi S, Obata Y *et al.*JACC Study Group (2008). Cigarette smoking, alcohol drinking and the risk of gallbladder cancer death: a prospective cohort study in Japan. *Int J Cancer*, 122: 924–929. doi:10.1002/ijc.23159 PMID:17955487

Yamasaki E & Ames BN (1977). Concentration of mutagens from urine by absorption with the nonpolar resin XAD-2: cigarette smokers have mutagenic urine. *Proc Natl Acad Sci U S A*, 74: 3555–3559. doi:10.1073/pnas.74.8.3555 PMID:333441

Yang J, Qian LX, Wu HF *et al.* (2006). Genetic polymorphisms in the cytochrome P450 1A1 and 2E1 genes, smoking, drinking and prostate cancer susceptibility: a case-control study in a Han nationality population in Southern China. *Int J Urol*, 13: 773–780. doi:10.1111/j.1442-2042.2006.01401.x PMID:16834659

Yang M, Kim S, Lee E *et al.* (2003). Sources of polycyclic aromatic hydrocarbon exposure in non-occupationally exposed Koreans. *Environ Mol Mutagen*, 42: 250–257. doi:10.1002/em.10196 PMID:14673870

Yang M, Koga M, Katoh T, Kawamoto T (1999). A study for the proper application of urinary naphthols, new biomarkers for airborne polycyclic aromatic hydrocarbons. *Arch Environ Contam Toxicol*, 36: 99–108. doi:10.1007/s002449900447 PMID:9828267

Yang P, Cunningham JM, Halling KC *et al.* (2000). Higher risk of mismatch repair-deficient colorectal cancer in alpha(1)-antitrypsin deficiency carriers and cigarette smokers. *Mol Genet Metab*, 71: 639–645. doi:10.1006/mgme.2000.3089 PMID:11136557

Yang P, Sun Z, Krowka MJ *et al.* (2008). Alpha1-antitrypsin deficiency carriers, tobacco smoke, chronic obstructive pulmonary disease, and lung cancer risk. *Arch Intern Med*, 168: 1097–1103. doi:10.1001/archinte.168.10.1097 PMID:18504338

Yauk CL, Berndt ML, Williams A *et al.* (2007). Mainstream tobacco smoke causes paternal germ-line DNA mutation. *Cancer Res*, 67: 5103–5106. doi:10.1158/0008-5472.CAN-07-0279 PMID:17545587

Ye WM, Ye YN, Lin RD *et al.* (1995). Case control study on nasopharyngeal cancer in southern region of Fujian province. *Chin J Prev Control Chronic Dis*, 3: 158–161.

Ye Z, Song H, Higgins JP *et al.* (2006). Five glutathione s-transferase gene variants in 23,452 cases of lung cancer and 30,397 controls: meta-analysis of 130 studies. *PLoS Med*, 3: 524–534 doi:10.1371/journal.pmed.0030091 PMID:16509765

Yen TT, Lin WD, Wang CP *et al.* (2008). The association of smoking, alcoholic consumption, betel quid chewing and oral cavity cancer: a cohort study. *Eur Arch Otorhinolaryngol*, 265: 1403–1407. doi:10.1007/s00405-008-0659-z PMID:18389268

Yoo KY, Tajima K, Miura S *et al.* (1997). Breast cancer risk factors according to combined estrogen and progesterone receptor status: a case-control analysis. *Am J Epidemiol*, 146: 307–314. PMID:9270409

Young E, Leatherdale S, Sloan M *et al.* (2009). Age of smoking initiation and risk of breast cancer in a sample of Ontario women. *Tob Induc Dis*, 5: 4 doi:10.1186/1617-9625-5-4 PMID:19222858

Yu GP, Ostroff JS, Zhang ZF *et al.* (1997). Smoking history and cancer patient survival: a hospital cancer registry study. *Cancer Detect Prev*, 21: 497–509. PMID:9398990

Yu MC, Garabrant DH, Huang TB, Henderson BE (1990). Occupational and other non-dietary risk factors for nasopharyngeal carcinoma in Guangzhou, China. *Int J Cancer*, 45: 1033–1039. doi:10.1002/ijc.2910450609 PMID:2351484

Yu MC, Ho JH, Lai SH, Henderson BE (1986). Cantonese-style salted fish as a cause of nasopharyngeal carcinoma: report of a case-control study in Hong Kong. *Cancer Res*, 46: 956–961. PMID:3940655

Yuan JM, Koh WP, Murphy SE *et al.* (2009). Urinary levels of tobacco-specific nitrosamine metabolites in relation to lung cancer development in two prospective cohorts of cigarette smokers. *Cancer Res*, 69: 2990–2995. doi:10.1158/0008-5472.CAN-08-4330 PMID:19318550

Yuan JM, Ross RK, Wang XL *et al.* (1996). Morbidity and mortality in relation to cigarette smoking in Shanghai, China. A prospective male cohort study. *JAMA*, 275: 1646–1650. doi:10.1001/jama.275.21.1646 PMID:8637137

Yuan JM, Wang XL, Xiang YB *et al.* (2000). Non-dietary risk factors for nasopharyngeal carcinoma in Shanghai, China. *Int J Cancer*, 85: 364–369. doi:10.1002/(SICI)1097-0215(20000201)85:3<364::AID-IJC12>3.0.CO;2-C PMID:10652428

Yun YH, Jung KW, Bae JM *et al.* (2005). Cigarette smoking and cancer incidence risk in adult men: National Health Insurance Corporation Study. *Cancer Detect Prev*, 29: 15–24. doi:10.1016/j.cdp.2004.08.006 PMID:15734213

Zahm SH, Heineman EF, Vaught JB (1992). Soft tissue sarcoma and tobacco use: data from a prospective cohort study of United States veterans. *Cancer Causes Control*, 3: 371–376. doi:10.1007/BF00146891 PMID:1617125

Zak-Prelich M, Narbutt J, Sysa-Jedrzejowska A (2004). Environmental risk factors predisposing to the development of basal cell carcinoma. *Dermatol Surg*, 30: s2248–252. doi:10.1111/j.1524-4725.2004.30089.x PMID:14871217

Zang EA & Wynder EL (1996). Differences in lung cancer risk between men and women: examination of the evidence. *J Natl Cancer Inst*, 88: 183–192. doi:10.1093/jnci/88.3-4.183 PMID:8632492

Zanieri L, Galvan P, Checchini L *et al.* (2007). Polycyclic aromatic hydrocarbons (PAHs) in human milk from Italian women: influence of cigarette smoking and residential area. *Chemosphere*, 67: 1265–1274. doi:10.1016/j.chemosphere.2006.12.011 PMID:17258279

Zaridze D, Borisova E, Maximovitch D, Chkhikvadze V (2000). Alcohol consumption, smoking and risk of gastric cancer: case-control study from Moscow, Russia. *Cancer Causes Control*, 11: 363–371. doi:10.1023/A:1008907924938 PMID:10843447

Zatonski W, Becher H, Lissowska J, Wahrendorf J (1991). Tobacco, alcohol, and diet in the etiology of laryngeal cancer: a population-based case-control study. *Cancer Causes Control*, 2: 3–10. doi:10.1007/BF00052355 PMID:1873431

Zendehdel K, Nyrén O, Luo J *et al.* (2008). Risk of gastroesophageal cancer among smokers and users of Scandinavian moist snuff. *Int J Cancer*, 122: 1095–1099. doi:10.1002/ijc.23076 PMID:17973262

Zhang J, Ichiba M, Hara K *et al.* (2001). Urinary 1-hydroxypyrene in coke oven workers relative to exposure, alcohol consumption, and metabolic enzymes. *Occup Environ Med*, 58: 716–721. doi:10.1136/oem.58.11.716 PMID:11600727

Zhang L, Rothman N, Li G *et al.* (2007). Aberrations in chromosomes associated with lymphoma and therapy-related leukemia in benzene-exposed workers. *Environ Mol Mutagen*, 48: 467–474. doi:10.1002/em.20306 PMID:17584886

Zhang L, Steinmaus C, Eastmond DA *et al.* (2009c). Formaldehyde exposure and leukemia: a new meta-analysis and potential mechanisms. *Mutat Res*, 681: 150–168. doi:10.1016/j.mrrev.2008.07.002 PMID:18674636

Zhang S, Wang M, Villalta PW *et al.* (2009a). Quantitation of pyridyloxobutyl DNA adducts in nasal and oral mucosa of rats treated chronically with enantiomers of *N'*-nitrosonornicotine. *Chem Res Toxicol*, 22: 949–956. doi:10.1021/tx900040j PMID:19405515

Zhang S, Wang M, Villalta PW *et al.* (2009b). Analysis of pyridyloxobutyl and pyridylhydroxybutyl DNA adducts in extrahepatic tissues of F344 rats treated chronically with 4-(methylnitrosamino)-1-(3-pyridyl)-1-butanone and enantiomers of 4-(methylnitrosamino)-1-(3-pyridyl)-1-butanol. *Chem Res Toxicol*, 22: 926–936. doi:10.1021/tx900015d PMID:19358518

Zhang X, Su T, Zhang QY *et al.* (2002). Genetic polymorphisms of the human *CYP2A13* gene: identification of single-nucleotide polymorphisms and functional characterization of an Arg257Cys variant. *J Pharmacol Exp Ther*, 302: 416–423. PMID:12130698

Zhang Y, Coogan PF, Palmer JR *et al.* (2004). Cigarette smoking and increased risk of mucinous epithelial ovarian cancer. *Am J Epidemiol*, 159: 133–139. doi:10.1093/aje/kwh015 PMID:14718214

Zhang ZF, Kurtz RC, Sun M *et al.* (1996). Adenocarcinomas of the esophagus and gastric cardia: medical conditions, tobacco, alcohol, and socioeconomic factors. *Cancer Epidemiol Biomarkers Prev*, 5: 761–768. PMID:8896886

Zhao B, Seow A, Lee EJ *et al.* (2001). Dietary isothiocyanates, glutathione S-transferase -M1, -T1 polymorphisms and lung cancer risk among Chinese women in Singapore. *Cancer Epidemiol Biomarkers Prev*, 10: 1063–1067. PMID:11588132

Zhao C, Tyndyk M, Eide I, Hemminki K (1999). Endogenous and background DNA adducts by methylating and 2-hydroxyethylating agents. *Mutat Res*, 424: 117–125. PMID:10064855

Zheng T, Holford T, Chen Y *et al.* (1997). Risk of tongue cancer associated with tobacco smoking and alcohol consumption: a case-control study. *Oral Oncol*, 33: 82–85. doi:10.1016/S0964-1955(96)00056-5 PMID:9231164

Zheng T, Holford TR, Zahm SH *et al.* (2002). Cigarette smoking, glutathione-s-transferase M1 and t1 genetic polymorphisms, and breast cancer risk (United States). *Cancer Causes Control*, 13: 637–645. doi:10.1023/A:1019500109267 PMID:12296511

Zheng TZ, Boyle P, Hu HF *et al.* (1990). Tobacco smoking, alcohol consumption, and risk of oral cancer: a case-control study in Beijing, People's Republic of China. *Cancer Causes Control*, 1: 173–179. doi:10.1007/BF00053170 PMID:2102288

Zheng W, Blot WJ, Shu XO *et al.* (1992). Diet and other risk factors for laryngeal cancer in Shanghai, China. *Am J Epidemiol*, 136: 178–191. PMID:1415140

Zheng W, Blot WJ, Shu XO *et al.* (1992b). Diet and other risk factors for laryngeal cancer in Shanghai, China. *Am J Epidemiol*, 136: 178–191. PMID:1415140

Zheng W, Blot WJ, Shu XO *et al.* (1992c). A population-based case-control study of cancers of the nasal cavity and paranasal sinuses in Shanghai. *Int J Cancer*, 52: 557–561. doi:10.1002/ijc.2910520410 PMID:1399136

Zheng W, McLaughlin JK, Chow WH *et al.* (1993a). Risk factors for cancers of the nasal cavity and paranasal sinuses among white men in the United States. *Am J Epidemiol*, 138: 965–972. PMID:8256781

Zheng W, McLaughlin JK, Gridley G *et al.* (1993). A cohort study of smoking, alcohol consumption, and dietary factors for pancreatic cancer (United States). *Cancer Causes Control*, 4: 477–482. doi:10.1007/BF00050867 PMID:8218880

Zheng YM, Tuppin P, Hubert A *et al.* (1994). Environmental and dietary risk factors for nasopharyngeal carcinoma: a case-control study in Zangwu County, Guangxi, China. *Br J Cancer*, 69: 508–514. PMID:8123482

Zhu BT & Conney AH (1998). Functional role of estrogen metabolism in target cells: review and perspectives. *Carcinogenesis*, 19: 1–27. doi:10.1093/carcin/19.1.1 PMID:9472688

Zhu K, Levine RS, Brann EA *et al.* (1995). A population-based case-control study of the relationship between cigarette smoking and nasopharyngeal cancer (United States). *Cancer Causes Control*, 6: 507–512. doi:10.1007/BF00054158 PMID:8580298

Zienolddiny S, Campa D, Lind H *et al.* (2008). A comprehensive analysis of phase I and phase II metabolism gene polymorphisms and risk of non-small cell lung cancer in smokers. *Carcinogenesis*, 29: 1164–1169. doi:10.1093/carcin/bgn020 PMID:18258609

Zivaljevic V, Vlajinac H, Marinkovic J *et al.* (2004). Cigarette smoking as a risk factor for cancer of the thyroid in women. *Tumori*, 90: 273–275. PMID:15315303

Znaor A, Brennan P, Gajalakshmi V *et al.* (2003). Independent and combined effects of tobacco smoking, chewing and alcohol drinking on the risk of oral, pharyngeal and esophageal cancers in Indian men. *Int J Cancer*, 105: 681–686. doi:10.1002/ijc.11114 PMID:12740918

Zu K & Giovannucci E (2009). Smoking and aggressive prostate cancer: a review of the epidemiologic evidence. *Cancer Causes Control*, Epub ahead of printPMID: 19562492.

SECOND-HAND TOBACCO SMOKE

Second-hand tobacco smoke was considered by a previous IARC Working Group in 2002 as "involuntary smoking" (IARC, 2004). Since that time, new data have become available, these have been incorporated into the *Monograph*, and taken into consideration in the present evaluation.

1. Exposure Data

Second-hand tobacco smoke comprises the smoke released from the burning tip of a cigarette (or other burned tobacco product) between puffs (called sidestream smoke (SM)) and the smoke exhaled by the smoker (exhaled mainstream smoke (MS)). Small additional amounts are contributed from the tip of the cigarette and through the cigarette paper during a puff, and through the paper and from the mouth end of the cigarette between puffs (Jenkins *et al.*, 2000).

Second-hand tobacco smoke is also referred as 'environmental tobacco smoke', 'passive smoking' or 'involuntary smoking' (IARC, 2004). The terms 'passive smoking' or 'involuntary smoking' suggest that while involuntary or passive smoking is not acceptable, voluntary or active smoking is acceptable. In this document, we use the term second-hand tobacco smoke (WHO, 2010).

1.1 Chemical composition

Many studies have examined the concentrations of cigarette smoke constituents in mainstream and sidestream smoke. The composition of mainstream and sidestream smoke is qualitatively similar but quantitatively different. The ratios of sidestream to mainstream smoke vary greatly depending on the constituent. Some representative SS:MS ratios are: nicotine, 7.1; carbon monoxide, 4.8; ammonia, 455; formaldehyde, 36.5; acrolein, 18.6; benzo[*a*]pyrene, 16.0; *N*′-nitrosonornicotine (NNN), 0.43; (methylnitrosamino)-1-(3-pyridyl)-1-butanone (NNK), 0.40 (Jenkins *et al.*, 2000; IARC, 2004).

The physicochemical properties of second-hand tobacco smoke are different from those of mainstream smoke and sidestream smoke because of its rapid dilution and dispersion into the indoor environment (IARC, 2004). Concentrations of individual constituents in second-hand tobacco smoke can vary with time and environmental conditions. Field studies of these constituents and representative data have been extensively summarized (Jenkins *et al.*, 2000; IARC, 2004). Some representative data are presented in Table 1.1 (Jenkins *et al.*, 2000; IARC, 2004; US Department of Health and Human Services, 2006).

Table 1.1 Concentration of selected constituents in second-hand tobacco smoke

Constituent	Concentration
Nicotine	10–100 µg/m^3
Carbon monoxide	5–20 ppm
Benzene	15–30 µg/m^3
Formaldehyde	100–140 µg/m^3
Acetaldehyde	200–300 µg/m^3
1,3-Butadiene	20–40 µg/m^3
Benzo[*a*]pyrene	0.37–1.7 ng/m^3
NNK	0.2–29.3 ng/m^3
NNN	0.7–23 ng/m^3

1.2 Sources of exposure

Second-hand tobacco smoke is present in virtually all places where smoking takes place (Navas-Acien *et al.*, 2004): at home, in the workplace, in bars, restaurants, public buildings, hospitals, public transport and educational institutions. The setting that represents the most important source of exposure differs depending on the population. For example in children, the home environment may constitute a significant source of exposure, while other sources that may contribute are schools and public transportation. Likewise, for most women, the home environment is the primary source of second-hand tobacco smoke, which may be enhanced by exposure at the workplace.

Biomarker studies have evaluated carcinogen uptake in non-smokers to second-hand tobacco smoke. The NNK metabolites NNAL and its glucuronides (total NNAL) are consistently elevated in non-smokers exposed to second-hand tobacco smoke, in studies conducted in various living and occupational environments, and from infancy through adulthood (Hecht *et al.*, 2006; Hecht, 2008). Levels of the biomarker of PAHs, urinary 1-hydroxypyrene, were significantly elevated in a large study of non-smokers exposed to second-hand tobacco smoke (Suwan-ampai *et al.*, 2009).

1.3 Measures of exposure

A conceptual framework for considering exposure to second-hand tobacco smoke is the "microenvironmental model," which takes the weighted sum of the concentrations of second-hand tobacco smoke in the microenvironments where time is spent, with the weights the time spent in each, as a measure of personal exposure (Jaakkola & Jaakkola, 1997). Direct measures of exposure use concentrations of second-hand tobacco smoke components in the air in the home, workplace, or other environments, combined with information on the time spent in the microenvironments where exposure took place. Measurements of tobacco smoke biomarker(s) in biological specimens also represent a direct measure of exposure to second-hand smoke (Samet & Yang, 2001; Table 1.2). Indirect measures are generally obtained by survey questionnaires. These include self-reported exposure and descriptions of the source of second-hand tobacco smoke in relevant microenvironments, most often the home and workplace (Samet & Yang, 2001).

One useful surrogate measure, and the only available in many countries, is the prevalence of smoking among men and women. It provides a measure of the likelihood of exposure. In most countries in Asia and the Middle East,

Table 1.2 Types of indicators measuring exposure to second-hand tobacco smoke

Measure	Suggested indicators
Direct	Concentration of second-hand tobacco smoke components in the air:
	- Nicotine
	- Respirable particles
	- Other markers
	Biomarker concentrations:
	- Cotinine
	- Carboxyhaemoglobin
Indirect	Report of second-hand tobacco smoke exposure at:
	Home
	- Number of smokers
	- Smoking of parents
	- Intensity (number of cigarettes smoked)
	Workplace
	- Presence of second-hand tobacco smoke
	- Number of smokers
Surrogate	Pre Prevalence of smoking tobacco in men and in women
	Sel Self reported smoking habits of parents
	Nic Nicotine concentration in house dust

From Samet & Yang (2001) and Whitehead *et al.* (2009)

for example, the very high prevalence of smoking among men combined with the low prevalence among women would imply that most women are exposed to second-hand tobacco smoke at home (Samet & Yang, 2001).

To measure exposure to second-hand tobacco smoke in children, self-reported smoking habits of their parents are used as a surrogate (US Department of Health and Human Services, 2006). More recently, other surrogate measures such as nicotine concentrations in house dust have been considered less biased than parental smoking as they reflect cumulative smoking habits and long-term exposure rather than current patterns of smoking (Whitehead *et al.*, 2009).

1.4 Prevalence of exposure

1.4.1 Exposure among children

(a) Overview

The most extensive population-based data on exposure to second-hand tobacco smoke among children are available through the Global Youth Tobacco Survey (GYTS) (CDC/WHO, 2009). GYTS is part of the Global Tobacco Surveillance System (GTSS), developed by the WHO and the United States' Centers for Disease Control and Prevention (CDC) in 1998. The GYTS is a school-based survey designed to measure tobacco use and some key tobacco control measures among youth (13–15 years) using a common methodology and core questionnaire. While most GYTS are national surveys, in some countries they are limited to subnational locations. Further, countries conduct the GYTS in different years, rendering comparison across countries for the same year difficult. The GYTS questionnaire

Fig. 1.1 Average prevalence (in%) of 13–15 year old children living in a home where others smoke, by WHO region, 2007

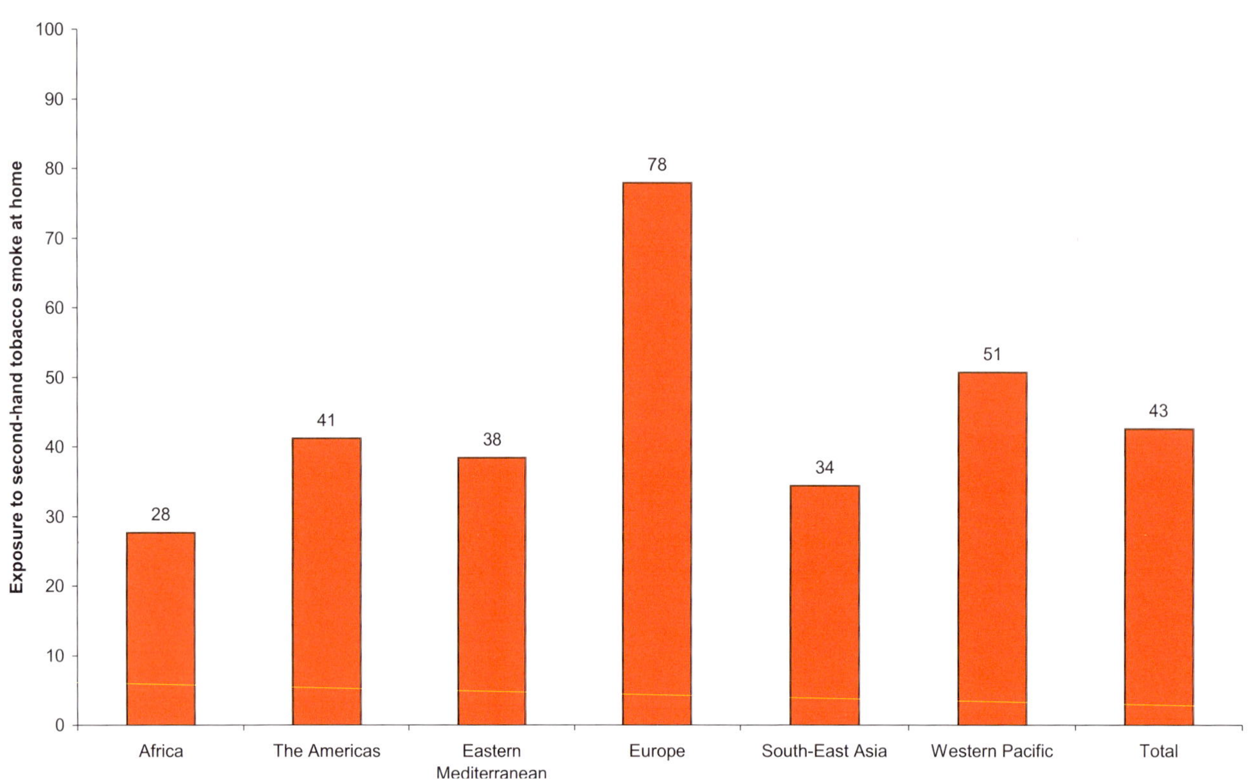

From CDC (2008)

asks about children's exposure to second-hand tobacco smoke in their home or in other places in the last 7 days preceding the survey. Since its inception in 1999, over 2 million students in 160 countries representing all six WHO regions have participated in the GYTS (WHO, 2008, 2009a).

Country-level estimates on second-hand tobacco smoke exposure at home and in public places among youth are available in the WHO Reports on the global tobacco epidemic (WHO, 2008, 2009a, 2011).

(b) Exposure at home

Nearly half of youth aged 13–15 years are exposed to second-hand tobacco smoke in their homes (Fig. 1.1; CDC, 2008). Among the six WHO regions, exposure to second-hand tobacco smoke at home was highest in the European Region (77.8%) and lowest in the African region (27.6%). In the other four regions, exposure to second-hand tobacco smoke at home ranged from 50.6% in the Western Pacific Region to 34.3% in the South East Asian Region.

Fig. 1.2 shows the range of exposure to second-hand tobacco smoke at home by WHO region for boys and girls and for both sexes combined. The largest variations are observed in the Eastern Mediterranean Region and the European Region irrespective of sex. These variations are predominantly due to differences in parental smoking prevalence between countries, as well as the impact of the smoke-free places campaigns in place in various countries.

Country-level estimates from the Global Youth Tobacco Survey (1999–2009) are presented in Table 1.3.

Fig. 1.2 Range of prevalence (in%) of exposure of 13–15 year old children to second-hand tobacco smoke at home, by WHO region, 2009

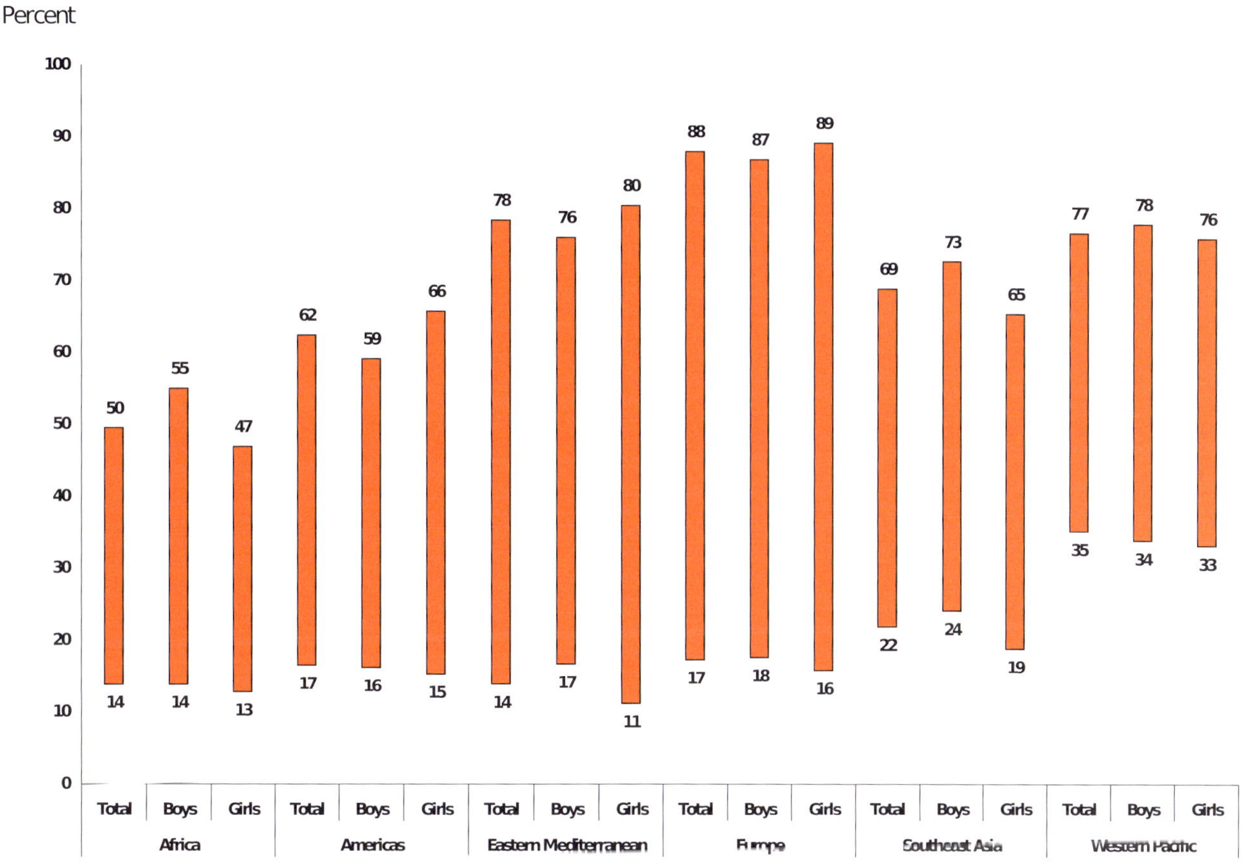

From CDC/WHO (2009)

Öberg and colleagues have estimated the worldwide exposure to second-hand tobacco smoke among children by using parent's current smoking status as an indicator of exposure among children (WHO, 2010). Four out of ten children (approximately 700 million children globally) have at least one parent who currently smokes, predisposing them to exposure to second-hand tobacco smoke at home (Table 1.4). Children in the Western Pacific Region had the highest level of potential exposure (68%) while Africa had the lowest, with about 13% of children having at least one parent who smoked. In the 2010 WHO Report on global estimate of the burden of disease from second-hand smoke (WHO, 2010), country-level estimates were collected or modelled from various sources. [Data partially overlap with those of the Global Youth Tobacco Survey].

(c) Exposure outside home

Similar to second-hand tobacco smoke exposure at home, almost half of the youth are exposed to second-hand tobacco smoke in public places, according to estimates from the Global Youth Tobacco Survey (Fig. 1.3; CDC, 2008). Exposure was highest in Europe (86.1%); for the other five regions, exposure to second-hand tobacco smoke in public places ranged from 64.1% in the Western Pacific to 43.7% in Africa.

Table 1.3 Prevalence of exposure to second-hand tobacco smoke at home and outside home among 13–15 year olds, by country and sex, from the Global Youth Tobacco Survey (participating countries only) — 1999–2009

Country	WHO region	National survey, or jurisdiction where survey conducted	Year	Exposed to second-hand tobacco smoke at home			Exposed to second-hand tobacco smoke outside their homes		
				Total	Boys	Girls	Total	Boys	Girls
Afghanistan	EMRO	Kabul	2004	38.8	43.4	33.3	45.0	60.2	23.6
Albania	EURO	National	2009	49.7	48.6	50.9	64.5	65.3	63.9
Algeria	AFRO	Constantine	2007	38.7	39.8	37.9	60.2	66.0	56.2
Antigua and Barbuda	AMRO	National	2009	26.7	22.5	29.7	47.5	45.0	49.6
Argentina	AMRO	National	2007	54.7	51.7	57.7	68.6	66.4	70.7
Armenia	EURO	National	2009	70.6	69.2	71.6	78.3	80.7	76.4
Bahamas	AMRO	National	2009	25.1	23.4	27.0	51.0	50.8	52.7
Bahrain	EMRO	National	2002	38.7	37.2	39.5	45.3	49.7	40.9
Bangladesh	SEARO	National	2007	34.7	37.8	32.4	42.2	47.1	38.7
Barbados	AMRO	National	2007	25.9	25.9	26.0	59.6	59.7	59.6
Belize	AMRO	National	2008	25.7	26.2	25.1	50.4	52.1	48.6
Benin	AFRO	Atlantique Littoral	2003	21.5	23.7	18.3	38.0	41.3	33.5
Bhutan	SEARO	National	2009	29.5	29.2	29.5	59.4	58.6	59.7
The Plurinational State of Bolivia	AMRO	La Paz	2003	34.3	34.3	34.4	52.9	54.4	51.4
Bosnia and Herzegovina	EURO	National	2008	77.3	74.0	80.3	84.0	82.3	85.6
Botswana	AFRO	National	2008	38.5	38.2	38.6	62.1	60.0	63.7
Brazil	AMRO	São Paulo	2009	35.5	31.9	38.7	51.3	48.2	54.1
Bulgaria	EURO	National	2008	63.9	61.5	66.3	70.1	66.7	73.7
Burkina Faso	AFRO	Ouagadougou	2009	29.2	28.9	29.2	47.5	53.5	42.2
Burundi	AFRO	National	2008	33.9	35.2	31.7	49.3	54.0	45.3
Cambodia	WPRO	National	2003	47.0	48.9	44.5	58.5	60.6	56.5
Cameroon	AFRO	Yaounde	2008	21.7	25.0	19.1	45.8	49.3	42.4
Cape Verde	AFRO	National	2007	13.9	13.9	13.7	25.4	27.0	24.2
Central African Republic	AFRO	Bangui	2008	35.2	29.9	40.7	52.4	49.9	53.8
Chad	AFRO	National	2008	33.9	34.1	31.2	55.1	54.0	56.2
Chile	AMRO	Santiago	2008	51.7	48.9	54.4	68.3	63.4	73.0
China	WPRO	Shanghai	2005	47.0	46.6	47.4	35.2	34.2	36.2
Colombia	AMRO	Bogota	2007	26.2	25.3	27.0	56.1	55.1	56.9
Comoros	AFRO	National	2007	35.2	35.7	34.9	58.3	66.7	52.9
Congo	AFRO	National	2009	22.3	24.7	19.6	44.4	46.8	41.5
Cook Islands	WPRO	National	2008	61.9	58.8	64.5	73.8	70.3	76.8

Table 1.3 (continued)

Country	WHO region	National survey, or jurisdiction where survey conducted	Year	Exposed to second-hand tobacco smoke at home			Exposed to second-hand tobacco smoke outside their homes		
				Total	Boys	Girls	Total	Boys	Girls
Costa Rica	AMRO	National	2008	21.6	20.8	22.1	41.5	40.0	42.8
Côte d'Ivoire	AFRO	National	2009	33.1	33.1	33.0	74.4	75.9	72.3
Croatia	EURO	National	2007	73.4	71.4	75.7	82.5	81.2	84.2
Cuba	AMRO	Havana	2004	62.4	59.1	65.7	65.0	64.6	65.8
Cyprus	EURO	National	2005	87.9	86.8	89.1	87.8	85.4	90.4
Czech Republic	EURO	National	2007	38.0	37.3	38.9	75.2	71.6	79.5
Democratic Republic of the Congo	AFRO	Kinshasa	2008	30.2	32.5	27.0	36.8	37.4	34.7
Djibouti	EMRO	National	2009	36.0	36.2	35.3	44.7	44.8	44.8
Dominica	AMRO	National	2009	26.9	25.2	27.4	62.3	61.4	62.5
Dominican Republic	AMRO	National	2004	33.1	31.1	34.5	41.9	38.5	44.9
Ecuador	AMRO	Quito	2007	28.9	27.5	30.2	52.5	49.5	54.6
Egypt	EMRO	National	2009	47.6	50.1	45.9	52.2	57.7	47.5
El Salvador	AMRO	National	2009	17.9	19.3	16.5	33.7	36.7	30.7
Equatorial Guinea	AFRO	National	2008	47.5	47.8	45.8	61.7	64.0	59.8
Eritrea	AFRO	National	2006	18.4	20.4	14.8	37.3	40.4	32.3
Estonia	EURO	National	2007	41.1	39.3	42.8	68.5	68.2	68.7
Ethiopia	AFRO	Addis Ababa	2003	14.9	15.5	12.8	41.2	45.1	37.4
Fiji	WPRO	National	2009	42.1	45.4	39.6	55.1	55.2	54.9
Gambia	AFRO	Banjul	2008	45.8	45.8	44.4	59.2	61.6	57.2
Georgia	EURO	National	2008	62.7	62.4	62.8	74.4	75.5	73.4
Ghana	AFRO	National	2009	19.1	19.6	17.9	32.3	33.9	30.4
Greece	EURO	National	2005	...	...	...	...	...	...
Grenada	AMRO	National	2009	27.3	24.9	29.7	53.1	50.5	55.7
Guatemala	AMRO	National	2008	23.1	23.9	22.1	40.8	43.8	37.9
Guinea	AFRO	National	2008	27.7	27.6	28.1	52.3	57.0	48.1
Guinea-Bissau	AFRO	Bissau	2008	31.0	32.1	29.7	35.3	36.6	34.1
Guyana	AMRO	National	2004	33.4	36.6	30.6	61.1	62.9	59.1
Haiti	AMRO	Port-au-Prince	2005	32.3	34.7	29.6	43.2	46.2	40.4
Honduras	AMRO	Tegucigalpa	2003	29.6	26.2	31.6	42.2	46.9	38.4
Hungary	EURO	National	2008	43.0	39.9	45.3	72.6	70.0	74.7
India	SEARO	National	2009	21.9	24.1	18.8	36.6	39.0	33.1
Indonesia	SEARO	National	2009	68.8	72.6	65.3	78.1	83.7	73.1

Table 1.3 (continued)

Country	WHO region	National survey, or jurisdiction where survey conducted	Year	Exposed to second-hand tobacco smoke at home			Exposed to second-hand tobacco smoke outside their homes		
				Total	Boys	Girls	Total	Boys	Girls
Islamic Republic of Iran	EMRO	National	2007	35.4	38.1	32.7	44.8	49.8	39.6
Iraq	EMRO	Baghdad	2008	32.3	30.3	34.4	29.2	27.8	30.7
Jamaica	AMRO	National	2006	32.5	32.2	32.5	60.5	59.9	61.6
Jordan	EMRO	National	2009	53.6	50.6	55.5	50.5	50.6	49.7
Kenya	AFRO	National	2007	24.7	25.4	23.6	48.2	48.6	47.6
Kiribati	WPRO	National	2009	68.3	68.7	68.3	65.8	67.9	64.0
Kuwait	EMRO	National	2009	49.8	46.9	52.0	53.3	54.3	52.4
Kyrgyzstan	EURO	National	2008	33.4	35.1	31.9	57.7	58.7	56.8
Lao People's Democratic Republic	WPRO	Vientiane Capital	2007	40.3	41.2	39.5	55.4	57.7	53.2
Latvia	EURO	National	2007	55.2	55.1	55.1	72.7	73.2	72.3
Lebanon	EMRO	National	2005	78.4	76.0	80.4	74.4	73.9	74.7
Lesotho	AFRO	National	2008	36.9	34.2	37.3	52.6	50.2	53.2
Liberia	AFRO	Monrovia	2008	23.6	22.2	24.5	45.5	45.1	45.4
Lithuania	EURO	National	2009	38.3	34.1	42.6	64.9	66.5	63.3
Madagascar	AFRO	National	2008	49.5	55.0	44.9	62.9	69.5	57.5
Malawi	AFRO	National	2009	19.7	25.0	14.0	29.5	32.9	26.1
Malaysia	WPRO	National	2009	48.7	49.6	47.6	64.1	67.7	60.2
Maldives	SEARO	National	2007	48.3	49.4	47.1	68.0	70.6	65.4
Mali	AFRO	National	2008	48.5	50.1	46.9	81.4	83.1	79.2
Marshall Islands	WPRO	National	2009	52.1	54.7	50.5	59.7	60.5	60.6
Mauritania	AFRO	National	2009	37.5	39.8	35.0	50.9	55.4	47.1
Mauritius	AFRO	National	2008	36.1	38.5	34.1	73.6	77.2	70.7
Mexico	AMRO	Mexico City	2006	46.2	46.3	45.5	60.2	61.6	59.0
Federated States of Micronesia	WPRO	National	2007	60.7	60.4	59.6	71.3	73.3	68.7
Mongolia	WPRO	National	2007	54.4	53.7	54.3	55.5	60.7	50.7
Montenegro	EURO	National	2008	76.8	73.5	79.9	69.9	68.8	70.8
Morocco	EMRO	National	2006	27.1	24.7	29.2	41.1	41.1	40.9
Mozambique	AFRO	Maputo	2007	22.5	25.2	19.6	26.2	28.6	23.0
Myanmar	SEARO	National	2007	34.1	38.8	29.4	46.4	51.2	42.1
Namibia	AFRO	National	2008	38.1	38.0	37.9	49.9	47.7	51.5
Nepal	SEARO	National	2007	35.3	38.5	31.7	47.3	49.5	44.7
New Zealand	WPRO	National	2008	36.0	38.5	33.1	67.2	63.3	71.3

Table 1.3 (continued)

Country	WHO region	National survey, or jurisdiction where survey conducted	Year	Exposed to second-hand tobacco smoke at home			Exposed to second-hand tobacco smoke outside their homes		
				Total	Boys	Girls	Total	Boys	Girls
Nicaragua	AMRO	Centro Managua	2003	43.7	43.9	43.2	54.1	56.4	51.9
Niger	AFRO	National	2009	24.1	28.1	20.4	54.3	58.8	50.2
Nigeria	AFRO	Abuja	2008	21.7	29.2	12.8	39.7	43.6	36.0
Oman	EMRO	National	2007	13.9	16.7	11.2	27.4	29.8	25.2
Pakistan	EMRO	Islamabad	2003	26.6	32.1	21.7	33.9	42.5	26.4
Palau	WPRO	National	2009	...	...	...	79.2	70.4	85.3
Panama	AMRO	National	2008	21.9	22.2	21.5	40.3	38.9	41.4
Papua New Guinea	WPRO	National	2007	73.9	75.4	72.2	86.4	87.0	85.6
Paraguay	AMRO	National	2008	32.5	35.1	30.1	55.3	57.3	53.4
Peru	AMRO	National	2007	25.5	26.2	24.2	46.8	46.9	46.4
Philippines	WPRO	National	2007	54.5	55.7	53.1	64.8	67.2	62.8
Poland	EURO	Warsaw	2009	49.1	42.8	54.6	76.8	75.5	77.8
Qatar	EMRO	National	2007	35.7	36.3	35.2	45.9	52.1	42.8
Republic of Korea	WPRO	National	2008	37.6	33.8	41.6	70.8	67.3	74.8
Republic of Moldova	EURO	National	2008	20.3	20.6	20.1	57.0	59.4	54.8
Romania	EURO	National	2009	52.8	50.0	55.4	59.1	57.1	61.3
Russian Federation	EURO	National	2004	76.4	74.3	78.5	89.4	89.0	89.9
Rwanda	AFRO	National	2008	19.2	19.9	18.0	...	...	...
Saint Kitts and Nevis	AMRO	National	2002	16.5	16.2	15.3	48.8	48.0	49.0
Saint Lucia	AMRO	National	2007	25.2	28.4	22.6	64.0	61.1	65.7
Saint Vincent and the Grenadines	AMRO	National	2007	31.5	31.7	30.9	59.7	56.5	61.8
Samoa	WPRO	National	2007	59.1	60.8	56.4	62.8	64.8	60.5
San Marino	EURO	National	2009	32.9	31.8	34.0	65.8	62.8	69.3
Saudi Arabia	EMRO	National	2007	27.9	28.9	26.4	38.2	45.1	31.6
Senegal	AFRO	National	2007	47.6	49.9	42.5	48.3	48.3	45.0
Serbia	EURO	National	2008	76.9	73.4	80.0	71.9	68.1	74.8
Seychelles	AFRO	National	2007	42.3	38.2	46.1	57.1	54.3	60.6
Sierra Leone	AFRO	National	2008	44.2	46.3	42.9	56.5	59.9	53.4
Singapore	WPRO	National	2000	35.1	34.8	35.2	65.1	64.0	66.0
Slovakia	EURO	National	2007	44.9	42.4	46.9	69.3	68.0	70.5
Somalia	EMRO	Somaliland	2007	29.1	30.8	21.9	48.7	50.2	41.8
South Africa	AFRO	National	2008	32.1	32.7	31.5	41.1	43.5	39.4

Table 1.3 (continued)

Country	WHO region	National survey, or jurisdiction where survey conducted	Year	Exposed to second-hand tobacco smoke at home			Exposed to second-hand tobacco smoke outside their homes		
				Total	Boys	Girls	Total	Boys	Girls
Sri Lanka	SEARO	National	2007	35.4	37.6	33.4	65.9	66.5	65.1
Sudan	EMRO	National	2009	27.6	26.0	28.7	33.1	33.8	32.0
Suriname	AMRO	National	2009	46.6	44.2	47.7	53.3	51.4	53.8
Swaziland	AFRO	National	2009	23.3	21.8	24.3	55.6	52.1	58.0
Syrian Arab Republic	EMRO	National	2010	60.1	58.7	61.7	58.4	61.1	55.7
Thailand	SEARO	National	2009	45.7	46.6	44.7	67.6	68.0	67.1
The former Yugoslav Republic of Macedonia	EURO	National	2008	67.5	64.7	70.5	66.0	63.7	68.3
Timor-Leste	SEARO	National	2009	59.4	66.7	52.1	61.3	66.7	56.0
Togo	AFRO	National	2007	20.2	23.5	15.7	41.6	45.1	36.7
Trinidad and Tobago	AMRO	National	2007	40.1	36.3	43.6	64.2	62.8	65.9
Tunisia	EMRO	National	2007	51.9	53.1	50.6	65.2	69.7	61.0
Turkey	EURO	National	2009	48.6	43.8	53.0	79.9	80.1	79.6
Tuvalu	WPRO	National	2006	76.6	77.8	75.8	76.7	72.0	79.3
Uganda	AFRO	National	2007	20.0	20.7	18.8	45.6	46.1	45.2
United Arab Emirates	EMRO	National	2005	25.3	24.3	25.4	31.6	34.3	28.4
United Republic of Tanzania	AFRO	Arusha	2008	15.7	16.4	14.9	34.7	35.2	33.9
United States of America	AMRO	National	2009	35.7	35.3	36.1	42.8	38.2	47.6
Uruguay	AMRO	National	2007	50.5	47.6	52.5	68.6	64.0	72.1
Uzbekistan	EURO	Tashkent	2008	17.3	17.6	15.8	46.7	47.5	42.4
Vanuatu	WPRO	National	2007	59.3	62.8	56.7	75.9	78.7	73.9
Venezuela (Bolivarian Republic of)	AMRO	National	1999	43.5	40.7	45.3	47.8	47.0	48.4
Viet Nam	WPRO	National	2007	58.5	59.0	58.0	71.2	71.4	71.0
West Bank*	EMRO	West Bank	2009	63.0	61.6	64.4	61.6	67.6	55.8
Gaza Strip*	EMRO	Gaza Strip	2005	47.4	48.0	46.5	46.1	51.9	40.6
Yemen	EMRO	National	2008	44.9	48.2	37.8	42.7	49.8	30.7
Zambia	AFRO	Lusaka	2007	23.1	21.2	24.3	45.5	43.2	47.1
Zimbabwe	AFRO	Harare	2008	20.9	22.0	19.4	40.1	40.5	39.5

* Refers to a territory
From WHO (2008, 2009a)

Table 1.4 Proportion of children under 15 years with one or more parent who smokes, by WHO subregion (based on survey data and modeling)

Subregion	Parental smoking (%)
Africa (D)	13
Africa (E)	13
The Americas (A)	25
The Americas (B)	29
The Americas (D)	22
Eastern Mediterranean (B)	37
Eastern Mediterranean (D)	34
Europe (A)	51
Europe (B)	61
Europe (C)	61
South-eastern Asia (B)	53
South-eastern Asia (D)	36
Western Pacific (A)	51
Western Pacific (B)	68
GLOBAL	41

WHO subregional country grouping (adapted from WHO, 2002):
Africa. ***Region D***: Algeria, Angola, Benin, Burkina Faso, Cameroon, Cape Verde, Chad, Comoros, Equatorial Guinea, Gabon, The Gambia, Ghana, Guinea, Guinea-Bissau, Liberia, Madagascar, Mali, Mauritania, Mauritius, Niger, Nigeria, Sao Tome and Principe, Senegal, Seychelles, Sierra Leone, Togo; ***Region E***: Botswana, Burundi, Central African Republic, Congo, Côte d'Ivoire, Democratic Republic of the Congo, Eritrea, Ethiopia, Kenya, Lesotho, Malawi, Mozambique, Namibia, Rwanda, South Africa, Swaziland, Uganda, United Republic of Tanzania, Zambia, Zimbabwe
The Americas. ***Region A***: Canada, Cuba, USA; ***Region B***: Antigua and Barbuda, Argentina, Bahamas, Barbados, Belize, Brazil, Chile, Colombia, Costa Rica, Dominica, Dominican Republic, El Salvador, Grenada, Guyana, Honduras, Jamaica, Mexico, Panama, Paraguay, Saint Kitts and Nevis, Saint Lucia, Saint Vincent and the Grenadines, Suriname, Trinidad and Tobago, Uruguay, Venezuela; ***Region D***: Bolivia, Ecuador, Guatemala, Haiti, Nicaragua, Peru
Eastern Mediterranea. ***Region B***: Bahrain, Islamic Republic of Iran, Jordan, Kuwait, Lebanon, Libyan Arab Jamahirya, Oman, Qatar, Saudi Arabia, Syrian Arab Republic, Tunisia, United Arab Emirates; ***Region D***: Afghanistan, Djibouti, Egypt, Iraq, Morocco, Pakistan, Somalia, Sudan, Yemen
Europe. ***Region A***: Andorra, Austria, Belgium, Croatia, Cyprus, Czech Republic, Denmark, Finland, France, Germany, Greece, Iceland, Ireland, Israel, Italy, Luxembourg, Malta, Monaco, Netherlands, Norway, Portugal, San Marino, Slovenia, Spain, Sweden, Switzerland, United Kingdom; ***Region B***: Albania, Armenia, Azerbaijan, Bosnia and Herzegovina, Bulgaria, Georgia, Kyrgyzstan, Poland, Romania, Serbia and Montenegro, Slovakia, Tajikistan, Former Yugoslav Republic of The former Yugoslav Republic of Macedonia, Turkey, Turkmenistan, Uzbekistan; ***Region C***: Belarus, Estonia, Hungary, Kazakhstan, Latvia, Lithuania, Republic of the Republic of Moldova, Russian Federation, Ukraine
South-eastern Asia. ***Region B***: Indonesia, Sri Lanka, Thailand; ***Region D***: Bangladesh, Bhutan, Democratic People's Republic of Korea, India, Maldives, Myanmar (Burma), Nepal, Timor-Leste
Western Pacific. ***Region A***: Australia, Brunei Darussalam, Japan, New Zealand, Singapore; ***Region B***: Cambodia, China, Cook Islands, Fiji, Kiribati, Lao People's Democratic Republic, Malaysia, Marshall Islands, Federated States of Micronesia, Mongolia, Nauru, Niue, Palau, Papua New Guinea, Philippines, Republic of Korea, Samoa, Solomon Islands, Tonga, Tuvalu, Vanuatu, Viet Nam
Regions are categorized as follows (WHO-approved classifications): A = very low child mortality and very low adult mortality; B = low child mortality and low adult mortality; C = low child mortality and high adult mortality; D = high child mortality and high adult mortality; E = high child mortality and very high adult mortality.

Fig. 1.3 Average prevalence (in%) of exposure of 13–15 year old children to second-hand tobacco smoke in public places, by WHO region, 2007

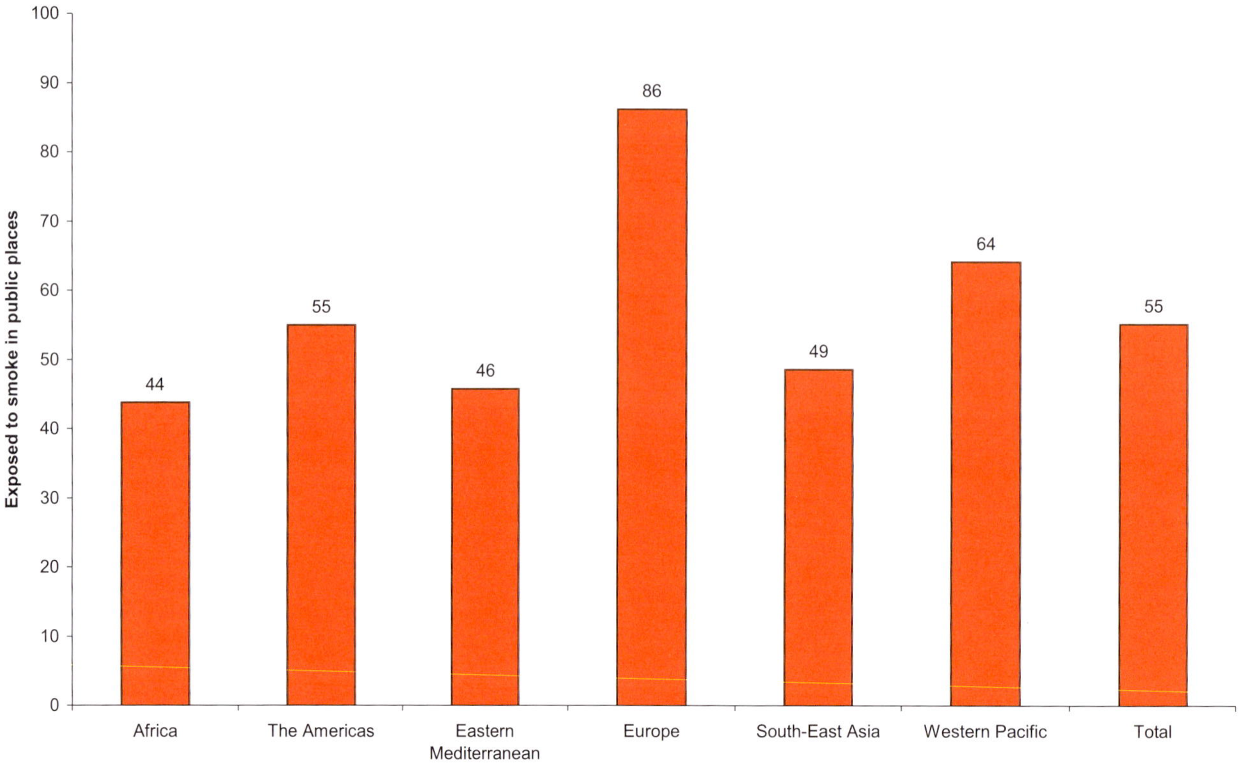

Exposed to smoke in public places
Africa 44
The Americas 55
Eastern Mediterranean 46
Europe 86
South-East Asia 49
Western Pacific 64
Total 55

From CDC (2008)

Fig. 1.4 presents the range of exposure to second-hand tobacco smoke outside home by WHO region for boys and girls and for both sexes combined. There are wide variations in second-hand tobacco smoke exposure outside home within each region. The largest variations are observed in the African region and the Western Pacific region irrespective of sex. This is largely influenced by the presence of smoke-free legislation for public paces in the countries, as well as levels of enforcement and public's compliance with these laws.

1.4.2. Exposure among adults

(a) Overview

While the GYTS offers a valuable global source for estimating exposure to second-hand tobacco smoke among children, there is no such extensive source of data for adults. Estimates of second-hand tobacco smoke exposure among adults have used the definitions of exposure based on having a spouse who smokes or exposure to tobacco smoke at work. For the countries lacking such data, exposure was estimated using a model based on smoking prevalence among men from the WHO Global InfoBase.

About one third of adults worldwide are regularly exposed to second-hand tobacco smoke (Table 1.5). The highest exposure was estimated in European Region C with 66% of the population

Fig. 1.4 Range of prevalence (in%) of exposure of 13–15 year old children to second-hand tobacco smoke outside their home, by WHO region, 2009

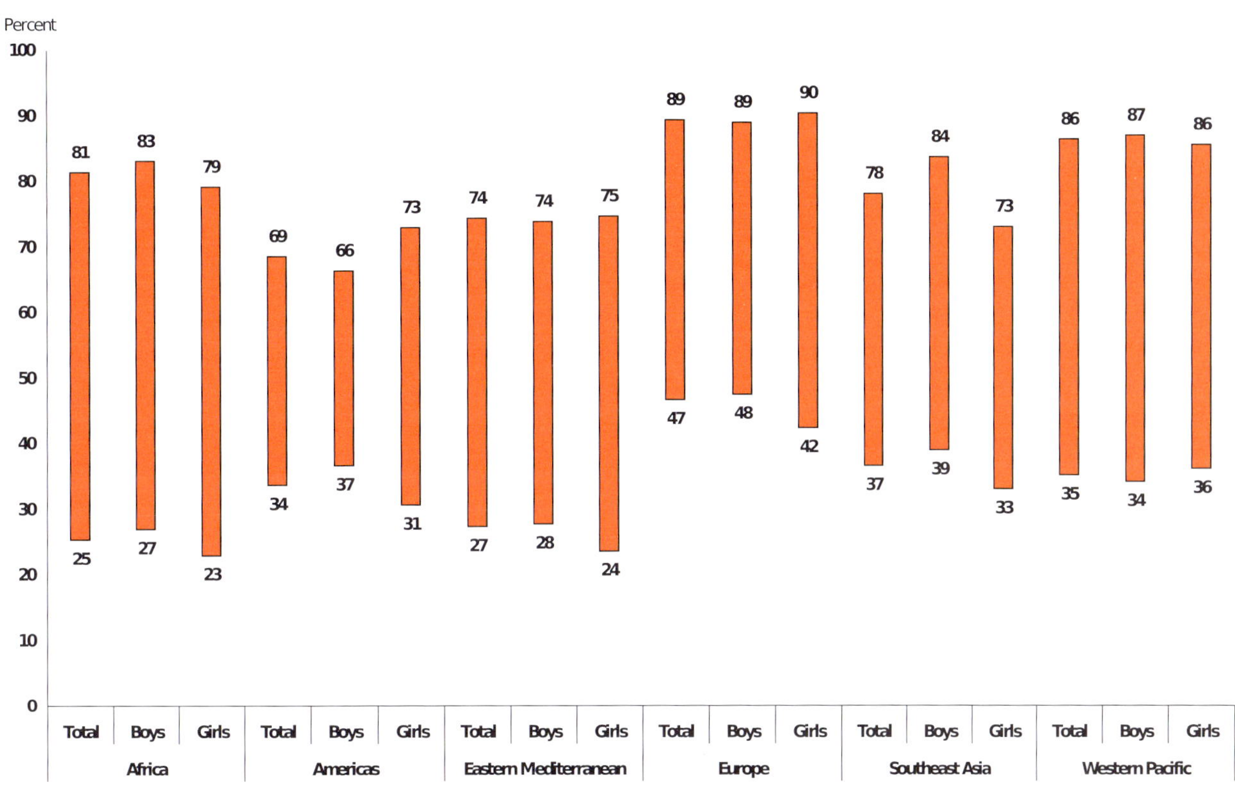

From CDC/WHO (2009)

being regularly exposed to second-hand tobacco smoke. The lowest regional exposure was estimated in the African region (4%). Differences between men and women were generally small, except in Eastern Mediterranean Region D and South East Asia Region B.

(b) Exposure at home

The Global Tobacco Surveillance System, through its adult household survey "Global Adult Tobacco Survey" (GATS), collects information on key tobacco control indicators including information on second-hand tobacco smoke exposure at home, at work and several public places (WHO, 2009b). GATS is a nationally representative survey conducted among persons aged ≥ 15 years using a standardized questionnaire, sample design, data collection method, and analysis protocol. GATS results are available from 14 countries with a high tobacco burden. Additionally since 2008, The WHO STEPwise approach to surveillance (STEPS) surveys have started to collect information on exposure to second-hand tobacco smoke at home and at work, now available for 7 countries (WHO, 2009c).

In the 21 countries that have reported data on exposure to second-hand tobacco smoke, large numbers of people are exposed at home (Fig. 1.5). Exposure was highest in Sierra Leone (74%) and lowest in the British Virgin Islands (3%). Overall, differences between men and women were relatively small in most countries; in China, Cambodia and Mongolia, more women reported being exposed to second-hand tobacco smoke

Table 1.5 Proportion of non-smoking adults exposed regularly to second-hand tobacco smoke, by WHO region (based on survey data and modeling)

WHO Subregion	Exposure in men (%)	Exposure in women (%)
Africa (D)	7	11
Africa (E)	4	9
The Americas (A)	16	16
The Americas (B)	13	21
The Americas (D)	15	18
Eastern Mediterranean (B)	24	22
Eastern Mediterranean (D)	21	34
Europe (A)	34	32
Europe (B)	52	53
Europe (C)	66	66
South-eastern Asia (B)	58	41
South-eastern Asia (D)	23	18
Western Pacific (A)	50	54
Western Pacific (B)	53	51
GLOBAL	33	31

From WHO (2010)
For the WHO subregional country grouping, see footnote of Table 1.4.

in their homes then men. This lack of difference implies that even when prevalence of smoking among women is low, they are exposed to second-hand tobacco smoke at home as much as men.

(c) Exposure at the workplace

The same magnitude of second-hand tobacco smoke exposure at the workplace was reported as at home (Fig. 1.6). Exposure to second-hand tobacco smoke at the workplace was highest in Sierra Leone (74%) and lowest in the British Virgin Islands (3%). However, more men reported being exposed to others' smoke at their workplace as compared to women in all countries. This difference was most significant in Libyan Arab Jamahirya and Bangladesh. These differences could be explained by the fact that women either tend to work in places where smoking is banned, such as education or health facilities, or work predominantly with other women.

1.5 Regulations

The World Health Organization's Framework Convention on Tobacco Control (WHO FCTC) is a multilateral treaty with legally binding obligations for its 174 Parties (as of November 2011) (WHO, 2003). This comprehensive treaty contains supply and demand reduction measures available to countries to counter the tobacco epidemic. Article 8 of the Treaty specifically addresses the need for protection from second-hand tobacco smoke, and articulates the "adoption and implementation of effective legislative, executive, administrative and /or other measures" by Parties to the Convention to this effect. Guidelines to Article 8 specify key elements needed in legislation to help countries meet the highest standards of protection from second-hand tobacco smoke and provide a clear timeline for Parties to adopt appropriate measures (within five years after entry into Force of the WHO FCTC) (WHO, 2007).

Fig. 1.5 Prevalence of adults exposed to second-hand tobacco smoke in their homes, in the countries that completed the Global Adult Tobacco Survey (GATS) and WHO STEPwise approach to surveillance (STEPS) surveys, 2008–2009

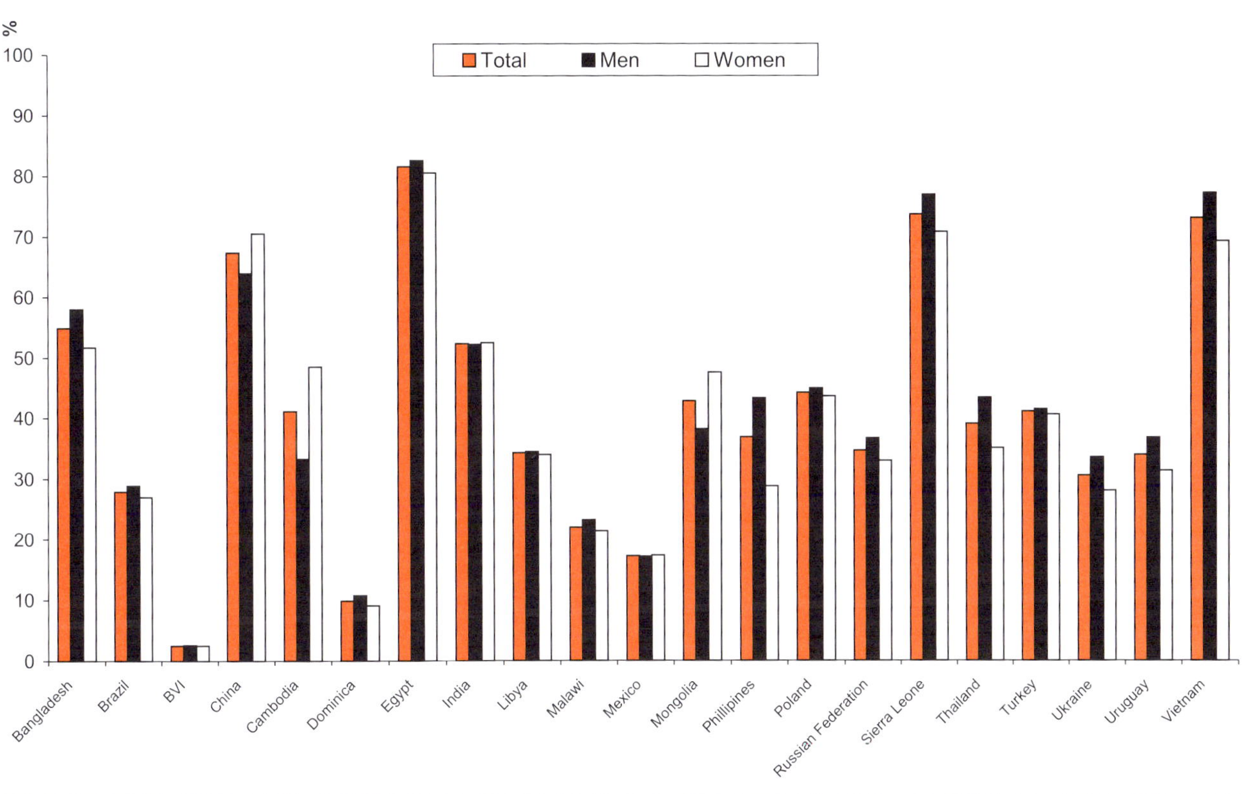

From WHO (2009b, c)
GATS defines second hand tobacco smoke exposure at home as reporting that smoking inside their home occurs daily, weekly, or monthly.
STEPS defines second-hand tobacco smoke exposure at home as reporting exposure in the home on one or more days in the past 7 days.

All countries, regardless of their FCTC ratification status, are taking steps to reduce second-hand tobacco smoke in public places, through either planning the steps to or implementing national smoke-free laws for public places or workplaces. In 2008, approximately 5% of the world's population (354 million) had national smoke-free laws. Fig. 1.7 provides details on the number of public places with national smoke-free legislation for all WHO Member States.

As of December 2008, fifteen countries across the globe have legislation that provide the highest level of protection against second-hand tobacco smoke exposure. These include: Albania, Australia, Bhutan, Canada, Colombia, Guatemala, Islamic Republic of Iran, Ireland, Marshall Islands, New Zealand, Panama, Turkey, Turkmenistan, United Kingdom of Great Britain and Northern Ireland and Uruguay.

2 Cancer in Humans

2.1 Cancer of the lung

More than 50 epidemiological studies since 1981 have examined the association between second-hand tobacco smoke and lung cancer resulting in the conclusion that exposure of non-smokers to second-hand tobacco smoke

Fig. 1.6 Prevalence of adults exposed to second-hand tobacco smoke in their workplaces, in the countries that completed the Global Adult Tobacco Survey and WHO STEPwise approach to surveillance (STEPS) surveys, 2008–2009

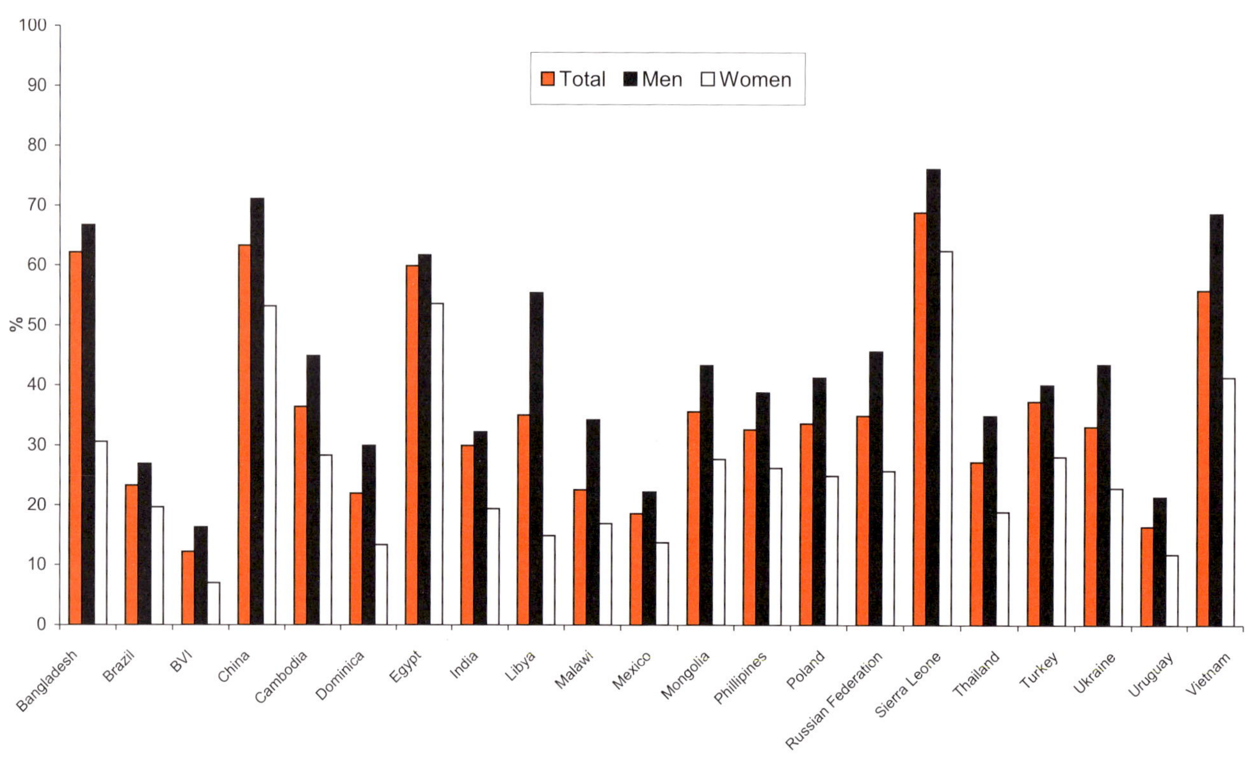

GATS defines second-hand tobacco smoke exposure at work as indoor workers who were exposed at work in the past 30 days.
STEPS defines second-hand tobacco smoke exposure at work as reporting exposure in the workplace on one or more days in the past 7 days
From WHO (2009b, c)

is causally associated with lung cancer risk (IARC, 2004). Many studies previously available assessed the lung cancer risk among the nonsmoking spouses of smokers since it is one of the sources of adult exposure to second-hand tobacco smoke that is less likely to be subject to exposure misclassification or other bias. Several important new, cohort, case–control studies and meta-analyses have been published since 2004 that provide additional evidence confirming the causal association (Table 2.1 available at http://monographs.iarc.fr/ENG/Monographs/vol100E/100E-02-Table2.1.pdf, Table 2.2 available at http://monographs.iarc.fr/ENG/Monographs/vol100E/100E-02-Table2.2.pdf, and Table 2.3 available at http://monographs.iarc.fr/ENG/Monographs/vol100E/100E-02-Table2.3.pdf). These new studies also expand our assessment of the effect of second-hand tobacco smoke in the workplace allowing for more refined estimates of lung cancer risk. Preliminary data also suggest significant interactions between several genetic polymorphisms, second-hand tobacco smoke and lung cancer risk.

In a meta-analysis of 55 studies, including 7 cohort, 25 population based case–control studies and 23 hospital based case–control studies the pooled relative risk (RR) for lung cancer for never smoking women exposed to second-hand tobacco smoke from spouses was 1.27 (95%CI: 1.17–1.37). The relative risk for studies in North America was 1.15 (95%CI: 1.03–1.28), in Asia 1.31

Fig. 1.7 Number and percentage of countries with number of public places covered by smoke free legislations, by income status (as of 31 December 2008)

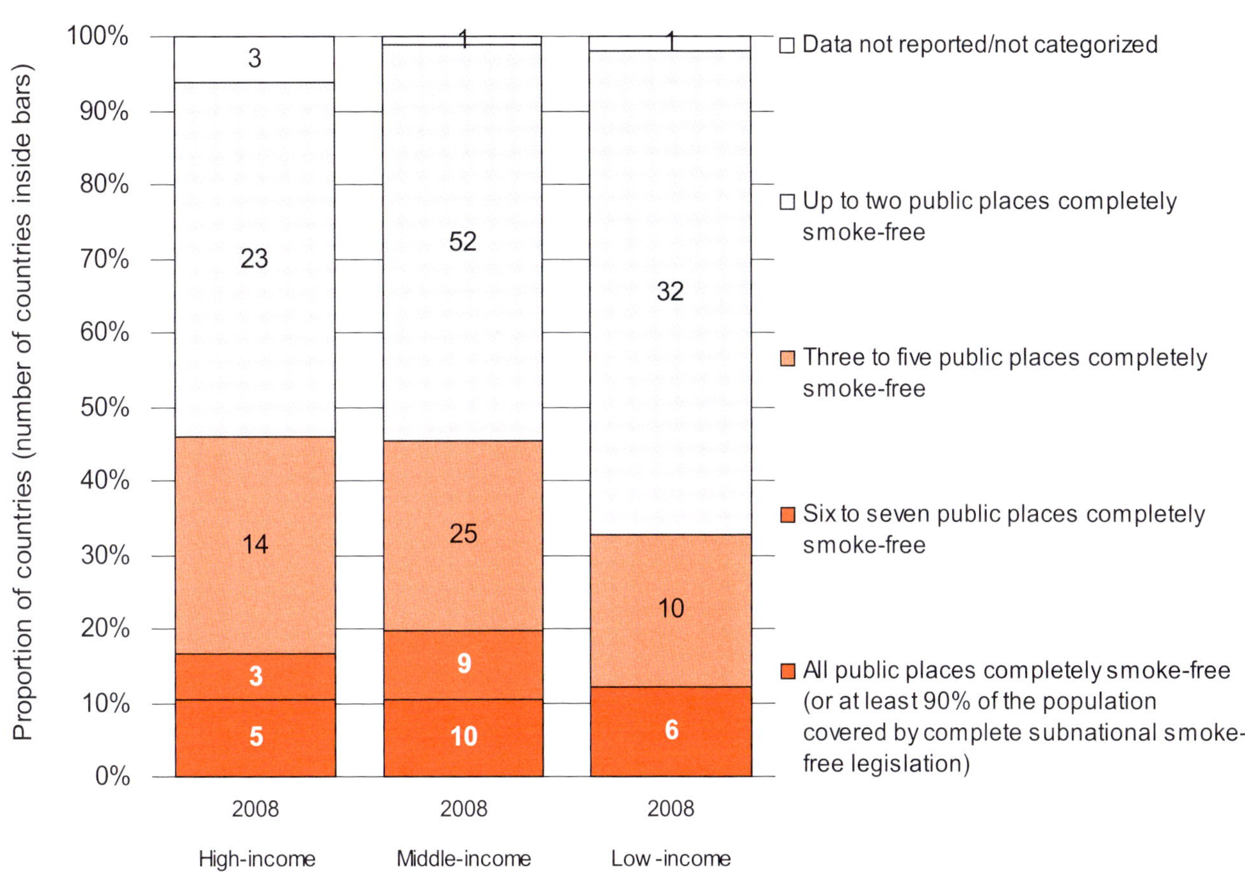

From WHO (2009a)

(95%CI: 1.16–1.48) and Europe 1.31 (1.24–1.52) (Taylor *et al.*, 2007).

In a meta-analysis of 22 studies that assessed the effect of second-hand tobacco smoke exposures at work, the relative risk for lung cancer among exposed non-smokers was 1.24 (95%CI: 1.18–1.29) and among those workers classified as highly exposed to second-hand tobacco smoke at work 2.01 (95%CI: 1.33–2.60) compared to those with no exposure at work (Stayner *et al.*, 2007).

In a large cohort study conducted in 10 European countries (European Prospective Investigation into Cancer and Nutrition, EPIC), it was estimated that the hazard ratio (HR) for lung cancer risk from second-hand tobacco smoke exposure at home and/or at work for never smokers and ex-smokers (at least 10 years) was 1.34 (0.85–2.13) (Vineis *et al.*, 2007a). The main component of this risk was attributable to exposure at the workplace, resulting in a hazard ratio of 1.65 (1.04–2.63). The overall hazard ratio between childhood exposure and the risk of lung cancer in adulthood was 2.00 (0.94–4.28); among children with daily exposure for many hours each day the hazard ratio was 3.63 (1.19–11.12). In a separate analysis of workplace exposure to second-hand tobacco smoke in this cohort women were observed to have a lung cancer hazard ratio of 2.13 (1.6–3.4) (Veglia *et al.*, 2007).

In a large population-based cohort study conducted in Japan, findings confirmed that exposure to second-hand tobacco smoke is a risk factor for lung cancer among Japanese women (Kurahashi *et al.*, 2008). Compared with women married to never smokers, the hazard ratio for all lung cancer incidence was 1.34 (95%CI:0.81–2.21) and for adenocarcinoma 2.03 (95%CI:1.07–3.86). For adenocarcinoma dose–response relationships were seen for both intensity (*P* for trend = 0.02) and total amount (*P* for trend = 0.03) of the husband's smoking. Exposure to second-hand tobacco smoke at the workplace also increased the risk of lung cancer (HR, 1.32; 95%CI: 0.85–2.04).

Data from a cohort study of women from Shanghai, China also found that exposure to second-hand tobacco smoke is associated with lung cancer mortality. Exposure to second-hand tobacco smoke at work was associated with a significantly increased mortality to lung cancer (HR 1.79, 95%CI: 1.09–2.93) but the risk was not significant for exposure to husband's second-hand tobacco smoke (HR 1.09, 95%CI: 0.74–1.61) (Wen *et al.*, 2006). In a case–control study of lung cancer among lifetime non-smoking Chinese men living in Hong Kong Special Administrative Region a non-significant association between all lung cancer and ever being exposed to household and/or workplace second-hand tobacco smoke was observed (OR, 1.11, 95%CI: 0.74–1.67) but a significant increase was observed for adenocarcinoma (OR, 1.68, 95%CI: 1.00–2.38) (Tse *et al.*, 2009).

In a long-term case–control study of lung cancer cases at the Massachusetts General Hospital, study participants exposed to second-hand tobacco smoke at work and at leisure were at a significantly greater risk (OR, 1.30, 95%CI: 1.08–1.57) if the exposure occurred between birth and 25 years of age. If the exposures occurred after the age of 25 years the risk was not elevated (OR, 0.66, 95%CI: 0.21–1.57) but the confidence limits are wide for this subgroup analysis (Asomaning *et al.*, 2008).

In two other cohort studies, one conducted in California (Enstrom & Kabat, 2003) and another in New Zealand (Hill *et al.*, 2007) no excess risk was observed among lifelong non-smokers exposed to second-hand tobacco smoke. In the California study the relative risk was 0.99 (95%CI: 0.72–1.37) based on 126 lung cancer cases. [The confidence intervals in this study are relatively wide and they include the current IARC estimate of lung cancer risk from second-hand tobacco smoke exposure. In addition the opportunity for substantial misclassification of second-hand tobacco smoke exposure is great because exposures outside the home were not assessed and the second-hand tobacco smoke exposures were not re-evaluated after enrollment into the study.] Hill *et al.* (2007) observed no association between second-hand tobacco smoke exposure in a census enumeration of current second-hand tobacco smoke exposure at home and linkage to cancer registries three years later. The authors suggest that this may be a result of either the misclassification of total second-hand tobacco smoke exposure since exposures outside the home were not assessed and/or the fact that a 3-year follow-up after exposure ascertainment may have been too short to capture important exposures before the diagnosis of lung cancer.

One case–control study (Wenzlaff *et al.*, 2005) and one case-only study (Bonner *et al.*, 2006) assessed lung cancer risk associated with second-hand tobacco smoke exposure and several polymorphisms. In the case–control study, individuals were stratified by household second-hand tobacco smoke exposure (yes/no), those with *CYP1B1 Leu*^{432}*Val* genotype alone or in combination with Phase II enzyme polymorphisms were more strongly associated with lung cancer risk if they also were exposed to at least some household second-hand tobacco smoke exposure compared to those that had no exposure. In the case-only study a significant interaction was observed between lung cancer risk, second-hand tobacco smoke and a GSTM1 (null) genotype (OR, 2.28, 95%CI:1.15–4.51).

2.2 Cancer of the breast

2.2.1 Overview of studies

The relationship between exposure to second-hand tobacco smoke and breast cancer has been comprehensively reviewed in the peer reviewed literature (Johnson, 2005; Miller *et al.*, 2007) and in reports from national and international committees (IARC, 2004, 2009; California Environmental Protection Agency, 2005; US. Department of Health and Human Services, 2006; Collishaw *et al.*, 2009). These reviews have drawn different conclusions. IARC (2004) characterized the evidence as "inconsistent," based on studies published or in press by June, 2002. A US Surgeon General Report (2006) concluded that the evidence was "suggestive but not sufficient" to infer a causal relationship between second-hand tobacco smoke and breast cancer, whereas reviews by the California Environmental Protection Agency (CalEPA) in 2005 and by a panel of researchers in this area convened in Canada (Collishaw *et al.*, 2009) designated the evidence for second-hand tobacco smoke as "consistent with a causal association in younger primarily premenopausal women."

A total of 16 new studies have been published since the previous *IARC Monograph* (IARC, 2004). These include three cohort studies (Reynolds *et al.*, 2004; Hanaoka *et al.*, 2005; Pirie *et al.*, 2008) (Table 2.4 available at http://monographs.iarc.fr/ENG/Monographs/vol100E/100E-02-Table2.4.pdf), and 13 new case–control studies (Lash & Aschengrau, 2002; Alberg *et al.*, 2004; Gammon *et al.*, 2004; Shrubsole *et al.*, 2004; Bonner *et al.*, 2005; Sillanpää *et al.*, 2005; Lissowska *et al.*, 2006; Mechanic *et al.*, 2006; Roddam *et al.*, 2007; Rollison *et al.*, 2008; Slattery *et al.*, 2008; Ahern *et al.*, 2009; Young *et al.*, 2009) (Table 2.5 available at http://monographs.iarc.fr/ENG/Monographs/vol100E/100E-02-Table2.5.pdf). Table 2.5 also presents two case–control studies not discussed previously (Zhao *et al.*, 1999; Liu *et al.*, 2000). Several meta-analyses have also been published as new data became available (California Environmental Protection Agency, 2005; Johnson, 2005; US. Department of Health and Human Services, 2006; Pirie *et al.*, 2008; IARC, 2009).

The largest of the cohort studies, identified 2518 incident breast cancers among 224917 never smokers followed for an average of 3.5 years in the British Million Women Study (Pirie *et al.*, 2008). The cohort was drawn from women, age 50–64 years, participating in mammography screening programmes. Nearly all cases were post-menopausal and the overall analyses pertain to postmenopausal breast cancer. No relationship was observed between breast cancer risk and smoking by a parent at the time of birth and/or age 10 years (HR, 0.98; 95%CI: 0.88–1.08); the results were also null for smoking by a current partner (HR, 1.02; 95%CI: 0.89–1.16) or exposure to the combination of parental and spousal smoking (HR, 1.03; 95%CI: 0.90–1.19). Pirie *et al.* (2008) also present a meta-analysis of studies of second-hand smoke and breast cancer risk, separating studies by cohort or case–control design. No overall association was observed in the cohort studies. These largely represent post-menopausal breast cancer, so the analysis was not stratified by menopausal status. An overall association was seen in the case–control studies, similar to the findings of other meta-analyses (California Environmental Protection Agency, 2005; US. Department of Health and Human Services, 2006; IARC, 2009). [Pirie *et al.* (2008) focus on the discrepancy between the cohort and case–control results and propose that the associations observed in early case–control studies can likely be explained by recall bias. The study has been criticized for the lack of information on occupational exposures to second-hand smoke (Collishaw *et al.*, 2009).]

A second large cohort study (Reynolds *et al.*, 2004) identified 1998 women diagnosed with breast cancer during five years of follow-up of the California Teachers Study. Analyses were based on 433 women with pre/peri-menopausal breast cancer and 1361 women with postmenopausal cancer. No association was observed between post-menopausal breast cancer and residential exposure to second-hand tobacco smoke in childhood or adulthood. No association was initially reported with pre/peri-menopausal breast cancer in analyses based on menopausal status at enrollment (RR 0.93, 95%CI: 0.71–1.22). When menopausal status was defined by age at diagnosis rather than by age at enrollment, the hazard ratio for premenopausal breast cancer among women exposed in both childhood and adulthood increased to 1.27 (95%CI: 0.84–1.92) (Reynolds *et al.*, 2006).

Hanaoka *et al.* (2005) identified 162 incident breast cancer cases during a nine-year follow-up of 20169 Japanese women, age 40–59 years, who reported no history of active smoking when enrolled in the Japan Public Health Center (JPHC) study in 1990. Nearly three quarters (72%) of the women reported exposure to second-hand tobacco smoke. About half of the women were premenopausal when enrolled in the study, although there were only nine unexposed cases among the pre-menopausal women. The multivariate-adjusted relative risk for breast cancer among all exposed women irrespective of menopausal status was 1.1 (95%CI: 0.8–1.6) compared to those classified as unexposed. The corresponding relative risks for women who were pre- or postmenopausal at baseline were 2.6 (95%CI: 1.3–5.2) and 0.7 (95%CI: 0.4–1.0), respectively.

Six of the 13 new population-based case–control studies included more than 1000 cases each (Shrubsole *et al.*, 2004; Bonner *et al.*, 2005; Lissowska *et al.*, 2006; Mechanic *et al.*, 2006; Slattery *et al.*, 2008; Young *et al.*, 2009; Table 2.5 on-line). None of these 13 studies showed an overall increase in breast cancer risk associated with second-hand tobacco smoke exposure in Caucasians. The incidence of premenopausal breast cancer was associated with one or more indices of second-hand tobacco smoke exposure in all four studies that stratified the results by menopausal status (Gammon *et al.*, 2004; Shrubsole *et al.*, 2004; Bonner *et al.*, 2005; Slattery *et al.*, 2008) although the association was not always statistically significant (Gammon *et al.*, 2004; Bonner *et al.*, 2005; Fig. 2.1). Associations were also reported between second-hand tobacco smoke exposure and overall breast cancer risk in African Americans (Mechanic *et al.*, 2006) and with premenopausal breast cancer in Hispanics/American Indians (Slattery *et al.*, 2008). The associations observed in these case–control studies are generally weaker than those reported in earlier case–control studies. Whereas the relative risk estimates reported in the earlier studies often equalled or exceeded 2.0 (Sandler *et al.*, 1985a; Lash & Aschengrau, 1999; Zhao *et al.*, 1999; Johnson & Repace, 2000; Liu *et al.*, 2000) or 3.0 (Smith *et al.*, 1984; Morabia *et al.*, 1996; Liu *et al.*, 2000; Morabia *et al.*, 2000), the estimates in the later studies were mostly under 1.5, even in studies that reported positive associations.

2.2.2 Issues affecting the interpretation of studies

One important consideration in evaluating these data has been the lack of a strong and convincing relationship between active smoking and breast cancer. Several theories have been advanced to explain why second-hand tobacco smoke might have a stronger effect on breast cancer than active smoking (California Environmental Protection Agency, 2005; Johnson, 2005; Collishaw *et al.*, 2009). Central to these is the hypothesis that active smoking may have counterbalancing protective and detrimental effects on breast cancer risk

Fig. 2.1 Relative risk of pre-menopausal breast cancer associated with second-hand tobacco smoke. Ever versus never.

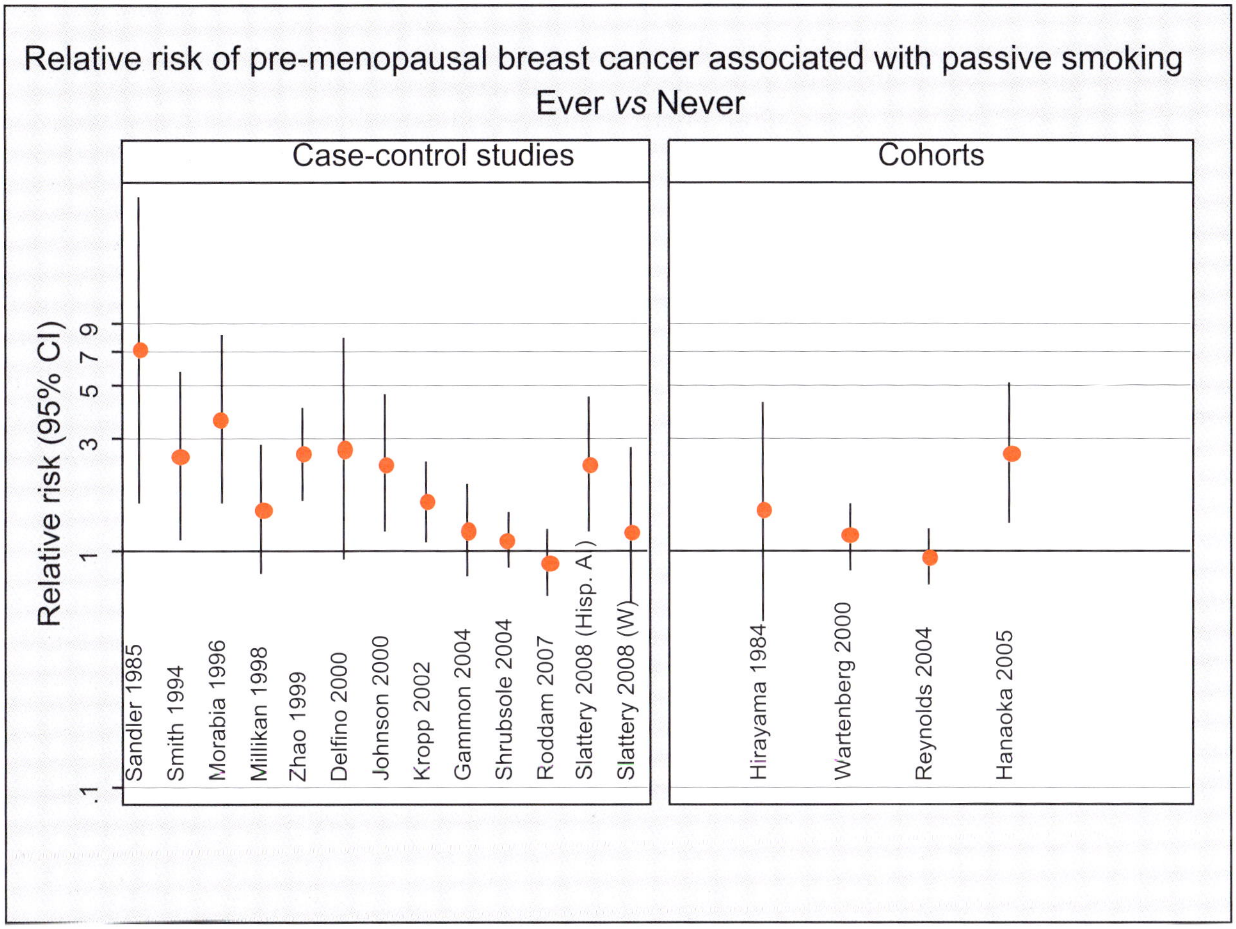

Relative risk of pre-menopausal breast cancer associated with passive smoking
Ever *vs* Never

Study sorted by calendar year

that, in combination, produce little or no overall association, whereas second-hand tobacco smoke may have only an adverse effect on risk. The weakness of this theory is that there is little direct evidence (see Section 4) identifying the mechanism by which active smoking may cause the proposed [protective] antiestrogenic effects. Without knowing the mechanism, it has been impossible to prove that active smoking has this effect but exposure to second-hand tobacco smoke does not. A second hypothesis that has been advanced is that second-hand tobacco smoke may have a greater effect on pre- than on postmenopausal breast cancer. This theory was proposed by CalEPA in 2005 (Johnson & Glantz, 2008) based on analyses of studies available at the time, and was subsequently questioned by some (US. Department of Health and Human Services, 2006) but not all (Collishaw *et al.*, 2009) subsequent reviews. [Because this arose as an a posteriori observation rather than as an a priori hypothesis, it must be confirmed by independent studies.] The strongest support for the hypothesis comes from a cohort study in Japan (Hanaoka *et al.*, 2005), which reported significantly increased risk (RR 2.6, 95%CI: 1.3–5.2) of premenopausal breast cancer in women who previously reported having ever lived with a regular smoker or ever being exposed to second-hand tobacco smoke for at least one hour per day in settings outside the home. However, the referent group in this analysis included only nine unexposed cases. No associations were observed with post-menopausal breast cancer. A weak association between second-hand tobacco smoke exposure and premenopausal breast cancer was reported in the California Teachers cohort, when menopausal status was defined by age at diagnosis rather than age at entry into the study (Reynolds *et al.*, 2006). In case–control studies published since the CalEPA review (California Environmental Protection Agency, 2005) that reported results stratified by menopausal status, Bonner *et al.* (2005) and Slattery *et al.* (2008) reported stronger associations with pre- than with post-menopausal breast cancer, although the only statistically significant association with premenopausal breast cancer was in Hispanic or American Indian women who had second-hand tobacco smoke exposure of more than ten hours per week (OR, 2.3, 95%CI:1.2–4.5) (Slattery *et al.*, 2008). In a case–control study of breast cancer in women age 36–45 years Roddam *et al.* (2007) observed no increased risk in premenopausal women who, since age 16, were married to or lived with a boyfriend who smoked for at least one year.

Two other explanations for inconsistencies in the evidence relate to the fundamental design differences between cohort and case–control studies. A critical advantage of cohort studies is that they collect information on exposures before the disease of interest is diagnosed, thus preventing knowledge of disease status influencing how participants recall and/or report their exposures. Recall bias is especially challenging in case–control studies of exposures that are difficult to measure, when recollection of the frequency and intensity of exposure is necessarily subjective. In counterpart, an important advantage of case–control studies is that they can collect more detailed information on the exposure of interest than is usually possible in cohort studies. Together, these factors create what has been described as "a tension" between the potential for recall or selection bias in case–control studies, and the reduced possibility of collecting full "lifetime exposure histories" in cohort studies (Collishaw *et al.*, 2009). The discrepancy in the results from case–control and cohort studies is seen especially in the earlier case–control studies, which found much stronger associations than those observed in most recent studies. Five studies in particular (Smith *et al.*, 1984; Morabia *et al.*, 1996; Zhao *et al.*, 1999; Johnson & Repace, 2000; Kropp & Chang-Claude, 2002) were considered by Collishaw *et al.* (2009) as having the most complete information on lifetime exposure to second-hand tobacco smoke from all sources. At the same time, these studies are among the most susceptible to recall bias for two reasons. The first is a general problem of case–control studies, in that cases are more likely to remember and report potentially hazardous exposures than controls. Second, recall bias is potentially more problematic when subjective considerations can influence reporting. It is easier to report smoking by a parent or spouse than it is to remember exposures from other sources that possibly occurred many years ago in daily life. Exposure to second-hand tobacco smoke was highly prevalent in the decades following World War II in Europe and North America. It would be unusual for someone not to be exposed. The studies that the California Environmental Protection Agency (2005) considered to have the best information on exposure to second-hand tobacco smoke are also those which rely more heavily on recall of past exposures outside the home. Moreover, inclusion in the referent group in these studies is also vulnerable to recall bias. Previous reviews by IARC (2004) and the US Surgeon General (US. Department of Health and Human Services, 2006) have expressed concern about potential biases that may be introduced by relying on a small and unusual subgroup (the unexposed to active smoking and second-hand tobacco smoke) as the referent category in these studies. Recall bias remains a plausible explanation for why the association with second-hand tobacco smoke is stronger in studies that collect "lifetime exposure histories" than in those that rely on parental or spousal smoking. In addition, publication bias cannot be ruled out because the reporting of association limited by subgroup (pre-menopausal) could have been selective.

[The Working Group noted that adjustment for potential confounders using the questionnaire data on other established risk factors for breast cancer did not eliminate the association with second-hand tobacco smoke in these studies. However, this does not resolve concerns about the possibility of recall or publication bias.]

Several meta-analyses have been published, largely showing similar results but leading to substantially different interpretations of the evidence (California Environmental Protection Agency, 2005; US Department of Health and Human Services, 2006; Johnson, 2007; IARC, 2009). The California Environmental Protection Agency (2005) calculated a pooled estimate for second-hand tobacco smoke and breast cancer risk of 1.11 (95%CI: 1.04–1.19) in all women and 1.38 (95%CI: 1.21–1.56) in premenopausal women, based on 19 studies and a fixed effects model. These estimates increased to 1.89 (95%CI: 1.57–2.27) for all women and 2.18 (95%CI: 1.70–2.79) in premenopausal women when the analysis was restricted to the subset of studies considered to have the best exposure data.

Based on these analyses, the California Environmental Protection Agency (2005) and Collishaw *et al.* (2009) emphasized the positive association with premenopausal breast cancer in their conclusion that the evidence is "consistent with a causal relationship" whereas the US Surgeon General (US Department of Health and Human Services, 2006) was more cautious in characterizing the evidence as "suggestive but not sufficient."

[The Working Group noted that the criterion used by IARC specifies "sufficient evidence of carcinogenicity in which chance, bias and confounding could be ruled out with reasonable confidence." This is a more stringent definition than "consistent with a causal relationship."]

2.3 Cancers of the upper aerodigestive tract

2.3.1 Upper areodigestive tract combined

Cancers of the upper aerodigestive tract traditionally comprise cancers of the oral cavity, pharynx, larynx and oesophagus. However, some epidemiological studies have examined only head and neck cancers restricted to tumours of the oral cavity, pharynx and larynx. Four case–control studies (Tan *et al.*, 1997; Zhang *et al.*, 2000; Lee *et al.*, 2008; Ramroth *et al.*, 2008) assessed the effects of second-hand tobacco smoke on head and neck cancers combined and separately for oral cavity, oropharynx or larynx cancers (Table 2.6 available at http://monographs.iarc.fr/ENG/Monographs/vol100E/100E-02-Table2.6.pdf).

In a hospital-based case–control study in the USA, including only non smoking cases and controls, Tan *et al.* (1997) detected high risk of head and neck cancer among those ever exposed to second-hand tobacco smoke at home or at work. Women presented higher risk at home (OR, 7.3; $P < 0.001$) than men (OR, 1.1; $P < 0.79$). On the other hand, men showed higher risk at work (OR, 11.6; $P < 0.001$) than women (OR, 8.9; $P < 0.002$). [The authors did not provide the percentages of the telephone interviews done with the spouses of cases and controls. Probably, this is the main weakness of this study and differential misclassification of exposure to second-hand tobacco smoke could not be excluded. The analysis was performed without adjustment for potential confounding variables.] In a study in the USA,

Zhang *et al.* (2000) observed an increased risk (OR, 2.4; 95%CI: 0.9–6.8) with lifetime second-hand tobacco smoke exposure (ever/never) for head and neck cancers, adjusted for age, sex, ethnicity, education, alcohol drinking, pack-years of cigarette smoking, and marijuana consumption.

Lee *et al.* (2008) pooled the data from several studies including cases of head and neck cancers and controls (population and hospital) from central Europe, Latin America and United States. Two groups were examined separately, never tobacco users and never tobacco and alcohol users. Among never tobacco users, no association was observed between ever exposure to second-hand tobacco smoke at home or at work and the risk for head and neck cancers. Among never tobacco and alcohol users, a non-statistically significant risk (or 1.30; 95%ci: 0.94–1.81) was observed. When considering specific anatomical sites, only laryngeal cancer risk was increased when ever exposed to second-hand tobacco smoke in a lifetime, detected among never tobacco users (OR, 1.71; 95%CI: 0.98–3.00) and among never tobacco and alcohol users (OR, 2.90; 95%CI: 1.09–7.73).

In Germany, in a population-based case–control study on laryngeal cancer, Ramroth *et al.* (2008) observed a non-statistically significant risk (OR, 2.0; 95%CI: 0.39–10.7) for exposure to second-hand tobacco smoke (ever/never) at home and in workplaces among nonsmokers.

(a) Evidence of a dose–response

Zhang *et al.* (2000) observed a dose–response relationship with the intensity of exposure to second-hand tobacco smoke (never, moderate and heavy) on head and neck cancers ($P = 0.025$); those at heavy level of exposure at home or at work showed highest risk for head and neck cancer (OR, 3.6; 95%CI: 1.1–11.5). However, the classification of exposure to second-hand tobacco smoke at work as never, occasionally or regularly did not show any dose–response effect; and the risk for the groups of occasionally or regularly exposed at home were similar and non statistically significant.

Lee *et al.* (2008) explored the intensity and duration of sexposure to second-hand tobacco smoke. For intensity the number of hours of exposure per day was considered at home (0–3 hours, > 3 hours) or at the workplace (never, 1–3 hours and > 3 hours). Among both groups of never tobacco users and never tobacco and alcohol users non-statistically significant risks of head and neck cancers were observed for those exposed for > 3 hours per day at home or at work. For duration the number of years of exposure at home and at work was considered (never, 1–15 years, and > 15 years). Among never tobacco users, there was a trend of increase in risk for head and neck cancers with greater number of years of exposure at home, but not at work. Among never tobacco and alcohol users, the duration of exposure showed a trend for exposure both at work or at home.

Considering specific anatomical sites, for cancer of the oral cavity no dose–response effect was observed with increasing number of years of exposure to second-hand tobacco smoke at home or at work. For cancer of the pharynx, a dose–response effect was observed with increasing number of years of exposure to second-hand tobacco smoke with only at home, in both never tobacco users and never tobacco and alcohol users. For cancer of the larynx, a dose–response effect was noted with increasing number of years of exposure to second-hand tobacco smoke at home among never tobacco users and at work among never tobacco and alcohol users. Among never tobacco and alcohol users, all the odd ratios (OR) were statistically significantly elevated for > 15 years of exposure at home or at work for head and neck cancers overall and separately for cancer of the pharynx, and only at work for cancer of the larynx.

2.3.2 Cancers of the nasopharynx, and nasal cavity and sinonasal cavity

The relationship between exposure to second-hand tobacco smoke and risk for these rare cancers of the upper respiratory tract has been examined in one cohort study (Hirayama, 1984; Table 2.7 available at http://monographs.iarc.fr/ENG/Monographs/vol100E/100E-02-Table2.7.pdf) and five case–controls studies (Fukuda & Shibata, 1990; Yu *et al.*, 1990; Zheng *et al.*, 1993; Cheng *et al.*, 1999; Yuan *et al.*, 2000; Table 2.6 on-line). A positive association was found in most of these studies.

Hirayama (1984) found an increased risk of sinonasal cancer in women (histology not noted) associated with increasing numbers of cigarettes smoked by husbands of nonsmoking women. When compared with nonsmoking women married to nonsmokers, wives whose husbands smoked had a relative risk of 1.7 (95%CI: 0.7–4.2) for 1–14 cigarettes per day, 2.0 (95%CI: 0.6–6.3) for 15–19 cigarettes per day and 2.55 (95%CI: 1.0–6.3) for ≥ 20 cigarettes per day (*P* for trend = 0.03).

Fukuda & Shibata (1990) reported the results of a Japanese case–control study based on 169 cases of squamous-cell carcinoma of the maxillary sinus and 338 controls matched on sex, age and residence in Hokkaido, Japan. Among nonsmoking women, a relative risk of 5.4 ($P < 0.05$) was associated with exposure in the household to second-hand tobacco smoke from one or more smokers. Active smoking was associated with an increased risk for squamous-cell carcinoma of the maxillary sinus in men in the same study.

Zheng *et al.* (1993) used data from the 1986 US National Mortality Followback Survey to assess risk for cancer of the nasal cavity and sinuses in relation to exposure to second-hand tobacco smoke in white men. A total of 147 deaths from cancer of the nasal cavity and sinuses was compared to 449 controls who had died from other causes (excluding any causes strongly linked to alcohol and/or tobacco use). Data were obtained from postal questionnaires completed by next-of-kins. Among nonsmokers, patients with nasal cancer were more likely to have a spouse who smoked cigarettes (RR, 3.0; 95%CI: 1.0–8.9) after adjustment for age and alcohol use. When the analysis of cases was restricted to those with cancer of the maxillary sinus, the risk was somewhat higher (RR 4.8; 95%CI: 0.9–24.7). The risks reported for active smoking and exposure to second-hand tobacco smoke were of similar magnitude in this study.

Neither second-hand tobacco smoke exposure during childhood nor exposure during adulthood were positively associated with an increased risk for nasopharyngeal cancer in a study in Taiwan, China (Cheng *et al.*, 1999). Although histological type was not specified, all cases were histologically confirmed. Among never-smokers, the risk estimates for cumulative exposure to second-hand tobacco smoke (pack-person-years) in childhood declined as exposure increased (*P* for trend = 0.05); a similar but non-significant inverse relationship was found for exposure during adulthood. Significant elevations in risk for nasopharyngeal cancer were observed for active smokers in this study. [The Working Group noted that the exposure assessment was relatively detailed and that the estimates of relative risk were adjusted for age, sex, education and family history of nasopharyngeal cancer.]

A large population-based case–control study conducted in Shanghai, China, included 935 cases of nasopharyngeal carcinoma and 1032 population controls randomly selected from a population-registry and frequency-matched by sex and 5-year age group (Yuan *et al.*, 2000). All cases were histologically confirmed, but the cell type was not specified. The study subjects were interviewed face to face, and the response rates were 84% for cases and 99% for controls. In female never-smokers, a consistent increase in risk related to exposure to second-hand tobacco smoke during childhood was noted. The relative risk was 3.4 (95%CI: 1.4–8.1) if the mother smoked; 3.0 (95%CI: 1.4–6.2) if the father smoked; 2.7 (95%CI: 1.1–6.9) if another household member smoked and 3.0 (95%CI: 1.4–6.2) if any household member smoked. Risks associated with exposure to second-hand tobacco smoke during adulthood in women were also statistically significantly increased. For male never-smokers, the associations were weaker and were not statistically significantly elevated for exposure during childhood and adulthood. [The Working Group noted that this was a large, well conducted study that included a detailed exposure assessment and adjustment for numerous potential confounders.]

2.4 Leukaemia and lymphomas

Kasim *et al.* (2005) analysed the risk of leukaemia in adults after exposure to second-hand tobacco smoke (Table 2.8 available at http://monographs.iarc.fr/ENG/Monographs/vol100E/100E-02-Table2.8.pdf). This case–control study was based on postal questionnaires. There was a slightly increased risk (*P* for trend = 0.001) with increasing duration of exposure to second-hand tobacco smoke. The association was limited to chronic lymphocytic leukaemia and was stronger for occupational exposures to second-hand tobacco smoke.

2.5 Other cancers in adults

2.5.1 All cancer combined

Hirayama (1984), Sandler *et al.* (1985b), and Miller (1990) observed a significant association between exposure to second-hand tobacco smoke and overall cancer incidence or mortality. Nishino *et al.* (2001) also studied all cancers combined and reported a relative risk of 1.1 (95%CI: 0.92–1.4) associated with husband's smoking.

2.5.2 Cancers of the gastrointestinal tract

In addition to the studies reviewed previously (Sandler *et al.* 1988; Gerhardsson de Verdier *et al.*, 1992; Mao et.al., 2002), ten new studies have been identified: two cohort (Nishino *et al.*, 2001; Hooker *et al.*, 2008; Table 2.13 available at http://monographs.iarc.fr/ENG/Monographs/vol100E/100E-02-Table2.13.pdf); seven case–control (Sandler *et al.*, 1985a, b; Slattery *et al.*, 2003; Lilla *et al.*, 2006; Wang *et al.*, 2006; Duan *et al.*, 2009; Verla-Tebit *et al.*, 2009; Table 2.14 available at http://monographs.iarc.fr/ENG/Monographs/vol100E/100E-02-Table2.14.pdf) and one case-only study (Peppone *et al.*, 2008; Table 2.15 available at http://monographs.iarc.fr/ENG/Monographs/vol100E/100E-02-Table2.15.pdf). Two studies (Sandler *et al.*, 1985a; Wang *et al.*, 2006) did not provide risk estimates of gastrointestinal cancers for never smokers and are not discussed further. [No data for these studies are included in the tables.]

Sandler *et al.* (1985b) observed a relative risk of 0.7 and 1.3 for cancer of the digestive system from exposure to maternal and paternal passive smoke, respectively. [No CIs were provided and the numbers of never smokers exposed were small.] Verla-Tebit *et al.* (2009) found no evidence of an increased risk for colorectal cancer associated with exposure to second-hand tobacco smoke overall.

(a) Cancer of the colorectum

Nishino *et al.* (2001) observed no association with husband's smoking for cancer of the colon (RR 1.3; CI: 0.65–2.4) or of the rectum (RR 1.8; 0.85–3.9).

Four studies investigated risk for cancer or the colon and/or rectum by sex. Sandler *et al.* (1988) reported an increased risk for colorectal cancer in men (RR 3.0; 95%CI: 1.8–5.0) but a protective effect in women (RR 0.7; 95%CI: 0.6–1.0). Slattery *et al.* (2003) noted that rectal cancer was significantly associated with exposure to second-hand tobacco smoke in men (OR, 1.5; 95%CI: 1.1–2.2 for never smokers) but not in women. Hooker *et al.* (2008) reported an effect among men only, with a significantly increased risk for rectal cancer in the 1963 cohort (RR 5.8, 95%CI: 1.8–18.4) but not the 1975 cohort. Gerhardsson de Verdier *et al.* (1992) found an increased risk for rectal cancer in men (RR 1.9; 95%CI: 1.0–3) and for colon cancer in women (RR 1.8; 95%CI: 1.2–2.8). [The Working Group noted that it is unclear whether the analysis was restricted to never-smokers.]

When analysing different sources of exposure to second-hand tobacco smoke, Verla-Tebit *et al.* (2009) found no evidence of an increased risk for cancer of the colorectum associated with exposure to second-hand tobacco smoke specifically during childhood or at work, but observed a significant increase in risk associated with spousal exposure.

Peppone *et al.* (2008) noted that considerable exposure to second-hand tobacco smoke, especially during childhood, was more likely to lead to an earlier-age diagnosis of cancer of the colorectum.

In exploring the association of cancer of the colorectum with exposure to second-hand tobacco smoke and NAT1 and NAT2 status, Lilla *et al.* (2006) noted that risk may only be relevant among genetically susceptible (NAT1 and NAT2 status) individuals.

(b) Cancer of the stomach

Nishino *et al.* (2001) observed no association with husband's smoking for cancer of the stomach (RR, 0.95; 95%CI: 0.58–1.6).

The two studies on the association of exposure to second-hand tobacco smoke with stomach cancer by subsite (cardia versus distal) gave contradictory results. In one study (Mao *et al.*, 2002) a positive trend ($P = 0.03$) in risk for cancer of the gastric cardia was associated with lifetime exposure to second-hand tobacco smoke (residential plus occupational) in never smoking men, with a relative risk of 5.8 (95%CI: 1.2–27.5) at the highest level of exposure (≥ 43 years); no increased risks or trends were observed for distal gastric cancer. In the other study, Duan *et al.* (2009) an increased risk for distal gastric cancer was found, but not for gastric cardia [Data were not analysed by sex due to small sample size].

2.5.3 Cancer of the pancreas

Six studies have been identified on the association of exposure to second-hand tobacco smoke with cancer of the pancreas: three cohort (Nishino *et al.*, 2001; Gallicchio *et al.*, 2006; Bao *et al.*, 2009; the latter two are summarized in Table 2.17 available at http://monographs.iarc.fr/ENG/Monographs/vol100E/100E-02-Table2.17.pdf) and three case–control (Villeneuve *et al.*, 2004; Hassan *et al.*, 2007; Lo *et al.*, 2007; the former two studies are summarized in Table 2.18 available at http://monographs.iarc.fr/ENG/Monographs/vol100E/100E-02-Table2.18.pdf).

(a) Exposure in adulthood

Data from the majority of the studies (Nishino *et al.*, 2001; Villeneuve *et al.*, 2004; Gallicchio *et al.*, 2006; Hassan *et al.*, 2007; Bao *et al.*, 2009) suggested lack of an association of cancer of the pancreas with never smokers exposed to second-hand tobacco smoke in adulthood at home or at work. (RR 1.2 (95%CI: 0.45–3.1) and 1.21 (95%CI: 0.60–2.44) respectively).

Lo *et al.* (2007) reported an odd ratio of 6.0 (95%CI: 2.4 –14.8) for never smokers (both sexes combined) exposed to second-hand tobacco smoke in Egypt. [The Working Group noted the small numbers of cases, the use of hospital controls and the small proportion of the cases (35%) with histopathological confirmation. Data are not included in Table 2.18 on-line].

(b) Exposure during childhood

In the Nurses' Health Study, Bao *et al.* (2009) noted an increased risk for cancer of the pancreas (RR 1.42; 95%CI: 1.07–1.89) for maternal but not for paternal smoking (RR 0.97; 95%CI: 0.77–1.21) during childhood.

2.5.4 Cancer of the kidney (renal cell carcinoma)

Two case–control studies have been published on the association of exposure to second-hand tobacco smoke with cancer of the kidney (specifically renal cell carcinoma) since IARC (2004) (Hu *et al.*, 2005; Theis *et al.*, 2008; Table 2.19 available at http://monographs.iarc.fr/ENG/Monographs/vol100E/100E-02-Table2.19.pdf). In both studies a significantly increased risk associated with exposure to second-hand tobacco smoke among never smokers was reported.

2.5.5 Cancer of the urinary bladder

A total of seven studies and one meta-analysis have considered the association between exposure to second-hand tobacco smoke and cancer of the urinary bladder: three cohort studies (Zeegers *et al.*, 2002; Bjerregaard *et al.*, 2006; Alberg *et al.*, 2007; Table 2.9, available at http://monographs.iarc.fr/ENG/Monographs/vol100E/100E-02-Table2.9.pdf), four case–control studies (Burch *et al.*, 1989; Chen *et al.*, 2005a; Samanic *et al.*, 2006; Jiang *et al.*, 2007; Table 2.10 available at http://monographs.iarc.fr/ENG/Monographs/vol100E/100E-02-Table2.10.pdf), and one meta-analysis (Van Hemelrijck *et al.*, 2009).

(a) Population-based exposure-response relationship

Burch *et al.* (1989) and Zeegers *et al.* (2002) reported no increased risk for cancer of the urinary bladder [Data are not included in the Tables]. Van Hemelrijck *et al.* (2009) reported a meta-relative risk of 0.99 (95%CI: 0.86–1.14) for never smokers exposed to second-hand tobacco smoke. [Data not included in Table. The Working Group noted the marked variation in risk in the analyses by sex and by timing of exposure to second-hand tobacco smoke during adulthood or childhood].

In the European Prospective Investigation into Cancer and Nutrition (EPIC) study, Bjerregaard *et al.* (2006) compared ever versus never exposed to second-hand tobacco smoke as an adult or a child: the risk for cancer of the urinary bladder increased for exposures during childhood (OR, 1.38; 95%CI: 1.00–1.90), and was stronger for never-smokers (OR, 2.02; 95%CI: 0.94–4.35).

Alberg *et al.* (2007) analysed data from two cohorts of non-smoking women in the USA exposed to second-hand smoke at home. An association with exposure to second-hand tobacco smoke was found in the 1963 cohort (RR, 2.3; 95%CI: 1.0–5.4) but not in the 1975 cohort (RR, 0.9; 95%CI: 0.4–2.3). [The Working Group noted the small number of cases available for some of the risk estimates.]

In a study assessing occupational exposure to second-hand tobacco smoke (Samanic *et al.*, 2006), the risk for cancer of the urinary bladder was increased in the highest exposure category among women (RR, 3.3; 95%CI: 1.1–9.5) but not among men (RR, 0.6; 95%CI: 0.2–1.4).

(b) Molecular-based exposure-response relationship

4-aminobiphenyl (4-ABP) can form DNA adducts and induce mutations, and cigarette smoke is the most prominent source of exposure to 4-aminobiphenyl in humans (see Section 4). Jiang *et al.* (2007) used variation in 4-ABP-haemoglobin adducts levels to assess exposure to second-hand tobacco smoke and reported a significantly increased risk with increasing lifetime exposure among never-smoking women exposed in adulthood or childhood.

Chen *et al.* (2005a) hypothesized that the ability to detoxify arsenic (a risk factor urinary bladder cancer) through methylation may modify risk related to second-hand tobacco smoke exposure. Results of the adjusted analyses show that a high primary methylation index associates with lower risk of cancer of the urinary bladder (OR, 0.37; 95%CI: 0.14–0.96, p interaction = 0.11) in second-hand tobacco smoke exposed subjects compared to unexposed. In endemic area the ability to methylate arsenic may play a role in reducing the risk of cancer of the urinary bladder associated with second-hand tobacco smoke exposure. [The Working Group noted that the small number of cases and the use of hospital controls limit the validity of inferences from this study].

Using case–control data for never and former smokers nested within the EPIC study Vineis *et al.* (2007b) examined susceptibility in genes involved in oxidative stress (such as *NQO1*, *MPO*, *COMT*, *MnSOD*), in phase I (such as *CYP1A1* and *CYP1B1*) and phase II (such as *GSTM1*, and *GSTT1*) metabolizing genes, and in methylene-tetrahydrofolate (*MTHFR*). *GSTM1* deletion was strongly associated with risk for urinary bladder cancer in never smokers (OR, 1.75; 95%CI: 0.89–3.43), and a similar association was noted for former smokers and for men.

2.5.6 Cancer of the cervix

The cohort studies evaluated previously (Hirayama, 1984; Jee *et al.*, 1999; Nishino *et al.*, 2001) consistently indicated the lack of association between exposure to second-hand tobacco smoke and cancer of the uterine cervix, while the informative case–control studies (Sandler *et al.*, 1985b; Slattery *et al.*, 1989; Scholes *et al.*, 1999) suggested a non-statistically significant increase in risk.

A total of 10 new studies have been identified: one cohort study (Table 2.11 available at http://monographs.iarc.fr/ENG/Monographs/vol100E/100E-02-Table2.11.pdf) and nine case–control studies (Buckley *et al.*, 1981; Brown *et al.*, 1982; Hellberg *et al.*, 1986; Hirose *et al.*, 1996; Coker *et al.*, 2002; Wu *et al.*, 2003; Tay & Tay, 2004; Sobti *et al.*, 2006; Tsai *et al.*, 2007; Table 2.12 available at http://monographs.iarc.fr/ENG/Monographs/vol100E/100E-02-Table2.12.pdf). Three early case–control studies (Buckley *et al.*, 1981; Brown *et al.*, 1982; Hellberg *et al.*, 1986) did not look at risk of exposure to second-hand tobacco smoke in never smoking women, and are not further discussed.

(a) Squamous cell carcinoma of the cervix

A significant increase risk for invasive cancer of the uterine cervix associated with exposure to second-hand tobacco smoke during adulthood was found in three case–control studies (Hirose *et al.*, 1996; Wu *et al.*, 2003; Tay & Tay, 2004) and one cohort study (Trimble *et al.*, 2005).

(b) Cervical intraepithelial lesions and neoplasia

An earlier case–control study (Coker *et al.*, 1992) found no statistically significant association between exposure to second-hand tobacco smoke and CIN II/III in non-smokers, after adjustment for age, race, education, number of partners, contraceptive use, history of sexually transmitted disease and history of Pap smear. A later study (Coker *et al.*, 2002) looked at risk of low grade and high grade cervical squamous intraepithelial lesions (LSIL and HSIL, respectively) in HPV positive never-smokers and reported a significant association with exposure to second-hand tobacco smoke. In a community-based case–control study, Tsai *et al.* (2007) observed a markedly increased risk for both CIN1 and CIN2 in both HPV-positive and HPV-negative women exposed to second-hand tobacco smoke. Only Coker *et al.* (2002) and Tsai *et al.* (2007) controlled for HPV status in women.

Sobti *et al.* (2006) reported that cervical cancer risk is increased in individuals exposed to second-hand tobacco smoke with *GSTM1* (null), *GSTT1* (null) and *GSTP1* ($Ile^{105}Val$) genotypes, with odd ratios ranging from 6.4 to 10.2.

2.5.7 Cancer of the ovary

One cohort study (Nishino *et al.*, 2001) and two case–control studies (Goodman & Tung, 2003; Baker *et al.*, 2006; Table 2.16 available at http://monographs.iarc.fr/ENG/Monographs/vol100E/100E-02-Table2.16.pdf) have been published on the association of exposure to second-hand tobacco smoke with cancer of the ovary. In all three studies a null or inverse association of cancer of the ovary for never smokers exposed to second-hand tobacco smoke was found. Nishino *et al.* (2001) observed no association with husband's smoking (RR 1.7; 95%CI: 0.6- 5.2). Goodman & Tung (2003) reported no association of exposure to second-hand tobacco smoke during childhood with risk of cancer of the ovary. Baker *et al.* (2006) reported a decreased risk of cancer of the ovary for never smokers exposed to second-hand tobacco smoke (OR, 0.68; 95%CI: 0.46–0.99), with similar findings for former and current smokers.

2.5.8 Tumours of the brain and CNS

A total of three case–control studies (Ryan *et al.*, 1992; Hurley *et al.*, 1996; Phillips *et al.*, 2005) have considered the association of second-hand tobacco smoke and cancers of the brain and central nervous system. Ryan *et al.* (1992) reported an increased risk of meningioma associated with spousal exposure, particularly among women (RR 2.7; 95%CI: 1.2–6.1). In a case–control study of gliomas in Australia no association was found for exposure to second-hand tobacco smoke in never smokers (RR 0.97, 95%CI: 0.61–1.53) (both sexes combined) (Hurley *et al.*, 1996). However Phillips *et al.* (2005) found that spousal smoking was associated with an increased risk for intracranial meningioma in both sexes combined (OR, 2.0; 95%CI: 1.1–3.5), the risk increased with increasing duration of exposure (*P* for trend = 0.02).

2.5.9 Other cancers

One case–control study on hepatocellular cancer (Hassan *et al.*, 2008) and one on cancer of the testis (McGlynn *et al.*, 2006) were published since IARC (2004). Hassan *et al.* (2008) did not find an association with exposure to second-hand tobacco smoke and hepatocellular cancer, while that of McGlynn *et al.* (2006) did not support the hypothesis that maternal smoking is related to the development of cancer of the testis (Table 2.20 available at http://monographs.iarc.fr/ENG/Monographs/vol100E/100E-02-Table2.20.pdf). However, these studies provide limited information on the association of exposure to second-hand tobacco smoke with the risk of these cancers.

2.6 Parental tobacco smoking and childhood cancers

2.6.1. Overview

A large number of studies have evaluated the association of cancer risk in childhood with exposure to parental smoking. However, childhood cancers are extremely heterogeneous, both between major cancer sites and within subtypes. In addition, given the rarity of childhood cancers, studies of specific cancer sites and subtypes that have adequate sample sizes and detailed exposure assessments are difficult to achieve.

(a) Smoking exposure assessment

Parental smoking before and during pregnancy exposes germ cells (spermatozoa and ova) and/or the fetus to the same chemical mixture and levels of tobacco smoke as during active smoking, while post-natal exposure to parental tobacco smoking exposes the offspring to second-hand tobacco smoke. Some studies distinguish whether exposure to parental smoking was preconceptional, *in utero* or postnatal. Even when a study reports only on one time period, exposure may have occurred at all three periods. Exposures to tobacco smoking during each of these periods tend to correlate, in particular, paternal smoking is less likely to change during and after pregnancy. In addition, paternal and maternal smoking habits are highly correlated (Boffetta *et al.*, 2000).

Most studies assessed the number of cigarettes smoked per day (e.g. 0–10, 11–20, 20+) and, when data were available, some assessed continuous consumption of cigarettes per day. One study reported exposure in pack-years (Lee *et al.*, 2009). The SEARC international case–control study assessed polycyclic aromatic hydrocarbons (PAHs) as the main exposure of interest and obtained information on both tobacco smoke and occupational exposures (Cordier *et al.*, 2004).

(b) Bias and confounding

Whitehead *et al.* (2009) evaluated the adequacy of self-reported smoking histories on 469 homes of leukaemia cases and controls and found that nicotine concentrations derived from interview responses to a structured questionnaire strongly correlated to measured levels in dust samples.

The major confounders for the relationship between parental smoking and childhood cancers were markers of socioeconomic status, race or ethnicity, birth weight or gestational age, parental age, sex and age of the case child. In most studies matching or adjusting for these confounders was performed as appropriate. In some studies matching was performed for birth order and centre of diagnosis.

2.6.2 All childhood cancers combined

In addition to the four cohort and 10 case–control studies reviewed by IARC (2004), three case–control studies have examined the role of second-hand tobacco smoke in relation to risk for all childhood cancers combined (Sorahan *et al.*, 2001; Pang *et al.*, 2003; Sorahan & Lancashire, 2004; Table 2.21 available at http://monographs.iarc.fr/ENG/Monographs/vol100E/100E-02-Table2.21.pdf).

(a) Intensity and timing of parental smoking

In a follow-up of the Inter-Regional Epidemiological Study of Childhood Cancer (IRESCC) by McKinney *et al.* (1987), a statistically significant positive trend with daily paternal smoking before pregnancy was observed when cases were compared with controls selected from General Practitioners' (GPs') lists, but not from hospitals; an inverse trend was noted for maternal smoking before pregnancy when cases were compared with hospital, but not with General Practitioners, controls (Sorahan *et al.*, 2001).

In the United Kingdom Childhood Cancer Study (UKCCS), Pang *et al.* (2003) observed a similar pattern of increasing risk with increasing intensity of paternal preconception smoking, and of decreasing risk for increasing maternal smoking before and during pregnancy for all diagnoses combined, and for most individual diagnostic groups.

In the most recent report from the Oxford Survey of Childhood Cancers (OSCC), the risk of death from all childhood cancers combined was not associated with maternal smoking, but was consistently associated with paternal smoking alone or in combination with maternal smoking, in both adjusted and unadjusted analyses [Ex-smokers of more than 2 years before birth of the survey child were assimilated to non-smokers] (Sorahan & Lancashire, 2004).

(b) Bias and confounding

The significant trends observed by Sorahan *et al.* (2001) and Pang & Birch (2003) did not diminish when adjusted for potential confounding covariates or with simultaneous analysis of parental smoking habits. The relationship between maternal smoking and birth weight reported by Sorahan *et al.* (2001) suggested that self-reported maternal smoking was equally reliable for cases and for controls. However, comparisons of smoking patterns with national data suggested that control parents in this study were heavier smokers.

2.6.3 Leukaemias and lymphomas

Since IARC (2004), one cohort study (Mucci *et al.*, 2004) (Table 2.22 available at http://monographs.iarc.fr/ENG/Monographs/vol100E/100E-02-Table2.22.pdf), eleven case–control studies (Table 2.23 available at http://monographs.iarc.fr/ENG/Monographs/vol100E/100E-02-Table2.23.pdf), and one meta-analysis (Lee *et al.*, 2009) (Table 2.24 available at http://monographs.iarc.fr/ENG/Monographs/vol100E/100E-02-Table2.24.pdf) have evaluated the association of parental tobacco smoking with the risk for lymphatic and haematopoietic cancers.

(a) Duration and intensity of exposure

From a meta-analysis of 30 studies published before 1999 Boffetta *et al.* (2000) reported no statistically significant association for all lymphatic and haematopoietic neoplasms and noted evidence of publication bias for the available data.

Lee *et al.* (2009) performed a meta-analysis of twelve studies on paternal smoking and risk of childhood leukaemia. Paternal smoking before conception of the index child was significantly associated with the risk for acute leukaemia (AL) and acute lymphoblastic leukaemia (ALL) (Fig. 2.2).

In a cohort study, maternal smoking was associated with a lower risk of acute lymphoblastic leukaemia, a higher risk of acute myeloid leukaemia (AML) particularly among heavy smokers, and a slight excess risk for non-Hodgkin lymphoma (NHL) (Mucci *et al.*, 2004).

Because of the diversity of types of exposure (paternal, maternal, parental), of timing of exposure (preconception, *in utero*, post-natally) and of the outcome, the case–control studies are briefly summarized individually.

Schüz *et al.* (1999) showed that the risk for acute childhood leukaemias was inversely related to maternal smoking during pregnancy. Paternal smoking before pregnancy showed no association with leukaemia risk for any smoking category. Sorahan *et al.* (2001) reported a non-significant positive association between risk for acute lymphoblastic leukaemia and daily cigarette smoking by fathers before pregnancy, and a non-significant inverse association between risk for acute lymphoblastic leukaemia and daily smoking by mothers before pregnancy. Down Syndrome children are highly susceptible to the development of acute leukaemia. In a case–control study of 27 children with acute leukaemia and Down Syndrome compared with 58 Down Syndrome children without acute leukaemia Mejía-Aranguré *et al.* (2003) found that paternal smoking of more than 10 cigarettes/day, both preconception and after birth of the index child was associated with acute leukaemia. In the UKCC case–control study (Pang *et al.*, 2003), paternal but not maternal preconception tobacco smoking of 1–19 cigarettes/day was associated with an increased risk of leukaemia, and a similar pattern was reported for lymphoma. Menegaux *et al.* (2005) reported no increased risk of acute lymphoblastic leukaemia or acute nonlymphocytic leukaemia (ANLL) associated with any category of post-natal exposure to tobacco smoking (i.e. maternal smoking during breastfeeding or after, paternal smoking after birth, other smokers at home), except for an increased risk of acute nonlymphocytic leukaemia with paternal smoking. In a later study, (Menegaux *et al.*, 2007) reported no association between acute and parental smoking, by subtype (acute myeloid leukaemia or acute lymphoblastic leukaemia) or by time of exposure, with the exception of an increased risk of acute lymphoblastic leukaemia associated with maternal smoking during pregnancy. Chang *et al.* (2006) reported

Fig. 2.2 Meta-analysis of the association between paternal smoking and childhood leukaemia

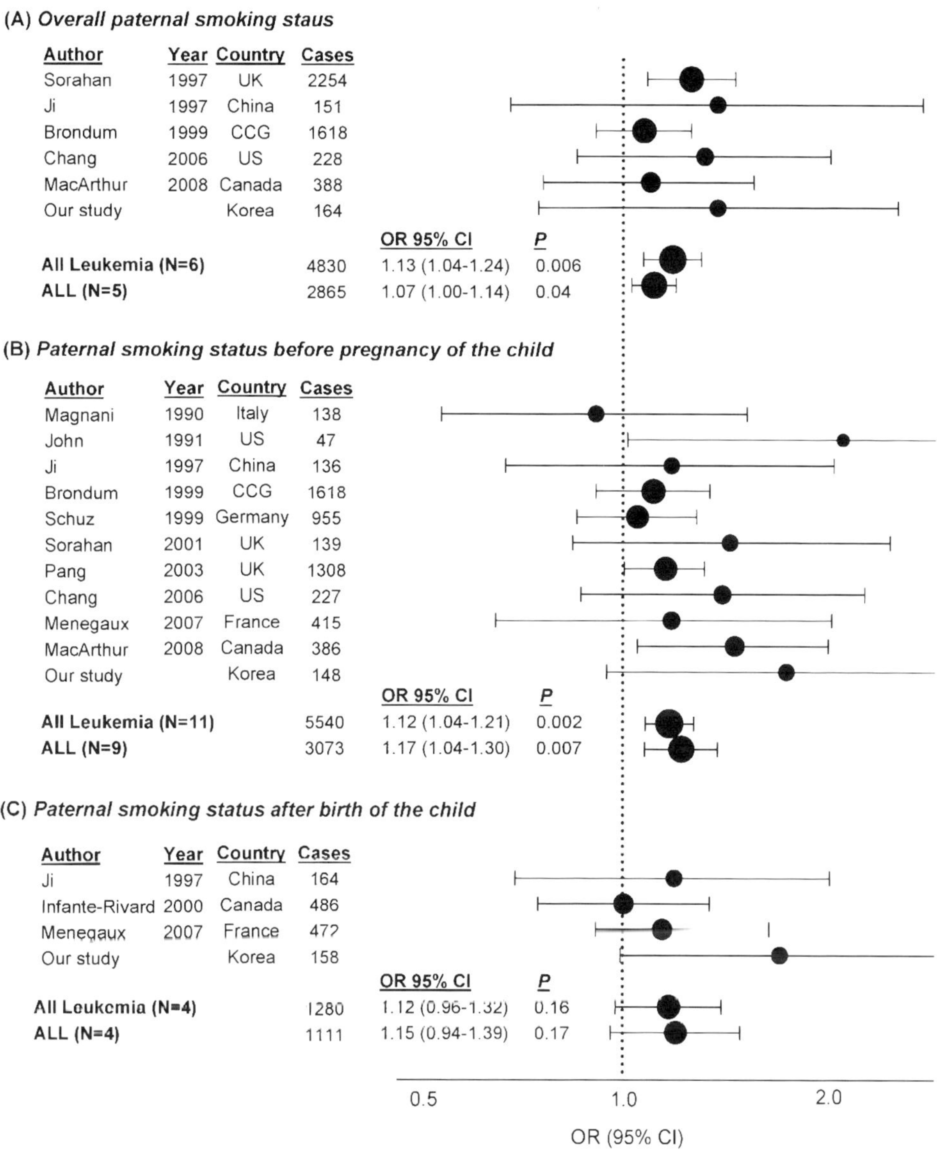

no risk for acute leukaemia, acute lymphoblastic leukaemia or acute myeloid leukaemia associated with maternal smoking either by period of smoking (preconception, during pregnancy, post-natally) or by amount smoked. Paternal preconception smoking was strongly associated with risk for acute myeloid leukaemia both by period and intensity of smoking. When both paternal preconception smoking and maternal postnatal smoking were considered, the risk for acute lymphoblastic leukaemia was stronger. Rudant *et al.* (2008) reported a significant positive association between paternal smoking and acute lymphoblastic leukaemia, acute myeloid leukaemia, Burkitt lymphoma, and anaplastic large cell non-Hodgkin lymphoma, with increasing relative risks (RR) with increasing number of cigarettes smoked. No associations with Hodgkin lymphoma or other types of non-Hodgkin lymphoma were observed. Non-significantly elevated risks were observed for maternal smoking during pregnancy for acute lymphoblastic leukaemia and non-Hodgkin lymphoma, but not in the highest category of 10 or more cigarettes/day. MacArthur *et al.* (2008) reported non-significantly elevated risk estimates for acute lymphoblastic leukaemia and acute myeloid leukaemia with maternal smoking, but not with paternal smoking, before and during pregnancy. Lee *et al.* (2009) in Seoul, Republic of Korea, reported that paternal smoking was associated with a significantly increased risk of acute leukaemia and acute lymphoblastic leukaemia in a dose–response manner. The proportion of mothers who smoked was too low (6.1% in controls) to analyse risk in association with maternal smoking.

(b) Potential confounders

In the study of Down Syndrome children (Mejía-Aranguré *et al.*, 2003), the adjustment models did not show any interaction between paternal alcoholism and smoking. Menegaux *et al.* (2005) examined the association of parental smoking and maternal alcohol and coffee intake during pregnancy with the risk for childhood leukaemia. They found no association of acute lymphoblastic leukaemia or acute nonlymphocytic leukaemia with maternal smoking during pregnancy but an association with maternal alcohol and coffee consumption.

(c) Effect modification

Cigarette smoke is a known germ-cell mutagen in mice (Yauk *et al.*, 2007), a likely germ-cell mutagen in humans (see Section 4.1.3a) and alters gene expression (see Section 4.1.4). Infante-Rivard *et al.* (2000) first assessed the role of parental smoking and *CYP1A1* genetic polymorphisms with leukaemia and reported no statistically significant association with leukaemia overall. However, a case-only subanalysis suggested that the effect of parental smoking may be modified by variant alleles in the *CYP1A1* gene: *CYP1A1*2B* tended to decrease risks and *CYP1A1*2A* and *CYP1A1*4* increased the risks associated with smoking in the second and third trimesters of pregnancy. Clavel *et al.* (2005) examined the role of metabolic polymorphisms in the *CYP1A1*, *GSTM1*, *GSTP1*, *GSTT1* and *NQO1* genes. The slow *EPHX1* allele (exon 3 homozygous genotype) was negatively associated with leukaemia, in particular acute lymphoblastic leukaemia, whereas the fast *EPHX1* allele (exon 4 homozygous genotype) was positively associated with leukaemia overall. A non-significant association with acute lymphoblastic leukaemia was noted for the homozygous *NQO1*2* genotype. There was a significant interaction of the *CYP1A1*2A* allele with smoking in the case-only analysis and a not significant interaction, but similar in magnitude, in the case–control analysis. A significant interaction was also observed with the *GSTM1* deletion in the case-only analysis, but not in the case–control analysis. Lee *et al.* (2009) genotyped five single-nucleotide *CYP1A1* polymorphisms: acute lymphoblastic leukaemia risk was significantly increased for cases without the *CGACC* haplotype and with paternal smoking or the presence of at least one smoker in the home.

RAS is the second most mutated gene in smoking-associated lung tumours (Section 4.1.3b). *RAS* mutations have been consistently correlated with myeloid leukaemias in adults and children, in particular with occupationally-associated adult myeloid leukemias (Taylor *et al.*, 1992; Barletta *et al.*, 2004). Wiemels *et al.* (2005) studied the relationship of *RAS* mutations, hyperdiploidy (> 50 chromosomes) and smoking in a case series of 191 acute leukaemia. Smoking was negatively associated with hyperdiploidy (possibly due to the sensitivity of the hyperdiploid clone and consequent differential survival) and hyperdiploid acute leukaemia cases had the highest rates of *RAS* mutations. [Paternal smoking in the three months before pregnancy was less frequent among hyperdiploids than among non-hyperdiploids.]

2.6.4 Cancers of the brain and central nervous system

Since IARC (2004), the association of exposure to parental smoking and risk for childhood brain and central nervous system (CNS) tumours has been examined in one cohort study (Brooks *et al.*, 2004; Table 2.25 available at http://monographs.iarc.fr/ENG/Monographs/vol100E/100E-02-Table2.25.pdf), six case–control studies (Schüz *et al.*, 1999; Sorahan *et al.*, 2001; Filippini *et al.*, 2002; Pang *et al.*, 2003; Cordier *et al.*, 2004; Plichart *et al.*, 2008; Table 2.26 available at http://monographs.iarc.fr/ENG/Monographs/vol100E/100E-02-Table2.26.pdf), and one meta-analysis (Huncharek *et al.*, 2002; Table 2.27 available at http://monographs.iarc.fr/ENG/Monographs/vol100E/100E-02-Table2.27.pdf).

A meta-analysis of 30 studies published before 1999 indicated no significant increase in risk for CNS tumours associated with maternal smoking during pregnancy and an increased risk for brain tumours with paternal smoking (Boffetta *et al.*, 2000).

Huncharek *et al.* (2002) included one cohort and eleven case–control studies in a meta-analysis and found no clear association of maternal smoking during pregnancy with risk for childhood brain tumours, and a null risk estimate for all CNS tumours (even when the analysis was restricted to astrocytomas, the main brain tumour type). The results were comparable and consistently null for all sensitivity analyses conducted (Table 2.27 on-line).

Brooks *et al.* (2004) analysing the Swedish birth cohort study observed that children, in particular those aged 2–4 years, whose mother smoked during pregnancy, had an increased incidence of childhood brain tumours; the increase in risk was similar for benign and malignant brain tumours and most apparent for astrocytomas (Table 2.25 on-line).

Schüz *et al.* (1999) evaluated parental smoking and CNS tumour risk in children < 15 years from the German Childhood Cancer Registry (see Table 2.26 on-line). No association with risk of CNS tumours was observed for either maternal smoking during pregnancy or paternal smoking before pregnancy. Sorahan *et al.* (2001) found no significant association or trends of risk of CNS tumours with either paternal or maternal smoking, except for low level of maternal exposure [the latter analysis is based on only eleven exposed cases and one control, yielding a very wide confidence interval]. Filippini *et al.* (2002) observed no association between risk of childhood brain tumours and parental smoking before pregnancy, maternal smoking, regular maternal exposure to second-hand tobacco smoke during pregnancy, or exposure of the child to second-hand tobacco smoke during its first year of life. The results did not vary by child's age at diagnosis, type of CNS tumour or study centre. Plichart *et al.* (2008) reported no association for maternal smoking during pregnancy with CNS tumours, while paternal smoking preconception showed a significant association, especially for astrocytomas. When assessing parental exposure to PAHs, Cordier *et al.* (2004) observed an association of paternal exposure to occupational PAHs preconception with all childhood brain tumours and with astroglial tumours, but no trend of increasing risk with increased exposure. Paternal smoking alone was associated with a risk for astroglial tumours when compared with non-smoking, non-occupationally-exposed fathers. Pang *et al.* (2003) found a decreased CNS risk with maternal smoking of more than 20 cigarettes/day preconception, in both unadjusted and adjusted analyses. In the analyses by histological subgroups a statistically significant decreased risk was associated with maternal smoking during pregnancy for primitive neuroectodermal tumours.

2.6.5 Hepatoblastoma

Hepatoblastoma is an embryonal tumour presumably of fetal origin and prenatal exposures are likely more important than post-natal. In some children, a diagnosis of hepatoblastoma is evident at birth or shortly thereafter, with a median age at diagnosis of 12 months. The ability of hepatoblastoma tumour cells to synthesize α-fetoprotein (AFP), a major serum protein synthesized by fetal liver cells, also suggests a fetal origin. Also, hepatoblastomas, like many other embryonal tumours, are associated with Beckwith-Wiedemann syndrome and hemihypertrophy, further suggesting a gestational oncogenic event (DeBaun & Tucker, 1998). Data were available for both maternal and paternal exposures from two studies (Pang *et al.*, 2003; Sorahan & Lancashire, 2004) while two other studies (McLaughlin *et al.*, 2006; Pu *et al.*, 2009) were limited to data on maternal smoking, available from birth certificates and medical records, respectively (Table 2.28). Most of these studies had limited sample sizes given the extreme rarity of these tumours.

(a) Parental smoking exposure

After adjustment for relevant covariates, Pang *et al.* (2003) observed a statistically significant increased risk of hepatoblastoma in association with maternal preconception smoking (OR, 2.68; 95%CI: 1.16–6.21, $P = 0.02$) in a somewhat dose-dependent manner ($P = 0.058$). The association with parental smoking was strongest (relative to neither parent smoking) when both parents smoked (OR, 4.74; 95%CI: 1.68–13.35, $P = 0.003$). Sorahan & Lancashire (2004) found no increased risk associated with maternal or paternal smoking alone compared to non-smokers, in both adjusted and unadjusted analyses. In contrast, parental smoking (paternal and maternal smoking combined) was strongly and consistently associated with an increased risk for hepatoblastoma in both adjusted and unadjusted analyses.

In a record-based case–cohort study only maternal smoking was examined (McLaughlin *et al.*, 2006). Extremely low birth weight (< 1000 g) was strongly associated with hepatoblastoma. After adjustement for birth weight, a statistically significant elevated risk for hepatoblastoma was found with maternal smoking (RR 2.1; 95%CI: 1.0–4.2). The increased risk was stronger for children diagnosed at the age of two years or older (RR 6.0 versus 1.4). Also, the relarive risk for maternal smoking and hepatoblastoma was stronger for children with normal birth weight [> 2500 g] than for low birth weight children. For cases of hepatoblastoma diagnosed after the age of two years, the relative risk for maternal smoking among children with normal birth weight was also stronger than that among children with low birth weight.

Another study on maternal smoking only was conducted in Chonquing, China (Pu *et al.*, 2009). After adjustment for birth weight, a significantly increased risk for hepatoblastoma was found for maternal smoking (RR 2.9; 95%CI: 1.1–4.2). Adjustments for maternal age, maternal body mass index and sex of the baby did not change the odd ratios. When analyses were stratified by birth weight, the odd ratio associated with maternal smoking for children with a birth weight greater than 2500 g was increased almost fourfold. Stratification by age at diagnosis showed that the risk increased almost fivefold with diagnosis at the age of two years or over. [The Working Group noted that since information regarding mother's smoking status for both cases and controls was obtained before diagnosis the potential for biased recall of maternal exposures during pregnancy is reduced].

(b) Bias and confounding

The known risk factors for hepatoblastoma include low and very low birth weights (< 2000 g and < 1000 g, respectively), maternal age and

Table 2.28 Studies of parental tobacco smoking and childhood hepatoblastoma

Reference, study location and period	Characteristics of cases	Characteristics of controls	Exposure assessment	Exposure categories (case/control)	(Cases/ controls)	OR (95% CI)* * $P < 0.05$ ** $P < 0.01$	Adjustment for potential confounders	Comments
Pang *et al.* (2003) United Kingdom	3838 childhood cancer cases, of which 28 hepatoblastoma; Hospital based; < 15 yr of age; 1991–94 in Scotland; 1992–94 in England and Wales	7581 controls; matched for sex, date of birth and geographical area of residence at diagnosis; randomly selected from Family Health Services Authorities in England and Wales and Health boards in Scotland	Face-to-face structured interviews; Computerized self-administered questionnaires to parents of index child	*Parental smoking*			Deprivation and parental age at birth of index child	Underreporting of smoking by case mothers
				Neither parent	(8/3142)	1.00 (ref)		
				Mother only	(2/574)	2.02 (0.40–10.2)		
				Father only	(3/1008)	1.86 (0.46–7.55)		
				Both parents	(10/1249) **	4.74 (1.68–13.35)		
				Paternal preconception smoking (cigarettes per d)				
				0	(11/3082)	1 (ref)		
				1–19	(6/1003)	1.88 (0.67–5.26)		
				20+	(7/1440)	1.65 (0.61–4.45)		
				Trend *P*	0.272			
				Maternal preconception smoking (cigarettes per d)				
				0	(10/3916)	1 (ref)		
				1–19	(9/1490)	2.99 (1.15–7.76)*		
				20+	(4/882)	2.17 (0.65–7.20)		
				P for trend	0.058			
Pang & Birch (2003) United Kingdom	Birch and Kelsey diagnostic subgroups, which group biologically similar tumours together (UKCCS Investigators, 2000) excluding diagnostic subgroups with less than 10 cases			*Maternal preconception smoking*	(28/7581)	2.68 (1.16–6.21)*	§ As above, additionally adjusted for birth weight	
				Both parents preconception smoking	(27/6987)	4.74**		
				§ *Maternal preconception smoking*		2.50*		
				§ *Both parents preconception smoking*		4.97**		

Table 2.28 (continued)

Reference, study location and period	Characteristics of cases	Characteristics of controls	Exposure assessment	Exposure categories (case/control)	(Cases/ controls)	OR (95% CI)* * $P < 0.05$ ** $P < 0.01$	Adjustment for potential confounders	Comments
Sorahan & Lancashire (2004) United Kingdom, 1953–84	43 deaths from hepatoblastoma < 16 yr of age	5777 matched controls, (analysed as unmatched series)	Parental smoking during yr 1953–55, 1971–76, 1977–81	*Maternal cigarette smoking*			Sex, age at death, yr of death, social class, sibship position, age of mother and father at birth of child, obstetric radiography	
				Non-smoker	(19/3191)	1 (ref)		
				Smoker	(24/2524)	1.73 (0.93–3.21)		
				Paternal cigarette smoking				
				Non-smoker	(12/2267)	1 (ref)		
				Smoker	(28/3359)	2.10 (1.03–4.25)*		
				Parental cigarette smoking				
				Neither parent	(9/1601)	1.0 (ref)		
				Mother only	(3/662)	0.85 (0.23–3.19)		
				Father only	(8/1545)	1.23 (0.46–3.28)		
				Both parents	(20/1800)	2.69 (1.18–6.13)*		
McLaughlin *et al.* (2006), New York, USA, 1985–2001	58 cases of hepatoblastoma, identified from New York State Cancer Registry	Matched on yr of birth, electronic birth records for 1985–2001 from New York State	Routinely recorded data on birth certificate	*Maternal smoking*			Birth yr and birth weight	Association of maternal smoking was stronger in children with birth weights over 2.5kg.
				Non-smoker	(36/3439)	1 (ref)		
				Smoker	(12/742)	2.1 (1.0–4.2)		
				Birth weight > 2500 g		2.7 (1.2–5.5)		
				Birth weight > 2500 g and age > 2 yr		5.8 (1.4–25.1)		
Pu *et al.* (2009), Chongquing China, 1990–97	58 cases	92 controls, appendicitis patients, matched on age, sex, yr	Medical record of mother or follow-up interviews as needed	*Maternal smoking*			Birth weight	
				Non-smoker	(43/84)	1 (ref)		
				Smoker	(15/8)	2.9 (1.1–4.2)		

d, day or days; yr, year or years

use of assisted reproductive technologies. All studies adjusted for maternal age, and low birth weight was addressed in three of them (Pang & Birch, 2003; McLaughlin *et al.*, 2006; Pu *et al.*, 2009). Assisted reproductive technologies were not considered to be an important potential confounder of these studies.

Spector & Ross (2003) argued that the association of hepatoblastoma with parental smoking observed by Pang *et al.* (2003) might be confounded by birth weight. In their response, Pang & Birch (2003) showed evidence supporting their initial conclusion: the comparable results for maternal smoking, smoking by both parents and maternal smoking for cases diagnosed at an older age, i.e. one year or older, before and after adjustment for birth weight, appear to rule out low birth weight as an explanation for the association.

Also, both later studies (McLaughlin *et al.*, 2006; Pu *et al.*, 2009) reported higher relative risks for children with normal birth weight compared to those with low birth weight, particularly in cases diagnosed after the age of two years.

2.6.6 Other childhood cancers

Several other childhood cancers have been studied in relation to parental tobacco smoke exposures, namely neuroblastoma, nephroblastoma, bone tumours, Wilms tumour, soft tissue sarcomas, other neoplasms of the reticuloendothelial system, and childhood germ cell tumours. The data are few and inconsistent (Schüz *et al.*, 1999; Sorahan *et al.*, 2001; Chen *et al.*, 2005b; Table 2.28).

2.7 Synthesis

2.7.1 Lung

The totality of evidence available to date firmly establishes that exposure to second-hand tobacco smoke at home and at the workplace is causally associated with lung cancer risk in both men and women. This association has been observed in studies from North America, Europe, and Asia. Emerging evidence is also suggesting that exposure to second-hand tobacco smoke among children significantly enhances the risk of lung cancer in adulthood.

2.7.2 Breast

A large number of cohort studies, case–control studies and meta-analyses have assessed the association between exposure to second-hand tobacco smoke and breast cancer. Recent large cohort studies in Europe and North America showed no association between second-hand tobacco smoke and breast cancer. Positive associations in one or more subgroups were reported from some case–control studies; however, these associations were weaker in more recent studies compared with earlier studies.

Explorative analyses focusing on premenopausal breast cancer have suggested that second-hand tobacco smoke may preferentially cause premenopausal breast cancer. Positive associations were largely reported from case–control studies, in which both recall and publication bias cannot be ruled out. Case–control studies that collect a lifetime exposure history are particularly vulnerable to subjective and differential reporting of exposures that occurred long in the past from sources that are difficult to quantify. Overall, the results for an association with premenopausal breast cancer are also inconsistent.

2.7.3 Upper aerodigestive tract combined

Most evidence of the association between second-hand tobacco smoke and upper aerodigestive tract cancers, and the subsites of the oral cavity, pharynx and larynx, comes from a pooled analysis. Overall, the association between second-hand tobacco smoke exposure and cancers of the larynx and pharynx is less than causal.

2.7.4 Nasopharynx, and nasal cavity and accesory sinuses

There is some evidence from a cohort and case–control study that exposure to second-hand tobacco smoke increases the risk of sinonasal cancer; for cancer of the nasopharynx, the evidence is contradictory.

2.7.5 Others sites

Overall, data are conflicting and sparse for the association of exposure to second-hand tobacco smoke with all cancers combined, cancers of the gastrointestinal tract combined, and cancers of the stomach, colon, rectum, pancreas, liver (hepatocellular carcinoma), kidney (renal cell carcinoma), urinary bladder, cervix, ovary, testes, and brain and central nervous system.

2.7.6 Childhood cancers

(a) All childhood cancers combined

Four cohort studies, 13 case–control studies and one meta-analysis have assessed the association of parental tobacco smoking with childhood cancers, all sites combined, in offspring. Most of the early studies only assessed the contribution of maternal smoking, whereas recent studies generally assessed both paternal and maternal smoking, and at various time periods (preconception, during pregnancy, post-natally). Overall, the evidence for an association between parental smoking and childhood cancer (all sites combined) remains inconsistent and may be subject to bias. Nevertheless, a fairly consistent association of paternal tobacco smoking with childhood cancers is beginning to emerge, which is stronger in studies with more specific exposure assessments.

(b) Leukaemias and lymphomas

Two cohort studies, 27 case–control studies and 2 meta-analyses have examined the association of childhood haematopoietic malignancies (leukaemia and lymphoma) with exposure to parental smoking (paternal, maternal or both). All studies examined leukaemia, and a large number of these addressed non-Hodgkin lymphoma.

The body of evidence suggests a consistent association of leukaemia (and lymphoma) with paternal smoking preconception and with combined parental smoking, with risk ratios ranging from 1.5 to 4.0. Maternal tobacco smoking during pregnancy generally showed modest increases in risk, or null or inverse relationships. The combined effects of preconception and post-conception exposures to tobacco smoke were highly significant.

Several studies on lymphoma risk associated with parental smoking showed significantly elevated risks associated with paternal tobacco smoking preconception. The analyses had small samples sizes, and biases due to participation, recall and response, especially related to exposure, cannot be ruled out.

(c) Brain and central nervous system

The association of childhood tumours of the brain and central nervous system with parental smoking was assessed in two cohort studies, 21 case–control studies and 2 meta-analyses. Overall these studies do not show an association with either paternal smoking, largely preconception, or maternal smoking prior, during or after pregnancy, or by CNS types, gliomas and primitive neuroectodermal tumours. The strongly positive associations noted in some studies for paternal tobacco smoking with astrocytomas are offset by the lack of association with childhood brain tumours reported by the large UK Childhood Cancer Study.

(d) Hepatoblastoma

Four informative case–control studies provided data on the association between parental smoking and hepatoblastomas. Two studies reported on both maternal and paternal smoking, while the two others assessed only maternal smoking. In one study where a large number of categories of childhood cancers ($n = 25$) were assessed, the only childhood cancer that showed an association with parental smoking was hepatoblastoma. This original observation was confirmed in three later studies, with relative risks ranging from 2.0 to 5.5. Chance, bias and confounding were adequately addressed in the data from the studies available. The evidence for the association of parental smoking with hepatoblastoma is convincing, with an emphasis on prenatal exposures.

(e) Other childhood cancers

Most of the associations reported for the other childhood cancers, notably soft tissue sarcomas, rhabdomyosarcomas, Ewing's sarcoma, neuroblastoma, Wilms tumour, reticuloendothelial sarcomas and germ cell tumours were null, with a few isolated and inconsistent positive observations.

3. Cancer in Experimental Animals

3.1 Simulated second-hand tobacco smoke

Simulated second-hand tobacco smoke, frequently a mixture of 89% sidestream and 11% mainstream smoke, generated from cigarettes by smoking machines (Teague *et al.*, 1994) has been tested for carcinogenicity in adult mice of strains that are genetically susceptible to induction of lung tumours (Malkinson, 1992). Mice were exposed in inhalation chambers. Several studies reported no increase in lung tumour incidence or multiplicity in mice exposed to simulated second-hand tobacco smoke for 5–9 months and killed immediately thereafter (Witschi *et al.*, 1995, 1997a; Finch *et al.*, 1996). It was suggested that the lack of tumour response in simulated second-hand tobacco smoke-exposed mice might be due to treatment-induced stress (as determined by the increased plasma corticosterone level) that has been shown to attenuate lung tumorigenesis (Stinn *et al.*, 2005a).

In subsequent studies from several laboratories (Table 3.1), an increased multiplicity and often increased incidence of lung tumours was reported in male and female A/J mice exposed for five months and kept in filtered air for another four months (Witschi *et al.*, 1997a, b, 1998, 1999; D'Agostini *et al.*, 2001) or longer (Witschi *et al.*, 2006) before the mice were killed. Similar results were obtained with Swiss albino mice (Witschi *et al.*, 2002). In these studies, no nasal tumours were observed in smoke-exposed mice.

In one study, male and female transgenic mice with a dominant negative *p53* mutation on an A/J background were exposed to simulated second-hand tobacco smoke for 9.5 continuous months or for 5 months followed by recovery in air for 4.5 months. Transgenic mice exposed by either regimen developed significantly higher incidence and multiplicity of lung tumours than sham-exposed control transgenic mice (DeFlora *et al.*, 2003). Neither lung tumour incidence nor multiplicity was increased in smoke-exposed wild-type control mice in this study.

In one study, male and female rats exposed to room-aged sidestream cigarette smoke by nose-only inhalation for 24 months and then killed had no increased incidence of lung or other tumours in comparison with fresh-air controls. Lung tumours were not significantly increased in rats exposed for 24 months and kept until 30 months of age (Stinn *et al.*, 2005b).

Table 3.1 Carcinogenicity studies of inhalation exposure to simulated second-hand tobacco smoke[a] in A/J mice, transgenic mice with a dominant negative *p53* mutation, and Wistar rats as a function of length of the post-exposure recovery period

Species, strain (sex) Reference	Animals/group at start Dosing regimen Duration	Results Target organ Incidence and/or multiplicity of tumours (%)	Significance	Comments
Mice, A/J (M) Witschi *et al.* (1997a)	48 animals/group Chamber concentration, 0 or 87 mg/m³ total suspended particulates; 6 h/d, 5 d/wk for 5 mo followed by 0 or 4 mo post-exposure recovery 9 mo	5 mo: 2/24 (8%, 0.1 ± 0.1); 6/24 (25%, 0.3 ± 0.1) 9 mo: 9/24 (38%, 0.5 ± 0.2); 20/24 (83%, 1.4 ± 0.2)	NS Incidence: $P < 0.05$ Multiplicity: $P < 0.05$	> 80% of tumours were adenomas; the rest were adenocarcinomas
Mice, A/J (F) D'Agostini *et al.* (2001)	20 animals/group Chamber concentration, 0 or 120 mg/m³ total suspended particulates; 6 h/d, 5 d/wk, for 5 mo followed by 4 mo post-exposure recovery 9 mo	5/20 (25%, 0.25 ± 0.10); 15/20 (75%, 1.05 ± 0.17)	Incidence: $P < 0.01$ Multiplicity: $P < 0.01$	
A/J mice (sex NR) Witschi *et al.* (2006)	24, 25 controls (12 mo) 19, 17 controls (24 mo) Chamber concentration, 0 (control) or 158 mg/m³ total suspended particulates; 6 h/d, 5 d/wk, for 6 mo followed by 4 or 16 mo post-exposure recovery 24 mo	12 mo: 13/24 (54%, 0.9 ± 0.2); 24/25 (96%, 1.8 ± 0.2) 24 mo: 8/9 (89%, 2.1 ± 0.5); 10/10 (100%, 4.3 ± 0.7)	Incidence: $P < 0.05$ Multiplicity: $P < 0.05$ Incidence: NS Multiplicity: $P < 0.05$	80% of tumours were adenomas
(UL53-3xA/J)F_1, Transgenic mice (M, F) De Flora *et al.* (2003)	222 (108; 114 controls) Chamber concentration, 0 (control) or 113 mg/m³ total suspended particulates; 6 h/d for 5 mo or 9.5 mo followed by 0 or 4.5 mo post-exposure recovery 9.5 mo	No recovery: NR; 17/30 (57%, 0.93 ± 0.18) With recovery: 5/26 (19%, 0.27 ± 0.10); 15/23 (65%, 0.74 ± 0.11)	Incidence: $P < 0.01$ Multiplicity: $P < 0.01$ Incidence: $P < 0.01$ Multiplicity: $P < 0.01$	
Wistar rats (M, F) Stinn *et al.* (2005b)	99 rats/group Nose-only exposure; concentration, 0 (controls) or low dose 3 mg/m³ or high dose 10 mg/m³; 6 h/d, 7 d/wk, 24 mo followed by 0 or 6 mo post-exposure recovery 30 mo	24 mo: controls–0/16 Low dose–0/16 High dose–0/16 30 mo: controls–2/99 (2%) Low dose–4/98 (4%) High dose–5/94 (5%)	NS	

[a] Simulated second-hand tobacco smoke: 89% sidestream and 11% mainstream smoke from Kentucky 1R4F or 2R1 reference cigarettes
d, day or days; F, female; h, hour or hours; M, male; mo, month or months; NR, not reported; NS, not significant; wk, week or weeks

3.2 Sidestream smoke condensate

In one study, sidestream cigarette smoke condensate applied to the shaved skin of female NMRI mice lower back, at total weekly doses of 5, 10 and 15 mg, for 3 months caused benign and malignant skin tumours and mammary carcinomas in mice observed for their lifespan and was more potently carcinogenic in this assay than mainstream smoke condensate. No cutaneous or subcutaneous tumours developed in any of three control groups ($P < 0.001$) (Mohtashamipur *et al.*, 1990). In one study, fractionated sidestream cigarette smoke condensates were implanted into the lungs of female rats. The fraction containing PAHs with four and more rings (dose, 1.06 mg/rat) induced 5 lung carcinomas in 35 treated rats; fractions containing no PAHs or PAHs with two or three rings (16 mg/rat) had little or no carcinogenic effect (Grimmer *et al.*, 1988).

3.3 Observational studies of companion animals

In one study, sinonasal cancers occurred more frequently in pet dogs of long-nosed breeds which lived in homes with at least one smoker (Reif *et al.*, 1998), but no such excess risk was seen in a second study (Bukowski *et al.*, 1998). A marginal excess risk of lung cancer was observed in dogs aged 10 years or less and exposed to household tobacco smoke in one study (Reif *et al.*, 1992). Risk of bladder cancer in dogs was not related to exposure to household cigarette smoke in another study (Glickman *et al.*, 1989).

Risk of malignant lymphoma was increased in pet cats exposed to household tobacco smoke in one study (Bertone *et al.*, 2002), but the conclusion that this association was causal has been questioned (Denson, 2003). In another study by the same group (Bertone *et al.*, 2003), exposure of pet cats to household tobacco smoke was also associated with a non-significant 2-fold increase in risk of oral squamous cell carcinoma.

3.4 Synthesis

Several studies showed consistent increases in lung tumour multiplicity and often lung tumour incidence in inbred strain A/J mice and in transgenic mice with a dominant negative *p53* tumour suppressor gene exposed by inhalation. In addition, in one report, skin and mammary tumours were induced in NMRI mice exposed to sidestream cigarette smoke condensate applied topically to the skin.

4. Other Relevant Data

See Section 4 of the *Monograph* on Tobacco Smoking in this volume.

5. Evaluation

There is *sufficient evidence* in humans for the carcinogenicity of second-hand tobacco smoke. Second-hand tobacco smoke causes cancer of the lung. Also, a positive association has been observed between exposure to second-hand tobacco smoke and cancers of the larynx and the pharynx.

There is *sufficient* evidence in experimental animals for the carcinogenicity of mixtures of mainstream and sidestream tobacco smoke.

There is *sufficient* evidence in experimental animals for the carcinogenicity of sidestream tobacco smoke condensates.

Second-hand tobacco smoke is *carcinogenic to humans (Group 1).*

References

Ahern TP, Lash TL, Egan KM, Baron JA (2009). Lifetime tobacco smoke exposure and breast cancer incidence. *Cancer Causes Control*, 20: 1837–1844. doi:10.1007/s10552-009-9376-1 PMID:19533391

Alberg AJ, Daudt A, Huang HY *et al.* (2004). N-acetyltransferase 2 (NAT2) genotypes, cigarette smoking, and the risk of breast cancer. *Cancer Detect Prev*, 28: 187–193. doi:10.1016/j.cdp.2004.04.001 PMID:15225898

Alberg AJ, Kouzis A, Genkinger JM *et al.* (2007). A prospective cohort study of bladder cancer risk in relation to active cigarette smoking and household exposure to secondhand cigarette smoke. *Am J Epidemiol*, 165: 660–666. doi:10.1093/aje/kwk047 PMID:17204516

Asomaning K, Miller DP, Liu G *et al.* (2008). Second hand smoke, age of exposure and lung cancer risk. *Lung Cancer*, 61: 13–20. doi:10.1016/j.lungcan.2007.11.013 PMID:18191495

Baker JA, Odunuga OO, Rodabaugh KJ *et al.* (2006). Active and passive smoking and risk of ovarian cancer. *Int J Gynecol Cancer*, 16: Suppl 1211–218. doi:10.1111/j.1525-1438.2006.00473.x PMID:16515593

Bao Y, Giovannucci E, Fuchs CS, Michaud DS (2009). Passive smoking and pancreatic cancer in women: a prospective cohort study. *Cancer Epidemiol Biomarkers Prev*, 18: 2292–2296. doi:10.1158/1055-9965.EPI-09-0352 PMID:19602702

Barletta E, Gorini G, Vineis P *et al.* (2004). Ras gene mutations in patients with acute myeloid leukaemia and exposure to chemical agents. *Carcinogenesis*, 25: 749–755. doi:10.1093/carcin/bgh057 PMID:14688017

Bertone ER, Snyder LA, Moore AS (2002). Environmental tobacco smoke and risk of malignant lymphoma in pet cats. *Am J Epidemiol*, 156: 268–273. doi:10.1093/aje/kwf044 PMID:12142262

Bertone ER, Snyder LA, Moore AS (2003). Environmental and lifestyle risk factors for oral squamous cell carcinoma in domestic cats. *J Vet Intern Med*, 17: 557–562. doi:10.1111/j.1939-1676.2003.tb02478.x PMID:12892308

Bjerregaard BK, Raaschou-Nielsen O, Sørensen M *et al.* (2006). Tobacco smoke and bladder cancer–in the European Prospective Investigation into Cancer and Nutrition. *Int J Cancer*, 119: 2412–2416. doi:10.1002/ijc.22169 PMID:16894557

Boffetta P, Trédaniel J, Greco A (2000). Risk of childhood cancer and adult lung cancer after childhood exposure to passive smoke: A meta-analysis. *Environ Health Perspect*, 108: 73–82. doi:10.1289/ehp.0010873 PMID:10620527

Bonner MR, Bennett WP, Xiong W *et al.* (2006). Radon, secondhand smoke, glutathione-S-transferase M1 and lung cancer among women. *Int J Cancer*, 119: 1462–1467. doi:10.1002/ijc.22002 PMID:16642467

Bonner MR, Nie J, Han D *et al.* (2005). Secondhand smoke exposure in early life and the risk of breast cancer among never smokers (United States). *Cancer Causes Control*, 16: 683–689. doi:10.1007/s10552-005-1906-x PMID:16049807

Brooks DR, Mucci LA, Hatch EE, Cnattingius S (2004). Maternal smoking during pregnancy and risk of brain tumors in the offspring. A prospective study of 1.4 million Swedish births. *Cancer Causes Control*, 15: 997–1005. doi:10.1007/s10552-004-1123-z PMID:15801484

Brown DC, Pereira L, Garner JB (1982). Cancer of the cervix and the smoking husband. *Can Fam Physician*, 28: 499–502. PMID:21286079

Buckley JD, Harris RW, Doll R *et al.* (1981). Case-control study of the husbands of women with dysplasia or carcinoma of the cervix uteri. *Lancet*, 2: 1010–1015. doi:10.1016/S0140-6736(81)91215-0 PMID:6118477

Bukowski JA, Wartenberg D, Goldschmidt MJohn A. Bukowski Daniel Wartenberg (1998). Environmental causes for sinonasal cancers in pet dogs, and their usefulness as sentinels of indoor cancer risk. *J Toxicol Environ Health A*, 54: 579–591. doi:10.1080/009841098158719 PMID:9726781

Burch JD, Rohan TE, Howe GR *et al.* (1989). Risk of bladder cancer by source and type of tobacco exposure: a case-control study. *Int J Cancer*, 44: 622–628. doi:10.1002/ijc.2910440411 PMID:2793235

California Environmental Protection Agency (2005). *Health Effects Assessment for ETS: Final.* California Environmental Protection Agency, Office of Environmental Health Hazard Assesment: Sacramento, CA.

CDC (2008). Centers for Disease Control and Prevention. Global Youth Tobacco Surveillance, 2000–2007. *Morbidity and Mortality Weekly Report.*, 57: 1–21. PMID:18185492

CDC/WHO (2009). Centers for Disease Control and Prevention (CDC) and World Health Organization (WHO). Global Youth Tobacco Survey (GYTS). Atlanta GA. (http://www.cdc.gov/tobacco/global/gyts/index.htm, (accessed 27 November 2011).

Chang JS, Selvin S, Metayer C *et al.* (2006). Parental smoking and the risk of childhood leukemia. *Am J Epidemiol*, 163: 1091–1100. doi:10.1093/aje/kwj143 PMID:16597704

Chen YC, Su HJ, Guo Y-LL *et al.* (2005a). Interaction between environmental tobacco smoke and arsenic methylation ability on the risk of bladder cancer. *Cancer Causes Control*, 16: 75–81. doi:10.1007/s10552-004-2235-1 PMID:15868449

Chen Z, Robison L, Giller R *et al.* (2005b). Risk of childhood germ cell tumors in association with parental smoking and drinking. *Cancer*, 103: 1064–1071. doi:10.1002/cncr.20894 PMID:15685619

Cheng YJ, Hildesheim A, Hsu MM *et al.* (1999). Cigarette smoking, alcohol consumption and risk of nasopharyngeal carcinoma in Taiwan. *Cancer Causes Control*, 10: 201–207. doi:10.1023/A:1008893109257 PMID:10454065

Clavel J, Bellec S, Rebouissou S *et al.* (2005). Childhood leukaemia, polymorphisms of metabolism enzyme genes, and interactions with maternal tobacco, coffee and alcohol consumption during pregnancy. *Eur J Cancer Prev*, 14: 531–540. doi:10.1097/00008469-200512000-00007 PMID:16284498

Coker AL, Bond SM, Williams A *et al.* (2002). Active and passive smoking, high-risk human papillomaviruses and cervical neoplasia. *Cancer Detect Prev*, 26: 121–128. doi:10.1016/S0361-090X(02)00039-9 PMID:12102146

Coker AL, Rosenberg AJ, McCann MF, Hulka BS (1992). Active and passive cigarette smoke exposure and cervical intraepithelial neoplasia. *Cancer Epidemiol Biomarkers Prev*, 1: 349–356. PMID:1305466

Collishaw NE *et al.* (2009). *Canadian Expert Panel on Tobacco Smoke and Breast Cancer Risk*, in *OTRU Special Report Series*. Ontario Tobacco Research Unit: Toronto.

Cordier S, Monfort C, Filippini G *et al.* (2004). Parental exposure to polycyclic aromatic hydrocarbons and the risk of childhood brain tumors: The SEARCH International Childhood Brain Tumor Study. *Am J Epidemiol*, 159: 1109–1116. doi:10.1093/aje/kwh154 PMID:15191928

D'Agostini F, Balansky RM, Bennicelli C *et al.* (2001). Pilot studies evaluating the lung tumor yield in cigarette smoke-exposed mice. *Int J Oncol*, 18: 607–615. PMID:11179494

De Flora S, Balansky RM, D'Agostini F *et al.* (2003). Molecular alterations and lung tumors in p53 mutant mice exposed to cigarette smoke. *Cancer Res*, 63: 793–800. PMID:12591728

DeBaun MR & Tucker MA (1998). Risk of cancer during the first four years of life in children from The Beckwith-Wiedemann Syndrome Registry. *J Pediatr*, 132: 398–400. doi:10.1016/S0022-3476(98)70008-3 PMID:9544889

Denson KW (2003). Re: Environmental tobacco smoke and risk of malignant lymphoma in pet cats. *Am J Epidemiol*, 158: 1227–1228, author reply 1227–1228. PMID:14692044

Duan L, Wu AH, Sullivan-Halley J, Bernstein L (2009). Passive smoking and risk of oesophageal and gastric adenocarcinomas. *Br J Cancer*, 100: 1483–1485. doi:10.1038/sj.bjc.6605023 PMID:19352383

Enstrom JE & Kabat GC (2003). Environmental tobacco smoke and tobacco related mortality in a prospective study of Californians, 1960–98. *BMJ*, 326: 1057 doi:10.1136/bmj.326.7398.1057 PMID:12750205

Filippini G, Maisonneuve P, McCredie M *et al.* (2002). Relation of childhood brain tumors to exposure of parents and children to tobacco smoke: the SEARCH international case-control study. Surveillance of Environmental Aspects Related to Cancer in Humans. *Int J Cancer*, 100: 206–213. doi:10.1002/ijc.10465 PMID:12115571

Finch GL, Nikula KJ, Belinsky SA *et al.* (1996). Failure of cigarette smoke to induce or promote lung cancer in the A/J mouse. *Cancer Lett*, 99: 161–167. doi:10.1016/0304-3835(95)04059-5 PMID:8616820

Fukuda K & Shibata A (1990). Exposure-response relationships between woodworking, smoking or passive smoking, and squamous cell neoplasms of the maxillary sinus. *Cancer Causes Control*, 1: 165–168. doi:10.1007/BF00053168 PMID:2102286

Gallicchio L, Kouzis A, Genkinger JM *et al.* (2006). Active cigarette smoking, household passive smoke exposure, and the risk of developing pancreatic cancer. *Prev Med*, 42: 200–205. doi:10.1016/j.ypmed.2005.12.014 PMID:16458957

Gammon MD, Eng SM, Teitelbaum SL *et al.* (2004). Environmental tobacco smoke and breast cancer incidence. *Environ Res*, 96: 176–185. doi:10.1016/j.envres.2003.08.009 PMID:15325878

Gerhardsson de Verdier M, Plato N, Steineck G, Peters JM (1992). Occupational exposures and cancer of the colon and rectum. *Am J Ind Med*, 22: 291–303. doi:10.1002/ajim.4700220303 PMID:1519614

Glickman LT, Schofer FS, McKee LJ *et al.* (1989). Epidemiologic study of insecticide exposures, obesity, and risk of bladder cancer in household dogs. *J Toxicol Environ Health*, 28: 407–414. doi:10.1080/15287398909531360 PMID:2593174

Goodman MT & Tung KH (2003). Active and passive tobacco smoking and the risk of borderline and invasive ovarian cancer (United States). *Cancer Causes Control*, 14: 569–577. doi:10.1023/A:1024828309874 PMID:12948288

Grimmer G, Brune H, Dettbarn G *et al.* (1988). Contribution of polycyclic aromatic compounds to the carcinogenicity of sidestream smoke of cigarettes evaluated by implantation into the lungs of rats. *Cancer Lett*, 43: 173–177. doi:10.1016/0304-3835(88)90167-X PMID:3203336

Hanaoka T, Yamamoto S, Sobue T *et al.*Japan Public Health Center-Based Prospective Study on Cancer and Cardiovascular Disease Study Group (2005). Active and passive smoking and breast cancer risk in middle-aged Japanese women. *Int J Cancer*, 114: 317–322. doi:10.1002/ijc.20709 PMID:15540214

Hassan MM, Abbruzzese JL, Bondy ML *et al.* (2007). Passive smoking and the use of noncigarette tobacco products in association with risk for pancreatic cancer: a case-control study. *Cancer*, 109: 2547–2556. doi:10.1002/cncr.22724 PMID:17492688

Hassan MM, Spitz MR, Thomas MB *et al.* (2008). Effect of different types of smoking and synergism with hepatitis C virus on risk of hepatocellular carcinoma in American men and women: case-control study. *Int J Cancer*, 123: 1883–1891. doi:10.1002/ijc.23730 PMID:18688864

Hecht SS (2008). Progress and challenges in selected areas of tobacco carcinogenesis. *Chem Res Toxicol*, 21: 160–171. doi:10.1021/tx7002068 PMID:18052103

Hecht SS, Carmella SG, Le KA *et al.* (2006). 4-(methylnitrosamino)-1-(3-pyridyl)-1-butanol and its glucuronides in the urine of infants exposed to environmental tobacco smoke. *Cancer Epidemiol Biomarkers Prev*, 15: 988–992. doi:10.1158/1055-9965.EPI-05-0596 PMID:16702381

Hellberg D, Valentin J, Nilsson S (1986). Smoking and cervical intraepithelial neoplasia. An association independent of sexual and other risk factors? *Acta Obstet Gynecol Scand*, 65: 625–631. doi:10.3109/00016348609158400 PMID:3799159

Hill SE, Blakely T, Kawachi I, Woodward A (2007). Mortality among lifelong nonsmokers exposed to secondhand smoke at home: cohort data and sensitivity analyses. *Am J Epidemiol*, 165: 530–540. doi:10.1093/aje/kwk043 PMID:17172631

Hirayama T (1984). Cancer mortality in nonsmoking women with smoking husbands based on a large-scale cohort study in Japan. *Prev Med*, 13: 680–690. doi:10.1016/S0091-7435(84)80017-1 PMID:6536942

Hirose K, Tajima K, Hamajima N *et al.* (1996). Subsite (cervix/endometrium)-specific risk and protective factors in uterus cancer. *Jpn J Cancer Res*, 87: 1001–1009. doi:10.1111/j.1349-7006.1996.tb02132.x PMID:8878465

Hooker CM, Gallicchio L, Genkinger JM *et al.* (2008). A prospective cohort study of rectal cancer risk in relation to active cigarette smoking and passive smoke exposure. *Ann Epidemiol*, 18: 28–35. doi:10.1016/j.annepidem.2007.06.010 PMID:17900927

Hu J & Ugnat AMCanadian Cancer Registries Epidemiology Research Group (2005). Active and passive smoking and risk of renal cell carcinoma in Canada. *Eur J Cancer*, 41: 770–778. doi:10.1016/j.ejca.2005.01.003 PMID:15763654

Huncharek M, Kupelnick B, Klassen H (2002). Maternal smoking during pregnancy and the risk of childhood brain tumors: a meta-analysis of 6566 subjects from twelve epidemiological studies. *J Neurooncol*, 57: 51–57. doi:10.1023/A:1015734921470 PMID:12125967

Hurley SF, McNeil JJ, Donnan GA *et al.* (1996). Tobacco smoking and alcohol consumption as risk factors for glioma: a case-control study in Melbourne, Australia. *J Epidemiol Community Health*, 50: 442–446. doi:10.1136/jech.50.4.442 PMID:8882229

IARC (2009). *Evaluating the effectiveness of smoke-free policies*. IARC Handbook of Cancer Prevention. Vol. 13. Lyon: International Agency for Research on Cancer. http://www.iarc.fr/en/publications/pdfs-online/prev/index1.php

IARC (2004). Tobacco smoke and involuntary smoking. *IARC Monogr Eval Carcinog Risks Hum*, 83: 1–1438. PMID:15285078

Infante-Rivard C, Krajinovic M, Labuda D, Sinnett D (2000). Parental smoking, CYP1A1 genetic polymorphisms and childhood leukemia (Québec, Canada). *Cancer Causes Control*, 11: 547–553. doi:10.1023/A:1008976116512 PMID:10880037

Jaakkola MS & Jaakkola JJK (1997). Assessment of exposure to environmental tobacco smoke. *Eur Respir J*, 10: 2384–2397. doi:10.1183/09031936.97.10102384 PMID:9387970

Jee SH, Ohrr H, Kim IS (1999). Effects of husbands' smoking on the incidence of lung cancer in Korean women. *Int J Epidemiol*, 28: 824–828. doi:10.1093/ije/28.5.824 PMID:10597977

Jenkins RA, Guerin MR, Tomkins BA (2000) *The Chemistry of Environmental Tobacco Smoke: Composition and Measurement, Second Edition.*, Jenkins RA, Guerin MR, Tomkins BA, editors. London: Lewis Boca Raton.

Jiang X, Yuan JM, Skipper PL *et al.* (2007). Environmental tobacco smoke and bladder cancer risk in never smokers of Los Angeles County. *Cancer Res*, 67: 7540–7545. doi:10.1158/0008-5472.CAN-07-0048 PMID:17671226

Johnson KC (2005). Accumulating evidence on passive and active smoking and breast cancer risk. *Int J Cancer*, 117: 619–628. doi:10.1002/ijc.21150 PMID:15929073

Johnson KC (2007). Re: more data regarding the effects of passive smoking on breast cancer risk among younger women. *Int J Cancer*, 120: 2519–2520. doi:10.1002/ijc.22611 PMID:17304510

Johnson KC & Glantz SA (2008). Evidence second-hand smoke causes breast cancer in 2005 stronger than for lung cancer in 1986. *Prev Med*, 46: 492–496. doi:10.1016/j.ypmed.2007.11.016 PMID:18182169

Johnson KC & Repace J (2000). Lung cancer and passive smoking. Turning over the wrong stone. *BMJ*, 321: 1221–, author reply 1222–1223. doi:10.1136/bmj.321.7270.1221 PMID:11073521

Kasim K, Levallois P, Abdous B *et al.*Canadian Cancer Registries Epidemiology Research Group (2005). Environmental tobacco smoke and risk of adult leukemia. *Epidemiology*, 16: 672–680. doi:10.1097/01.ede.0000173039.79207.80 PMID:16135944

Kropp S & Chang-Claude J (2002). Active and passive smoking and risk of breast cancer by age 50 years among German women. *Am J Epidemiol*, 156: 616–626. doi:10.1093/aje/kwf093 PMID:12244030

Kurahashi N, Inoue M, Liu Y *et al.*JPHC Study Group (2008). Passive smoking and lung cancer in Japanese non-smoking women: a prospective study. *Int J Cancer*, 122: 653–657. doi:10.1002/ijc.23116 PMID:17935128

Lash TL & Aschengrau A (1999). Active and passive cigarette smoking and the occurrence of breast cancer. *Am J Epidemiol*, 149: 5–12. PMID:9883788

Lash TL & Aschengrau A (2002). A null association between active or passive cigarette smoking and breast cancer risk. *Breast Cancer Res Treat*, 75: 181–184. doi:10.1023/A:1019625102365 PMID:12243511

Lee KM, Ward MH, Han S *et al.* (2009). Paternal smoking, genetic polymorphisms in CYP1A1 and childhood leukemia risk. *Leuk Res*, 33: 250–258. doi:10.1016/j.leukres.2008.06.031 PMID:18691756

Lee YC, Boffetta P, Sturgis EM *et al.* (2008). Involuntary smoking and head and neck cancer risk: pooled analysis in the International Head and Neck Cancer Epidemiology Consortium. *Cancer Epidemiol Biomarkers Prev*, 17: 1974–1981. doi:10.1158/1055-9965.EPI-08-0047 PMID:18708387

Lilla C, Verla-Tebit E, Risch A *et al.* (2006). Effect of NAT1 and NAT2 genetic polymorphisms on colorectal cancer risk associated with exposure to tobacco smoke and meat consumption. *Cancer Epidemiol Biomarkers Prev*, 15: 99–107. doi:10.1158/1055-9965.EPI-05-0618 PMID:16434594

Lissowska J, Brinton LA, Zatonski W *et al.* (2006). Tobacco smoking, NAT2 acetylation genotype and breast cancer risk. *Int J Cancer*, 119: 1961–1969. doi:10.1002/ijc.22044 PMID:16721725

Liu L, Wu K, Lin X *et al.* (2000). Passive Smoking and Other Factors at Different Periods of Life and Breast Cancer Risk in Chinese Women who have Never Smoked - A Case-control Study in Chongqing, People's Republic of China. *Asian Pac J Cancer Prev*, 1: 131–137. PMID:12718680

Lo AC, Soliman AS, El-Ghawalby N *et al.* (2007). Lifestyle, occupational, and reproductive factors in relation to pancreatic cancer risk. *Pancreas*, 35: 120–129. doi:10.1097/mpa.0b013e318053e7d3 PMID:17632317

MacArthur AC, McBride ML, Spinelli JJ *et al.* (2008). Risk of childhood leukemia associated with parental smoking and alcohol consumption prior to conception and during pregnancy: the cross-Canada childhood leukemia study. *Cancer Causes Control*, 19: 283–295. doi:10.1007/s10552-007-9091-8 PMID:18283545

Malkinson AM (1992). Primary lung tumors in mice: an experimentally manipulable model of human adenocarcinoma. *Cancer Res*, 52: Suppl2670s–2676s. PMID:1562998

Mao Y, Hu J, Semenciw R, White KCanadian Cancer Registries Epidemiology Research Group (2002). Active and passive smoking and the risk of stomach cancer, by subsite, in Canada. *Eur J Cancer Prev*, 11: 27–38. doi:10.1097/00008469-200202000-00005 PMID:11917206

McGlynn KA, Zhang Y, Sakoda LC *et al.* (2006). Maternal smoking and testicular germ cell tumors. *Cancer Epidemiol Biomarkers Prev*, 15: 1820–1824. doi:10.1158/1055-9965.EPI-06-0389 PMID:17035387

McKinney PA, Cartwright RA, Saiu JM *et al.* (1987). The inter-regional epidemiological study of childhood cancer (IRESCC): a case control study of aetiological factors in leukaemia and lymphoma. *Arch Dis Child*, 62: 279–287. doi:10.1136/adc.62.3.279 PMID:3646026

McLaughlin CC, Baptiste MS, Schymura MJ *et al.* (2006). Maternal and infant birth characteristics and hepatoblastoma. *Am J Epidemiol*, 163: 818–828. doi:10.1093/aje/kwj104 PMID:16510543

Mechanic LE, Millikan RC, Player J *et al.* (2006). Polymorphisms in nucleotide excision repair genes, smoking and breast cancer in African Americans and whites: a population-based case-control study. *Carcinogenesis*, 27: 1377–1385. doi:10.1093/carcin/bgi330 PMID:16399771

Mejía-Aranguré JM, Fajardo-Gutiérrez A, Flores-Aguilar H *et al.* (2003). Environmental factors contributing to the development of childhood leukemia in children with Down's syndrome. *Leukemia*, 17: 1905–1907. doi:10.1038/sj.leu.2403047 PMID:12970794

Menegaux F, Ripert M, Hémon D, Clavel J (2007). Maternal alcohol and coffee drinking, parental smoking and childhood leukaemia: a French population-based case-control study. *Paediatr Perinat Epidemiol*, 21: 293–299. doi:10.1111/j.1365-3016.2007.00824.x PMID:17564585

Menegaux F, Steffen C, Bellec S *et al.* (2005). Maternal coffee and alcohol consumption during pregnancy, parental smoking and risk of childhood acute leukaemia. *Cancer Detect Prev*, 29: 487–493. doi:10.1016/j.cdp.2005.06.008 PMID:16289502

Miller GH (1990). The impact of passive smoking: cancer deaths among nonsmoking women. *Cancer Detect Prev*, 14: 497–503. PMID:2224913

Miller MD, Marty MA, Broadwin R *et al.*California Environmental Protection Agency (2007). The association between exposure to environmental tobacco smoke and breast cancer: a review by the California Environmental Protection Agency. *Prev Med*, 44: 93–106. doi:10.1016/j.ypmed.2006.08.015 PMID:17027075

Mohtashamipur E, Mohtashamipur A, Germann PG *et al.* (1990). Comparative carcinogenicity of cigarette mainstream and sidestream smoke condensates on the mouse skin. *J Cancer Res Clin Oncol*, 116: 604–608. doi:10.1007/BF01637081 PMID:2254379

Morabia A, Bernstein M, Héritier S, Khatchatrian N (1996). Relation of breast cancer with passive and active exposure to tobacco smoke. *Am J Epidemiol*, 143: 918–928. PMID:8610705

Morabia A, Bernstein MS, Bouchardy I *et al.* (2000). Breast cancer and active and passive smoking: the role of the N-acetyltransferase 2 genotype. *Am J Epidemiol*, 152: 226–232. doi:10.1093/aje/152.3.226 PMID:10933269

Mucci LA, Granath F, Cnattingius S (2004). Maternal smoking and childhood leukemia and lymphoma risk among 1,440,542 Swedish children. *Cancer Epidemiol Biomarkers Prev*, 13: 1528–1533. PMID:15342456

Navas-Acien A, Peruga A, Breysse P *et al.* (2004). Secondhand tobacco smoke in public places in Latin America, 2002–2003. *JAMA*, 291: 2741–2745. doi:10.1001/jama.291.22.2741 PMID:15187056

Nishino Y, Tsubono Y, Tsuji I *et al.* (2001). Passive smoking at home and cancer risk: a population-based prospective study in Japanese nonsmoking women. *Cancer Causes Control*, 12: 797–802. doi:10.1023/A:1012273806199 PMID:11714107

Pang D & Birch JM (2003). Reply: smoking and hepatoblastoma:confounding by birth weight? *Br J Cancer*, 89: 603 doi:10.1038/sj.bjc.6601144

Pang D, McNally R, Birch JM (2003). Parental smoking and childhood cancer: results from the United Kingdom Childhood Cancer Study. *Br J Cancer*, 88: 373–381. doi:10.1038/sj.bjc.6600774 PMID:12569379

Peppone LJ, Mahoney MC, Cummings KM *et al.* (2008). Colorectal cancer occurs earlier in those exposed to tobacco smoke: implications for screening. *J Cancer Res Clin Oncol*, 134: 743–751. doi:10.1007/s00432-007-0332-8 PMID:18264728

Phillips LE, Longstreth WT Jr, Koepsell T *et al.* (2005). Active and passive cigarette smoking and risk of intracranial meningioma. *Neuroepidemiology*, 24: 117–122. doi:10.1159/000082998 PMID:15637448

Pirie K, Beral V, Peto R *et al.*Million Women Study Collaborators (2008). Passive smoking and breast cancer in never smokers: prospective study and meta-analysis. *Int J Epidemiol*, 37: 1069–1079. doi:10.1093/ije/dyn110 PMID:18544575

Plichart M, Menegaux F, Lacour B *et al.* (2008). Parental smoking, maternal alcohol, coffee and tea consumption during pregnancy and childhood malignant central nervous system tumours: the ESCALE study (SFCE). *Eur J Cancer Prev*, 17: 376–383. doi:10.1097/CEJ.0b013e3282f75e6f PMID:18562965

Pu CL, Guo CB, Jin XQ *et al.* (2009). [Retrospective analysis of maternal and infant birth features of hepatoblastoma patients] *Zhonghua Gan Zang Bing Za Zhi*, 17: 459–461. PMID:19567028

Ramroth H, Dietz A, Becher H (2008). Environmental tobacco smoke and laryngeal cancer: results from a population-based case-control study. *Eur Arch Otorhinolaryngol*, 265: 1367–1371. doi:10.1007/s00405-008-0651-7 PMID:18379814

Reif JS, Bruns C, Lower KS (1998). Cancer of the nasal cavity and paranasal sinuses and exposure to environmental tobacco smoke in pet dogs. *Am J Epidemiol*, 147: 488–492. PMID:9525536

Reif JS, Dunn K, Ogilvie GK, Harris CK (1992). Passive smoking and canine lung cancer risk. *Am J Epidemiol*, 135: 234–239. PMID:1546698

Reynolds P, Hurley S, Goldberg DCalifornia Teachers Study Steering Committee (2006). Accumulating evidence on passive and active smoking and breast cancer risk. *Int J Cancer*, 119: 239–1, author reply 240–241. doi:10.1002/ijc.21776 PMID:16432834

Reynolds P, Hurley S, Goldberg DE *et al.* (2004). Active smoking, household passive smoking, and breast cancer: evidence from the California Teachers Study. *J Natl Cancer Inst*, 96: 29–37. doi:10.1093/jnci/djh002 PMID:14709736

Roddam AW, Pirie K, Pike MC *et al.* (2007). Active and passive smoking and the risk of breast cancer in women aged 36–45 years: a population based case-control study in the UK. *Br J Cancer*, 97: 434–439. doi:10.1038/sj.bjc.6603859 PMID:17579618

Rollison DE, Brownson RC, Hathcock HL, Newschaffer CJ (2008). Case-control study of tobacco smoke exposure and breast cancer risk in Delaware. *BMC Cancer*, 8: 157 doi:10.1186/1471-2407-8-157 PMID:18518960

Rudant J, Menegaux F, Leverger G *et al.* (2008). Childhood hematopoietic malignancies and parental use of tobacco and alcohol: the ESCALE study (SFCE). *Cancer Causes Control*, 19: 1277–1290. doi:10.1007/s10552-008-9199-5 PMID:18618277

Ryan P, Lee MW, North B, McMichael AJ (1992). Risk factors for tumors of the brain and meninges: results from the Adelaide Adult Brain Tumor Study. *Int J Cancer*, 51: 20–27. doi:10.1002/ijc.2910510105 PMID:1563840

Samanic C, Kogevinas M, Dosemeci M *et al.* (2006). Smoking and bladder cancer in Spain: effects of tobacco type, timing, environmental tobacco smoke, and gender. *Cancer Epidemiol Biomarkers Prev*, 15: 1348–1354. doi:10.1158/1055-9965.EPI-06-0021 PMID:16835335

Samet J, Yang G (2001) *Passive smoking, women and children*. In: *Women and the Tobacco Epidemic, Challenges for the 21st Century*, Samet, J. and Yoon, S.-Y., editors. (WHO/NMH/TF1/ 01.1), Geneva: World Health Organization

Sandler DP, Everson RB, Wilcox AJ (1985a). Passive smoking in adulthood and cancer risk. *Am J Epidemiol*, 121: 37–48. PMID:3964991

Sandler DP, Everson RB, Wilcox AJ, Browder JP (1985b). Cancer risk in adulthood from early life exposure to parents' smoking. *Am J Public Health*, 75: 487–492. doi:10.2105/AJPH.75.5.487 PMID:3985235

Sandler RS, Sandler DP, Comstock GW *et al.* (1988). Cigarette smoking and the risk of colorectal cancer in women. *J Natl Cancer Inst*, 80: 1329–1333. doi:10.1093/jnci/80.16.1329 PMID:3172257

Scholes D, McBride C, Grothaus L *et al.* (1999). The association between cigarette smoking and low-grade cervical abnormalities in reproductive-age women. *Cancer Causes Control*, 10: 339–344. doi:10.1023/A:1008993619060 PMID:10530602

Schüz J, Kaatsch P, Kaletsch U *et al.* (1999). Association of childhood cancer with factors related to pregnancy and birth. *Int J Epidemiol*, 28: 631–639. doi:10.1093/ije/28.4.631 PMID:10480689

Shrubsole MJ, Gao YT, Dai Q *et al.* (2004). Passive smoking and breast cancer risk among non-smoking Chinese women. *Int J Cancer*, 110: 605–609. doi:10.1002/ijc.20168 PMID:15122595

SMOKELESS TOBACCO

Smokeless tobacco was considered by a previous IARC Working Group in 2004 (IARC, 2007a). Since that time, new data have become available, these have been incorporated into the *Monograph*, and taken into consideration in the present evaluation.

1. Exposure Data

1.1 Smokeless tobacco products

The term smokeless tobacco implies use of unburned tobacco in the finished products. A variety of smokeless tobacco products are available, for oral or nasal use. Products intended for oral use are sucked, chewed (dipped), gargled or applied to the gums or teeth, while fine tobacco mixtures are usually inhaled into the nostrils.

Table 1.1 summarizes for each smokeless tobacco product its mode of use, the main ingredients included, the WHO regions in which the product is used, and some specification of the countries is which the product is used most commonly or specifically (DHHS, 2001; IARC, 2007a; European Commission, 2008). Smokeless tobacco products that contain areca nut are commonly used in India, other countries in South Asia, and in migrant populations from these countries. These products may be mentioned here for comparison but are reviewed in the *Monograph* on Betel Quid and Areca Nut in this volume.

1.2 Chemical composition of smokeless tobacco

The tobacco used in a particular product has a decisive influence on its chemical composition, and varies with tobacco species, growing, curing, processing and storage. During product manufacture, tobacco is blended to achieve a specific nicotine content and pH. The pH strongly influences the concentration of unprotonated nicotine, the bioavailable form of nicotine, while the nitrite/nitrate content strongly influences the levels of carcinogenic nitrosamines in the product. Other tobacco components are alkaloids which include nicotine (85–95% of total alkaloids), terpenes, polyphenols, phytosterols, carboxylic acids, aromatic hydrocarbons, aldehydes, ketones, amines, nitriles, *N*- and *O*-heterocyclic hydrocarbons, pesticides, and metallic compounds. Flavour-type additives are also present (Bates *et al.*, 1999). Ammonia, ammonium carbonate and sodium carbonate are applied to control nicotine delivery by raising pH and subsequently the level of unprotonated nicotine which is most readily absorbed through the mouth into the bloodstream (Djordjevic *et al.*, 1995).

Table 1.1 Smokeless tobacco products, ingredients, and use by WHO region

Tobacco product	Mode of use	Ingredients	WHO Region					
			AFRO	AMRO	EMRO	EURO	SEARO	WPRO
Oral use								
Betel quid with tobacco[a]	Chewing	Betel leaf, areca nut, slaked lime, tobacco in various forms			X		X	X
Chimó	Sucking	Paste of crushed and boiled tobacco leaves, sodium bicarbonate, sugar, wood ash, flavourings		X[b]				
Chewing tobacco	Chewing	See Tobacco chewing gum						
Chewing tobacco twist/roll	Chewing	Dark, air- or fire-cured tobacco leaves treated with tobacco extract, flavourings		X[c]				
Creamy snuff	Other	Finely ground tobacco with aromatic substances (manufactured commercially)					X	
Dry snuff	Sucking	Fire- or air-cured, fermented powdered tobacco	X[d]	X[c]	X[e]	X[f]	X[g]	
Gudhaku	Other	Paste of powdered tobacco and molasses					X[g]	
Gul	Other	Powdered tobacco, molasses and other ingredients					X[g]	
Gutka[a]	Sucking	Sun-dried finely chopped tobacco, areca nut, slaked lime, catechu, flavourings, sweeteners (manufactured commercially)					X	
Iq'mik	Chewing	Fire-cured tobacco leaves with punk ash		X[h]				
Khaini	Sucking	Sun-dried or fermented coarsely crushed tobacco leaves					X[i]	
Khiwam	Chewing	Paste of tobacco extract, spices, additives					X[j]	
Loose leaf	Chewing	Small strips of air-cured, shredded cigar tobacco leaves (manufactured commercially)		X[c]		X		
Maraş	Sucking	Sun-dried powdered tobacco leaves, wood ash, water				X[k]		
Mawa[a]	Chewing	Sun-cured areca nut, crushed tobacco leaves, slaked lime					X[j]	
Mishri	Sucking	Tobacco toasted on hot metal plate and powdered					X[g]	
Moist snuff	Sucking	Air- or fire-cured tobacco, processed into fine particles (fine-cut) or strips (long-cut), with stem and seeds		X[c]		X[l]		
Naswar/nass	Sucking	Sun-dried, powdered tobacco, ash, oil, flavourings, colourings, slaked lime (optional)	X[d]		X[m]	X		
Plug chewing tobacco	Chewing	Heavy-grade or cigar tobacco top leaves immersed in liquorice or sugar, pressed into a plug		X[c]				
Red tooth powder	Other	Fine tobacco powder, many additional ingredients (manufactured commercially)					X	
Shammah	Sucking	Powdered tobacco, lime, ash, black pepper, oils, flavourings			X[n]	X		
Snus	-	See moist stuff		X[c]		X[l]		

Table 1.1 (continued)

Tobacco product	Mode of use	Ingredients	WHO Region					
			AFRO	AMRO	EMRO	EURO	SEARO	WPRO
Saffa	-	*Toomback* rolled into a ball	X[q]					
Tobacco tablet	Sucking	Compressed powdered tobacco, mint, eucalyptus		X[c]				
Toombak	Sucking	Dried, fermented, ground and matured tobacco leaves, sodium bicarbonate	X[q]					
Tuibur	Other	Tobacco water					X[r]	
Zarda	Chewing	Tobacco leaves boiled with lime and spices until dry, colourings; chewed with areca nut and spices			X		X	
Nasal use								
Dry snuff	Sniffing	Fire-cured, fermented and powdered tobacco	X[s]		X	X[t]	X	
Liquid snuff	Sniffing	Powered tobacco mixed with ash from plants, oil, lemon juice, herbs	X[u]					

[a] These products contain areca nut and are reviewed in the*Monograph* on Betel Quid and Areca Nut in this volume.
[b] Specific to Venezuela, used by young boys and urban teenagers
[c] Used in the USA
[d] Used principally in South Africa; dry snuff is mostly inhaled.
[e] Common in North Africa, notably in Tunisia as*neffa*
[f] Used in Germany, Georgia and the United Kingdom
[g] Used as dentifrice, mostly by women, in various parts of India
[h] Specific to native American tribes of North-West Alaska
[i] Used in India, Bangladesh and Nepal
[j] Specific to India
[k] Specific to remote regions of Turkey
[l] Used in Sweden, Norway and Finland
[m] Common in Afghanistan, Islamic Republic of Iran, Pakistan and central Asia
[n] Common in the Middle East, particularly in Saudi Arabia and Yemen
[o] Used in Sweden and Denmark
[p] Specific to Japan (new product)
[q] Specific to Sudan, used by men
[r] Specific to eastern States of India
[s] Used by several tribes in South Africa, namely Bantus
[t] Used in the United Kingdom
[u] Specific to tribes in East Africa
AFRO, African Region; AMRO, Regions of the Americas; EMRO, Eastern Mediterranean Region; EURO, European Region; SEARO, South East Asian Region, WPRO, Western Pacific Region; the countries included in each region are available at http://www.who.int/about/regions/en/

1.2.1 Nicotine content in smokeless tobacco

The majority of commercial tobacco products are made from *N. tabacum* species, grown throughout the world with an alkaloid content that varies greatly. In randomly cultivated varieties examined, the alkaloid content ranged between 0.17 and 4.93%.

N. rustica species is cultivated in eastern Europe, Asia Minor and Africa, and the cured leaves may contain up to 12% nicotine. *Toombak* from Sudan, which contains *N. rustica* tobacco, had the highest reported levels of nicotine (Idris *et al.*, 1991; Prokopczyk *et al.*, 1995). In 17 brands of moist snuff from the USA, the nicotine content ranged from 0.47 to 3.43%.The nicotine content of Swedish snus ranges from 0.5–1.7% (Idris *et al.*, 1998; Stepanov *et al.*, 2008).

1.2.2 Carcinogenic compounds in smokeless tobacco

Multiple carcinogens have been identified in smokeless tobacco (IARC, 2007a) including:

(a) Tobacco-specific N-nitrosamines

Tobacco-specific *N*-nitrosamines include the carcinogens *N'*-nitrosonornicotine (NNN), and 4-(methylnitrosamino)-1-(3-pyridyl)-1-butanone (NNK).

Tobacco-specific *N*-nitrosamines are formed from tobacco alkaloids (nicotine, nornicotine, anatabine, anabasine, and nitrite) primarily during tobacco curing, fermentation and ageing. The nitrate or nitrite content, the mode of curing and the various steps of processing are the main determining factors for the yields of tobacco-specific *N*-nitrosamines in tobacco.

IARC (2007a) compiled an international comparison of the concentrations of NNN and NNK in smokeless tobacco products. The ranges vary widely and are product- and country-specific. In some moist snuff brands in the USA, the highest concentrations of NNN and NNK measured were 135 and 17.8 μg/g tobacco, respectively. In home-made *toombak* from Sudan, values as high as 3085 and 7870 μg/g dry wt tobacco, respectively, have been reported (Idris *et al.*, 1991; Prokopczyk *et al.*, 1995).

(b) N-Nitrosamino acids

The amino acids present in tobacco, and probably also the proteins with secondary amino groups, are amenable to *N*-nitrosation. Since 1985, numerous studies have reported the presence of *N*-nitrosamino acids in smokeless tobacco products (IARC, 2007a).

To date, 11 *N*-nitrosamino acids have been identified in smokeless tobacco: *N*-nitrososarcosine (NSAR), *N*-nitrosoazetidine-4-carboxylic acid (NAzCA), 3-(methylnitrosamino)propionic acid (MNPA), 4-(methylnitrosamino) butyric acid (MNBA), *N*-nitrosoproline (NPRO), *N*-nitrosohydroxyproline (NHPRO), *N*-nitrosopipecolic acid (NPIC), *N*-nitrosothiazolidine-4-carboxylic acid (NTCA), *N*-nitroso-2-methylthiazolidine-4-carboxylic acid (MNTCA), 4-(methylnitrosamino)-4-(3-pyridyl)butyric acid (*iso*-NNAC) and 2-(methylnitrosamino)-3-phenylpropionic acid (MNPhPA) (Ohshima *et al.*, 1985; Tricker & Preussmann, 1988; Hoffmann *et al.*, 1995). Of these, NSAR, MNPA, MNBA and NAzCA have been established as carcinogens in experimental animals.

The concentration of *N*-nitrosamino acids depends on the nitrate or nitrite content of tobacco; they are formed during prolonged storage, particularly under adverse conditions of temperature and relative humidity. The concentrations reported in USA moist snuff samples were in the range of 5.7 to 13.45 μg/g dry wt. Highest amounts of MNPA were found in Indian *zarda* (up to 18 μg/g) and in moist snuff (up to 70 μg/g).

Table 1.2 PAHs in moist snuff brands marketed in the USA

Compound	Mean ± SD of 23 brands (ng/g dry weight)
Naphthalene	1726 ± 392.3
Acenaphthylene	110.5 ± 42.9
Acenaphthene	105.1 ± 53.8
Fluorene	826.5 ± 287.0
Phenanthrene	4700 ± 1571
Anthracene	844.2 ± 277.8
Fluoranthene	1404 ± 537.4
Pyrene	1292 ± 428.5
Benz[*a*]anthracene	193.6 ± 71.3
Chrysene	232.1 ± 109.8
Methylchrysenes	92.6 ± 35.0
Benzo[*b*]fluoranthene + Benzo[*f*]fluoranthene	107.0 ± 69.5
Benzo[*k*]fluoranthene	19.6 ± 6.6
Benzo[*e*]pyrene	52.4 ± 23.8
Benzo[*a*]pyrene	55.8 ± 21.5
Indeno[*c*,*d*]pyrene	20.5 ± 12.1
Benzo[*g*,*h*,*i*]perylene	18.0 ± 8.3
Dibenz[*a*,*h*]anthracene	7.5 ± 1.9

From Stepanov *et al.* (2010)

(c) *Volatile N-nitrosamines*

These include *N*-nitrosodimehtylamine (NDMA), *N*-nitrosopyrrolidine (NPYR) and *N*-nitrosopiperidine (NPIP).

Levels of volatile *N*-nitrosamines formed from volatile amines and nitrosating agents in smokeless tobacco products worldwide have been summarized (IARC, 2007a). The highest amounts were found in moist snuff (NDMA up to 265 ng/g dry wt and NPYR up to 860 ng/g dry wt).

(d) *PAHs*

These include benzo[a]pyrene, benz[a] anthracene, chrysene, benzofluoranthenes, and dibenz[a,h]anthracene.

Levels of various PAHs in 23 moist snuff brands marketed in the USA were determined by Stepanov *et al.* (2010) and are summarized in Table 1.2.

(e) *Other carcinogenic compounds and constituents*

Levels of the volatile aldehydes formaldehyde, acetaldehyde, acrolein and crotonaldehyde in smokeless tobacco products ranged from 0.207–10.6, 0.97–72.3, 0.27–7.85, and 0.55–19.4 μg/g dry weight tobacco, respectively (Stepanov *et al.*, 2010).

Uranium was reported in Indian snuff at a concentration of about 3 pCi/g tobacco (Sharma *et al.*, 1985). Levels of polonium-210 in commercial moist and dry snuff in the USA were reported to be 0.16–1.22 and 0.23–0.39 pCi/g, respectively.

In several parts of the world, smokeless tobacco is invariably chewed with lime which is responsible for highly alkaline pH (Nair *et al.*, 1990, 1992), facilitating absorption of nicotine in the oral mucosa.

1.2.3 *Comparison of new and traditional smokeless tobacco products*

Newer types of smokeless tobacco products are appearing on the market. These products are sold as small pouches and do not require spitting. Similar to Swedish snus, they have been manufactured with additional controls to inhibit nitrosamine formation, and are being promoted as reduced risk products. Levels of carcinogens in these newer products are compared to those in traditional products in Table 1.3 (Stepanov *et al.*, 2008).

1.3 Prevalence of use

1.3.1 *Prevalence of smokeless tobacco use among adults*

Several surveys have evaluated the prevalence of smokeless tobacco use at different times and targeting different populations in the WHO regions (AFRO, African Region; AMRO, Region of the Americas; EURO, European Region; EMRO, Eastern Mediterranean Region; SEARO,

Table 1.3 Mean levels of selected carcinogens in newer and traditional smokeless tobacco products

	Newer products (n = 12)	Traditional products (n = 5)
NNN (µg/g dry weight)	2.05	4.41
NNK (µg/g dry weight)	0.231	1.20
Benzo[*a*]pyrene (ng/g dry weight)	3.12	38.2
Fluoranthene	10.0	400
Benzo[*b*]fluoranthene + Benzo[*k*]fluoranthene (ng/g dry weight)	2.76	38.3
Formaldehyde (µg/g dry weight)	3.23	8.43
Acetaldehyde (µg/g dry weight)	6.16	35.7
Crotonaldehyde (µg/g dry weight)	9.12	2.98

NNN, *N*′-nitrosonornicotine; NNK, 4-(methylnitrosamino)-1-(3-pyridyl)-1-butanone
From Stepanov *et al.* (2008)

South-East Asian Region; WPRO, Western Pacific Region). The major surveys that form the basis of this report are (Table 1.4):

- the Global Adult Tobacco Survey conducted during 2009–10 among adults aged 15 years or more in 14 middle and low-income countries in AMRO, SEARO, EURO, EMRO and WPRO;
- the national level STEPS noncommunicable risk factor survey (2006–09) was conducted in 8 countries in AFRO, and a few countries in SEARO, EURO (Georgia), EMRO and WPRO (Mongolia), in adults aged 15–64 years, except for AFRO (age group, 25–64 years);
- the Demographic and Health Surveys (2003–10) provide prevalence on smokeless tobacco use among adults aged 15–49 years in countries in AFRO (16), EURO (4), EMRO (2), WPRO (8);
- some other surveys such as the Behavioural Risk Factor Survey, the National Smoking/Tobacco/Drug use Survey, health cost studies, and national health, public health or morbidity surveys.

The prevalence of smokeless tobacco use reported in the various surveys are not directly comparable because of the different methodologies and time periods; however, they provide a snapshot of the global smokeless tobacco burden. Large variations are observed between countries (Table 1.5), between sex within a country, and sometimes within a country (Table 1.6). Those countries with a high prevalence (≥ 10%) represent about 25% of the global adult population. They include, by WHO region:

- in AFRO: Benin (men, 13%), Madagascar (men 23%; women, 20%), Mauritania (women, 28%), South Africa (women, 11%);
- in EMRO: Yemen (men, 15%);
- in EURO: Norway (men, 17.0%; women, 5.0%), Sweden (men, 26%), Uzbekistan (men, 22.5%);
- in SEARO: Bangladesh (men, 26%; women, 28%), India (men, 33%; women 11–18%), Myanmar (men, 51.4%; women, 16.1%), Nepal (men, 31%), Sri Lanka (men, 24.9%);
- in WPRO: Cambodia (women, 12.7%).

A few countries have medium prevalence (between 5% and 10%); these include:

- in AFRO: Benin, Cape Verde, Malawi in women; Lesotho, Mali, Mauritania, Swaziland, Zimbabwe in men;
- in AMRO: USA in men;

- in EMRO: Tunisia in men; Yemen in women;
- in EURO: Finland, Iceland and Kyrgyzstan in men; Norway and Sweden in women;
- in SEARO: Sri Lanka and Thailand in women.

In most countries, current prevalence of smokeless tobacco use is higher among men than among women. Some exceptions are found at all levels of prevalence (in women and men, respectively): Bangladesh (27.9, 26.9), Barbados (0.6, 0), Cambodia (12.7, 0.7), Cape Verde (5.8, 3.5), Malaysia (3.1, 0.5), Mauritania (28.3, 5.7), South Africa (10.9, 2.4), Thailand (6.3, 1.3) and Viet Nam (2.3, 0.3).

Demographic health survey data indicate that in countries in AFRO and SEARO smokeless tobacco is more prevalent in rural compared to urban areas, and higher among low-income compared to high-income groups. Also, prevalence generally increases with increasing age.

Some countries warrant more detailed information of their pattern of smokeless tobacco use, and are presented below.

1.3.2 Country specific data

(a) India

The India Global Adult Tobacco Survey (2009–10) revealed that 26% of all adults use smokeless tobacco in some form, 21.4% daily and 4.5% occasionally. Prevalence in men (32.9%) is higher than in women (18.4%), and is higher in rural (29.3%) than urban areas (17.7%). Large variations are observed between States, from around 5% in Himachal Pradesh, Goa and Chandigarh to 49% in Bihar (India GATS Report, 2009–10).

Khaini is the most commonly used smokeless tobacco product (11.6%), followed by *gutka* (8.2%). Prevalence of *khaini* chewing is significantly higher among men (18%) than among women (5%); 13.1% men and 2.9% women chew *gutka*; 6.2% (7.5% men, 4.9% women) of adults use betel quid with tobacco; 4.7% (3.3% men, 6.3% women) use tobacco products such as *mishri, gul, gudakhu* for oral application (dentifrice); and 4.4% uses some other products, such as snuff for nasal application and some local products. The pattern of use of smokeless tobacco products also varies widely in different States of India (Table 1.6) (India GATS Report, 2009–10).

Proportion of dual tobacco users (smoking+smokeless) is 19.4% among men and 5.3% among women (Sinha *et al.*, 2011).

(b) Bangladesh

In Bangladesh the most prevalent form of smokeless tobacco is betel quid with tobacco (24.3%), followed by *gul* (5.3%), *sada pata* (1.8%), *khaini* (1.5%) and others (1.4%) (BAN GATS Report, 2009). Use decreases with increasing education and socioeconomic level in both men and women, by a steeper rate among women compared to men. Among current users, those with the highest prevalence of use of *gul* and *khaini* were labourers among men (7.5% and 2.8%, respectively) and homemaker among women (5.7% and 1.4%, respectively) (BAN GATS Report, 2009).

Proportion of dual tobacco users (smoking+smokeless) is 22.5% among men and 2.5% among women (Sinha *et al.*, 2011).

(c) Canada

Unchanged from surveys conducted in 2008 and 2009, 8% of Canadians aged 15 years and older reported having ever tried smokeless tobacco products in 2010. In 2009, 11% of young adults aged 20 to 24 years reported ever using smokeless tobacco and 1% having used it within the past 30 days. There has been a shift in the distribution of past-30-day smokeless tobacco users from youth towards older adults: in 2003, 23% of users were aged 15–19 years and 14% were older than 45 years, whereas in 2009, 16% of smokeless tobacco users were 15 to 19 years old and 33% were aged 45 and older.

Table 1.4 Surveys and articles used to compile the information presented*

Bangladesh GATS report Government of the People's Republic of Bangladesh, Ministry of Health and Family Welfare; World Health Organization, Country Office for Bangladesh. Global Adult Tobacco Survey: Bangladesh Report 2009. Dhaka, 2009. http://www.searo.who.int/LinkFiles/Regional_Tobacco_Surveillance_System_GATSBAN_FullReport2009.pdf

Canada CTUMS Canadian Tobacco Use Monitoring Survey (CTUMS) 2010, http://www.hc-sc.gc.ca/hc-ps/tobac-tabac/research-recherche/stat/_ctums-esutc_2010/ann_summary-sommaire-eng.php

Central Statistical Office (CSO) [Swaziland], and Macro International Inc. 2008. *Swaziland Demographic and Health Survey 2006–07.* Mbabane, Swaziland: Central Statistical Office and Macro International Inc. http://www.measuredhs.com/pubs/pdf/FR202/FR202.pdf

Central Statistical Office (CSO) [Zimbabwe] and Macro International Inc. 2007. *Zimbabwe Demographic and Health Survey 2005–06.* Calverton, Maryland: CSO and Macro International Inc. http://www.measuredhs.com/pubs/pdf/FR186/FR186.pdf

Central Statistical Office (CSO), Ministry of Health (health ministry), Tropical Diseases Research Centre (TDRC), University of Zambia, and Macro International Inc. 2009. *Zambia Demographic and Health Survey 2007.* Calverton, Maryland, USA: CSO and Macro International Inc. http://www.measuredhs.com/pubs/pdf/FR211/FR211[revised-05-12-2009].pdf

Department of Health, Medical Research Council, OrcMacro. 2007. *South Africa Demographic and Health Survey 2003. Pretoria: Department of Health.* http://www.measuredhs.com/pubs/pdf/FR206/FR206.pdf

Ghana Statistical Service (GSS), Ghana Health Service (GHS), and ICF Macro. 2009. *Ghana Demographic and Health Survey 2008.* Accra, Ghana: GSS, GHS, and ICF Macro. http://www.measuredhs.com/publications/publication-FR221-DHS-Final-Reports.cfm

Global Tobacco epidemic report World Health Organization. World Report on the Global Tobacco Epidemic, 2009: Implementing Smoke-Free Environments. Geneva: WHO, 2009.

Global Tobacco epidemic report World Health Organization. World Report on the Global Tobacco Epidemic, 2011 Geneva: WHO, 2011.

India GATS report Government of India, Ministry of Health and Family Welfare. Global Adult Tobacco Survey: GATS India 2009–2010. Mumbai, 2010. http://www.searo.who.int/LinkFiles/Regional_Tobacco_Surveillance_System_GATS_India.pdf

Institut National de la Statistique (INSTAT) et ICF Macro. 2010. *Enquête Démographique et de Santé de Madagascar 2008–2009.* Antananarivo, Madagascar: INSTAT et ICF Macro. http://www.measuredhs.com/pubs/pdf/FR236/FR236.pdf

Institut National de la Statistique et de l'Analyse Économique (INSAE) [Bénin] et Macro International Inc. 2007: *Enquête Démographique et de Santé (EDSB-III) – Bénin 2006.* Calverton, Maryland, USA: Institut National de la Statistique et de l'Analyse Économique et Macro International Inc. http://www.measuredhs.com/publications/publication-FR197-DHS-Final-Reports.cfm

Kenya National Bureau of Statistics (KNBS) and ICF Macro. 2010. *Kenya Demographic and Health Survey 2008–09.* Calverton, Maryland: KNBS and ICF Macro. http://www.measuredhs.com/publications/publication-FR229-DHS-Final-Reports.cfm

Liberia Institute of Statistics and Geo-Information Services (LISGIS) [Liberia], Ministry of Health and Social Welfare [Liberia], National AIDS Control Program [Liberia], and Macro International Inc. 2008. *Liberia Demographic and Health Survey 2007.* Monrovia, Liberia: Liberia Institute of Statistics and Geo-Information Services (LISGIS) and Macro International Inc. http://www.measuredhs.com/publications/publication-FR201-DHS-Final-Reports.cfm

Lund M, Lindbak R. *Norwegian Tobacco Statistics 1973–2006.* Oslo: Norwegian Institute for Alcohol and Drug Research; 2007. Sirus skrifter No. 3/2007.

Lundqvist G, Sandström H, Ohman A, Weinehall L. Patterns of tobacco use: a 10-yr follow-up study of smoking and snus habits in a middle-aged Swedish population, Scand J Public Health. 2009, 37:161–7

Ministry of Health and Social Services (MoHSS) [Namibia] and Macro International Inc. 2008. *Namibia Demographic and Health Survey 2006–07.* Windhoek, Namibia and Calverton, Maryland, USA: MoHSS and Macro International Inc. http://www.measuredhs.com/publications/publication-FR204-DHS-Final-Reports.cfm

Ministry of Health and Social Welfare (MOHSW) [Lesotho] and ICF Macro. 2010. *Lesotho Demographic and Health Survey 2009.* Maseru, Lesotho: MOHSW and ICF Macro. http://www.measuredhs.com/publications/publication-FR241-DHS-Final-Reports.cfm

Table 1.4 (continued)

MMWR August 27, 2010, 59(33), 487–92, Tobacco use among Middle and High school students –USA 2000–2009

MMWR August 6, 2010/59(30);946–950, Any tobacco use in 13 states-Behavioural Risk factor Surveillance System 2008

National Bureau of Statistics (NBS) [United Republic of Tanzania] and ICF Macro. 2011. *United Republic of Tanzania Demographic and Health Survey 2010*. Dar es Salaam, United Republic of Tanzania: NBS and ICF Macro. http://www.measuredhs.com/pubs/pdf/FR243/FR243[24June2011].pdf

National Institute of Population Research and Training (NIPORT), Mitra and Associates, and Macro International. 2009. *Bangladesh Demographic and Health Survey 2007*. Dhaka, Bangladesh and Calverton, Maryland, USA: National Institute of Population Research and Training, Mitra and Associates, and Macro International. http://www.measuredhs.com/pubs/pdf/FR207/FR207[April-10-2009].pdf

National Population Commission (NPC) [Nigeria] and ICF Macro. 2009. *Nigeria Demographic and Health Survey 2008*. Abuja, Nigeria: National Population Commission and ICF Macro. http://www.measuredhs.com/publications/publication-FR222-DHS-Final-Reports.cfm

National Statistics Directorate (NSD) [Timor-Leste], Ministry of Finance [Timor-Leste], and ICF Macro. 2010. *Timor-Leste Demographic and Health Survey 2009–10*. Dili, Timor-Leste: NSD [Timor-Leste] and ICF Macro. http://www.measuredhs.com/pubs/pdf/FR235/FR235.pdf

Sinha DN, Palipudi KM, Rolle I *et al.* (2011). Tobacco use among youth and adults in member countries of South-East Asia region: Review of findings from surveys under the global tobacco surveillance system. Indian J Public Health, 55:169–176. PMID:22089684

Statistics Indonesia (Badan Pusat Statistik—BPS) and Macro International. 2008. *Indonesia Demographic and Health Survey 2007*. Calverton, Maryland, USA: BPS and Macro International. http://www.measuredhs.com/pubs/pdf/FR218/FR218[27August2010].pdf

Statistics Sierra Leone (SSL) and ICF Macro. 2009. *Sierra Leone Demographic and Health Survey 2008*. Calverton, Maryland, USA: Statistics Sierra Leone (SSL) and ICF Macro. http://www.measuredhs.com/pubs/pdf/FR225/FR225.pdf

Uganda Bureau of Statistics (UBOS) and Macro International Inc. 2007. *Uganda Demographic and Health Survey 2006*. Calverton, Maryland, USA: UBOS and Macro International Inc. http://www.measuredhs.com/pubs/pdf/FR194/FR194.pdf

*, Exceptionally, the most recent updates of well established ongoing surveys and reports, published after the meeting, were included in this *Monograph*. The methodology and data available at the time of the meeting were reviewed by the Working Group; the updates reflect the most current estimates of prevalence of exposure and therefore have no influence on the final evaluation.

Table 1.5 Highest and lowest prevalence of smokeless tobacco use by WHO regions and by sex

	Men		Women	
WHO region	Lowest	Highest	Lowest	Highest
AFRO	0.8% in Gambia	22.6% in Madagascar	0.2% in Ghana	28.3% in Mauritania
AMRO	0.0% in Barbados	6.9% in USA	0.2% in Guyana & Dominican Republic	0.6% in Barbados
EMRO	1.3% in Saudi Arabia	15.1% in Yemen	0.1% in Libyan	6.2% in Yemen
EURO	0.2% in Switzerland & Latvia	26.0% in Sweden	0% in Switzerland & Ukraine	5% in Kyrgyzstan
SEARO	1.3% in Thailand	51.4% in Myanmar	0.3% in Indonesia	27.9% in Bangladesh
WPRO	0.3% in Viet Nam	2.8% in Mongolia & Philippines	0.1% in the People's Republic of China	12.7% in Cambodia

(d) USA

According to the Behavioural Risk Factor Surveillance System survey (2008), conducted in 13 States, prevalence varied from 0.5% (New Jersey) to 8.8% (West Virginia). Dual use of cigarette and smokeless tobacco products varied from 0.2% (Delaware) to 1.8% (West Virginia).

In an overall analysis of users' demographic characteristics, prevalence of smokeless tobacco use was higher among men (6.3%) than women (0.3%); more prevalent among non-Hispanic whites (4.1%) compared to other ethnic groups; highest in the youngest age group (18–24 years) and decreased steadily with age. Users of smokeless tobacco were almost equally distributed between the sextiles of annual income (3.0 to 3.8%).

(e) Europe

In Europe, countries with a high prevalence of smokeless tobacco use are Norway, Sweden and Uzbekistan.

In Sweden, a 10-year follow-up study of smoking and snus [Swedish moist snuff] habits in a middle-aged Swedish population showed that use of snus increased from 3.1% to 6.0% among women and from 24.6% to 26.3% among men. The number of people who used both snus and cigarettes was stable: 0.5% to 0.8% from baseline to follow-up for women and 4.1% to 3.3% for men. Whereas nearly all snus users in Sweden are daily users, almost half of snus users in Norway use it only occasionally.

1.3.3 Prevalence of smokeless tobacco use among youth

The Global Youth Tobacco Survey (GYTS) is a school-based survey of students aged 13–15 years that uses a two-stage sampling design. In a first stage, schools are selected based on the probability proportional to the enrolment of students in schools. In a second stage, classes are selected randomly. It uses standard questionnaire, field methodology and analysis. The Survey has core questions that spans seven thematic areas pertinent to tobacco. In addition, countries can include country-specific questions that allow assessment of tobacco unique to the country [smokeless tobacco use may include betel quid with tobacco.]

In AFRO, all countries surveyed reported a prevalence of smokeless tobacco use among youth above 5%, ranging from 5.4% in Swaziland to 16.4% in Congo. Among boys, it varied from 5.2% in Seychelles to 18.3% in Congo, whereas among girls, from 4.8% in Togo to 15.8% in Namibia. Prevalence was higher among boys than girls in most countries, except in Uganda where

Table 1.6 Highest and lowest prevalence of use of selected smokeless tobacco products in India, by State

	Lowest	Highest
Betel quid	0.5% in Punjab, Himachal Pradesh, Chandigarh and Uttrakhand	32.8% in Tripura
Dentifrice	0.4% in Tripura	28.35 in Chattishgarh
Khaini	0.5% in Tamil Nadu	32.6% in Jharkhand
Gutka	0.6% in Puducherry	17.0% in Madhya Pradesh

it was higher among girls (9.6% versus 8.6%) (Asma *et al.*, 2011). Four countries (Botswana, Congo, Lesotho and Namibia) are particularly noteworthy: these countries reported the highest prevalence in both sexes (11.3–16.4%), the highest prevalence in boys (11.3–18.3%), the highest prevalence in girls (11.4–15.8%), and similar prevalence in boys and girls.

In AMRO, prevalence of smokeless tobacco use among youth varied from 3.5% in Panama to 9.8% in Barbados. Among boys, it varied from 3.8% in Panama to 11.5% in Barbados, whereas among girls, it varies from 2.6% in Venezuela to 8.5% in Jamaica. Most notably, smokeless tobacco use among boys was above 10% in Barbados, Dominican Republic and Grenada. Girls in most countries used less smokeless tobacco than boys, except in Jamaica (8.5% for both) and Peru (boys, 4.3%; girls, 4.8%) where boys and girls had comparable prevalence (Asma *et al.*, 2011).

In SEARO, all countries surveyed reported a prevalence of smokeless tobacco use among youth above 5%, ranging from 4.9% in Bangladesh to 9.4% in Bhutan. Among boys, it ranged from 5.8% in Bangladesh to 14.1% in Bhutan whereas among girls, it varies from 2.7% in Myanmar to 6% in India. In all countries more boys than girls used smokeless tobacco products (Asma *et al.*, 2011).

In EURO, prevalence of smokeless tobacco use among youth is lower than in other WHO regions, ranging from 1.1% in Montenegro to 6.9% in Estonia. While it ranged from 1.1% in Montenegro to 9.4% in Estonia among boys, it varied from 0.7% in Serbia to 4.5% in Estonia among girls. Except for Estonia (6.9%), all countries reported a prevalence among youth below 5%. Also, in all countries boys used more smokeless tobacco than girls (Asma *et al.*, 2011).

In EMRO, prevalence of smokeless tobacco use among youth varied from 1.6% in Oman to 12.6% Djibouti. Among boys, it varied from 2% in Libyan Arab Jamahirya to 15.2% in Djibouti, whereas among girls, it varied from 0.9% in Oman and Tunisia to 9% in Djibouti. Prevalence of smokeless tobacco use among youth was highest in Djibouti (12.6%), where it is also highest among boys and girls separately. Boys generally used more smokeless tobacco than girls, except in Libyan Arab Jamahirya and Yemen where girl users slightly outnumbered boy users (Asma *et al.*, 2011).

In WPRO, prevalence of smokeless tobacco use among youth varies from 2.1% in Macau to 8.7% in Cook Islands. Among boys, it varies from 2.2% in Macau to 10.5% in Cook Islands, whereas among girls, it varies from 2.1% in Macau to 7.3% in Cook Islands. Prevalence of smokeless tobacco use among youth in Cook Island and Republic of Korea is above 5% for boys and girls combined, as well as separately for boys and girls. Prevalence among boys was generally higher than among girls (Asma *et al.*, 2011).

In summary, among the countries included in the GYTS survey 2007–2010, the prevalence of smokeless tobacco use among youth aged 13–15 years exceeds 5% in all or most countries in AFRO, AMRO and SEARO, in Djibouti, Islamic Republic of Iran, Qatar, Syrian Arab Republic and Yemen in EMRO, and in the Cook Islands and Republic of Korea in WPRO (Asma *et al.*, 2011).

In general, prevalence among boys was higher than among girls, although in several countries prevalence was similar, or higher among girls.

In several countries, smokeless tobacco use among 13 to 15 year-old men is higher than that among adult men (aged 15 years or more). These include Albania, Argentina, Brazil, the Dominican Republic, Guyana, Lesotho, Mexico, Namibia, Saudi Arabia, Tunisia and Uganda. Similarly, in Albania, Argentina, Barbados, Brazil, Dominican Republic, Guyana, Kyrgyzstan, Libyan Arab Jamahirya, Mexico, Saudi Arabia, Swaziland, Uganda and Yemen, smokeless tobacco use among 13–15 year women is higher than that in adult women.

2. Cancer in Humans

2.1 Oral use

2.1.1 Cancers of the oral cavity and pharynx

(a) Overview of studies

Studies of smokeless tobacco and oral and pharyngeal cancer have been conducted in North and South America, Europe, Asia, and Africa. All of the studies reported here examined oral cancer risks associated with use of unsmoked tobacco that was not part of a betel quid. Evidence regarding betel quid is presented in the *Monograph* on Betel Quid in this volume. This section focuses on the predominant smokeless tobacco products and behaviours in the countries in which the studies were conducted, for example on chewing tobacco and snuff in North America, snus in northern Europe, *shammah* in Saudi Arabia and Yemen, *toombak* in Sudan, and a variety of types in South Asia (see Table 1.1 for their mode of use, ingredients and region of use). The studies typically examine cancers arising in intra-oral sites, which are predominantly squamous cell in origin (Canto & Devesa, 2002), but some include other sites as well, such as the oropharynx, hypopharynx, or larynx. Studies involving smokeless tobacco and nasopharyngeal cancer are discussed in another chapter.

The previous *Monograph* (IARC, 2007a) concluded that there was *sufficient evidence* in humans that smokeless tobacco causes cancer of the oral cavity. Studies published since include updates on mortality and incidence for one of the cohorts reviewed previously (Accortt *et al.*, 2002, 2005), two new cohort studies (Luo *et al.*, 2007; Roosaar *et al.*, 2008); case–control studies from Sweden (Rosenquist, 2005; Rosenquist *et al.*, 2005) and India (Sapkota *et al.*, 2007); and three meta-analyses (Weitkunat *et al.*, 2007; Boffetta *et al.*, 2008; Lee & Hamling, 2009).

Because tobacco smoking is a risk factor for oral and pharyngeal cancers (IARC, 2004), and tobacco smoking is often positively correlated with smokeless tobacco use (Tomar, 2002), addressing confounding by smoking is important in the examination of causality related to smokeless tobacco. Heavy alcohol use is another important risk factor and can potentially confound the relationship between tobacco use and risk of oral and pharyngeal cancer (IARC, 2010, 2012).

While analysis restricted to non-smokers and non-alcohol drinkers eliminates the possibility of confounding due to smoking and alcohol drinking, the sample sizes can be small in study populations in regions where these behaviours are common. Adjusting statistically for smoking and alcohol can alternatively be used to address confounding by these factors in populations where these behaviours are common and can provide unbiased estimates that may be more stable if there is no residual confounding within smoking/drinking categories used in the adjustment. There is *sufficient evidence* that human papillomavirus (HPV) 16 causes oral cancer in humans (IARC, 2007b). Studies have shown that the prevalence of HPV DNA is negatively correlated with tobacco smoking and alcoholic beverage consumption (Gillison *et al.*, 2000), suggesting that positive confounding by HPV is not likely to account for a spurious association between smokeless tobacco and oral cancer.

The specific name of the smokeless tobacco product will be used whenever available. In the USA, where moist snuff and chewing tobacco are both common, the term “smokeless tobacco” refers to use of either. Most publications provide data on “ever” versus “never” use of these products, usually defined as using the product or not for some minimal length of time such as a year. Due to the large body of evidence, this *Monograph* will focus on studies published since IARC (2007a).

(i) Cohort studies

Ever lifetime use or ever daily use of smokeless tobacco and risk of oral and pharyngeal cancers was examined in six cohort studies conducted in the USA (Zahm *et al.*, 1992; Accortt *et al.*, 2002, 2005; Henley *et al.*, 2005), Sweden (Luo *et al.*, 2007; Roosaar *et al.*, 2008), and Norway (Boffetta *et al.*, 2005). Mortality data were analysed in four studies (Zahm *et al.*, 1992; Accortt *et al.*, 2002; Henley *et al.*, 2005; Roosaar *et al.*, 2008), four (Accortt *et al.*, 2005; Boffetta *et al.*, 2005; Luo *et al.*, 2007; Roosaar *et al.*, 2008) analysed cancer incidence. None of the studies excluded persons diagnosed in the first 1 or 2 years of follow-up nor did they collect information on changes in behaviours, such as smokeless tobacco or smoking cessation or initiation, after the baseline (Table 2.1 available at http://monographs.iarc.fr/ENG/Monographs/vol100E/100E-03-Table2.1.pdf).

Ever use of smokeless tobacco was associated with a statistically significant threefold increased risk of death from oral cancer and an 8.7 fold increased risk of death from pharyngeal cancer in one study from the USA (Zahm *et al.*, 1992). Risks were greater among those with more frequent use, but adjustment was not performed for tobacco smoking and therefore this study will not be considered further in this section.

Ever use of smokeless tobacco was not associated with risk for cancer in four cohorts (Accortt *et al.*, 2005; Boffetta *et al.*, 2005; Henley *et al.*, 2005; Luo *et al.*, 2007). In one cohort the age-adjusted standardized mortality ratio for oral cancer associated with ever smokeless tobacco use was not elevated (Accortt *et al.*, 2002) and the age-adjusted standardized incidence ratio for smokeless tobacco use and oral cancer was statistically lower than expected (Accortt *et al.*, 2005). The expected number of oral cancer deaths among ever smokeless tobacco users in this cohort was zero, suggesting limited statistical power to detect elevated risks.

In the Cancer Prevention Study I and II cohorts (Henley *et al.*, 2005; CPS-I and CPS-II, respectively), the hazard ratio (HR) for death from oral and pharyngeal cancer in CPS-I for current use of smokeless tobacco versus never use among men who never used any other form of tobacco was 2.0 (95%CI: 0.5–7.7), based on four deaths adjusting for alcohol consumption, fruit/vegetable intake and other factors. The corresponding HR in CPS-II was 0.9 (95%CI: 0.1–6.7), based on one death adjusting for similar factors as CPS-I.

In the Norwegian cohort (Boffetta *et al.*, 2005), the HR for ever use of smokeless tobacco was 1.1 (95%CI: 0.5–2.4), for oral, pharynx or salivary gland cancer after adjusting for age and smoking. Among non-smokers in a cohort of 280 000 Swedish male construction workers, the relative risk of developing oral cancer was 0.8 (95%CI: 0.4–1.7), adjusting for attained age and body mass index (BMI) (Luo *et al.*, 2007).

One cohort study in Sweden involved 9 860 men who participated in an oral examination (Roosaar *et al.*, 2008). An elevated relative risk (RR) of 3.1 (95%CI: 1.5–6.6) was found for ever daily use of snus compared to never daily use of snus controlling for calendar period, area of residence, alcohol consumption, smoking, and an interaction variable for age and smoking. Among the never-smokers in the cohort, the relative risk for ever daily use of snus was 2.3 (95%CI: 0.7–8.3).

All cohort studies had at least 12 years of follow-up. No increased risk of oral cancer was observed for the three cohorts with 12–26 years of follow-up (Accortt *et al.*, 2002, 2005; Henley *et al.*, 2005; Luo *et al.*, 2007). One study with 35 years follow-up found no association of smokeless tobacco and oral cancer risk (Boffetta *et al.*, 2005) and another study with 27–29 years follow-up had significant positive findings among smokers only (Roosaar *et al.*, 2008).

(ii) Case–control studies

Many case–control studies examined smokeless tobacco and oral and pharyngeal cancer (Broders, 1920; Moore *et al.*, 1953; Wynder & Bross, 1957; Wynder *et al.*, 1957a, b; Peacock *et al.*, 1960; Chandra, 1962; Vogler *et al.*, 1962; Vincent & Marchetta, 1963; Martinez, 1969; Keller, 1970; Browne *et al.*, 1977; Jafarey *et al.*, 1977; Williams & Horm, 1977; Wynder & Stellman, 1977; Westbrook, 1980; Winn *et al.*, 1981a; Wynder *et al.*, 1983; Stockwell & Lyman, 1986; Young *et al.*, 1986; Blot *et al.*, 1988; Spitz *et al.*, 1988; Franco *et al.*, 1989; Goud *et al.*, 1990; Blomqvist *et al.*, 1991; Maden *et al.*, 1992; Marshall *et al.*, 1992; Mashberg *et al.*, 1993; Spitz *et al.*, 1993; Kabat *et al.*, 1994; Bundgaard *et al.*, 1995; Idris *et al.*, 1995a; Muscat *et al.*, 1996; Lewin *et al.*, 1998; Muscat & Wynder, 1998; Schildt *et al.*, 1998; Schwartz *et al.*, 1998; Wasnik *et al.*, 1998; Chelleng *et al.*, 2000; Merchant *et al.*, 2000; Rosenquist *et al.*, 2005; Rosenquist, 2005; Sapkota *et al.*, 2007). Two studies were of cancer of the salivary gland (Keller, 1969; Muscat & Wynder, 1998), one reported on hypopharyngeal cancer (Sapkota *et al.*, 2007), and one on nasopharyngeal cancer (Chelleng *et al.*, 2000). The same study was reported on twice in two instances (Wynder & Bross, 1957; Wynder *et al.*, 1957a; Rosenquist, 2005; Rosenquist *et al.*, 2005). Additionally, one cross-sectional study was conducted, but the comparability of the two surveys analysed to yield risk estimates was uncertain (Sterling *et al.*, 1992).

Nearly half the studies addressed potential confounding by tobacco smoking. In three (Broders, 1920; Stockwell & Lyman, 1986; Keller, 1970), smokeless tobacco information was probably obtained from medical records and, if ascertainment of smokeless tobacco use was more likely from cases than from controls, measurement error might account for the findings and these studies will not be considered further. The remaining 15 studies were conducted in the USA (Vogler *et al.*, 1962; Martinez, 1969; Williams & Horm, 1977; Winn *et al.*, 1981a; Blot *et al.*, 1988; Mashberg *et al.*, 1993; Kabat *et al.*, 1994), Sweden (Lewin *et al.*, 1998; Schildt *et al.*, 1998; Rosenquist, 2005; Rosenquist *et al.*, 2005), India (Chandra, 1962; Wasnik *et al.*, 1998; Sapkota *et al.*, 2007), Pakistan (Merchant *et al.*, 2000), and Sudan (Idris *et al.*, 1995a) (Table 2.2 available at http://monographs.iarc.fr/ENG/Monographs/vol100E/100E-03-Table2.2.pdf).

Five studies were population-based (Williams & Horm, 1977; Blot *et al.*, 1988; Lewin *et al.*, 1998; Schildt *et al.*, 1998; Rosenquist *et al.*, 2005); positive findings were observed in the majority of them (Williams & Horm, 1977; Blot *et al.*, 1988; Lewin *et al.*, 1998) and in all of the hospital-based studies except one (Mashberg *et al.*, 1993). One study (Winn *et al.*, 1981a) also included death certificate cases and controls.

Several case–control studies of oral cancer addressed potential confounding by tobacco smoking either by statistically controlling for tobacco smoking or by restricting to non-smokers. Odds ratios (OR) for ever versus never use of smokeless tobacco overall, or for at least one of the major cancer subtypes, was statistically significantly elevated in eight studies, with odds ratios for oral cavity cancer ranging from 3.9 to 34.5 (Vogler *et al.*, 1962; Martinez, 1969; Williams & Horm, 1977; Winn *et al.*, 1981a; Blot *et al.*, 1988; Kabat *et al.*, 1994; Idris *et al.*, 1995a; Wasnik *et al.*, 1998; Merchant *et al.*, 2000) and in one study of hypopharyngeal cancer in India (Sapkota *et al.*, 2007). In case–control studies conducted in Sweden, there was no association with use of smokeless tobacco in 2 studies (Schildt *et al.*, 1998; Rosenquist, 2005) or in another study (Lewin *et al.*, 1998) that controlled for smoking and alcohol intake. However, when Lewin *et al.*, 1998 restricted the analysis to non-smokers the odds ratio for head and neck cancer associated with ever use of smokeless tobacco was 4.7 (95%CI: 1.6–13.8). [Rosenquist (2005) was based on a relatively small sample size of 132 cases and 320 controls.]

In one case–control study conducted in the USA (Vogler *et al.*, 1962) and another of *toombak* users in Sudan (Idris *et al.*, 1995a), neither statistical adjustment for tobacco smoking nor restriction to non-smokers was done. However, confounding by smoking was not likely to have a major effect on the risk estimates from these studies. The proportions of smokers in the case and control groups were low in the rural women in the study of Vogler *et al.* (1962) among whom positive findings were found. In the study in Sudan less than 10–12% of the two case groups and in a hospital-based control groups smoked; in the population-based control group 21% were smokers, but most had smoked for less than one year (Idris *et al.*, 1995a).

In a meta-analysis Boffetta *et al.* (2008) included studies published through 2007 that provided information about non-smokers and studies that adjusted for tobacco smoking. The summary estimate for the 11 studies of oral cancer (6 of them also including pharyngeal cancer) was 1.8 (95%CI: 1.1–2.9) overall. For the USA, it was 2.6 (95%CI: 1.3–5.2) and for northern European countries, 1.0 (95%CI: 0.7–1.3) (Table 2.3 available at http://monographs.iarc.fr/ENG/Monographs/vol100E/100E-03-Table2.3.pdf).

Another meta-analysis included 40 studies published through May 2008 (Table 2.4 available at http://monographs.iarc.fr/ENG/Monographs/vol100E/100E-03-Table2.4.pdf) but excluded studies in Asian or African populations (Lee & Hamling, 2009). In addition to the studies in the meta-analysis by Boffetta *et al.* (2008), 15 other studies were included: (Moore *et al.*, 1953; Wynder & Bross, 1957; Wynder *et al.*, 1957, 1983; Peacock *et al.*, 1960; Vincent & Marchetta, 1963; Martinez, 1969; Keller, 1970; Browne *et al.*, 1977; Wynder & Stellman, 1977; Young *et al.*, 1986; Spitz *et al.*, 1988; Franco *et al.*, 1989; Blomqvist *et al.*, 1991; Maden *et al.*, 1992; Marshall *et al.*, 1992; Sterling *et al.*, 1992; Zahm *et al.*, 1992; Spitz *et al.*, 1993; Bundgaard *et al.*, 1995; Muscat *et al.*, 1996; Schwartz *et al.*, 1998) and one unpublished study by Perry and colleagues in 1993. Among never-smokers the odds ratio was 1.72 (95%CI: 1.01–2.94) based on 9 studies; further adjustment for alcohol in the three studies where this was possible yielded an odds ratio among never-smokers of 1.87 (95%CI: 0.82–4.27). The estimate for never-smokers among the studies conducted in the USA was 3.33 (95%CI: 1.76–6.32), and decreased with additional adjustment for alcohol drinking (1.58; 95%CI: 0.52–4.81), based on two studies among never-smokers. Corresponding estimates for snuff use in never-smokers in Scandinavia were 1.01 (95%CI: 0.71–1.45; 4 studies) and 2.30 (95%CI: 0.67–7.92; 1 study) adjusted for alcohol drinking. For studies published since 1990, the corresponding estimates were 1.24 (95%CI: 0.80–1.90; 7 studies) in never-smokers and 1.87 (95%CI: 0.82–4.27; 3 studies) adjusted for alcohol drinking.

Lee & Hamling (2009) updated an earlier meta-analysis (Weitkunat *et al.*, 2007) of 32 studies through 2005, excluding studies conducted in Asian populations. Weitkunat *et al.* (2007) did not include three studies (Rosenquist *et al.*, 2005; Luo *et al.*, 2007; Roosaar *et al.*, 2008), but provided sex- and tobacco type- specific estimates not reported by Lee & Hamling (2009). For smokeless tobacco, the overall smoking-adjusted relative risk was 1.35 (95%CI: 1.04–1.76), and for chewing tobacco and snuff, the estimates were 1.42 (95%CI: 0.99–2.03; 6 studies) and

1.28 (95%CI: 0.76–2.14; 7 studies). For men the smoking-adjusted estimate was 1.15 (95%CI: 0.97–1.37) and for women 2.51 (95%CI: 1.73–3.64). For case–control studies with hospital-based controls, the estimates were 1.41 (95%CI: 1.18–1.68) and for studies with population-based controls 0.99 (95%CI: 0.69–1.42). Smoking-adjusted relative risks for smokeless tobacco were elevated only for studies conducted before 1980: 2.02 (95%CI: 1.28–3.20) for earlier than 1969, 2.67 (95%CI: 1.83–3.90) for 1970–1979, compared with 0.97 (95%CI: 0.71–1.31) for 1980–1989, and 1.10 (95%CI: 0.88–1.37) for 1990 or later.

(b) Dose–response evidence

In this and subsequent sections, the relative risks and odds ratios are either among non-smokers or are adjusted for tobacco smoking. Dose–response relationships were observed in several studies.

(i) Duration and intensity

Williams & Horm (1977) found that the odds ratio for oral cavity cancers in men associated with heavy use of smokeless tobacco was higher than for moderate use. Lewin *et al.* (1998) also reported relative risks for head and neck cancer that increased with increasing intensity of oral snuff use. Of the case–control studies that examined duration, higher risks of oral cancer with greater numbers of years of snuff use were noted for cancers of the gum/buccal mucosa, but not for other cancers of the mouth/pharynx category (Winn *et al.*, 1981a). No increase with years of snus use was observed in two Swedish case–control studies (Lewin *et al.*, 1998; Rosenquist *et al.*, 2005). In a study in Sudan (Idris *et al.*, 1995a), the odds ratio for use of *toombak* for more than 11 years was greater than that for fewer years of use.

(ii) Cessation

In two cohort (Boffetta *et al.*, 2005; Luo *et al.*, 2007) and three case–control studies (Lewin *et al.*, 1998; Schildt *et al.*, 1998; Rosenquist *et al.*, 2005), risks were not significantly elevated in either current or former smokeless tobacco users. No studies provided information on time since stopping.

(c) Comparison of types of smokeless tobacco by geographical location

(i) Northern Europe

Four studies from this area found no overall association between use of snus and oral cancer (Lewin *et al.*, 1998; Schildt *et al.*, 1998; Boffetta *et al.*, 2005; Rosenquist, 2005). One case–control study (Rosenquist, 2005) examined users of fermented and not fermented snuff and observed no risk for either type. In Sweden before 1983, snuff was fermented as part of the manufacturing process, and this process is conducive to formation of tobacco-specific *N*-nitrosamines. In one cohort study (Roosaar *et al.*, 2008) the relative risk for ever daily use of snus was 3.1 (95%CI: 1.5–6.6, adjusted for smoking, calendar period, area of residence, alcohol consumption and a variable to account for the interaction between age and smoking) and 2.3 (95%CI: 0.7–8.3) among non-smokers with adjustment for calendar period, area of residence and alcohol consumption. In a case–control study, among non-smokers, the odds ratio for cancers of the oral cavity, pharynx and oesophagus combined was 4.7 (95%CI: 1.6–13.8) (Lewin *et al.*, 1998).

(ii) USA

In the USA chewing tobacco and moist snuff are the predominant forms of smokeless tobacco. In five case–control studies of oral cancer, the odds ratio for ever use of smokeless tobacco were statistically significantly elevated overall for use of one or other type, ranging from 4.2 to 34.5 (Martinez, 1969; Williams & Horm, 1977; Williams *et al.*, 1977; Winn *et al.*, 1981a; Blot *et al.*, 1988; Kabat *et al.*, 1994). No association with use of either of these products was observed in 2 cohort studies (Accortt *et al.*, 2002; 2005;

Henley *et al.*, 2005) and one case–control study (Mashberg *et al.*, 1993).

The odds ratio for chewing tobacco was not statistically significantly elevated in two studies (Mashberg *et al.*, 1993; Kabat *et al.*, 1994); but was in a third (Martinez, 1969). For snuff, one study found no association (Mashberg *et al.*, 1993) and in three others statistically significant elevated risks were observed, ranging from 4.2 to 34.5 (Winn *et al.*, 1981a; Blot *et al.*, 1988; Kabat *et al.*, 1994). In one case–control study in the southern USA positive associations were observed among non-smoking women who were snuff dippers, but a significant association was observed for white, but not black women; dry snuff was the predominant form of snuff used by women in that area (Winn *et al.*, 1981a). Elevated odds ratios persisted with control for poor dentition (Winn *et al.*, 1981b), use of mouthwashes (Blot *et al.*, 1983), fruits and vegetables (Winn *et al.*, 1984), type of respondent (self versus proxy), and alcohol consumption (Winn, 1986).

(iii) Africa, Middle East, and Asia

In Sudan the majority of a consecutively accrued series of oral cancer cases used *saffa*, an oral snuff, a moistened, powdered tobacco treated with sodium sesquicarbonate (Elbeshir *et al.*, 1989). Also, in Sudan *toombak* use was higher in oral cancer cases with squamous cell-carcinomas in sites with direct contact with the quid (e.g. floor of mouth) than cases with less or no contact (e.g. palate) (Idris *et al.*, 1995b). The odds ratio for *toombak* use was 7.3 (4.3–12.4) comparing hospital-based cases with oral cancers in direct contact with the quid versus hospital controls, and 1.4 (0.8–2.5) for cases with oral cancers not usually in direct contact with the quid (Idris *et al.*, 1995a), adjusting for age, sex, tribe and residence. Ten to twelve percent of the cases and hospital controls smoked. Twenty-one percent of population controls smoked, although most had smoked for less than one year.

Case series from Saudi Arabia have noted a high frequency of use of *shammah* or *al-shammah* in series of oral, pharyngeal, and laryngeal cancer cases (Amer *et al.*, 1985; Ibrahim *et al.*, 1986; al-Idrissi, 1990; Allard *et al.*, 1999).

In Pakistan, ever using *naswar* was associated with an odds ratio of 9.5 (95%CI: 1.7–52.5; adjusted for cigarette smoking and alcohol consumption) (Merchant *et al.*, 2000). Reports based on small series of users in which potential confounding by tobacco smoking could not be ruled out also noted higher frequencies of *naswar* use in oral cancer cases than controls or oral cancers among *naswar* users (Aleksandrova, 1970; Nugmanov & Baimakanov, 1970).

In India, a case–control study of buccal mucosa cancer observed an odds ratio of [2.7] for men and [2.5] for women associated with tobacco chewing among non-smokers (Chandra, 1962). In a cross-sectional survey, the period prevalence of oral and oropharyngeal cancer among persons who used *pattiwala*, sun-cured tobacco leaf only, was 1.17 per 100 persons compared to 0.36 among non-chewers of tobacco (Wahi, 1968) [tobacco smoking was not accounted for]. A case–control study of oropharyngeal cancer, using a smokeless tobacco product for teeth cleaning was associated with an odds ratio of 5.2 (95%CI: 2.5–11.8), adjusted for smoking (Wasnik *et al.*, 1998). In another case–control study in India, snuffing tobacco nasally or orally, generally using *naswar*, was associated with elevated odds ratios for hypopharyngeal cancer in never-smokers and in analyses adjusted for tobacco smoking and alcohol consumption (Sapkota *et al.*, 2007). [The Working Group noted that in the Sapkota *et al.* (2007) study, snuff use was nasal as well as oral so the role of oral use could not be separately determined.] In the same study, odds ratios for hypopharyngeal cancer among never-smokers were significantly elevated for *zarda* and non-significantly elevated for *khaini*, after adjusting for centre, age, sex, socioeconomic status, alcohol consumption and tobacco snuffing.

(d) Interactions

In one study in the USA that provided odds ratios for smokers only, smokeless tobacco users only, and smokers who also used smokeless tobacco, each compared to non-users of either, there was no evidence of an interaction between smokeless tobacco use and smoking (Winn *et al.*, 1981a), nor was there any evidence of an interaction between smokeless tobacco use and alcohol consumption in a similar analysis of that study population (Winn, 1986).

2.1.2 Precancerous lesions of the oral cavity

(a) Overview of studies

Studies on the natural history of oral cancer suggest that several types of potentially malignant lesions and conditions precede the development of cancer of the oral cavity. Oral precancerous lesions of relevance are leukoplakia and erythroplakia. The term leukoplakia will be used below to describe white lesions and erythroplakia to describe red lesions. Several classification systems for the lesions have been used (Axéll *et al.*, 1976; Pindborg, 1980, Greer & Poulson, 1983; Pindborg *et al.*, 1996), all involving visual inspection of the oral cavity and a diagnosis based on clinical appearance of the lesions to identify the causes of the white and red oral lesions. Smokeless tobacco use has previously been identified as a risk factor for oral premalignant lesions (IARC, 2007a). Histological and clinical changes occur in the mucosa of snuff users in as few as 2–7 days after initiation of use (Payne *et al.*, 1998). Furthermore, the location of the lesion in the mouth has been shown to correspond to where the smokeless tobacco is typically placed (Salem *et al.*, 1984; Zaridze *et al.*, 1986; Ernster *et al.*, 1990; Tomar *et al.*, 1997; Martin *et al.*, 1999; Ayo-Yusuf *et al.*, 2000).

Since IARC (2007a) one cross-sectional study has been published in the USA (Fisher *et al.*, 2005), one from Sweden (Roosaar *et al.*, 2008), and one from Yemen (Scheifele *et al.*, 2007). Cross-sectional studies and case series from many parts of the world have reported that leukoplakia occurs more commonly among smokeless tobacco users and that persons with lesions are more frequently smokeless tobacco users. Many cross-sectional studies were conducted in the USA (Greer & Poulson, 1983; Poulson *et al.*, 1984; Offenbacher & Weathers, 1985; Wolfe & Carlos, 1987; Creath *et al.*, 1988; Cummings *et al.*, 1989; Stewart *et al.*, 1989; Ernster *et al.*, 1990; Grady *et al.*, 1990; Creath *et al.*, 1991; Daniels *et al.*, 1992; Sinusas *et al.*, 1992; Grasser & Childers, 1997; Tomar *et al.*, 1997; Martin *et al.*, 1999; Lee *et al.*, 2000; Shulman *et al.*, 2004; Fisher *et al.*, 2005; Sinusas & Coroso, 2006). The types of smokeless tobacco implicated are snus in Sweden (Salonen *et al.*, 1990; Rolandsson *et al.*, 2005), Finland (Jungell & Malmström, 1985), and Denmark (Roed-Petersen *et al.*, 1972; Roed-Petersen & Pindborg, 1973; Rolandsson *et al.*, 2005), chewing tobacco in the United Kingdom (Tyldesley, 1971) and India (Jacob *et al.*, 2004), *nass* (*naswar*) in Uzbekistan (Zaridze *et al.*, 1985, 1986; Evstifeeva & Zaridze, 1992), *toombak* in Sudan (Idris *et al.*, 1996; Ahmed *et al.*, 2003; Ahmed & Mahgoob, 2007), snuff (finely ground fermented tobacco leaf with the wet ash of an Amaranthus species plant) in South Africa (Ayo-Yusuf *et al.*, 2000), *shammah* in Yemen (Scheifele *et al.*, 2007) and Saudi Arabia (Salem *et al.*, 1984; Mani, 1985).

Table 2.5 (available at http://monographs.iarc.fr/ENG/Monographs/vol100E/100E-03-Table2.5.pdf) includes cross-sectional and case–control studies of smokeless tobacco and leukoplakia, listed by country. Eight reports from the USA adjusted for tobacco smoking, either through statistical adjustment or restriction to non-smokers, one in schoolchildren (Tomar *et al.*, 1997) and the others in adults (Shulman *et al.*, 2004; Ernster *et al.*, 1990; Grady *et al.*, 1990; Daniels *et al.*, 1992; Greene *et al.*, 1992; Martin *et al.*, 1999; Fisher *et al.*, 2005). The prevalence rate ratio or odds ratio for oral leukoplakia in current smokeless tobacco users exceeded those of non-users for smokeless tobacco overall in four studies from the USA (Ernster *et al.*, 1990; Tomar *et al.*, 1997; Martin *et al.*, 1999; Fisher *et al.*, 2005) for snuff in four studies (Ernster *et al.*, 1990; Tomar *et al.*, 1997; Martin *et al.*, 1999; Fisher *et al.*, 2005) and for chewing tobacco in two (Ernster *et al.*, 1990; Tomar *et al.*, 1997) but not in a third (Fisher *et al.*, 2005).

In Uzbekistan *nass* (*naswar*) use was positively associated with oral leukoplakia in non-smokers (Zaridze *et al.*, 1986) and after adjusting for smoking, alcoholic beverage consumption, and age (Evstifeeva & Zaridze, 1992). In India, oral precancerous lesions (oral leukoplakia, submucous fibrosis, erythroplakia, and multiple lesions) were associated with tobacco chewing after adjusting for age, sex, BMI, pack–years of smoking, and years of drinking alcohol (Thomas *et al.*, 2003; Jacob *et al.*, 2004).

(b) Dose–response evidence

(i) Duration and intensity

Strong dose–response relationships have been observed in studies in the USA with intensity and duration of use of smokeless tobacco, snuff or chewing tobacco. The prevalence odds ratio for mucosal lesions increased with increasing intensity (amounts used per day or week) and duration (months, years, minutes or hours per day with tobacco in the mouth; shorter time since last used) of use of smokeless tobacco (chewing tobacco and snuff) (Ernster *et al.*, 1990; Tomar *et al.*, 1997; Martin *et al.*, 1999; Fisher *et al.*, 2005). Baseball players who used smokeless tobacco only during the playing season had a lower prevalence rate of oral lesions than year-long users, but higher than non-users (Greene *et al.*, 1992).

In Uzbekistan there was a trend of greater odds ratios for pre-leukoplakia and leukoplakia with the number of times *nass* was used per day, earlier age at initiation of the habit, years used, and lifetime intake (Evstifeeva & Zaridze, 1992). In Yemen, there was a dose–response relationship with number of minutes *shammah* was kept in the mouth and the risk was reduced if the mouth was rinsed after using the product (Scheifele *et al.*, 2007).

(ii) Cessation

The prevalence or prevalence odds ratio for oral lesions were higher in current than in former users in studies in the USA (Ernster *et al.*, 1990; Tomar *et al.*, 1997; Shulman *et al.*, 2004; Fisher *et al.*, 2005). Former users generally had higher prevalence or prevalence odds ratio (although not always statistically significantly elevated) than never users (Ernster *et al.*, 1990; Tomar *et al.*, 1997; Fisher *et al.*, 2005). In Uzbekistan, both former (OR, 3.00; 95%CI: 1.08–8.32) and current users (OR, 3.86; 95%CI: 2.60–5.72) had statistically significantly elevated odds ratios associated with *nass* use (Evstifeeva & Zaridze, 1992).

(c) Severity of lesions

The percentage of more severe leukoplakia lesions (degree 3 and 4) was higher with increasing amount of use, longer duration of use, shorter time since last use of snuff, and exposure time in the mouth in studies in the USA (Ernster *et al.*, 1990; Grady *et al.*, 1990; Daniels *et al.*, 1992; Greene *et al.*, 1992; Tomar *et al.*; 1997; Martin *et al.*, 1999). Basal-cell hyperplasia was observed in 4% of 132 lesion biopsies from snuff users, while no hyperplasia was found in the 6 biopsies from chewing tobacco users (Daniels *et al.*, 1992). Severe epithelial atypia was observed in *toombak* users (38%) in a case series in Sudan (Ahmed *et al.*, 2003). Also in Sudan greater duration of *toombak* use was associated with greater severity of the lesions (Idris *et al.*, 1996). In a South African study, lesions were more severe among those with more minutes per day of use and the users of the commercial brand compared to home-made snuff (Ayo-Yusuf *et al.*, 2000).

(d) Types

The prevalence of lesions was higher among snuff users compared with tobacco chewers in several studies (Ernster *et al.*, 1990; Greene *et al.*, 1992; Tomar *et al.*, 1997; Martin *et al.*, 1999). Among snuff users, the prevalence of lesions and the relative risk varied depending on the brand used (Grady *et al.*, 1990; Greene *et al.*, 1992; Martin *et al.*, 1999). In Yemen (Scheifele *et al.*, 2007) the prevalence odds ratio was higher for using black *shammah* compared to white *shammah*. Greater frequency of more severe lesions has been found in users of loose snus compared to men using portion-bag snus (Andersson & Axéll, 1989; Andersson *et al.*, 1994; Rolandsson *et al.*, 2005).

(e) Reversal or progression of lesions

Table 2.6 (available at http://monographs.iarc.fr/ENG/Monographs/vol100E/100E-03-Table2.6.pdf) provides information from studies that examined reversal or progression of lesions. In men with leukoplakia that were re-examined 1–21 days after the first examination, 15% of the lesions resolved and 18% improved by one degree (Grady *et al.*, 1991). Smaller lesions were most likely to have resolved in men who decreased or stopped smokeless tobacco use, among users of chewing tobacco compared with those of snuff, among light users, and among seasonal users only. Disappearance or regression of lesions was not associated with duration of smokeless tobacco use or the number of days between the initial examination and follow-up. In a study of military recruits, 97% of the oral lesions observed at the initial examination had completely resolved six weeks after they ceased using tobacco (Martin *et al.*, 1999). In a study in Denmark, there was a lower percentage of snuff users whose lesions transformed to dysplasia or malignancy compared to patients with leukoplakia who did not use snuff (Roed-Petersen & Pindborg, 1973).

Men in Sweden with snus-induced lesions followed over 27–29 years did not have a higher risk of oral cancer (not smoking adjusted) compared to the entire Swedish population (Roosaar *et al.*, 2006). A subset of men had a repeat oral examination 19–22 years after the baseline. Among those who stopped snus entirely or used it less than once per day, 6.1% had a lesion at the follow-up exam. Lesions were still present with the same or lesser severity in 91% of the men who continued use of loose snuff or changed to portion-bag snuff and 8.7% had a worse lesion. Of those who used snus for more hours per day at the follow-up than at baseline, 12.1% had a worse lesion. In an earlier study, after 3–6 months, snus users with oral lesions who used portion-bag snus were more likely to have less severe lesions and users who stopped using snus or who changed to portion bags and changed the placement of the snus in the mouth had no lesions at the original site (Larsson *et al.*, 1991). Snus users who changed to snus with a lower pH and lower nicotine concentrations had less severe lesions after 24 weeks (Andersson & Warfvinge, 2003).

In a 10 year follow up study in India, Gupta *et al.* (1980) reported significantly higher malignant transformation in a group of smokeless tobacco users with precancer.

2.1.3 Cancer of the oesophagus

(a) Overview of studies

Studies of smokeless tobacco and oesophageal cancer have been conducted in North America, Europe and Asia. All of the studies reported here examined oesophageal cancer risks associated with use of unsmoked tobacco that was not part of a betel quid. Evidence regarding betel quid is presented in the *Monograph* on Betel Quid in this volume. These studies generally focused on the predominant smokeless tobacco products and behaviours in the countries in which the studies were conducted.

Two studies (Zendehdel *et al.*, 2008; Nasrollahzadeh *et al.*, 2008) have been published since the previous *Monograph* (IARC, 2007a).

Major risk factors for oesophageal cancers are tobacco smoking, betel quid chewing, heavy alcohol consumption (only for squamous cell carcinomas of the oesophagus) (IARC, 2004, IARC, 2010) and BMI (for adenocarcinoma of the oesophagus) (Kubo & Corley, 2006), making these factors potential confounders in studies of smokeless tobacco. [The Working Group notes that betel quid chewing and smokeless tobacco use are nearly always mutually exclusive in certain geographic regions.]

In two cohort studies (Boffetta *et al.*, 2005; Zendehdel *et al.*, 2008) smokeless tobacco use and oesophageal cancer has been examined (Table 2.7 available at http://monographs.iarc.fr/ENG/Monographs/vol100E/100E-03-Table2.7.pdf); both addressed potential confounding by smoking and included incident cases occurring in the first few years of follow-up.

One of the cohort studies was conducted in Norway and study participants were followed for 35 years for cancer incidence (Boffetta *et al.*, 2005). The relative risk for oesophageal cancer was 1.4 (95%CI: 0.6–3.2) for ever use of snuff compared to never use, adjusted for age and smoking. In a Swedish cohort study (Zendehdel *et al.*, 2008) the relative risk for squamous cell carcinoma of the oesophagus among non-smoking men who used only snuff compared to never users of tobacco was 3.5 (95%CI: 1.6–7.6) adjusting for age and BMI.

Several case–control studies in the USA have been conducted that did not include odds ratio among non-smokers or did not adjust statistically for smoking behaviours (Wynder *et al.*, 1957; Wynder & Bross, 1961; Wynder & Stellman, 1977; Pottern *et al.*, 1981). Of the seven case–control studies of smokeless tobacco and oesophageal cancer that did so (Table 2.8 available at http://monographs.iarc.fr/ENG/Monographs/vol100E/100E-03-Table2.8.pdf), two were conducted in Sweden (Lewin *et al.*, 1998; Lagergren *et al.*, 2000), three in the USA (Martinez, 1969; Williams & Horm, 1977; Williams *et al.*, 1977; Brown *et al.*, 1988), one in India (Phukan *et al.*, 2001) and one in the Islamic Republic of Iran (Nasrollahzadeh *et al.*, 2008). Because the survival rate for oesophageal cancer is poor (Crew & Neugut, 2004), case–control studies may be susceptible to selection bias from not interviewing study cases who died before the time of interview or measurement error due to obtaining information from proxy interviews (Winn, 1986).

Three case–control studies from the USA (one from Puerto Rico) showed no association between use of smokeless tobacco and oesophageal cancer (Martinez, 1969; Williams & Horm, 1977; Williams *et al.*, 1977; Brown *et al.*, 1988) after adjusting for smoking or restricting the analysis to non-smokers. The proportion of proxy interviews needed to ascertain smokeless tobacco use in these studies was 45% (Williams & Horm, 1977; Williams *et al.*, 1977), at least 69% (Brown *et al.*, 1988), and 12% (Martinez, 1969).

Both of the Swedish case–control studies were population-based and adjusted the analyses for smoking and alcohol intake (Lewin *et al.*, 1998; Lagergren *et al.*, 2000). In one of them that involved both squamous cell and adenocarcinoma, no proxy interviews were permitted (Lagergren *et al.*, 2000). The odds ratio for users of smokeless tobacco only compared to non-users of tobacco was 1.4 (95%CI: 0.9–2.3) for squamous cell carcinoma of the oesophagus and 1.2 (95%CI: 0.7–2.0) for adenocarcinoma of the oesophagus adjusting for age, tobacco smoking, alcohol drinking and other factors. In the other Swedish study (Lewin *et al.*, 1998) on squamous cell carcinoma, most were interviewed about a month after the case's diagnosis date. The odds ratio for ever use of snuff was 1.2 (95%CI: 0.7–2.2), adjusting for age, region, tobacco smoking and alcoholic beverages.

In a hospital-based case–control study from India an association between smokeless tobacco and oesophageal cancer was found (Phukan *et al.*, 2001). Relative to persons who neither used smokeless tobacco nor smoked, the odds ratio for persons who used only *chadha* (a type of smokeless tobacco) but did not chew betel quid nor smoke was 3.2 (95%CI: 1.6–9.5) for men and 6.2 (95%CI: 2.4–12.1) for women, adjusting for alcohol. In a study in the Islamic Republic of Iran cases were interviewed at the time of diagnosis (there were no proxy interviews), and only histologically confirmed squamous cell carcinoma were included (Nasrollahzadeh *et al.*, 2008); when use of different tobacco products was examined in a multivariate model, there was a significant positive association with *nass* use only compared to never users of any tobacco product, after adjustment for education, ethnicity, and total intake of fruit and vegetables.

In a meta-analysis of studies published through 2007 (Boffetta *et al.*, 2008; Table 2.9, available at http://monographs.iarc.fr/ENG/Monographs/vol100E/100E-03-Table2.9.pdf), only studies from Europe and the USA that provided information about non-smokers and studies that included smokers but adjusted for tobacco smoking were included. The overall estimate of effect for the five studies of oesophageal cancer was 1.6 (95%CI: 1.1–2.3). In a second meta-analysis Lee & Hamling (2009) included studies from Europe and the USA of smokeless tobacco and oesophageal cancer through May 2008, including and two studies that did not adjust for smoking (Wynder & Bross, 1961; Wynder & Stellman, 1977; Table 2.10, available at http://monographs.iarc.fr/ENG/Monographs/vol100E/100E-03-Table2.10.pdf). The overall relative risk among never-smokers was 1.91 (95%CI: 1.15–3.17) and the smoking-adjusted relative risk 1.13 (95%CI: 0.95–1.36). For Scandinavian studies, the summary relative risk in never-smokers was 1.92 (95%CI: 1.00–3.68; one study) and 1.10 (95%CI: 0.92–1.33) when smoking adjusted. For studies from the USA, the relative risks restricted to never-smokers or adjusted for smoking were identical, 1.89 (95%CI: 0.84–4.25).

(b) Dose–response evidence

(i) Duration and intensity

In one case–control study (Lagergren *et al.*, 2000), there were no significant increases in risk for years of use up to 25 years, adjusted for smoking, alcohol, and other factors. For more than 25 years of use, the odds ratio for snuff use controlling for smoking, alcohol intake and other factors was 2.0 (95%CI: 0.9–4.1) for squamous cell carcinoma of the oesophagus and 1.9 (95%CI: 0.9–4.0) for adenocarcinoma of the oesophagus. The odds ratio for use of 15–35 quids per week for squamous cell carcinoma was 2.1 (95%CI: 1.0–4.4) and for adenocarcinoma, 2.0 (95%CI: 1.0–4.3). Corresponding estimates for using more than 35 quids per week were 1.0 (95%CI: 0.4–2.4) and 0.8 (95%CI: 0.3–2.0), respectively. In another case–control study (Lewin *et al.*, 1998), the odds ratio for smokeless tobacco users of more than 50 g per week was 1.9 (95%CI: 0.8–3.9) adjusting for smoking and alcohol intake among other factors. In the Islamic Republic of Iran study (Nasrollahzadeh *et al.*, 2008), there were significant positive exposure-response relationships for frequency of use per day of *nass*, cumulative use (frequency times duration), and duration of *nass* use. However, these findings were not controlled for tobacco smoking.

(ii) Cessation

In one case–control study of oesophageal cancer (Lewin *et al.*, 1998), there was no association with snuff use for former or current smokeless tobacco users compared to never smokeless tobacco users.

(c) Types

In northern Europe, the predominant form of smokeless tobacco is snus. Of the four studies from that geographic region – two cohort

(Boffetta *et al.*, 2005; Zendehdel *et al.*, 2008) and two case–control (Lewin *et al.*, 1998; Lagergren *et al.*, 2000) – all of the odds ratios were greater than 1.0, but statistically significantly elevated only in one study (Zendehdel *et al.*, 2008). The odds ratios in the three studies from the USA where snuff and chewing tobacco are used, were not statistically significantly elevated (Martinez, 1969; Williams & Horm, 1977; Brown *et al.*, 1988).

In India, among non-smokers, statistically significantly elevated odds ratios associated with chewing *chadha* were reported for both men and women adjusting for alcohol consumption (Phukan *et al.*, 2001). In a study in the Islamic Republic of Iran, *nass* users had a significantly increased risk of oesophageal cancer (Nasrollahzadeh *et al.*, 2008).

It was noted in a report on a case series in Sudan that use of tobacco in the form of *toombak* under the tongue or in the labiodental groove was common in an area where oesophageal cancer incidence rates were high (Babekir *et al.*, 1989).

(d) Histology

Two studies analysed squamous cell cancer and adenocarcinoma separately (Lagergren *et al.*, 2000; Zendehdel *et al.*, 2008); in the other studies (Brown *et al.*, 1988; Phukan *et al.*, 2001; Nasrollahzadeh *et al.*, 2008), most (if not all) of the cases had squamous cell carcinomas. Statistically significantly elevated odds ratios were found for ever use of smokeless tobacco and squamous cell carcinomas in one study (Zendehdel *et al.*, 2008), in another study (Lagergren *et al.*, 2000) for users of 15–35 quids per week, and in a third study of predominantly squamous cell carcinomas (Phukan *et al.*, 2001). In a fourth study from the Islamic Republic of Iran that assessed squamous cell carcinomas, *nass* use was found to have a significant positive association with oesophageal cancer (Nasrollahzadeh *et al.*, 2008).

Two studies provided odds ratios for use of smokeless tobacco and adenocarcinoma of the oesophagus; in one the odds ratio was statistically significantly elevated for ever users (Zendehdel *et al.*, 2008) and in the other (Lagergren *et al.*, 2000) users of 15–35 quids per week had an increased risk for adenocarcinoma of the oesophagus.

(e) Population characteristics

In the study in India (Phukan *et al.*, 2001), significantly elevated odds ratios were observed in both men and women.

(f) Subsites of cancers of the upper aerodigestive tract

In some studies smokeless tobacco-associated risks were examined only for oral cancer or provided oral cavity cancer-specific findings. Of these studies, statistically significantly elevated odds ratios for ever use of smokeless tobacco were noted in seven (Chandra, 1962; Williams & Horm, 1977; Blot *et al.*, 1988; Idris *et al.*, 1995a; Merchant *et al.*, 2000) but no association in two (Schildt *et al.*, 1998; Accortt *et al.*, 2002, 2005; Luo *et al.*, 2007). Some other studies provided estimates for the oral cavity plus one or more of the pharynx, lip, salivary gland, oesophagus, and larynx. Of these four had positive findings (Kabat *et al.*, 1994; Lewin *et al.*, 1998; Wasnik *et al.*, 1998; Roosaar *et al.*, 2008) and four had relative risks below one or close to approximately equal to one (Mashberg *et al.*, 1993; Boffetta *et al.*, 2005; Henley *et al.*, 2005; Rosenquist, 2005). In studies providing information separately for the pharynx, estimates were positive for women with 20 or more years of snuff use in the USA (Winn *et al.*, 1981a); for hypopharyngeal cancer, estimates were positive in one study in India (Sapkota *et al.*, 2007) and below one in two other studies (Williams & Horm, 1977; Lewin *et al.*, 1998).

2.1.4 Cancer of the pancreas

Three cohort studies (Zheng *et al.*, 1993; Boffetta *et al.*, 2005; Luo *et al.* 2007), three population-based case–control studies (Williams & Horm 1977; Farrow & Davis, 1990; Alguacil & Silverman, 2004) and two hospital based case–control studies (Muscat *et al.*, 1997; Hassan *et al.*, 2007) in North America and in Europe investigated the association between the use of smokeless tobacco and pancreatic cancer.

(a) North America

(i) Cohort study

In the Lutheran Brotherhood Insurance Society cohort with 20 years follow-up, a relative risk of 1.7 (95%CI: 0.9–3.1, based on 16 deaths) adjusted for age, alcoholic beverages and smoking was found for male ever users of smokeless tobacco (Zheng *et al.*, 1993).

(ii) Case–control studies

No association was found with smokeless tobacco in two population-based case–control studies (Williams & Horm 1977; Farrow & Davis, 1990). In a population-based case–control study that restricted analyses to lifelong non-smokers of cigarettes, a non-significantly 40% increase in risk for pancreatic cancer (95%CI: 0.5–3.6) was found in those who used smokeless tobacco regularly compared to non-users of tobacco (Alguacil & Silverman, 2004). Among tobacco chewers who were not current cigarette smokers, an elevated risk of 3.6 (CI: 1.0–12.8) was seen when compared to never-smokers and long-term quitters (≥ 20 years) in one hospital-based case–control study (Muscat *et al.*, 1997) and no association with chewing tobacco or using snuff was noted in an another hospital-based case–control study (Hassan *et al.*, 2007). None of the studies adjusted for BMI or alcohol, which are potentially important risk factors for pancreatic cancer (Table 2.11, available at http://monographs.iarc.fr/ENG/Monographs/vol100E/100E-03-Table2.11.pdf).

In a meta-analysis of four studies from the USA, the summary relative risk for pancreatic cancer among users of smokeless tobacco was 1.4 (95%CI: 0.7–2.7) (Boffetta *et al.*, 2008).

(iii) Duration and intensity

Only a few studies assessed risk in relation to duration and intensity of use, assessing oz per week or grams per day and duration of use. In one study (Alguacil & Silverman, 2004), the odds ratio for those who used > 2.5 oz of smokeless tobacco a week compared to non-users of tobacco was 3.5 (95%CI: 1.1–10.6) and for those who used smokeless tobacco for more than 20 years was 1.5 (95%CI: 0.6–4.0), adjusted for age, sex, race, cigar smoking and study area.

(b) Europe

In the Norwegian Cohort Study followed up for 35 years the relative risk for pancreatic cancer for ever use of snuff (snus) was 1.67 (95%CI: 1.12–2.50; 45 cases), adjusted for smoking and age (Boffetta *et al.*, 2005). Among ever users of snuff, the relative risk was 0.85 (95%CI: 0.24–3.07, based on three cases) in never-smokers. In the Swedish construction worker cohort study, analyses were restricted to never smoking men at the time of entry into the study (Luo *et al.*, 2007). Average follow-up was 20 years and 83 pancreatic cancers were recorded. Compared to never users of any tobacco product, and after adjustment for age and BMI, the relative risk for never smoking current users of snus was 2.1 (95%CI: 1.2–3.6; 18 cases) and in never-smokers who used ≥ 10 g/day snus was 2.1 (95%CI: 1.1–3.8) (Table 2.12, available at http://monographs.iarc.fr/ENG/Monographs/vol100E/100E-03-Table2.12.pdf).

A meta-analysis showed a summary relative risk for pancreatic cancer among users of smokeless tobacco based on the two above cohort studies of 1.8 (95%CI: 1.3–2.5) (Boffetta *et al.*, 2008).

2.1.5 Other cancers

(a) Cancer of the stomach

Four cohort studies (Kneller *et al.*, 1991; Chao *et al.*, 2002; Boffetta *et al.*, 2005; Zendehdel *et al.* 2008) and 4 case–control studies (Williams & Horm, 1977; Hansson *et al.*, 1994; Ye *et al.*, 1999; Phukan *et al.*, 2005) investigated the association between stomach cancer and use of smokeless tobacco. Phukan *et al.* (2005) also reported exposure to *tuibur* (Table 1.1).

(i) Cohort studies

In the USA, non-significantly elevated risks associated with smokeless tobacco use were observed among never-smokers compared to men who never used tobacco in the Lutheran Brotherhood cohort study with 20 years follow-up (Kneller *et al.*, 1991) and in the CPS-II cohort study with 18 years follow-up (Chao *et al.*, 2002). In the cohort study from Norway (35 years follow-up), a non-significantly elevated risk for snuff use was found (Boffetta *et al.*, 2005). A total of 343 822 men were analysed in the construction worker cohort study from Sweden (33 years follow-up) and a significant positive relative risk was seen among non-smoking snus users aged 70 and over for cancer in the non-cardia region of the stomach when compared to never users of any tobacco product (Zendehdel *et al.*, 2008; Table 2.13, available at http://monographs.iarc.fr/ENG/Monographs/vol100E/100E-03-Table2.13.pdf).

(ii) Case–control studies

Williams & Horm (1977), Hansson *et al.* (1994) and Ye *et al.* (1999) found no significant associations with the use of smokeless tobacco products or snuff. The study by Phukan *et al.* (2005) showed a significantly elevated risk for chewing tobacco alone among non-betel quid users (adjusted for tobacco smoking, alcohol drinking, *tuibur*, education, occupation, income) and for *tuibur* use (adjusted for tobacco smoking, alcohol drinking, education, occupation, income) (Table 2.14, available at http://monographs.iarc.fr/ENG/Monographs/vol100E/100E-03-Table2.14.pdf).

(iii) Dose–response evidence

In one study, risk increased with cumulative dose of tobacco chewing and for *tuibur* use (p for trend < 0.001), each adjusted for other confounding factors (Phukan *et al.*, 2005).

(iv) Cessation

Phukan *et al.* (2005) found that risk decreased with years of cessation of *tuibur* use, although the test for trend was not significant.

(b) Cancer of the colon and rectum

In the US Veterans' cohort study with 26 years follow-up (Heineman *et al.*, 1995), smokeless tobacco users had a relative risk of 1.2 (95%CI: 0.9–1.7; based on 39 deaths) for cancer of the colon and 1.9 (95%CI: 1.2–3.1; based on 17 deaths) for cancer of the rectum compared to those who had never used tobacco. No new data have been published since the previous *IARC Monograph* (IARC, 2007a).

(c) Cancer of the extra-hepatic bile duct

In a population-based case–control study in Los Angeles County, USA (Chow *et al.*, 1994) an odds ratio of 18 (95%CI: 1.4–227.7; based on 3 cases) was found for chewing tobacco and cancer of the ampulla of Vater. [All cases of cancer of the ampulla of Vater who chewed tobacco also smoked.] There have been no new studies published since the previous *IARC Monograph* (IARC, 2007a).

(d) Cancers of the digestive system combined

A reduced risk with use of smokeless tobacco was seen in the case–control study by Sterling *et al.* (1992) and in the National Health and Nutrition Examination Survey (NHANES I) follow-up study that analysed 6805 men and women aged

45–75 years at baseline (1971–75) (Accortt *et al.*, 2002). The entire NHANES I cohort was reassessed between 1982 and 1984 and analysed 7787 subjects aged 45 and over at baseline. The results showed non-significantly elevated risks for those aged 65 years and over in men and aged 45–64 years in women (Accortt *et al.*, 2005). [The analysis was limited to incident diseases that required an overnight stay in health care facility. Hence, there is a possibility of underrepresentation of the actual number of cancer cases that occurred in the cohort. Analysis was based on a small sample size, 414 exclusive smokeless tobacco users, and chewing tobacco and snuff use were not analysed separately. Pipe and cigar use was not controlled for in the analysis.]

The hazard ratio for men who reported current use of smokeless tobacco and never used other tobacco products was significantly elevated after adjustment for age, race, educational level, BMI, exercise, alcoholic beverage consumption, fat consumption, fruit and vegetable intake and aspirin use in the CPS I cohort but not in the CPS II cohort (additionally adjusted for status and type of employment) (Henley *et al.*, 2005).

(e) Cancer of the gall bladder

One case–control study in India found positive associations with chewing *khaini* [raw tobacco with lime] and cancer of the gall bladder (OR, 1.65; 95%CI: 0.78–3.49) or chewing tobacco alone (OR, 2.71, 95%CI: 1.22–6.02), unadjusted for other potential confounding factors (Shukla *et al.*, 2008).

(f) Cancers of the respiratory tract

(i) Nasal cavities

Brinton *et al.* (1984) in a case–control study found non-significant sex-adjusted odds ratios for tobacco chewers or snuff users while Stockwell & Lyman (1986) found an odds ratio for smokeless tobacco of 3.3 (95%CI,0.4–25.9), adjusted for age, race, sex and tobacco use. [The Working Group noted that information about tobacco use was obtained from medical records and ascertainment bias cannot be ruled out.] No new studies were identified since the previous *IARC Monograph* (IARC, 2007a).

(ii) Larynx

In a case–control study in Florida, USA, a significantly elevated odds ratio for smokeless tobacco use, adjusted for age, race, sex and tobacco smoking was found (Stockwell & Lyman, 1986). [The Working Group noted that information about tobacco use was obtained from medical records and ascertainment bias cannot be ruled out.] From a case–control study in Sweden Lewin *et al.* (1998) reported no significant association for current and former use of snuff, adjusted for age, smoking and alcoholic beverages. No new studies were identified since the previous *IARC Monograph* (IARC, 2007a).

(iii) Lung

The NHANES follow-up study ascertained incident cases (Accortt *et al.*, 2005) and deaths from lung cancer (Accortt *et al.*, 2002). Never-smoking women who ever used smokeless tobacco had significantly higher mortality compared to never tobacco users. In men, no deaths from lung cancer occurred among those who were never-smokers and used smokeless tobacco. Estimates of the relative risk were adjusted for age, race, poverty index ratio, region of residence, alcoholic beverages, recreational physical exercise and fruit/vegetable intake. The results for cancer incidence (Accortt *et al.*, 2005) showed significantly elevated risks in women aged 65 years and over, based on small numbers of cases among exclusive smokeless tobacco users ($n < 4$ cases). No incident cases of lung cancer occurred in men who used smokeless tobacco. Risk was adjusted for age, race and poverty index ratio. [The Working Group noted limitations to this study. See section on cancers of the digestive system *(d)*.]

In the Cancer Prevention Study I (CPS-I) in the USA, the hazard ratio for lung cancer for current smokeless tobacco users who never used other tobacco products was non-significantly elevated and the corresponding hazard ratio in the CPS-II cohort was significantly elevated, after adjusting for age, race, level of education, BMI, exercise, alcoholic beverage consumption, fat consumption, fruit and vegetable intake, aspirin use and status and type of employment (for CPS-II only) (Henley *et al.*, 2005). The magnitude of effect was similar for those who chewed tobacco but never used snuff and for those who used snuff but never chewed tobacco. In the Norwegian cohort study the relative risk adjusted for age and smoking was non-significantly reduced for ever users of snus compared to never users (Boffetta *et al.*, 2005). In the Swedish construction worker cohort study with 279 897 men followed for an average of 20 years there was no significant association for snus use among never-smokers (Luo *et al.*, 2007).

Henley *et al.* (2007) used CPS II data to compare mortality among former cigarette smokers who switched to smokeless tobacco (switchers) with those who quit using tobacco entirely (quitters), based on tobacco use ascertained at baseline and followed-up for 20 years. In a subset of the cohort that examined uptake of tobacco after baseline, the proportions of persons taking up cigarette smoking was very low. Compared with quitters, the relative risk of lung cancer was 1.5 (95%CI: 1.2–1.7) for all switchers, 1.3 (95%CI: 1.1–1.6) for switchers to tobacco chewing only, 1.8 (95%CI: 1.2–2.5) for snuff only, and 1.9 (95%CI: 1.2–2.9) for tobacco chewing and snuff combined. Compared with men who never used any tobacco product, the relative risk of lung cancer was 3.9 for quitters and 5.6 for switchers (statistically significant but 95% confidence intervals were not provided). Risk estimates were adjusted for age, number of cigarettes formerly smoked per day, number of years smoking cigarettes, age at which they quit smoking cigarettes, race, educational level, BMI, exercise level, alcohol consumption, employment type, employment status, fat consumption, fruit and vegetable intake and aspirin use. The analysis was restricted to men because women were not asked whether or not they used smokeless tobacco.

The case–control study of lung cancer by Williams & Horm (1977) reported non-significant risk for smokeless tobacco use in men, adjusted for age, race, and smoking.

(g) Sarcoma

In the US Veterans' cohort, the relative risk for soft-tissue sarcomas associated with smokeless tobacco use compared to persons who never used tobacco products was 1.5 (95%CI: 0.8–2.7) (Zahm *et al.*, 1992). In a population-based case–control study conducted in the USA, the unadjusted odds ratio for ever use of smokeless tobacco was 1.8 (95%CI: 1.1–2.9); the risk was highest for those diagnosed at age 80 years or above (3.2; 95%CI: 1.0–10.1). Risks were elevated but not significantly so when analysed by anatomical site of the soft-tissue sarcoma (upper gastrointestinal; lung, pleura and thorax; head, neck and face) or by cell type (fibromatous; adipose, myomatous) (Zahm *et al.*, 1989). No new studies were identified since the previous *IARC Monograph* (IARC, 2007a).

(h) Cancer of the breast

Spangler *et al.* (2001, 2002) conducted a case–control study in Cherokee Native American women and reported a non-significant elevated risk of breast cancer for use of smokeless tobacco. [There was no medical verification of breast cancer and the time relationship between use of smokeless tobacco and breast cancer diagnosis was not reported.] A prospective cohort study of the US population (NHANES I) showed a positive but non-significant association with smokeless tobacco (snuff or chewing tobacco) in women aged 45 years and over based on five breast cancer cases, however the hazard ratios were below one when stratified by age (Accortt *et al.*, 2005). [The Working Group noted limitations to this study. See Section on cancer of the digestive system, 2.1.5 *(d)*.]

(i) Cancer of the uterine cervix

In a population-based case–control study elevated risks for cervical cancer, adjusted for smoking, age and race, for use of chewing tobacco or snuff were reported (Williams & Horm, 1977). No new studies were identified since the previous *IARC Monograph* (IARC, 2007a).

(j) Cancer of the prostate

In two cohort studies significantly elevated risks were found among users of smokeless tobacco compared to never users of tobacco (Hsing *et al.*, 1990, 1991). Putnam *et al.* (2000) reported no association with use of snuff and chewing tobacco. [The Working Group noted that data were not presented to support this.] In one case–control study (Hayes *et al.*, 1994) and one cohort study (Accortt *et al.*, 2005) non-significantly elevated risks of prostate cancer associated with chewing tobacco were found.

(k) Cancer of the penis

In a case–control study of cancer and the penis in India, the relative risk for snuff users was 4.2 (95%CI: 1.6–11.3), adjusted for smoking, tobacco chewing and phimosis (Harish & Ravi, 1995). [It was not clear whether snuff was used orally or nasally.] No new studies were identified since the previous *IARC Monograph* (IARC, 2007a).

(l) Cancer of the urinary bladder

Population-based case–control studies conducted in three provinces of Canada (Howe *et al.*, 1980), in the USA (Hartge *et al.*, 1985; Slattery *et al.*, 1988) and in Alberta and Ontario provinces of Canada (Burch *et al.*, 1989) did not show a significant association between chewing tobacco and bladder cancer. No association with snuff use was seen in the Norwegian cohort (Boffetta *et al.*, 2005).

(m) Cancer of the kidney

Four case–control studies (Goodman *et al.*, 1986; McLaughlin *et al.*, 1995; Muscat *et al.*, 1995; Asal *et al.*, 1988) and one cohort study (Boffetta *et al.*, 2005) evaluated the risk associated with smokeless tobacco use. The adjusted risk for chewing tobacco in non-smokers was not significantly elevated in two case–control studies (Goodman *et al.*, 1986; McLaughlin *et al.*, 1995) and in one cohort study in Norway (Boffetta *et al.*, 2005). In two studies, a significant association was reported for ever use of smokeless tobacco (Asal *et al.*, 1988; Muscat *et al.*, 1995) but there was no adjustment for potential confounders in either study. A dose–response relationship was observed: odds ratio 2.5 (95%CI: 1.0–6.1) for chewing 10 times or fewer per week and 6.0 (95%CI: 1.9–18.7) for chewing 11 or more times per week (Muscat *et al.*, 1995), although there was no adjustment for smoking and other potentially confounding factors.

(n) Cancer of the brain

From a population-based case–control study in the USA (Zheng *et al.*, 2001), no significantly increased risk of brain cancer was reported for either men or women with the use of snuff or chewing tobacco. [Data to support this were not presented.] No new studies were identified since the previous *IARC Monograph* (IARC, 2007a).

(o) Non-Hodgkin lymphoma

Two population-based case–control studies of non-Hodgkin lymphoma in men were conducted in the USA (Brown *et al.*, 1992a; Schroeder *et al.*, 2002). Schroeder *et al.* (2002) found an increased risk for t(14;18)-positive non-Hodgkin lymphoma cases who started chewing tobacco ≤ 18 years of age, after adjusting for age and state (OR, 2.5;

95%CI: 1.0–6.0). No significant associations were observed in the study by Brown *et al.*, (1992a) for any non-Hodgkin lymphoma subtype or overall.

Bracci & Holly (2005) from a population-based case–control study of non-Hodgkin lymphoma conducted in the USA reported significantly elevated risks for non-Hodgkin lymphoma and for follicular and diffuse large cell types in those who used smokeless tobacco. Risk estimates were adjusted for age, level of education and level of average weekly alcohol consumption. [The results are based on only seven cases and six controls.]

(p) Leukaemia

Brown *et al.* (1992b) conducted a population-based case–control study in the USA of chewing tobacco/snuff only and risk for leukaemia. Non-significant elevated risks were seen for all leukaemias, chronic myelogenous leukaemia, chronic lymphocytic leukaemia and myelodysplasia. In the Swedish construction worker cohort study (average follow-up 22.2 years), non-significantly elevated risks for acute lymphocytic and chronic myelogenous leukaemias and no association in men for snuff dipping and acute myelogenous leukaemia and multiple myeloma were found (Fernberg *et al.*, 2007).

(q) Myeloma

In a population-based case–control study in the USA, Brown *et al.* (1992a) compared users of smokeless tobacco only with never users of tobacco and found an odds ratio of 1.9 (95%CI: 0.5–6.6; based on 5 cases). A Swedish construction worker cohort study showed no association for myeloma in men with snuff dipping (Fernberg *et al.*, 2007).

(r) Cutaneous squamous cell carcinoma

Odenbro *et al.* (2005) analysed the Swedish cohort study and found a relative risk of 0.64 (95%CI: 0.44–0.95) for the association between snuff dipping and the incidence of cutaneous squamous cell carcinoma.

2.2 Nasal use

There are no cohort or case–control studies that examined the association between nasal snuff use and nasal cancer.

2.2.1 Cancers of the oral cavity and pharynx

(a) Overview of studies

Three case–control studies from India investigated the association between nasal snuff use and cancer of oral and pharyngeal subsites (Table 2.15, available at http://monographs.iarc.fr/ENG/Monographs/vol100E/100E-03-Table2.15.pdf).

Sankaranarayanan *et al.* (1989a) focused on cancer of the anterior two-thirds of tongue and floor of the mouth; the age-adjusted odds ratio was 4.27 (95%CI: 1.24–14.67; men only) for occasional nasal snuff users and 3.02 (95%CI: 0.94–9.60) for daily snuff users. For cancer of the gingiva the odds ratio for regular snuff use was 3.04 (95%CI: 0.67–12.65) after adjustment for daily frequency of use of betel quid, *bidi* smoking and alcoholic beverage use (Sankaranarayanan *et al.*, 1989b). For cancer of the buccal and labial mucosa, the age-adjusted odds ratio was 3.98 (95%CI: 1.53–10.34) for regular nasal snuff users and 2.28 (95%CI: 0.74–7.03) for occasional nasal snuff users (Sankaranarayanan *et al.*, 1990a). After adjusting for daily frequency of use of betel quid, *bidi* smoking and alcoholic beverage use, the odds ratio associated with ever snuff use was 2.93 (95%CI: 0.98–8.77).

In a multicentre case–control study of cancer of the hypopharynx in India, Sapkota *et al.* (2007) found an odds ratio of 2.85 (95%CI: 1.15–7.08) for tobacco snuffing among never-smokers who did not chew tobacco or a non-tobacco product, adjusting for alcohol use, and other factors [The Working Group noted that snuff use was oral as well as nasal so the role of nasal use could not be determined separately.]

(b) Dose–response evidence

In the study of cancer of the gingiva (Sankaranarayanan *et al.*, 1989b), the age-adjusted odds ratio for daily nasal snuff use was 3.90 (95%CI: 1.19–12.70) and that for occasional use was 3.78 (95%CI: 1.05–13.54). When categories of high versus low defective nasal snuff use were compared, the odds ratios were significantly elevated for the category of lower intensity for cancers of the tongue (Sankaranarayanan *et al.*, 1989a) and of the buccal and labial mucosa (Sankaranarayanan *et al.*, 1990a).

2.2.2 Other cancers

No new studies were identified since the previous *IARC Monograph* (IARC, 2007a) for the sites listed except for cancer of the nostril.

(a) Cancer of the oesophagus

A case–control study of oesophageal cancer form India showed an age-adjusted odds ratio for daily snuff use of 2.39 (95%CI: 0.81–7.04) and that for occasional use of 3.59 (95%CI: 1.20–10.67) (Sankaranarayanan *et al.*, 1991). [Estimates were not adjusted for smoking or betel quid chewing.]

(b) Cancer of the paranasal sinuses

Shapiro *et al.* (1955) studied Bantu cases of paranasal sinus cancer from radiation therapy department records from 1949–51 of a group of hospitals in South Africa. The authors noted that a high proportion (80%) of the antral cancer cases reported 'prolonged and heavy' use of snuff in contrast to 34% of Bantu men with cancer at other sites. The product snuffed by Bantus typically contained powdered tobacco leaves and an ash from aloe plants or other species, with the occasional addition of oil, lemon juice and herbs; typical use was 'one teaspoonful' per day (Keen *et al.*, 1955). [The Working Group noted that the source and nature of the control group was not described.]

(c) Cancer of the larynx

A case–control study from India (Sankaranarayanan *et al.*, 1990b) of laryngeal cancer showed a non-significant risk for snuff use.

(d) Cancer of the lung

Hsairi *et al.* (1993) conducted a case–control study of bronchial cancer in Tunisia. The odds ratio for ever use of inhaled snuff ('tabac à priser'), adjusted for age, sex, cigarette use, water pipe and cannabis use was 2.2 (95%CI: 0.9–5.6).

(e) Carcinoma of the nostril

Sreedharan *et al.* (2007) reported a case of squamous cell carcinoma in the right nostril in a 69-year-old woman in Karnataka, south India, with a history of daily snuff usage of more than 2 g for a duration of 30 years.

2.3 Synthesis

2.3.1 Oral use

(a) Oral cavity and pharynx

Smokeless tobacco was positively associated with cancers of the oral cavity in a cohort study in northern Europe and several case–control studies, some of which that adjusted for smoking and others that adjusted both for smoking and alcohol. There were elevated risks for every type of smokeless tobacco studied: snuff and chewing tobacco in the USA, snus in northern Europe, *toombak* in Sudan, smokeless tobacco used as a dentifrice in India and *naswar* in Pakistan. Case series implicate *shammah* used in Saudi Arabia as a risk factor for oral cancer. Not all reports were positive, namely some studies in Scandinavia and the USA, including two cohorts with small sample sizes. The evidence is strongest for the oral cavity, with some indication of increased risks for the hypopharynx, or oropharynx and hypopharynx combined. Dose–response relationships with intensity of use were noted in one study and with duration in another. It is unclear whether risks are elevated in former smokeless tobacco users. Three meta-analyses of studies from northern Europe and the USA were generally consistent. In one meta-analysis an overall relative risk of 1.8 (95%CI: 1.1–2.9) was computed for studies that adjusted for smoking or among non-smokers; in another the relative risk was 1.72 (95%CI: 1.01–2.94) among never-smokers and 1.87 (95%CI: 0.82–4.27) when further adjusted for alcohol among never-smokers. In conclusion, there is strong evidence in humans that smokeless tobacco causes cancer of the oral cavity.

(b) Precancerous lesions

Studies in many countries have observed that oral lesions are more common in smokeless tobacco users than non-users, regardless of the type of smokeless tobacco used. The types include snus, snuff, chewing tobacco, smokeless tobacco used as a dentifrice, *naswar*, *toombak*, and *shammah*. In many studies the oral lesions were observed to be in the place in the mouth where users in that geographic region typically place the smokeless tobacco. The prevalence of the lesions increased with various exposure metrics of increasing intensity and duration of use, such as amounts used per day, time kept in mouth, duration of use in months or years. Although some lesions in young persons resolve, the prevalence of lesions in older adult users of these products remains elevated even in former users. There is some evidence from three studies that a small proportion of the lesions among smokeless tobacco users can progress to oral cancer over a period of years, although the rates vary, are not adjusted for any medical intervention to remove the lesions, smoking has not been taken into account, and the follow-up periods are highly variable. Use of smokeless tobacco causes leukoplakia and erythroplakia, both considered precancerous, with a much higher risk of progressing to cancer than normal mucosa.

(c) Oesophagus

Nine studies evaluated the association between smokeless tobacco use and oesophageal cancer. The risks for ever use of smokeless tobacco compared to never use were statistically significantly elevated in one cohort study from Sweden and case–control studies from the Islamic Republic of Iran and India. In a Swedish case–control study, increased risks were observed with 15–35 quids used per week. Smoking could be ruled out as a potential confounder in all of the studies, as well as alcohol intake in two. No increased risk was observed in the three studies from the USA, which included a significant proportion of proxy respondents. Two meta-analyses found that, overall and for the Nordic countries, the estimates of effect for smokeless tobacco use were significantly elevated. The two studies published since the previous *Monograph* on Smokeless Tobacco showed a positive significant association with oesophageal cancer and were adjusted for major confounders. Four of five studies of squamous cell carcinomas and both studies of adenocarcinoma showed significantly positive results.

(d) Pancreas

In North America, 3 case–control studies showed no association, one cohort study and two case–control studies showed a non-significant increased risk and one case–control study showed a borderline significant increase in risk. While these studies accounted for smoking, none adjusted for BMI or alcohol, potentially important risk factors for pancreatic cancer. In Europe, two cohort studies showed a significant increase in risk of pancreatic cancer associated with snuff use. Both studies controlled for smoking; one study adjusted for BMI and also showed that the highest risks were seen in the highest exposure

Table 3.1 Carcinogenicity studies of application of smokeless tobacco to the skin of experimental animals

Species, strain (sex) Reference	Animals/group at start Dosing regimen Duration	Results Target organ Incidence and/or multiplicity of tumours (%)	Significance	Comments
Mouse, CAF1 and Swiss (sex NR) Wynder & Wright (1957)	40, 30 controls Skin application 3 × /wk of unburnt cigarette tobacco 50% methanol extract, (dose NR), controls received whole tar extract; 24 mo	Skin (papillomas): CAF1–11/40 (27%), 16/30 (53%) in controls (8 converted to carcinoma)	NR	No adequate control groups
		Swiss–3/40 (7%) (1 converted to carcinoma), 16/30 (53%) in controls (3 converted to carcinoma)	NR	

mo, month or months; NR, not reported

category. There is good evidence to support a causal association between smokeless tobacco use and pancreatic cancer.

(e) Stomach

One cohort study in Sweden showed a significantly higher risk among non-smoking snus users aged 70 years and over for cancer in the non-cardia region of the stomach, not adjusted for alcohol use. One case–control study in India showed significantly higher risks for chewing tobacco alone and for *tuibur* users, with dose-dependent increases in risk. Risk decreased with cessation of *tuibur* use. The risk was not statistically significant in the other studies. Despite some positive findings for chewing tobacco in two different countries and for tobacco smoke-infused water, it was not considered strong enough to conclude for a causal association.

(f) Lung

In summary, in two cohort studies significant positive associations between smokeless tobacco use and lung cancer were found while in three cohort studies and one case–control study there was no association. In one of the positive cohort studies switching from cigarette smoking to smokeless tobacco significantly increased the risk for lung cancer compared to never-tobacco users, and the risk was of greater magnitude than for quitting all together (RR, 3.9 versus 5.6).

2.3.2 Nasal use

Strong positive associations for cancers of the tongue and floor of mouth, gingiva and buccal and labial mucosa were observed in one study in India. In one positive study snuff use was oral as well as nasal so the role of nasal use could not be determined separately.

3. Cancer in Experimental Animals

Since the previous *IARC Monograph* on Smokeless Tobacco (IARC, 2007a), only one new study has been published. The collective evidence for the carcinogenicity of smokeless tobacco in experimental animals is summarized below.

3.1 Chewing tobacco, unburned cigarette tobacco, *mishri* and *naswar*

3.1.1 Mouse

Topical application of unburned cigarette tobacco induced skin papillomas in mice (Wynder & Wright, 1957; Table 3.1). Similar treatment with

Table 3.2 Carcinogenicity studies on administration of smokeless tobacco with known carcinogens or modifiers to the skin of experimental animals

Species, strain (sex) Reference	Animals/group at start Dosing regimen Duration	Results Target organ Incidence and/or multiplicity of tumours (%)	Significance
Mouse, Paris albino XVII x 57 black (sex NR) Ranadive *et al.* (1963)	11–36 animals/ group Totally alkaloid free extract, twice/wk for 95 wk + croton oil/dose and duration not specified, controls received acetone	Papillomas: 22/35 (63%) Controls–3/19 (16%) Carcinomas: 10/35 (27%) Controls–0/19	 $P > 0.001$ $P = 0.0097$
Mouse, ICR Swiss (F) Bock *et al.* (1964, 1965)	30 animals/group A single DMBA application of 125 µg DMBA in 0.25 mL acetone + 0.25 mL acetone extract of unburnt tobacco 2.5 from cigarettes/d, 5 × / wk; controls received a single application of DMBA 125 µg 36 wk	16 papillomas in 7/30 (23%) mice Controls–0/30	$P > 0.01$
Mouse, ICR Swiss (F) Van Duuren *et al.* (1966)	20 animals/group 150 µg DMBA in 0.1 ml acetone once + (after 2–3 wk) reconstituted extract of flue-cured cigarette tobacco leaf, 25 mg in 0.1 ml solvent, tobacco extract, 3 × /wk; 52 wk	Papillomas: 5/14 (36%) Controls–0/12	$P = 0.04$

d, day or days; F, female; NR, not reported; wk, week or weeks

chewing tobacco extract for 95 weeks followed by croton oil increased the incidence of skin papillomas and carcinomas in mice (Ranadive *et al.*, 1963; Table 3.2). Application of chewing tobacco extract to benzo[*a*]pyrene-initiated mouse skin promoted development of a few skin papillomas and carcinomas in mice (Ranadive *et al.*, 1963). In mice initiated with 7,12-dimethylbenz[a]anthracene (DMBA) applied topically, application of a barium hydroxide extract of unburned tobacco promoted skin papilloma development (Bock *et al.*, 1964; Table 3.2). Skin-tumour-promoting activity of unburned tobacco was reported in some DMBA-initiated mice in two additional studies (Bock *et al.*, 1965; Van Duuren *et al.*, 1966; Table 3.2). Application of brown or black *mishri* extracts to DMBA-initiated skin increased significantly the total incidence of papilloma and carcinoma in Swiss mice (Kulkarni *et al.*, 1989; Table 3.3). Administration of chewing tobacco extracts to the oral mucosa (Mody & Ranadive, 1959), skin painting with chewing tobacco extracts (Mody & Ranadive, 1959; Ranadive *et al.*, 1976), or intravesicular or intravaginal application of *jarda* (Randeria, 1972) did not induce tumours in mice.

Inhalation of powdered tobacco leaves led to a significant increase in the incidence of tumours of the lung and liver in strain A mice (Hamazaki & Murao, 1969; Table 3.4). Mice given chewing tobacco extract by oral intubation developed lung adenocarcinoma and hepatocellular carcinoma in one study [with incomplete reporting of the distribution of different neoplasms] (Bhide *et al.*, 1984). Adding black or brown *mishri* in the diet increased significantly the incidence of forestomach papilloma in Swiss mice (Kulkarni *et al.*, 1988; Table 3.5).

Table 3.3 Carcinogenicity studies of *mishri* alone or with known carcinogens or modifiers to the skin of experimental animals

Species, strain (sex) Reference	Animals/group at start Dosing regimen Duration	Results Target organ Incidence and/or multiplicity of tumours (%)	Significance
Mouse Swiss (M) Kulkarni *et al.*, (1989)	30 animals Topical/a single application of 200 nmol DMBA; 24 mo	No tumours	
	29 animals 200 nmol DMBA + 2.5 mg per application of black *mishri* extract, 5 d/wk for 20 wk; 24 mo	Skin papillomas: 4/29 (14%)	$P < 0.05$
	30 animals Topical application of black *mishri* extract, 2.5 mg per application, 5 d/wk for 20 wk; 24 mo	No skin tumours	
	30 animals 200 nmol DMBA + 2.5 mg per application of brown *mishri* extract, 5 d/wk for 20 wk; 24 mo	Skin papillomas: 4/30 (13%)	$P < 0.05$

d, day or days; M, male; mo, month or months; wk, week or weeks

3.1.2 Rat

Administration of chewing tobacco extract by gavage to vitamin-A-sufficient rats induced benign tumours in the lung and forestomach while similarly treated vitamin-A-deficient rats developed benign tumours in the stomach and pituitary gland and "lymphoma" in the lung [extremely rare tumour in rats] (Bhide *et al.*, 1991; Table 3.6).

Administration of *mishri* by gavage to vitamin-A-sufficient or vitamin-A-deficient rats increased significantly the proportion of tumour-bearing rats in both groups. Lung adenomas and forestomach papillomas developed in vitamin-A-sufficient animals while multiple neoplasms including lung lymphoma [an extremely rare tumour in rats] pituitary adenoma and forestomach papilloma occurred in vitamin-A-deficient animals. Control animals did not develop tumours (Ammigan *et al.*, 1991; Table 3.5). No tumours appeared when chewing tobacco extract was applied to the oral mucosa (Gothoskar *et al.*, 1975). Adding black or brown *mishri* in the diet increased significantly the incidence of forestomach papillomas in male and female Sprague-Dawley rats (Kulkarni *et al.*, 1988; Table 3.5).

3.1.3 Hamster

Application of a chewing tobacco extract to the cheek pouch of Syrian golden hamsters produced squamous cell papillomas and/or carcinomas in a small number of animals (Rao, 1984; Table 3.7). Adding black or brown *mishri* in the diet significantly increased the incidence of forestomach papillomas (Kulkarni *et al.*, 1988; Table 3.5). Implantation of chewing tobacco in the cheek pouch (Peacock & Brawley, 1959; Peacock *et al.*, 1960; Dunham & Herrold, 1962; Summerlin *et al.*, 1992), or application of chewing tobacco extract (Suri *et al.*, 1971; Ranadive *et al.*, 1976) or *jarda* (Kandarkar *et al.*, 1981) to the cheek pouch did not induce tumours.

Application of *naswar* to the cheek pouch for life increased incidence of tumours in treated

Table 3.4 Carcinogenicity studies of inhalation of smokeless tobacco in experimental animals

Species, strain (sex) Reference	Animals/group at start Dosing regimen Duration	Results Target organ Incidence and/or multiplicity of tumours (%)	Significance	Comments
Mouse, Strain A (M) Hamazaki & Murao (1969)	80 animals/group Inhalation of powdered tobacco leaf, dose (NR), alternate days, controls were untreated; 30 mo	Treated– Lung tumours 12/75 (16%; alveologenic carcinomas 6, squamous cell carcinomas 3, malignant adenomas 3) Leukaemia 11/80 (15%) Hepatocellular carcinomas 3/75 (4%) Controls– Malignant lung adenomas 1/80 Leukaemia 2/80 Hepatocellular carcinomas 0/80 Controls– Malignant lung adenomas 1/80 Leukaemia 2/80 Hepatocellular carcinomas 0/80	Lung tumours: $P < 0.001$ Leukaemias: $P < 0.01$ $P < 0.01$	The incidence of lung tumours and leukaemia was significantly increased in treated animals, the incidence of lung and liver tumours in the untreated controls was unusually low

M, male; mo, month or months, NR, not reported

Table 3.5 Carcinogenicity studies of oral administration of *mishri* alone or with modifiers to experimental animals

Species, strain (sex) Reference	Animals/group at start Dosing regimen Duration	Results Target organ Incidence and/or multiplicity of tumours (%)	Significance
Mouse, Swiss (M, F) Kulkarni *et al.* (1988)	26 animals/sex/group Black *mishri* 10% in diet for 20 mo; 25 mo	Forestomach (papillomas): M–11/24 (46%) F–11/26 (42%)	$P < 0.01$ *vs* controls
	26 animals/sex/group Brown *mishri* 10% in diet for 20 mo; 25 mo	Forestomach (papillomas): M–14/26 (54%) F–11/26 (42%)	$P < 0.01$ *vs* controls
	27 M, 31 F (controls) No *mishri* tobacco, standard diet only; 25 mo	Forestomach (papillomas): M–3/27 (11%) F–1/31 (3%)	$P < 0.01$ *vs* controls
Rat Sprague Dawley (M, F) Kulkarni *et al.* (1988)	27 M, 24 F Brown *mishri* 10% in diet for 20 mo; 25 mo	Forestomach (papillomas): M–10/27 (37%) F–9/24 (37%)	$P < 0.01$ *vs* controls
	25 M, 30 F No *mishri* tobacco, standard diet only; 25 mo	Forestomach (papillomas): M, F–0%	$P < 0.01$ *vs* controls
Hamster Syrian Golden (M, F) Kulkarni *et al.* (1988)	23 M, 26 F Black *mishri* 10% in diet for 20 mo; 25 mo	Forestomach (papillomas): M–10/23 (43%) F–7/26 (27%)	 $P < 0.01$ *vs* controls $P < 0.02$ *vs* controls
	28M, 20F Brown *mishri* 10% in diet for 20 mo; 25 mo	Forestomach (papillomas): M–12/28 (43%) F–5/20 (25%)	 $P < 0.01$ *vs* controls $P < 0.01$ *vs* controls
	23 animals/sex No *mishri* tobacco, standard diet only; 25 mo	Forestomach (papillomas): M–2/23 (9%) F–1/23 (4%)	
Rat Sprague Dawley (M) Ammigan *et al.* (1991)	30 or 31 animals/group VitA sufficient diet + 3 mg *mishri* extract per application by gavage 5 × /wk; 21 mo Controls received VitA sufficient diet + 0.0.5 ml per application DMSO by gavage 5 × /wk; 21 mo	Lung (adenomas and stomach papillomas): 8/30 (27%) Controls–0/31	Total tumour incidence treated *vs* controls $P < 0.001$
	30 animals/group Vit A deficient diet + 3 mg *mishri* extract per application by gavage 5 × /wk; 21 mo Controls received Vit A deficient diet + 0.05 ml per application DMSO by gavage 5 × /wk; 21 mo	28/30 (93%) Controls–0/30	Total tumour incidence Vit deficient *vs* controls $P < 0.001$

F, female; M, male; mo, month or months; *vs*, versus; wk, week or weeks

Table 3.6 Carcinogenicity studies of oral administration of chewing tobacco in experimental animals

Species, strain (sex) Reference	Animals/group at start Dosing regimen Duration	Results Target organ Incidence and/or multiplicity of tumours (%)	Significance	Comments
Rat Sprague Dawley (M) Bhide *et al.* (1991)	29, 31 controls Diet containing shark liver oil + tobacco by gavage, 3mg tobacco extract (vaccum dried powder of 100 g tobacco extracted with 1L dichloromethane) in 0.05 ml DMSO, 5 × /wk; controls received diet containing shark liver oil + 0.05 ml DMSO 5 d/wk; 21 mo	Lung (adenomas):3/29 (10%) Forestomach (papillomas): 3/29 (10%) Controls–0/31	$P < 0.05$ χ^2 test	
	31, 30 controls Diet containing shark liver oil + tobacco by gavage, diet without shark liver oil + tobacco by gavage; controls received diet without shark liver oil + 0.05 ml DMSO, 5 × /wk; 21 mo	Lung (lymphomas): 22/31 (71%) Pituitary (adenomas): 19/31 (61%) Stomach (papillomas): 24/31 (77%) Controls–0/30	$P < 0.001$ χ^2 test	Primary lymphoma of the lung is extremely rare in rats

d, day or days; mo, month or months; wk, week or weeks

Table 3.7 Carcinogenicity studies of application of smokeless tobacco to the oral mucosa or cheek pouch of experimental animals

Species, strain (sex) Reference	Animals/group at start Dosing regimen Duration	Results Target organ Incidence and/or multiplicity of tumours (%)	Significance	Comments
Hamster Syrian golden (M) Suri *et al.* (1971)	11–12 animals/group Banarasi Tobacco-DMSO extract/not specified; application to the cheek pouch 3 × /wk for 21 wk; controls received DMSO; 21 wk	No tumours found in treated and control animals Leukoplakia: 8/12 (67%)		Short duration of exposure, tobacco/DMSO dose not specified
Hamster Syrian golden (F) Rao (1984)	20, 10 controls Topical application to the cheek pouch of lyophilised aqueous tobacco extract, 1 mg in 0.05 mL water twice/d for 6 mo; controls received topical application of 0.05 mL water; 12 mo	Squamous cell papillomas and carcinomas: 3/17 (18%) Controls–no tumours	NR	Statistics not provided

D, day or days; F, female; M, male; mo, month or months; NR, not reported; wk, week or weeks

Table 3.8 Carcinogenicity studies of administration of naswar with known carcinogens or modifiers to the skin of experimental animals

Species, strain (sex) Reference	Animals/group at start Dosing regimen Duration	Results Target organ Incidence and/or multiplicity of tumours (%)	SSignificance	Comments
Hamster Syrian golden (M, F) Kiseleva *et al.* (1976)	33 M, 28 F *Naswar* introduced as dry powder in the left buccal pouch (mixture of tobacco 45%, lime 8%, ash 30%, plant oil 12% and water 5%, dose (NR); life time	13 animals with tumours: Liver–6 Mixed–1 Adrenal gland–3 Forestomach–1 Uterus/ovary–1 Skin (melanoma)–1 Large intestine–1	Tumour frequency higher than in controls $P < 0.05$	Dose of *naswar* not specified Tumour type not specified genderwise
	24 M, 13 F *Nas* introduced as sunflower oil suspension in the left buccal pouch	Liver: 1 Uterus/ovary: 2 Skin (Papilloma): 1	Tumour frequency higher than in controls, $P < 0.05$	
	46 M, 40 F *Nas* introduced as sunflower oil suspension in the left buccal pouch	13 animals with tumours: Liver–4 Mixed–1 Adrenal gland–3 Forestomach (papillomas)–4 Uterus/ovary–1 Skin (papilloma)–1 Pancreas–1	Tumour frequency higher than in controls $P < 0.05$	
	41 M, 9 F *Nas* suspension in sunflower oil introduced in oesophagus	No tumours		
	31 M, 19 F *Nas* suspension in sunflower oil applied to dorsal skin	3 animals with tumours: Liver–1 Adrenal gland–1 Forestomach (papilloma)–1		
	41 M, 69 F Untreated controls	2 animals with tumours: Stomach–1 Adrenal gland–1		

Table 3.8 (continued)

Species, strain (sex) Reference	Animals/group at start Dosing regimen Duration	Results Target organ Incidence and/or multiplicity of tumours (%)	SSignificance	Comments
Hamster Syrian golden (M, F) Milievskaja & Kiseleva (1976)	184 animals *Naswar* introduced in the buccal pouch as dry powder or 50% suspension in sunflower oil; life time	Buccal pouch: 0 Forestomach: 5 Liver: 13 Adrenal gland: 6 Others: 9	NR	The number of animals that survived at the time of first tumour appearance was small High mortality was seen even in control animals
	30 animals DMBA only introduced in the buccal pouch once	Buccal pouch: 1 Stomach: 2		
	30 animals 0.1 g DMBA only + *naswar* introduced in the buccal pouch as dry powder or 50% suspension in sunflower oil; life time	Buccal pouch: 0 Stomach: 5 Others: 1		
	110 untreated controls	Stomach: 1 Adrenal gland: 1		

F, female; M, male; NR, not reported

Table 3.9 Carcinogenicity studies of oral administration of snuff to experimental animals

Reference Species, strain (sex)	Animals/group at start Dosing regimen Duration	Results Target organ Incidence and/or multiplicity of tumours (%)	Significance	Comments
Stenström *et al.* (2007)	5.9% snuff diet (snus mixed with powdered standard mouse show); 6 mo	Gastric carcinoma in situ		
Mouse, wild type, FVB (M)	8, 11 controls	0/8 Controls: 0/11	NR	
Wild type, FVB *Helicobacter pylori* infected (M)	20, 8 controls	9/17 Controls: 0/11	NR	Gastric carcinoma in situ invading the mucosa and submucosa
INS-GAS (M)	8 animals/group	4/8 Controls: 2/8	NR	
INS-GAS (M) *Helicobacter pylori*-infected (M)	22, 8 controls	12/12 Controls: 2/8	NR	Gastric carcinoma in situ invading the mucosa

M, male; mo, month or months; NR, not reported

Table 3.10 Carcinogenicity studies of snuff to the oral mucosa or cheek pouch of experimental animals

Species, strain (sex) Reference	Animals/group at start Dosing regimen Duration	Results Target organ Incidence and/or multiplicity of tumours (%)	Significance
Rat, Sprague Dawley (M) Johansson *et al.* (1989)	30 animals/group Snuff insertion in lip canal, 100 mg per application twice/d, 5 d/wk, controls received cotton pellet dipped in saline; 108 wk	Squamous cell carcinomas: 5 (lip–1, hard palate–2, nasal cavity–1, forestomach–1)	All squamous cell tumours
		Squamous cell carcinomas in situ: hard palate–1	$P < 0.01$
		Squamous cell papillomas: 3 (lip–1, hard palate–1, nasal cavity–1) Undifferentiated lip sarcomas: 2 Controls: no tumours	Malignant squamous cell tumours $P < 0.05$
Rat, Sprague-Dawley (M) Johansson *et al.* (1991)	38, 30 controls Snuff inserted in surgically created lip canal, moist snuff,150–200 mg/ application twice/d, 5 d/wk for 104 wk, controls received a cotton pellet dipped in saline once/d 5 d/wk for 100 wk	Sarcoma of the lip: 10/38 (26%)	Comparison of sarcoma $P < 0.01$
		Squamous cell carcinomas and papillomas of the oral cavity: 3/38 (8%) (lip palate and buccal mucosa), Controls–1/30 (3%) sarcoma of the lip	Comparison of all tumours $P < 0.01$

d, day or days; M, male; wk, week or weeks

hamsters compared to controls (Kiseleva *et al.*, 1976; Milievskaja & Kiseleva, 1976; Table 3.8).

3.2 Snuff

3.2.1 Mouse

Addition of snuff (snus) to the diet induced stomach tumours in gastrin transgenic mice but not in wild-type mice unless they were infected with *Helicobacter pylori* (*H. pylori*). Feeding snuff to *H. pylori*-infected transgenic mice increased gastric carcinoma incidence 2-fold versus control transgenic mice (Stenström *et al.*, 2007; Table 3.9).

3.2.2 Rat

Application of snuff to the oral mucosa (Chen, 1989) or swabbing of lips and oral cavity with a snuff extract (Hecht *et al.*, 1986) did not induce tumours.

In one study, the administration of snuff in a surgically created lip canal did not induce tumours in the oral cavity (Hirsch *et al.*, 1984) while a squamous cell carcinoma of the oral mucosa developed in one rat in another study (Hirsch & Johansson, 1983). Insertion of snuff in a surgically prepared lip canal induced a squamous cell carcinoma in the lip canal, a papilloma in the oral cavity and an olfactory tumour (Hecht *et al.*, 1986).

Insertion of snuff in a surgically prepared lip canal induced squamous cell carcinoma in the lip, hard palate, nasal cavity and forestomach and a carcinoma in situ in the hard palate. In addition, the treated animals developed squamous cell papillomas in the lip, hard palate and nasal cavity and two undifferentiated lip sarcomas. The incidence of all squamous cell tumours, squamous cell carcinomas and the total number of tumours in the treated group were significantly greater than in controls (Johansson *et al.*, 1989; Table 3.10).

In another independent study, the insertion of snuff in the surgically prepared lip canal induced two squamous cell papillomas in the lip,

Table 3.11 Carcinogenicity studies of snuff with known carcinogens or modifiers to experimental animals

Species, strain (sex) Reference	Animals/group at start Dosing regimen Duration	Results Target organ Incidence and/or multiplicity of tumours (%)	Significance
Rat, Sprague-Dawley (M) Johansson *et al.* (1991)	40 animals/group with surgically created lip canal Group 1: DMBA in mineral oil – 70 mg solution + a cotton pellet containing saline 1 × /d, 5 d/wk + snuff 150–200 mg/application. Group 2: DMBA initiation as for control group + snuff in the lip canal twice/d, 5 d/wk. Group 3: Controls initiated with cotton pellets containing 0.1% DMBA in mineral oil in lip canal 3 × / wk for 4 wk only, 104 wk	Sarcomas of the lip: 9/40 (22%) Squamous cell carcinomas and papillomas of the oral cavity (lip, palate, and buccal mucosa): 3/40 (7%) Controls: 0/40	Significant increase in lip sarcoma over Group 1
	38, 40 controls Group 4: Initiation with 4 NQO as for control group + snuff in the lip canal twice/d, 5 d/wk, 70 mg 4NQO sol + cotton pellet containing saline 1 × /d, 5 d/wk + snuff 150 – 200 mg/application. Group 5: Controls initiated with 4 NQO (0.5% in propylene glycol) in cotton pellet placed in lip canal 3 × / wk for 4 wk only, 70 mg 4NQO sol + cotton dipped in saline inserted in the lip canal once/d, 5d/wk; 100 wk	Sarcoma of the lip: 25/38 (66%) Controls–1/40 (2%) Squamous cell carcinomas and papillomas of the oral cavity (lip, palate, and buccal mucosa): 8/38 (21%) Controls–9/40 (22%)	Significant increase in lip sarcoma over control
Hamster Syrian golden (M) Park *et al.* (1986)	15–20 animals/group Cheek pouches inoculated with HSV1 or HSV2 (groups 1 and 1'), once/mo for 6 mo (no snuff); 6 mo	No tumours 0/19 (HSV1) No tumours 0/16 (HSV2)	
	Cheek pouches inoculated with HSV1 once/mo + snuff 150 mg/pouch, in both pouches twice/d, 5 d/wk for 6 mo; 6 mo (Group 2)	Invasive squamous cell buccal pouch carcinomas: 10/20 (50%)	Increase in carcinoma $P < 0.05$ Group 2 *vs* Group 1
	Cheek pouches inoculated with HSV2 once a mo + Snuff 150 mg/pouch in both pouches twice/d, 5 d/wk for 6 mo; 6 mo (Group 3)	Invasive squamous cell buccal pouch carcinoma: 11/20 (55%)	Increase in carcinoma $P < 0.05$ Group 3 *vs* Group 1'

Table 3.11 (continued)

Species, strain (sex) Reference	Animals/group at start Dosing regimen Duration	Results Target organ Incidence and/or multiplicity of tumours (%)	Significance
Hamster Syrial golden (M) Gijare *et al.* (1990)	15 or 20 animals/group Application of 0.125 mg DMBA in 50 µl oil, twice/wk for 1 mo to both cheek pouches 0.25% in liquid paraffin; 6 mo	Cheek pouch tumours: 10/15 (66%) Forestomach tumours: 15/15 (100%)	NR
	Application of 0.125 mg DMBA in 50 ml oil, twice/wk for 1 mo + 50 µl snuff in liquid paraffin 20 mg per cheek pouch twice/wk to both cheek pouches 0.25% in liquid paraffin + Manglorian snuff; 6 mo	Cheek pouch tumours: 3/20 (15%) Forestomach tumours: 20/20 (100%)	NR
	Application of 50 µl snuff in liquid paraffin, 20 mg per cheek pouch twice/wk to both cheek pouches; 6 mo	Cheek pouch tumours: 0/20 Forestomach tumours: 17/20 (85%)	NR
	Application of 0.125 mg DMBA in 50 ml oil, twice/wk for 1 mo + 50 µl scented snuff in liquid paraffin 20 mg per cheek pouch twice/wk to both cheek pouches 0.25% in liquid paraffin + Scented snuff; 6 mo	Cheek pouch tumours: 2/20 (10%) Forestomach tumours: 19/20 (95%)	NR
	Untreated controls	No tumours	

d, day or days; M, male; mo, month or months; NR, not reported; *vs*, versus; wk, week or weeks

10 lip sarcomas and three squamous cell carcinomas in the hard palate. In the control group, a lip sarcoma occurred in one rat. The total incidence of epithelial and mesenchymal tumours of the lip and oral cavity and the incidence of lip sarcoma was significantly greater in snuff-treated rats than in controls (Johansson *et al.*, 1991; Table 3.10).

In one study, animals were repeatedly administered snuff extracts by the subcutaneous route. No local tumours developed in either treated or control groups (Schmähl, 1965).

Application of snuff to the surgically created lip canal of rats infected with HSV 1 resulted in the development of squamous cell carcinoma of the oral cavity in 2/7 (28%) rats and a retroperitoneal sarcoma developed in one rat. In the group exposed to snuff alone, one rat each developed a squamous cell carcinoma of the anus and a retroperitoneal sarcoma (Hirsch *et al.*, 1984).

In animals whose hard palate was treated with 4-Nitroquinoline 1-oxide (4NQO), repeated application of snuff did not enhance the incidence of benign and malignant oral cavity tumours over that in animals treated with 4NQO alone (Johansson *et al.*, 1989). However, in another study, application of snuff to a 4NQO-treated surgically created lip canal increased the incidence of lip sarcoma (Johansson *et al.*, 1991; Table 3.10).

3.2.3 Hamster

In hamsters infected with HSV1 or HSV2, insertion of snuff in the cheek pouch increased significantly the incidence of squamous cell carcinoma over that in animals infected with HSV1 or HSV2 and not administered snuff (Park *et al.*, 1986; Table 3.11). Application of a snuff suspension alone to the cheek pouch resulted in the development of stomach papillomas but did not increase the forestomach papilloma incidence in animals initiated with DMBA (Gijare *et al.*, 1990). In one study, chronic feeding of snuff and calcium hydroxide induced a pancreatic carcinoid in one animal only (Dunham *et al.*, 1975) but did not induce any tumours in another study (Homburger *et al.*, 1976). Snuff instillation in the cheek pouch did not induce tumours in six studies (Peacock & Brawley, 1959; Peacock *et al.*, 1960, Dunham & Herrold, 1962; Dunham *et al.*, 1975; Homburger *et al.*, 1976; Park *et al.*, 1986).

3.3 Synthesis

In animals administered various smokeless tobacco preparations, consistent increases were observed for forestomach, lung, oral cavity and nasal tumours in rats; lung, skin, forestomach and liver tumours in mice; and oral cavity (cheek pouch) and forestomach tumours in hamsters.

4. Other Relevant Data

See Section 4 of the *Monograph* on Tobacco Smoking in this volume.

5. Evaluation

There is *sufficient evidence* in humans for the carcinogenicity of smokeless tobacco. Smokeless tobacco causes cancers of the oral cavity, oesophagus and pancreas.

There is *sufficient evidence* in experimental animals for the carcinogenicity of smokeless tobacco.

Smokeless tobacco is *carcinogenic to humans (Group 1).*

References

Accortt NA, Waterbor JW, Beall C, Howard G (2002). Chronic disease mortality in a cohort of smokeless tobacco users. *Am J Epidemiol*, 156: 730–737. doi:10.1093/aje/kwf106 PMID:12370161

Accortt NA, Waterbor JW, Beall C, Howard G (2005). Cancer incidence among a cohort of smokeless tobacco users (United States). *Cancer Causes Control*, 16: 1107–1115. doi:10.1007/s10552-005-0247-0 PMID:16184477

Ahmed HG, Idris AM, Ibrahim SO (2003). Study of oral epithelial atypia among Sudanese tobacco users by exfoliative cytology. *Anticancer Res*, 23: 2C1943–1949. PMID:12820484

Ahmed HG & Mahgoob RM (2007). Impact of Toombak dipping in the etiology of oral cancer: gender-exclusive hazard in the Sudan. *J Cancer Res Ther*, 3: 127–130. PMID:17998740

al-Idrissi HY (1990). Head and neck cancer in Saudi Arabia: retrospective analysis of 65 patients. *J Int Med Res*, 18: 515–519. PMID:2292333

Aleksandrova HM (1970) [Role of nass in the development of pathological changes in the mouth] In Russian. In:*Epidemiology of Malignant Tumours* Alma-Ata: Nauka Publishing House, 243–246.

Alguacil J & Silverman DT (2004). Smokeless and other noncigarette tobacco use and pancreatic cancer: a case-control study based on direct interviews. *Cancer Epidemiol Biomarkers Prev*, 13: 55–58. doi:10.1158/1055-9965.EPI-03-0033 PMID:14744733

Allard WF, DeVol EB, Te OB (1999). Smokeless tobacco (shamma) and oral cancer in Saudi Arabia. *Community Dent Oral Epidemiol*, 27: 398–405. PMID:10600072

Amer M, Bull CA, Daouk MN *et al.* (1985). Shamma usage and oral cancer in Saudi Arabia. *Ann Saudi Med*, 5: 135–140.

Ammigan N, Nair UJ, Lalitha VS, Bhide SV (1991). Carcinogenicity studies of masheri: pyrolysed tobacco product, in vitamin-A-deficient Sprague Dawley rats. *J Cancer Res Clin Oncol*, 117: 50–54. PMID:1997470

Andersson G & Axéll T (1989). Clinical appearance of lesions associated with the use of loose and portion-bag packed Swedish moist snuff: a comparative study. *J Oral Pathol Med*, 18: 2–7. PMID:2746515

Andersson G, Björnberg G, Curvall M (1994). Oral mucosal changes and nicotine disposition in users of Swedish smokeless tobacco products: a comparative study. *J Oral Pathol Med*, 23: 161–167. PMID:8046653

Andersson G & Warfvinge G (2003). The influence of pH and nicotine concentration in oral moist snuff on mucosal changes and salivary pH in Swedish snuff users. *Swed Dent J*, 27: 67–75. PMID:12856395

Asal NR, Risser DR, Kadamani S *et al.* (1988). Risk factors in renal cell carcinoma: I. Methodology, demographics, tobacco, beverage use, and obesity. *Cancer Detect Prev*, 11: 359–377. PMID:3390857

Asma S, Palipudi K, Sinha DN (2011).* Smokeless tobacco and public health in India, a scientific monograph presented during Stakeholders Meeting; New Delhi, India, October 17

Axéll T, Mörnstad H, Sundström B (1976). The relation of the clinical picture to the histopathology of snuff dipper"s lesions in a Swedish population. *J Oral Pathol*, 5: 229–236. PMID:820845

Ayo-Yusuf OA, Swart TJ, Ayo-Yusuf IJ (2000). Prevalence and pattern of snuff dipping in a rural South African population. *SADJ*, 55: 610–614. PMID:12608224

Babekir AR, el Fahal AH, Alla AH (1989). Oesophageal cancer in Sudan. *Trop Doct*, 19: 33–34. PMID:2922814

Bates C, Jarvis M, Connolly G (1999) *Tobacco Additives: cigarette engineering and nicotine addiction.Action on Smoking and Health.*, http://www.ash.org.uk/html/regulation/html/additives.html

Bhide SV, Ammigan N, Nair UJ, Lalitha VS (1991). Carcinogenicity studies of tobacco extract in vitamin A-deficient Sprague-Dawley rats. *Cancer Res*, 51: 3018–3023. PMID:2032240

Bhide SV, Shah AS, Nair J, Nagarajrao D (1984). Epidemiological and experimental studies on tobacco-related oral cancer in India. *IARC Sci Publ*, 851–857. PMID:6398309

Blomqvist G, Hirsch JM, Alberius P (1991). Association between development of lower lip cancer and tobacco habits. *J Oral Maxillofac Surg*, 49: 1044–1047, discussion 1048–1049. PMID:1653824

Blot WJ, McLaughlin JK, Winn DM *et al.* (1988). Smoking and drinking in relation to oral and pharyngeal cancer. *Cancer Res*, 48: 3282–3287. PMID:3365707

Blot WJ, Winn DM, Fraumeni JF Jr (1983). Oral cancer and mouthwash. *J Natl Cancer Inst*, 70: 251–253. PMID:6571933

Bock FG, Moore GE, Crouch SK (1964). Tumor promoting activity of extracts of unburned tobacco. *Science*, 145: 831–833. PMID:14163329

Bock FG, Shamberger RJ, Myers HK (1965). Tumour-promoting agents in unburned cigarette tobacco. *Nature*, 208: 584–585.

Boffetta P, Aagnes B, Weiderpass E, Andersen A (2005). Smokeless tobacco use and risk of cancer of the pancreas and other organs. *Int J Cancer*, 114: 992–995. doi:10.1002/ijc.20811 PMID:15645430

Boffetta P, Hecht S, Gray N *et al.* (2008). Smokeless tobacco and cancer. *Lancet Oncol*, 9: 667–675. doi:10.1016/S1470-2045(08)70173-6 PMID:18598931

Bracci PM & Holly EA (2005). Tobacco use and non-Hodgkin lymphoma: results from a population-based case-control study in the San Francisco Bay Area, California. *Cancer Causes Control*, 16: 333–346. doi:10.1007/s10552-004-4324-6 PMID:15953976

Brinton LA, Blot WJ, Becker JA *et al.* (1984). A case-control study of cancers of the nasal cavity and paranasal sinuses. *Am J Epidemiol*, 119: 896–906. PMID:6731431

Broders AC (1920). Squamous-cell epithelioma of the lip. A study of five hundred and thirty-seven cases. *JAMA*, 74: 656–664.

Brown LM, Blot WJ, Schuman SH *et al.* (1988). Environmental factors and high risk of esophageal cancer among men in coastal South Carolina. *J Natl*

Cancer Inst, 80: 1620–1625. doi:10.1093/jnci/80.20.1620 PMID:3193480

Brown LM, Everett GD, Gibson R *et al.* (1992a). Smoking and risk of non-Hodgkin's lymphoma and multiple myeloma. *Cancer Causes Control*, 3: 49–55. doi:10.1007/BF00051912 PMID:1536913

Brown LM, Gibson R, Blair A *et al.* (1992b). Smoking and risk of leukemia. *Am J Epidemiol*, 135: 763–768. PMID:1595675

Browne RM, Camsey MC, Waterhouse JA, Manning GL (1977). Etiological factors in oral squamous cell carcinoma. *Community Dent Oral Epidemiol*, 5: 301–306. PMID:272257

Bundgaard T, Wildt J, Frydenberg M *et al.* (1995). Case-control study of squamous cell cancer of the oral cavity in Denmark. *Cancer Causes Control*, 6: 57–67. PMID:7718736

Burch JD, Rohan TE, Howe GR *et al.* (1989). Risk of bladder cancer by source and type of tobacco exposure: a case-control study. *Int J Cancer*, 44: 622–628. doi:10.1002/ijc.2910440411 PMID:2793235

Canto MT & Devesa SS (2002). Oral cavity and pharynx cancer incidence rates in the United States, 1975–1998. *Oral Oncol*, 38: 610–617. PMID:12167440

Chandra A (1962). Different habits and their relation with cheek cancer. *Chittaranjan Cancer Hosp Calcutta natl Cancer Res Cent Bull*, 33–36.

Chao A, Thun MJ, Henley SJ *et al.* (2002). Cigarette smoking, use of other tobacco products and stomach cancer mortality in US adults: The Cancer Prevention Study II. *Int J Cancer*, 101: 380–389. doi:10.1002/ijc.10614 PMID:12209964

Chelleng PK, Narain K, Das HK *et al.* (2000). Risk factors for cancer nasopharynx: a case-control study from Nagaland, India. *Natl Med J India*, 13: 6–8. PMID:10743368

Chen SY (1989). Effects of smokeless tobacco on the buccal mucosa of HMT rats. *J Oral Pathol Med*, 18: 108–112. PMID:2746519

Chow WH, McLaughlin JK, Menck HR, Mack TM (1994). Risk factors for extrahepatic bile duct cancers: Los Angeles County, California (USA). *Cancer Causes Control*, 5: 267–272. doi:10.1007/BF01830247 PMID:8061176

Creath CJ, Cutter G, Bradley DH, Wright JT (1991). Oral leukoplakia and adolescent smokeless tobacco use. *Oral Surg Oral Med Oral Pathol*, 72: 35–41. PMID:1891243

Creath CJ, Shelton WO, Wright JT *et al.* (1988). The prevalence of smokeless tobacco use among adolescent male athletes. *J Am Dent Assoc*, 116: 43–48. PMID:3422665

Crew KD & Neugut AI (2004). Epidemiology of upper gastrointestinal malignancies. *Semin Oncol*, 31: 450–464. doi:10.1053/j.seminoncol.2004.04.021 PMID:15297938

Cummings KM, Michalek AM, Carl W *et al.* (1989). Use of smokeless tobacco in a group of professional baseball players. *J Behav Med*, 12: 559–567. PMID:2634109

Daniels TE, Hansen LS, Greenspan JS *et al.* (1992). Histopathology of smokeless tobacco lesions in professional baseball players. Associations with different types of tobacco. *Oral Surg Oral Med Oral Pathol*, 73: 720–725. PMID:1279496

DHHS; Department of Health and Human Services (2001). Summary of Findings from the 2000 National Household Survey on Drug Abuse. Substance Abuse and Mental Health Services Administration, Office of Applied Studies, NHSDA Series H-13, DHHS Publication No. (SMA) 01-3549. Rockville, MD.

Djordjevic MV, Hoffmann D, Glynn T, Connolly GN (1995). US commercial brands of moist snuff, 1994. I. Assessment of nicotine, moisture, and pH. *Tob Control*, 4: 62–66. doi:10.1136/tc.4.1.62

Dunham LJ & Herrold KM (1962). Failure to Produce Tumors in the Hamster Cheek Pouch by Exposure to Ingredients of Betel Quid; Histopathologic Changes in the Pouch and Other Organs by Exposure to Known Carcinogens. *J Natl Cancer Inst*, 29: 1047–1059.

Dunham LJ, Snell KC, Stewart HL (1975). Argyrophilic carcinoids in two Syrian hamsters (Mesocricetus auratus). *J Natl Cancer Inst*, 54: 507–513. PMID:46277

Elbeshir EI, Abeen HA, Idris AM, Abbas K (1989). Snuff dipping and oral cancer in Sudan: a retrospective study. *Br J Oral Maxillofac Surg*, 27: 243–248. PMID:2742810

Ernster VL, Grady DG, Greene JC *et al.* (1990). Smokeless tobacco use and health effects among baseball players. *JAMA*, 264: 218–224. PMID:2355443

European Commission (2008). SCENIHR (Scientific Committee on Emerging and Newly-Identified Health Risks), Scientific opinion on the Health Effects of Smokeless Tobacco Products

Evstifeeva TV & Zaridze DG (1992). Nass use, cigarette smoking, alcohol consumption and risk of oral and oesophageal precancer. *Eur J Cancer B Oral Oncol*, 28B: 29–35. PMID:1422467

Farrow DC & Davis S (1990). Risk of pancreatic cancer in relation to medical history and the use of tobacco, alcohol and coffee. *Int J Cancer*, 45: 816–820. doi:10.1002/ijc.2910450504 PMID:2335385

Fernberg P, Odenbro A, Bellocco R *et al.* (2007). Tobacco use, body mass index, and the risk of leukemia and multiple myeloma: a nationwide cohort study in Sweden. *Cancer Res*, 67: 5983–5986. doi:10.1158/0008-5472.CAN-07-0274 PMID:17575169

Fisher MA, Bouquot JE, Shelton BJ (2005). Assessment of risk factors for oral leukoplakia in West Virginia. *Community Dent Oral Epidemiol*, 33: 45–52. PMID:15642046

Franco EL, Kowalski LP, Oliveira BV *et al.* (1989). Risk factors for oral cancer in Brazil: a case-control study. *Int J Cancer*, 43: 992–1000. PMID:2732011

Gijare PS, Rao KV, Bhide SV (1990). Modulatory effects of snuff, retinoic acid, and beta-carotene on DMBA-induced hamster cheek pouch carcinogenesis in relation to keratin expression. *Nutr Cancer*, 14: 253–259. PMID:1707524

Gillison ML, Koch WM, Capone RB *et al.* (2000). Evidence for a causal association between human papillomavirus and a subset of head and neck cancers. *J Natl Cancer Inst*, 92: 709–720. doi:10.1093/jnci/92.9.709 PMID:10793107

Goodman MT, Morgenstern H, Wynder EL (1986). A case-control study of factors affecting the development of renal cell cancer. *Am J Epidemiol*, 124: 926–941. PMID:3776975

Gothoskar SV, Sant SM, Ranadive KJ (1975). Effect of ‘tobacco and lime on oral mucosa of rats’ fed on vitamin B deficient diet. *Indian J Cancer*, 12: 424–429. PMID:1221046

Goud ML, Mohapatra SC, Mohapatra P *et al.* (1990). Epidemiological correlates between consumption of Indian chewing tobacco and oral cancer. *Eur J Epidemiol*, 6: 219–222. PMID:2361546

Grady D, Greene J, Daniels TE *et al.* (1990). Oral mucosal lesions found in smokeless tobacco users. *J Am Dent Assoc*, 121: 117–123. PMID:2370378

Grady D, Greene J, Ernster VL *et al.* (1991). Short term changes a surprise with smokeless tobacco. Oral lesions. *J Am Dent Assoc*, 122: 62–64. PMID:1999587

Grasser JA & Childers E (1997). Prevalence of smokeless tobacco use and clinical oral leukoplakia in a military population. *Mil Med*, 162: 401–404. PMID:9183161

Greene JC, Ernster VL, Grady DG *et al.* (1992) *Oral mucosal lesions: Clinical findings in relation to smokeless tobacco use among US baseball players. In: Smokeless tobacco or health: An International Perspective.* Bethesda, MD: National Institutes of Health.

Greer RO Jr & Poulson TC (1983). Oral tissue alterations associated with the use of smokeless tobacco by teenagers. Part I. Clinical findings. *Oral Surg Oral Med Oral Pathol*, 56: 275–284. PMID:6195576

Gupta PC, Mehta FS, Daftary DK *et al.* (1980). Incidence rates of oral cancer and natural history of oral precancerous lesions in a 10-year follow-up study of Indian villagers. *Community Dent Oral Epidemiol*, 8: 283–333. doi:10.1111/j.1600-0528.1980.tb01302.x PMID:6937277

Hamazaki Y & Murao T (1969). On the Carcinogenic Factors of Tobacco Leaf Powder. I. Inhalation of tobacco leaf powder. *J Karyopathol Esp Tumor Tumorvirus*, 12: 163–178.

Hansson LE, Baron J, Nyrén O *et al.* (1994). Tobacco, alcohol and the risk of gastric cancer. A population-based case-control study in Sweden. *Int J Cancer*, 57: 26–31. doi:10.1002/ijc.2910570106 PMID:8150537

Harish K & Ravi R (1995). The role of tobacco in penile carcinoma. *Br J Urol*, 75: 375–377. doi:10.1111/j.1464-410X.1995.tb07352.x PMID:7735804

Hartge P, Hoover R, Kantor A (1985). Bladder cancer risk and pipes, cigars, and smokeless tobacco. *Cancer*, 55: 901–906. doi:10.1002/1097-0142(19850215)55:4<901::AID-CNCR2820550432>3.0.CO;2-Q PMID:3967183

Hassan MM, Abbruzzese JL, Bondy ML *et al.* (2007). Passive smoking and the use of noncigarette tobacco products in association with risk for pancreatic cancer: a case-control study. *Cancer*, 109: 2547–2556. doi:10.1002/cncr.22724 PMID:17492688

Hayes RB, Pottern LM, Swanson GM *et al.* (1994). Tobacco use and prostate cancer in blacks and whites in the United States. *Cancer Causes Control*, 5: 221–226. doi:10.1007/BF01830240 PMID:8061169

Hecht SS, Rivenson A, Braley J *et al.* (1986). Induction of oral cavity tumors in F344 rats by tobacco-specific nitrosamines and snuff. *Cancer Res*, 46: 4162–4166. PMID:3731083

Heineman EF, Zahm SH, McLaughlin JK, Vaught JB (1995). Increased risk of colorectal cancer among smokers: results of a 26-year follow-up of US veterans and a review. *Int J Cancer*, 59: 728–738. doi:10.1002/ijc.2910590603 PMID:7989109

Henley SJ, Connell CJ, Richter P *et al.* (2007). Tobacco-related disease mortality among men who switched from cigarettes to spit tobacco. *Tob Control*, 16: 22–28. doi:10.1136/tc.2006.018069 PMID:17297069

Henley SJ, Thun MJ, Connell C, Calle EE (2005). Two large prospective studies of mortality among men who use snuff or chewing tobacco (United States). *Cancer Causes Control*, 16: 347–358. doi:10.1007/s10552-004-5519-6 PMID:15953977

Hirsch JM & Johansson SL (1983). Effect of long-term application of snuff on the oral mucosa: an experimental study in the rat. *J Oral Pathol*, 12: 187–198. PMID:6410027

Hirsch JM, Johansson SL, Thilander H, Vahlne A (1984). Effect of long-term application of snuff and herpes simplex virus 1 on rat oral mucosa. Possible association with development of oral cancer. *IARC Sci Publ*, 829–836. PMID:6099829

Hoffmann D, Djordjevic MV, Fan J *et al.* (1995). Five leading U.S. commercial brands of moist snuff in 1994: assessment of carcinogenic N-nitrosamines. *J Natl Cancer Inst*, 87: 1862–1869. doi:10.1093/jnci/87.24.1862 PMID:7494230

Homburger F, Hsueh SS, Russfield AB *et al.* (1976). Absence of carcinogenic effects of chronic feeding of snuff in inbred syrian hamsters. *Toxicol Appl Pharmacol*, 35: 515–521. PMID:944469

Howe GR, Burch JD, Miller AB *et al.* (1980). Tobacco use, occupation, coffee, various nutrients, and bladder cancer. *J Natl Cancer Inst*, 64: 701–713. PMID:6928984

Hsairi M, Achour N, Zouari B *et al.* (1993). Etiologic factors in primary bronchial carcinoma in Tunisia*Tunis Med*, 71: 265–268. PMID:8212345

Hsing AW, McLaughlin JK, Hrubec Z *et al.* (1991). Tobacco use and prostate cancer: 26-year follow-up of US veterans. *Am J Epidemiol*, 133: 437–441. PMID:2000853

Hsing AW, McLaughlin JK, Schuman LM *et al.* (1990). Diet, tobacco use, and fatal prostate cancer: results from the Lutheran Brotherhood Cohort Study. *Cancer Res*, 50: 6836–6840. PMID:2208150

IARC (2004). Tobacco smoke and involuntary smoking. *IARC Monogr Eval Carcinog Risks Hum*, 83: 1–1438. PMID:15285078

IARC (2007a). Smokeless tobacco and some tobacco-specific N-nitrosamines. *IARC Monogr Eval Carcinog Risks Hum*, 89: 1–592. PMID:18335640

IARC (2007b). Human papillomaviruses. *IARC Monogr Eval Carcinog Risks Hum*, 90: 1–636. PMID:18354839

IARC (2010). Alcohol consumption and ethyl carbamate. *IARC Monogr Eval Carcinog Risks Hum*, 96: 1–1428.

IARC (2012). Chemical agents and related occupations. *IARC Monogr Eval Carcinog Risks Hum*, 100F.

Ibrahim EM, Satti MB, Al Idrissi HY *et al.* (1986). Oral cancer in Saudi Arabia: the role of alqat and alshammah. *Cancer Detect Prev*, 9: 215–218.

Idris AM, Ahmed HM, Malik MO (1995a). Toombak dipping and cancer of the oral cavity in the Sudan: a case-control study. *Int J Cancer*, 63: 477–480. PMID:7591252

Idris AM, Ahmed HM, Mukhtar BI *et al.* (1995b). Descriptive epidemiology of oral neoplasms in Sudan 1970–1985 and the role of toombak. *Int J Cancer*, 61: 155–158. PMID:7705940

Idris AM, Ibrahim SO, Vasstrand EN *et al.* (1998). The Swedish snus and the Sudanese toombak: are they different? *Oral Oncol*, 34: 558–566. doi:10.1016/S1368-8375(98)00047-5 PMID:9930371

Idris AM, Nair J, Ohshima H *et al.* (1991). Unusually high levels of carcinogenic tobacco-specific nitrosamines in Sudan snuff (toombak). *Carcinogenesis*, 12: 1115–1118. doi:10.1093/carcin/12.6.1115 PMID:2044192

Idris AM, Warnakulasuriya KA, Ibrahim YE *et al.* (1996). Toombak-associated oral mucosal lesions in Sudanese show a low prevalence of epithelial dysplasia. *J Oral Pathol Med*, 25: 239–244. PMID:8835821

Jacob BJ, Straif K, Thomas G *et al.* (2004). Betel quid without tobacco as a risk factor for oral precancers. *Oral Oncol*, 40: 697–704. PMID:15172639

Jafarey NA, Mahmood Z, Zaidi SH (1977). Habits and dietary pattern of cases of carcinoma of the oral cavity and oropharynx. *J Pak Med Assoc*, 27: 340–343. PMID:413946

Johansson SL, Hirsch JM, Larsson PA *et al.* (1989). Snuff-induced carcinogenesis: effect of snuff in rats initiated with 4-nitroquinoline N-oxide. *Cancer Res*, 49: 3063–3069. PMID:2497972

Johansson SL, Saidi J, Osterdahl BG, Smith RA (1991). Promoting effect of snuff in rats initiated by 4-nitroquinoline-N-oxide or 7,12-dimethylbenz(a) anthracene. *Cancer Res*, 51: 4388–4394. PMID:1907884

Jungell P & Malmström M (1985). Snuff-induced lesions in Finnish recruits. *Scand J Dent Res*, 93: 442–447. PMID:3864218

Kabat GC, Chang CJ, Wynder EL (1994). The role of tobacco, alcohol use, and body mass index in oral and pharyngeal cancer. *Int J Epidemiol*, 23: 1137–1144. PMID:7721514

Kandarkar SV, Hasgekar NN, Sirsat SM (1981). Optical and ultrastructural pathology of vitamin A pretreated hamster cheek pouch–exposed to lime (Ca(OH)2) and tobacco over total life span. *Neoplasma*, 28: 729–737. PMID:7339502

Keen P, De Moor NG, Shapiro MP *et al.* (1955). The artiology of respiratory tract cancer in the South African Bantu; clinical aspects. *Br J Cancer*, 9: 528–538. doi:10.1038/bjc.1955.54 PMID:13304212

Keller AZ (1969). Residence, age, race and related factors in the survival and associations with salivary tumors. *Am J Epidemiol*, 90: 269–277. PMID:5823440

Keller AZ (1970). Cellular types, survival, race, nativity, occupations, habits and associated diseases in the pathogenesis of lip cancers. *Am J Epidemiol*, 91: 486–499. PMID:5438996

Kiseleva NS, Milievskaja IL, Căklin AV (1976). Development of tumours in Syrian hamsters during prolonged experimental exposure to nas. *Bull World Health Organ*, 54: 597–605. PMID:1088508

Kneller RW, McLaughlin JK, Bjelke E *et al.* (1991). A cohort study of stomach cancer in a high-risk American population. *Cancer*, 68: 672–678. doi:10.1002/1097-0142(19910801)68:3<672::AID-CNCR2820680339>3.0.CO;2-T PMID:2065291

Kubo A & Corley DA (2006). Body mass index and adenocarcinomas of the esophagus or gastric cardia: a systematic review and meta-analysis. *Cancer Epidemiol Biomarkers Prev*, 15: 872–878. doi:10.1158/1055-9965.EPI-05-0860 PMID:16702363

Kulkarni J, Lalitha VS, Bhide S (1989). Weak carcinogenic effect of masheri, a pyrolysed tobacco product, in mouse skin tumor models. *J Cancer Res Clin Oncol*, 115: 166–169. PMID:2497102

Kulkarni JR, Lalitha VS, Bhide SV (1988). Carcinogenicity studies of masheri, a pyrolysed product of tobacco. *Carcinogenesis*, 9: 2137–2138. PMID:3180350

Lagergren J, Bergström R, Lindgren A, Nyrén O (2000). The role of tobacco, snuff and alcohol use in the aetiology of cancer of the oesophagus and gastric cardia. *Int J Cancer*, 85: 340–346. doi:10.1002/(SICI)1097-0215(20000201)85:3<340::AID-IJC8>3.0.CO;2-N PMID:10652424

Larsson A, Axéll T, Andersson G (1991). Reversibility of snuff dippers' lesion in Swedish moist snuff users: a clinical and histologic follow-up study. *J Oral Pathol Med*, 20: 258–264. PMID:1890661

Lee JJ, Hong WK, Hittelman WN *et al.* (2000). Predicting cancer development in oral leukoplakia: ten years of translational research. *Clin Cancer Res*, 6: 1702–1710. PMID:10815888

Lee PN & Hamling JS (2009). Systematic review of the relation between smokeless tobacco and cancer in Europe and North America. *BMC Med*, 7: 36 doi:10.1186/1741-7015-7-36 PMID:19638245

Lewin F, Norell SE, Johansson H *et al.* (1998). Smoking tobacco, oral snuff, and alcohol in the etiology of squamous cell carcinoma of the head and neck: a population-based case-referent study in Sweden. *Cancer*, 82: 1367–1375. doi:10.1002/(SICI)1097-0142(19980401)82:7<1367::AID-CNCR21>3.0.CO;2-3 PMID:9529030

Luo J, Ye W, Zendehdel K *et al.* (2007). Oral use of Swedish moist snuff (snus) and risk for cancer of the mouth, lung, and pancreas in male construction workers: a retrospective cohort study. *Lancet*, 369: 2015–2020. doi:10.1016/S0140-6736(07)60678-3 PMID:17498797

Maden C, Beckmann AM, Thomas DB *et al.* (1992). Human papillomaviruses, herpes simplex viruses, and the risk of oral cancer in men. *Am J Epidemiol*, 135: 1093–1102. PMID:1321561

Mani NJ (1985). Preliminary report on prevalence of oral cancer and precancerous lesions among dental patients in Saudi Arabia. *Community Dent Oral Epidemiol*, 13: 247–248. PMID:3862510

Marshall JR, Graham S, Haughey BP *et al.* (1992). Smoking, alcohol, dentition and diet in the epidemiology of oral cancer. *Eur J Cancer B Oral Oncol*, 28B: 9–15. PMID:1422474

Martin GC, Brown JP, Eifler CW, Houston GD (1999). Oral leukoplakia status six weeks after cessation of smokeless tobacco use. *J Am Dent Assoc*, 130: 945–954. PMID:10422398

Martinez I (1969). Factors associated with ccer of the esophagus, mouth, and pharynx in Puerto Rico. *J Natl Cancer Inst*, 42: 1069–1094. PMID:5793187

Mashberg A, Boffetta P, Winkelman R, Garfinkel L (1993). Tobacco smoking, alcohol drinking, and cancer of the oral cavity and oropharynx among U.S. veterans. *Cancer*, 72: 1369–1375. PMID:8339227

McLaughlin JK, Lindblad P, Mellemgaard A *et al.* (1995). International renal-cell cancer study. I. Tobacco use. *Int J Cancer*, 60: 194–198. doi:10.1002/ijc.2910600211 PMID:7829215

Merchant A, Husain SS, Hosain M *et al.* (2000). Paan without tobacco: an independent risk factor for oral cancer. *Int J Cancer*, 86: 128–131. PMID:10728606

Milievskaja IL & Kiseleva NS (1976). Comparative study of the carcinogenic activities of nas and some chemical carcinogens when introduced into the buccal pouch of the Syrian hamster. *Bull World Health Organ*, 54: 607–614. PMID:829414

Mody JK & Ranadive KJ (1959). Biological study of tobacco in relation to oral cancer. *Indian J Med Sci*, 13: 1023–1037. PMID:14423157

Moore GE, Bissinger LL, Proehl EC (1953). Intraoral cancer and the use of chewing tobacco. *J Am Geriatr Soc*, 1: 497–506. PMID:13069216

Muscat JE, Hoffmann D, Wynder EL (1995). The epidemiology of renal cell carcinoma. A second look. *Cancer*, 75: 2552–2557. doi:10.1002/1097-0142(19950515)75:10<2552::AID-CNCR2820751023>3.0.CO;2-1 PMID:7736400

Muscat JE, Richie JP Jr, Thompson S, Wynder EL (1996). Gender differences in smoking and risk for oral cancer. *Cancer Res*, 56: 5192–5197. PMID:8912856

Muscat JE, Stellman SD, Hoffmann D, Wynder EL (1997). Smoking and pancreatic cancer in men and women. *Cancer Epidemiol Biomarkers Prev*, 6: 15–19. PMID:8993792

Muscat JE & Wynder EL (1998). A case/control study of risk factors for major salivary gland cancer. *Otolaryngol Head Neck Surg*, 118: 195–198. PMID:9482552

Nair UJ, Friesen M, Richard I *et al.* (1990). Effect of lime composition on the formation of reactive oxygen species from areca nut extract in vitro. *Carcinogenesis*, 11: 2145–2148. doi:10.1093/carcin/11.12.2145 PMID:2176136

Nair UJ, Obe G, Friesen M *et al.* (1992). Role of lime in the generation of reactive oxygen species from betel-quid ingredients. *Environ Health Perspect*, 98: 203–205. doi:10.2307/3431271 PMID:1486850

Nasrollahzadeh D, Kamangar F, Aghcheli K *et al.* (2008). Opium, tobacco, and alcohol use in relation to oesophageal squamous cell carcinoma in a high-risk area of Iran. *Br J Cancer*, 98: 1857–1863. doi:10.1038/sj.bjc.6604369 PMID:18475303

Nugmanov SN, Baimakanov SS (1970) [The results of an epidemiological study of oro-pharyngeal tumours in Kazakhstan following the WHO project] In Russian. In:*Epidemiology of Malignant Tumours* Alma-Ata: Nauka Publishing House, 227–231.

Odenbro A, Bellocco R, Boffetta P *et al.* (2005). Tobacco smoking, snuff dipping and the risk of cutaneous squamous cell carcinoma: a nationwide cohort study in Sweden. *Br J Cancer*, 92: 1326–1328. doi:10.1038/sj.bjc.6602475 PMID:15770206

Offenbacher S & Weathers DR (1985). Effects of smokeless tobacco on the periodontal, mucosal and caries status of adolescent males. *J Oral Pathol*, 14: 169–181. PMID:3920367

Ohshima H, Nair J, Bourgade MC *et al.* (1985). Identification and occurrence of two new N-nitrosamino acids in tobacco products: 3-(N-nitroso-N-methylamino) propionic acid and 4-(N-nitroso-N-methylamino) butyric acid. *Cancer Lett*, 26: 153–162. doi:10.1016/0304-3835(85)90021-7 PMID:3978605

Park NH, Sapp JP, Herbosa EG (1986). Oral cancer induced in hamsters with herpes simplex infection and simulated snuff dipping. *Oral Surg Oral Med Oral Pathol*, 62: 164–168. PMID:3462612

Payne JB, Johnson GK, Reinhardt RA, Schmid M (1998). Histological alterations following short term smokeless tobacco exposure in humans. *J Periodontal Res*, 33: 274–279. PMID:9777594

Peacock EE Jr & Brawley BW (1959). An evaluation of snuff and tobacco in the production of mouth cancer. *Plast Reconstr Surg Transplant Bull*, 23: 628–635. PMID:13667478

Peacock EE Jr, Greenberg BG, Brawley BW (1960). The effect of snuff and tobacco on the production of oral carcinoma: an experimental and epidemiological study. *Ann Surg*, 151: 542–550. PMID:14431201

Phukan RK, Ali MS, Chetia CK, Mahanta J (2001). Betel nut and tobacco chewing; potential risk factors of cancer of oesophagus in Assam, India. *Br J Cancer*, 85: 661–667. doi:10.1054/bjoc.2001.1920 PMID:11531248

Phukan RK, Zomawia E, Narain K *et al.* (2005). Tobacco use and stomach cancer in Mizoram, India. *Cancer Epidemiol Biomarkers Prev*, 14: 1892–1896. doi:10.1158/1055-9965.EPI-05-0074 PMID:16103433

Pindborg JJ (1980) *Oral cancer and precancer.* Bristol: John Wright.

Pindborg JJ, Reichart PA, Smith CJ *et al.* (1996) *Histological typing of cancer and precancer of the oral mucosa. In: International Histological Classification of Tumours.*2nd Ed., Sobin LH (ed) Geneva: World Health Organaization.

Pottern LM, Morris LE, Blot WJ *et al.* (1981). Esophageal cancer among black men in Washington, D.C. I. Alcohol, tobacco, and other risk factors. *J Natl Cancer Inst*, 67: 777–783. PMID:6944547

Poulson TC, Lindenmuth JE, Greer RO Jr (1984). A comparison of the use of smokeless tobacco in rural and urban teenagers. *CA Cancer J Clin*, 34: 248–261. PMID:6432238

Prokopczyk B, Wu M, Cox JE *et al.* (1995). Improved Methodology for the Quantitative Assessment of Tobacco-Specific N-Nitrosamines in Tobacco by Supercritical-Fluid Extraction. *J Agric Food Chem*, 43: 916–922. doi:10.1021/jf00052a013

Putnam SD, Cerhan JR, Parker AS *et al.* (2000). Lifestyle and anthropometric risk factors for prostate cancer in a cohort of Iowa men. *Ann Epidemiol*, 10: 361–369. doi:10.1016/S1047-2797(00)00057-0 PMID:10964002

Ranadive KJ, Gothoskar SV, Khanolkar VR (1963). Experimental studies on the etiology of cancer types specific to India (a)oral cancer (b) Kangri cancer. *Acta Unio Int Contra Cancrum*, 19: 634–639. PMID:14050624

Ranadive KJ, Gothoskar SV, Rao AR *et al.* (1976). Experimental studies on betel nut and tobacco carcinogenicity. *Int J Cancer*, 17: 469–476. PMID:1279039

Randeria JD (1972). Tobacco induced changes in the bladder buccal and vaginal mucosae. *Indian J Med Res*, 60: 694–698. PMID:4663237

Rao AR (1984). Modifying influences of betel quid ingredients on B(a)P-induced carcinogenesis in the buccal pouch of hamster. *Int J Cancer*, 33: 581–586. PMID:6327538

Roed-Petersen B, Gupta PC, Pindborg JJ, Singh B (1972). Association between oral leukoplakia and sex, age, and tobacco habits. *Bull World Health Organ*, 47: 13–19. PMID:4538900

Roed-Petersen B & Pindborg JJ (1973). A study of Danish snuff-induced oral leukoplakias. *J Oral Pathol*, 2: 301–313. doi:10.1111/j.1600-0714.1973.tb01848.x PMID:4136500

Rolandsson M, Hellqvist L, Lindqvist L, Hugoson A (2005). Effects of snuff on the oral health status of adolescent males: a comparative study. *Oral Health Prev Dent*, 3: 77–85. PMID:16173384

Roosaar A, Johansson AL, Sandborgh-Englund G *et al.* (2006). A long-term follow-up study on the natural course of snus-induced lesions among Swedish snus users. *Int J Cancer*, 119: 392–397. PMID:16470839

Roosaar A, Johansson AL, Sandborgh-Englund G *et al.* (2008). Cancer and mortality among users and nonusers of snus. *Int J Cancer*, 123: 168–173. PMID:18412245

Rosenquist K (2005). Risk factors in oral and oropharyngeal squamous cell carcinoma: a population-based case-control study in southern Sweden. *Swed Dent J Suppl*, 1791–66. PMID:16335030

Rosenquist K, Wennerberg J, Schildt EB *et al.* (2005). Use of Swedish moist snuff, smoking and alcohol consumption in the aetiology of oral and oropharyngeal squamous cell carcinoma. A population-based case-control study in southern Sweden. *Acta Otolaryngol*, 125: 991–998. PMID:16193590

Salem G, Juhl R, Schiødt T (1984). Oral malignant and premalignant changes in 'Shammah'-users from the Gizan region, Saudi Arabia. *Acta Odontol Scand*, 42: 41–45. PMID:6585122

Salonen L, Axéll T, Helldén L (1990). Occurrence of oral mucosal lesions, the influence of tobacco habits and an estimate of treatment time in an adult Swedish population. *J Oral Pathol Med*, 19: 170–176. PMID:2366203

Sankaranarayanan R, Duffy SW, Day NE *et al.* (1989a). A case-control investigation of cancer of the oral tongue and the floor of the mouth in southern India. *Int J Cancer*, 44: 617–621. doi:10.1002/ijc.2910440410 PMID:2793234

Sankaranarayanan R, Duffy SW, Nair MK *et al.* (1990b). Tobacco and alcohol as risk factors in cancer of the larynx in Kerala, India. *Int J Cancer*, 45: 879–882. doi:10.1002/ijc.2910450517 PMID:2335391

Sankaranarayanan R, Duffy SW, Padmakumary G *et al.* (1989b). Tobacco chewing, alcohol and nasal snuff in cancer of the gingiva in Kerala, India. *Br J Cancer*, 60: 638–643. doi:10.1038/bjc.1989.330 PMID:2803939

Sankaranarayanan R, Duffy SW, Padmakumary G *et al.* (1990a). Risk factors for cancer of the buccal and labial mucosa in Kerala, southern India. *J Epidemiol Community Health*, 44: 286–292. doi:10.1136/jech.44.4.286 PMID:2277249

Sankaranarayanan R, Duffy SW, Padmakumary G *et al.* (1991). Risk factors for cancer of the oesophagus in Kerala, India. *Int J Cancer*, 49: 485–489. doi:10.1002/ijc.2910490402 PMID:1917146

Sapkota A, Gajalakshmi V, Jetly DH *et al.* (2007). Smokeless tobacco and increased risk of hypopharyngeal and laryngeal cancers: a multicentric case-control study from India. *Int J Cancer*, 121: 1793–1798. doi:10.1002/ijc.22832 PMID:17583577

Scheifele C, Nassar A, Reichart PA (2007). Prevalence of oral cancer and potentially malignant lesions among shammah users in Yemen. *Oral Oncol*, 43: 42–50. PMID:16759897

Schildt EB, Eriksson M, Hardell L, Magnuson A (1998). Oral snuff, smoking habits and alcohol consumption in relation to oral cancer in a Swedish case-control study. *Int J Cancer*, 77: 341–346. PMID:9663593

Schmähl D (1965). Examination of chewing tobaco extract for cancerogenic effects in rats*Arzneimittelforschung*, 15: 704–705. PMID:5899252

Schroeder JC, Olshan AF, Baric R *et al.* (2002). A case-control study of tobacco use and other non-occupational risk factors for t(14;18) subtypes of non-Hodgkin's lymphoma (United States). *Cancer Causes Control*, 13: 159–168. doi:10.1023/A:1014397920185 PMID:11936822

Schwartz SM, Daling JR, Doody DR *et al.* (1998). Oral cancer risk in relation to sexual history and evidence of human papillomavirus infection. *J Natl Cancer Inst*, 90: 1626–1636. PMID:9811312

Shapiro MP, Keen P, Cohen L, De Moor NG (1955). Malignant disease in the Transvaal. II. Tumours of the musculo-skeletal system. III. Cancer of the respiratory tract; first statistical report of the radiation therapy department of the Johannesburg group of hospitals. *S Afr Med J*, 29: 95–101. PMID:14358867

Sharma PK, Lal N, Nagpaul KK (1985). Study of trace amounts of U in snuff. *Health Phys*, 48: 811–812. PMID:4039716

Shukla VK, Chauhan VS, Mishra RN, Basu S (2008). Lifestyle, reproductive factors and risk of gallbladder cancer. *Singapore Med J*, 49: 912–915. PMID:19037558

Shulman JD, Beach MM, Rivera-Hidalgo F (2004). The prevalence of oral mucosal lesions in U.S. adults: data from the Third National Health and Nutrition Examination Survey, 1988–1994. *J Am Dent Assoc*, 135: 1279–1286. PMID:15493392

Sinha DN, Palipudi KM, Rolle I *et al.* (2011).* Tobacco use among youth and adults in member countries of South-East Asia region: Review of findings from surveys under the global tobacco surveillance system. *Indian J Public Health*, 55: 169–176. doi:10.4103/0019-557X.89946 PMID:22089684

Sinusas K & Coroso JG (2006). A 10-yr study of smokeless tobacco use in a professional baseball organization. *Med Sci Sports Exerc*, 38: 1204–1207. PMID:16826015

Sinusas K, Coroso JG, Sopher MD, Crabtree BF (1992). Smokeless tobacco use and oral pathology in a professional baseball organization. *J Fam Pract*, 34: 713–718. PMID:1593245

Slattery ML, West DW, Robison LM (1988). Fluid intake and bladder cancer in Utah. *Int J Cancer*, 42: 17–22. doi:10.1002/ijc.2910420105 PMID:3391705

Spangler JG (2002). Corrections to Spangler *et al.* 2001b *Ethn Dis*, 12: 158–159.

Spangler JG, Michielutte R, Bell RA *et al.* (2001). Association between smokeless tobacco use and breast cancer among Native-American women in North Carolina. *Ethn Dis*, 11: 36–43.

Spitz MR, Fueger JJ, Goepfert H *et al.* (1988). Squamous cell carcinoma of the upper aerodigestive tract. A case comparison analysis. *Cancer*, 61: 203–208. PMID:3334949

Spitz MR, Fueger JJ, Halabi S *et al.* (1993). Mutagen sensitivity in upper aerodigestive tract cancer: a case-control analysis. *Cancer Epidemiol Biomarkers Prev*, 2: 329–333. PMID:7688625

Sreedharan S, Hegde MC, Pai R *et al.* (2007). Snuff-induced malignancy of the nasal vestibule: a case report. *Am J Otolaryngol*, 28: 353–356. doi:10.1016/j.amjoto.2006.10.008 PMID:17826541

Stenström B, Zhao CM, Rogers AB *et al.* (2007). Swedish moist snuff accelerates gastric cancer development in Helicobacter pylori-infected wild-type and gastrin transgenic mice. *Carcinogenesis*, 28: 2041–2046. PMID:17389611

Stepanov I, Jensen J, Hatsukami D, Hecht SS (2008). New and traditional smokeless tobacco: comparison of toxicant and carcinogen levels. *Nicotine Tob Res*, 10: 1773–1782. doi:10.1080/14622200802443544 PMID:19023828

Stepanov I, Villalta PW, Knezevich A *et al.* (2010). Analysis of 23 polycyclic aromatic hydrocarbons in smokeless tobacco by gas chromatography-mass spectrometry. *Chem Res Toxicol*, 23: 66–73. doi:10.1021/tx900281u PMID:19860436

Sterling TD, Rosenbaum WL, Weinkam JJ (1992). Analysis of the relationship between smokeless tobacco and cancer based on data from the National Mortality Followback Survey. *J Clin Epidemiol*, 45: 223–231. doi:10.1016/0895-4356(92)90082-X PMID:1569419

Stewart CM, Baughman RA, Bates RE (1989). Smokeless tobacco use among Florida teenagers: prevalence, attitudes, and oral changes. *Fla Dent J*, 60: 38–42. PMID:2599145

Stockwell HG & Lyman GH (1986). Impact of smoking and smokeless tobacco on the risk of cancer of the head and neck. *Head Neck Surg*, 9: 104–110. doi:10.1002/hed.2890090206 PMID:3623935

Summerlin DJ, Dunipace A, Potter R (1992). Histologic effects of smokeless tobacco and alcohol on the pouch mucosa and organs of the Syrian hamster. *J Oral Pathol Med*, 21: 105–108. PMID:1583594

Suri K, Goldman HM, Wells H (1971). Carcinogenic effect of a dimethyl sulphoxide extract of betel nut on the mucosa of the hamster buccal pouch. *Nature*, 230: 383–384. PMID:4927728

Thomas G, Hashibe M, Jacob BJ *et al.* (2003). Risk factors for multiple oral premalignant lesions. *Int J Cancer*, 107: 285–291. PMID:12949809

Tomar SL (2002). Snuff use and smoking in U.S. men: implications for harm reduction. *Am J Prev Med*, 23: 143–149. PMID:12350445

Tomar SL, Winn DM, Swango PA *et al.* (1997). Oral mucosal smokeless tobacco lesions among adolescents in the United States. *J Dent Res*, 76: 1277–1286. PMID:9168861

Tricker AR & Preussmann R (1988). The occurrence of N-nitrosocompounds [corrected] in zarda tobacco. *Cancer Lett*, 42: 113–118. doi:10.1016/0304-3835(88)90247-9 PMID:3242503

Tyldesley WR (1971). Tobacco chewing in english coal miners. A preliminary report. *Br J Oral Surg*, 9: 21–28. PMID:5286076

Van Duuren BL, Sivak A, Segal A *et al.* (1966). The tumor-promoting agents of tobacco leaf and tobacco smoke condensate. *J Natl Cancer Inst*, 37: 519–526. PMID:5923502

Vincent RG & Marchetta F (1963). The relationship of the use of tobacco and alcohol to cancer of the oral cavity, pharynx or larynx. *Am J Surg*, 106: 501–505. PMID:14062955

Vogler WR, Lloyd JW, Milmore BK (1962). A retrospective study of etiological factors in cancer of the mouth, pharynx, and larynx. *Cancer*, 15: 246–258. PMID:13926472

Wahi PN (1968). The epidemiology of oral anc oropharyngeal cancer. A report of the study in Mainpuri district, Uttar Pradesh, India. *Bull World Health Organ*, 38: 495–521. PMID:5302449

Wasnik KS, Ughade SN, Zodpey SP, Ingole DL (1998). Tobacco consumption practices and risk of oro-pharyngeal cancer: a case-control study in Central India. *Southeast Asian J Trop Med Public Health*, 29: 827–834. PMID:10772572

Weitkunat R, Sanders E, Lee PN (2007). Meta-analysis of the relation between European and American smokeless tobacco and oral cancer. *BMC Public Health*, 7: 334 PMID:18005437

Westbrook KC (1980) *Snuff dipper's carcinoma. Fact or Fiction? In: Prevention and Detection of Cancer.*, Nieburg HE (ed) New York: Marcel Dekker.

Williams RR & Horm JW (1977). Association of cancer sites with tobacco and alcohol consumption and socioeconomic status of patients: interview study from the Third National Cancer Survey. *J Natl Cancer Inst*, 58: 525–547. PMID:557114

Williams RR, Stegens NL, Horm JW (1977). Patient interview study from the Third National Cancer Survey: overview of problems and potentials of these data. *J Natl Cancer Inst*, 58: 519–524. PMID:839554

Winn DM (1986) *Smokeless tobacco and oral/pharynx cancer: The role of cofactors.* In: *Mechanisms in Tobacco Carcinogenesis.*, Hoffmann D, Harris CC (eds) Cold Spring Harbor, NY: Cold Spring Harbor Laboratory, No. Banbury Report No. 23, 361–375.

Winn DM, Blot WJ, Shy CM *et al.* (1981a). Snuff dipping and oral cancer among women in the southern United States. *N Engl J Med*, 304: 745–749. PMID:7193288

Winn DM, Blot WJ, Shy CM *et al.* (1981b). Snuff dipping and oral cancer among women in the southern United States. *N Engl J Med*, 304: 745–749. doi:10.1056/NEJM198103263041301 PMID:7193288

Winn DM, Ziegler RG, Pickle LW *et al.* (1984). Diet in the etiology of oral and pharyngeal cancer among women from the southern United States. *Cancer Res*, 44: 1216–1222. PMID:6692405

Wolfe MD & Carlos JP (1987). Oral health effects of smokeless tobacco use in Navajo Indian adolescents. *Community Dent Oral Epidemiol*, 15: 230–235. PMID:3476250

Wynder EL & Bross IJ (1957). Aetiological factors in mouth cancer; an approach to its prevention. *Br Med J*, 1: 1137–1143. PMID:13426561

Wynder EL & Bross IJ (1961). A study of etiological factors in cancer of the esophagus. *Cancer*, 14: 389–413. doi:10.1002/1097-0142(196103/04)14:2<389::AID-CNCR2820140220>3.0.CO,2-E PMID:13786981

Wynder EL, Bross IJ, Feldman RM (1957a). A study of the etiological factors in cancer of the mouth. *Cancer*, 10: 1300–1323. PMID:13489682

Wynder EL, Hultberg S, Jacobsson F, Bross IJ (1957). Environmental factors in cancer of the upper alimentary tract; a Swedish study with special reference to Plummer-Vinson (Paterson-Kelly) syndrome. *Cancer*, 10: 470–487. doi:10.1002/1097-0142(195705/06)10:3<470::AID-CNCR2820100309>3.0.CO;2-7 PMID:13460941

Wynder EL, Hultberg S, Jacobsson F, Bross IJ (1957b). Environmental factors in cancer of the upper alimentary tract; a Swedish study with special reference to Plummer-Vinson (Paterson-Kelly) syndrome. *Cancer*, 10: 470–487. PMID:13460941

Wynder EL, Kabat G, Rosenberg S, Levenstein M (1983). Oral cancer and mouthwash use. *J Natl Cancer Inst*, 70: 255–260. PMID:6571934

Wynder EL & Stellman SD (1977). Comparative epidemiology of tobacco-related cancers. *Cancer Res*, 37: 4608–4622. PMID:562711

Wynder EL & Wright G (1957). A study of tobacco carcinogenesis. I. The primary fractions. *Cancer*, 10: 255–271. PMID:13426984

Ye W, Ekström AM, Hansson LE *et al.* (1999). Tobacco, alcohol and the risk of gastric cancer by sub-site and histologic type. *Int J Cancer*, 83: 223–229. doi:10.1002/(SICI)1097-0215(19991008)83:2<223::AID-IJC13>3.0.CO;2-M PMID:10471531

Young TB, Ford CN, Brandenburg JH (1986). An epidemiologic study of oral cancer in a statewide network. *Am J Otolaryngol*, 7: 200–208. PMID:3728828

Zahm SH, Blair A, Holmes FF *et al.* (1989). A case-control study of soft-tissue sarcoma. *Am J Epidemiol*, 130: 665–674. PMID:2773915

Zahm SH, Heineman EF, Vaught JB (1992). Soft tissue sarcoma and tobacco use: data from a prospective cohort study of United States veterans. *Cancer Causes Control*, 3: 371–376. doi:10.1007/BF00146891 PMID:1617125

Zaridze DG, Blettner M, Matiakin EG *et al.* (1986). The effect of nass use and smoking on the risk of oral leukoplakia. *Cancer Detect Prev*, 9: 435–440. PMID:3779705

Zaridze DG, Kuvshinov JP, Matiakin E *et al.* (1985). Chemoprevention of oral and esophageal cancer in Uzbekistan, Union of Soviet Socialist Republics. *Natl Cancer Inst Monogr*, 69: 259–262. PMID:2939349

Zendehdel K, Nyrén O, Luo J *et al.* (2008). Risk of gastroesophageal cancer among smokers and users of Scandinavian moist snuff. *Int J Cancer*, 122: 1095–1099. doi:10.1002/ijc.23076 PMID:17973262

Zheng T, Cantor KP, Zhang Y *et al.* (2001). Risk of brain glioma not associated with cigarette smoking or use of other tobacco products in Iowa. *Cancer Epidemiol Biomarkers Prev*, 10: 413–414. PMID:11319186

Zheng W, McLaughlin JK, Gridley G *et al.* (1993). A cohort study of smoking, alcohol consumption, and dietary factors for pancreatic cancer (United States). *Cancer Causes Control*, 4: 477–482. doi:10.1007/BF00050867 PMID:8218880

* Exceptionally, the most recent updates of well-established ongoing surveys and reports, published after the meeting, were included in this *Monograph*. The methodology and data available at the time of the meeting were reviewed by the Working Group; the updates reflect the most current estimates of prevalence of exposure and therefore have no influence on the final evaluation.

N′-NITROSONORNICOTINE AND 4-(METHYLNITROSAMINO)-1-(3-PYRIDYL)-1-BUTANONE

N′-Nitrosonornicotine (NNN) and 4-(methylnitrosamino)-1-(3-pyridyl)-1-butanone (NNK) were considered by previous IARC Working Groups in 1984 and 2004 (IARC, 1985, 2007). Since that time, new data have become available, these have been incorporated into the *Monograph*, and taken into consideration in the present evaluation.

1. Exposure Data

1.1. Chemical and physical data

1.1.1 4-(Methylnitrosamino)-1-(3-pyridyl)-1-butanone

(a) Synonyms and trade names

Chem. Abstr. Services Reg. No.: 64091-91-4
Chem. Abstr. Name: 1-Butanone, 4-(methylnitrosoamino)-1-(3-pyridinyl)-
IUPAC Systematic Name: 4-(Methylnitrosamino)-1-(3-pyridyl)-1-butanone
Synonym: 4-(N-Methyl-N-nitrosamino)-1-(3-pyridyl)-1-butanone

(b) Structural and molecular formulae and relative molecular mass

O
N — CH3
N = O
N

$C_{10}H_{13}N_3O_2$
Relative molecular mass: 207.2

(c) Chemical and physical properties of the pure substance

From IARC (2007)
Description: Light-yellow crystalline solid
Melting-point: 61–63 °C
Spectroscopy data: Infrared, nuclear magnetic resonance and mass spectra have been reported.
Solubility: Soluble in dichloromethane, dimethyl sulfoxide (DMSO), dimethylformamide, ethyl acetate and methanol
Stability: Sensitive to light

1.1.2 N′-Nitrosonornicotine

(a) Synonyms and trade names

Chem. Abstr. Services Reg. Nos: 80508-23-2; 16543-55-8; 84237-38-7
Chem. Abstr. Names: Pyridine, 3-(1-nitroso-2-pyrrolidinyl)-; pyridine,

3-(1-nitroso-2-pyrrolidinyl)-,(S)-; pyridine, 3-(1-nitroso-2-pyrrolidinyl)-, (+,–)-
IUPAC Systematic Name:
1′-Demethyl-1′-nitrosonicotine
Synonyms: 1′-Demethyl-1′-nitrosonicotine; 1′-desmethyl-1′-nitrosonicotine; 1′-nitroso-1′-demethylnicotine; nitrosonornicotine; *N*-nitrosonornicotine; 1′-nitrosonornicotine; 1-nitroso-2-(3-pyridyl)pyrrolidine; 3-(1-nitroso-2-pyrrolidinyl)pyridine

Note: the chemical abstracts services registry number 16543-55-8 and name refer to the (s) stereoisomer; the chemical abstracts services registry number 84237-38-7 and name refer to the racemic mixture that was synthesized and used in the biological studies reported in this *Monograph*.

(b) Structural and molecular formulae and relative molecular mass

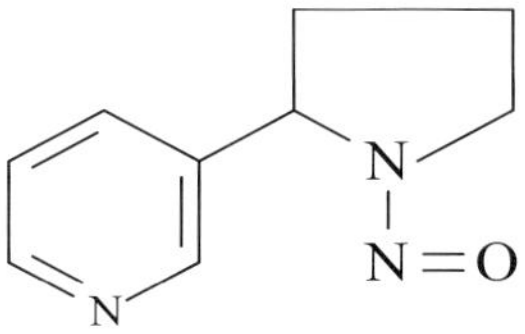

$C_9H_{11}N_3O$
Relative molecular mass: 177.2

(c) Chemical and physical properties of the pure substance

From IARC (2007)
Description: Light-yellow oil
Boiling-point: 154 °C at 0.2 mm
Melting-point: 47 °C; 42–45 °C
Spectroscopy data: Mass, ultraviolet, infrared and nuclear magnetic resonance spectra have been reported.
Solubility: Soluble in acetone and chloroform
Stability: Hygroscopic

1.2 Occurrence in tobacco products

Virtually all commercial tobacco products contain NNN and NNK, and they always occur together. They are mainly formed during the curing of tobacco. There is a great variation in levels of these compounds in mainstream smoke and sidestream smoke of cigarettes and in smokeless tobacco products. This is mainly due to differences in tobacco types used for the various products, in agricultural practices, curing methods, and in manufacturing processes. Factors that lead to relatively high levels of NNN and NNK in cured tobacco include the use of Burley tobacco, the use of midribs from air-cured tobacco or lamina from flue-cured tobacco, storage of tobacco leaves under humid conditions or in bales, processes that encourage bacterial growth thus leading to increased nitrite, and heating with propane during curing (IARC, 2007).

Since the first reports of NNN and NNK in tobacco (Hoffmann *et al.*, 1974; Hecht *et al.*, 1978), many studies have quantified their levels in various tobacco products. Extensive compilations of data may be found in previous *IARC Monographs* (IARC, 2004, 2007). Levels of NNN ranged from 20 to 58000 ng per cigarette and NNK from 19 to 10745 ng per cigarette in tobacco from commercial cigarettes sold in different parts of the world; and from 4 to 2830 ng per cigarette (NNN) and 3 to 1749 ng per cigarette (NNK) in mainstream smoke of internationally available commercial cigarettes. Levels of NNN ranged from 19 to 3080000 ng per gram tobacco and NNK from 10 to 7870000 ng per gram tobacco in smokeless tobacco products worldwide.

Several recent studies have examined levels of NNN and NNK in cigarette tobacco and mainstream smoke, and in smokeless tobacco. Hammond & O'Connor (2008) reported data for 247 brands sold in Canada, and tested in 2004. Mean (± standard deviation (SD)). levels of NNN were significantly higher in the tobacco of imported (1776.2 ± 817.2 ng/cigarette) than domestic Canadian brands (286.9 ± 118.3 ng/cigarette) while those of NNK were similar (437.2 ± 376.1 ng/cigarette imported and 448.5 ± 237.4 ng/cigarette domestic). Using the Canadian Intense smoking conditions, levels of NNN (353.3 ± 91.3 ng/cigarette) were significantly higher in mainstream smoke of imported cigarettes than if Canadian brands (53.1 ± 12.6 ng/cigarette), as were levels of NNK (212.1 ± 90.8 ng/cigarette imported; 110.3 ± 33.2 domestic Canadian). These differences are caused by the exclusive use of Virginia flue-cured tobacco in Canadian brands while imported brands – mainly from the USA – use a blend of tobacco types.

The impact of curing using indirect-fired barns instead of direct-fired methods on levels of NNK and NNN in cigarette tobacco and mainstream smoke was examined in a study of Canadian brands. Reductions of 65–78% in tobacco NNN levels and 60–85% in NNK levels were observed while the corresponding reductions in mainstream smoke levels (under ISO conditions) were 57–69% for NNN and 59–72% for NNK (Rickert *et al.*, 2008).

Levels of NNN and NNK were quantified in the smoke of research cigarettes made from different tobacco varieties, using the ISO method (Ding *et al.*, 2008). Levels of NNN and NNK were greatest in Burley tobacco smoke, with substantially lower amounts in the smoke of Oriental and Bright cigarettes. Nitrate content of the tobacco was significantly related to levels of smoke NNK (but not NNN), and was inversely proportional to PAH levels. These results are completely consistent with earlier studies (IARC, 1986, 2004).

Based on currently available data, NNN and NNK in smokeless tobacco products, expressed per g dry weight, can be divided arbitrarily into three levels:

Level I: less than 2 µg per g NNN plus NNK;

Level II: 2–10 µg per g NNN plus NNK;

Level III: greater than 10 µg per g NNN plus NNK.

The "new" products Taboka, Marlboro Snus, and Camel Snus were introduced in test markets in the USA and probably use pasteurization-like processing parameters designed to reduce levels of NNN and NNK, similar to those used by Swedish Match for products sold in Sweden. The NNN plus NNK levels in these products mostly fall into Level I, while "traditional" smokeless tobacco products manufactured in the USA fall into Level II (Stepanov *et al.*, 2008a).

Another study reported tobacco-specific nitrosamine levels in 40 top selling brands of USA moist snuff manufactured by four different companies, which collectively held over 97% of the US market in the year in which they were purchased (Richter *et al.*, 2008). The results for NNN plus NNK demonstrate that 12 brands were in Level II while 27 were in Level III. None were in Level I. In this study, amounts of NNN ranged from 2.2–42.5 µg/g wet weight while those of NNK ranged from 0.38–9.9 µg/g wet weight. The amounts in the brand with the highest levels of NNN and NNK are reminiscent of tobacco-specific nitrosamine levels in smokeless tobacco products of the 1970s.

While NNN and NNK have not been detected in oral gum nicotine-replacement therapy products, two recent studies demonstrate that NNN can be formed endogenously in trace amounts in some users of these products (Stepanov *et al.*, 2009a, b).

2. Cancer in Humans

Two molecular epidemiology studies investigated the relationship of NNK to lung cancer in smokers using nested case–control designs. In one, urinary levels of NNAL plus its glucuronides (total NNAL), metabolites of NNK, were significantly associated with risk for lung cancer in a dose-dependent manner (Yuan *et al.*, 2009). Relative to the lowest tertile, risks associated with the second and third tertiles of total NNAL were 1.4 (95%CI: 0.9–2.4) and 2.1 (95%CI: 1.2–3.5), respectively (*P* for trend = 0.005) after adjustment for smoking history and total cotinine. In a second study, after adjustment for sex, age at randomization, family history of lung cancer, cotinine, *r*-1,*t*-2,3,*c*-4-tetrahydroxy-1,2,3,4-tetrahydrophenanthrene (PheT), and years of cigarette smoking, total NNAL was significantly associated with risk for lung cancer (odds ratio (OR), 1.6 per unit SD increase; 95%CI: 1.1–2.3) (Church *et al.*, 2009). A similar statistically significant result was obtained for adenocarcinoma risk, but not for nonadenocarcinoma. Although these results demonstrate an association of NNK metabolites with lung cancer in smokers, it is impossible to exclude the potential confounding effect of other carcinogens present in tobacco smoke.

3. Cancer in Experimental Animals

NNK and NNN have been tested for carcinogenicity by various routes of administration in adult mice, rats, and Syrian hamsters, and in limited experiments in mink and ferrets. NNK has also been tested for carcinogenicity in neonatal and infant mice and transplacentally in hamsters. NNK and NNN in combination have been tested in rats and minks. Of all the numerous studies on tumour development in animal models, a selection is presented in this *Monograph*. Table 3.1 includes the studies considered the most representative of the carcinogenicity of NNK and NNN.

3.1 Administration of NNN and NNK

3.1.1 Oral administration

(a) Mouse

Mice given NNK or NNN orally developed both lung and forestomach tumours and a few liver tumours in one study (Padma *et al.*, 1989).

(b) Rat

Oral administration of NNK in drinking-water caused tumours of the lung, nasal cavity, and liver (Rivenson *et al.*, 1988; Prokopczyk *et al.*, 1991). In two studies, tumours of the exocrine pancreas were observed following administration of NNK in drinking-water (Rivenson *et al.*, 1988; Hoffmann *et al.*, 1993). Rats given NNN orally developed tumours of the oesophagus and of the nasal cavity (Hoffmann *et al.*, 1975; Hecht *et al.*, 1983).

3.1.2 Subcutaneous administration

(a) Rat

NNK given to rats subcutaneously caused tumours of the lung, nasal cavity, and liver (Hoffmann *et al.*, 1984; Hecht *et al.*, 1986a; Belinsky *et al.*, 1990). Rats given NNN subcutaneously developed tumours of the oesophagus and of the nasal cavity (Castonguay *et al.*, 1984; Hoffmann *et al.*, 1984).

(b) Hamster

NNK given subcutaneously to Syrian hamsters caused lung tumours (Hoffmann *et al.*, 1981; Schüller *et al.*, 1990). NNN given subcutaneously to hamsters caused tumours of the trachea (Hilfrich *et al.*, 1977).

(c) Mink

In one study, NNK caused malignant tumours of the nasal cavity after subcutaneous injection (Koppang *et al.*, 1997). Subcutaneously injected NNN caused malignant tumours of the nasal cavity in mink (Koppang *et al.*, 1992, 1997).

Table 3.1 Selected carcinogenicity studies of subcutaneous (sc) or oral exposure to NNK, NNN, and NNK + NNN in rats

Species, strain (sex) Reference	No/group at start Dosing regimen Duration	Results Target organ Incidence and/or multiplicity of tumours (%)	Significance	Comments
NNN				
Rat, F344 (M) Rivenson *et al.* (1988)	80, 80, 80, 30 0, 0.5, 1.0, 5.0 ppm in drinking-water, daily 108–128 wk	*Nasal cavity* 0, 1, 2, 5[a] *Lung* adenomas: 3, 5, 16[a], 2 carcinomas: 3, 4, 4, 25[a] total: 6, 9, 20[a], 27[a] *Liver* adenomas: 6, 2, 9, 10[a] carcinomas: 0, 1, 2, 2 total: 6, 3, 11, 12[a] *Exocrine pancreas* adenomas: 1, 5, 8[b], 1 carcinomas: 0, 0, 1, 1 total: 1, 5, 9[a], 2	 [a]$P < 0.01$ [a]$P < 0.01$ [a]$P < 0.01$ [a]$P < 0.01$ [b]$P < 0.05$	Purity > 99% Lung carcinomas included adenocarcinomas, adenosquamous carcinomas, and squamous cell carcinomas. Pancreatic tumours were acinar adenomas and acinar or ductal carcinomas
Rat, F344 (M) Prokopczyk *et al.* (1991)	30 animals/group 0, 15 mmolar aqueous solution; 0.3 mL by oral swabbing, 3 ×/wk (wk 1), daily (wk 2–4), and twice/d (wk 5–61) Up to 61 wk	*Nasal cavity* adenomas or papillomas: 0/30, 13/29 (45%) carcinomas: 0/30, 2/29 (7%) *Lung* adenomas: 0/30, 5/29 (17%) carcinomas: 0/30, 23/29 (79%) *Liver* adenomas: 0/30, 9/29 (31%) carcinomas: 0/30, 3/29 (10%) *Oral cavity* papilloma: 0/20, 1/29 (3%)	NR NR	Purity > 99% Lung carcinomas were adenocarcinomas and adenosquamous carcinomas.

Table 3.1 (continued)

Species, strain (sex) Reference	No/group at start Dosing regimen Duration	Results Target organ Incidence and/or multiplicity of tumours (%)	Significance	Comments
NNK				
Rat, F344 (M) Hoffmann *et al.* (1984)	27, 27, 15, 15 SC, 3 × /wk, 20 wk: total average doses 0, 0.312, 0.936, 2.81 mmole (1.0, 3.0, 9.0 mmole/kg) Lifespan (70–120 wk)	*Nasal cavity* benign: 0, 19, 6, 4 malignant: 0, 1, 7, 10 total: 0, 20[a], 13[a], 14[a] *Lung* benign: 0, 7, 1, 7 malignant: 0, 16, 12, 7 total: 0, 23[a], 13[a], 14[a] *Liver* benign: 3, 2, 1, 2 malignant: 0, 1, 3, 4 total: 3, 3, 4, 6[b] *Oesophagus* benign: 0, 1, 1, 0	[a]$P < 0.01$ [a]$P < 0.01$ [b]$P < 0.05$	NNK analysed for purity by HPLC Benign nasal cavity tumours included papillomas and polyps. Malignant nasal cavity tumours included anaplastic and squamous cell carcinomas, esthesioneuroepitheliomas and a sarcoma. Lung carcinomas included adenocarcinomas and squamous cell carcinomas
Rat, F344 (F) Hoffmann *et al.* (1984)	27, 27, 15, 15 SC, 3 × /wk, 20 wk: total average doses 0, 0.18, 0.54, 1.62 mmole (1.0, 3.0, 9.0 mmole/kg) Lifespan (60–120 wk)	*Nasal cavity* benign: 0, 10, 9, 3 malignant: 0, 0, 3, 11 total: 0, 10[a], 12[a], 14[a] *Lung* benign: 1, 5, 4, 8 malignant: 0, 3, 3, 1 total: 1, 8[b], 7[a], 9[a] *Liver* benign: 1, 3, 2, 2 malignant: 0, 1, 2, 3 total: 1, 4, 4, 5[b] *Oesophagus* benign: 0, 0, 0, 0	[a]$P < 0.01$ [a]$P < 0.01$ [b]$P < 0.05$ [b]$P < 0.05$	

Table 3.1 (continued)

Species, strain (sex) Reference	No/group at start Dosing regimen Duration	Results Target organ Incidence and/or multiplicity of tumours (%)	Significance	Comments
NNN				
Rat, F344 (M) Hoffmann *et al.* (1975)	19, 20 0, 0.02% NNN in drinking-water 5 d/wk for 30 wk 11 mo	*Oesophagus* papillomas: 0, 11 carcinomas: 0, 3 *Nasal cavity* carcinomas: 0, 3 *Pharynx* papilloma 0, 1	$P < 0.0001$	
Rat, F344 (M) Hoffmann *et al.* (1984)	27, 27, 15, 15 SC, 3 × /wk, 20 wk: total average doses 0, 0.312, 0.936, 2.81 mmole (1.0, 3.0, 9.0 mmole/kg) Lifespan (50–120 wk)	*Nasal cavity* benign: 0, 11, 3, 0 malignant: 0, 4, 8, 12 total: 0, 15[a], 11[a], 12[a] *Lung* benign 0, 2, 5, 0 malignant: 0, 0, 0, 0 total: 0, 2, 5[a], 0 *Liver* benign: 3, 0, 2, 0 malignant: 0, 0, 0, 0 total: 3, 0, 2, 0 *Oesophagus* benign: 0, 1, 5[a], 4[a]	[a]$P < 0.01$ [a]$P < 0.01$ [a]$P < 0.01$	NNN analysed for purity by HPLC Benign nasal cavity tumours included papillomas and polyps. Malignant nasal cavity tumours included anaplastic and squamous cell carcinomas, esthesioneuroepitheliomas and a sarcoma. Lung carcinomas included adenocarcinomas and squamous cell carcinomas

Table 3.1 (continued)

Species, strain (sex) Reference	No/group at start Dosing regimen Duration	Results Target organ Incidence and/or multiplicity of tumours (%)	Significance	Comments
Rat, F344 (F) Hoffmann *et al.* (1984)	27, 27, 15, 15 SC, 3 × /wk, 20 wk: total average doses 0, 0.18, 0.54, 1.62 mmole (1.0, 3.0, 9.0 mmole/kg) Lifespan (50–120 wk)	*Nasal cavity* benign: 0, 12, 4, 0 malignant: 0, 0, 5, 15 total: 0, 12[a], 9[a], 15[a] *Lung* benign: 1, 2, 1, 1 malignant: 0, 1, 0, 0 total: 1, 3, 1, 1 *Liver* benign: 1, 2, 0, 0 malignant: 0, 0, 0, 0 total: 1, 2, 0, 0 *Oesophagus* benign: 0, 1, 2, 3[b]	[a]$P < 0.01$ [b]$P < 0.05$	
NNN + NNK				
Rat, F344 (M) Hecht *et al.* (1986b)	21, 30 0, 68µg NNN + 14µg NNK in 0.5 mL aqueous solution by oral swabbing, twice/d 131 wk	*Lung* adenomas: 1/21 (5%), 1/30 (3%) carcinomas: 0/21, 4/30 (13%) *Oral cavity* papillomas: 0/21, 8/30 (27%) (9 tumours in 8 animals)	NS $P < 0.05$	Purity NR

d, day or days; F, female; M, male; mo, month or months; NNK, 4-(methylnitrosamino)-1-(3-pyridyl)-1-butanone; NNN, *N′*-nitrosonornicotine; NR, not reported; NS, not significant; SC. subcutaneous; wk, week or weeks

3.1.3 Intraperitoneal administration

(a) Mouse

NNK or NNN given to mice intraperitoneally increased the incidence of lung adenomas and carcinomas after less than one year (Hecht *et al.*, 1978, 1988, 1989; Rivenson *et al.*, 1989; Belinsky *et al.*, 1992; Amin *et al.*, 1996; Castonguay *et al.*, 1983).

(b) Hamster

NNN given intraperitoneally to hamsters caused tumours of the trachea and nasal cavity (McCoy *et al.*, 1981).

3.1.4 Skin application

When applied topically to SENCAR mice, NNK was weakly active as a skin tumour initiator, but lung tumours were observed, while NNN was inactive (LaVoie *et al.*, 1987). A few skin tumours developed in mice given NNN by skin application for 104 weeks (Deutsch-Wenzel *et al.*, 1985).

3.1.5 Perinatal administration

NNK increased both lung and liver tumours when given intraperitoneally to neonatal and infant mice (Anderson *et al.*, 1991) but was not a transplacental carcinogen when given intraperitoneally to pregnant females (Beebe *et al.*, 1993). NNK injected subcutaneously to pregnant Syrian hamsters caused tumours of the nasal cavity, larynx, and trachea in offspring in one experiment (Correa *et al.*, 1990).

3.1.6 Administration with known carcinogens

In one study, NNK and NNN in combination caused oral cavity papillomas and lung carcinomas when administered to rats by swabbing the lips and oral cavity with an aqueous solution of the nitrosamines (Hecht *et al.*, 1986b); oral cavity tumours were rarely observed in rats given NNK alone. In one study, NNK and NNN in combination caused nasal cavity tumours in mink of both sexes (Koppang *et al.*, 1997). Offspring of Syrian hamsters given ethanol in drinking-water during pregnancy and NNK by intratracheal instillation on day 15 of pregnancy developed tumours of the nasal cavity, exocrine pancreas, and adrenal medulla (Schüller *et al.*, 1994, 2002). In a single study of limited duration, NNK given by injection concurrently with cigarette smoke by inhalation caused lung tumours in 6 of 12 ferrets within six months (Kim *et al.*, 2006).

3.2 NNK and NNN metabolites

NNN-1-*N*-oxide given in drinking-water caused tumours of the oesophagus and nasal cavity in rats but not in hamsters (Hecht *et al.*, 1983). In a short-term study, NNK-1-*N*-oxide and 4-(methylnitrosamino)-1-(3-pyridyl) butan-1-ol (NNAL) given intraperitoneally caused lung tumours in mice and was as effective as NNK. Similarly, in a lifetime study in rats, NNAL was equally as effective as NNK in inducing lung tumours (Rivenson *et al.*, 1988). 4′-Hydroxy-NNN given intraperitoneally slightly increased the incidence and multiplicity of lung tumours, while 3′-hydroxy-NNN and NNN-1-*N*-oxide had no significant carcinogenic effect (Castonguay *et al.*, 1983).

3.3 Synthesis

NNK by various routes of administration consistently caused tumours of the lung in mice, hamsters and rats, and tumours of the nasal cavity in rats and mink. NNN given by various routes and particularly in drinking-water consistently caused tumours of the oesophagus in rats, and in many studies caused tumours of the nasal cavity in multiple species. NNN and NNK administered in combination caused tumours of the oral cavity in rats and nasal cavity in mink. Table 3.2 summarizes the reports of tumours induced in

Table 3.2 Summary of reports of tumours induced in experimental animals by NNK and NNN

Compound/ species	Lung	Nasal cavity	Oral cavity	Trachea	Oesophagus	Fore-stomach	Pancreas (exocrine)	Liver	Adrenal gland	Skin
NNK										
Mouse	x					x		x		x[a]
infants	x							x		
Rat	x	x					x	x		
Hamster	x									
progeny		x		x			x[c]		x	
Mink		x								
Ferret	x[b]									
NNN										
Mouse	x					x				x
Rat		x			x					
Hamster		x		x						
Mink		x								
NNK + NNN										
Rat	x		x							
Mink		x								

[a] Initiator only (SENCAR mouse skin)
[b] Co-exposure to NNK and cigarette smoke
[c] Transplacental co-exposure to NNK and ethanol
NNK, 4-(methylnitrosamino)-1-(3-pyridyl)-1-butanone; NNN, *N′*-nitrosonornicotine
From IARC (2007)

experimental animals after exposure to NNK and/or NNN.

4. Other Relevant Data

See Section 4 of the *Monograph* on Tobacco Smoking in this volume.

5. Evaluation

There is *inadequate evidence* in humans for the carcinogenicity of *N′*-nitrosonornicotine (NNK) and 4-(methylnitrosamino)-1-(3-pyridyl)-1-butanone (NNN).

There is *sufficient evidence* in experimental animals for the carcinogenicity of 4-(methylnitrosamino)-1-(3-pyridyl)-1-butanone.

There is *sufficient evidence* in experimental animals for the carcinogenicity of *N′*-nitrosonornicotine.

4-(Methylnitrosamino)-1-(3-pyridyl)-1-butanone and *N′*-nitrosonornicotine are *carcinogenic to humans (Group 1).*

In making the overall evaluation, the Working Group took into consideration the following mechanistic evidence, detailed in Section 4 of the *Monograph* on Tobacco Smoking in this volume.

NNK and NNN are the most abundant strong carcinogens in smokeless tobacco; their uptake and metabolic activation has been clearly documented in smokeless tobacco users. Combined application of NNN and NNK to the oral mucosa of rats induced oral tumours, consistent with their induction by smokeless tobacco. One of the mechanisms of carcinogenicity is cytochrome-P450-mediated α-hydroxylation, which leads to the formation of DNA and haemoglobin adducts that have been detected in users of tobacco.

References

Amin S, Desai D, Hecht SS, Hoffmann D (1996). Synthesis of tobacco-specific N-nitrosamines and their metabolites and results of related bioassays. *Crit Rev Toxicol*, 26: 139–147. doi:10.3109/10408449609017927 PMID:8688157

Anderson LM, Hecht SS, Kovatch RM *et al.* (1991). Tumorigenicity of the tobacco-specific carcinogen 4-(methyl-nitrosamino)-1-(3-pyridyl)-1-butanone in infant mice. *Cancer Lett*, 58: 177–181. doi:10.1016/0304-3835(91)90097-2 PMID:1855194

Beebe LE, Kim YE, Amin S *et al.* (1993). Comparison of transplacental and neonatal initiation of mouse lung and liver tumors by N-nitrosodimethylamine (NDMA) and 4-(methylnitrosamino)-1-(3-pyridyl)-1-butanone (NNK) and promotability by a polychlorinated biphenyls mixture (Aroclor 1254). *Carcinogenesis*, 14: 1545–1548. doi:10.1093/carcin/14.8.1545 PMID:8353839

Belinsky SA, Devereux TR, Foley JF *et al.* (1992). Role of the alveolar type II cell in the development and progression of pulmonary tumors induced by 4-(methylnitrosamino)-1-(3-pyridyl)-1-butanone in the A/J mouse. *Cancer Res*, 52: 3164–3173. PMID:1591728

Belinsky SA, Foley JF, White CM *et al.* (1990). Dose-response relationship between O6-methylguanine formation in Clara cells and induction of pulmonary neoplasia in the rat by 4-(methylnitrosamino)-1-(3-pyridyl)-1-butanone. *Cancer Res*, 50: 3772–3780. PMID:2340522

Castonguay A, Lin D, Stoner GD *et al.* (1983). Comparative carcinogenicity in A/J mice and metabolism by cultured mouse peripheral lung of N'-nitrosonornicotine, 4-(methylnitrosamino)-1-(3-pyridyl)-1-butanone, and their analogues. *Cancer Res*, 43: 1223–1229. PMID:6825093

Castonguay A, Rivenson A, Trushin N *et al.* (1984). Effects of chronic ethanol consumption on the metabolism and carcinogenicity of N'-nitrosonornicotine in F344 rats. *Cancer Res*, 44: 2285–2290. PMID:6722769

Church TR, Anderson KE, Caporaso NE *et al.* (2009). A prospectively measured serum biomarker for a tobacco-specific carcinogen and lung cancer in smokers. *Cancer Epidemiol Biomarkers Prev*, 18: 260–266. doi:10.1158/1055-9965.EPI-08-0718 PMID:19124507

Correa E, Joshi PA, Castonguay A, Schüller HM (1990). The tobacco-specific nitrosamine 4-(methylnitrosamino)-1-(3-pyridyl)-1-butanone is an active transplacental carcinogen in Syrian golden hamsters. *Cancer Res*, 50: 3435–3438. PMID:2334940

Deutsch-Wenzel RP, Brune H, Grimmer G, Misfeld J (1985). Local application to mouse skin as a carcinogen specific test system for non-volatile nitroso compounds. *Cancer Lett*, 29: 85–92. doi:10.1016/0304-3835(85)90127-2 PMID:3933815

Ding YS, Zhang L, Jain RB *et al.* (2008). Levels of tobacco-specific nitrosamines and polycyclic aromatic hydrocarbons in mainstream smoke from different tobacco varieties. *Cancer Epidemiol Biomarkers Prev*, 17: 3366–3371. doi:10.1158/1055-9965.EPI-08-0320 PMID:19064552

Hammond D & O'Connor RJ (2008). Constituents in tobacco and smoke emissions from Canadian cigarettes. *Tob Control*, 17: Suppl 1i24–i31. doi:10.1136/tc.2008.024778 PMID:18768456

Hecht SS, Abbaspour A, Hoffman D (1988). A study of tobacco carcinogenesis. XLII. Bioassay in A/J mice of some structural analogues of tobacco-specific nitrosamines. *Cancer Lett*, 42: 141–145. doi:10.1016/0304-3835(88)90251-0 PMID:3180033

Hecht SS, Chen CB, Hirota N *et al.* (1978). Tobacco-specific nitrosamines: formation from nicotine in vitro and during tobacco curing and carcinogenicity in strain A mice. *J Natl Cancer Inst*, 60: 819–824. PMID:633391

Hecht SS, Morse MA, Amin S *et al.* (1989). Rapid single-dose model for lung tumor induction in A/J mice by 4-(methylnitrosamino)-1-(3-pyridyl)-1-butanone and the effect of diet. *Carcinogenesis*, 10: 1901–1904. doi:10.1093/carcin/10.10.1901 PMID:2791206

Hecht SS, Rivenson A, Braley J *et al.* (1986b). Induction of oral cavity tumors in F344 rats by tobacco-specific nitrosamines and snuff. *Cancer Res*, 46: 4162–4166. PMID:3731083

Hecht SS, Trushin N, Castonguay A, Rivenson A (1986a). Comparative tumorigenicity and DNA methylation in F344 rats by 4-(methylnitrosamino)-1-(3-pyridyl)-1-butanone and N-nitrosodimethylamine. *Cancer Res*, 46: 498–502. PMID:3940627

Hecht SS, Young R, Maeura Y (1983). Comparative carcinogenicity in F344 rats and Syrian golden hamsters of N'-nitrosonornicotine and N'-nitrosonornicotine-1-N-oxide. *Cancer Lett*, 20: 333–340. doi:10.1016/0304-3835(83)90032-0 PMID:6627230

Hilfrich J, Hecht SS, Hoffmann D (1977). A study of tobacco carcinogenesis. XV. Effects of N'-nitrosonornicotine and N'-nitrosoanabasine in Syrian golden hamsters. *Cancer Lett*, 2: 169–175. doi:10.1016/S0304-3835(77)80007-4 PMID:837363

Hoffmann D, Castonguay A, Rivenson A, Hecht SS (1981). Comparative carcinogenicity and metabolism of 4-(methylnitrosamino)-1-(3-pyridyl)-1-butanone and N'-nitrosonornicotine in Syrian golden hamsters. *Cancer Res*, 41: 2386–2393. PMID:7237437

Hoffmann D, Hecht SS, Ornaf RM, Wynder EL (1974). N'-nitrosonornicotine in tobacco. *Science*, 186: 265–267. doi:10.1126/science.186.4160.265 PMID:4414773

Hoffmann D, Raineri R, Hecht SS *et al.* (1975). A study of tobacco carcinogenesis. XIV. Effects of N'-nitrosonornicotine and N'-nitrosonanabasine in rats. *J Natl Cancer Inst*, 55: 977–981. PMID:1237631

Hoffmann D, Rivenson A, Abbi R, Wynder EL (1993). A study of tobacco carcinogenesis: effect of the fat content of the diet on the carcinogenic activity of 4-(methylnitrosamino)-1-(3-pyridyl)-1-butanone in F344 rats. *Cancer Res*, 53: 2758–2761. PMID:8389244

Hoffmann D, Rivenson A, Amin S, Hecht SS (1984). Dose-response study of the carcinogenicity of tobacco-specific N-nitrosamines in F344 rats. *J Cancer Res Clin Oncol*, 108: 81–86. doi:10.1007/BF00390978 PMID:6746721

IARC (1985). Tobacco habits other than smoking; betel-quid and areca-nut chewing; and some related nitrosamines. *IARC Monogr Eval Carcinog Risk Chem Hum*, 37: 1–268. PMID:3866741

IARC (1986). Tobacco smoking. *IARC Monogr Eval Carcinog Risk Chem Hum*, 38: 1–421. PMID:3866741

IARC (2004). Tobacco smoke and involuntary smoking. *IARC Monogr Eval Carcinog Risks Hum*, 83: 1–1438. PMID:15285078

IARC (2007). Smokeless tobacco and some tobacco-specific N-nitrosamines. *IARC Monogr Eval Carcinog Risks Hum*, 89: 1–592. PMID:18335640

Kim Y, Liu XS, Liu C *et al.* (2006). Induction of pulmonary neoplasia in the smoke-exposed ferret by 4-(methylnitrosamino)-1-(3-pyridyl)-1-butanone (NNK): a model for human lung cancer. *Cancer Lett*, 234: 209–219. doi:10.1016/j.canlet.2005.03.052 PMID:15894421

Koppang N, Rivenson A, Dahle HK, Hoffmann D (1997). A study of tobacco carcinogenesis, LIII: carcinogenicity of N'-nitrosonornicotine (NNN) and 4-(methylnitrosamino)-1-(3-pyridyl)-1-butanone (NNK) in mink (Mustela vison). *Cancer Lett*, 111: 167–171. doi:10.1016/S0304-3835(96)04507-7 PMID:9022142

Koppang N, Rivenson A, Reith A *et al.* (1992). A study of tobacco carcinogenesis XLVIII. Carcinogenicity of N'-nitrosonornicotine in mink (Mustela vison). *Carcinogenesis*, 13: 1957–1960. doi:10.1093/carcin/13.11.1957 PMID:1423862

LaVoie EJ, Prokopczyk G, Rigotty J *et al.* (1987). Tumorigenic activity of the tobacco-specific nitrosamines 4-(methylnitrosamino)-1-(3-pyridyl)-1-butanone (NNK), 4-(methylnitrosamino)-4-(3-pyridyl)-1-butanol (iso-NNAL) and N'-nitrosonornicotine (NNN) on topical application to Sencar mice. *Cancer Lett*, 37: 277–283. doi:10.1016/0304-3835(87)90112-1 PMID:3677059

McCoy GD, Hecht SS, Katayama S, Wynder EL (1981). Differential effect of chronic ethanol consumption on the carcinogenicity of N-nitrosopyrrolidine and N'-nitrosonornicotine in male Syrian golden hamsters. *Cancer Res*, 41: 2849–2854. PMID:7248945

Padma PR, Lalitha VS, Amonkar AJ, Bhide SV (1989). Carcinogenicity studies on the two tobacco-specific N-nitrosamines, N'-nitrosonornicotine and 4-(methylnitrosamino)-1-(3-pyridyl)-1-butanone. *Carcinogenesis*, 10: 1997–2002. doi:10.1093/carcin/10.11.1997 PMID:2680142

Prokopczyk B, Rivenson A, Hoffmann D (1991). A study of betel quid carcinogenesis. IX. Comparative carcinogenicity of 3-(methylnitrosamino)propionitrile and 4-(methylnitrosamino)-1-(3-pyridyl)-1-butanone upon local application to mouse skin and rat oral mucosa. *Cancer Lett*, 60: 153–157. doi:10.1016/0304-3835(91)90222-4 PMID:1933838

Richter P, Hodge K, Stanfill S *et al.* (2008). Surveillance of moist snuff: total nicotine, moisture, pH, un-ionized nicotine, and tobacco-specific nitrosamines. *Nicotine Tob Res*, 10: 1645–1652. doi:10.1080/14622200802412937 PMID:18988077

Rickert WS, Joza PJ, Sharifi M *et al.* (2008). Reductions in the tobacco specific nitrosamine (TSNA) content of tobaccos taken from commercial Canadian cigarettes and corresponding reductions in TSNA deliveries in mainstream smoke from such cigarettes. *Regul Toxicol Pharmacol*, 51: 306–310. doi:10.1016/j.yrtph.2008.04.009 PMID:18508168

Rivenson A, Djordjevic MV, Amin S, Hoffmann R (1989). A study of tobacco carcinogenesis XLIV. Bioassay in A/J mice of some N-nitrosamines. *Cancer Lett*, 47: 111–114. doi:10.1016/0304-3835(89)90185-7 PMID:2636026

Rivenson A, Hoffmann D, Prokopczyk B *et al.* (1988). Induction of lung and exocrine pancreas tumors in F344 rats by tobacco-specific and Areca-derived N-nitrosamines. *Cancer Res*, 48: 6912–6917. PMID:3180100

Schüller HM, Jorquera R, Lu X *et al.* (1994). Transplacental carcinogenicity of low doses of 4-(methylnitrosamino)-1-(3-pyridyl)-1-butanone administered subcutaneously or intratracheally to hamsters. *J Cancer Res Clin Oncol*, 120: 200–203. doi:10.1007/BF01372556 PMID:8288673

Schüller HM, Witschi HP, Nylen E *et al.* (1990). Pathobiology of lung tumors induced in hamsters by 4-(methylnitrosamino)-1-(3-pyridyl)-1-butanone and the modulating effect of hyperoxia. *Cancer Res*, 50: 1960–1965. PMID:2306745

Schüller HM, Zhang L, Weddle DL *et al.* (2002). The cyclooxygenase inhibitor ibuprofen and the FLAP inhibitor MK886 inhibit pancreatic carcinogenesis induced in hamsters by transplacental exposure to ethanol and the tobacco carcinogen NNK. *J Cancer Res Clin Oncol*, 128: 525–532. doi:10.1007/s00432-002-0365-y PMID:12384795

Stepanov I, Carmella SG, Briggs A *et al.* (2009a). Presence of the carcinogen N'-nitrosonornicotine in the urine of some users of oral nicotine replacement therapy products. *Cancer Res*, 69: 8236–8240. doi:10.1158/0008-5472.CAN-09-1084 PMID:19843845

Stepanov I, Carmella SG, Han S *et al.* (2009b). Evidence for endogenous formation of N'-nitrosonornicotine in some long-term nicotine patch users. *Nicotine Tob Res*, 11: 99–105. doi:10.1093/ntr/ntn004 PMID:19246447

Stepanov I, Jensen J, Hatsukami D, Hecht SS (2008a). New and traditional smokeless tobacco: comparison of toxicant and carcinogen levels. *Nicotine Tob Res*, 10: 1773–1782. doi:10.1080/14622200802443544 PMID:19023828

Yuan JM, Koh WP, Murphy SE *et al.* (2009). Urinary levels of tobacco-specific nitrosamine metabolites in relation to lung cancer development in two prospective cohorts of cigarette smokers. *Cancer Res*, 69: 2990–2995. doi:10.1158/0008-5472.CAN-08-4330 PMID:19318550

BETEL QUID AND ARECA NUT

Betel quid and areca nut were considered by previous IARC Working Groups in 1984, 1987 and 2003 (IARC, 1985, 1987, 2004). Since that time, new data have become available, these have been incorporated into the *Monograph*, and taken into consideration in the present evaluation.

1. Exposure Data

1.1 Constituents of betel quid

1.1.1 Definitions

Betel quid chewing is an ancient practice in the Indian subcontinent and many parts of Asia, and is still prevalent today. In modern times the term "betel quid" for most people is synonymous with "*pan*," a chewing item used in India and neighbouring countries.

The term "quid" denotes a substance or a mixture of substances that is placed and retained in the mouth, and often swallowed. Apart from areca nut it may contain a variety of ingredients, including betel leaf and tobacco (Zain *et al.*, 1999; IARC, 2004).

In India and neighbouring countries, dry areca nut pieces or tobacco may be chewed alone, as a mixture of areca nut, tobacco and slaked lime, or tobacco and slaked lime. Dry powdered ready-to-chew mixtures containing areca nut, catechu, lime, unspecified spices without betel leaf and with or without tobacco are sold commercially in India (Ramchandani *et al.*, 1998). The product that does not contain tobacco is called *pan masala* while the term *gutka* is used for the product that contains tobacco in addition to the ingredients of *pan masala* (Nair *et al.*, 2004). In the south-eastern part of China, unprocessed fresh areca nut is treated with maltose and lime. It is cut into pieces and chewed with a few drops of cassia oil (Tang *et al.*, 1997).

A *pan* comprises mainly betel leaf (Piper betel), areca nut (areca catechu), catechu and slaked lime. The basic ingredients may be supplemented with condiments, sweetening agents and tobacco as per individual preference (IARC, 1985). The ingredients are placed on the betel leaf and the leaf is folded into a triangular-shaped object to obtain a betel quid with or without tobacco. Like slaked lime, thick paste of catechu may be smeared on the betel leaf or small bits of dry catechu may be placed on the betel leaf before it is folded to form a *pan*. Three types of betel quid are consumed in Taiwan, China. These are *lao-hwa* quid, betel quid and stem quid (Yang *et al.*, 2001). *Lao-hwa* quid is prepared by inserting a piece of inflorescence of Piper betel L. and red lime into an unripe areca nut. Another variety of Taiwanese betel quid is prepared by wrapping two halves of an unripe areca nut and white slaked lime in a betel leaf. The third variety is similar to the *lao-hwa* quid except that stems

Table 1.1 Composition of the different types of areca-containing chewing substances

	Areca nut[a]	Betel[b]			Catechu[d]	Tobacco[e]	Slaked lime
		Leaf	Inflorescence	Stem[c]			
Areca nut	X						
Betel quid without tobacco	X	X			(X)[f]		X
Betel quid with tobacco	X	X			(X)[f]	X	X
Gutka	X				X	X	X
Pan masala[g]	X				X		X
Mawa	X					X	X
Mainpuri tobacco	X					X	X
Lao-hwa (Taiwan, China)	X[g]		X				X
Betel quid (Taiwan, China)	X[g]	X					X
Stem quid (Taiwan, China)	X[g]			X			X

[a] May be used unripe, raw or processed by baking, roasting or baking with sweetening, flavouring and decorative agents (see Table 1.2)
[b] In place of the leaf, the inflorescence or its stem may also be used (see Table 1.2)
[c] Stem of inflorescence
[d] In powdered or paste form (see Table 1.2)
[e] In flaked, powdered or paste form, with or without processing, with or without sweetening (see Table 1.2)
[f] (X) means optional
[g] Used in unripe form
Adapted from IARC (2004)

of Piper betel L. are used in place of the inflorescence (IARC, 2004). While flavouring agents may be added to the Taiwanese betel quid, it does not contain tobacco. Different types of areca nut-containing chewing products and their ingredients are listed in Table 1.1.

1.1.2 Main ingredients of a quid

Areca nut, the major constituent of a betel quid, is the fruit of the Areca catechu L., a palm tree that grows in South and South-East Asia and the Pacific islands.

The chemical composition of areca nut has been reported in many studies (Raghavan & Baruah, 1958; Shivashankar *et al.*, 1969; Arjungi, 1976; Jayalakshmi & Mathew, 1982). The major constituents are carbohydrates, fats, proteins, crude fibre, polyphenols, alkaloids and minerals. The concentrations of various constituents vary between raw and ripe areca nuts (Jayalakshmi & Mathew, 1982). Arecaidine, arecoline, guvacine and guvacoline are the four alkaloids conclusively identified in areca nut (Raghavan & Baruah, 1958; Huang & McLeish, 1989; Lord *et al.*, 2002). Areca nut also contains sodium, magnesium, calcium, vanadium, manganese and copper (Wei & Chung, 1997; Ridge *et al.*, 2001).

Betel leaf (Piper betel L.) is a vine cultivated in many South-Asian countries including India. It contains betel oil, which includes phenolic compounds such as hydroxychevicol, euginol phenol, and chevicol. Trace elements, vitamin C and carotenes are also present in betel leaf (Wang & Wu, 1996; Zaidi *et al.*, 2002).

Slaked lime is prepared from seashells or quarried from limestone in regions that are far from the sea. Seashells are roasted, finely powdered and water is added to make slaked lime paste. The pH of slaked lime obtained from seashells or limestone is similar (Bhonsle *et al.*, 1992).

Catechu is a common ingredient of betel quid. It is a reddish brown substance derived from the heartwood of the Acacia Catechu tree, which is indigenous to India and Myanmar. It is obtained from the resins extracted from the matrix of Acacia catechu or Acacia suma (Muir

Table 1.2 Forms of different betel quids that contain areca nut and regions where they are used

Some common names and spellings	Major ingredients	Country where used
Betel quid	Areca nut (fresh, unripe) alone or with lime	Southern China, Pacific Islands
	Areca nut (dried, unripe) alone or with lime	Hunan Province in China
	Areca nut (cured, ripe) alone or with lime	South Asia
	Areca nut (fresh, unripe) with lime and betel leaves	Taiwan, China, Hainan Island, Papua New Guinea and Pacific Islands
Lao-hwa quid	Areca nut (fresh, unripe) with lime and betel inflorescence	Taiwan, China (lao-hwa quid), Papua New Guinea
Stem quid	Areca nut (fresh, unripe) with lime and betel stem	Taiwan, China
	Areca nut (fresh, unripe) with betel leaves	Guam
	Areca nut (cured, ripe) with lime and betel leaves	South Asia
Pan or *paan*	Areca nut (cured, ripe) with lime, an additional source of catechins, flavourings and betel leaves	South Asia
Pan or *paan* with tobacco, (the most common form)	Areca nut (cured, ripe) with lime, an additional source of catechins, flavourings, tobacco and betel leaves	South Asia, parts of South-eastern Asia
Pan masala or *chaalia*	Areca nut (cured, ripe) with lime, catechu, flavourings and other chemicals	India (paan masala), Pakistan (chaalia)
Mawa, kharra	Areca nut (cured, ripe) with lime, catechu, flavourings and other chemicals and tobacco – a variant of pan masala – usually called gutka; similar products with different proportions and shavings of areca nut	India

& Kirk, 1960). The main constituents of catechu are catechin, catechu tannic acid, quercetin and catechu red (IARC, 2004). Catechu contains a variety of trace elements as well (Zaidi *et al.*, 2002).

The chewing tobacco added to a betel quid is prepared from sun-dried and partly fermented coarse leaves of *Nicotiana tabacum* and *Nicotiana rustica* (IARC 2004).

A list of different forms in which areca nut is used is given in Table 1.2 (Gupta & Warnakulasuriya, 2002; IARC, 2004).

1.2 Prevalence of use

1.2.1 Distribution of betel quid chewing worldwide

It has been estimated that betel quid is used by about 10–20% of the world's population and that globally up to 600 million users chew areca nut (Gupta & Warnakulasuriya, 2002). Users are distributed around the world, but concentrated in South and South-eastern Asia, including South-eastern China, Hainan Island and Taiwan, China, and the Pacific Islands, as well as in areas of immigration of peoples from South Asia, e.g. in the Malay peninsula, eastern and southern Africa, Europe and North America. Concern among health professionals over increasing use of areca nut among South Asians and in Taiwan, China, have led to increasing numbers of prevalence surveys in the past several years.

In South Asia, South-eastern Asia, and parts of the Pacific Islands, the most common way of chewing betel quid is by inserting smokeless tobacco in the quid. Betel quid is chewed exclusively without tobacco in Southern China, Taiwan, China and Papua New Guinea, but in these areas, most chewers are also cigarette smokers. Emigrants from these areas have carried their betel quid practices to the countries of immigration.

In South Asia, dry mixtures of areca nut and betel quid related ingredients (minus the betel leaf) are prepared industrially and sold in sachets. The most popular form contains tobacco and is usually called *gutka*, a variant of *pan masala*. These forms are now being exported from India to over 50 countries. Surveys on the prevalence of areca nut use across the world are summarized in Table 1.3 (available at http://monographs.iarc.fr/ENG/Monographs/vol100E/100E-05-Table1.3.pdf) and Table 1.4 (available at http://monographs.iarc.fr/ENG/Monographs/vol100E/100E-05-Table1.4.pdf).

1.2.2 Prevalence by country or region

(a) Adults

Information from several countries, especially in South-eastern Asia, has indicated that areca nut usage may be dying out in Cambodia, Indonesia, Thailand, and Viet Nam as it has declined considerably and become confined to the older middle aged and elderly groups. In contrast, rapidly increasing prevalence of areca nut usage has been registered in India and Taiwan, China (IARC, 2004). This corresponds, in India, to the introduction of industrially manufactured areca nut products, especially *pan masala*, *gutka* and *mawa*, while betel quid use has declined; and in Taiwan, China, to changes in marketing of betel quid, where young women sell betel quid and cigarettes on roadsides.

Surveys on prevalence of areca nut use have been conducted in India, Pakistan, Taiwan, China, the People's Republic of China, Thailand, the United Kingdom and the United States.

(i) India

In India, prevalence of areca nut chewing nationwide can be estimated at around 30% of men and 7% of women, since the National Family Health Survey found 36.5% of men and 8.4% of women aged 15–49 years chewing some form of tobacco, "including *pan masala*, *gutka*, and other tobacco" (IIPS, 2007). [The Working Group noted that *pan masala* does not contain tobacco.] Since in many states of India tobacco is mainly chewed in the form of betel quid, and betel quid is mainly chewed with tobacco, the prevalence of "tobacco chewing" is only slightly higher than that of areca nut use. Local surveys have found betel quid use to be as high as 80% among both male and female adult school personnel in Mizoram; *gutka* was used by 44.8% of male school personnel in Sikkim (Sinha *et al.*, 2003). Reasons for use of tobacco products, including those containing areca nut (*gutka, mawa,* and *pan*, i.e. betel quid), among non teaching university personnel in Mumbai included peer pressure, the media (TV, advertisements, films, sports) as well as family influence (Bansode, 2002). In Chitrakoot, Madhya Pradesh, on the border with Uttar Pradesh, 46% of dental outpatients were current *gutka* users (Anwar *et al.*, 2005). In two districts of Uttar Pradesh in 2001, the prevalence of betel quid with tobacco use was only 2.0% (2.3% men, 1.4% women) (Chaudhry *et al.*, 2001). Fig. 1.1 and 1.2 present the age and sex distribution of use of betel quid with tobacco in Karnataka and Uttar Pradesh, respectively (Chaudhry *et al.*, 2001).

A statewide survey in 63 districts of Uttar Pradesh found that among 1209 *pan* [betel quid] and *pan masala* users, 94.4% (1141) used *pan* while 59.1% (n = 714) used both *pan* and *pan masala*, mostly by incorporating *pan masala* into *pan*. Additionally, 5.6% (n = 68) were exclusive *pan masala* users (Tripathi *et al.*, 2006).

(ii) Pakistan

A few recent studies in low-income urban areas of Karachi, Pakistan, have found 30–40% use of areca nut use among adults, as betel quid, areca nut by itself (*chaalia*), *gutka* and packaged *chaalia*, the equivalent of Indian *pan masala* (Mazahir *et al.*, 2006; Nisar *et al.*, 2007; Tanwir *et al.*, 2008). Among the ethnic groups in Karachi,

Fig. 1.1 Current use of betel quid with tobacco by age and sex in Karnataka

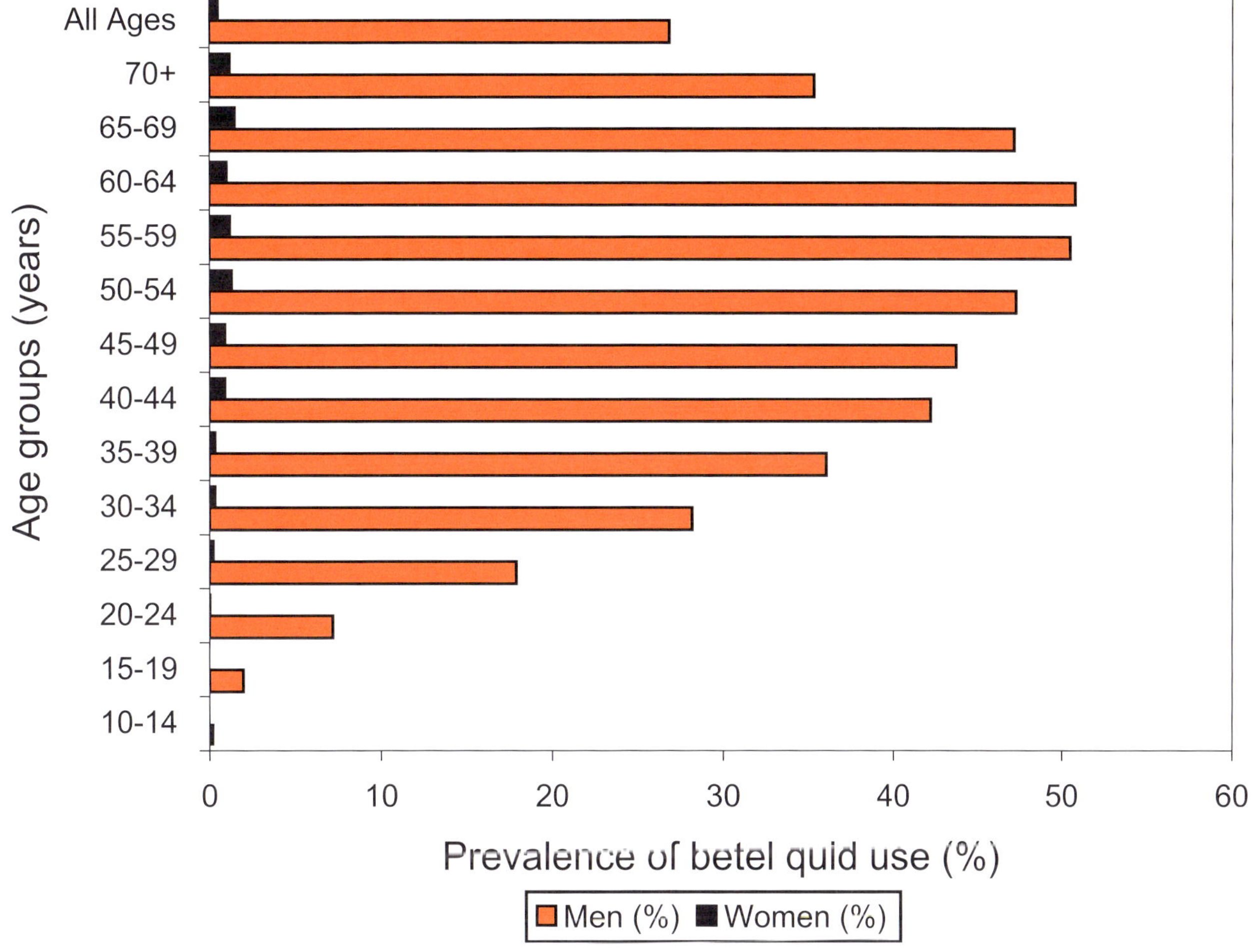

From Chaudhry *et al.* (2001)

the Mohajir appear to have a higher prevalence of use of areca nut products (Mazahir *et al.*, 2006). Adolescents prefer *chaalia* (Mazahir *et al.*, 2006), while adults over 30 years prefer betel quid (Tanwir *et al.*, 2008).

(iii) Bangladesh

A rural oral screening study in Bangladesh found that 40% of adult villagers of Kishore Ganj used areca nut with slaked lime and tobacco in various combinations (Eswar, 2002).

(iv) Thailand

In a survey of 4955 rural adults aged 30–89 years in Thailand, 17% reported using betel quid (Chatrchaiwiwatana, 2007). Betel quid chewing has been reported to be on the decline in Thailand as early as 1955 as a result of educational campaigns, and to be more common in the older population (Reichart, 1995).

(v) China

National surveys in Taiwan, China, indicate that 20.9% of men and 1.2% of women chew betel quid. Prevalence was highest in the aboriginal population: 54.3% of men and 33.8%

Fig. 1.2 Current use of betel quid with tobacco by age and sex in Uttar Pradesh

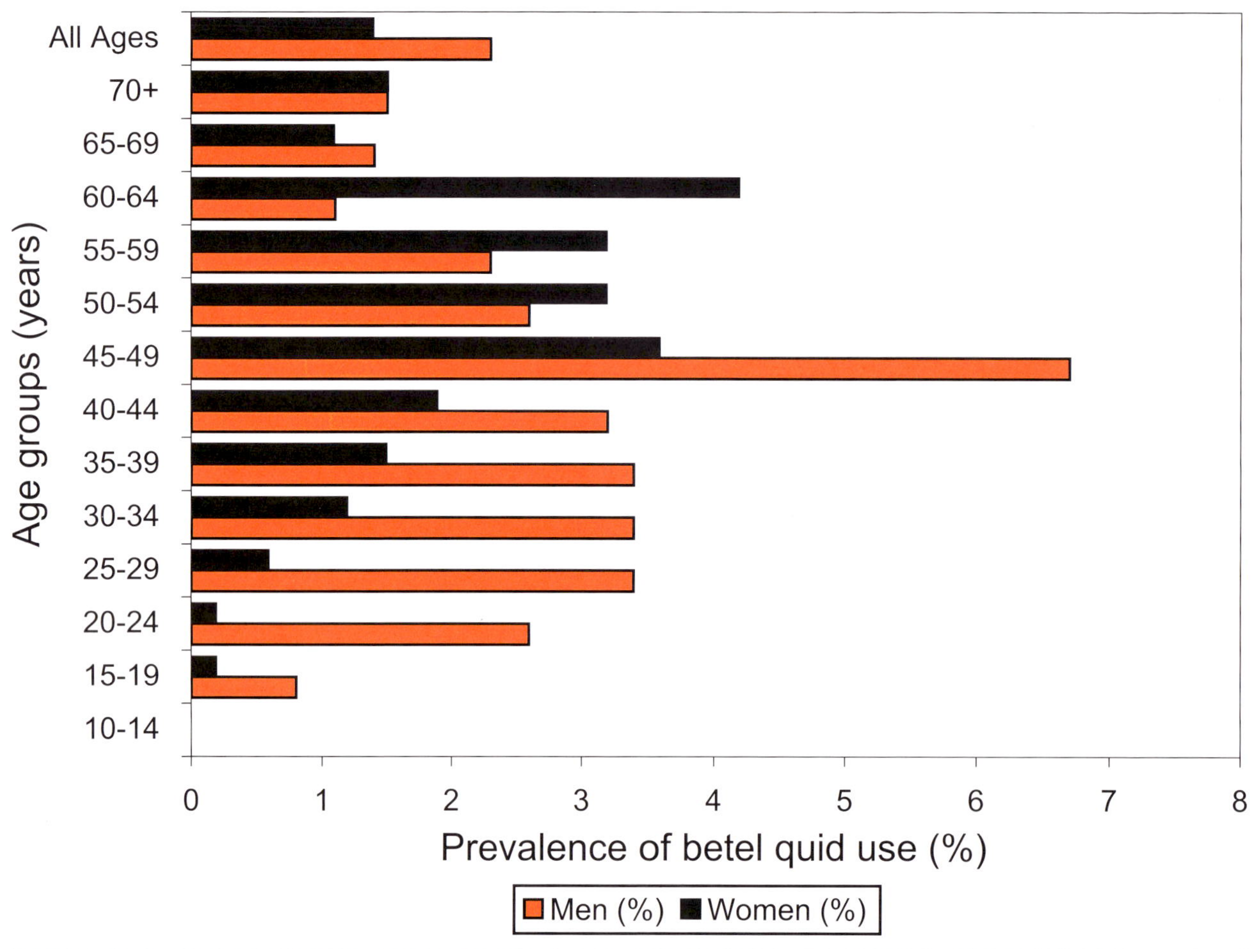

The age-wise *pan*-tobacco usage pattern of men and women differs significantly, but prevalence may be too low to be interesting.
From Chaudhry *et al.* (2001)

of women (Yap *et al.*, 2008). Betel quid chewing is more common among those who consume alcohol or who smoke. In another study, betel quid was chewed by 34.7% of aboriginal pregnant women (Chou *et al.*, 2009). Almost all betel quid chewers started chewing after they started smoking, particularly so among people over 25 years (Wen *et al.*, 2005a). Two thirds of the increase in betel quid chewing in the past decade has been attributed to the opening of the market to foreign cigarette brands in 1987, after which these cigarettes began to be placed in betel quid stalls. Betel quid sales increased dramatically as smokers turned to betel quid stalls to purchase cigarettes. Notably, 34% of betel quid chewers smoke, while 3% of non-smokers chew. Per capita consumption of betel quid increased 5 fold from 1981 to 1996 (Wen *et al.*, 2005b).

In the People's Republic of China, betel quid chewing is most common in, but not confined to, Yunnan and Hunan provinces and Hainan Island, all located in the south-eastern part of China. In Hunan, a land locked province where areca nut is not grown, the nuts are cut in half with the husk and dried, flavoured and industrially packaged. Reports on prevalence of betel quid chewing from China are limited; a review of the Chinese literature from the late 1980s and early 1990s showed that prevalence in Hunan at that time was between 64.5% and 82.7% (Zhang & Reichart, 2007).

(vi) Pacific Islands

In the Pacific islands, betel quid chewing is high among adults: 72% of men and 80% of women in Palau (Ysaol *et al.*, 1996); and 76.8% of adults (83.0% men, 68.4% women) in the Solomon Islands (Tovosia *et al.*, 2007) use betel quid.

(vii) Immigrants

In areas of immigration of South Asians, such as the United Kingdom, people of Bangladeshi origin appear to have the highest prevalence of betel quid use (mostly with tobacco) from around 30% to over 90% in both men and women (IARC, 2004). In a recent study of Bangladeshi women in the United Kingdom aged 18–39 years, prevalence of betel quid chewing was 25–35% (Núñez-de la Mora *et al.*, 2007).

Changrani *et al.* (2006) from the United States found 25% current use of betel quid and 6% *gutka* use among people of Bangladeshi origin, but a reverse pattern among people of Indian-Gujarati origin, with 2% current betel quid use and 24% *gutka* use. Areca nut and betel quid chewing without tobacco have been reported from South Africa for many years among the population of Indian origin, but no recent studies are available.

(b) Children and youth

In India *pan masala* use and *gutka* use have increased among children, also in rural areas, as a mouth freshener and a status symbol. Even after an educational intervention and a local ban on *gutka* sales near schools, 46% of 986 rural schoolchildren aged 10–15 years in Madhya Pradesh were using *gutka* regularly (Chaturvedi *et al.*, 2002). In a state-wide survey in Uttar Pradesh in 2002, 9.9% of students in 8th through 10th grades (mostly 13–15 years) were currently using *gutka* (at least once in 30 days) (Sinha & Gupta, 2005). In a survey of 385 rural adolescents (15–19 years) in villages of Wardha, Maharashtra in 2008, 17.1% were using *gutka* (31.7% boys, 4.0% girls) and 26.2% (54.1% boys, 1.0% girls) were using *kharra* [*mawa*] (Dongre *et al.*, 2008). In a very small unpublished survey in a small town in Gujarat in 1999, 16% of boys in 8th and 9th grades were using *gutka* (Gupta & Ray, 2002). In a survey in Delhi, 10.2% of 2387 urban students aged 10–18 years were using betel quid with tobacco (Kapil *et al.*, 2005a).

Male college students (16–23 years) in Karnataka in 1998 who smoked cigarettes said they sometimes substituted *gutka* for a cigarette when and where it was inappropriate to smoke. Though believed it to be very harmful and addictive, some students used *gutka* to help themselves quit smoking and then switched to *pan masala* to wean themselves off *gutka*. Those who believed that *gutka* was more addictive than cigarettes thought this strategy was unwise (Nichter *et al.*, 2004).

Use of areca nut products is prevalent among youth in other South Asian countries. In a deprived area of Karachi, Pakistan, 47.2% of school boys aged 10–16 years were using areca nut by itself; [12.6%] used betel quid without tobacco and 16.1% used *gutka* or other smokeless tobacco products (Rozi & Akhtar, 2007). In Pokhara City, Nepal, ever use of *pan masala* and *gutka* by adolescents aged 13–15 years was found to be 51.4% in boys and 30.3% in girls (Paudel, 2003).

Among adolescent students in Taiwan, China, overall use of betel quid was 3.9% (6.6% boys, 1.5% girls), and ranged from 0.8% in cities to 4.3% in towns and 7.6% in villages (Wang *et al.*, 2003a). The most variance in prevalence of betel quid use is found by type of school, ranging from 10.3% boys and 1.4% girls in general schools to 20.6% in boys and 4.7% in girls in agricultural schools (Wang *et al.*, 2004). It was found that 26.9% of ex-chewers and 22.3% of current chewers tried betel quid for the first time in elementary school. Peer pressure was the most important influence, followed by fathers giving the nuts to their child (Wang *et al.*, 2003a). A survey of fourth grade elementary students in northern Taiwan, China, found ever chewers to be 10.8% in city schools and 56.6% in mountain schools, reflecting a higher prevalence in aboriginal population in mountainous areas (Huang *et al.*, 2009).

Areca nut and tobacco practices and products from India are also becoming popular among children in countries of immigration, especially but not exclusively among children of Asian origin. A study from United Republic of Tanzania found that *gutka* and other packaged oral products imported from India were beginning to be used by adolescent students there, including those not of Indian origin (Kaduri *et al.*, 2008). In the United Kingdom, betel quid chewing is known to be taken up by students of South Asian origin, and *gutka* is available and has been reportedly used among them (Warnakulasuriya, 2002). In East London, three quarters of the students of Bangladeshi origin in ninth grade had ever tried betel quid [apparently no question was asked about *gutka*] (Jayakody *et al.*, 2006).

2. Cancer in Humans

2.1 *Cancer of the oral cavity*

Studies on betel quid and oral cavity cancers have been conducted in India, Pakistan, Sri Lanka, Thailand, Taiwan, China, South Africa, and Papua New Guinea. These populations differ in their patterns of betel quid use and the products and ingredients added to the quid (Yang *et al.*, 2001; Gupta & Warnakulasuriya, 2002). Betel quid is defined as any chewing substance that contains areca nut. In evaluating betel quid exposure, the main distinction is whether or not tobacco is added to the betel quid. When this was not explicitly stated, tobacco was considered to be absent from the betel quid only if the study was conducted in a region/ethnicity where it is uncommon/unlikely for tobacco to be added to the betel quid (i.e. Taiwan, China). However if there was good background information that the habit of betel quid chewing was very prevalent in a region/ethnicity (i.e. India, Sri Lanka, persons of Indian descent), studies that assessed "tobacco chewing" and mentioned betel quid chewing in the exposure assessment were considered as exposure to betel quid with added tobacco. If this background information was not available, studies that assessed tobacco chewing without mention of betel quid chewing were excluded from both this *Monograph* and the *Monograph* on Smokeless Tobacco in this volume. Studies that evaluated genetic polymorphisms as a main effect and their interaction with betel quid chewing were also excluded even if a crude relative risk for betel quid chewing could be calculated.

2.1.1 *Overview of studies*

When the carcinogenicity of betel quid was first evaluated in 1984 (IARC, 1985), the relationship between betel quid chewing and cancer of the oral cavity had been investigated in four cohort studies (Wahi, 1968; Mehta *et al.*, 1972; Bhargava *et al.*, 1975; Gupta *et al.*, 1980) and many case–control studies (Orr, 1933; Sanghvi *et al.*, 1955; Sarma, 1958; Khanolkar, 1959; Shanta & Krishnamurthi, 1959, 1963; Chandra, 1962; Wahi *et al.*, 1965; Hirayama, 1966; Jussawalla & Deshpande, 1971; Khanna *et al.*, 1975; Kwan, 1976; Notani & Sanghvi, 1976; Simarak *et al.*, 1977; Jafarey *et al.*, 1977). The effect of betel quid without added tobacco was investigated in only a few studies.

When the available evidence was evaluated in 2003 (IARC, 2004), 15 additional case–control studies had been published (Sankaranarayanan *et al.*, 1989a, b, 1990a; Nandakumar *et al.*, 1990; van Wyk *et al.*, 1993; Rao *et al.*, 1994; Ko *et al.*, 1995; Lu *et al.*, 1996; Rao & Desai, 1998; Wasnik *et al.*, 1998; Dikshit & Kanhere, 2000; Merchant *et al.*, 2000; Balaram *et al.*, 2002; Chen *et al.*, 2002; Znaor *et al.*, 2003).

The case–control studies of cancer of the oral cavity that clearly distinguish betel quid without and with added tobacco are summarized in Table 2.1 (available at http://monographs.iarc.fr/ENG/Monographs/vol100E/100E-05-Table2.1.pdf) and Table 2.2 (available at http://monographs.iarc.fr/ENG/Monographs/vol100E/100E-05-Table2.2.pdf) respectively. The derived relative risk estimates ranged from 1.5 to 58.4 for use of betel quid without tobacco and from 0.7 to 45.9 for betel quid with tobacco. Most of these studies adjusted for potential confounders such as tobacco smoking, use of smokeless tobacco, alcohol use, and HPV infection.

Since then there have been several publications assessing the association between betel quid chewing and cancer of the oral cavity (Wen *et al.*, 2005a; Yang *et al.*, 2005a; Subapriya *et al.*, 2007; Thomas *et al.*, 2007; Muwonge *et al.*, 2008; Yen *et al.*, 2008b; Jayalekshmi *et al.*, 2009). The relative risk estimates from the three case–control studies ranged from 2.03 to 5.4 for use of betel quid without tobacco and from 3.19 to 11.8 for betel quid with tobacco.

2.1.2 Risk by type of agent

(a) Betel quid without added tobacco

An increased risk of statistical (or borderline) significance associated with betel quid chewing without tobacco was reported from all case–control studies of cancer of the oral cavity that considered this after adjusting for smoking and/or alcohol intake (Nandakumar *et al.*, 1990; Ko *et al.*, 1995; Lu *et al.*, 1996; Wasnik *et al.*, 1998; Dikshit & Kanhere, 2000; Merchant *et al.*, 2000; Balaram *et al.*, 2002; Chen *et al.*, 2002; Znaor *et al.*, 2003; Subapriya *et al.*, 2007; Thomas *et al.*, 2007; Muwonge *et al.*, 2008; Table 2.1 online). Znaor *et al.* (2003) reported an increased risk for cancer of the oral cavity associated with the use of betel quid without added tobacco in non-smoking and non-drinking men that had no other known risk factors (OR, 3.39; 95%CI: 2.04–5.66) after adjustment for age, centre and education level. In a study in Pakistan (Merchant *et al.*, 2000) an increased risk for oral cancer was associated with the use of betel quid without added tobacco, after adjusting for smoking and alcohol. Data from Taiwan, China and Papua New Guinea, where betel quid is generally used without tobacco, also support this association.

In three cohort studies (Bhargava *et al.*, 1975; Yang *et al.*, 2005a; Yen *et al.*, 2008b) increased risks of cancer of the oral cavity among betel quid chewers were found (IARC, 2004; Table 2.3 available at http://monographs.iarc.fr/ENG/Monographs/vol100E/100E-05-Table2.3.pdf); in two of these studies (Bhargava *et al.*, 1975; Yang *et al.*, 2005a), incident cancers only occurred among betel quid chewers. Yen *et al.* (2008b) reported that the use of betel quid was significantly associated with cancer of the oral cavity in subjects who were neither smokers nor drinkers (OR, 10.97; 95%CI: 3.22–37.34). In a nested case–control study conducted in India, betel quid use without added tobacco was associated with cancer of the oral cavity overall (Muwonge *et al.*, 2008). Among women [with a low prevalence of smoking in this population], the risk was highly significant after adjusting for smoking and drinking.

In a meta-analysis Thomas *et al.* (2007) included 11 independent studies that examined risk of cancer of the oral cavity associated with chewing betel quid without added tobacco (Chandra, 1962; Hirayama, 1966; Jafarey *et al.*, 1977; Ko *et al.*, 1995; Lu *et al.*, 1996; Dikshit & Kanhere, 2000; Merchant *et al.*, 2000; Balaram *et al.*, 2002; Chen *et al.*, 2002; Znaor *et al.*, 2003; Thomas *et al.*, 2007). These studies either excluded smokers or controlled for smoking. The overall odds ratio estimated for betel quid without tobacco was 2.14 (95%CI: 1.06–4.32) among non-smokers and 3.50 (95%CI: 2.16–5.65) in studies that adjusted for smoking.

(b) Betel quid with added tobacco

Significantly increased risks for cancer of the oral cavity associated with chewing betel quid with added tobacco were observed in all of the case–control studies that considered this (Orr, 1933; Sanghvi *et al.*, 1955; Sarma, 1958; Khanolkar, 1959; Shanta & Krishnamurthi, 1959, 1963; Chandra, 1962; Hirayama, 1966; Wahi *et al.*, 1965; Wahi, 1968; Jussawalla & Deshpande, 1971; IARC, 1985; Sankaranarayanan *et al.*, 1989a, b, 1990a; Nandakumar *et al.*, 1990; van Wyk *et al.*, 1993; Rao *et al.*, 1994; Rao & Desai, 1998; Wasnik *et al.*, 1998; Dikshit & Kanhere, 2000; Merchant *et al.*, 2000; Balaram *et al.*, 2002; Znaor *et al.*, 2003; Subapriya *et al.*, 2007; Muwonge *et al.*, 2008; Table 2.2 online) and in two cohort studies (Wahi, 1968; Gupta *et al.*, 1980). All of the case–control studies adjusted for smoking and some studies additionally adjusted for alcohol use.

(c) Areca nut and betel inflorescence

The risk of chewing areca nut alone without other ingredients (particularly tobacco) was examined in one Indian study (Wasnik *et al.*, 1998), a suggestive increased risk of cancer of the oropharynx was reported (OR, 2.6; 95%CI: 0.9–7.7).

In a study in Taiwan, China, the risk for cancer of the oral cavity was highest among those who chewed only unripe areca nut (OR, 11.6; 95%CI: 3.7–36.9; 41 exposed cases) compared with those who chewed betel leaf alone (OR, 0.1; 95%CI: 0.0–6.3; 1 exposed case) or a mixture of the two (OR, 8.5; 95%CI: 2.7–26.3; 34 exposed cases) after adjustment for education, occupation, smoking and drinking (Ko *et al.*, 1995).

2.1.3 Exposure–response relationship

(a) Intensity and duration

An exposure–response relationship (by various metrics of exposure such as intensity, duration, age at starting or betel quid-years) between betel quid chewing and oral cancer was demonstrated in several studies (Orr, 1933; Sankaranarayanan *et al.*, 1989a, b, 1990a; Nandakumar *et al.*, 1990; Rao *et al.*, 1994; Lu *et al.*, 1996; Rao & Desai, 1998; Wasnik *et al.*, 1998; Dikshit & Kanhere, 2000; Merchant *et al.*, 2000; Balaram *et al.*, 2002; Znaor *et al.*, 2003; Thomas *et al.*, 2007; Muwonge *et al.*, 2008; Jayalekshmi *et al.*, 2009; IARC, 1985; Table 2.4 available at http://monographs.iarc.fr/ENG/Monographs/vol100E/100E-05-Table2.4.pdf). Not all reports distinguished whether or not tobacco was added to the betel quid, though many controlled for smoking, consumption of alcoholic beverages, or both. [Merchant *et al.* (2000) did not present odds ratios and corresponding 95% confidence intervals were not present for the tertiles of paan-years (P for trend = 0.004 for paan-years with tobacco and P for trend = 0.0008 for paan-years without tobacco.]

(b) Cessation

The effect of cessation has not been examined extensively. In one study, having quit chewing betel quid with added tobacco 10 years earlier or within 10 years did not demonstrate a beneficial effect in either sex (Balaram *et al.*, 2002). Znaor *et al.* (2003), however, were able to demonstrate a decrease of risk for cancer of the oral cavity after 10 years or more of quitting. [Znaor *et al.* (2003) did not distinguish whether or not tobacco was added to the quid for this analysis.]

2.1.4 Anatomical subsites of cancer

Some authors reported site-specific (gingiva, tongue, mouth) differences in relative risk (Sanghvi *et al.*, 1955; Khanolkar, 1959; Shanta

& Krishnamurthi, 1959, 1963; Chandra, 1962; Hirayama, 1966; Wahi, 1968; Jussawalla & Deshpande, 1971; Kwan, 1976; Sankaranarayanan *et al.*, 1989b; Rao & Desai, 1998; Znaor *et al.*, 2003). In non-smokers and non-drinkers, Wahi (1968) reported the highest risks for the buccal mucosa, gingiva and lip combined associated with chewing betel quid with tobacco. After adjusting for smoking and alcohol, Znaor *et al.* (2003) reported higher risks for the mouth compared to the tongue, for betel quid use both with or without tobacco.

2.1.5 Population characteristics

In most studies, markedly higher estimates of risk for cancer of the oral cavity were found in women than in men for betel quid chewing, with or without tobacco (Sanghvi *et al.*, 1955; Chandra, 1962; Shanta & Krishnamurthi, 1963; Hirayama, 1966; Wahi, 1968; Notani & Sanghvi, 1976; Jafarey *et al.*, 1977; Simarak *et al.*, 1977; Sankaranarayanan *et al.*, 1989a, b, 1990a; Nandakumar *et al.*, 1990; van Wyk *et al.*, 1993; Rao *et al.*, 1994; Rao & Desai, 1998; Dikshit & Kanhere, 2000; Balaram *et al.*, 2002; Znaor *et al.*, 2003; Muwonge *et al.*, 2008; Yen *et al.*, 2008b; Jayalekshmi *et al.*, 2009).

2.1.6 Interactions

Among the many studies of cancer of the oral cavity that have examined multiple habits with 2- and 3-way combinations among tobacco smoking, alcohol drinking and betel quid chewing, only a few studies formally tested for interaction. Table 2.5 (available at http://monographs.iarc.fr/ENG/Monographs/vol100E/100E-05-Table2.5.pdf) and Table 2.6 (available at http://monographs.iarc.fr/ENG/Monographs/vol100E/100E-05-Table2.6.pdf) provide data from studies reporting combined odds ratios for combination of habits. Findings are not consistent across studies. In general interaction is at an additive level only.

In three studies the interaction between betel quid chewing without added tobacco and tobacco smoking was examined (Ko *et al.*, 1995; Znaor *et al.*, 2003; Thomas *et al.*, 2007) and it was found that risk was highest in those who smoked, drank alcohol and chewed betel quid. For subjects consuming betel quid (with or without added tobacco) there was an interaction with smoking among non-alcohol drinkers by Znaor *et al.* (2003) ($P = 0.00$). However, in another study from India, there was no suggestion of an interaction between betel quid chewing with or without added tobacco and tobacco smoking (Muwonge *et al.*, 2008). For those chewing betel quid with tobacco, interactions with tobacco smoking were found in a few other studies (Sankaranarayanan *et al.*, 1989a, b, 1990a; Dikshit & Kanhere, 2000), and were significant in some (Sankaranarayanan *et al.*, 1989a, b, 1990a). In a study that examined 2-way interactions between betel quid chewing and consumption of alcoholic beverages, evidence suggestive of a synergistic effect was observed in men who chewed betel quid with tobacco (Znaor *et al.*, 2003). However, in another study from India, there was no suggestion of an interaction between betel quid chewing with or without added tobacco and consumption of alcoholic beverages (Muwonge *et al.*, 2008).

The 3-way interaction of betel quid chewing, tobacco smoking and consumption of alcoholic beverages was considered in few studies (Table 2.7 available at http://monographs.iarc.fr/ENG/Monographs/vol100E/100E-05-Table2.7.pdf). While the interactions were found significant in two studies (Sankaranarayanan *et al.*, 1989a; Znaor *et al.*, 2003) and, in 2 other studies from India there was no suggestion of an interaction (Sankaranarayanan *et al.*, 1990a; Muwonge *et al.*, 2008).

2.1.7 *Population attributable risk*

The population attributable risk fraction of cancer of the oral cavity was observed to be 66% for chewers of betel quid with tobacco in Bhopal, India (Dikshit & Kanhere, 2000). In a study in Trivandrum, India, the adjusted population attributable risk fraction estimated for women for having ever chewed (81.2%) was nearly double that of men (42.6%) (Muwonge *et al.*, 2008).

2.2 Precancerous lesions of the oral cavity

Precancerous lesions or potentially malignant disorders of the oral cavity precede cancer development and largely contribute to the burden of cancer of the oral cavity in South Asia. In the restricted geographic locations where people consume betel quid, the disorders of concern are leukoplakia, erythroplakia, erythroleukoplakia, and oral submucous fibrosis (Warnakulasuriya *et al.*, 2007).

In India, betel quid or areca nut use either alone or in combination with tobacco account for most of the leukoplakia cases (Smith *et al.*, 1975; Gupta *et al.*, 1980). The studies examining the association between betel quid chewing and oral precancerous lesions undertaken before 2004 were reviewed in previous *IARC Monographs* (IARC, 1985, 2004). The relative risk estimates for oral leukoplakia (Hashibe *et al.*, 2000a; Shiu *et al.*, 2000; Yang *et al.*, 2001; Lee *et al.*, 2003), erythroplakia (Hashibe *et al.*, 2000b), oral submucous fibrosis (Sinor *et al.*, 1990; Maher *et al.*, 1994; Gupta *et al.*, 1998; Hazare *et al.*, 1998; Shah & Sharma, 1998; Hashibe *et al.*, 2002) ranged from 7 to around 30. Other studies of oral submucous fibrosis reported high risks associated with betel quid use: RR 32 (95%CI: 6–177) for betel quid without tobacco and RR 154 (95%CI: 34–693) for areca nut alone (Maher *et al.*, 1994); RR 75.6 among users of mawa (a mixture of areca nut, tobacco and slaked lime) (Gupta *et al.*, 1998) and RR 49.2 (95%CI: 24.3–99.6) among betel quid chewers (with and without added tobacco) (Hashibe *et al.*, 2002).

Since then new evidence has accumulated on the association between betel quid and areca nut use and oral pre-cancer. Some of these studies evaluated the risks for combinations of oral mucosal disorders grouped together (oral precancer; oral potentially malignant disorders) or separately for leukoplakia, erythroplakia or oral submucous fibrosis. Data from these new studies are summarized in Table 2.8 (available at http://monographs.iarc.fr/ENG/Monographs/vol100E/100E-05-Table2.8.pdf). In two cross-sectional studies from Sri Lanka and Taiwan, China, where betel quid is used without added tobacco, significant associations for areca quid/betel quid chewing with oral precancerous lesions were found. The risks were 8.40 (95%CI: 5.13–13.75) in Taiwan, China (Chung *et al.*, 2005) and 3.01 (95%CI: 2.25–4.0) in Sri Lanka (betel quid with or without added tobacco) (Ariyawardana *et al.*, 2007). Both studies were adjusted for tobacco smoking and alcohol drinking. In several case–control studies (in India, Sri Lanka, Taiwan, China and Papua New Guinea), use of betel quid without added tobacco in non tobacco smokers and/or non alcohol drinkers was associated with an increased risk in oral precancerous lesions (Jacob *et al.*, 2004; Yang *et al.*, 2005b; Thomas *et al.*, 2008). The risks for oral leukoplakia and erythroplakia were significantly elevated in betel quid chewers with tobacco, as well as in those chewing betel quid without tobacco in an Indian population (Jacob *et al.*, 2004) and among Taiwan, China, Chinese populations, who do not add tobacco to their betel quid (Shiu *et al.*, 2000; Chen *et al.*, 2006; Yen *et al.*, 2007). In some of these studies significant exposure–response relationships were found (Jacob *et al.*, 2004; Yang *et al.*, 2005b; Yen *et al.*, 2008a). Shiu *et al.* (2000) found that betel quid use without added tobacco is a significant factor influencing malignant transformation of oral leukoplakia (OR, 4.59;

95%CI: 1.25–16.86). Ho *et al.* (2009) however found no positive association with betel quid use without added tobacco and malignant transformation of existing premalignant disorders (OR, 0.98; 95%CI: 0.36–2.97). Yang *et al.* (2005b) reported a significant positive association for betel quid chewing without tobacco (among non smokers) with oral submucous fibrosis from a case–control study in Taiwan, China (OR, 4.51; 95%CI: 1.20–16.94). In a further study from Sri Lanka, Ariyawardana *et al.* (2006) found that betel quid chewing with and without tobacco was the only significantly associated risk factor in oral submucous fibrosis (OR, 171.8; 95%CI: 36.35–812.25) and there was no interaction with either tobacco smoking or alcohol use. However, alcohol drinking had a significant effect on the malignant transformation in oral submucous fibrosis, while areca/betel quid chewing showed no association (Ho *et al.*, 2007). In a study from the People's Republic of China, duration of betel quid use without added tobacco was associated with a significantly increased risk (OR for longest duration, 10.15; 95%CI: 2.72–37.79) for malignant transformation of oral submucous fibrosis, (*P* for trend = 0.008) (Zhou *et al.*, 2008). [The Working Group noted that interpretation of these results may be hampered by the use of oral submucous fibrosis controls]. In a further case–control study (Ahmad *et al.*, 2006), *gutka* and other areca nut products had a highly significant association with oral submucous fibrosis ($\chi^2 = 188.14$, $P < 0.001$). [The Working Group noted that oral submucous fibrosis is not associated with tobacco use or alcohol drinking.]

Intervention studies demonstrated that reduction in the use of betel quid with added tobacco resulted in lowering the incidence of precancerous lesions (Gupta *et al.*, 1986, 1992) and cessation resulted in development of no new precancerous lesions (Gupta *et al.*, 1995).

Thomas *et al.* (2008) included 6 studies in a meta-analysis that examined risk of oral precancerous disorders associated with betel quid without tobacco. These studies either excluded smokers or controlled for smoking. Among non-smokers with oral precancerous lesions their overall odds ratio estimated for betel quid without tobacco was 10.13 (95%CI:4.09–25.08) and in studies that adjusted for smoking the combined odds ratio was 5.17 (95%CI: 2.79–9.57).

2.3 Other cancers of the upper aerodigestive tract

2.3.1 Cancers of the pharynx

(a) Nasopharynx

In a cohort study from Taiwan, China, where tobacco is never added to betel quid (Wen *et al.*, 2005a), betel quid chewers who smoked had an increased risk of death from cancer of the nasopharynx (RR, 4.2; 95%CI: 1.5–11.4) after adjusting for age, alcohol use and education (Table 2.9 available at http://monographs.iarc.fr/ENG/Monographs/vol100E/100E-05-Table2.9.pdf). [There has been no publication from Taiwan, China where betel quid chewing was reported separately from smoking, because most betel quid chewers smoke.] Positive associations with 20 or more years of area nut use were found in a case–control study of cancer of the nasopharynx from Taiwan, China (Yang *et al.*, 2005; Table 2.10 available at http://monographs.iarc.fr/ENG/Monographs/vol100E/100E-05-Table2.10.pdf). [The models were adjusted for age and sex but it was unclear if they were further adjusted for other factors such as cigarette smoking, Guangdong salted fish consumption during childhood, and cumulative wood dust exposure]. Two case–control studies of cancer of the nasopharynx from India, where tobacco is commonly added to the betel quid, also found positive associations with betel quid chewing (Jussawalla & Deshpande, 1971; Chelleng *et al.*, 2000).

(b) Oropharynx

Cancer of the oropharynx has been associated with chewing betel quid with added tobacco (Sanghvi *et al.*, 1955; Khanolkar, 1959; Shanta & Krishnamurthi, 1963; Hirayama, 1966; Jussawalla & Deshpande, 1971; Wasnik *et al.*, 1998; Dikshit & Kanhere, 2000; Znaor *et al.*, 2003) and without added tobacco (Shanta & Krishnamurthi, 1963; Hirayama, 1966; Jussawalla & Deshpande, 1971; Wasnik *et al.*, 1998; Znaor *et al.*, 2003) in all of the studies in which it was assessed (IARC (2004) and Table 2.10 online. [The Working Group noted that the title of the study by Dikshit & Kanhere (2000) mentioned 'oropharyngeal' but the authors made occasional references to 'oral cavity' in the article]. None of the studies controlled for HPV, an important risk factor for cancer of the oropharynx. All of the studies were conducted in India, and Hirayama (1966) additionally enrolled subjects from Sri Lanka.

(c) Hypopharynx

Several positive associations between cancer of the hypopharynx and chewing betel quid (with or without added tobacco or unspecified) have been reported (Sanghvi *et al.*, 1955; Shanta & Krishnamurthi, 1963; Jussawalla & Deshpande, 1971; Simarak *et al.*, 1977; Znaor *et al.*, 2003; Sapkota *et al.*, 2007; IARC (2004) and Table 2.10 online. Most analyses accounted for tobacco use and two additionally adjusted for alcohol drinking (Znaor *et al.*, 2003; Sapkota *et al.*, 2007). For users of products containing both tobacco and areca nut (*mawa*, *pan* with tobacco and *gutka*), statistically significant results were seen for each of those behaviours (separately evaluated) for never smokers only, with adjustment for snuff use (nasal or oral), alcohol, drinking and smoking (Sapkota *et al.*, 2007).

(d) Pharynx

In several case–control studies a positive association between chewing betel quid with added tobacco and cancer of the pharynx has been found after controlling for tobacco smoking (Sanghvi *et al.*, 1955; Shanta & Krishnamurthi, 1963; Jussawalla & Deshpande, 1971; Simarak *et al.*, 1977; Wasnik *et al.*, 1998; Dikshit & Kanhere, 2000; Znaor *et al.*, 2003; Sapkota *et al.*, 2007; IARC, 2004; Table 2.10 online). Znaor *et al.* (2003) and Sapkota *et al.* (2007) additionally adjusted for alcohol drinking. Znaor *et al.* (2003) also found dose-dependent increases in risk of combined oro-, hypo- and unspecified pharyngeal cancers by amount used, duration of use and cumulative use of unspecified betel quid (considered to be mostly with added tobacco).

In two studies chewing of betel quid without added tobacco was found to be positively associated with cancer of the pharynx (Znaor *et al.*, 2003; Lee *et al.*, 2005a), after adjusting for tobacco smoking and alcohol drinking. Lee *et al.* (2005a) showed dose-dependent increases in risk of combined hypo- and oro-pharyngeal cancers by age of chewing initiation and amount chewed. The highest odds ratios were for people who used betel inflorescence and for those who swallowed the juice of the quid (Lee *et al.*, 2005a).

2.3.2 Cancer of the oesophagus

The risk of cancer of the oesophagus associated with chewing betel quid with added tobacco has been assessed in several studies (IARC, 2004; Table 2.10 online). These included studies carried out in India that specifically assessed betel quid with added tobacco (Shanta & Krishnamurthi, 1963; Jussawalla & Deshpande, 1971; Jayant *et al.*, 1977; Sankaranarayanan *et al.*, 1991; Znaor *et al.*, 2003); others carried out in India that did not specify as to whether tobacco was added to the betel quid (Sanghvi *et al.*, 1955; Nandakumar *et al.*, 1996; Chitra *et al.*, 2004); and studies in Thailand (Phukan *et al.*, 2001; Boonyaphiphat *et al.*, 2002) where tobacco is typically added to the quid. The majority of studies reported positive associations but only three (Nandakumar *et al.*, 1996; Boonyaphiphat *et al.*, 2002; Znaor *et al.*, 2003) controlled for both smoking and alcohol use. In a case–control study in Kerala, India no association of cancer of the oesophagus with chewing betel quid with added tobacco was found but there was no control for smoking (Sankaranarayanan *et al.*, 1991). In the case–control study in Thailand odds ratios increased with increasing number of quids chewed from 1.47 (95%CI: 0.9–2.3) with chewing less than 10 quids per day to 5.6 (95%CI: 2.7–11.8) for chewing more than 10 quids per day (Boonyaphiphat *et al.*, 2002).

The association between betel quid without added tobacco and cancer of the oesophagus has been evaluated in eight studies (Shanta & Krishnamurthi, 1963; Jussawalla & Deshpande, 1971; Wu *et al.*, 2001, 2004a, 2006; Znaor *et al.*, 2003; Lee *et al.*, 2005b, 2007); five analyses controlled for tobacco smoking and alcohol drinking (Znaor *et al.* 2003; Wu *et al.* 2004a, 2006; Lee *et al.* 2005b, 2007). Positive associations were found in all studies, of which six (Jussawalla & Deshpande, 1971; Wu *et al.*, 2001, 2004a; Znaor *et al.*, 2003; Lee *et al.*, 2005b, 2007) were statistically significant. Significant dose–response relationships after controlling for smoking and alcohol were observed by Lee *et al.* (2005b, 2007). In a cohort study based on a national survey and community, Wen *et al.* (2005a) could not separate the effect of chewing betel quid without added tobacco and tobacco smoking since currently most betel quid chewers smoke in Taiwan, China (Table 2.9 online). The highest relative risks were reported in Taiwan, China among those who chewed betel inflorescence (Wu *et al.*, 2004a, Lee *et al.*, 2005b, 2007; Wu *et al.*, 2006). [Betel inflorescence contains a high concentration of safrole, a possible human carcinogen (IARC Group 2B)].

In two studies risk was evaluated for cancer at subsites of the oesophagus. The highest magnitude of effect associated with chewing betel quid were reported for the upper third of the oesophagus in Taiwan, China (Lee *et al.*, 2007) and for the middle-third of the oesophagus in India (Nandakumar *et al.*, 1996). Both studies controlled for tobacco smoking and alcohol drinking.

2.3.3 Cancer of the larynx

In India, where tobacco is commonly added to the betel quid, positive associations with chewing betel quid were found in two case–control studies of cancer of the larynx (Jussawalla & Deshpande, 1971; Kapil *et al.*, 2005b) while in two other case–control studies there was no association (Sankaranarayanan *et al.*, 1990b; Sapkota *et al.*, 2007; IARC, 2004; Table 2.10 online). [Jussawalla & Deshpande (1971), Sankaranarayanan *et al.* (1990b) and Kapil *et al.* (2005b) did not adjust for smoking or drinking habits.] In Taiwan, China (Lee *et al.*, 2005a), chewing betel quid without added tobacco was positively but not significantly associated with the risk of cancer of the larynx, after adjusting for smoking and alcohol (OR, 1.3; 95%CI: 0.7–2.5).

2.3.4 Interactions

Several studies have reported the joint effects of chewing betel quid, adding chewing tobacco, smoking tobacco and/or drinking alcohol. A re-analysis of the data from Jussawalla & Deshpande (1971) found that chewing and smoking practices interacted synergistically for cancers of the oral cavity, oropharynx, hypopharynx, larynx and oesophagus (Jayant *et al.*, 1977). Znaor *et al.* (2003) also showed a synergistic relationship between betel quid chewing, tobacco smoking and alcohol consumption for cancer of the pharynx. These findings are similar to those on smoking and betel quid chewing from a cohort study in Taiwan, China with nasopharyngeal and oesophageal cancer as reported outcomes (Wen *et al.*, 2005a). The common occurrence of dual or multiple substance use (chewing betel quid, adding chewing tobacco, smoking tobacco and drinking alcohol) in populations makes these findings important, as the magnitude of effect is highest for those who combine these habits.

2.4 Cancer of the liver

2.4.1 Cohort studies

Three cohort studies conducted in Taiwan, China, investigated the association between betel quid use [without added tobacco] and cancer of the liver (Sun *et al.*, 2003; Wang *et al.*, 2003b; Wen *et al.*, 2005a; Table 2.11 available at http://monographs.iarc.fr/ENG/Monographs/vol100E/100E-05-Table2.11.pdf). Sun *et al.* (2003) found a synergistic association between hepatocellular carcinoma and betel quid chewing without added tobacco in those with hepatitis C virus (HCV) infection. [The number of cases was small (2 cases among betel quid chewers with HCV infection; 8 cases among betel quid chewers without HCV infection) and there was no adjustment for tobacco smoking and alcohol consumption.]

Wang *et al.* (2003b) found high and statistically significant relative risks for hepatocellular carcinoma associated with betel quid chewing without added tobacco. Compared to Hepatitis B surface Antigen (HBsAg) seronegative men who did not chew betel quid, chewing betel quid without added tobacco conferred a relative risk of 3.43 (95%CI: 1.19–9.89), with a dose–response relationship for quantity chewed per day (*P* trend = 0.007). [The Working Group noted that the authors adjusted for liver function at baseline but did not adjust for tobacco smoking and alcohol consumption.] Wen *et al.* (2005a) conducted a cohort study in Taiwan, China and found a statistically significant positive association with liver cancer and cirrhosis of the liver, after adjusting for HBsAg, for those who both smoked cigarettes and chewed betel quid without added tobacco (RR, 1.8; 95%CI: 1.1–2.8). The magnitude of effect observed was much higher than that observed for those who only smoked but did not chew betel quid. [The Working Group noted that there were too few non smoking betel chewers to calculate a relative risk for them in this study].

2.4.2 Case–control studies

Two case–control studies (Tsai *et al.*, 2001, 2004) and one cross-sectional study (Wu *et al.*, 2009a) from Taiwan, China, and one case–control study from Thailand (Srivatanakul *et al.*, 1991) showed significant associations between chewing betel quid without added tobacco and hepatocellular carcinoma (Table 2.12 available at http://monographs.iarc.fr/ENG/Monographs/vol100E/100E-05-Table2.12.pdf). [It was not specified whether or not tobacco was added to the betel quid in Srivatanakul *et al.*, 1991]. Tsai *et al.* (2001) reported an exposure-response relationship and a synergy with viral infection after adjusting for infection with hepatitis virus (HBV and HCV), tobacco smoking, alcohol consumption and socio-demographic variables. Tsai *et al.* (2004) showed significant associations of hepatocellular carcinoma with betel quid chewing, using two separate control groups (healthy population-based controls and cirrhosis patients). Furthermore, an exposure-response relationship was observed with the duration and quantity of betel quid chewed (*P* for trend < 0.0001). There was also a positive association between betel quid chewing without tobacco and cirrhosis, a precursor to liver cancer (La Vecchia *et al.*, 1998).

Betel quid appears to act synergistically with viral infections in causing liver cancer. When comparing hepatocellular carcinoma patients to healthy controls, the odds ratio associated with chewing betel quid without tobacco among persons positive for a hepatitis virus (HBV or HCV) was statistically significantly elevated and orders of magnitude higher than the odds ratio associated with being hepatitis virus positive and a non-chewer or being a chewer and hepatitis virus negative. [No formal test for interaction was presented and the 95% confidence intervals were wide due to the small sample size. It was not possible to determine whether these models were adjusted for alcohol consumption, tobacco smoking or other confounding factors. There was some overlap in cases between Tsai *et al.* (2001) and Tsai *et al.* (2004).]

A population-based study of liver cirrhosis and hepatocellular carcinoma combined was conducted in Keelung, northern Taiwan, China on 60 326 persons aged 30 years and above who were enrolled in a screening programme (Wu *et al.*, 2009a). [Prevalent and incident cases were combined.] There was a statistically significant positive association with chewing betel quid without added tobacco and significant exposure-response relationships for the number of quids chewed daily, number of years of chewing, cumulative exposure (portion-days), and age at initiation (*P* for trend < 0.01) after adjusting for sex, HBsAg, anti-HCV antibodies, cumulative exposure to alcohol consumption and cigarette smoking. Betel quid chewers who were seronegative for both HBsAg and anti-HCV had a hazard ratio of 5.09 (95%CI: 2.87–9.03); a synergistic association was observed for betel quid chewing and seropositivity for one or both viral markers (hazard ratios ranged from 25–29). [The Working Group noted that the most popular type of betel quid in Keelung includes unripe nuts, betel inflorescence and red lime paste and is swallowed after chewing. It was mentioned that aflatoxin is commonly present in areca nuts, but this was according to a reference from India, where ripe nuts are used for chewing and may be stored for long periods, making them susceptible to mould. Both prevalent and incident cases were included and hepatocellular carcinoma and liver cirrhosis cases were combined, which limits the interpretation of the data for the carcinogenicity of betel quid chewing.]

2.5 Other cancers

2.5.1 *Cancer of the stomach*

In a case–control study on stomach cancer from Taiwan, China Wu *et al.* (2004b) found a positive association with cumulative chewing of betel quid without added tobacco (betel-years): the odds ratios increased with higher consumption, after adjusting for alcohol consumption, tobacco smoking and *H. pylori* infection (*P* for trend = 0.03). In a hospital-based case–control study from Chennai, India (Gajalakshmi & Shanta, 1996), elevated odds ratios (not statistically significant) of similar magnitude (range 1.2–1.4) were observed for chewing areca nut only, betel quid only, and betel quid with added tobacco, although the risk disappeared after adjusting for tobacco smoking, alcohol consumption and diet. From a hospital-based case–control study of stomach cancer in Mizoram, India Phukan *et al.* (2005) reported elevated odds ratios for chewing betel quid with or without added tobacco, with significant trends for increasing odds ratios with increasing exposure (according to various exposure metrics) after adjusting for alcohol drinking, smoking, use of *tuibur*, level of education, occupation and income group.

2.5.2 *Cancer of the cervix*

One study described the association between betel quid chewing (with or without added tobacco) and cervical cancer in which nearly all women were non-smokers and in which all cases, but one, were HPV positive (Rajkumar *et al.*, 2003). There was an association between the use of betel quid without tobacco and cervical cancer; among women who reported using betel quid more than 5 times per day the odds ratio was 4.0

(95%CI: 1.20–13.33) with a significant trend with increasing number of times used per day.

A cross-sectional study derived from a screening programme (Chakrabarti *et al.*, 1990) showed an association between betel quid chewing with and without tobacco and cervical dysplasia. [Women with cytoepidemiological evidence of infection with HPV, HSV, *Trichomonas vaginalis* and *Chlamydia trachomatis* were excluded from the study.]

2.5.3 Cancers of thelung, colon and gallbladder

Several studies have assessed the association between chewing betel quid with or without added tobacco and cancer of the lung (Wen *et al.*, 2005a), colon (Wu *et al.*, 2009b) and gallbladder (Pandey & Shukla, 2003; Shukla *et al.*, 2008).

2.6 Synthesis

2.6.1 Oral cavity

Chewing betel quid, both with and without added tobacco, causes cancer of the oral cavity (IARC, 2004). Recent studies, many of which were adjusted for tobacco smoking, consumption of alcoholic beverages, and/or HPV infection, the major risk factors for oral cancer, confirmed this evaluation. Additionally, positive exposure–response relationships were reported in some studies.

2.6.2 Precancerous lesions of the oral cavity

Many cohort, case–control and cross-sectional studies from a wide range of countries have noted a high prevalence of oral precancerous disorders (leukoplakia, erythroplakia, oral submucous fibrosis) among users of betel quid and areca nut compared to non-users. Among betel quid users with added tobacco in Sri Lanka and India, significant associations were reported in four studies after adjusting for or stratifying by tobacco smoking or consumption of alcoholic beverages. The association between betel quid without added tobacco and precancerous disorders was examined in 6 studies from India, Taiwan, China and Papua New Guinea. A significant positive association was found in all studies and a significant dose–response was observed in 2 of them. Among users of areca nut only, significant associations were reported after adjusting for stratifying by tobacco smoking or consumption of alcoholic beverages. A significant positive association was reported from three studies in Pakistan and India that examined the association between areca nut use and oral submucous fibrosis.

2.6.3 Pharynx

Numerous studies, some of cohort and many of case–control design, have been performed on chewing betel quid, with or without tobacco, and the risk for cancers of the naso-, oro- and hypopharynx, or of the pharynx not otherwise specified. Chewing betel quid with added tobacco is causally associated with cancers of the pharynx and its subsites. Positive exposure–response relationships were noted in some studies, strengthening the credibility of a causal association. In some studies it was possible to demonstrate a synergistic relationship between betel quid chewing, tobacco smoking and consumption of alcoholic beverages on the risk of cancer of the pharynx.

2.6.4 Oesophagus

One cohort and several case–control studies have been performed on chewing betel quid and the risk for cancer of the oesophagus. Chewing betel quid, both with and without added tobacco, causes cancer of the oesophagus. Positive exposure–response relationships were reported in some studies, strengthening the credibility of a causal association. A synergistic relationship between betel quid chewing, tobacco smoking and consumption of alcoholic beverages on the risk of cancer of the oesophagus was demonstrated in some studies.

2.6.5 Liver

The association between betel quid without added tobacco and cancer of the liver has been evaluated in six studies: 3 cohort studies, 2 case–control and 1 cross-sectional study. Five studies were from Taiwan, China, where betel quid is chewed without added tobacco, and one study was from Thailand, in which the use of betel quid with or without added tobacco was not specified. Significant positive associations were observed in 4 of the 5 Taiwanese studies, although confounding by tobacco smoking, alcohol consumption, hepatitis B or C virus positivity could not be ruled out. Significant positive dose–response relationships with the amount of betel quid chewed were observed in two studies, although confounding could not be ruled out.

2.6.6 Other sites

Several epidemiological studies assessed cancers at other sites but there are not enough data to permit a conclusion.

3. Cancer in Experimental Animals

Several studies investigating the carcinogenicity of betel quid and areca nut in experimental animal have inadequate numbers of animals per group, inadequate frequency and duration of treatment, absence of appropriate controls, ambiguous description of lesions, low survival of animals and inadequate reporting of survival data. Studies that were considered uninformative are not included in the present evaluation.

Representative studies are reported below and are described in Tables 3.1, 3.2, 3.3.

3.1 Mouse

Administration of either areca nut, areca nut and tobacco, arecoline or *pan masala* by skin application did not produce tumours in some studies (Ranadive *et al.*, 1976; Pai *et al.*, 1981; Ramchandani *et al.*, 1998). Topical application of an extract of areca nut extract and tobacco produced epidermoid carcinomas in a small number (2/23) of C17 mice (Ranadive *et al.*, 1976).

A group of 21 male Swiss mice was administered 0.1 mL of an aqueous extract of areca nut (containing 1.5 mg arecoline and 1.9 mg polyphenol) by gavage on five days a week for life. Twelve out of 21 treated mice developed tumours (five hepatocellular carcinomas [$P < 0.05$], two liver haemangiomas, two lung adenocarcinomas, one adenocarcinoma, one squamous cell carcinoma of the stomach, and one leukaemia). No tumour was observed in 20 untreated controls (Bhide *et al.*, 1979).

Administration of 0.1 mL of an aqueous extract of areca nut (containing 1.5 mg arecoline) on five days a week for life by gavage produced lung adenocarcinomas in 47% (9/19, $P < 0.05$) of male Swiss mice. One untreated control mouse of 20 developed a lung adenocarcinoma (Shirname *et al.*, 1983).

Administration by gavage of arecoline hydrochloride, a component of areca nut, induced three squamous cell carcinomas of the stomach, four lung adenocarcinomas and eight liver haemangiomas [not significant] in 43% (15/35) male Swiss mice. One untreated control mouse of 20 developed an unspecified tumour (Bhide *et al.*, 1984).

Dietary feeding of unprocessed areca nut or application of a paste of unprocessed areca nut to the oral cavity of male and female Swiss mice induced squamous cell carcinomas and papillomas in the oesophagus of a small number of

Table 3.1 Carcinogenicity studies of administration of areca nut or betel quid in experimental animals

Species, strain (sex) Duration Reference	Route Dosing regimen Animals/group at start	Incidence and/or multiplicity of tumours	Significance	Comments
Mouse, Swiss (M, F) Lifetime Ranadive *et al.* (1976)	Subcutaneous injection	Fibrosarcomas:		
	Areca nut (hot aqueous extract), 50 mg/mL, 0.2 mL, once/wk for 6 wk; 20/group	14/20	[$P < 0.0001$]	
	Areca nut (cold aqueous extract), 50 mg/mL, 0.2 mL, once/wk for 6 wk; 20/group	10/20	[$P < 0.001$]	
	Distilled water, 0.2 mL, once/wk for 10 wk; 25/group	0/25	-	
Mouse, Swiss (M, F) Lifetime Ranadive *et al.* (1976)	Topical application	Skin tumours:		
	Areca nut/DMSO extract, 30 g areca nut in 20 mL DMSO, 0.1 mL, 3 × /wk; 10M+8F/group	0/18	NS	
	Tobacco/DMSO extract, 5 g tobacco in 20 mL DMSO, 0.1 mL, 3 × /wk; 10M+6F/group	0/16	NS	
	Areca nut + tobacco/DMSO extract, 30 g areca nut + 5 g tobacco in 20 mL DMSO, 0.1 mL, 3 × /wk; 11M+12F/group	1/23 (papillomas), 2/23 (carcinomas)	NS	
	DSMO 0.1 mL, 3 × /wk; 9M+12F/group	0/21	-	
Mouse, Swiss (M) Lifetime Shivapurkar *et al.* (1980)	Subcutaneous injection			Age not specified
	Areca nut/polyphenol fraction, 0.1 mL, once/wk for 13 wk (total dose, 24.7 mg polyphenol)	20/20 (fibrosarcoma, 16/20; hepatoma, 1/20; lung adenocarcinoma, 3/20)	[$P < 0.0001$] (fibrosarcomas)	
	Betel quid aqueous extract, 0.2 mL, once/wk for 13 wk (total dose, 38.4 mg alkaloid + 46.0 mg polyphenol)	7/20 (fibrosarcoma)	[$P < 0.01$]	
	Distilled water, 0.1 mL, once/wk for 13 wk 20/group	0/20	-	
Rat, NIH Black (M, F) 68 wk Kapadia *et al.* (1978)	Subcutaneous injection	Fibrosarcomas:		
	Areca nut/tannin rich areca nut extract, 0.5 mL, once/wk for 56 wk	30/30	Significant	
	Saline, 0.5 mL, once/wk for 56 wk 30/group	0/30	-	

Table 3.1 (continued)

Species, strain (sex) Duration Reference	Route Dosing regimen Animals/group at start	Incidence and/or multiplicity of tumours	Significance	Comments
Hamster, Syrian golden (M) 21 wk Suri *et al.* (1971)	Cheek pouch application	Cheek pouch squamous cell carcinomas:		
	DMSO extract of areca nut, 3 × /wk	8/21	[$P < 0.05$]	
	DMSO extract of areca nut + tobacco, 3 × /wk	16/21	[$P < 0.0001$]	
	DMSO-treated control, 3 × /wk 11–21/group	0/11	-	
Hamster, Syrian golden & white mutant (M, F) 21 mo Ranadive *et al.* (1979)	Cheek pouch application	Forestomach carcinomas–Cheek pouch carcinomas:		Lack of information on sex and strain distribution.
	Areca nut aqueous extract, 3 × /wk	4/21–1/21	[$P < 0.05$]–[NS]	
	Polyphenol fraction of areca nut, 3 × /wk	4/20–1/20	[$P < 0.05$]–[NS]	
	Areca nut pieces + aqueous extract of areca nut, 3 × /wk	6/13–0/13	[$P < 0.001$]–[NS]	
	Betel quid aqueous extract, 3 × /wk	5/20–0/20	[$P < 0.01$]–[NS]	
	Betel quid aqueous extract + tobacco, 3 × /wk	4/13–0/13	[$P < 0.01$]–[NS]	
	Untreated control 13–30/group	0/30–0/30	-	
Hamster, Syrian golden & white mutant (M, F) 21 mo Ranadive *et al.* (1979)	Cheek pouch implantation	Forestomach carcinomas–Cheek pouch carcinomas:		Lack of information on sex and strain distribution.
	Areca nut powder, in capsule, 1 × /2wk	6/19–4/19	[NS]–[NS]	
	Capsule control	0/9–0/9	-	
	Betel quid, 0.8–13 mg of material in wax pellet, once/2wk	8/18–4/18	[$P < 0.001$]–[$P < 0.05$]	
	Betel quid + tobacco, 0.8–13 mg of test material in wax pellet, once/2wk	6/21–3/21	[$P < 0.01$]–[NS]	
	Wax pellet control 9–25/group	0/25–0/25	-	

DMSO, dimethyl sulfoxide; F, female; M, male; mo, month or months. NS, not significant; wk, week or weeks

Table 3.2 Carcinogenicity studies of administration of *pan masala* in mice

Species, strain (sex) Duration Reference	Route Dosing regimen Animals/group at start	Incidence and/or multiplicity of tumours	Significance	Comments
Mouse, Swiss S/RVCri (M, F) Lifetime Bhisey et al. (1999)	Diet		Positive trend for lung adenocarcinoma ($P < 0.004$)	
	Normal diet	0/108		
	Pan masala 2.5% in diet, lifetime	Liver haemangioma, 7/108; lung adenocarcinoma, 3/108; liver adenocarcinoma, 1/108; hepatoma, 1/108; forestomach papilloma, 1/108		
	Pan masala 5% in diet, lifetime 108/group	Liver haemangioma, 1/108; lung adenocarcinoma, 5/108; forestomach carcinoma, 1/108; testicular lymphoma, 1/108		
Mouse, Swiss (M, F) 56 wk Nigam et al. (2001)	Diet		NS	
	Pan masala 2% in diet, 56 wk	Lung tumour, 2/12; haemangioma, 1/12; haemangioendothelioma, 1/12		
	Normal diet, 56 wk 12/group	Lung tumour, 1/12		
Mouse, ICRC (M, F) 6 mo Ramchandani et al. (1998)	Gavage		$P < 0.001$; $P < 0.01$	EPME tested as promoter
	NDEA in drinking-water for 4 d (16 mg/kg bw) followed by EPME by gavage (25 mg/treatment) 5 × /wk for 6 mo	Forestomach papilloma, 17/26; esophageal papilloma, 11/26		
	NDEA in drinking-water for 4 d (16 mg/kg bw) followed by distilled water by gavage 5 × /wk for 6 mo 30/group	Forestomach papilloma, 5/27; esophageal papilloma, 3/27	-;-	

Table 3.2 (continued)

Species, strain (sex) Duration Reference	Route Dosing regimen Animals/group at start	Incidence and/or multiplicity of tumours	Significance	Comments
Mouse, Swiss Bare (F) 40 wk Ramchandani et al. (1998)	Topical application DMBA (20 nmol in 100 µl acetone) followed by EPME (25 mg in 100 µl acetone) 2x/wk for 40 wk	Skin papilloma: 6.8/mouse	$P < 0.05$	EPME tested as promoter
	DMBA (20 nmol in 100 µl acetone) followed by 100 µl acetone twice/wk for 40 wk 15/group	Skin papilloma: 4.2/mouse	-	

bw, body weight; d, day or days; DMBA, 7,12-dimethylbenz[*a*]anthracene; EPME, Ethanolic *pan masala* extract; F, female; M, male; mo, month or months; NDEA, *N*-nitrosodiethylamine; NS, not significant; wk, week or weeks

Table 3.3 Carcinogenicity studies of administration of areca nut, betel quid or betel leaf with known carcinogens or modifiers of cancer risk in experimental animals

Species, strain (sex) Duration Reference	Route Dosing regimen Animals/group at start	Incidence and/or multiplicity of tumours (%)	Significance	Comments
Mouse, Swiss (M) 180 d Padma *et al.* (1989)	Intragastric instillation		*P* < 0.005, tumour multiplicity inhibition	
	BLE (1 mg/d, 5 × /wk) for 2 wk, followed by B[*a*]P by gavage (1 mg/d, 2 × /wk) for 4 wk, followed by BLE (1 mg/d, twice/wk) for 2 wk	Forestomach papilloma: 0.9/mouse		
	B[*a*]P by gavage (1 mg/d, twice/wk) for 4 wk 20/group	Forestomach papilloma: 4.9/mouse	-	
Mouse, Swiss (M) 180 d Padma *et al.* (1989)	Drinking-water		-	
	NNN, application to tongue (22 mg/mouse)	Total: 13/19 (lung, 4/19; stomach, 5/19; Lung + stomach, 3/19; Liver + stomach, 1/19)		
	NNN, application to tongue (22 mg/mouse); BLE in drinking-water 5 × /wk (2.5 mg/d)	Total: 3/21 (lung)	[*P* < 0.005], inhibition of stomach tumourigenesis	
	NNK, application to tongue (22 mg/mouse)	Total: 10/13 (lung, 8/13; stomach, 1/13;lung + liver, 1/13)	-	
	NNK, application to tongue (22 mg/mouse); BLE in drinking-water 5 × /wk (2.5 mg/d)	Total: 7/15 (lung, 5/15; stomach, 1/15; lung + LIVER, 1/15)	NS	
	Untreated control 20/group	Total: 2/18 (lung)	-	
Hamster, Syrian golden (M) 30 wk Wong *et al.* (1992)	Cheek pouch insertion	Cheek pouch		
	DMBA 0.5%, 3 × /wk for 4 wk	Squamous cell carcinoma: 1/9	-	
	DMBA 0.5%, 3 × /wk for 4 wk, followed by betel quid twice/wk for 24 wk 10/group	Squamous cell carcinoma: 6/9	*P* < 0.05	
Hamster, Syrian golden (M) 18 wk Wong *et al.* (1992)	Cheek pouch insertion	Cheek pouch		
	DMBA 0.5%, 3 × /wk for 6 wk	Squamous cell carcinoma: 1/9	-	
	DMBA 0.5%, 3 × /wk for 6 wk, followed by betel quid twice/wk for 12 wk 10/group	Squamous cell carcinoma: 7/7	*P* < 0.01	

Table 3.3 (continued)

Species, strain (sex) Duration Reference	Route Dosing regimen Animals/group at start	Incidence and/or multiplicity of tumours (%)	Significance	Comments
Hamster, Syrian golden (M) 35 wk Jin *et al.* (1996)	Cheek pouch insertion or painting DMBA 0.5%, 3 × /wk for 4 wk DMBA 0.5%, 3 × /wk for 4 wk, followed by areca nut fibre 3 × /wk for 24 wk DMBA 0.5%, 3 × /wk for 4 wk, followed by cold aqueous extract of areca nut 3 × /wk for 24 wk 10/group	Cheek pouch Squamous cell carcinoma: 2/9 Squamous cell carcinoma: 9/10 Squamous cell carcinoma: 7/10	 - $P < 0.01$ $P < 0.05$	

BLE, Betel leaf extract; B[*a*]P, benzo[*a*]pyrene; d, day or days; DMBA, 7,12-dimethylbenz[*a*]anthracene; M, male; NNN, *N'*-Nitrosonornicotine; NNK, 4-(*N*-Nitrosomethylamino)-1-(3-pyridyl)-1-butanone; NS, not significant; wk, week or weeks animals. No oesophageal tumours were observed in control mice (Rao & Das, 1989).

Subcutaneous injections of hot and cold areca nut extracts to Swiss mice increased the incidence of fibrosarcomas at the injection site (Ranadive *et al.*, 1976). Subcutaneous injections of a polyphenol fraction of areca nut to Swiss mice produced fibrosarcomas in 80% (16/20) of the animals (Shivapurkar *et al.*, 1980). In the same study, 35% (7/20) of mice concurrently treated with an aqueous extract of betel quid developed fibrosarcomas.

In a skin tumourigenesis experiment using 7,12-dimethylbenz[*a*]anthracene (DMBA) plus croton oil, feeding of areca nut did not influence the incidence of skin papilloma in Swiss mice (Singh & Rao, 1995).

Betel leaf extract given to mice treated with benzo[*a*]pyrene (B[*a*]P) by gavage reduced the incidence and multiplicity of B[*a*]P-induced forestomach papillomas (Padma *et al.*, 1989; Bhide *et al.*, 1991). It also reduced stomach tumour incidence in mice treated with *N*′-nitrosonornicotine or 4-(*N*-nitrosomethylamino)-1-(3-pyridyl)-1-butanone (Padma *et al.*, 1989).

Lifetime feeding of a diet containing either 2.5% or 5% *pan masala* to Swiss mice induced a variety of benign and malignant tumours in the liver, stomach and lung. No tumours were found in controls. A significant positive trend ($P = 0.004$) with dose was observed in the number of mice with lung adenocarcinoma (Bhisey *et al.*, 1999).

Administration of *pan masala* in the diet produced liver haemangiomas and papillary adenomas of the lung in Swiss mice [not significant]. A few lung adenomas, liver tumours, and benign tumours at some other sites were also observed in mice receiving *pan masala* and tobacco in the diet (Nigam *et al.*, 2001).

Topical application of an extract of *pan masala* to the skin of DMBA-initiated Swiss mice increased significantly the tumour multiplicity of skin papillomas. In the same study, administration of a *pan masala* extract by gavage to ICRC mice given *N*-nitrosodiethylamine (NDEA) in the drinking-water increased the incidence of squamous cell papillomas of the forestomach and oesophagus (Ramchandani *et al.*, 1998).

3.2 Rat

Subcutaneous injection of a tannin rich-extract of areca nut produced fibrosarcomas at the injection site in 30/30 NIH Black rats. No tumours were observed in 30 saline-treated controls (Kapadia *et al.*, 1978).

Dietary administration of areca nut to ACI rats fed vitamin A-sufficient or -deficient diets did not increase tumour incidence (Tanaka *et al.*, 1983).

In ACI rats treated with 4-nitroquinoline-1-oxide in the drinking-water followed by areca nut in the diet, the incidence of squamous cell carcinoma of the tongue was significantly greater (12/17 versus 4/14, $P < 0.0205$) than in animals given 4-nitroquinoline-1-oxide alone (Tanaka *et al.*, 1986).

Oral administration to Holtzman rats of an aqueous extract of betel leaf inhibited DMBA-induced mammary carcinogenesis (6/26 versus 17/27, $P < 0.05$) when given concurrently with DMBA (Rao *et al.*, 1985).

3.3 Hamster

A topical application of either DMSO extracts of areca nut or areca nut with tobacco on the cheek-pouch mucosa increased the incidence of squamous cell carcinoma and leukoplakia in Syrian golden hamster (Suri *et al.*, 1971).

Implantation in the cheek pouch of either (i) areca nut powder or (ii) betel quid with or without tobacco produced cheek-pouch carcinomas and forestomach carcinomas in Syrian golden hamsters and white mutant hamsters. In the same study, topical application of extracts of betel quid with or without tobacco increased the incidence of forestomach carcinomas. Also, application of either (i) areca nut, (ii) a polyphenol fraction of areca nut, or (iii) areca nut pieces with extract of areca nut increased the incidence of forestomach carcinomas (Ranadive *et al.*, 1979). [The Working Group noted the lack of information on sex and strain distribution.]

Application of an extract of areca nut to the B[*a*]P-initiated cheek pouch of Syrian golden hamsters led to a slight increase in the incidence of squamous cell papillomas and carcinomas compared to B[*a*]P-only-treated animals. In the same study, application of betel leaf extract to B[*a*]P-initiated hamster cheek pouch reduced significantly the incidence of squamous cell papillomas and carcinomas (Rao, 1984).

Administration to the hamsters cheek-pouch of either areca nut fibre or areca nut extract by insertion (Jin *et al.*, 1996) or arecaidine by painting (Lin *et al.*, 1996) increased significantly the incidence of cheek pouch squamous cell carcinomas initiated by application of DMBA.

Concomitant treatment of hamster cheek pouch with DMBA and with an extract of betel quid, by insertion or painting, increased significantly the incidence (Wong *et al.*, 1992) or multiplicity (Lin *et al.*, 1997) of cheek pouch squamous cell carcinomas.

3.4 Baboon

Insertion into a surgically created buccal pouch for 42 months of a betel quid preparation with tobacco in seven baboons or without tobacco in five baboons did not lead to tumour formation (Hamner, 1972).

3.5 Synthesis

In mice, administration by gavage of areca nut extracts containing arecholine increased the incidence of lung adenocarcinoma in one study and of hepatocellular carcinomas in another study. Subcutaneous injections of hot and cold areca nut extracts in one study and of a polyphenol fraction of areca nut in another study increased the incidence of fibrosarcoma. In one study in rats, subcutaneous injection of an areca nut extract also produced fibrosarcomas.

In mice, subcutaneous injection of an extract of betel quid increased the incidence of fibrosarcoma in one study.

In one study in hamsters, topical application of extracts of areca nut or areca nut with tobacco increased the incidence of cheek pouch squamous cell carcinoma. In another similar study, betel quid and betel quid plus tobacco extracts, and areca nut pieces, extracts and polyphenol fractions, increased the incidence of forestomach carcinomas. In a third study, cheek pouch implantation of betel quid increased the incidence of forestomach and cheek pouch carcinomas; implantation of betel quid plus tobacco increased the incidence of forestomach carcinomas. Areca nut or betel quid also promoted DMBA-induced cheek pouch squamous cell carcinomas.

In one study in mice, feeding of a diet containing *pan masala* increased the incidence of lung adenocarcinomas. *Pan masala* also enhanced DMBA-induced skin papillomas and NDEA-induced forestomach and oesophagus papillomas.

Betel leaf extracts reduced the incidence of B[*a*]P-induced squamous cell tumours of the oral cavity in hamsters, of B[*a*]P-induced forestomach papillomas and NNN- and NNK-induced stomach tumours in mice, and of DMBA-induced mammary tumours in rats.

4. Other Relevant Data

For the effects of chewing betel quid and areca nut with tobacco, we refer the reader to Section 4 of the *Monograph* on Tobacco Smoking in this volume.

4.1 Distribution and metabolism of the constituents of betel quid

Metabolism, toxicity, genotoxicity, mutation induction in cancer-related genes, immunomodulatory effects and gene–environment interactions have been investigated for arecoline, the major alkaloid in areca nut, and for other betel-quid ingredients, e.g. catechu, betel leaf and slaked lime. In addition, reactive oxygen species and areca nut-derived nitrosamines are produced in situ in saliva during betel-quid chewing, and their adverse effects have been studied in the oral cavity of betel-quid chewers and in experimental systems.

Areca nut contains several alkaloids and tannins (polyphenols). Arecoline is the most abundant alkaloid, whereas arecaidine, guvacine and guvacoline occur in smaller quantities (Fig. 4.1). In rodents, arecoline is rapidly metabolized in both liver and kidney. In rats, arecoline is de-esterified in the liver to arecaidine, and both arecoline and arecaidine are excreted as the mercapturic acid (Boyland & Nery, 1969). The metabolism of arecoline and arecaidine was investigated in the mouse using a metabolomic approach (Giri *et al.*, 2006). The major metabolite of both alkaloids, *N*-methylnipecotic acid, is a newly discovered metabolite (see Fig. 4.1). A total of 11 metabolites of arecoline were identified. Arecaidine shares six of these with arecoline.

4.1.1 Formation of N-nitroso compounds in the oral cavity

Areca nut contains secondary and tertiary amines that can be nitrosated in saliva during betel-quid chewing by reaction with nitrite in the presence of thiocyanate as a nitrosation catalyst (Fig. 4.1).

Three areca nut-derived nitrosamines, i.e. 3-methylnitrosaminopropionitrile (MNPN; a rodent carcinogen), *N*-nitrosoguvacine (NGC) and *N*-nitrosoguvacoline (NGL) have been detected in the saliva of betel-quid chewers (Nair *et al.*, 1985; Prokopczyk *et al.*, 1987; IARC, 2004). The formation of these nitrosamines can be mimicked *in vitro* by nitrosation with nitrite, thiocyanate and arecoline, which are all present in saliva. Endogenous nitrosation reactions in the oral cavity have been demonstrated in chewers of betel quid mixed with proline (a probe for ingested secondary amines), by measuring increased levels of *N*-nitrosoproline in saliva and urine (Nair *et al.*, 1987a). As chewers often swallow the quid – which contains nitrosamine precursors – the intragastric nitrosation reaction of secondary and tertiary amines may occur at higher rates due to the low pH in the stomach (Nair *et al.*, 1985).

4.1.2 Formation of reactive oxygen species in the oral cavity

Direct evidence that oxidative stress and reactive oxygen species such as the hydroxyl radical ($HO^{\bullet}$) are generated in the oral cavity during betel-quid chewing was provided by measuring the formation of *ortho*- and *meta*-tyrosines from L-phenylalanine in human saliva (Nair *et al.*, 1995). Auto-oxidation of polyphenols in areca nut and catechu generates the superoxide anion ($O_2^{\bullet -}$), especially at the high pH of slaked lime. The superoxide anion is converted to H_2O_2, which reacts in the presence of copper and iron ions (present in µg/gram amounts in

Fig. 4.1 Relationship of areca-nut alkaloids to areca-nut-derived nitrosamines (formed by nitrosation) and a urinary metabolite of *N*-nitrosoguvacoline and *N*-nitrosoguvacine

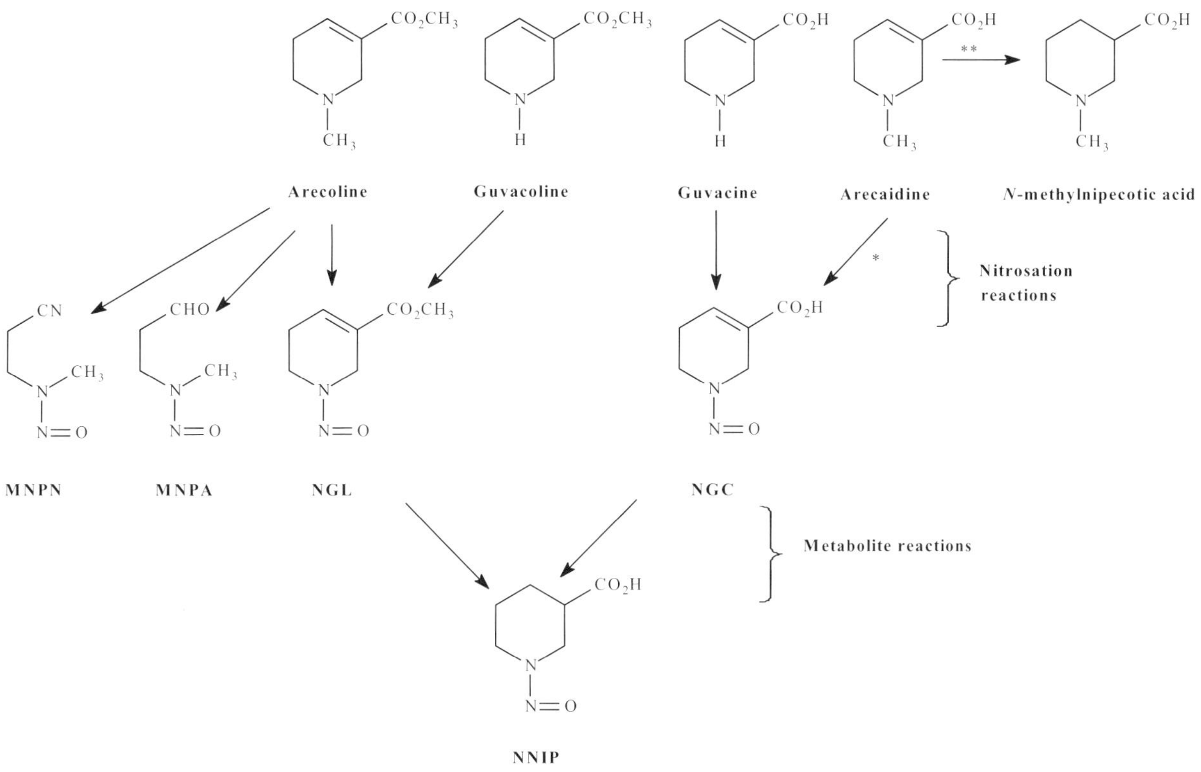

Arecoline · Guvacoline · Guvacine · Arecaidine · *N*-methylnipecotic acid

Nitrosation reactions

MNPN · MNPA · NGL · NGC

Metabolite reactions

NNIP

Adapted from Wenke & Hoffmann (1983), Nair *et al.* (1985), and Ohshima *et al.* (1989)

MNPA, 3-methylnitrosaminopropionaldehyde; MNPN, 3-methylnitrosaminopropionitrile; NGC, *N*-nitrosoguvacine; NGL, *N*-nitrosoguvacoline; NNIP, *N*-nitrosonipecotic acid

* It is likely that nitrosation of arecaidine would produce NGC but this has not been demonstrated.

** *N*-methylnipecotic acid is a recently isolated metabolite of arecoline; nitrosation reactions on this metabolite have not been studied (Giri *et al.*, 2006).

areca nut, catechu and slaked lime) to generate hydroxyl radicals (Nair *et al.*, 1987b). These can induce oxidation of deoxyguanosine to yield 8-hydroxydeoxyguanosine 8-(OH-dG) and DNA strand-breaks (IARC, 2004). Areca-nut extract and arecoline treatment led to depletion of glutathione (GSH) and reduction of glutathione-*S*-transferase (GST) activity in human oral cells and in rodent liver; both processes are known to increase cellular damage and DNA lesions (Chang *et al.*, 2001a, b).

4.2 Genetic and related effects

The genetic and related effects of areca nut and the various constituents of betel quid without tobacco were reviewed in detail by IARC (2004) and are summarized below.

4.2.1 Humans

Elevated formation of micronuclei has been reported in oral exfoliated cells in chewers of betel quid without tobacco. Micronucleus formation has been observed in precancerous lesions in the oral cavity of chewers of betel quid alone (Dave *et al.*, 1991; Kayal *et al.*, 1993), and betel quid with tobacco (Stich *et al.*, 1989, 1991; Nair *et al.*, 1991).

Elevated sister-chromatid exchange and micronucleus formation have been demonstrated in cultured peripheral lymphocytes collected from chewers of areca nut without tobacco and slaked lime (Dave *et al.*, 1991, 1992; Desai *et al.*, 1996) and with tobacco (Adhvaryu *et al.*, 1986).

In subjects chewing betel quid without tobacco accumulation of p53 protein was observed (Kaur *et al.*, 1994, 1998; Yan *et al.*, 1996; Thongsuksai & Boonyaphiphat, 2001; Chang *et al.*, 2002a). *TP53 m*RNA was frequently downregulated in betel quid chewing associated oral cancer (Tsai *et al.*, 2008).

Arecoline modulates matrix metalloproteinases (MMPs) and their tissue inhibitors (TIMPs), as well as the activity of lysyl oxidase, which leads to the accumulation of collagen in oral mucosal fibroblasts (Trivedy *et al.*, 1999a, 2001; Chang *et al.*, 2002b). Areca-nut polyphenols inhibit collagenases and increase the cross-linkage of collagen, reducing its degradation (Scutt *et al.*, 1987). These events may underlie the generation of oral submucous fibrosis in betel-quid chewers (Chang *et al.*, 2002b), which could be further enhanced by the release of copper ions, present in areca nut, catechu and slaked lime into the oral cavity of the chewers; inorganic copper salts increased the production of collagen by oral fibroblasts (Trivedy *et al.*, 1999b, 2001).

Cyclooxygenase-2 (COX2) is an inducible enzyme responsible for prostaglandin synthesis in certain inflammatory diseases. Its expression was significantly higher in oral submucous fibrosis specimens than in buccal mucosal fibroblasts (Tsai *et al.*, 2003).

In an oral epithelial cell line, arecoline was found to elevate the expression of the heat-shock protein HSP70 and haem oxygenase HO-1 mRNA in a dose- and time-dependent manner (Lee *et al.*, 2008a, b). Expression of HSP70 and HO-1 was significantly higher in specimens of human oral squamous cell carcinoma associated with areca-quid chewing. Areca-nut extracts increased the expression of inflammatory cytokines, tumour necrosis factor-α, interleukin-1-β, interleukin-6, and interleukin-8, in peripheral blood mononuclear cells (Chang *et al.*, 2009).

Collagen-related genes (*COLA1* and *COLA2*) and collagenase-1 lysil oxidase, transforming growth factor β (TGF-β1) and cystatin C involved in oral submucous fibrosis and DNA-repair genes (X-ray repair cross complementing 1 *XRCC1*) have been investigated in small studies in India, Taiwan, China, in relation to oral and oesophageal cancer and premalignant lesions (Lee *et al.*, 2001; Chiu *et al.*, 2002). No clear gene-environment interactions could be established because of the concurrent confounding by tobacco chewing and smoking or alcohol consumption (IARC, 2004).

4.2.2 Experimental systems

(a) Areca nut extracts

Extracts of betel quid and *pan masala* induced sister chromatid exchange and sperm abnormalities in mice. Betel quid extracts were mutagenic in bacteria and induced chromosomal aberrations, sister chromatid exchange and micronucleus formation in Chinese hamster ovary cells.

Aqueous extracts of areca nut produced gene conversion in yeast, DNA strand-breaks, gene mutation, chromosomal aberrations, sister chromatid exchange and micronucleus formation in rodent cells, both *in vitro* and *in vivo*. It also induced cell transformation in mouse C3H10T1/2 cells and DNA strand-breaks, unscheduled DNA synthesis and DNA–protein crosslinks in cultured human buccal and laryngeal epithelial cells.

(b) Areca nut alkaloids

Arecoline and other areca-nut alkaloids gave positive responses in most bacterial mutagenicity assays, and induced chromosomal aberrations, micronucleus formation and sister chromatid exchange in mammalian cells, both *in vitro* and *in vivo*. Arecoline inhibited *Tp53* mRNA expression and its transactivating function, repressed DNA repair and triggered DNA damage response in human epithelial cells (Tsai *et al.*, 2008).

(a) Areca-nut-derived nitrosamines

Three areca-nut-derived nitrosamines, i.e. *N*-nitrosoguvacoline (NGL), *N*-nitrosoguvacine (NGC) and 3-methylnitrosaminopropionitrile (MNPN), were detected in the saliva of chewers of betel quid without tobacco. Genotoxic effects of these nitrosamines and of 3-methylnitrosaminopropionaldehyde (MNPA) can be summarized as follows: NGL but not NGC was mutagenic to bacteria. MNPN did not induced DNA single-strand breaks in human buccal epithelial cells (Sundqvist *et al.*, 1989). MNPN formed the DNA adducts 7-methylguanine and O^6-methylguanine (a pro-mutagenic DNA adduct) as well as (2-cyanoethyl)guanines in treated rats (Prokopczyk *et al.*, 1987, 1988). MNPA was not mutagenic in the presence of a metabolic activating system but caused single-strand breaks and DNA crosslinks in human buccal epithelial cells (Sundqvist *et al.*, 1989; Sundqvist & Grafström, 1992).

In Taiwan, China, areca nut is often chewed with fresh betel inflorescence). Betel inflorescence contains safrole and hydroxychavicol at relatively high concentrations (10–15 mg/g fresh nut) (IARC, 2004). Safrole is a possible human carcinogen (IARC, 1987). Taiwanese betel quid-chewers had 3-fold higher urinary excretion of hydroxychavicol, a metabolite of safrole, than non-chewers (Chang *et al.*, 2002c). They also had a high frequency of safrole-like DNA adducts (detected by ^{32}P-postlabelling) in the oral cavity that co-eluted with synthetic safrole-2′deoxyguanosine 3′-monophosphate adducts (Chen *et al.*, 1999). In HBsAg/HCV seronegative hepatocarcinoma, safrole-type DNA adducts were found in hepatic tissues of hepatocarcinoma patients who had chewed betel quid for > 10 years (Chung *et al.*, 2008).

4.3 Mechanistic considerations

Betel quid and areca-nut ingredients and extracts exert a variety of genetic and related effects (Section 4.2.1). Continuous local irritation of buccal epithelial cells caused by betel quid and its ingredients, particularly areca nut and slaked lime, can generate chronic inflammation, oxidative stress and cytokine production. Reactive oxygen species generated during chewing of betel quid and other genotoxic reactants formed from arecoline and areca nut-derived nitrosamines, can lead to DNA- and genetic damage in exposed oral keratinocytes. Persistent oxidative stress can drive affected cells to uncontrolled proliferation and hyperplastic/dysplastic lesions. Chronic occurrence of these toxic insults in the oral cavity of chewers could drive these pre-neoplastic cells towards full malignancy.

4.4 Synthesis

These mechanistic data support the causal associations for carcinogenicity observed in humans at several target sites (indicated in Section 2 of this *Monograph*) for chewers of betel quid without tobacco, and areca nut.

5 Evaluation

There is *sufficient* evidence in humans for the carcinogenicity of betel quid with added tobacco. Betel quid with added tobacco causes cancers of the oral cavity, pharynx and oesophagus.

There is *sufficient* evidence in humans for the carcinogenicity of betel quid without added tobacco. Betel quid without added tobacco causes cancers of the oral cavity and oesophagus. Also, a positive association has been observed between exposure to betel quid without added tobacco and cancer of the liver.

There is *sufficient* evidence in experimental animals for the carcinogenicity of betel quid with added tobacco.

There is *sufficient* evidence in experimental animals for the carcinogenicity of betel quid without added tobacco.

There is *sufficient* evidence in experimental animals for the carcinogenicity of areca nut.

There is *limited* evidence in experimental animals for the carcinogenicity of *pan masala.*

There is *evidence suggesting lack of carcinogenicity* of betel leaf in experimental animals.

Betel quid with added tobacco is *carcinogenic to humans (Group 1).*

Betel quid without added tobacco is *carcinogenic to humans (Group 1).*

Areca nut is *carcinogenic to humans (Group 1).*

References

Adhvaryu SG, Bhatt RG, Dayal PK *et al.* (1986). SCE frequencies in lymphocytes of tobacco/betel nut chewers and patients with oral submucous fibrosis. *Br J Cancer*, 53: 141–143. doi:10.1038/bjc.1986.20 PMID:3947511

Ahmad MS, Ali SA, Ali AS, Chaubey KK (2006). Epidemiological and etiological study of oral submucous fibrosis among gutkha chewers of Patna, Bihar, India. *J Indian Soc Pedod Prev Dent*, 24: 84–89. PMID:16823233

Anwar S, Williams SA, Scott-Smith J *et al.* (2005). A comparison of attitudes and practices of *gutka* users and non-users in Chitrakoot, India. A pilot. *Prim Dent Care*, 12: 5–10. PMID:15703153

Ariyawardana A, Athukorala AD, Arulanandam A (2006). Effect of betel chewing, tobacco smoking and alcohol consumption on oral submucous fibrosis: a case-control study in Sri Lanka. *J Oral Pathol Med*, 35: 197–201. PMID:16519765

Ariyawardana A, Sitheeque MA, Ranasinghe AW *et al.* (2007). Prevalence of oral cancer and pre-cancer and associated risk factors among tea estate workers in the central Sri Lanka. *J Oral Pathol Med*, 36: 581–587. PMID:17944750

Arjungi KN (1976). Areca nut: a review. *Arzneimittelforschung*, 26: 951–956. PMID:786304

Balaram P, Sridhar H, Rajkumar T *et al.* (2002). Oral cancer in southern India: the influence of smoking, drinking, paan-chewing and oral hygiene. *Int J Cancer*, 98: 440–445. PMID:11920597

Bansode NN (2002). An exploratory study on gutkha and smokeless tobacco consumption. *Nurs J India*, 93: 127–128. PMID:12649939

Bhargava K, Smith LW, Mani NJ *et al.* (1975). A follow up study of oral cancer and precancerous lesions in 57,518 industrial workers of Gujarat, India. *Indian J Cancer*, 12: 124–129. PMID:1184078

Bhide SV, Gothoskar SV, Shivapurkar NM (1984). Arecoline tumorigenicity in Swiss strain mice on normal and vitamin B deficient diet. *J Cancer Res Clin Oncol*, 107: 169–171. doi:10.1007/BF01032602 PMID:6736104

Bhide SV, Shivapurkar NM, Gothoskar SV, Ranadive KJ (1979). Carcinogenicity of betel quid ingredients: feeding mice with aqueous extract and the polyphenol fraction of betel nut. *Br J Cancer*, 40: 922–926. doi:10.1038/bjc.1979.286 PMID:526433

Bhide SV, Zariwala MB, Amonkar AJ, Azuine MA (1991). Chemopreventive efficacy of a betel leaf extract against benzo[a]pyrene-induced forestomach tumors in mice. *J Ethnopharmacol*, 34: 207–213. doi:10.1016/0378-8741(91)90039-G PMID:1795525

Bhisey RA, Ramchandani AG, D'Souza AV *et al.* (1999). Long-term carcinogenicity of pan masala in Swiss mice. *Int J Cancer*, 83: 679–684. doi:10.1002/(SICI)1097-0215(19991126)83:5<679::AID-IJC19>3.0.CO;2-E PMID:10521807

Bhonsle RB, Murti PR, Gupta PC (1992). *Tobacco Habits in India*. In: *Control of Tobacco- related Cancers and other diseases (Proceeding of an International Symposium January 15–19, 1990, TIFR, Bombay)*. Hamner JE III, Gupta PC, Murti PR, editors. Oxford: Oxford University Press, pp. 25–46.

Boonyaphiphat P, Thongsuksai P, Sriplung H, Puttawibul P (2002). Lifestyle habits and genetic susceptibility and the risk of esophageal cancer in the Thai population. *Cancer Lett*, 186: 193–199. doi:10.1016/S0304-3835(02)00354-3 PMID:12213289

Boyland E & Nery R (1969). Mercapturic acid formation during the metabolism of arecoline and arecaidine in the rat. *Biochem J*, 113: 123–130. PMID:5806385

Chakrabarti RN, Dutta K, Ghosh K, Sikdar S (1990). Uterine cervical dysplasia with reference to the betel quid chewing habit. *Eur J Gynaecol Oncol*, 11: 57–59. PMID:2347336

Chandra A (1962). Different habits and their relation with cancer cheek. *Chittaranjan Cancer Hosp Calcutta natl Cancer Res Cent Bull*, 33–36.

Chang KC, Su IJ, Tsai ST *et al.* (2002a). Pathological features of betel quid-related oral epithelial lesions in taiwan with special emphasis on the tumor progression and human papillomavirus association. *Oncology*, 63: 362–369. doi:10.1159/000066227 PMID:12417791

Chang LY, Wan HC, Lai YL *et al.* (2009). Areca nut extracts increased expression of inflammatory cytokines, tumor necrosis factor-alpha, interleukin-1beta, interleukin-6 and interleukin-8, in peripheral blood mononuclear cells. *J Periodontal Res*, 44: 175–183. PMID:18973534

Chang MC, Ho YS, Lee PH *et al.* (2001a). Areca nut extract and arecoline induced the cell cycle arrest but not apoptosis of cultured oral KB epithelial cells: association of glutathione, reactive oxygen species and mitochondrial membrane potential. *Carcinogenesis*, 22: 1527–1535. doi:10.1093/carcin/22.9.1527 PMID:11532876

Chang MJ, Ko CY, Lin RF, Hsieh LL (2002c). Biological monitoring of environment exposure to safrole and the Taiwanese betel quid chewing. *Arch Environ Contam Toxicol*, 43: 432–437. doi:10.1007/s00244-002-1241-0 PMID:12399914

Chang YC, Hu CC, Tseng TH *et al.* (2001b). Synergistic effects of nicotine on arecoline-induced cytotoxicity in human buccal mucosal fibroblasts. *J Oral Pathol Med*, 30: 458–464. doi:10.1034/j.1600-0714.2001.030008458.x PMID:11545236

Chang YC, Yang SF, Tai KW *et al.* (2002b). Increased tissue inhibitor of metalloproteinase-1 expression and inhibition of gelatinase A activity in buccal mucosal fibroblasts by arecoline as possible mechanisms for oral submucous fibrosis. *Oral Oncol*, 38: 195–200. doi:10.1016/S1368-8375(01)00045-8 PMID:11854068

Changrani J, Gany FM, Cruz G *et al.* (2006). Paan and *Gutka* Use in the United States: A Pilot Study in Bangladeshi and Indian-Gujarati Immigrants in New York City. *J Immigr Refug Stud*, 4: 99–110. PMID:17492057

Chatrchaiwiwatana S (2007). Factors affecting tooth loss among rural Khon Kaen adults: analysis of two data sets. *Public Health*, 121: 106–112. PMID:17005217

Chaturvedi P, Chaturvedi U, Sanyai B (2002). Prevalence of tobacco consumption in schoolchildren in rural India–an epidemic of tobaccogenic cancers looming ahead in the Third World. *J Cancer Educ*, 17: 6 PMID:12000110

Chaudhry K, Prabhakar AK, Prabhakaran PS *et al.* (2001). *Prevalence of Tobacco Use in Karnataka and Uttar Pradesh in India*. New Delhi: Indian Council of Medical Research and WHO South East Asian Regional Office.

Chelleng PK, Narain K, Das HK *et al.* (2000). Risk factors for cancer nasopharynx: a case-control study from Nagaland, India. *Natl Med J India*, 13: 6–8. PMID:10743368

Chen CL, Chi CW, Chang KW, Liu TY (1999). Safrole-like DNA adducts in oral tissue from oral cancer patients with a betel quid chewing history. *Carcinogenesis*, 20: 2331–2334. doi:10.1093/carcin/20.12.2331 PMID:10590228

Chen PC, Kuo C, Pan CC, Chou MY (2002). Risk of oral cancer associated with human papillomavirus infection, betel quid chewing, and cigarette smoking in Taiwan–an integrated molecular and epidemiological study of 58 cases. *J Oral Pathol Med*, 31: 317–322. PMID:12190813

Chen PC, Pan CC, Kuo C, Lin CP (2006). Risk of oral nonmalignant lesions associated with human papillomavirus infection, betel quid chewing, and cigarette smoking in Taiwan: an integrated molecular and epidemiologic study. *Arch Pathol Lab Med*, 130: 57–61. PMID:16390239

Chitra S, Ashok L, Anand L *et al.* (2004). Risk factors for esophageal cancer in Coimbatore, southern India: a hospital-based case-control study. *Indian J Gastroenterol*, 23: 19–21. PMID:15106710

Chiu CJ, Chang ML, Chiang CP *et al.* (2002). Interaction of collagen-related genes and susceptibility to betel quid-induced oral submucous fibrosis. *Cancer Epidemiol Biomarkers Prev*, 11: 646–653. PMID:12101112

Chou FH, Yang YH, Kuo SH *et al.* (2009). Relationships among smoking, drinking, betel quid chewing and pregnancy-related nausea and vomiting in Taiwanese aboriginal women. *Kaohsiung J Med Sci*, 25: 62–69. PMID:19321408

Chung CH, Yang YH, Wang TY *et al.* (2005). Oral precancerous disorders associated with areca quid chewing, smoking, and alcohol drinking in southern Taiwan. *J Oral Pathol Med*, 34: 460–466. PMID:16091112

Chung YT, Chen CL, Wu CC *et al.* (2008). Safrole-DNA adduct in hepatocellular carcinoma associated with betel quid chewing. *Toxicol Lett*, 183: 21–27. doi:10.1016/j.toxlet.2008.09.013 PMID:18938230

Dave BJ, Trivedi AH, Adhvaryu SG (1991). Cytogenetic studies reveal increased genomic damage among 'pan masala' consumers. *Mutagenesis*, 6: 159–163. doi:10.1093/mutage/6.2.159 PMID:2056918

Dave BJ, Trivedi AH, Adhvaryu SG (1992). Role of areca nut consumption in the cause of oral cancers. A cytogenetic assessment. *Cancer*, 70: 1017–1023. doi:10.1002/1097-0142(19920901)70:5<1017::AID-CNCR2820700502>3.0.CO;2-# PMID:1515978

Desai SS, Ghaisas SD, Jakhi SD, Bhide SV (1996). Cytogenetic damage in exfoliated oral mucosal cells and circulating lymphocytes of patients suffering from precancerous oral lesions. *Cancer Lett*, 109: 9–14. doi:10.1016/S0304-3835(96)04390-X PMID:9020897

Dikshit RP & Kanhere S (2000). Tobacco habits and risk of lung, oropharyngeal and oral cavity cancer: a population-based case-control study in Bhopal, India. *Int J Epidemiol*, 29: 609–614. doi:10.1093/ije/29.4.609 PMID:10922335

Dongre A, Deshmukh P, Murali N, Garg B (2008). Tobacco consumption among adolescents in rural Wardha: where and how tobacco control should focus its attention? *Indian J Cancer*, 45: 100–106. PMID:19018113

Eswar N (2002). Oral health status among the tobacco and betel nut chewers in the Kishore Ganj District of

Bangladesh. A statistical study. *Indian J Dent Res*, 13: 167–171. PMID:12765097

Gajalakshmi CK & Shanta V (1996). Lifestyle and risk of stomach cancer: a hospital-based case-control study. *Int J Epidemiol*, 25: 1146–1153. doi:10.1093/ije/25.6.1146 PMID:9027518

Giri S, Idle JR, Chen C *et al.* (2006). A metabolomic approach to the metabolism of the areca nut alkaloids arecoline and arecaidine in the mouse. *Chem Res Toxicol*, 19: 818–827. doi:10.1021/tx0600402 PMID:16780361

Gupta PC, Mehta FS, Daftary DK *et al.* (1980). Incidence rates of oral cancer and natural history of oral precancerous lesions in a 10-year follow-up study of Indian villagers. *Community Dent Oral Epidemiol*, 8: 283–333. PMID:6937277

Gupta PC, Mehta FS, Pindborg JJ *et al.* (1986). Intervention study for primary prevention of oral cancer among 36 000 Indian tobacco users. *Lancet*, 1: 1235–1239. PMID:2872391

Gupta PC, Mehta FS, Pindborg JJ *et al.* (1992). Primary prevention trial of oral cancer in india: a 10-year follow-up study. *J Oral Pathol Med*, 21: 433–439. PMID:1460581

Gupta PC, Murti PR, Bhonsle RB *et al.* (1995). Effect of cessation of tobacco use on the incidence of oral mucosal lesions in a 10-yr follow-up study of 12,212 users. *Oral Dis*, 1: 54–58. PMID:7553382

Gupta PC & Ray C (2002). Tobacco and youth in the South-East Asian region. *Indian J Cancer*, 39: 5–35.

Gupta PC, Sinor PN, Bhonsle RB *et al.* (1998). Oral submucous fibrosis in India: a new epidemic? *Natl Med J India*, 11: 113–116. PMID:9707699

Gupta PC & Warnakulasuriya S (2002). Global epidemiology of areca nut usage. *Addict Biol*, 7: 77–83. PMID:11900626

Hamner JE 3rd (1972). Betel quid inducement of epithelial atypia in the buccal mucosa of baboons. *Cancer*, 30: 1001–1005. doi:10.1002/1097-0142(197210)30:4<1001::AID-CNCR2820300422>3.0.CO;2-U PMID:4627988

Hashibe M, Mathew B, Kuruvilla B *et al.* (2000b). Chewing tobacco, alcohol, and the risk of erythroplakia. *Cancer Epidemiol Biomarkers Prev*, 9: 639–645. PMID:10919731

Hashibe M, Sankaranarayanan R, Thomas G *et al.* (2000a). Alcohol drinking, body mass index and the risk of oral leukoplakia in an Indian population. *Int J Cancer*, 88: 129–134. PMID:10962450

Hashibe M, Sankaranarayanan R, Thomas G *et al.* (2002). Body mass index, tobacco chewing, alcohol drinking and the risk of oral submucous fibrosis in Kerala, India. *Cancer Causes Control*, 13: 55–64. PMID:11899118

Hazare VK, Goel RR, Gupta PC (1998). Oral submucous fibrosis, areca nut and pan masala use: a case-control study. *Natl Med J India*, 11: 299 PMID:10083804

Hirayama T (1966). An epidemiological study of oral and pharyngeal cancer in Central and South-East Asia. *Bull World Health Organ*, 34: 41–69. PMID:5295564

Ho PS, Chen PL, Warnakulasuriya S *et al.* (2009). Malignant transformation of oral potentially malignant disorders in males: a retrospective cohort study. *BMC Cancer*, 9: 260 PMID:19640311

Ho PS, Yang YH, Shieh TY *et al.* (2007). Consumption of areca quid, cigarettes, and alcohol related to the comorbidity of oral submucous fibrosis and oral cancer. *Oral Surg Oral Med Oral Pathol Oral Radiol Endod*, 104: 647–652. PMID:17449298

Huang HL, Lee CH, Yen YY *et al.* (2009). School-level contextual factors associated with betel quid chewing among schoolchildren in Taiwan. *Community Dent Oral Epidemiol*, 37: 58–67. PMID:19191820

Huang JL & McLeish MJ (1989). High performance liquid chromatographic determination of the alkaloids in betel nut. *J Chromatogr A*, 475: 447–450.

IARC (1985). Tobacco habits other than smoking; betel-quid and areca-nut chewing; and some related nitrosamines. IARC Working Group. Lyon, 23–30 October 1984. *IARC Monogr Eval Carcinog Risk Chem Hum*, 37: 1–268. PMID:3866741

IARC (1987). Overall evaluations of carcinogenicity: an updating of IARC Monographs volumes 1 to 42. *IARC Monogr Eval Carcinog Risks Hum Suppl*, 7: 1–440. PMID:3482203

IARC (2004). Betel-quid and areca-nut chewing and some areca-nut derived nitrosamines. *IARC Monogr Eval Carcinog Risks Hum*, 85: 1–334. PMID:15635762

IIPS; International Institute for Population Sciences and ORC Macro International (2007). *National Family Health Survey (NFHS-3), 2005–06: India.*, Mumbai *IIPS, No.*, II: 426–429.

Jacob BJ, Straif K, Thomas G *et al.* (2004). Betel quid without tobacco as a risk factor for oral precancers. *Oral Oncol*, 40: 697–704. PMID:15172639

Jafarey NA, Mahmood Z, Zaidi SH (1977). Habits and dietary pattern of cases of carcinoma of the oral cavity and oropharynx. *J Pak Med Assoc*, 27: 340–343. PMID:413946

Jayakody AA, Viner RM, Haines MM *et al.* (2006). Illicit and traditional drug use among ethnic minority adolescents in East London. *Public Health*, 120: 329–338. PMID:16543028

Jayalakshmi A, Mathew AG (1982). *Chemical composition and processing.* In: *The arecanut Palm.* Bavappa KVA, Nair MK, Kumar TP, editors. Kerala, India: Central plantation Crops Research Institute, pp. 225–244.

Jayalekshmi PA, Gangadharan P, Akiba S *et al.* (2009). Tobacco chewing and female oral cavity cancer risk in Karunagappally cohort, India. *Br J Cancer*, 100: 848–852. doi:10.1038/sj.bjc.6604907 PMID:19259098

Jayant K, Balakrishnan V, Sanghvi LD, Jussawalla DJ (1977). Quantification of the role of smoking and chewing tobacco in oral, pharyngeal, and oesophageal cancers. *Br J Cancer*, 35: 232–235. doi:10.1038/bjc.1977.31 PMID:836760

Jin YT, Tsai ST, Wong TY *et al.* (1996). Studies on promoting activity of Taiwan betel quid ingredients in hamster buccal pouch carcinogenesis. *Eur J Cancer B Oral Oncol*, 32B: 343–346. doi:10.1016/0964-1955(96)00018-8 PMID:8944839

Jussawalla DJ & Deshpande VA (1971). Evaluation of cancer risk in tobacco chewers and smokers: an epidemiologic assessment. *Cancer*, 28: 244–252. doi:10.1002/1097-0142(197107)28:1<244::AID-CNCR2820280150>3.0.CO;2-H PMID:5110639

Kaduri P, Kitua H, Mbatia J *et al.* (2008). Smokeless tobacco use among adolescents in Ilala Municipality, Tanzania. *Tanzania J Health Res*, 10: 28–33. PMID:18680962

Kapadia GJ, Chung EB, Ghosh B *et al.* (1978). Carcinogenicity of some folk medicinal herbs in rats. *J Natl Cancer Inst*, 60: 683–686. PMID:625070

Kapil U, Goindi G, Singh V *et al.* (2005a). Consumption of tobacco, alcohol and betel leaf amongst school children in Delhi. *Indian J Pediatr*, 72: 993 PMID:16391460

Kapil U, Singh P, Bahadur S *et al.* (2005b). Assessment of risk factors in laryngeal cancer in India: a case-control study. *Asian Pac J Cancer Prev*, 6: 202–207. PMID:16101334

Kaur J, Srivastava A, Ralhan R (1994). Overexpression of p53 protein in betel- and tobacco-related human oral dysplasia and squamous-cell carcinoma in India. *Int J Cancer*, 58: 340–345. doi:10.1002/ijc.2910580305 PMID:8050814

Kaur J, Srivastava A, Ralhan R (1998). Prognostic significance of p53 protein overexpression in betel- and tobacco-related oral oncogenesis. *Int J Cancer*, 79: 370–375. doi:10.1002/(SICI)1097-0215(19980821)79:4<370::AID-IJC11>3.0.CO;2-9 PMID:9699529

Kayal JJ, Trivedi AH, Dave BJ *et al.* (1993). Incidence of micronuclei in oral mucosa of users of tobacco products singly or in various combinations. *Mutagenesis*, 8: 31–33. doi:10.1093/mutage/8.1.31 PMID:8450765

Khanna NN, Pant GC, Tripathi FM *et al.* (1975). Some observations on the etiology of oral cancer. *Indian J Cancer*, 12: 77–83. PMID:1184070

Khanolkar VR (1959). Oral cancer in India. *Acta Unio Int Contra Cancrum*, 15: 67–77. PMID:13649428

Ko YC, Huang YL, Lee CH *et al.* (1995). Betel quid chewing, cigarette smoking and alcohol consumption related to oral cancer in Taiwan. *J Oral Pathol Med*, 24: 450–453. PMID:8600280

Kwan HW (1976). A statistical study on oral carcinomas in Taiwan with emphasis on the relationship with betel nut chewing: a preliminary report. *Taiwan Yi Xue Hui Za Zhi*, 75: 497–505. PMID:1070520

La Vecchia C, Negri E, Cavalieri d'Oro L, Franceschi S (1998). Liver cirrhosis and the risk of primary liver cancer. *Eur J Cancer Prev*, 7: 315–320. doi:10.1097/00008469-199808000-00007 PMID:9806120

Lee CH, Ko YC, Huang HL *et al.* (2003). The precancer risk of betel quid chewing, tobacco use and alcohol consumption in oral leukoplakia and oral submucous fibrosis in southern Taiwan. *Br J Cancer*, 88: 366–372. PMID:12569378

Lee CH, Lee JM, Wu DC *et al.* (2005b). Independent and combined effects of alcohol intake, tobacco smoking and betel quid chewing on the risk of esophageal cancer in Taiwan. *Int J Cancer*, 113: 475–482. doi:10.1002/ijc.20619 PMID:15455377

Lee CH, Wu DC, Lee JM *et al.* (2007). Anatomical subsite discrepancy in relation to the impact of the consumption of alcohol, tobacco and betel quid on esophageal cancer. *Int J Cancer*, 120: 1755–1762. doi:10.1002/ijc.22324 PMID:17230518

Lee JM, Lee YC, Yang SY *et al.* (2001). Genetic polymorphisms of *XRCC1* and risk of the esophageal cancer. *Int J Cancer*, 95: 240–246. doi:10.1002/1097-0215(20010720)95:4<240::AID-IJC1041>3.0.CO;2-1 PMID:11400117

Lee KW, Kuo WR, Tsai SM *et al.* (2005a). Different impact from betel quid, alcohol and cigarette: risk factors for pharyngeal and laryngeal cancer. *Int J Cancer*, 117: 831–836. doi:10.1002/ijc.21237 PMID:15957167

Lee SS, Tsai CH, Ho YC, Chang YC (2008a). The upregulation of heat shock protein 70 expression in areca quid chewing-associated oral squamous cell carcinomas. *Oral Oncol*, 44: 884–890. doi:10.1016/j.oraloncology.2007.11.004 PMID:18234541

Lee SS, Yang SF, Tsai CH *et al.* (2008b). Upregulation of heme oxygenase 1 expression in areca-quid-chewing-associated oral squamous cell carcinoma. *J Formos Med Assoc*, 107: 355–363. doi:10.1016/S0929-6646(08)60100-X PMID:18492619

Lin LM, Chen YK, Lai DL, Huang YL (1996). Minimal arecaidine concentrations showing a promotion effect during DMBA-induced hamster cheek pouch carcinogenesis. *J Oral Pathol Med*, 25: 65–68. doi:10.1111/j.1600-0714.1996.tb00194.x PMID:8667258

Lin LM, Chen YK, Lai DR *et al.* (1997). Cancer-promoting effect of Taiwan betel quid in hamster buccal pouch carcinogenesis. *Oral Dis*, 3: 232–235. doi:10.1111/j.1601-0825.1997.tb00047.x PMID:9643218

Lord GA, Lim CK, Warnakulasuriya S, Peters TJ (2002). Chemical and analytical aspects of areca nut. *Addict Biol*, 7: 99–102. PMID:11900628

Lu CT, Yen YY, Ho CS *et al.* (1996). A case-control study of oral cancer in Changhua County, Taiwan. *J Oral Pathol Med*, 25: 245–248. PMID:8835822

Maher R, Lee AJ, Warnakulasuriya KA *et al.* (1994). Role of areca nut in the causation of oral submucous fibrosis: a case-control study in Pakistan. *J Oral Pathol Med*, 23: 65–69. PMID:8164155

Mazahir S, Malik R, Maqsood M *et al.* (2006). Socio-demographic correlates of betel, areca and smokeless tobacco use as a high risk behavior for head and neck cancers in a squatter settlement of Karachi, Pakistan. *Subst Abuse Treat Prev Policy*, 1: 10 PMID:16722535

Mehta FS, Shroff BC, Gupta PC, Daftary DK (1972). Oral leukoplakia in relation to tobacco habits. A ten-year follow-up study of Bombay policemen. *Oral Surg Oral Med Oral Pathol*, 34: 426–433. doi:10.1016/0030-4220(72)90319-2 PMID:4505755

Merchant A, Husain SS, Hosain M *et al.* (2000). Paan without tobacco: an independent risk factor for oral cancer. *Int J Cancer*, 86: 128–131. PMID:10728606

Muir CS & Kirk R (1960). Betel, tobacco, and cancer of the mouth. *Br J Cancer*, 14: 597–608. PMID:13773626

Muwonge R, Ramadas K, Sankila R *et al.* (2008). Role of tobacco smoking, chewing and alcohol drinking in the risk of oral cancer in Trivandrum, India: a nested case-control design using incident cancer cases. *Oral Oncol*, 44: 446–454. PMID:17933578

Nair J, Nair UJ, Ohshima H *et al.* (1987a). Endogenous nitrosation in the oral cavity of chewers while chewing betel quid with or without tobacco. *IARC Sci Publ*, 84465–469. PMID:3679424

Nair J, Ohshima H, Friesen M *et al.* (1985). Tobacco-specific and betel nut-specific N-nitroso compounds: occurrence in saliva and urine of betel quid chewers and formation in vitro by nitrosation of betel quid. *Carcinogenesis*, 6: 295–303. doi:10.1093/carcin/6.2.295 PMID:3971493

Nair U, Bartsch H, Nair J (2004). Alert for an epidemic of oral cancer due to use of the betel quid substitutes gutkha and *pan masala*: a review of agents and causative mechanisms. *Mutagenesis*, 19: 251–262. PMID:15215323

Nair U, Obe G, Nair J *et al.* (1991). Evaluation of frequency of micronucleated oral mucosa cells as a marker for genotoxic damage in chewers of betel quid with or without tobacco. *Mutat Res*, 261: 163–168. doi:10.1016/0165-1218(91)90063-R PMID:1719407

Nair UJ, Floyd RA, Nair J *et al.* (1987b). Formation of reactive oxygen species and of 8-hydroxydeoxyguanosine in DNA in vitro with betel quid ingredients. *Chem Biol Interact*, 63: 157–169. doi:10.1016/0009-2797(87)90095-0 PMID:3664791

Nair UJ, Nair J, Friesen MD *et al.* (1995). *Ortho*- and *meta*-tyrosine formation from phenylalanine in human saliva as a marker of hydroxyl radical generation during betel quid chewing. *Carcinogenesis*, 16: 1195–1198. doi:10.1093/carcin/16.5.1195 PMID:7767985

Nandakumar A, Anantha N, Pattabhiraman V *et al.* (1996). Importance of anatomical subsite in correlating risk factors in cancer of the oesophagus–report of a case–control study. *Br J Cancer*, 73: 1306–1311. doi:10.1038/bjc.1996.249 PMID:8630297

Nandakumar A, Thimmasetty KT, Sreeramareddy NM *et al.* (1990). A population-based case-control investigation on cancers of the oral cavity in Bangalore, India. *Br J Cancer*, 62: 847–851. PMID:2245179

Nichter M, Nichter M, Van Sickle D (2004). Popular perceptions of tobacco products and patterns of use among male college students in India. *Soc Sci Med*, 59: 415–431. PMID:15110430

Nigam SK, Kumar A, Sheikh S, Saiyed HN (2001). Toxicological evaluation of pan masala in pure inbred swiss mice: a preliminary report on long term exposure study. *Curr Sci*, 80: 1306–1309.

Nisar N, Qadri MH, Fatima K, Perveen S (2007). A community based study about knowledge and practices regarding tobacco consumption and passive smoking in Gadap Town, Karachi. *J Pak Med Assoc*, 57: 186–188. PMID:17489526

Notani PN & Sanghvi LD (1976). Role of diet in the cancers of the oral cavity. *Indian J Cancer*, 13: 156–160. PMID:987991

Núñez-de la Mora A, Jesmin F, Bentley GR (2007). Betel nut use among first and second generation Bangladeshi women in London, UK. *J Immigr Minor Health*, 9: 299–306. PMID:17431783

Ohshima H, Friesen M, Bartsch H (1989). Identification in rats of N-nitrosonipecotic acid as a major urinary metabolite of the areca-nut alkaloid-derived nitrosamines, N-nitrosoguvacoline and N-nitrosoguvacine. *Cancer Lett*, 44: 211–216. doi:10.1016/0304-3835(89)90063-3 PMID:2924287

Orr IM (1933). Oral cancer in betel nut chewers in travancore. *Lancet*, 222: 575–580. doi:10.1016/S0140-6736(01)18622-8

Padma PR, Lalitha VS, Amonkar AJ, Bhide SV (1989). Anticarcinogenic effect of betel leaf extract against tobacco carcinogens. *Cancer Lett*, 45: 195–202. doi:10.1016/0304-3835(89)90077-3 PMID:2731162

Pai SR, Shirke AJ, Gothoskar SV (1981). Long-term feeding study in C17 mice administered saccharin coated betel nut and 1,4-dinitrosopiperazine in combination. *Carcinogenesis*, 2: 175–177. doi:10.1093/carcin/2.3.175 PMID:7273302

Pandey M & Shukla VK (2003). Lifestyle, parity, menstrual and reproductive factors and risk of gallbladder cancer. *Eur J Cancer Prev*, 12: 269–272. doi:10.1097/00008469-200308000-00005 PMID:12883378

Paudel D *(2003).* Tobacco use among adolescent students in secondary schools of Pokhara - Summary Report. Thesis for Master's Degree in Public Health, Institute of Medicine Tribhuvan University, Nepal.

Phukan RK, Ali MS, Chetia CK, Mahanta J (2001). Betel nut and tobacco chewing; potential risk factors of cancer of oesophagus in Assam, India. *Br J Cancer*, 85: 661–667. doi:10.1054/bjoc.2001.1920 PMID:11531248

Phukan RK, Zomawia E, Narain K *et al.* (2005). Tobacco use and stomach cancer in Mizoram, India.

Cancer Epidemiol Biomarkers Prev, 14: 1892–1896. doi:10.1158/1055-9965.EPI-05-0074 PMID:16103433

Prokopczyk B, Bertinato P, Hoffmann D (1988). Cyanoethylation of DNA *in vivo* by 3-(methylnitrosamino)propionitrile, an *Areca*-derived carcinogen. *Cancer Res*, 48: 6780–6784. PMID:3180087

Prokopczyk B, Rivenson A, Bertinato P *et al.* (1987). 3-(Methylnitrosamino)propionitrile: occurrence in saliva of betel quid chewers, carcinogenicity, and DNA methylation in F344 rats. *Cancer Res*, 47: 467–471. PMID:3791234

Raghavan V & Baruah HK (1958). Areca nut, India's popular masticatory history, chemistry and utilisation. *Econ Botany*, 12: 315–325.

Rajkumar T, Franceschi S, Vaccarella S *et al.* (2003). Role of paan chewing and dietary habits in cervical carcinoma in Chennai, India. *Br J Cancer*, 88: 1388–1393. doi:10.1038/sj.bjc.6600902 PMID:12778066

Ramchandani AG, D'Souza AV, Borges AM, Bhisey RA (1998). Evaluation of carcinogenic/co-carcinogenic activity of a common chewing product, pan masala, in mouse skin, stomach and esophagus. *Int J Cancer*, 75: 225–232. doi:10.1002/(SICI)1097-0215(19980119)75:2<225::AID-IJC10>3.0.CO;2-C PMID:9462712

Ranadive KJ, Gothoskar SV, Rao AR *et al.* (1976). Experimental studies on betel nut and tobacco carcinogenicity. *Int J Cancer*, 17: 469–476. doi:10.1002/ijc.2910170409 PMID:1279039

Ranadive KJ, Ranadive SN, Shivapurkar NM, Gothoskar SV (1979). Betel quid chewing and oral cancer: experimental studies on hamsters. *Int J Cancer*, 24: 835–843. doi:10.1002/ijc.2910240623 PMID:544535

Rao AR (1984). Modifying influences of betel quid ingredients on B(a)P-induced carcinogenesis in the buccal pouch of hamster. *Int J Cancer*, 33: 581–586. doi:10.1002/ijc.2910330506 PMID:6327538

Rao AR & Das P (1989). Evaluation of the carcinogenicity of different preparations of areca nut in mice. *Int J Cancer*, 43: 728–732. doi:10.1002/ijc.2910430431 PMID:2703277

Rao AR, Sinha A, Selvan RS (1985). Inhibitory action of Piper betle on the initiation of 7,12-dimethylbenz[a]anthracene-induced mammary carcinogenesis in rats. *Cancer Lett*, 26: 207–214. doi:10.1016/0304-3835(85)90028-X PMID:3919938

Rao DN & Desai PB (1998). Risk assessment of tobacco, alcohol and diet in cancers of base tongue and oral tongue–a case control study. *Indian J Cancer*, 35: 65–72. PMID:9849026

Rao DN, Ganesh B, Rao RS, Desai PB (1994). Risk assessment of tobacco, alcohol and diet in oral cancer–a case-control study. *Int J Cancer*, 58: 469–473. PMID:8056441

Reichart PA (1995). Oral cancer and precancer related to betel and miang chewing in Thailand: a review. *J Oral Pathol Med*, 24: 241–243. PMID:7562658

Ridge C, Akanle O, Spyrou NM (2001). Elemental composition of betel nut associated chewing material. *J Radioanal Nucl Chem*, 249: 67–70.

Rozi S & Akhtar S (2007). Prevalence and predictors of smokeless tobacco use among high-school males in Karachi, Pakistan. *East Mediterr Health J*, 13: 916–924. PMID:17955775

Sanghvi LD, Rao KC, Khanolkar VR (1955). Smoking and chewing of tobacco in relation to cancer of the upper alimentary tract. *BMJ*, 1: 1111–1114. doi:10.1136/bmj.1.4922.1111 PMID:14363805

Sankaranarayanan R, Duffy SW, Day NE *et al.* (1989b). A case-control investigation of cancer of the oral tongue and the floor of the mouth in southern India. *Int J Cancer*, 44: 617–621. PMID:2793234

Sankaranarayanan R, Duffy SW, Nair MK *et al.* (1990b). Tobacco and alcohol as risk factors in cancer of the larynx in Kerala, India. *Int J Cancer*, 45: 879–882. doi:10.1002/ijc.2910450517 PMID:2335391

Sankaranarayanan R, Duffy SW, Padmakumary G *et al.* (1989a). Tobacco chewing, alcohol and nasal snuff in cancer of the gingiva in Kerala, India. *Br J Cancer*, 60: 638–643. PMID:2803939

Sankaranarayanan R, Duffy SW, Padmakumary G *et al.* (1990a). Risk factors for cancer of the buccal and labial mucosa in Kerala, southern India. *J Epidemiol Community Health*, 44: 286–292. PMID:2277249

Sankaranarayanan R, Duffy SW, Padmakumary G *et al.* (1991). Risk factors for cancer of the oesophagus in Kerala, India. *Int J Cancer*, 49: 485–489. doi:10.1002/ijc.2910490402 PMID:1917146

Sapkota A, Gajalakshmi V, Jetly DH *et al.* (2007). Smokeless tobacco and increased risk of hypopharyngeal and laryngeal cancers: a multicentric case-control study from India. *Int J Cancer*, 121: 1793–1798. doi:10.1002/ijc.22832 PMID:17583577

Sarma SN (1958). A study into the incidence and etiology of cancer of the larynx and adjacent parts in Assam. *Indian J Med Res*, 46: 525–533. PMID:13562893

Scutt A, Meghji S, Canniff JP, Harvey W (1987). Stabilisation of collagen by betel nut polyphenols as a mechanism in oral submucous fibrosis. *Experientia*, 43: 391–393. doi:10.1007/BF01940422 PMID:3032668

Shah N & Sharma PP (1998). Role of chewing and smoking habits in the etiology of oral submucous fibrosis (OSF): a case-control study. *J Oral Pathol Med*, 27: 475–479. PMID:9831959

Shanta V & Krishnamurthi S (1959). A study of aetiological factors in oral squamous cell carcinoma. *Br J Cancer*, 13: 381–388. doi:10.1038/bjc.1959.43 PMID:14445489

Shanta V & Krishnamurthi S (1963). Further study in aetiology of carcinomas of the upper alimentary tract. *Br J Cancer*, 17: 8–23. doi:10.1038/bjc.1963.2 PMID:13976794

Shirname LP, Menon MM, Nair J, Bhide SV (1983). Correlation of mutagenicity and tumorigenicity of betel quid and its ingredients. *Nutr Cancer*, 5: 87–91. doi:10.1080/01635588309513783 PMID:6647042

Shiu MN, Chen TH, Chang SH, Hahn LJ (2000). Risk factors for leukoplakia and malignant transformation to oral carcinoma: a leukoplakia cohort in Taiwan. *Br J Cancer*, 82: 1871–1874. PMID:10839305

Shivapurkar NM, Ranadive SN, Gothoskar SV *et al.* (1980). Tumorigenic effect of aqueous & polyphenolic fractions of betel nut in Swiss strain mice. *Indian J Exp Biol*, 18: 1159–1161. PMID:7216269

Shivashankar S, Dhanaraj S, Mathew AG *et al.* (1969). Physical and chemical characteristics of processed arecanuts. *J Food Sci Technol*, 41: 113–116.

Shukla VK, Chauhan VS, Mishra RN, Basu S (2008). Lifestyle, reproductive factors and risk of gallbladder cancer. *Singapore Med J*, 49: 912–915. PMID:19037558

Simarak S, de Jong UW, Breslow N *et al.* (1977). Cancer of the oral cavity, pharynx/larynx and lung in North Thailand: case-control study and analysis of cigar smoke. *Br J Cancer*, 36: 130–140. doi:10.1038/bjc.1977.163 PMID:19028

Singh A & Rao AR (1995). Modulatory influence of arecanut on the mouse hepatic xenobiotic detoxication system and skin papillomagenesis. *Teratog Carcinog Mutagen*, 15: 135–146. doi:10.1002/tcm.1770150306 PMID:8584985

Sinha DN & Gupta PC (2005). Tobacco use among students in Orissa and Uttar Pradesh. *Indian Pediatr*, 42: 846–847. PMID:16141500

Sinha DN, Gupta PC, Pednekar MS (2003). Tobacco use among school personnel in eight North-eastern states of India. *Indian J Cancer*, 40: 3–14. PMID:14716126

Sinor PN, Gupta PC, Murti PR *et al.* (1990). A case-control study of oral submucous fibrosis with special reference to the etiologic role of areca nut. *J Oral Pathol Med*, 19: 94–98. PMID:2341977

Smith LW, Bhargava K, Mani NJ *et al.* (1975). Oral cancer and precancerous lesions in 57,518 industrial workers of Gujarat, India. *Indian J Cancer*, 12: 118–123. PMID:1184077

Srivatanakul P, Parkin DM, Khlat M *et al.* (1991). Liver cancer in Thailand. II. A case-control study of hepatocellular carcinoma. *Int J Cancer*, 48: 329–332. doi:10.1002/ijc.2910480303 PMID:1645698

Stich HF, Brunnemann KD, Mathew B *et al.* (1989). Chemopreventive trials with vitamin A and beta-carotene: some unresolved issues. *Prev Med*, 18: 732–739. doi:10.1016/0091-7435(89)90044-3 PMID:2616546

Stich HF, Mathew B, Sankaranarayanan R, Nair MK (1991). Remission of precancerous lesions in the oral cavity of tobacco chewers and maintenance of the protective effect of beta-carotene or vitamin A. *Am J Clin Nutr*, 53: Suppl298S–304S. PMID:1985402

Subapriya R, Thangavelu A, Mathavan B *et al.* (2007). Assessment of risk factors for oral squamous cell carcinoma in Chidambaram, Southern India: a case-control study. *Eur J Cancer Prev*, 16: 251–256. PMID:17415096

Sun CA, Wu DM, Lin CC *et al.* (2003). Incidence and cofactors of hepatitis C virus-related hepatocellular carcinoma: a prospective study of 12,008 men in Taiwan. *Am J Epidemiol*, 157: 674–682. doi:10.1093/aje/kwg041 PMID:12697571

Sundqvist K & Grafström RC (1992). Effects of areca nut on growth, differentiation and formation of DNA damage in cultured human buccal epithelial cells. *Int J Cancer*, 52: 305–310. doi:10.1002/ijc.2910520225 PMID:1521917

Sundqvist K, Liu Y, Nair J *et al.* (1989). Cytotoxic and genotoxic effects of areca nut-related compounds in cultured human buccal epithelial cells. *Cancer Res*, 49: 5294–5298. PMID:2766297

Suri K, Goldman HM, Wells H (1971). carcinogenic effect of diethyl sulfoxide extract of betel nut on the mucosa of the hamster Buccal pouch. *Nature*, 230: 383–384. PMID:4927728 doi:10.1038/230383a0

Tanaka T, Kuniyasu T, Shima H *et al.* (1986). Carcinogenicity of betel quid. III. Enhancement of 4-nitroquinoline-1-oxide- and N-2-fluorenylacetamide-induced carcinogenesis in rats by subsequent administration of betel nut. *J Natl Cancer Inst*, 77: 777–781. PMID:3091901

Tanaka T, Mori H, Fujii M *et al.* (1983). Carcinogenicity examination of betel quid. II. Effect of vitamin A deficiency on rats fed semipurified diet containing betel nut and calcium hydroxide. *Nutr Cancer*, 4: 260–266. doi:10.1080/01635588209513766 PMID:6878046

Tang JG, Jian XF, Gao ML *et al.* (1997). Epidemiological survey of oral submucous fibrosis in Xiangtan City, Hunan Province, China. *Community Dent Oral Epidemiol*, 25: 177–180. PMID:9181294

Tanwir F, Altamash M, Gustafsson A (2008). Influence of betel nut chewing, dental care habits and attitudes on perceived oral health among adult Pakistanis. *Oral Health Prev Dent*, 6: 89–94. PMID:18637386

Thomas SJ, Bain CJ, Battistutta D *et al.* (2007). Betel quid not containing tobacco and oral cancer: a report on a case-control study in Papua New Guinea and a meta-analysis of current evidence. *Int J Cancer*, 120: 1318–1323. PMID:17163423

Thomas SJ, Harris R, Ness AR *et al.* (2008). Betel quid not containing tobacco and oral leukoplakia: a report on a cross-sectional study in Papua New Guinea and a meta-analysis of current evidence. *Int J Cancer*, 123: 1871–1876. PMID:18688850

Thongsuksai P & Boonyaphiphat P (2001). Lack of association between p53 expression and betel nut chewing in oral cancers from Thailand. *Oral Oncol*, 37: 276–281. doi:10.1016/S1368-8375(00)00127-5 PMID:11287282

Tovosia S, Chen PH, Ko AM *et al.* (2007). Prevalence and associated factors of betel quid use in the Solomon Islands: a hyperendemic area for oral and pharyngeal cancer. *Am J Trop Med Hyg*, 77: 586–590. PMID:17827384

Tripathi M, Khanna SK, Das M (2006). Usage of saccharin in food products and its intake by the population of Lucknow, India. *Food Addit Contam*, 23: 1265–1275. PMID:17118869

Trivedy C, Meghji S, Warnakulasuriya KA *et al.* (2001). Copper stimulates human oral fibroblasts *in vitro*: a role in the pathogenesis of oral submucous fibrosis. *J Oral Pathol Med*, 30: 465–470. doi:10.1034/j.1600-0714.2001.030008465.x PMID:11545237

Trivedy C, Warnakulasuriya KA, Hazarey VK *et al.* (1999a). The upregulation of lysyl oxidase in oral submucous fibrosis and squamous cell carcinoma. *J Oral Pathol Med*, 28: 246–251. doi:10.1111/j.1600-0714.1999.tb02033.x PMID:10426196

Trivedy C, Warnakulasuriya S, Hazarey VK *et al.* (1999b). *The role of copper in the aetiopathogenesis of oral submucous fibrosis.* In: *Oral Oncology, Proceedings of the 6th International Congress on Oral Cancer.* Varma AK, editor. New Delhi: Macmillan Press, pp. 7–10.

Tsai CH, Chou MY, Chang YC (2003). The up-regulation of cyclooxygenase-2 expression in human buccal mucosal fibroblasts by arecoline: a possible role in the pathogenesis of oral submucous fibrosis. *J Oral Pathol Med*, 32: 146–153. doi:10.1034/j.1600-0714.2003.00004.x PMID:12581384

Tsai JF, Chuang LY, Jeng JE *et al.* (2001). Betel quid chewing as a risk factor for hepatocellular carcinoma: a case-control study. *Br J Cancer*, 84: 709–713. doi:10.1054/bjoc.1999.1597 PMID:11237396

Tsai JF, Jeng JE, Chuang LY *et al.* (2004). Habitual betel quid chewing and risk for hepatocellular carcinoma complicating cirrhosis. *Medicine (Baltimore)*, 83: 176–187. doi:10.1097/01.md.0000126971.80227.a4 PMID:15118544

Tsai YS, Lee KW, Huang JL *et al.* (2008). Arecoline, a major alkaloid of areca nut, inhibits p53, represses DNA repair, and triggers DNA damage response in human epithelial cells. *Toxicology*, 249: 230–237. doi:10.1016/j.tox.2008.05.007 PMID:18585839

van Wyk CW, Stander I, Padayachee A, Grobler-Rabie AF (1993). The areca nut chewing habit and oral squamous cell carcinoma in South African Indians. A retrospective study. *S Afr Med J*, 83: 425–429. PMID:8211462

Wahi PN (1968). The epidemiology of oral anc oropharyngeal cancer. A report of the study in Mainpuri district, Uttar Pradesh, India. *Bull World Health Organ*, 38: 495–521. PMID:5302449

Wahi PN, Kehar U, Lahiri B (1965). Factors influencing oral and oropharyngeal cancers in India. *Br J Cancer*, 19: 642–660. doi:10.1038/bjc.1965.80 PMID:5867785

Wang CK & Wu MJ (1996[The separation of phenolics from Piper betle leaf and the effect on the mutagenicity of arecoline.]). *J Chin Agric Chem Soc*, 34: 638–647.

Wang LY, You SL, Lu SN *et al.* (2003b). Risk of hepatocellular carcinoma and habits of alcohol drinking, betel quid chewing and cigarette smoking: a cohort of 2416 HBsAg-seropositive and 9421 HBsAg-seronegative male residents in Taiwan. *Cancer Causes Control*, 14: 241–250. doi:10.1023/A:1023636619477 PMID:12814203

Wang SC, Tsai CC, Huang ST, Hong YJ (2003a). Betel nut chewing and related factors in adolescent students in Taiwan. *Public Health*, 117: 339–345. PMID:12909424

Wang SC, Tsai CC, Huang ST, Hong YJ (2004). Betel nut chewing: the prevalence and the intergenerational effect of parental behavior on adolescent students. *J Adolesc Health*, 34: 244–249. PMID:14967349

Warnakulasuriya S (2002). Areca nut use following migration and its consequences. *Addict Biol*, 7: 127–132. PMID:11900632

Warnakulasuriya S, Johnson NW, van der Waal I (2007). Nomenclature and classification of potentially malignant disorders of the oral mucosa. *J Oral Pathol Med*, 36: 575–580. PMID:17944749

Wasnik KS, Ughade SN, Zodpey SP, Ingole DL (1998). Tobacco consumption practices and risk of oro-pharyngeal cancer: a case-control study in Central India. *Southeast Asian J Trop Med Public Health*, 29: 827–834. PMID:10772572

Wei FC & Chung FL (1997). Trace elements in areca nut from Taiwan. *J Radioanal Nucl Chem*, 217: 45–51.

Wen CP, Cheng TY, Eriksen MP (2005b). How opening the cigarette market led to an increase in betel quid use in Taiwan. *Public Health*, 119: 940–944. PMID:15998528

Wen CP, Tsai SP, Cheng TY *et al.* (2005a). Uncovering the relation between betel quid chewing and cigarette smoking in Taiwan. *Tob Control*, 14: Suppl 1i16–i22. doi:10.1136/tc.2004.008003 PMID:15923442

Wenke G & Hoffmann D (1983). A study of betel quid carcinogenesis. 1. On the *in vitro* N-nitrosation of arecoline. *Carcinogenesis*, 4: 169–172. doi:10.1093/carcin/4.2.169 PMID:6825205

Wong TY, Jin YT, Chen HO *et al.* (1992). Studies on Taiwan betel quid carcinogenicity in hamster cheek-pouch. *Chinese Dent J*, 11: 155–162.

Wu IC, Lee CH, Kuo CH *et al.* (2009b). Consumption of cigarettes but not betel quid or alcohol increases colorectal cancer risk. *J Formos Med Assoc*, 108: 155–163. doi:10.1016/S0929-6646(09)60046-2 PMID:19251551

Wu IC, Lu CY, Kuo FC *et al.* (2006). Interaction between cigarette, alcohol and betel nut use on esophageal cancer risk in Taiwan. *Eur J Clin Invest*, 36: 236–241. doi:10.1111/j.1365-2362.2006.01621.x PMID:16620285

Wu MT, Chen MC, Wu DC (2004b). Influences of lifestyle habits and p53 codon 72 and p21 codon 31 polymorphisms on gastric cancer risk in Taiwan. *Cancer Lett*, 205: 61–68. doi:10.1016/j.canlet.2003.11.026 PMID:15036662

Wu MT, Lee YC, Chen CJ *et al.* (2001). Risk of betel chewing for oesophageal cancer in Taiwan. *Br J Cancer*, 85: 658–660. doi:10.1054/bjoc.2001.1927 PMID:11531247
Wu MT, Wu DC, Hsu HK *et al.* (2004a). Constituents of areca chewing related to esophageal cancer risk in Taiwanese men. *Dis Esophagus*, 17: 257–259. doi:10.1111/j.1442-2050.2004.00419.x PMID:15361101
Wu GH, Boucher BJ, Chiu YH *et al.* (2009a). Impact of chewing betel-nut (Areca catechu) on liver cirrhosis and hepatocellular carcinoma: a population-based study from an area with a high prevalence of hepatitis B and C infections. *Public Health Nutr*, 12: 129–135. doi:10.1017/S1368980008002073 PMID:18410705
Yan JJ, Tzeng CC, Jin YT (1996). Overexpression of p53 protein in squamous cell carcinoma of buccal mucosa and tongue in Taiwan: an immunohistochemical and clinicopathological study. *J Oral Pathol Med*, 25: 55–59. doi:10.1111/j.1600-0714.1996.tb00192.x PMID:8667256
Yang XR, Diehl S, Pfeiffer R *et al.*Chinese and American Genetic Epidemiology of NPC Study Team (2005). Evaluation of risk factors for nasopharyngeal carcinoma in high-risk nasopharyngeal carcinoma families in Taiwan. *Cancer Epidemiol Biomarkers Prev*, 14: 900–905. doi:10.1158/1055-9965.EPI-04-0680 PMID:15826929
Yang YH, Chen CH, Chang JS *et al.* (2005a). Incidence rates of oral cancer and oral pre-cancerous lesions in a 6-year follow-up study of a Taiwanese aboriginal community. *J Oral Pathol Med*, 34: 596–601. PMID:16202079
Yang YH, Lee HY, Tung S, Shieh TY (2001). Epidemiological survey of oral submucous fibrosis and leukoplakia in aborigines of Taiwan. *J Oral Pathol Med*, 30: 213–219. PMID:11302240
Yang YH, Lien YC, Ho PS *et al.* (2005b). The effects of chewing areca/betel quid with and without cigarette smoking on oral submucous fibrosis and oral mucosal lesions. *Oral Dis*, 11: 88–94. PMID:15752081
Yap SF, Ho PS, Kuo HC, Yang YH (2008). Comparing factors affecting commencement and cessation of betel quid chewing behavior in Taiwanese adults. *BMC Public Health*, 8: 199 PMID:18533044
Yen AM, Chen SC, Chang SH, Chen TH (2008a). The effect of betel quid and cigarette on multistate progression of oral pre-malignancy. *J Oral Pathol Med*, 37: 417–422. PMID:18410311
Yen AM, Chen SC, Chen TH (2007). Dose-response relationships of oral habits associated with the risk of oral pre-malignant lesions among men who chew betel quid. *Oral Oncol*, 43: 634–638. PMID:17466570
Yen TT, Lin WD, Wang CP *et al.* (2008b). The association of smoking, alcoholic consumption, betel quid chewing and oral cavity cancer: a cohort study. *Eur Arch Otorhinolaryngol*, 265: 1403–1407. PMID:18389268
Ysaol J, Chilton JI, Callagan P (1996). A survey of betel nut chewing in Palau. *Isla Journal of Micronesian Studies*, 4: 224–255.
Zaidi SH, Arif M, Fatima I (2002). Radiochemical neutron activation analysis for trace elements of basic ingredients of *pan*. *J Radioanal Nucl Chem*, 253: 459–464.
Zain RB, Ikeda N, Gupta PC *et al.* (1999). Oral mucosal lesions associated with betel quid, areca nut and tobacco chewing habits: consensus from a workshop held in Kuala Lumpur, Malaysia, November 25–27, 1996. *J Oral Pathol Med*, 28: 1–4. PMID:9890449
Zhang X & Reichart PA (2007). A review of betel quid chewing, oral cancer and precancer in Mainland China. *Oral Oncol*, 43: 424–430. PMID:17258497
Zhou S, Guo F, Li L *et al.* (2008). Multiple logistic regression analysis of risk factors for carcinogenesis of oral submucous fibrosis in mainland China. *Int J Oral Maxillofac Surg*, 37: 1094–1098. PMID:18684592
Znaor A, Brennan P, Gajalakshmi V *et al.* (2003). Independent and combined effects of tobacco smoking, chewing and alcohol drinking on the risk of oral, pharyngeal and esophageal cancers in Indian men. *Int J Cancer*, 105: 681–686. doi:10.1002/ijc.11114 PMID:12740918

CONSUMPTION OF ALCOHOLIC BEVERAGES

Consumption of alcoholic beverages was considered by previous IARC Working Groups in 1987 and 2007 (IARC, 1988, 2010). Since that time, new data have become available, these have been incorporated into the *Monograph*, and taken into consideration in the present evaluation.

1. Exposure Data

1.1 Types and ethanol content of alcoholic beverages

1.1.1 Types of alcoholic beverages

The predominant types of commercially produced alcoholic beverages are beer, wine and spirits. Basic ingredients for beer are malted barley, water, hops and yeast. Wheat may be used. Nearly all wine is produced from grapes, although wine can be also made from other fruits and berries. Spirits are frequently produced from cereals (e.g. corn, wheat), beet or molasses, grapes or other fruits, cane sugar or potatoes. Main beverage types (i.e. beer, wine and spirits) may be consumed in combination with each other to fortify the strength of an alcoholic beverage (e.g. fortified wine, in which spirits are added to wine) (WHO, 2004).

In addition to commercialized products, in many developing countries different types of home- or locally produced alcoholic beverages such as sorghum beer, palm wine or sugarcane spirits are consumed (WHO, 2004). Home- or locally produced alcoholic beverages are produced through fermentation of seed, grains, fruit, vegetables or parts of palm trees, by a fairly simple production process.

1.1.2 Ethanol content of alcoholic beverages

Percentage by volume (% vol) is used to indicate the ethanol content of beverages, which is also called the French or Guy-Lussac system. Alcohol content differs according to the main beverage type and may also vary by country. Commonly, 4–5% vol are contained in beer, about 12% vol in wine and about 40% vol in distilled spirits. However, lower or higher ethanol content in alcoholic beverages is also possible. The ethanol content in beer can range from 2.3% vol to over 10% vol (lower alcohol content in home- or locally produced alcoholic beverages such as sorghum beer), in wine from 8 to 15% vol, and in spirits from 20% vol (aperitifs) to well over 40% vol (e.g. 80% vol in some kinds of absinthe). There is a trend in recent years towards higher (13.5–14.5%) alcohol volume in consumed wines, associated with technology advances and increasing proportion in overall consumption of wines produced outside the traditional wine-growing regions of Europe (IARC, 2010).

To calculate the amount of ethanol contained in a specific drink, the amount (e.g. ml) of alcoholic beverage consumed for each type of beverage (e.g. a 330-mL bottle of beer) is multiplied by the precentage of alcohol by volume, i.e. the proportion of the total volume of the beverage that is alcohol (e.g. (330 mL) × (0.04) = 13.2 mL of ethanol in a bottle of beer). Conversion factors may be used to convert the volume of alcoholic beverage into grams of ethanol, or volumes of alcohol may be recorded in 'ounces'. Conversion factors for these different measures (WHO, 2000) are as follows:

- 1 mL ethanol = 0.79 g
- 1 UK oz = 2.84 cL = 28.4 mL = 22.3 g
- 1 US fluid oz = 2.96 cL = 29.6 mL = 23.2 g

1.2 Chemical composition

The main components of most alcoholic beverages are ethanol and water. Some physical and chemical characteristics of anhydrous ethanol are as follows (O'Neil, 2001):

Chem. Abstr. Services Reg. No.: 64–17.5
Formula: C_2H_5OH
Relative molecular mass: 46.07
Synonyms and trade name: Ethanol, ethyl alcohol, ethyl hydroxide, ethyl hydrate, absolute alcohol, anhydrous alcohol, dehydrated alcohol
Description: Clear, colourless, very mobile, flammable liquid, pleasant odour, burning taste
Melting-point: –114.1 °C
Boiling-point: 78.5 °C
Density: d_4^{20} 0.789
Refractive index: n_D^{20} 1.361

In addition to ethanol and water, wine, beer and spirits contain volatile and non-volatile compounds. Volatile compounds include aliphatic carbonyl compounds, alcohols, monocarboxylic acids and their esters, nitrogen- and sulfur-containing compounds, hydrocarbons, terpenic compounds, and heterocyclic and aromatic compounds. Non-volatile extracts of alcoholic beverages comprise unfermented sugars, di- and tribasic carboxylic acids, colouring substances, tannic and polyphenolic substances and inorganic salts (IARC, 2010).

Occasionally, toxic additives, that are not permitted for use in commercial production have been identified in alcoholic beverages. These include methanol, diethylene glycol (used as sweetener) and chloroacetic acid or its bromine analogue, sodium azide and salicylic acid, which are used as fungicides or bactericides (Ough, 1987).

Contaminants may also be present in alcoholic beverages. Contaminants are defined as substances that are not intentionally added but are present in alcoholic beverages due to production, manufacture, processing, preparation, treatment, packing, packaging, transport or holding, or as a result of environmental contamination. Contaminants and toxins found in alcoholic beverages are nitrosamines, mycotoxins, ethyl carbamate, pesticides, thermal processing contaminants, benzene, and inorganic contaminants such as lead, cadmium, arsenic, copper, chromium, inorganic anions, and organometals (IARC, 2010).

In view of the potential carcinogenicity of acetaldehyde and its known toxic properties, recent studies attempted to estimate exposure to acetaldehyde from alcoholic beverages outside ethanol metabolism at known levels of alcohol exposure. The average exposure to acetaldehyde as a result of consumption of alcoholic beverages, including "unrecorded alcohol," was estimated at 0.112 mg/kg body weight/day (Lachenmeier *et al.*, 2009a). Levels of acetaldehyde in alcoholic beverages vary from less than 1 g/hl of pure alcohol up to 600 g/hl, and high concentrations of acetaldehyde were documented in alcoholic beverages commonly consumed in many parts of the world, including distilled beverages from Brazil, the People's Republic of China, Guatemala, Mexico, and the Russian Federation, as well as calvados and fortified wines and fruit and marc spirits from Europe (Lachenmeier & Sohnius,

2008; Linderborg *et al.*, 2008; Kanteres *et al.*, 2009; Lachenmeier *et al.*, 2009b).

1.3 Trends in consumption of alcoholic beverages

Volume, pattern and quality of consumed alcohol are included in the description of differential exposure to alcohol.

In a development of the WHO Global Alcohol Database, WHO has developed the Global Information System on Alcohol and Health (WHO, 2008). In 2008–09, WHO conducted the Global Survey on Alcohol and Health, collecting data on alcohol consumption, alcohol-related harm and policy responses from its Member States.

Total adult per capita consumption in litres of pure alcohol is defined as the total amount of alcohol consumed per person, taking into account recorded consumption (i.e. alcoholic beverages consumed that are recorded in official statistics of production, trade or sales) and unrecorded consumption (i.e. alcoholic beverages consumed that are not recorded in official statistics and that can come from a variety of sources such as home- or informally produced alcohol, illegal production and sale, smuggling and cross-border shopping), and subtracting consumption by tourists, if possible. Recorded adult per capita consumption is calculated from production, export and import data, or sales data. Unrecorded consumption is computed from representative surveys, specific empirical investigations or expert opinion. The percentage of lifetime and past-year abstainers provide important information about drinking in a population and complement the indicator on total adult (15+ years) per capita consumption.

Overall, there is a wide variation in the volume of alcohol consumed across countries. As presented in Table 1.1 and Table 1.2 (available at http://monographs.iarc.fr/ENG/Monographs/vol100E/100E-06-Table1.2.pdf), the countries with the highest overall consumption of alcohol per capita among the adult (15+ years) population can be found in the the WHO Regional Office for European Region (12.2 L of pure alcohol per capita), and more specifically in eastern Europe. The next highest alcohol consumption is in the WHO Region of the Americas (8.7 L of pure alcohol per capita). Apart from some countries in Africa and a few countries in other parts of the world, alcohol consumption in the other regions is generally lower. The WHO Eastern Mediterranean Region ranks lowest with 0.7 litres of alcohol consumed per adult. Total adult (15+ years) per capita consumption in litres of pure alcohol by region and country is an indicator of the alcohol consumption level of the adult population, irrespective of the number of abstainers (i.e. people who do not drink alcohol) in the country.

Globally, men consume more alcohol than women. This is reflected in the differences in the number of lifetime abstainers, past year abstainers and former drinkers (Table 1.2 on-line). Lifetime abstainers are defined as the proportion of people (15+ years) in a given population who have not consumed any alcohol during their lifetime, assessed at a given point in time. Past year abstainers are people aged 15+ years who did not consume any alcohol during the past year. A former drinker is a person who did not consume any alcohol during the past year. Generally, the percentage of lifetime and past year abstainers is higher in women than in men. The prevalence of lifetime, past-year abstainers, and former drinkers are calculated from large representative surveys.

Table 1.2 (on-line) provides information about the trend (i.e. robust estimate of five-year change) in per capita consumption (2001–05) of recorded alcohol, that is, indicates if consumption remained stable, increased, decreased, or if no conclusion could be drawn. To estimate five-year change in recorded adult (15+ years) per

Table 1.1 Estimate for total adult (15+ years) per capita consumption, by WHO region, average 2003–05

WHO Region	Adult (15+) per capita consumption*, total (recorded and unrecorded), average 2003–05
African Region (AFRO)	6.2
Region of the Americas (AMRO)	8.7
Eastern Mediterranean Region (EMRO)	0.7
European Region (EURO)	12.2
South-East Asian Region (SEARO)	2.2
Western Pacific Region (WPRO)	6.3

* in litres of pure alcohol
Source: WHO (2008)
AFRO: Algeria, Angola, Benin, Botswana, Burkina Faso, Burundi, Cameroon, Cape Verde, Central African Republic, Chad, Comoros, Congo, Côte d'Ivoire, Democratic Republic of the Congo, Equatorial Guinea, Eritrea, Ethiopia, Gabon, Gambia, Ghana, Guinea, Guinea-Bissau, Kenya, Lesotho, Liberia, Madagascar, Malawi, Mali, Mauritania, Mauritius, Mozambique, Namibia, Niger, Nigeria, Rwanda, Sao Tome and Principe, Senegal, Seychelles, Sierra Leone, South Africa, Swaziland, Togo, Uganda, United Republic of Tanzania, Zambia, Zimbabwe
AMRO: Antigua and Barbuda, Argentina, Bahamas, Barbados, Belize, Bolivia, Brazil, Canada, Chile, Colombia, Costa Rica, Cuba, Dominica, Dominican Republic, Ecuador, El Salvador, Grenada, Guatemala, Guyana, Haiti, Honduras, Jamaica, Mexico, Nicaragua, Panama, Paraguay, Peru, Saint Kitts and Nevis, Saint Lucia, Saint Vincent and the Grenadines, Suriname, Trinidad and Tobago, United States of America, Uruguay, Venezuela (Bolivarian Republic of)
EMRO: Afghanistan, Bahrain, Djibouti, Egypt, Islamic Republic of Iran, Iraq, Jordan, Kuwait, Lebanon, Libyan Arab Jamahiriya, Morocco, Oman, Pakistan, Qatar, Saudi Arabia, Somalia, Sudan, Syrian Arab Republic, Tunisia, United Arab Emirates, Yemen
EURO: Albania, Andorra, Armenia, Austria, Azerbaijan, Belarus, Belgium, Bosnia and Herzegovina, Bulgaria, Croatia, Cyprus, Czech Republic, Denmark, Estonia, Finland, France, Georgia, Germany, Greece, Hungary, Iceland, Ireland, Israel, Italy, Kazakhstan, Kyrgyzstan, Latvia, Lithuania, Luxembourg, Malta, Monaco, Montenegro, Netherlands, Norway, Poland, Portugal, Republic of the Republic of Moldova, Romania, Russian Federation, San Marino, Serbia, Slovakia, Slovenia, Spain, Sweden, Switzerland, Tajikistan, The former Yugoslav Republic of Macedonia, Turkey, Turkmenistan, Ukraine, United Kingdom, Uzbekistan
SEARO: Bangladesh, Bhutan, Democratic People's Republic of Korea, India, Indonesia, Maldives, Myanmar, Nepal, Sri Lanka, Thailand, Timor-Leste
WPRO: Australia, Brunei Darussalam, Cambodia, China, Cook Islands, Fiji, Japan, Kiribati, Lao People's Democratic Republic, Malaysia, Marshall Islands, Federated States of Micronesia, Mongolia, Nauru, New Zealand, Niue, Palau, Papua New Guinea, Philippines, Republic of Korea, Samoa, Singapore, Solomon Islands, Tonga, Tuvalu, Vanuatu, Viet Nam

capita consumption, three-year moving averages were calculated for per capita consumption of recorded alcohol for each year in the five-year period from 2001 to 2005.

Recent data on trends in consumption of alcoholic beverages indicate that the European Region and the Region of the Americas maintain a steady high consumption of alcoholic beverages, with 20% of all countries showing an increase in consumption. Alcohol consumption remains low in the Eastern Mediterranean Region. In the African Region, out of 50 countries, 20% show a decrease and 20% an increase in consumption. There is a recent and continuing increase in alcohol consumption in several low and middle-income countries in the South-East Asia and Western Pacific Regions, which probably reflects economic development and increases in consumers' purchasing power as well as increases in the marketing of branded alcoholic beverages (WHO, 2007).

2. Cancer in Humans

2.1 Description of cohort studies

2.1.1 Studies in the general population

Cohort studies are classified by the country in which the study was conducted (Table 2.1 available at http://monographs.iarc.fr/ENG/Monographs/vol100E/100E-06-Table2.1.pdf). The majority of cohort studies have been conducted in the USA, western Europe and Japan. Since the previous *IARC Monograph* (IARC, 2010), data on the association between alcohol consumption and risk of cancer have been published from several cohorts, including updates of cohorts described previously (Bongaerts *et al.*, 2006, 2008; Li *et al.*, 2006, 2009b; Weinstein *et al.*, 2006; Ericson *et al.*, 2007; Ferrari *et al.*, 2007; Ishihara *et al.*, 2007; Ozasa, 2007; Sutcliffe *et al.*, 2007; Thygesen *et al.*, 2007, 2008a, b; Fan *et al.*, 2008; Ide *et al.*, 2008; Kabat *et al.*, 2008; Nielsen & Grønbaek, 2008; Rohrmann *et al.*, 2008, 2009; Shimazu *et al.*, 2008; Friberg & Wolk, 2009; Ishiguro *et al.*, 2009; Heinen *et al.*, 2009; Klatsky *et al.*, 2009; Rod *et al.*, 2009; Thun *et al.*, 2009; Weikert *et al.*, 2009) and reports from recently established cohorts and some older cohorts from which data on alcohol consumption and risk of cancer were not available (Nakaya *et al.*, 2005; Velicer *et al.*, 2006; Akhter *et al.*, 2007; Chlebowski *et al.*, 2007; Freedman *et al.*, 2007a, b; Friborg *et al.*, 2007; Gwack *et al.*, 2007; Khurana *et al.*, 2007; Lim *et al.*, 2007; Mørch *et al.*, 2007; Sung *et al.*, 2007; Tsong *et al.*, 2007; Visvanathan *et al.*, 2007; Zhang *et al.*, 2007a; Ansems *et al.*, 2008; Brinton *et al.*, 2008, 2009; Chao *et al.*, 2008; Lim & Park, 2008; Muwonge *et al.*, 2008; Ohishi *et al.*, 2008; Toriola *et al.*, 2008, 2009; Allen *et al.*, 2009; Duffy *et al.*, 2009; Engeset *et al.*, 2009; Gibson *et al.*, 2009; Gong *et al.*, 2009; Jiao *et al.*, 2009; Johansen *et al.*, 2009; Lew *et al.*, 2009; Setiawan *et al.*, 2009; Chao *et al.*, 2010).

2.1.2 Studies in special populations

This group of studies is characterized by the assumption that the study subjects have a pattern of consumption of alcoholic beverages that is different from that of the general population, e.g. alcoholics, brewery workers, members of a temperance organization (Table 2.2 available at http://monographs.iarc.fr/ENG/Monographs/vol100E/100E-06-Table2.2.pdf). Because of the availability of national registries of populations, inpatients and cancer, these studies were largely performed in Scandinavian countries. The estimation of risk in these individuals is not based upon a comparison of exposed and unexposed subjects within the cohort, but with the expected rates of cancer in the general population. Thygesen *et al.* (2009) is the only report from cohorts of special populations that has been published since IARC (2010).

2.2. Cancers of the upper aerodigestive tract

2.2.1. Cancer of the oral cavity and pharynx

It was concluded in the previous *IARC Monograph* (IARC, 2010) that consumption of alcoholic beverages is causally related to cancer of the oral cavity and pharynx, and that the risk increases in a dose-dependent manner.

(a) Overview of cohort and case–control studies

The association of consumption of alcoholic beverages and risk of cancer of the oral cavity and/or pharynx has been assessed in six cohort studies (Freedman *et al.*, 2007a; Friborg *et al.*, 2007; Ide *et al.*, 2008; Muwonge *et al.*, 2008; Allen *et al.*, 2009; Weikert *et al.*, 2009; Table 2.3 available at http://monographs.iarc.fr/ENG/Monographs/vol100E/100E-06-Table2.3.pdf). Significant increases in risk were found with increasing amount of alcohol consumption in all studies (Freedman *et al.*, 2007a; Friborg *et al.*, 2007; Ide *et al.*, 2008; Allen *et al.*, 2009; Weikert *et al.*, 2009), increasing frequency of consumption (Friborg *et al.*, 2007; Muwonge *et al.*, 2008), and duration of consumption (Muwonge *et al.*, 2008). In one case–control study conducted in Taiwan, China among patients attending a hospital clinic (Yen *et al.*, 2008) no association was found among non-smokers and a positive association among drinkers and smokers (Table 2.4 available at http://monographs.iarc.fr/ENG/Monographs/

vol100E/100E-06-Table2.4.pdf). [No information on the quantity of alcohol or tobacco consumption was available.] In a case–control study in Uruguay (De Stefani *et al.*, 2009) a significant positive association with a predominantly alcohol-based dietary pattern and cancer of the oral cavity and pharynx was found (data not shown). [No specific assessment of alcohol intake was presented and the contribution of other foods to this dietary pattern was not known.]

Undifferentiated nasopharyngeal carcinoma (NPC), which is common in parts of Southern Asia, North Africa and the Arctic, is associated with Epstein-Barr virus and preserved foods (see the *Monograph* on Chinese-style Salted Fish in this volume). Friborg *et al.* (2007) confirmed earlier results suggesting limited or no association between alcohol and undifferentiated NPC (Yu *et al.*, 2002). However, in a Western population where differentiated forms of NPC are more common, a significantly increased risk of NPC has been associated with heavy drinking (> 21 drinks per week) (Vaughan *et al.*, 1996), indicating a difference in ethiology between differentiated and undifferentiated types of NPC (Table 2.4 on-line).

Thygesen *et al.* (2009) reported a significantly higher rate of cancer of the oral cavity and pharynx among Danish alcohol abusers compared with national rates. [This cohort study provided no information on individual exposures or results adjusted for potential confounders.] See Table 2.5 available at http://monographs.iarc.fr/ENG/Monographs/vol100E/100E-06-Table2.5.pdf.

(b) Intensity and duration

Previous studies consistently showed that consumption of alcoholic beverages is associated with an increased risk of cancer of the oral cavity and/or pharynx, although the nature of the dose–response relationship is not fully understood (IARC, 2010). In most studies an approximate threefold increased risk was found at relatively high levels of intake (i.e. > 60 g/day). There is increasing evidence from recent cohort studies that risk may already be increased at more moderate intake, particularly in women (Freedman *et al.*, 2007a; Allen *et al.*, 2009; Weikert *et al.*, 2009).

A pooled analysis of the International Head and Neck Cancer Epidemiology Consortium, which specifically examined the association of alcohol consumption and duration, found that among drinkers of 10 drinks per day or less, the association with total drink-years increased with increasing drinks/day, indicating that more drinks/day for a shorter duration was more deleterious than fewer drinks/day for a longer duration (Lubin *et al.*, 2009).

(c) Effect of cessation

A meta-analysis of 13 case–control studies of cancer of the oral cavity and pharynx combined found that compared with current drinkers, risk did not decrease until 10 years or more after cessation of drinking (odds ratio (OR), 0.67; 95%CI: 0.63–0.73) (Rehm *et al.*, 2007) (Table 2.6 available at http://monographs.iarc.fr/ENG/Monographs/vol100E/100E-06-Table2.6.pdf). Consistent with many earlier studies, risks were found to be elevated among recent former drinkers, most likely due to ill health directly related to the cancer or its precursors.

(d) Types of alcoholic beverage

Some studies have assessed whether the association of consumption of alcoholic beverages on risk varies by beverage type, and have found broadly similar associations in wine, beer and spirit drinkers (Freedman *et al.*, 2007a; Allen *et al.*, 2009).

(e) Population characteristics

The association of consumption of alcoholic beverages with risk of cancer of the oral cavity and pharynx is increased in both men and women (Freedman *et al.*, 2007a; Weikert *et al.*, 2009).

Studies have been hampered with low numbers of women at the highest levels of exposure.

(f) Histological subtype

Very few studies have examined the association of consumption of alcoholic beverages by histological subtype for cancers of the oral cavity and pharynx. From a large-scale cohort study, Weikert *et al.* (2009) reported that both baseline and lifetime alcohol intake were associated with an increased risk of squamous cell carcinoma of the oral cavity and the pharynx, with an increased risk of 10% (95%CI: 8–13%) per 10 g per day increase in lifetime alcohol intake.

(g) Association among non-smokers

There is evidence from a pooled analysis of 15 case–control studies that increasing consumption of alcoholic beverages increases risk of cancer of the oral cavity and oropharynx/hypopharynx cancer among never smokers, with risk estimates of 1.23 (95%CI: 0.59–2.57) and 5.50 (95%CI: 2.26–13.36), for 5 or more drinks/day versus never drinkers, for the two cancer sites, respectively (Hashibe *et al.*, 2007; Table 2.6 on-line). One study in Taiwan, China found no association with alcohol consumption among non-smoking ever-drinkers for cancer of the oral cavity (Yen *et al.*, 2008). [No information was provided on the quantity of alcohol consumed.]

(h) Joint effect of alcoholic beverages and tobacco smoking

It is well established that there is a joint effect of tobacco smoking and consumption of alcoholic beverages on the risk of cancer of the oral cavity and pharynx, with very high risks observed in individuals who are both heavy drinkers and heavy smokers, corresponding to a greater than a multiplicative interaction (IARC, 2010). The joint effect of alcohol consumption and tobacco smoking on the risk of cancers of the oral cavity and pharynx is described in Section 2.20 of the *Monograph* on Tobacco Smoking in this volume.

2.2.2 Cancer of the larynx

It was concluded in the previous *IARC Monograph* (IARC, 2010) that consumption of alcoholic beverages is causally related to cancer of the larynx, and that the risk increases in a dose-dependent manner.

(a) Overview of cohort and case–control studies

Since IARC (2010), the association of consumption of alcoholic beverages and risk of cancer of the larynx has been assessed in three general-population cohort studies (Freedman *et al.*, 2007a; Allen *et al.*, 2009, Weikert *et al.*, 2009; Table 2.7 available at http://monographs.iarc.fr/ENG/Monographs/vol100E/100E-06-Table2.7.pdf) and one case–control study (Garavello *et al.*, 2006; Table 2.8 available at http://monographs.iarc.fr/ENG/Monographs/vol100E/100E-06-Table2.8.pdf), all of which found significant increases in risk associated with alcohol consumption. In one further case–control study in Uruguay (De Stefani *et al.*, 2009) a significant positive association with a predominantly alcohol-based dietary pattern and cancer of the larynx was found (data not shown). [No specific assessment of alcohol intake was presented and the contribution of other foods to this dietary pattern was not known.]

Thygesen *et al.* (2009) reported a significantly higher rate of cancer of the larynx among Danish alcohol abusers compared with national rates (Table 2.5 on-line). This study provided no information on individual exposures or results adjusted for potential confounders

(b) Intensity and duration

Previous studies consistently showed that increasing alcohol consumption is associated with an increased risk of cancer of the larynx (IARC, 2010). Bagnardi *et al.* (2001) reported risk estimates of 1.38 (95%CI: 1.32–1.45) for intake of 25 g alcohol per day, 1.94 (95%CI: 1.78–2.11) for 50 g per day, and 3.95 (95%CI: 3.43–4.57) for 100 g per day from a meta-analysis of 20 case–control studies, including over 3500 cases. An increased risk for cancer of the larynx was found for women drinking above one drink/day in a large cohort of United Kingdom women [equivalent to an increased risk of 1.44 (95%CI: 1.10–1.88) per 10 g alcohol per day] (Allen *et al.*, 2009). This is consistent with the 1.38 (95%CI: 1.10–1.73) estimate per 10 g per day reported among women in the European Prospective Investigation into Cancer and Nutrition (Weikert *et al.*, 2009). Compatible with this, Freedman *et al.* (2007a) reported a risk estimate of 2.15 (95%CI: 0.82–5.65) among women associated with 3 or more drinks/day from the NIH-AARP Diet and Health Study. Among men, the dose–response relationship is slightly weaker (Freedman *et al.*, 2007a; Weikert *et al.*, 2009), although it is difficult to determine whether these differences are due to chance because of the relatively low number of cases in women. In a large case–control study in Italy there was clear evidence of a dose–response relationship for men and women combined (Garavello *et al.*, 2006).

A pooled analysis of the International Head and Neck Cancer Epidemiology Consortium, which specifically examined the association of quantity and duration of alcohol consumption, found that among drinkers of 10 drinks per day or less, the association with total drink-years increased with increasing drinks/day, indicating that more drinks/day for a shorter duration was more deleterious than fewer drinks/day for a longer duration (Lubin *et al.*, 2009).

(c) Effect of cessation

Few studies have assessed whether the risk for cancer of the larynx declines since stopping drinking. Altieri *et al.* (2002) reported a risk estimate of 0.53 (95%CI: 0.15–1.94) for stopping drinking for 20 years or more ago compared with current drinkers; the risk for never-drinkers was 0.56 (95%CI: 0.31–0.99).

(d) Types of alcoholic beverage

Evidence suggests that the most frequently consumed beverage in a population tends to be associated with the highest risk of cancer of the larynx. Data published recently largely supports this view (Garavello *et al.*, 2006). The NIH-AARP Diet and Health Study found a stronger association for spirits than for beer or wine consumption among men (Freedman *et al.*, 2007a). [The Working Group noted the small number of cases.]

(e) Risk among non-smokers

There is evidence from a pooled analysis of 11 case–control studies, based on 121 cases of laryngeal cancer, that increasing alcohol consumption increases the risk for cancer of the larynx among never smokers, with a risk estimate of 2.98 (95%CI: 1.72–5.17) for 5 or more drinks/day versus never drinkers (Hashibe *et al.*, 2007; Table 2.6 on-line).

(f) Joint effect of alcoholic beverages and tobacco smoking

Evidence suggests that there exists a joint effect of tobacco smoking and consumption of alcoholic beverages on the risk of cancer of the larynx, with very high risks observed in individuals who are both heavy drinkers and heavy smokers. More recent studies that have examined the joint effect of alcohol consumption and tobacco smoking on the risk of cancer of the larynx are described in Section 2.20 of the *Monograph* on Tobacco Smoking in this volume.

2.2.3 Cancer of the oesophagus

It was concluded in the previous *IARC Monograph* (IARC, 2010) that consumption of alcoholic beverages is causally associated with cancer of the oesophagus. The increased risk is largely restricted to squamous cell carcinoma, with little or no association for adenocarcinoma of the oesophagus.

(a) Overview of cohort and case–control studies

Since IARC (2010), the association of consumption of alcoholic beverages and risk of cancer of the oesophagus has been assessed in six cohort studies (Freedman *et al.*, 2007b; Ozasa *et al.*, 2007; Fan *et al.*, 2008; Allen *et al.*, 2009; Ishiguro *et al.*, 2009; Weikert *et al.*, 2009; Table 2.9 available at http://monographs.iarc.fr/ENG/Monographs/vol100E/100E-06-Table2.9 pdf) and four case–control studies (Lee *et al.*, 2005; Vioque *et al.*, 2008; Benedetti *et al.*, 2009; Pandeya *et al.*, 2009; Table 2.10 available at http://monographs.iarc.fr/ENG/Monographs/vol100E/100E-06-Table2.10.pdf), all of which found significant increases in risk with alcohol consumption. A case–control study in Uruguay (De Stefani *et al.*, 2009) found a significant positive association with a predominantly alcohol-based dietary pattern and cancer of the oesophagus (data not shown). [No specific assessment of alcohol intake was presented and the contribution of other foods to this dietary pattern was not known.]

Thygesen *et al.* (2009) reported a significantly higher rate of cancer of the oesophagus among Danish alcohol abusers compared with national rates (Table 2.5 on-line). [This study provided no information on individual exposures or results adjusted for potential confounders.]

(b) Intensity and duration

Data reviewed previously (IARC, 2010) consistently showed that increasing consumption of alcoholic beverages is associated with an increased risk of cancer of the oesophagus. Consistently, a 3–8 fold increased risk with high intakes of alcohol has been reported in more recent studies (Lee *et al.*, 2005; Freedman *et al.*, 2007b; Ozasa *et al.*, 2007; Fan *et al.*, 2008; Vioque *et al.*, 2008; Ishiguro *et al.*, 2009; Pandeya *et al.*, 2009). Smaller increases in risk at lower amounts of alcohol intake have been found by analysis of large cohorts in Europe, with a significant increased risk of approximately 20% per 10 g alcohol per day (Allen *et al.*, 2009; Weikert *et al.*, 2009).

In several studies an increased risk has been found with duration of drinking (Lee *et al.*, 2005; Ozasa *et al.*, 2007; Fan *et al.*, 2008, Vioque *et al.*, 2008), frequency of drinking (Ozasa *et al.*, 2007), a lower age at starting drinking (Ozasa *et al.*, 2007; Fan *et al.*, 2008), or cumulative intake (Benedetti *et al.*, 2009). Risk is similar when alcohol consumption is based on measures of either baseline or lifetime alcohol consumption (Fan *et al.*, 2008; Weikert *et al.*, 2009).

(c) Effect of cessation

In several studies the risk for cancer of the oesophagus was reduced with increasing time since cessation of drinking. In a meta-analysis of 5 case–control studies Rehm *et al.* (2007) reported that compared with current drinkers, risk was not reduced until 5 years or more after cessation of drinking (OR, 0.85; 95%CI: 0.78–0.92) and approached that of nondrinkers after 15 years or more since quitting drinking (Table 2.6 on-line). Similar results were obtained from a cohort study (Ozasa *et al.*, 2007). Risks are elevated among more former drinkers, who most likely cease drinking due to ill health directly related to the cancer or its precursors (Rehm *et al.*, 2007; Vioque *et al.*, 2008; Ozasa *et al.*, 2007).

(d) Types of alcoholic beverage

Most previous studies found no material difference in the association of consumption of alcoholic beverages on risk of cancer of the oesophagus according to specific beverage types, with the most commonly consumed beverage tending to be associated with the highest risk. This is supported by data from more recent studies (Lee *et al.*, 2005; Freedman *et al.*, 2007b; Fan *et al.*, 2008; Vioque *et al.*, 2008; Allen *et al.*, 2009; Pandeya *et al.*, 2009).

(e) Population characteristics

All recent studies have found significant positive associations in both men (Fan *et al.*, 2008; Benedetti *et al.*, 2009; Ishiguro *et al.*, 2009) and women (Allen *et al.*, 2009), and in studies that have stratified by sex (Pandeya *et al.*, 2009).

(f) Risk associated with facial flushing response

One cohort study in Japan examined the association of consumption of alcoholic beverages with cancer of the oesophagus according to whether the cohort members experienced a facial flushing response. Although the risk associated with a high alcohol intake among men with a flushing response was higher than among those with no flushing response, the differences were not significant. Details of the association of alcohol consumption according to genetic variants in alcohol-metabolizing genes related to the flushing response are presented in Section 2.19.

(g) Histological subtypes

In the previous *IARC Monograph* it was concluded that consumption of alcoholic beverages is causally related to squamous cell carcinoma of the oesophagus (OSCC), with no or little association with adenocarcinoma of the oesophagus (IARC, 2010). Data published since a strong association with OSCC or non-adenocarcinoma (Lee *et al.*, 2005; Freedman *et al.*, 2007b; Fan *et al.*, 2008; Vioque *et al.*, 2008; Allen *et al.*, 2009; Benedetti *et al.*, 2009; Ishiguro *et al.*, 2009; Pandeya *et al.*, 2009; Weikert *et al.*, 2009), and no association with alcohol consumption and adenocarcinoma of the oesophagus (Freedman *et al.*, 2007b; Allen *et al.*, 2009; Benedetti *et al.*, 2009; Pandeya *et al.*, 2009).

(h) Association among non-smokers

Data on the association of consumption of alcoholic beverages with risk of cancer of the oesophagus among non-smokers are limited. Pandeya *et al.* (2009) reported higher risks with increasing alcohol consumption among current smokers compared to never smokers from a case–control study in Australia. [The low numbers of highly exposed cases among never smokers makes it difficult to draw any conclusions.]

(i) Joint effect of alcoholic beverages and tobacco smoking

Evidence suggests a joint effect of tobacco smoking and consumption of alcoholic beverages on the risk for cancer of the oesophagus, with very high risks observed in individuals who were both heavy drinkers and heavy smokers. Recent studies that have examined the joint effect of alcohol consumption and tobacco smoking on the risk of cancer of the oesophagus are described in Section 2.20 of the *Monograph* on Tobacco Smoking in this volume.

2.2.4. Cancers of the upper aerodigestive tract combined

(a) Overview of cohort and case–control studies

In the previous *IARC Monograph* (IARC, 2010) the association between consumption of alcoholic beverages and risk of cancer of the upper aerodigestive tract combined was not evaluated. Since then, three cohort studies (Thygesen *et al.*, 2007; Allen *et al.*, 2009; Weikert *et al.*, 2009; Table 2.11 available at http://monographs.iarc.fr/ENG/Monographs/vol100E/100E-06-Table2.11.pdf) and one case–control study (Zaridze *et al.*, 2009; Table 2.12 available at http://monographs.iarc.fr/ENG/Monographs/vol100E/100E-06-Table2.12.pdf) have examined the association of alcoholic beverage consumption and cancers of the upper aerodigestive tract (i.e. oral cavity, pharynx, larynx and oesophagus combined), and one reported on cancers of the oral cavity, pharynx and larynx combined (Freedman *et al.*, 2007a). All studies reported significant increases in risk with alcoholic beverage consumption, observed in both men and women (Freedman *et al.*, 2007a; Thygesen *et al.*, 2007; Allen *et al.*, 2009; Weikert *et al.*, 2009; Zaridze *et al.*, 2009).

(b) Intensity and duration

In one cohort study an increased risk for cancer of the upper aerodigestive tract combined was observed only among those who had a relatively high alcohol intake (i.e. 42 drinks/week or more) (Thygesen *et al.*, 2007). Other studies have reported increases in risk at more moderate levels of consumption, particularly among women (Freedman *et al.*, 2007a; Allen *et al.*, 2009; Weikert *et al.*, 2009).

(c) Types of alcoholic beverage

The association of consumption of alcoholic beverages on risk of cancer of the upper aerodigestive tract combined does not vary by beverage type, as found in a meta-analysis of 15 case–control studies (Purdue *et al.*, 2009; Table 2.6 on-line) and cohort studies (Allen *et al.*, 2009; Weikert *et al.*, 2009).

(d) Association among non-smokers

Few studies have had sufficient statistical power to assess reliably the association of consumption of alcoholic beverages by smoking status with cancers of the upper aerodigestive tract combined. Most previous studies (as outlined in IARC, 2010), as well as recent data from the European Prospective Investigation into Cancer and Nutrition have found similar increased risks with increasing alcohol intake among both non-smokers and smokers (Weikert *et al.*, 2009). In a large cohort study among women in the United Kingdom with a low to moderate alcohol intake, alcohol consumption was not associated with an increased risk of cancers of the upper aerodigestive tract in never smokers or former smokers, but was strongly associated with an increased risk among current smokers (Allen *et al.*, 2009).

2.3 Cancer of the colorectum

In the previous *IARC Monograph* (IARC, 2010) it was concluded that consumption of alcoholic beverages is causally related to cancer of the colorectum. This conclusion was largely based on a pooled analysis of eight cohort studies of alcohol intake and cancer of the colorectum conducted in Europe and North America, which found a relative risk (RR) of about 1.4 for cancer of the colorectum with regular consumption of high intakes of alcohol (≥ 45 g/d), compared to non-drinkers, in men and women combined, and which was not related to beverage type (Cho *et al.*, 2004).

2.3.1 Cohort studies and meta-analyses of cohort studies

Since IARC (2010), 12 cohort studies have evaluated the association between consumption of alcoholic beverages and risk of cancer of the colorectum and/or cancer of the colon and rectum separately (Table 2.13 available at http://monographs.iarc.fr/ENG/Monographs/vol100E/100E-06-Table2.13.pdf). Of the nine cohort studies that examined the association of consumption of alcoholic beverages and risk of cancer of the colorectum, seven confirmed a significant positive association (Akhter *et al.*, 2007; Ferrari *et al.*, 2007; Ishihara *et al.*, 2007; Tsong *et al.*, 2007; Bongaerts *et al.*, 2008; Thygesen *et al.*, 2008b; Toriola *et al.*, 2008). In only two cohort studies was no overall association reported, although both of these likely included very few cases with a high alcohol intake (Kabat *et al.*, 2008; Lim & Park, 2008). In one further study (Engeset *et al.*, 2009) no association with a predominantly alcohol-based dietary pattern and cancer of the colorectum was found. [No quantitative assessment of alcohol intake per se was provided and the contribution of other foods to this dietary pattern was not known.] Of the seven studies that evaluated cancer of the colon and rectum separately (Akhter *et al.*, 2007; Ferrari *et al.*, 2007; Ozasa, 2007; Tsong *et al.*, 2007; Thygesen *et al.*, 2008b; Bongaerts *et al.*, 2008; Allen *et al.*, 2009), three reported a significant increased risk with alcohol intake for both sites (Akhter *et al.*, 2007; Ferrari *et al.*, 2007; Tsong *et al.*, 2007). This is consistent with findings from one meta-analysis and one pooled analysis (Table 2.14 available at http://monographs.iarc.fr/ENG/Monographs/vol100E/100E-06-Table2.14.pdf). In a meta-analysis of 21 cohort studies a significant increased risk for cancer of the colorectum, and for colon and rectal cancer separately, for heavy drinkers compared to light or non-drinkers was found (Huxley *et al.*, 2009). There was also a significant positive association of consumption of alcoholic beverages for men and women with both cancer of the colon and of the rectum in a pooled analysis of five cohort studies in Japan (Mizoue *et al.*, 2008). Thygesen *et al.* (2008b) reported an increased risk for colon cancer and not for rectal cancer; in two other studies a significant increased risk for rectal cancer and a weaker, non-significant positive association for colon cancer was found (Ozasa, 2007; Bongaerts *et al.*, 2008). [Such inconsistency may be due to the small numbers of heavy drinkers in each subsite.] In the largest study to date, with over 4000 cases of colon and over 2000 cases of rectal cancer, no association of alcohol intake was found with colon cancer and a small, but statistically significant, increased risk for rectal cancer (Allen *et al.*, 2009). [The Working Group noted that the reason for the lack of association with colon cancer in this study of United Kingdom women is not clear, but may, in part, relate to the narrower range of alcohol intake (which was mostly low to moderate), resulting in limited power to detect an association at higher levels of alcohol intake]. Most of the studies in which the association of alcohol intake has been examined by more detailed subsite definitions within the colon are more consistent in showing a positive association with alcohol intake for cancer of the distal colon, but a weak or null association for cancer of the proximal colon (Akhter *et al.*, 2007; Ferrari *et al.*, 2007; Bongaerts *et al.*, 2008; Thygesen *et al.*, 2008b).

2.3.2 Cohort studies in special populations

Since IARC (2010), in one cohort study in the Netherlands a significantly higher rate of rectal cancer among male alcohol abusers compared with national rates, but no association with colon cancer was found (Table 2.15 available at http://monographs.iarc.fr/ENG/Monographs/vol100E/100E-06-Table2.15.pdf). Among women, rates of both colon and rectal cancer were similar among alcohol abusers and the national population, although there were relatively low numbers for each cancer site (Thygesen *et al.*, 2009). [This study provided no information on individual exposures or results adjusted for potential confounders.]

2.3.3 Case–control studies

Since IARC (2010), reports on the association of consumption of alcoholic beverages and cancer of the colorectum have come from 10 case–control studies. There was a significant positive association in five, three of which found an increased risk of cancer of the colorectum at relatively high levels of consumption (Gao *et al.*, 2008; Lightfoot *et al.*, 2008; Benedetti *et al.*, 2009) and for two studies in the Far East an increased risk among drinkers was reported (Sriamporn *et al.*, 2007; Wei *et al.*, 2009). [Information on quantity of intake was not available for these studies.] (Table 2.16 available at http://monographs.iarc.fr/ENG/Monographs/vol100E/100E-06-Table2.16.pdf). No association for consumption of alcoholic beverages and cancer of the colorectum was reported for five case–control studies (Wang *et al.*, 2006a; Murtaugh *et al.*, 2007; Pereira Serafim *et al.*, 2008; Ganesh *et al.*, 2009; Wu *et al.*, 2009). [These studies were conducted in populations with a low intake of alcoholic beverages (Wang *et al.*, 2006a; Murtaugh *et al.*, 2007; Ganesh *et al.*, 2009) and/or had a small sample size and limited exposure information (Pereira Serafim *et al.*, 2008; Ganesh *et al.*, 2009; Wu *et al.*, 2009).]

2.3.4 Dose–response relationship

One pooled analysis of eight cohort studies (Cho *et al.*, 2004) and several independent studies found an increased risk for cancer of the colorectum for an alcohol intake of 20 g/day or more (Gao *et al.*, 2008), 30 g/day or more (Ferrari *et al.*, 2007; Bongaerts *et al.*, 2008) or 45 g/day or more (Akhter *et al.*, 2007). A pooled analysis of five cohort studies conducted in Japan also found an increased risk for cancer of the colorectum above 23 g/day, evident for both cancer of the colon and of the rectum for both men and women (Mizoue *et al.*, 2008). Other studies found an increased risk for cancer of the colorectum or rectum only with lower amounts of alcohol (i.e. of the order of 1 drink/d or 10 g/d) (Tsong *et al.*, 2007; Thygesen *et al.*, 2008b; Allen *et al.*, 2009).

2.3.5 Types of alcoholic beverage

(a) Other metrics of exposure

Few studies have examined the association between cancer of the colorectum and other metrics of exposure (average alcohol intake, over a lifetime or specifically during early adulthood, age at starting, duration). The limited evidence suggests that there is no strong association with duration of drinking in years or age at started drinking (Ferrari *et al.*, 2007; Ozasa, 2007; Wu *et al.*, 2009). In most earlier studies and some recent studies the risk associated with a baseline measure of intake is similar to a measure of average lifetime intake (Ferrari *et al.*, 2007; Thygesen *et al.*, 2008b), Benedetti *et al.* (2009) reported an increased risk with increasing cumulative intake. There is also very limited information on whether the frequency of drinking is an important determinant of risk. In three studies no association with frequency of alcohol intake (drinks/day) was found (Ozasa, 2007; Lim & Park, 2008; Benedetti *et al.*, 2009), while in others the frequency of intake was associated with an increased risk among those with a high intake of alcohol (> 15 g/d), but not among those with lower intake of alcohol (Mizoue *et al.*, 2008; Thygesen *et al.*, 2008b).

The association of consumption of alcoholic beverages and cancer of the colorectum does not appear to differ by beverage type (Ferrari *et al.*, 2007; Tsong *et al.*, 2007; Bongaerts *et al.*, 2008; Thygesen *et al.*, 2008b).

2.3.6 Population characteristics

The association of consumption of alcoholic beverages and cancer of the colorectum appears to be similar for men and women (Ferrari *et al.*, 2007; Bongaerts *et al.*, 2008). There is a causal association between cigarette smoking and risk for cancer of the colorectum (see the *Monograph* on Tobacco Smoking in this volume). Most studies of consumption of alcoholic beverages have adjusted for smoking status. In studies that statified the analysis by smoking status most found an increased risk among both never and current smokers, with the risk estimates slightly higher in current or ever smokers compared to never smokers (Akhter *et al.*, 2007; Ferrari *et al.*, 2007; Tsong *et al.*, 2007).

Ferrari *et al.* (2007) did not find a statistically significant interaction term between alcohol drinking and smoking with regard to cancers of the colorectum. Tsong *et al.* (2007) reported that the interaction effect between alcohol and smoking was not statistically significant on risk of cancer of the colorectum overall and rectal cancer alone (both $P > 0.19$), while the interaction effect on colon cancer risk was of marginal statistical significance ($P = 0.051$).

Few studies have examined whether the association of alcohol with cancer of the colorectum varies by folate status; the European Prospective Investigation into Cancer and Nutrition found some evidence that the risk for colorectal cancer associated with alcohol intake was stronger in individuals with a low folate intake, but the interaction term was of marginal statistical significance (Ferrari *et al.*, 2007), and two other studies found no evidence that the association of alcohol intake with risk differed according to intake of folate, or intake of related nutrients such as vitamin B6, vitamin B12 or methionine (Ishihara *et al.*, 2007; Kabat *et al.*, 2008).

2.4 Cancer of the liver and hepatobiliary tract

In the previous *IARC Monograph* (IARC, 2010) it was concluded that consumption of alcoholic beverages is causally related to risk of cancer of the liver. This conclusion was based on a considerable number of cohort and case–control studies.

Chronic infection with hepatitis viruses B and C are the major causes of cancer of the liver. The increased risk associated with consumption of alcoholic beverages has been found consistently among individuals infected with hepatitis viruses as well as among uninfected individuals. Quantification of the effect of consumption of alcoholic beverages on the risk of cancer of the liver cannot be determined reliably since cirrhosis and other liver disorders that often predate cancer of the liver tend to lead to a decrease in or the cessation of consumption of alcoholic beverages many years before the occurrence of cancer of the liver.

The previous *IARC Monograph* did not separately evaluate the effect of consumption of alcoholic beverages on the risk of cholangiocarcinoma.

2.4.1 Hepatocellular carcinoma

Three cohort studies (Gwack *et al.*, 2007; Ohishi *et al.*, 2008; Allen *et al.*, 2009; Table 2.17 available at http://monographs.iarc.fr/ENG/Monographs/vol100E/100E-06-Table2.17.pdf) and three case–control studies (Hassan *et al.*, 2008; Benedetti *et al.*, 2009; Zaridze *et al.*, 2009; Table 2.18 available at http://monographs.iarc.fr/ENG/Monographs/vol100E/100E-06-Table2.18.pdf) on the general population and one cohort study on alcoholics (Thygesen *et al.*, 2009; Table 2.19 available at http://monographs.iarc.fr/ENG/Monographs/vol100E/100E-06-Table2.19.pdf) have been identified since IARC (2010). No new meta-analysis or studies on the joint effect of alcohol beverage and virus infection were found.

In the three cohort studies, Gwack *et al.* (2007) in Republic of Korea, Ohishi *et al.* (2008) in Japan, and Allen *et al.* (2009) in the United Kingdom, an association between consumption of alcoholic beverages and cancer of the liver was found. Hassan *et al.* (2008) reported from a study in USA an increased risk for cancer of the liver in women with increasing alcohol consumption. Among men, the risk for cancer of the liver was only increased among those with an ethanol intake of $\geq$ 60 ml per day. Zaridze *et al.* (2009) found an increased risk of cancer of the liver with consumption of alcoholic beverages (usually vodka) among both men and women in the Russian Federation as did Benedetti *et al.* (2009) from Canada. Thygesen *et al.* (2009) reported a higher risk of cancer of the liver among both alcoholic men and women compared to the general population. [There were only 8 cases among women.]

2.4.2 Cholangiocarcinoma

Ten studies on the association between consumption of alcoholic beverages and cholangiocarcinoma (CCA) in the general population were identified (Parkin *et al.*, 1991; Shin *et al.*,

1996, Donato *et al.*, 2001; Kuper *et al.*, 2001; Yamamoto *et al.*, 2004; Honjo *et al.*, 2005; Shaib *et al.*, 2007; Hsing *et al.*, 2008; Lee *et al.*, 2008a; Zhou *et al.*, 2008), all of which were case–control studies (Table 2.20 available at http://monographs.iarc.fr/ENG/Monographs/vol100E/100E-06-Table2.20.pdf). An increased risk for cholangiocarcinoma among heavy drinkers (≥ 80 g/day) was reported in two studies from the Republic of Korea (Shin *et al.*, 1996 for CCA; Lee *et al.*, 2008a for intrahepatic CCA) and one study from the USA (Shaib *et al.*, 2007 for both intrahepatic and extrahepatic CCA), among current drinkers in a study from China (Hsing *et al.*, 2008 for extrahepatic CCA), and among regular drinkers in Thailand (Honjo *et al.*, 2005 for CCA). In another study in Thailand a non-significant increased risk among regular drinkers was found (Parkin *et al.*, 1991 for CCA). There was no association in three studies on intrahepatic CCA from Italy (Donato *et al.*, 2001), Japan (Yamamoto *et al.*, 2004), and China (Zhou *et al.*, 2008) (Table 2.20 on-line). Kuper *et al.* (2001) did not find any association between consumption of alcoholic beverages and cholangiocarcinoma in a low-risk Caucasian population in Greece [data not shown due to only six cases].

Cholangiocarcinoma is a recognized complication of primary sclerosing cholangitis. A study among patients with primary sclerosing cholangitis (26 cases of CCA following primary sclerosing cholangitis, 87 controls with primary sclerosing cholangitis) reported alcohol drinking as one of the risk factor for developing CCA (Chalasani *et al.*, 2000).

2.5 Cancer of the stomach

In the previous *IARC Monograph* (IARC, 2010), results on the risk for cancer of the stomach associated with the consumption of alcoholic beverages were considered inconsistent. Since then, four cohort studies (Freedman *et al.*, 2007; Larsson *et al.*, 2007; Sung *et al.*, 2007; Allen *et al.*, 2009) and three case–control studies (Lucenteforte *et al.*, 2008; Benedetti *et al.*, 2009; Zaridze *et al.*, 2009) in the general population, and one cohort study in alcoholics (Thygesen *et al.*, 2009) have been published.

2.5.1 Cohort studies in the general population

Among cohort studies, no general association between alcohol intake and cancer of the stomach was found in three studies (Freedman *et al.*, 2007; Larsson *et al.*, 2007; Allen *et al.*, 2009), while Sung *et al.* (2007) reported a slight increase in risk (Table 2.21 available at http://monographs.iarc.fr/ENG/Monographs/vol100E/100E-06-Table2.21.pdf).

2.5.2 Cohort studies in special populations (alcohol abusers)

Thygesen *et al.* (2009) reported a higher risk of cancer of the stomach in alcoholics than in the general population (Table 2.22 available at http://monographs.iarc.fr/ENG/Monographs/vol100E/100E-06-Table2.22.pdf). The increase was statistically significant in men (68 cases) but not in women (7 cases). [This study provided no information on individual exposures or results adjusted for potential confounders.]

2.5.3 Case–control studies

None of the case–control studies (Lucenteforte *et al.*, 2008; Benedetti *et al.*, 2009; Zaridze *et al.*, 2009; Table 2.23 available at http://monographs.iarc.fr/ENG/Monographs/vol100E/100E-06-Table2.23.pdf) found an overall association between alcohol intake and risk for cancer of the stomach. Benedetti *et al.* (2009) reported a statistically significant increase in the risk of cancer of the stomach among those who consumed 1–6 drinks per week, but not among those who drank 7 or more per week.

2.5.4 Types of alcoholic beverage

Analyses by different types of alcoholic beverages are presented in Table 2.24 (available at http://monographs.iarc.fr/ENG/Monographs/vol100E/100E-06-Table2.24.pdf). Larsson *et al.* (2007) found an increased risk for cancer of the stomach with intake of medium or strong beer, while no effects were found with light beer, wine or hard liquor. Freedman *et al.* (2007) reported an increased risk for cancer of gastric cardia among those with high intake of hard liquor while no such association was found in the case of non-cardia gastric adenocarcinoma. Benedetti *et al.* (2009) reported a statistically significant increase in risk for cancer of the stomach among those who consumed 1–6 drinks per week of any of beer, wine or hard liquor, but not with those who drank 7 or more per week.

2.5.5 Confounding

In the previous Monograph, significantly increased risks were reported in some studies, including those from Japan, China, Poland and the Russian Federation. In no study was it possible to stratify or adjust fully for lifetime infection with *Helicobacter pylori*. It was concluded that since most of the population in areas where an association between consumption of alcoholic beverages and stomach cancer emerged had probably been infected by the bacterium, potential confounding by *H. pylori* infection was not a major concern. Of concern, however, was the likelihood that dietary deficiencies exist in those populations and that the consumption of alcoholic beverages might be accompanied by other unfavourable lifestyle factors, such as low socioeconomic class and low intake of fresh fruit, vegetables and various micronutrients (IARC, 2010).

New studies did not provide any additional information of potential confounders.

2.6 Cancer of the pancreas

In the previous *IARC Monograph* (IARC, 2010), it was concluded that there was not strong evidence for an association between the consumption of alcoholic beverages and risk of cancer of the pancreas.

2.6.1 Meta- and pooled analyses

A pooled analysis of 14 cohort studies (Genkinger *et al.*, 2009) and a meta-analysis of 21 case–control studies and 11 cohort studies (one of which was the pooled analysis) (Tramacere *et al.*, 2009) reported a small, statistically significant, increased risk for cancer of the pancreas associated with high intakes of alcoholic beverages (Table 2.25 available at http://monographs.iarc.fr/ENG/Monographs/vol100E/100E-06-Table2.25.pdf). In the pooled analysis, with over 2000 incident cases of cancer of the pancreas, a relative risk of 1.22 (95%CI: 1.03–1.45) for those drinking ≥ 30 g/day versus none was found, with no significant difference by beverage type (Genkinger *et al.*, 2009). Tramacere *et al.* (2009) reported a relative risk of 1.22 (95%CI: 1.12–1.34) for those drinking ≥ 3 drinks/day [approx. 30 g/day] versus none or occasional drinkers.

2.6.2 Cohort studies in the general population

In addition to the cohort studies included in the pooled analysis by Genkinger *et al.* (2009), the association of alcoholic beverage consumption and risk for cancer of the pancreas has been independently examined in six cohort studies (Table 2.26 available at http://monographs.iarc.fr/ENG/Monographs/vol100E/100E-06-Table2.26.pdf). A nested case–control study within the Veterans Health Administration Cohort [the control population consisted of all participants without cancer of the pancreas enrolled in the study] found a significant negative association between alcohol use and cancer of the pancreas.

[Only data on current alcohol use were collected by the clinical provider, and duration and intensity of alcohol use were not recorded. It is possible that patients might have stopped drinking due to ill health, thereby causing a spuriously high risk among the non-drinkers (Khurana *et al.*, 2007).] In another study, high alcohol consumption, defined according to a scoring system that was based on a self-administered questionnaire designed to detect alcoholism and on serum levels of γ-glutamyl transferase [a biomarker of excessive drinking], was associated with an increased risk for cancer of the pancreas (Johansen *et al.*, 2009). [Data on the amount of alcohol consumption were not available.] In the Million Women Study in the United Kingdom, with approximately 1300 incident cases, there was no association between alcohol intake and risk for cancer of the pancreas among this population of low to moderate drinkers (only 5% drank ≥ 15 drinks/week) (Allen *et al.*, 2009). In the European Prospective Investigation of nutrition and Cancer there was also no association with alcohol intake (Rohrmann *et al.*, 2009), although there was some suggestion of an increased risk among those with a high average lifetime intake of spirits (RR for ≥ 10 g/day versus 0.1–4.9 g/day: 1.40; 95%CI: 0.93–2.10). This finding is based on small numbers and should be interpreted with caution, in the NIH-AARP study (based on over 1000 incident cases) there was also a positive association between high alcohol intake and risk for cancer of the pancreas (RR for ≥ 3 versus > 0 – < 1 drinks/day: 1.45; 95%CI: 1.17–1.80), which was stronger among those with a high intake of spirits (RR for ≥ 3 drinks/day versus > 0 – < 1 drinks/day: 1.62, 95%CI: 1.24–2.10); there was no association for increasing intake of beer or wine, although few participants were heavy wine or beer drinkers (Jiao *et al.*, 2009). In the Netherlands Cohort Study the increased risk was limited to heavy drinkers (RR for ≥ 30 g/day versus none: 1.57; 95%CI: 1.03–2.39), and was similar in a subgroup of individuals who reported a stable alcohol intake for the previous five years (RR for ≥ 30 g/day versus none: 1.82, 95%CI: 1.05–3.15), but there was no association with a specific beverage type (Heinen *et al.*, 2009). The increased risk was observed only during the first 7 years of follow-up and not with longer follow-ups.

2.6.3 Cohort studies in special populations

In one cohort study conducted in the Netherlands there was a significantly higher rate of cancer of the pancreas among male alcohol abusers compared with the national average. Among women, rates of cancer of the pancreas were similar among alcohol abusers and the national population (Thygesen *et al.*, 2009; Table 2.27 available at http://monographs.iarc.fr/ENG/Monographs/vol100E/100E-06-Table2.27.pdf). [The Working Group noted the low number of cases. This study provided no information on individual exposures or results adjusted for potential confounders.]

2.6.4 Case–control studies

In the previous *IARC Monograph* (IARC, 2010) reports of 29 case–control studies with quantitative data on the association of alcoholic beverage intake and the risk for cancer of the pancreas were considered. Most of these found no association, although some suggested that heavy alcoholic beverage drinking (e.g. ≥ 15 drinks/week) may be associated with an increased risk, while others found significant reductions in risk with increasing alcoholic beverage intake. Since then, four further case–control studies have been published (Table 2.28 available at http://monographs.iarc.fr/ENG/Monographs/vol100E/100E-06-Table2.28.pdf). In a case–control study in the USA, with over 800 cases, a significant positive association with heavy consumption of alcoholic beverages and risk for cancer of the pancreas was found (≥ 60 versus < 60 mL ethanol/day: RR, 1.6;

95%CI: 1.1–2.5) (Hassan *et al.*, 2007). A positive association with high lifetime consumption of alcohol, and which was strongest for intake of spirits, was found in a small study in Canada (with 83 cases) (Benedetti *et al.*, 2009). In another study in Canada, with over 400 cases, no association with alcohol intake was found (Anderson *et al.*, 2009). [In this study the range of alcohol intake was narrow and the response rate among the cases was low (24% of all identified cases; 45% of contacted living cases), which may have led to some response bias.] In a study conducted in the Russian Federation with 366 pancreatic cancer deaths no significant association between a very high intake of vodka and death from cancer of the pancreas was found; however, the numbers were small (52 men and 4 women in the highest intake group) and exposure information was obtained from proxies of the decedents [which may have led to some misclassification of exposure] (Zaridze *et al.*, 2009). [Other studies with a high proportion of proxy respondents may also be prone to recall bias (Benedetti *et al.*, 2009). On the other hand, given the lethality of the disease, studies that only included self-respondents (Hassan *et al.*, 2007) may be prone to selection bias if alcohol consumption is associated with tumour aggressiveness.]

2.6.5 Patient characteristics

Some studies have shown higher risks in men than in women (Heinen *et al.*, 2009; Jiao *et al.*, 2009; Zaridze *et al.*, 2009) [there were too few women in the highest category of alcohol intake to drawn meaningful comparisons.] Most studies, including the meta- and pooled analyses, have found no significant difference in risk estimates between men and women (Genkinger *et al.*, 2009; Rohrmann *et al.*, 2009; Tramacere *et al.*, 2009). No evidence of a significant interaction between alcohol intake and pancreatic risk was found by either smoking status (Anderson *et al.* 2009; Genkinger *et al.*, 2009; Heinen *et al.*, 2009; Jiao *et al.*, 2009; Johansen *et al.*, 2009; Rohrmann *et al.*, 2009), folate intake (Genkinger *et al.*, 2009; Heinen *et al.*, 2009; Jiao *et al.*, 2009) or body mass index (Johansen *et al.*, 2009; Rohrmann *et al.*, 2009), although Genkinger *et al.* (2009) found that the association of alcohol consumption with risk was stronger among normal-weight individuals compared with overweight and obese individuals.

2.6.6 Potential confounders

Since individuals who consume high amounts of alcohol are also often smokers, it is possible that the positive association observed with alcohol intake may, in part, be due to residual confounding by smoking. In the pooled analysis no association with increasing alcohol consumption among non-smokers was found but a small increased risk among past and current smokers (Genkinger *et al.*, 2009). Although these differences were not statistically significant, it suggests that residual confounding by smoking cannot be ruled out. Evidence from other smaller studies is inconsistent, perhaps due to the low numbers of heavily exposed cases among non-smokers (Anderson *et al.*, 2009; Heinen *et al.*, 2009; Johansen *et al.*, 2009; Jiao *et al.*, 2009; Rohrmann *et al.*, 2009). [The Working Group noted that among smokers, it is difficult to disentangle the effects of alcohol from that of smoking due to differences in the amount of cigarettes consumed.]

2.7 Cancer of the lung

A possible link between consumption of alcoholic beverages and risk for cancer of the lung has long been speculated; in the previous *IARC Monograph* (IARC, 2010) it was concluded that the available data were inadequate to determine a causal association between the consumption of alcoholic beverages and lung cancer.

Two case–control studies (Kubík *et al.*, 2004; Benedetti *et al.*, 2009), eight cohort studies (Takezaki *et al.*, 2003; Nakaya *et al.*, 2005; Chao *et al.*, 2008; Shimazu *et al.*, 2008; Allen *et al.*, 2009; Thun *et al.*, 2009; Thygesen *et al.*, 2009; Toriola *et al.*, 2009), two meta-analyses (Chao, 2007; Fan & Cai, 2009) and one systematic review (Wakai *et al.*, 2007) were not considered in the previous *IARC Monograph* (IARC, 2010). More detailed analyses with regard to cancer of the lung for one of the case–control studies (Benedetti *et al.*, 2009) were available in an earlier publication (Benedetti *et al.*, 2006); therefore, the earlier publication is considered for this evaluation. This section reviews all available data.

A high correlation has been identified between tobacco smoking and alcohol drinking in many populations. As such, careful adjustment for smoking is one of the most important requirements for a valid interpretation for the association between alcohol drinking and cancer of the lung.

2.7.1 Overview of studies

(a) Cohort studies in the general population

Among 29 cohort studies of the general population that provided tobacco smoking-adjusted risk estimates for total alcoholic beverage use, of which one was a pooled analysis of seven cohort studies (Freudenheim *et al.*, 2005), a significant elevated risk for cancer of the lung associated with alcoholic beverage consumption was reported in 16 (Klatsky *et al.*, 1981; Pollack *et al.*, 1984; Stemmermann *et al.*, 1990; Chow *et al.*, 1992; Potter *et al.*, 1992; Doll *et al.*, 1994; Murata *et al.*, 1996; Prescott *et al.*, 1999; Lu *et al.*, 2000; Korte *et al.*, 2002 [which includes two separate studies: the Cancer Prevention Study (CPS) I and II]; Balder *et al.*, 2005; Nakaya *et al.*, 2005; Nishino *et al.*, 2006; Chao *et al.*, 2008; Toriola *et al.*, 2009) (the new studies are summarized in Table 2.29 available at http://monographs.iarc.fr/ENG/Monographs/vol100E/100E-06-Table2.29.pdf). In some of these studies an increased risk at high levels of consumption was found (Klatsky *et al.*, 1981; Pollack *et al.*, 1984; Potter *et al.*, 1992; Doll *et al.*, 1994; Murata *et al.*, 1996; Prescott *et al.*, 1999; Lu *et al.*, 2000; Korte *et al.*, 2002 [CPS I and II]; Balder *et al.*, 2005; Nakaya *et al.*, 2005; Chao *et al.*, 2008), while no association at the highest consumption category but with moderate consumption was found in other studies (Stemmermann *et al.*, 1990; Chao *et al.*, 2008, [only for drinking < 1 drink beer per week versus non-drinkers]), among former drinkers (Nakaya *et al.*, 2005; Nishino *et al.*, 2006), or among binge drinkers (Toriola *et al.*, 2009). No significant association was observed in the other cohort studies with results adjusted for smoking, including the pooled analysis of seven cohorts (Kvåle *et al.*, 1983; Kono *et al.*, 1986; Bandera *et al.*, 1997; Yong *et al.*, 1997; Woodson *et al.*, 1999; Breslow *et al.*, 2000; Djoussé *et al.*, 2002; Takezaki *et al.*, 2003; Freudenheim *et al.*, 2005; Rohrmann *et al.*, 2006; Shimazu *et al.*, 2008; Allen *et al.*, 2009; Thun *et al.*, 2009). In some of these studies, levels of alcohol intake among the participants were moderate (Kono *et al.*, 1986; Breslow *et al.*, 2000; Freudenheim *et al.*, 2005; Allen *et al.*, 2009).

(b) Cohort studies in special populations

The risk for cancer of the lung among alcoholics or patients with alcohol use disorders was examined in seven cohort studies (Schmidt & Popham, 1981; Adami *et al.*, 1992; Tønnesen *et al.*, 1994; Sigvardsson *et al.*, 1996; Sørensen *et al.*, 1998; Boffetta *et al.*, 2001; Thygesen *et al.*, 2009) are summarized in Table 2.30 available at http://monographs.iarc.fr/ENG/Monographs/vol100E/100E-06-Table2.30.pdf. All reported elevated risk of cancer of the lung. However, due to the lack of control for tobacco smoking in all of the studies, the observed association may be largely explained by the confounding effect of tobacco smoking.

(c) Case–control studies

In all, 22 case–control studies reported tobacco smoking-adjusted odds ratios for total consumption of alcoholic beverages and the risk for cancer of the lung (the new studies are summarized in Table 2.31 available at http://monographs.iarc.fr/ENG/Monographs/vol100E/100E-06-Table2.31.pdf). In seven population-based studies (Koo, 1988; Bandera *et al.*, 1992; Mayne *et al.*, 1994; Carpenter *et al.*, 1998; Hu *et al.*, 2002; Freudenheim *et al.*, 2003; Benedetti *et al.*, 2006) and 11 hospital-based studies (Williams & Horm, 1977; Herity *et al.*, 1982; Kabat & Wynder, 1984; Mettlin, 1989; Pierce *et al.*, 1989; Rachtan & Sokolowski, 1997; Zang & Wynder, 2001; De Stefani *et al.*, 2002; Pacella-Norman *et al.*, 2002; Ruano-Ravina *et al.*, 2004; Kubík *et al.*, 2004) no significant association between any level of alcoholic beverage consumption and the risk for cancer of the lung was found, while in four hospital-based studies (De Stefani *et al.*, 1993; Dosemeci *et al.*, 1997; Rachtan, 2002; Gajalakshmi *et al.*, 2003) an association was found.

(d) Meta- and pooled analyses

Korte *et al.* (2002) found an increased risk for lung cancer with an ethanol intake of at least 2000 g per month (≥ 5 drinks/day): the relative risk from cohort studies was 1.53 (95%CI: 1.04–2.25) and the odds ratio from case–control studies was 1.86 (95%CI: 1.39–2.49) [the estimated risks for intake of 2000 g/month or more were based on only one study for both cohort and case–control studies]; lower intakes were not associated with increased risk (Table 2.32 available at http://monographs.iarc.fr/ENG/Monographs/vol100E/100E-06-Table2.32.pdf). [The exposure studied most extensively was the frequency of drinking. Other parameters of alcoholic beverage exposure, such as duration and age at initiation of drinking and the relevant exposure period were not considered.] In another meta-analysis Fan & Cai (2009) provided estimates for total alcohol drinking, and did not find a significant association with risk of lung cancer. In a pooled analysis of 7 cohort studies, Freudenheim *et al.* (2005) found a slightly greater risk of cancer of the lung with the consumption of ≥ 30 g alcohol per day than with no alcohol consumption (RR, 1.21; 95%CI: 0.91–1.61 in men, RR, 1.16; 95%CI: 0.94–1.43 in women).

2.7.2 Types of alcoholic beverage

Findings from studies examining risk estimates for the consumption of different types of alcoholic beverages (i.e. beer, wine, and hard liquor) have been inconsistent (Pollack *et al.*, 1984; Mettlin, 1989; Bandera *et al.*, 1992; Chow *et al.*, 1992; De Stefani *et al.*, 1993; Carpenter *et al.*, 1998; Prescott *et al.*, 1999; Woodson *et al.*, 1999; De Stefani *et al.*, 2002; Hu *et al.*, 2002; Rachtan 2002; Kubík *et al.*, 2004; Ruano-Ravina *et al.*, 2004; Freudenheim *et al.*, 2005; Benedetti *et al.*, 2006) (the new studies are summarized in Table 2.31 on-line). Risk estimates for different types of alcoholic beverages were also reported in two meta-analyses (Chao, 2007; Fan & Cai, 2009) using results adjusted for smoking (Table 2.32 on-line). Both found a slightly increased risk associated with beer drinking; there was also a slight association between drinking of liquor (Chao, 2007) and spirits (Fan & Cai, 2009) and risk for cancer of the lung. However, when one of the meta-analyses included only the studies with more comprehensive adjustments for smoking (Chao, 2007), there was no significant association.

2.7.3 Smoking status

Several cohort studies have examined the effect of alcoholic beverage consumption among both never smokers and smokers, and the interaction between these two risk factors (Korte *et al.*, 2002; Freudenheim *et al.*, 2005; Nishino *et al.*, 2006; Rohrmann *et al.*, 2006; Chao *et al.*, 2008;

Shimazu *et al.*, 2008; Thun *et al.*, 2009; Toriola *et al.*, 2009; Table 2.33 available at http://monographs.iarc.fr/ENG/Monographs/vol100E/100E-06-Table2.33.pdf, and Table 2.34 available at http://monographs.iarc.fr/ENG/Monographs/vol100E/100E-06-Table2.34.pdf). Korte *et al.* (2002) found an increased risk for cancer of the lung associated with drinking ≥ 500 g of alcohol per month among both never smoker men and women in CPS I but not in CPS II. In a pooled study of seven cohorts, Freudenheim *et al.* (2005) found an elevated pooled relative risk for alcoholic beverage consumption among never-smoking men but not among never-smoking women. A dose–response was also observed among men with a sixfold increase in risk among never smokers who consumed ≥ 15 g/day (pooled multivariate RR, 6.38; 95%CI: 2.74–14.90; *P for trend* < 0.001).

In contrast, Nishino *et al.* (2006), Rohrmann *et al.* (2006), Shimazu *et al.* (2008), Thun *et al.* (2009), and Toriola *et al.* (2009) reported no association among never smokers. [These analyses may have the limitation that most of the cases of cancer of the lung were smokers.] In a detailed analysis examining the effect of consumption of alcoholic beverages by smoking behaviour, Woodson *et al.* (1999) found no differences in the relative risks across smoking categories (< 20, 20–29, ≥ 30 cigarettes/day) [results were on smokers only]. However, Shimazu *et al.* (2008) found an increased risk for cancer of the lung among current smokers who drank 300–449 g ethanol per week (hazard ratio (HR, 1.66; 95%CI: 1.04–2.65) as well as those who drank ≥ 450 g/wk (HR, 1.69; 95%CI: 1.05–2.72; *P* for trend = 0.02) compared to current smokers who drank occasionally. Toriola *et al.* (2009) also found a significant positive association among smokers that was independent of the number of cigarettes smoked or the duration of smoking. However, the analysis was limited to binge drinkers.

Three case–control studies based on populations of never smokers (Kabat & Wynder, 1984; Koo, 1988; Hu *et al.*, 2002) found no significant risks for consumption of alcoholic beverages [There is a lack of power to examine the risk associated with heavy drinking, as it is uncommon to find heavy drinkers among never smokers.] In contrast, Rachtan (2002) observed a significantly elevated risk associated with alcoholic beverage intake among women who never smoked and a strong positive dose–response. Other studies on total alcohol intake with results stratified by smoking status have found positive associations between alcohol drinking and risk for cancer of the lung among smokers and no association among non-smokers (Dosemeci *et al.*, 1997; Zang & Wynder, 2001) or found associations among heavy smokers and no association among non-smokers and low/moderate-smokers combined (Herity *et al.*, 1982; Bandera *et al.*, 1992; Benedetti *et al.*, 2006 [men only]).

There is also some evidence that consumption of alcoholic beverages results in an inverse association with risk of cancer of the lung. Two studies reported an inverse association between wine consumption and lung cancer, one case–control study among non-smokers (Kubík *et al.*, 2004) [results not adjusted for consumption of other alcoholic beverages], and one cohort study (Chao *et al.*, 2008) among smokers.

2.7.4 Histological subtypes

Two cohort studies (Rohrmann *et al.*, 2006; Shimazu *et al.*, 2008), one pooled analysis (Freudenheim *et al.*, 2005) and eight case–control studies (Koo, 1988; Dosemeci *et al.*, 1997; Carpenter *et al.*, 1998; Zang & Wynder, 2001; De Stefani *et al.*, 2002; Djoussé *et al.*, 2002; Rachtan, 2002; Benedetti *et al.*, 2006) presented smoking-adjusted risk estimates for consumption of alcoholic beverages by histological type of cancer of the lung (the new studies are summarized in Table 2.35 available at http://monographs.iarc.fr/ENG/Monographs/vol100E/100E-06-Table2.35.pdf). There appears to be no consistent pattern of effect estimates by histological type. [Estimates for subtype of cancer of the lung were mostly based on small numbers of cases, which leads to difficulties in interpreting results due to wide confidence intervals and the possibility of chance findings.] Few studies have reported results by histological type among never smokers (Koo, 1988).

2.7.5 Population characteristics

Several studies conducted analyses stratified by sex using the same exposure categories (Williams & Horm, 1977; Bandera *et al.*, 1997; Prescott *et al.*, 1999; Korte *et al.*, 2002; Pacella-Norman *et al.*, 2002; Freudenheim *et al.*, 2005; Benedetti *et al.*, 2006; Rohrmann *et al.*, 2006). No significant findings that differed by sex have been reported.

2.8 Cancer of the breast

2.8.1 Cancer of the female breast

The previous *IARC Monograph* (IARC, 2010) concluded that occurrence of cancer of the female breast was causally associated with the consumption of alcoholic beverages. This conclusion was based on data from more than 100 epidemiological studies, together with a pooled analysis of 53 studies on more than 58000 women with breast cancer, which found a linear increase in risk for breast cancer with increasing levels of alcoholic beverage consumption (increase per 10 g/d of 7.1%, 95%CI: 5.5–8.7%) (Hamajima *et al.*, 2002).

(a) Cohort studies in the general population

Since IARC (2010), thirteen cohort studies have examined the association of consumption of alcoholic beverages and risk of cancer of the breast (Table 2.36 available at http://monographs.iarc.fr/ENG/Monographs/vol100E/100E-06-Table2.36.pdf), eight of which showed a significant positive association (Ericson *et al.*, 2007; Mørch *et al.*, 2007; Zhang *et al.*, 2007a; Thygesen *et al.*, 2008a; Allen *et al.*, 2009; Duffy *et al.*, 2009; Lew *et al.*, 2009; Li *et al.*, 2009b), and four no significant association (Trentham-Dietz *et al.*, 2007; Visvanathan *et al.*, 2007; Kabat *et al.*, 2008; Gibson *et al.*, 2009), [In two of these latter studies the number of drinkers was small and there was no quantitative assessment of alcohol intake.] One further study found no association with a predominantly alcohol-based dietary pattern and risk of cancer of the breast (Engeset *et al.*, 2009) [No specific assessment of alcohol intake was presented and the contribution of other foods to this dietary pattern was not known.] The Million Women Study in the United Kingdom, with over 28 000 incident cancers, is the largest single study to estimate reliably the risk for cancer of the breast at low to moderate levels of alcohol consumption. A linear increase in risk of cancer of the breast with increasing alcohol intake (increase per 10 g/day [equivalent to about one drink regularly consumed per day] of 12%, 95%CI: 9–14%) was found (Allen *et al.*, 2009). This estimate is slightly higher than the 7.1% increase in risk reported in the pooled analysis by Hamajima *et al.* (2002). [Allen *et al.* (2009) were able to take measurement error into account by repeating the alcohol consumption measure approximately three years after recruitment].

(b) Cohort studies in special populations

Since IARC (2010), Thygesen *et al.* (2009) reported a significantly higher rate of cancer of the breast among female alcoholics compared with national rates from a cohort study among Danish alcohol abusers (Table 2.37 available at http://monographs.iarc.fr/ENG/Monographs/vol100E/100E-06-Table2.37.pdf). [This study provided no information on individual exposures or adjusted for potential confounders.]

(c) Case–control studies

The association of consumption of alcoholic beverages and risk for incident cancer of the female breast has been examined in 11 case–control studies (Table 2.38 available at http://monographs.iarc.fr/ENG/Monographs/vol100E/100E-06-Table2.38.pdf). A significant positive association has been reported from six studies (Beji & Reis, 2007; Kruk, 2007; Berstad *et al.*, 2008; Kocić *et al.*, 2008; Knight *et al.*, 2009; Newcomb *et al.*, 2009) and a significant inverse association in one (Zaridze *et al.*, 2009). [This latter study was conducted in the Russian Federation where alcohol consumption is very high relative to other populations and exposure information was obtained from proxies of the decedents (case and control status was based on death certification information). Reasons for the inverse association with very high intake are not clear and information on potential confounders was unavailable.] Null associations were found in four studies (Terry *et al.*, 2007; Bessaoud & Daurès, 2008; Dolle *et al.*, 2009; Brown *et al.*, 2010), although they either had a very low alcohol intake (Bessaoud & Daurès, 2008; Dolle *et al.*, 2009; Brown *et al.*, 2010) or did not adjust for potential confounding factors (Terry *et al.*, 2007).

(d) Other metrics of exposure

Very few investigators have examined whether the frequency of drinking, age at started drinking or the cumulative lifetime intake influences risk; in one cohort study in Denmark some evidence was found that binge drinking at the weekend may additionally increase risk (Mørch *et al.*, 2007). Another cohort study in Denmark found that risk was attenuated when using updated alcohol information (i.e. most recent intake measured after recruitment), with the suggestion that there may be a long latent period between consumption of alcoholic beverages and development of cancer of the breast (Thygesen *et al.*, 2008a). In contrast, Berstad *et al.* (2008) reported a positive association for recent intake (i.e. in the last five years), but no association with lifetime intake or intake at a young age from a case–control study in the USA.

(e) Types of alcoholic beverage

There is consistent evidence from both cohort and case–control studies that the risk for cancer of the female breast does not vary significantly by beverage type (Zhang *et al.*, 2007a; Berstad *et al.*, 2008; Bessaoud & Daurès, 2008; Allen *et al.*, 2009; Lew *et al.*, 2009; Li *et al.*, 2009b; Newcomb *et al.*, 2009). Among wine drinkers, the risk does not vary by intake of red wine, white wine or a mixture of both (Allen *et al.*, 2009; Newcomb *et al.*, 2009).

(f) Other factors affecting risk

There is consistent evidence that the association does not vary by folate intake (Zhang *et al.*, 2007a; Duffy *et al.*, 2009; Lew *et al.*, 2009) or by menopausal status (Mørch *et al.*, 2007; Terry *et al.*, 2007; Visvanathan *et al.*, 2007; Zhang *et al.*, 2007a; Kabat *et al.*, 2008), although in two case–control studies there was a slightly stronger association of consumption of alcoholic beverages and risk for cancer of the breast in postmenopausal than in premenopausal women (Kruk, 2007; Newcomb *et al.*, 2009).

It remains unclear whether the association of consumption of alcoholic beverages with risk of cancer of the breast varies by use of hormone-replacement therapy. In the Copenhagen City Heart Study, and to a lesser extent, the Women's Health Study, a positive association between alcohol intake and risk for cancer of the breast among current users, and no association among non-users of hormone-replacement therapy was found (Zhang *et al.*, 2007a; Nielsen & Grønbaek, 2008), whereas others have found no such differences (Bessaoud & Daurès, 2008; Allen *et al.*, 2009; Lew *et al.*, 2009).

Most of the data for an association of consumption of alcoholic beverages on risk for cancer of the breast comes from Caucasian populations; there is very limited data among Asian populations (Gibson *et al.*, 2009; Brown *et al.*, 2010), perhaps due to the generally low prevalence of alcohol consumption. Most studies that included different ethnic groups estimated risk after adjusting for ethnicity; in two studies that stratified by ethnic group there was no difference in the risk associated with consumption of alcoholic beverages (Berstad *et al.*, 2008; Li *et al.*, 2009b).

There is accumulating evidence that cigarette smoking may increase risk for cancer of the breast (see Monograph on Tobacco Smoking in this Volume), and because drinking and smoking are highly correlated, most studies that have evaluated the association of consumption of alcoholic beverages on risk for cancer of the breast have adjusted for smoking, to a greater or lesser extent. Hamajima *et al.* (2002) found that the association of consumption of alcoholic beverages with risk for cancer of the breast was similar in never, ever and current smokers. No subsequent studies have had sufficient statistical power to evaluate this in more detail, although the evidence to date suggests that the association of consumption of alcoholic beverages on risk of cancer of the breast is unlikely to be confounded by smoking. Another potentially important confounder is body size; in those studies that have examined potential effect modification by body mass index no significant differences have been found (Zhang *et al.*, 2007a; Berstad *et al.*, 2008; Lew *et al.*, 2009).

(g) Contralateral cancer of the breast

The association of consumption of alcoholic beverages with risk for contralateral cancer of the breast was not evaluated in IARC (2010). To date, four cohort (Table 2.39 available at http://monographs.iarc.fr/ENG/Monographs/vol100E/100E-06-Table2.39.pdf) and one case–control study (Table 2.40 available at http://monographs.iarc.fr/ENG/Monographs/vol100E/100E-06-Table2.40.pdf) have examined whether consumption of alcoholic beverages increases the risk of a subsequent contralateral cancer of the breast. In one cohort study alcohol consumption at the time of the first diagnosis and during the period between the first and second diagnosis was positively associated with the risk of contralateral cancer of the breast (Li *et al.*, 2009a), although no association was found in other cohort studies (Bernstein *et al.*, 1992; Li *et al.*, 2003b; Trentham-Dietz *et al.*, 2007). In the case–control study women with a contralateral breast cancer were more likely to have drunk regularly and to have drunk for a prolonged period of time compared with women who only had one diagnosis of cancer of the breast, although regular drinking during the period between the first and second diagnosis was not significantly associated with risk (Knight *et al.*, 2009).

(h) Tumour receptor status

The association of consumption of alcoholic beverages and risk for cancer of the breast by estrogen (ER) and progesterone (PR) receptor status has been examined in six cohort studies (Table 2.41 available at http://monographs.iarc.fr/ENG/Monographs/vol100E/100E-06-Table2.41.pdf). Similar associations for ER+ and ER- tumours were reported by Chlebowski *et al.* (2007), Visvanathan *et al.* (2007), Lew *et al.* (2009) and Setiawan *et al.* (2009). Lew *et al.* (2009) found a slightly stronger association with alcohol intake and ER+/PR+ tumours than for ER+/PR- or ER-/PR- tumours. Li *et al.* (2009b) and Zhang *et al.* (2007a) in contrast reported positive associations for ER+ and PR+ tumours (together with the subgroup of ER+/PR+) and no association with ER- or PR- tumours. Tumour receptor status has also been evaluated in five case–control studies (Table 2.42 available at http://monographs.iarc.fr/ENG/Monographs/vol100E/100E-06-Table2.42.pdf). In the largest, with approximately 1000 cases with information on receptor status, an increased risk for all

ER+ tumours, and no significant association for ER- tumours, irrespective of PR status, was found; the relative risk per 10 g alcohol/day for ER+/PR+ tumours was 1.14 (95%CI:1.07–1.20), that for ER+/PR- tumours was 1.07 (95%CI: 0.95–1.21) (Deandrea *et al.*, 2008). The association was slightly stronger among pre/perimenopausal women and among women with a high folate intake, although the numbers in these subgroups were small (Deandrea *et al.*, 2008). In a meta-analysis of 16 case–control studies and 3 cohort studies (Table 2.43 available at http://monographs.iarc.fr/ENG/Monographs/vol100E/100E-06-Table2.43.pdf) an increased risk per 10 g/day increase in alcohol intake for all ER+ tumours was found (12% increased risk), and for the subtypes of ER+/PR+ tumours (11%) and ER+/PR- tumours (15%), and a smaller positive association for all ER- (7%), but no association with ER-/PR- or ER-/PR+ tumours (Suzuki *et al.*, 2008).

There are limited data on the association of consumption of alcoholic beverages with tumours that are characterized as triple-negative or basal-like (defined as ER-/PR-/HER2-), largely because of the recency of available data on HER2 status (human epidermal growth factor receptor). From a case–control study among premenopausal women Dolle *et al.* (2009) reported no association between consumption of alcoholic beverages with triple-negative or non triple-negative tumours, and in another case–control study no significant association with triple-negative or luminal B tumours (ER+ and/or PR+/HER2+) was found, but a stronger positive association for luminal A tumours (ER+ and/or PR+/HER2-) and HER2+ overexpressing tumours (defined as ER-/PR-/HER2+) (Trivers *et al.*, 2009). [The small numbers in some of these subgroups limits interpretation]. No significant differences in drinking status between women with luminal A tumours (the most common tumour type) and women diagnosed with triple-negative or HER2+ overexpressing tumours were reported by Kwan *et al.* (2009) and Millikan *et al.* (2008) from case-only analyses; one found that women with luminal B tumours were less likely to be drinkers (Kwan *et al.*, 2009), while there was no difference in the other study (Millikan *et al.*, 2008). [The null associations seen for the rarer subtypes of ER+/PR- and ER-/PR+ tumours may reflect limited power of the studies.]

(i) Histological subtype

To date, the NIH-AARP (Lew *et al.*, 2009) is the only cohort study to have examined the association of consumption of alcoholic beverages by histological subtype among postmenopausal women; similar positive associations were reported for ductal, lobular and ductal-lobular subtypes (Table 2.44 available at http://monographs.iarc.fr/ENG/Monographs/vol100E/100E-06-Table2.44.pdf). This is consistent with findings from one case–control study (Nasca *et al.*, 1994; Table 2.45 available at http://monographs.iarc.fr/ENG/Monographs/vol100E/100E-06-Table2.45.pdf), while a slightly stronger positive association for alcohol intake with the risk for lobular tumours compared with ductal tumours, particularly among postmenopausal women, was found in two others (Li *et al.*, 2003a, 2006). [The low numbers of cases in some subgroups resulted in limited power to detect a significant difference, and these may be chance findings. In addition, it should be noted that the histological data from all of these studies was derived from hospital records and were not subject to central pathology review, leading to potential misclassification due to observer variability.]

2.8.2 Cancer of the male breast

It was concluded in the previous *IARC Monograph* (IARC, 2010) that the evidence for an association of consumption of alcoholic beverages and risk of cancer of the male breast was inconsistent.

(a) Cohort studies

Since IARC (2010), the association between consumption of alcoholic beverages and the risk for cancer of the male breast has been assessed in two cohort studies (Table 2.46 available at http://monographs.iarc.fr/ENG/Monographs/vol100E/100E-06-Table2.46.pdf). In the NIH-AARP Study no evidence was found that alcohol intake was associated with the risk for cancer of the male breast (Brinton *et al.*, 2008). In a large cohort of US Army Veterans no association with alcoholism as recorded from hospital records and risk for cancer of the male breast was found (Brinton *et al.*, 2009).

(b) Studies in special populations

Thygesen *et al.* (2009) reported similar rates of cancer of the breast among male Danish alcoholics compared with national rates (Table 2.47 available at http://monographs.iarc.fr/ENG/Monographs/vol100E/100E-06-Table2.47.pdf) [This was based on a very small number of cases and provided no information on individual exposures.]

2.9 Cancer of the uterine cervix

It was concluded in IARC (2010) that the evidence for an association between consumption of alcoholic beverages and risk for cancer of the uterine cervix was sparse. Although some studies of special populations showed positive associations, bias and confounding could not be excluded.

2.9.1 Cohort studies

The association between consumption of alcoholic beverages and risk for cancer of the uterine cervix has been examined in 8 cohort studies, seven of which were carried out in women who were treated for alcohol abuse or alcoholism (Prior, 1988; Adami *et al.*, 1992; Tønnesen *et al.*, 1994; Sigvardsson *et al.*, 1996; Weiderpass *et al.*, 2001; Thygesen *et al.*, 2009) or worked as waitresses (Kjaerheim & Andersen, 1994), and one in the general population (Allen *et al.*, 2009) (the new studies are summarized in Table 2.48 available at http://monographs.iarc.fr/ENG/Monographs/vol100E/100E-06-Table2.48.pdf).

The majority of studies were conducted in Scandinavia (Adami *et al.*, 1992; Kjaerheim & Andersen, 1994; Tønnesen *et al.*, 1994; Sigvardsson *et al.*, 1996; Weiderpass *et al.*, 2001; Thygesen *et al.*, 2009), where the use of the unique identification numbers makes it possible to work on large, registry based data. Two cohort studies were conducted in the United Kingdom (Prior, 1988; Allen *et al.*, 2009). In all seven studies conducted in special populations elevated risk estimates for invasive cancer of the uterine cervix among alcoholic women were found compared to the general population. [None of the studies adjusted for known risk factors for cancer of the uterine cervix, namely human papilloma virus (HPV) infection, number of sexual partners and tobacco smoking, or attendance at cervical cancer screening programmes. It is possible that women with alcohol abuse have other behavioural patterns that may affect risk for cancer of the uterine cervix, such as non-compliance to screening, tobacco smoking and having a higher prevalence of HPV than the general population in their respective countries.]

In the Million Women Study (Allen *et al.*, 2009) non-drinking women had an elevated risk for cancer of the uterine cervix compared to drinkers. Among drinkers, there was no association between the amount of alcohol consumed and risk for cancer of the uterine cervix. The analyses were adjusted for socioeconomic status, smoking, body mass index, physical activity, oral contraceptives and hormone replacement therapy use, but not for particular risk factors of cancer of the uterine cervix, including HPV infection and factors related to a sexual behaviour such as the number of lifetime sexual partners or age at first intercourse.

2.9.2 Case–control studies

The association between consumption of alcoholic beverages and cancer of the uterine cervix was evaluated in 12 case–control studies, seven of which were hospital-based (two from Italy, two from Thailand, one from Uganda, one from United Kingdom, one from the USA), three were register or cohort based (from the USA and Zimbabwe), and two were based on both hospital and population controls (one from Lesotho and one large multicentric study from Latin America). No or no significant increased risk for cancer of the uterine cervix among alcoholic drinkers was found in eight studies (Williams & Horm, 1977; Harris *et al.*, 1980; Marshall *et al.*, 1983; Cusimano *et al.*, 1989; Licciardone *et al.*, 1989; Thomas *et al.*, 2001a, b; Chiaffarino *et al.*, 2002). In the three studies from Africa (Martin & Hill, 1984; Parkin *et al.*, 1994; Newton *et al.*, 2007), women who drank alcohol had a significant or borderline significant elevated risk for cancer of the uterine cervix. [Adjustment for confounding in these studies was incomplete.] In the study from Latin America, in which adjustment for possible confounders was adequate, there was an elevated risk for cancer of the uterine cervix among occasional drinkers (confidence intervals not given) but no association with heavy drinking (Herrero *et al.*, 1989).

2.9.3 Evidence of a dose–response

The cohort studies on alcoholics did not provide convincing evidence of a dose–response between risk for cancer of the uterine cervix and duration of exposure, which was roughly estimated as years since cohort enrolment (first hospitalization/clinical treatment for alcoholism).

A case–control study from Latin America (Herrero *et al.*, 1989), which adjusted for important risk factors such as tobacco smoking and number of sexual partners, showed an inverse dose–response association. In four other case–control studies in which there was an indication of a higher risk for cancer of the uterine cervix with higher alcohol consumption, the observed association was weak in two (Harris *et al.*, 1980; Marshall *et al.*, 1983) and significant in two other studies (Martin & Hill, 1984; Parkin *et al.*, 1994), but adjustment for possible confounders was incomplete. In one study, a positive trend was observed among consumers in the category "wine and other alcoholic beverages" (Chiaffarino *et al.*, 2002).

2.9.4 Types of alcoholic beverage

The effect of specific types of alcoholic beverages (beer, wine and spirits) on risk for cancer of the uterine cervix was not investigated in the cohort studies.

In almost all case–control studies that evaluated specific types of alcoholic beverage (Marshall *et al.*, 1983; Martin & Hill, 1984; Chiaffarino *et al.*, 2002) no consistent differences in risk for cancer of the uterine cervix between drinkers and non-drinkers of a certain alcohol type were found. Williams & Horm (1977) found a non-significant higher risk for cancer of the uterine cervix among wine drinkers, while Marshall *et al.* (1983) found beer drinkers were at higher risk.

2.10 Cancer of the endometrium

In the previous *IARC Monograph* (IARC, 2010) it was concluded that the evidence for an association between consumption of alcoholic beverages and risk for cancer of the endometrium was inconsistent.

2.10.1 Cohort studies in the general population

The association between consumption of alcoholic beverages and cancer of the endometrium in the general population has been evaluated in eight cohort studies (Gapstur *et al.*, 1993; Terry *et al.*, 1999; Folsom *et al.*, 2003; Loerbroks *et al.*, 2007; Kabat *et al.*, 2008; Setiawan *et al.*, 2008; Allen *et al.*, 2009; Friberg & Wolk, 2009) (the new studies or updates are summarized in Table 2.49 available at http://monographs.iarc.fr/ENG/Monographs/vol100E/100E-06-Table2.49.pdf). These studies were conducted in North America (Gapstur *et al.*, 1993; Folsom *et al.*, 2003; Kabat *et al.*, 2008; Setiawan *et al.*, 2008) and in Europe, one in the Netherlands (Loerbroks *et al.*, 2007), one in the United Kingdom (Allen *et al.*, 2009) and two in Sweden (Terry *et al.*, 1999; Friberg & Wolk, 2009). Risk estimates adjusted for multiple possible confounders (body size and reproductive factors) were presented in seven reports (Gapstur *et al.* 1993; Terry *et al.*, 1999; Loerbroks *et al.*, 2007; Kabat *et al.*, 2008; Setiawan *et al.*, 2008; Allen *et al.*, 2009; Friberg & Wolk, 2009) while only five of these (Jain *et al.*, 2000a [an earlier report from the same study as Kabat *et al.* (2008) in which results were not adjusted for smoking]; Loerbroks *et al.*, 2007; Setiawan *et al.*, 2008; Allen *et al.*, 2009; Friberg & Wolk, 2009) adjusted the analysis of consumption of alcoholic beverages for smoking. Smoking showed non-significant negative association in almost all studies except for Friberg & Wolk (2009), where the risk estimates for cancer of the endometrium were decreased among never smokers, especially in women drinking more than 10 g of alcohol daily.

There was no clear evidence of association between consumption of alcoholic beverages and the risk for cancer of the endometrium in any of these studies. In four (Terry *et al.*, 1999; Loerbroks *et al.*, 2007; Kabat *et al.*, 2008; Setiawan *et al.*, 2008) some elevated risk for cancer of the endometrium among drinking women was found. Only Setiawan *et al.* (2008) reported a statistically significant association, which was among women who consumed more than 2 drinks per day. In one study (Folsom *et al.*, 2003), an inverse association was found. No association was found in the other studies (Gapstur *et al.*, 1993; Allen *et al.*, 2009; Friberg & Wolk, 2009).

2.10.2 Cohort studies in special populations

Three earlier cohort studies examined the association between alcoholic beverage intake and the risk for cancer of the endometrium in special populations, namely women hospitalized or being treated for alcohol dependence (Tønnesen *et al.*, 1994; Sigvardsson *et al.*, 1996; Weiderpass *et al.*, 2001, which was an update of Adami *et al.*, 1992). Thygesen *et al.* (2009) conducted the most recent study (Table 2.50 available at http://monographs.iarc.fr/ENG/Monographs/vol100E/100E-06-Table2.50.pdf).

Weiderpass *et al.* (2001) found an inverse association between alcoholic beverage consumption and cancer of the endometrium. [The analytical models did not include important covariates that may have confounded the association, such as cigarette smoking and body size.] In the other studies, there was no evidence of an association.

2.10.3 Case–control studies

Case–control studies that have investigated the relationship between alcoholic beverage consumption and the risk for cancer of the endometrium were carried out in North America, Japan and western Europe.Eight of these were hospital-based (La Vecchia *et al.*, 1986; Cusimano *et al.*, 1989; Austin *et al.*, 1993; Levi *et al.*, 1993; Parazzini *et al.*, 1995a; Kalandidi *et al.*, 1996; Petridou *et al.*, 2002; Hosono *et al.*, 2008), two were based on cases and controls from a cancer survey or registry database (Williams & Horm, 1977; Kato *et al.*, 1989) and eight were population-based (Webster *et al.*, 1989; Shu *et al.*, 1991; Swanson *et al.*, 1993; Goodman *et al.*, 1997; Newcomb *et al.*, 1997; Jain *et al.*, 2000b; McCann *et al.*, 2000; Weiderpass & Baron, 2001). The most recent study (Hosono *et al.*, 2008) is summarized in Table 2.51 (available at http://monographs.iarc.fr/ENG/Monographs/vol100E/100E-06-Table2.51.pdf)

Eleven studies (Cusimano *et al.*, 1989; Kato *et al.*, 1989; Webster *et al.*, 1989; Austin *et al.*, 1993; Swanson *et al.*, 1993; Parazzini *et al.*, 1995a; Kalandidi *et al.*, 1996; Newcomb *et al.*, 1997; Weiderpass & Baron, 2001; Petridou *et al.*, 2002; Hosono *et al.*, 2008) were designed to examine the association between consumption of alcoholic beverages, other lifestyle factors such as cigarette smoking, use of hormone replacement therapy and other risk factors in the etiology of cancer of the endometrium. Six studies (LaVecchia *et al.*, 1986; Shu *et al.*, 1991; Levi *et al.*, 1993; Goodman *et al.*, 1997; Jain *et al.*, 2000b; McCann *et al.*, 2000) were designed to evaluate nutritional factors. Potentially confounding factors were considered in all the studies except for one (Cusimano *et al.*, 1989), although adjustment may have been incomplete in three studies (Williams & Horm, 1977, [age, race and smoking]; Shu *et al.*, 1991, [pregnancies and weight]; Levi *et al.*, 1993, [only adjusted for age and centre]).

The results of case–control studies were not consistent. In 10 studies little or no association between consumption of alcoholic beverages and the risk for cancer of the endometrium was found (Kato *et al.*, 1989; Webster *et al.*, 1989; Austin *et al.*, 1993; Swanson *et al.*, 1993; Kalandidi *et al.*, 1996; Goodman *et al.*, 1997; Newcomb *et al.*, 1997; McCann *et al.*, 2000; Weiderpass & Baron, 2001; Petridou *et al.*, 2002). An inverse association was found in three (Williams & Horm, 1977; Jain *et al.*, 2000b; Hosono *et al.*, 2008), which was significant in two (Jain *et al.* 2000b; Hosono *et al.* 2008) among moderate drinking women. An increased risk for cancer of the endometrium with high consumption of alcoholic beverages was found by LaVecchia *et al.* (1986), Cusimano *et al.* (1989), Shu *et al.* (1991), Levi *et al.* (1993) and Parazzini *et al.* (1995a); in two the association was non-significant (Cusimano *et al.*, 1989; Shu *et al.*, 1991), in one it was significant (Parazzini *et al.*, 1995a) and one (Levi *et al.*, 1993) found a positive association relative to wine and liquor, but not to beer.

2.10.4 Evidence of a dose–response

There was no evidence of a trend of increasing risk for cancer of the endometrium with increasing consumption of alcoholic beverages in the cohort studies, nor a suggestion of a dose–response among long-term drinkers only (Friberg & Wolk, 2009).

In most case–control studies there was no dose–response relationship between consumption of alcoholic beverages and the risk for cancer of the endometrium. A negative dose–response association with significant trend was observed by Jain *et al.* (2000b) and Hosono *et al.* (2008), while one study showed a clear positive dose–response trend (Parazzini *et al.*, 1995a). In another study, there was an indication of a negative dose–response in the association but no formal test for trend was presented (Webster *et al.*, 1989).

2.10.5 Types of alcoholic beverage

The effect of specific types of alcoholic beverages (beer, wine, sprits) on the risk for cancer of the endometrium was investigated in three cohort studies, with no clear evidence of heterogeneity between different types of beverages (Gapstur *et al.*, 1993; Loerbroks *et al.*, 2007; Setiawan *et al.*, 2008).

Consumption of different alcoholic beverages in relation to risk for cancer of the endometrium was evaluated in seven case–control studies (Williams & Horm, 1977; Austin *et al.*, 1993; Levi *et al.*, 1993; Swanson *et al.*, 1993; Parazzini *et al.*, 1995a; Goodman *et al.*, 1997; Weiderpass & Baron, 2001). Levi *et al.* (1993) and Parazzini *et al.* (1995a) found increased risk for cancer of the endometrium with increasing consumption of wine and hard liquor, but not beer. Overall, there were no consistent patterns of association between any specific type of alcoholic beverage and risk for cancer of the endometrium.

2.10.6 Interactions

Only Setiawan *et al.* (2008) reported detailed results of interaction between other risk factors and consumption of alcoholic beverages for cancer of the endometrium. There was no clear effect modification by body mass index, post-menopausal hormone use, parity, oral contraceptive use or smoking status, though the power to detect such interactions was limited. The Million Women Study Collaborators (2005) investigated alcohol only as an interacting factor with hormone replacement therapy and found no evidence for an effect modification. Results from stratified analyses did not show any effect modification by age, smoking, body mass index, folic acid intake, or postmenopausal hormone use (Friberg & Wolk, 2009).

2.11 Cancer of the ovary

In the previous *IARC Monograph* (IARC, 2010), it was concluded that the evidence for an association between consumption of alcoholic beverages and risk for cancer of the ovary in both cohort and case–control studies was sparse and inconsistent. Since IARC (2010), one cohort study in alcoholics (Thygesen *et al.*, 2009) and one case–control study (Kolahdooz *et al.*, 2009) have evaluated the association between consumption of alcoholic beverages and risk of cancer of the ovary.

2.11.1 Cohort studies

A total of five cohort studies have examined the association between consumption of alcoholic beverages and the risk for cancer of the ovary in special populations, women hospitalized or being treated for alcohol dependence, four early (Adami *et al.*, 1992; Tønnesen *et al.*, 1994, Sigvardsson *et al.*, 1996; Lagiou *et al.*, 2001) and one more recent (Thygesen *et al.*, 2009; Table 2.52 available at http://monographs.iarc.fr/ENG/Monographs/vol100E/100E-06-Table2.52.pdf); the association in the general population has been examined in seven cohort studies (Kushi *et al.*, 1999; Kelemen *et al.*, 2004; Schouten *et al.*, 2004; Chang *et al.*, 2007; Kabat *et al.*, 2008; Tworoger *et al.*, 2008; Allen *et al.*, 2009). The studies were conducted in North America (USA and Canada) and Europe (the Netherlands, the United Kingdom and Scandinavia). The reports on studies in special populations presented results adjusted for age and calendar period only, whereas in the population based cohort studies results were adjusted for a large variety of factors.

There was no evidence of an overall association between consumption of alcoholic beverages and the risk for cancer of the ovary in these studies.

2.11.2 Case–control studies

Twenty-four case–control studies investigated the relationship between alcoholic beverage consumption and the risk for cancer of the ovary in North America, Japan, Australia, India, western Europe and Scandinavia, including one recent (Kolahdooz *et al.*, 2009; Table 2.53 available at http://monographs.iarc.fr/ENG/Monographs/vol100E/100E-06-Table2.53.pdf). Eleven were hospital-based (West, 1966; Williams & Horm, 1977; Byers *et al.*, 1983; Tzonou *et al.*, 1984; Mori *et al.*, 1988; Hartge *et al.*, 1989; LaVecchia *et al.*, 1992; Nandakumar *et al.*, 1995; Tavani *et al.*, 2001a; Yen *et al.*, 2003; Pelucchi *et al.*, 2005), one was based on cases and controls who were included in a cancer registry database (Kato *et al.*, 1989), 11 were population-based (Gwinn *et al.*, 1986; Polychronopoulou *et al.*, 1993; Godard *et al.*, 1998; Kuper *et al.*, 2000; Goodman & Tung, 2003; McCann *et al.*, 2003; Modugno *et al.*, 2003; Riman *et al.*, 2004; Webb *et al.*, 2004; Peterson *et al.*, 2006; Kolahdooz *et al.*, 2009) and one used controls chosen both among general population and hospital patients (Whittemore *et al.*, 1988). The recent study (Kolahdooz *et al.*, 2009) examined dietary patterns, including a predominantly snack and alcohol-based dietary pattern, and cancer of the ovary. [No specific assessment of alcohol intake was presented.] Confounding factors were considered in all studies, although adjustment was more extensive in more newly published studies than in studies published during the 1980s.

Overall, the results of case–control studies do not suggest any association between consumption of alcoholic beverages and risk for cancer of the ovary, although a few studies indicated either positive or negative associations.

2.11.3 Types of alcoholic beverage

In four population-based cohort studies the association with different types of alcoholic beverages was investigated (Kelemen *et al.*, 2004; Schouten *et al.*, 2004; Chang *et al.*, 2007; Tworoger *et al.*, 2008). Intake of wine during the year before baseline was associated with an increased risk for cancer of the ovary in one study (Chang *et al.*, 2007), but was not confirmed in the others (Kelemen *et al.*, 2004; Schouten *et al.*, 2004; Tworoger *et al.*, 2008).

Seven case–control studies evaluated different alcoholic beverages in relation to risk for cancer of the ovary (Gwinn *et al.*, 1986; LaVecchia *et al.*, 1992; Tavani *et al.*, 2001a; Goodman & Tung, 2003; Modugno *et al.*, 2003; Webb *et al.*, 2004; Peterson *et al.*, 2006). Overall, there were no consistent patterns of association between any specific type of alcoholic beverage (beer, wine and spirits) and risk for cancer of the ovary.

2.11.4 Interactions

Kelemen *et al.* (2004), Schouten *et al.* (2004) and Chang *et al.* (2007) evaluated their data for possible interaction between alcoholic beverage intake and other variables. Kelemen *et al.* (2004) found a statistically significant interaction between folate intake and alcohol consumption with regard to risk for cancer of the ovary. A similar association was observed by Chang *et al.* (2007) for women drinking more than one glass of wine daily. No other consistent interactions were reported. Among the case–control studies, there was no consistent evidence of interaction between alcoholic beverage consumption and different variables known or suspected to be associated with risk of cancer of the ovary, such as reproductive history, education, body size or diet.

2.12 Cancer of the prostate

In the previous *IARC Monograph* (IARC, 2010) it was concluded that the evidence for the association between consumption of alcoholic beverages and risk of cancer of the prostate is inconsistent. Increased risk for cancer of the prostate at elevated levels of consumption of alcoholic beverages was suggested from a few cohort studies, but there was no consistent dose–response relationship and in many cohort studies there was no association. The majority of case–control studies also showed no association between consumption of alcoholic beverages and cancer of the prostate.

2.12.1 Cohort studies in the general population

For studies of cancer of the prostate that were conducted more recently, there should be concern if no attempt is made to distinguish between cases that are detected by screening, with a possibility that many might not have presented clinically during the lifetime of the individual in the absence of screening, and those that present clinically and are more likely to be progressive. Among the 23 cohort studies six studies (Platz *et al.*, 2004; Baglietto *et al.*, 2006; Sutcliffe *et al.*, 2007; Rohrmann *et al.*, 2008; Gong *et al.*, 2009; Chao *et al.*, 2010; Table 2.54 available at http://monographs.iarc.fr/ENG/Monographs/vol100E/100E-06-Table2.54.pdf) have considered the stage or grade of the disease. None found any association between alcoholic beverage consumption and risk of advanced cases of cancer of the prostate. However in one study (Gong *et al.*, 2009) a strong association of increased risk of high-grade cancer of the prostate with heavy alcohol consumption in the whole study population was found (RR 2.01; 95%CI: 1.33–3.05), as well as among heavy beer drinkers (RR, 2.89; 95%CI: 1.76–3.76) compared to non-drinkers. In a few of the other cohort studies that did not make a distinction of cancer stage or grade there was an increased risk for cancer of the prostate at elevated levels of alcoholic beverage consumption (Hirayama, 1992; Schuurman *et al.*, 1999; Putnam *et al.*, 2000; Sesso *et al.*, 2001), but there was no consistent dose–response relationship. Many other cohort studies showed no association. The risk associated with different types of alcoholic beverages was inconsistent, with increased risks for both beer (Gong *et al.*, 2009) and white wine consumption (Velicer *et al.*, 2006), as well as null associations (Sutcliffe *et al.*, 2007; Chao *et al.*, 2010) for all alcoholic beverages. Most studies collected data on consumption of alcoholic beverages only at baseline. Two studies examined lifetime alcohol use up to baseline (Rohrmann *et al.*, 2008) and another alcohol use at ages 18 and 45 (Velicer *et al.*, 2006) and did not find associations.

2.12.2 Cohort studies in special populations

Two of the nine studies of special populations showed an association between alcoholic beverage consumption and cancer of the prostate. Tønnesen *et al.* (1994) and more recently Thygesen *et al.* (2009) (Table 2.55 available at http://monographs.iarc.fr/ENG/Monographs/vol100E/100E-06-Table2.55.pdf) studying Danish alcohol abusers observed greater numbers of cancers of the prostate compared with the number expected from the general population. None of the studies provided information on individual exposures or adjusted for potential confounders.

2.12.3 Case–control studies

Studies published since IARC (2010) are summarized in Table 2.56 available at http://monographs.iarc.fr/ENG/Monographs/vol100E/100E-06-Table2.56.pdf. Six of the 38 case–control studies considered aggressiveness of disease. In the study of Walker *et al.* (1992), 90% of the cases were advanced at presentation, and in the study by Li *et al.* (2008b), almost 50% of the cases were advanced and about 40% of moderately differentiated tumour presentation. The majority of the studies showed no association between consumption of alcoholic beverages and cancer of the prostate. Six studies found a positive association (De Stefani *et al.*, 1995; Hayes *et al.*, 1996; Sharpe & Siemiatycki, 2001; Chang *et al.*, 2005; Gallus *et al.*, 2007; Benedetti *et al.*, 2009). De Stefani *et al.*, (1995) found a borderline elevation of risk for high levels of consumption of beer, but the risk at high levels of total alcohol consumption was not significantly elevated. Hayes *et al.* (1996) found significant elevations in risk for 'heavy' and 'very heavy' consumers of alcoholic beverages, with higher risks among those with poorly or undifferentiated tumours, or with regional or distant metastases. Sharpe & Siemiatycki (2001) reported an elevation in risk for those with long duration of drinking, with the greatest elevation in risk for those who started drinking at age < 15 years. An elevated risk with increasing drink/year [with close to significant trend] was reported by Benedetti *et al.* (2009) among beer drinkers, as well as a borderline increased risk among moderate red wine drinkers. Gallus *et al.* (2007) reported an increased risk among men with poorly differentiated tumours (Gleason score ≥ 7). This association was not significant for all cancers of the prostate combined (regardless of the stage/differentiation status). Chang *et al.* (2005) found an association between consumption of alcoholic beverages (in g/week) and risk of cancer of the prostate with a borderline trend; there was no association with advanced cancer, whereas localized cancer showed significant association but without a dose–response relationship. De Stefani *et al.* (2009) analysed dietary patterns consisting of alcoholic beverages and processed meat and found no significant association with cancer of the prostate.

2.12.4 Meta-analyses

A meta-analysis that included six cohort and 27 case–control studies that were reported before July 1998 resulted in a relative risk estimate of 1.05 (95%CI: 0.98–1.11) for ever consumption of alcoholic beverages and of 1.05 (95%CI: 0.91–1.20) for each additional drink of alcohol per day (Dennis, 2000). The latter estimate was based on 15 studies reporting amount of alcohol consumed. Based on these 15 studies, the estimated relative risk for 4 drinks/day was 1.21 (95%CI: 1.05–1.39) (Table 2.57 available at http://monographs.iarc.fr/ENG/Monographs/vol100E/100E-06-Table2.57.pdf). Middleton-Fillmore *et al.* (2009) conducted a meta-analysis in which 14 cohorts and 21 case–control studies were included, reporting a weak but statistically significant association of incidence of cancer of the prostate with alcohol consumption levels in population case–control studies (RR, 1.24; 95%CI: 1.14–1.34), but meta-analyses of 7 hospital-based case–control studies and 14 cohort studies found no associations between consumption of alcoholic beverages and cancer of the prostate.

2.13 Cancer of the kidney

In the previous *IARC Monograph* (IARC, 2010) it was concluded that both cohort and case–control studies provide consistent evidence of no increase in risk for cancer of the kidney with consumption of alcoholic beverages (IARC, 2010). In several studies, increasing intake of alcoholic beverages was associated with a significantly lower risk for cancer of the kidney. These inverse trends were observed in both men and women and with multiple types of alcoholic beverage.

Since IARC (2010), one cohort (Table 2.58 available at http://monographs.iarc.fr/ENG/Monographs/vol100E/100E-06-Table2.58.pdf) and three case–control studies (Table 2.59 available at http://monographs.iarc.fr/ENG/Monographs/vol100E/100E-06-Table2.59.pdf) have been identified.

Allen *et al.* (2009) reported a decrease in risk for cancer of the kidney associated with moderate alcohol intake in women. The relative risk associated with ≥ 15 drinks per week was 0.66 (95%CI: 0.48–0.92); the reduction in risk per 10 g alcohol/day was 12% (95%CI: 1% to 22%).

Greving *et al.* (2007) (855 cases) reported an inverse association between alcohol intake measured as gram of ethanol per month and cancer of the kidney. Pelucchi *et al.* (2008) (1534 cases), in an update of a previous study (Pelucchi *et al.* (2002) together with a new study from the same area, found an inverse association between total alcohol intake or intake of wine measured as drinks per day and cancer of the kidney;

however, they did not find any effect of duration (years) of drinking or age of starting. Benedetti *et al.* (2009) (156 cases) found no effect of alcohol intake on the risk of cancer of the kidney.

2.14 Cancer of the urinary bladder

In the previous *IARC Monograph* (IARC, 2010) it was concluded that the evidence for an association between consumption of alcoholic beverages and risk for cancer of the urinary bladder was inconsistent.

One cohort (Allen *et al.*, 2009) and three case–control studies (Cao *et al.*, 2005; Jiang *et al.*, 2007; Zaridze *et al.*, 2009) on the general population and one cohort study on alcoholics (Thygesen *et al.*, 2009) have been identified since IARC (2010).

Allen *et al.* (2009) found no association between consumption of alcoholic beverages and cancer of the urinary bladder in women (Table 2.60 available at http://monographs.iarc.fr/ENG/Monographs/vol100E/100E-06-Table2.60.pdf). Likewise, Thygesen *et al.* (2009) reported no effect of alcohol on cancer of the urinary bladder among alcoholics (Table 2.61 available at http://monographs.iarc.fr/ENG/Monographs/vol100E/100E-06-Table2.61.pdf).

Two of the case–control studies (Cao *et al.*, 2005; Zaridze *et al.*, 2009) found no consistent association between consumption of alcoholic beverages and risk for cancer of the urinary bladder (Table 2.62 available at http://monographs.iarc.fr/ENG/Monographs/vol100E/100E-06-Table2.62.pdf). However, Jiang *et al.* (2007) in a large case–control study (1671 cases) found a statistically significant reduced risk both in relation to frequency of alcohol intake, duration (in years), and age of initiation. The reduction in risk was particularly large among those who urinated frequently. [The reduced risk for cancer of the urinary bladder among those who urinated frequently may to some extent be due to a high liquid intake and dilution of potential carcinogens.]

2.15 Cancers of the lymphatic and haematopoietic system

Lymphomas and haematopoietic malignancies comprise a heterogeneous group of malignancies and their respective etiologies are not fully understood. In the previous *IARC Monograph* (IARC, 2010) it was concluded that there was *evidence suggesting lack of carcinogenicity* in humans for alcoholic beverages and non-Hodgkin lymphoma (NHL). The results of cohort studies and evidence from some very large case–control studies showed an inverse association or no association between the consumption of alcoholic beverages and the risk for NHL. In general, there was no evidence of substantial differences in the effect of specific beverage types or for specific histological subtypes of NHL. The evidence for an association between consumption of alcoholic beverages and risk for Hodgkin disease was sparse, and no consistent pattern of association was observed for leukaemia and multiple myeloma (IARC, 2010).

2.15.1 Cohort studies in the general population

In seven cohort studies, associations of consumption of alcoholic beverages and the risk for lymphatic and/or haematopoietic cancers were examined (Boffetta *et al.*, 1989; Kato *et al.*, 1992; Chiu *et al.*, 1999; Lim *et al.*, 2006; Lim *et al.*, 2007; Allen *et al.*, 2009; Klatsky *et al.*, 2009). Studies published since the previous Monograph (IARC, 2010) are summarized in Table 2.63 (available at http://monographs.iarc.fr/ENG/Monographs/vol100E/100E-06-Table2.63.pdf)

For NHL specifically, Chiu *et al.* (1999) found a non-significant inverse association with consumption of alcoholic beverages among postmenopausal women in the USA. This relationship persisted after adjustment for several potential confounding factors including age, total energy intake, residence (farm, no farm), education, marital status, history of transfusion and diabetes, and intake of red meat and fruit. [The Working Group noted that the level of alcohol intake was very low in this study.] Lim *et al.* (2006) found weak evidence of an inverse association among Finnish male smokers in a multivariate analysis. The three cohort studies published recently and conducted among retired persons in the USA (Lim *et al.*, 2007), among middle-aged women in the United Kingdom (Allen *et al.*, 2009), and in a multiethnic USA population (Klatsky *et al.*, 2009) have shown significantly decreased risk of NHL among people with moderate alcohol intake A borderline significant inverse association was also shown for consumers of 7 or more drinks per week who were diagnosed with B-cell lymphoma, chronic lymphocytic lymphoma or small lymphocytic lymphoma, as well as an inverse (although non-significant) association of Hodgkin lymphoma risk with consumption of alcoholic beverages (Lim *et al.*, 2007).

In a study among American men of Japanese ancestry that also considered several potential lifestyle, medical and dietary confounding factors, consumption of ≥ 30 ml alcohol per day compared with non-drinkers was associated with a threefold higher risk for lymphoma and leukaemia combined (Kato *et al.*, 1992). In the multiethnic cohort in the USA (Klatsky *et al.*, 2009) risk for myelocytic leukaemia among regular drinkers compared with never-drinkers plus those reporting < 1 drink/month, and risk for lymphocytic leukaemia among people drinking more than 2 drinks per week versus drinkers who drank < 1 drink/week showed inverse associations (p for trend 0.01 and 0.03, respectively). Allen *et al.* (2009) did not find any association between alcohol intake and risk of all leukaemias combined.

In the four cohort studies that assessed consumption of alcoholic beverages and the risk for multiple myeloma, no association was found in three (Lim *et al.*, 2006; Allen *et al.*, 2009; Klatsky *et al.*, 2009) and in one a lower risk among ever regular drinkers compared with never regular drinkers was found (Boffetta *et al.*, 1989).

2.15.2 Cohort studies in special populations

Five studies among heavy alcoholic beverage users or brewery workers have investigated the risk for lymphatic and/or haematopoietic cancers (Hakulinen *et al.*, 1974; Jensen, 1979; Robinette *et al.*, 1979; Schmidt & Popham, 1981; Carstensen *et al.*, 1990).

Three studies examined lymphatic and haematopoietic cancers combined (Jensen, 1979; Robinette *et al.*, 1979; Carstensen *et al.*, 1990), Jensen (1979) found no significant differences between the observed number of cases among Danish brewery workers compared with the expected number of cases computed from age-, sex-, and area-specific rates. Carstensen *et al.* (1990) found slightly increased risk for these cancers among Swedish brewery workers compared to the expected cases calculated using age, follow-up time, and area-standardized rates of the Swedish male population. Robinette *et al.* (1979) found a non-significant decreased risk among chronic alcoholic male USA veterans compared with expected numbers computed from age- and time-specific rates for the US male population.

In two studies, the observed number of cases of lymphoma among alcoholics was lower than that expected based on rates for the local population (Hakulinen *et al.*, 1974; Schmidt & Popham, 1981).

In studies among alcoholics, the observed number of cases of leukaemia did not differ significantly from those expected in one study (Hakulinen *et al.*, 1974), and was non-significantly lower in two other studies (Robinette *et al.*, 1979; Schmidt & Popham, 1981). In studies among brewery workers, Jensen (1979) found no significant difference between the observed and expected number of leukaemia deaths, while Carstensen *et al.* (1990) found a 1.6-fold higher risk of mortality among brewery workers compared with those expected from the local population.

2.15.3 Case–control studies

(a) Lymphomas

Associations between consumption of alcoholic beverages and the risk for lymphoma were evaluated in 22 case–control studies (Williams & Horm, 1977; Cartwright *et al.*, 1988; Brown *et al.*, 1992; Nelson *et al.*, 1997; Tavani *et al.*, 1997; De Stefani *et al.*, 1998; Matsuo *et al.*, 2001a; Tavani *et al.*, 2001b; Briggs *et al.*, 2002; Chiu *et al.*, 2002; Morton *et al.*, 2003; Chang *et al.*, 2004; Willett *et al.*, 2004; Besson *et al.*, 2006a, b; Nieters *et al.*, 2006; Deandrea *et al.*, 2007; Casey *et al.*, 2007; Gorini *et al.*, 2007b; Willett *et al.*, 2007; Monnereau *et al.*, 2008; Benedetti *et al.*, 2009). Studies published since the previous Monograph (IARC, 2010) are summarized in Table 2.64 available at http://monographs.iarc.fr/ENG/Monographs/vol100E/100E-06-Table2.64.pdf).

Most case–control studies of consumption of alcoholic beverages and lymphoma focused specifically on NHL and/or its histological subtypes. Chang *et al.* (2004) found no overall association of NHL risk with moderate consumption of alcoholic beverages, although there was a suggestive possible increased risk of NHL among men. In that study, all cases and controls were free of human immunodeficiency viral infection and several potential confounding factors including age, tobacco smoking and occupational exposure to pesticides were considered. Briggs *et al.* (2002) also found no difference in the risk for NHL between drinkers and non-drinkers after adjustment for age, ethnicity and smoking status. Casey *et al.* (2007) found no significant associations of different characteristics of consumption of alcoholic beverages considering drinkers versus non drinkers, current and former drinking, age at drinking debut, drinking duration or daily intake for all lymphoid neoplasms and B-cell lymphomas. An inverse association for ever alcohol drinking and NHL was observed in a large multicentric study (Monnereau *et al.*, 2008) with 399 NHL cases (OR, 0.7; 95%CI: 0.5–1.0).

Most individual studies of NHL have limited power to conduct detailed analyses of consumption of alcoholic beverages and risk for this disease, particularly for specific beverage types and histological subtypes. Therefore, data from nine case–control studies conducted in Italy, Sweden, the United Kingdom and the USA were pooled to include 6492 cases of NHL and 8683 controls (Morton *et al.*, 2005). The analysis showed a significantly lower risk for NHL for ever drinkers when compared to non-drinkers; however, there was no consistent dose–response relationship between risk and frequency of consumption of alcoholic beverages, duration of alcoholic beverage consumption or age at starting drinking. The risk for NHL for current drinkers was lower than that for former drinkers. There was no difference in association by alcoholic beverage type or for the combination of beverages types consumed. For specific subtypes of NHL, no significantly elevated risks were found. The lowest risk associated with ever drinking versus non-drinker was that for Burkitt lymphoma (OR, 0.51; 95%CI: 0.33–0.77). Low risks for diffuse B-cell, follicular and T-cell lymphomas associated with ever drinking were also noted. The findings were unchanged when the analyses were restricted to studies that had a high response rate.

A multicentre case–control study of NHL and consumption of alcoholic beverages included data from five European countries and comprised 1742 cases and 2465 controls (Besson *et al.*, 2006a). Overall, there were no associations observed for ever drinking, age at starting drinking, duration of drinking or monthly consumption with risk for all NHL or with any histological subtype; similarly, no associations with risk of NHL were found with any specific type of alcoholic beverage. However, a lower risk associated with regular alcoholic beverage intake was observed for men (OR, 0.76; 95%CI: 0.62–0.93; 691 exposed cases) and for non-Mediterranean countries (OR, 0.73; 95%CI: 0.61–0.86).

Among the nine studies that examined Hodgkin lymphoma specifically (Williams & Horm, 1977; Tavani *et al.*, 1997; Besson *et al.*, 2006b; Nieters *et al.*, 2006; Deandrea *et al.*, 2007; Gorini *et al.*, 2007b; Willett *et al.*, 2007; Monnereau *et al.*, 2008; Benedetti *et al.*, 2009), a consistent inverse association was found almost in all. In the large multicentre European study, the odds ratio for Hodgkin lymphoma associated with ever regular drinking compared with never regular drinking was 0.61 (95%CI: 0.43–0.87; 81 exposed cases); this association was consistent for younger and older adults (Besson *et al.*, 2006b). Other multicentre studies have also shown an inverse association of Hodgkin lymphoma risk and frequent alcohol consumption of the order of 0.50 (Gorini *et al.*, 2007b; Monnereau *et al.*, 2008). Willett *et al.* (2007) found that the risk of Hodgkin lymphoma was higher among non-drinkers and persons with low alcohol consumption.

Inverse associations were also observed between specific alcoholic beverage types, namely wine and aperitif, and Hodgkin lymphoma (Gorini *et al.*, 2007b; Monnereau *et al.*, 2008).

(b) Leukaemia

The association of consumption of alcoholic beverages with risk for adult leukaemia was examined in eight case–control studies (Williams & Horm, 1977; Brown *et al.*, 1992; Wakabayashi *et al.*, 1994; Chang *et al.*, 2004; Pogoda *et al.*, 2004; Rauscher *et al.*, 2004; Gorini *et al.*, 2007a; Monnereau *et al.*, 2008). Studies published since the previous Monograph are summarized in Table 2.65 (available at http://monographs.iarc.fr/ENG/Monographs/vol100E/100E-06-Table2.65.pdf). No consistent patterns of associations between total consumption of alcoholic beverages and risk for all leukaemias combined were observed. In two studies a non-significant two- to threefold higher risk for acute lymphocytic leukaemia associated with heavy drinking (Wakabayashi *et al.*, 1994) or with any drinking (Brown *et al.*, 1992) was found, while in another no association of drinking with risk for this type of leukaemia was found (Gorini *et al.*, 2007a). Similarly, there was no consistent evidence of associations with acute non-lymphocytic leukaemia, chronic lymphocytic leukaemia or chronic myeloid leukaemia in these studies. Chang *et al.* (2004) found a positive significant association between high wine intake and risk for chronic lymphocytic leukaemia.

(c) Multiple myeloma

Associations between consumption of alcoholic beverages and the risk for multiple myeloma were examined in nine case–control studies, five in the USA, one in Canada, two in Italy and one in France (Williams & Horm, 1977; Gallagher *et al.*, 1983; Linet *et al.*, 1987; Brown *et al.*, 1992; Brown *et al.*, 1997; Deandrea *et al.*, 2007; Gorini *et al.*, 2007b; Hosgood *et al.*, 2007; Monnereau *et al.*, 2008). Studies published since the previous Monograph are summarized in Table 2.66 (available at http://monographs.iarc.fr/ENG/Monographs/vol100E/100E-06-Table2.66.pdf). In the largest studies, there was a statistically significant lower risk for multiple myeloma among drinkers compared with non-drinkers in white men (Hosgood *et al.*, 2007) and to a lesser extent in black men and white women (Brown *et al.*, 1997) and among both men and women (Gorini *et al.*, 2007b), but the latter associations were non-significant. Brown *et al.* (1997) found a non-significant 2.8-fold higher risk for multiple myeloma for white women who consumed ≥ 22 drinks per week. Non-significantly increased risk of multiple myeloma for consumption of alcoholic beverages was found by Deandrea *et al.* (2007)

and Monnereau *et al.* (2008) after adjustment for age, centre, sex and tobacco. No consistent association patterns were observed among the other case–control studies. Most studies collected data on alcoholic beverage consumption from proxy respondents, and some included prevalent cases. In addition, not all studies controlled for the potential confounding effects of tobacco smoking, and only two controlled for other factors such as farming, family history of cancer and occupational exposure to high-risk chemicals (Brown *et al.*, 1992; Monnereau *et al.*, 2008).

2.16 Other cancers

In the previous *IARC Monograph* (IARC, 2010) it was noted that the evidence for an association of consumption of alcoholic beverages with risk of other female cancers (vulva and vagina) and cancers of the testis, brain, thyroid, and skin melanoma was generally sparse and/or inconsistent.

2.16.1 Cancers of the vulva and vagina

In two cohort studies the association between consumption of alcoholic beverages and risk for other female cancers was examined. These were carried out in women being treated for alcohol abuse or alcoholism in Sweden (Sigvardsson *et al.*, 1996; Weiderpass *et al.*, 2001). In one study an elevated risk for vaginal cancer but not for vulva cancer was found (Weiderpass *et al.*, 2001). Sigvardsson *et al.* (1996) reported high relative risks for both vulva and vaginal cancers combined. In these studies relative risk estimates could not be adjusted for factors that may have confounded the association between alcoholic beverage consumption and vulva and vaginal cancers, such as HPV infections, number of sexual partners and tobacco smoking. It is possible that women who abuse alcohol have other behavioural patterns that may affect risks for these cancers.

Four case–control studies investigated the association between consumption of alcoholic beverages and risk for vulva cancer, conducted in Italy (Parazzini *et al.*, 1995b) and in the USA (Williams & Horm, 1977; Mabuchi *et al.*, 1985; Sturgeon *et al.*, 1991); one study from Denmark (Madsen *et al.*, 2008) investigated both cancer of the vulva and vagina. Studies published since the previous Monograph (IARC, 2010) are summarized in Table 2.67 available at http://monographs.iarc.fr/ENG/Monographs/vol100E/100E-06-Table2.67.pdf). Three were hospital-based studies (Williams & Horm, 1977; Mabuchi *et al.*, 1985; Parazzini *et al.*, 1995b), one was population-based (Sturgeon *et al.*, 1991), while Madsen *et al.* (2008) used two sets of controls, population- and hospital-based. Confounding factors were considered in four studies (Williams & Horm, 1977; Sturgeon *et al.*, 1991; Parazzini *et al.*, 1995b; Madsen *et al.*, 2008), but only two of these provided risk estimates adjusted for both smoking and sexual behaviour (Sturgeon *et al.*, 1991; Madsen *et al.*, 2008). Williams & Horm (1977), Mabuchi *et al.* (1985), Sturgeon *et al.* (1991) and Parazzini *et al.* (1995b) reported no association between alcoholic beverage consumption and risk for vulva cancer. Madsen *et al.* (2008) found a higher risk among drinkers compared to non-drinkers, for both vaginal and vulva cancers.

There was no evidence of dose–response for consumption of alcoholic beverages and vulva cancer, in any of these studies, either in terms of frequency of alcohol consumption (Parazzini *et al.*, 1995b), in terms of years of alcohol consumption (Madsen *et al.*, 2008), or when providing two defined levels of alcohol consumption (Williams & Horm, 1977). Williams & Horm (1977), Mabuchi *et al.* (1985) and Sturgeon *et al.* (1991) investigated risk of vulva cancer in relation to consumption of different alcoholic beverages. No significant associations were found with any type of alcoholic beverage.

2.16.2 *Other sites*

No new studies have been identified for cancer of testis, one on brain cancer and thyroid cancer, and three on skin cancer (malignant melanoma, basal cell carcinoma and squamous cell carcinoma).

In a large cohort study of women in the United Kingdom (Allen *et al.*, 2009) no association of consumption of alcoholic beverages was found with brain cancer (Table 2.68 available at http://monographs.iarc.fr/ENG/Monographs/vol100E/100E-06-Table2.68.pdf), but a significant inverse association with thyroid cancer (Table 2.69 available at http://monographs.iarc.fr/ENG/Monographs/vol100E/100E-06-Table2.69.pdf).

No association between consumption of alcoholic beverages and malignant melanomas was found by Allen *et al.* (2009) (Table 2.70 available at http://monographs.iarc.fr/ENG/Monographs/vol100E/100E-06-Table2.70.pdf) or by Benedetti *et al.* (2009) in a case–control study (Table 2.71 available at http://monographs.iarc.fr/ENG/Monographs/vol100E/100E-06-Table2.71.pdf). In a cohort study in Australia Ansems *et al.* (2008) found no significant association between overall basal cell carcinoma or squamous cell carcinoma risk and total alcohol intake or intake of beer, white wine, red wine or sherry and port (Table 2.70 on-line). Among those with a prior skin cancer history, there was a significant increase in risk of squamous cell carcinoma for above-median consumption of sherry and port compared with abstainers (multivariable adjusted RR, 2.46; 95%CI: 1.06–5.72).

2.17 Parental exposure and childhood cancers

Associations of paternal consumption of alcoholic beverages before pregnancy and/or maternal consumption of alcoholic beverages during pregnancy with risk for haematopoietic cancers in children were examined in nine case–control studies in Australia, Canada, France, the Netherlands, the United Kingdom and the USA (McKinney *et al.*, 1987; Severson *et al.*, 1993; van Duijn *et al.*, 1994; Shu *et al.*, 1996; Infante-Rivard *et al.*, 2002; Menegaux *et al.*, 2005; Menegaux *et al.*, 2007; MacArthur *et al.*, 2008; Rudant *et al.*, 2008). Studies published since the previous Monograph are summarized in Table 2.72 (available at http://monographs.iarc.fr/ENG/Monographs/vol100E/100E-06-Table2.72.pdf).

No association between maternal alcoholic beverage intake 1 month or 1 year before pregnancy with risk of any childhood leukaemia or lymphoma was reported by Severson *et al.* (1993), Shu *et al.* (1993) and van Duijn *et al.* (1994), whereas a borderline significant association for acute leukaemia and ALL was observed by MacArthur *et al.* (2008) and Infante-Rivard *et al.* (2002) found a positive association for ALL.

For maternal alcoholic beverage consumption during pregnancy, no association was found with leukaemia or lymphoma (McKinney *et al.*,1987) or with ALL (Rudant *et al.*, 2008), while Infante-Rivard *et al.* (2002) found a reduced risk for ALL when comparing any intake with no intake. Statistically significant two- to 2.4-fold increased risk for acute non-lymphocytic leukaemia were associated with any maternal alcoholic beverage consumption during pregnancy in two studies (van Duijn *et al.*, 1994; Menegaux *et al.*, 2005). Similarly, statistically significant positive associations between maternal alcoholic beverage consumption and risk for ALL (Shu *et al.*, 1993; Menegaux *et al.*, 2005, 2007; MacArthur *et al.*, 2008) and acute myeloid leukaemia (Severson *et al.*, 1993; Shu *et al.*, 1993) were observed. The strongest associations observed in the studies of alcoholic beverages and acute myeloid leukaemia were for children diagnosed at 10 years of age or younger (Severson *et al.*, 1993; Shu *et al.*, 1993). Overall, there was no consistent evidence of dose–response relationships for maternal or paternal alcoholic beverage intake or for intake of any specific type of alcohol beverage and risk for any childhood haematopoietic cancer. Most studies adjusted for potential confounding factors including maternal age, maternal smoking, and child's sex. Importantly, whether any of the observed associations between maternal or paternal consumption of alcoholic beverages and risk for childhood haematopoietic cancers are attributed to recall bias is unclear.

2.18 Polymorphisms and genetic susceptibility

Studies that identify associations between genetic polymorphisms and inter-individual differences in susceptibility to the agent(s) being evaluated may contribute to the identification of carcinogenic hazards to humans. If the polymorphism has been demonstrated experimentally to modify the functional activity of the gene product in a manner that is consistent with increased susceptibility, these data may be useful in making causal inferences. Similarly, studies that measure cell functions, enzymes or metabolites that are thought to be the basis of susceptibility may provide evidence that reinforces biological plausibility. If the known phenotype of a genetic polymorphism can explain the carcinogenic mechanism of the agent being evaluated, data on this phenotype may be useful in making causal inferences.

However, when data on genetic susceptibility originate from multiple comparisons in subgroup analyses, false-positive results and inconsistencies across studies can be generated. Furthermore, many of the identified susceptibility genes have no or unknown functional characterization; only for a few genes (e.g. ALDH2) are functional studies available; and generally induction of enzymes is not considered. Such data therefore require careful evaluation.

A challenge in the interpretation of the associations between the polymorphisms affecting alcohol and/or acetaldehyde metabolism and cancer is that the genes coding for more active alcohol oxidizing enzyme and/or less active acetaldehyde oxidizing enzyme, may both promote and inhibit the development of cancer. Carriers of genes enhancing alcohol oxidation and/or inhibiting acetaldehyde oxidation on average consume less alcohol (Matsuo *et al.*, 2006b, 2007; Zintzaras *et al.*, 2006) and thus may be protected from harmful chronic effects (e.g. cancer) induced by alcohol unless they drink heavily. Thus, in studying the mechanisms of the associations between these polymorphisms and cancer, it is essential to control for differences in alcohol drinking.

2.18.1 Alcohol dehydrogenase-1B (ADH1B)

ADH1B (previously called *ADH2*) is polymorphic, and its superactive *ADH1B*2* allele is highly prevalent among East Asians (54–96%; Goedde *et al.*, 1992), but relatively rare among Caucasians (1–23%). Individuals with the *ADH1B*1/*1* genotype code less active ADH, which is a risk factor for excessive alcohol consumption in both East Asians and Caucasians (Zintzaras *et al.*, 2006; Matsuo *et al.*, 2007).

(a) Cancer of the oesophagus

Individuals with the *ADH1B*1/*1* genotype were at increased risk for oesophageal cancer in 15 case–control studies among several populations (Hori *et al.*, 1997; Yokoyama *et al.*, 1998; Chao *et al.*, 2000; Matsuo *et al.* 2001b; Yokoyama *et al.*, 2001, 2002; Boonyaphiphat *et al.*, 2002; Yang *et al.*, 2005; Yang *et al.*, 2007; Guo *et al.*, 2008; Hashibe *et al.*, 2008; Lee *et al.*, 2008b; Cui *et al.*, 2009; Ding *et al.*, 2009) and in a cohort study in cancer-free Japanese alcoholics (Yokoyama *et al.*, 2006b) (Tables 2.73, 2.74). The difference was not significant in two Japanese studies (Tanabe *et al.* 1999; Yokoyama *et al.*, 2006a) and one study in South Africa (Li *et al.*, 2008a). [Many studies did not control for the amount of alcohol consumption, which makes it difficult to make firm conclusions about the etiology of the *ADH1B*1/*1* associated cancers.]

(b) Upper aerodigestive tract cancers combined

In four Japanese studies (Yokoyama *et al.*, 2001, 2006b; Asakage *et al.*, 2007; Hiraki *et al.*, 2007), one European study (Hashibe *et al.*, 2006) and one Indian study (Solomon *et al.*, 2008) an *ADH1B*1/*1*-associated increased risk for upper aerodigestive tract cancers was found in alcohol drinkers. No significant association was found in another European study (Risch *et al.*, 2003; Tables 2.74, 2.75).

A recent large multicentre study from Europe and Latin America of *ADH* genes and UADT cancer that focused on seven separate *ADH* variants known to change an amino acid (missense substitution) included a total of 3800 cases and 5200 controls (Hashibe *et al.*, 2008). One variant in *ADH1B* (rs1229984) that codes for fast ethanol metabolism was associated with a strong decreased risk for UADT cancer, after adjusting for amount of alcohol consumed (OR for dominant model, 0.56; 95%CI: 0.47–0.66, $P = 4 \times 10^{-11}$). The odds ratio was 0.45 (95%CI: 0.35–0.57) for oral/pharyngeal cancers combined and 0.71 (95%CI: 0.57–0.88) for laryngeal cancer.

(c) Cancers of the stomach, colorectum and pancreas

One Polish study showed no significant effects of the *ADH1B* polymorphism on risk for cancer of the stomach (Zhang *et al.*, 2007b; Table 2.76 available at http://monographs.iarc.fr/ENG/Monographs/vol100E/100E-06-Table2.76.pdf). For cancer of the colorectum, two Japanese case–control studies of alcohol drinkers found an increased risk in *ADH1B*1/*1* subjects compared with *ADH1B*2* carriers without stratification of *ALDH2* genotypes (Matsuo *et al.*, 2006a; Yin *et al.*, 2007). However, stratification by *ALDH2* genotypes rendered the association opposite within the *ALDH2*1/*1* subjects in one of the studies (Matsuo *et al.*, 2006a), while no such effect was seen in the other study (Yin *et al.*, 2007). In a Chinese study the *ADHB1*2/*2* genotype tended to increased the risk for cancer of the colorectum regardless of the *ALDH2* genotype (Gao *et al.*, 2008). Also, a study in Spain reported a non-significant decrease in risk for cancer of the colorectum for the *ADH1B*2/*2* versus *ADH1B*1/*1* (Landi *et al.*, 2005).

The *ADH1B*2* allele has been associated with an increase in risk for cancer of the pancreas and consumption of alcoholic beverages among Japanese (Kanda *et al.*, 2009).

(d) Hepatocellular cancer

In two studies in Japan and in a study in China it was concluded that the *ADH1B* polymorphism had no significant impact on the risk for hepatocellular carcinoma (Takeshita *et al.*, 2000b; Sakamoto *et al.*, 2006; Ding *et al.*, 2008; Table 2.76 on-line).

(e) Cancer of the breast

In a study in Germany (Lilla *et al.*, 2005), a decreased risk for cancer of the breast with consumption of alcoholic beverages ≥ 12 g ethanol/day compared with no intake was observed in women with the *ADH1B*2* allele, whereas no such association was found in women with the *ADH1B*1/*1* genotype. In four other studies from Japan, United Kingdom and the USA, no significant differences in the risk by *ADH1B* polymorphism were observed (Cox *et al.*, 2007; Terry *et al.*, 2007b; Visvanathan *et al.*, 2007; Kawase *et al.*, 2009; Table 2.76 on-line).

2.18.2 ADH1C

ADH1C (previously called *ADH3*) is a major gene polymorphism among Caucasians. The homodimer encoded by the *ADH1C*1* allele catalyses the production of acetaldehyde from ethanol at a rate 2.5 times faster than the

Table 2.73 Case-control studies and meta-analyses of *ALDH2, ADH1B* and *ADH1C* genotype-associated risk for cancer of the oesophagus

Reference, study location, period	Cancer site and/or type	Genes involved	No of cases/deaths	Relative risk (95% CI)[1]	Comments
Hori *et al.* (1997), Tokyo, Japan, study period NR	Squamous cell carcinoma	***ALDH2***			No adjustment was reported
		**1/*1*	20	1.0	
		**1/*2*	70	4.4 (2.5–7.7)	
		**2/*2*	3	0.9 (0.2–3.6)	
		ADH1B			
		**2/*2*	40	1.0	
		**1/*2*	33	1.7 (0.9–3.0)	
		**1/*1*	21	6.2 (2.6–14.7)	
Yokoyama *et al.* (1998), Kanagawa, Japan, 1987–97	Oesophagus NOS	***ALDH2***			Male alcoholics; because the differences in odds ratio between the incident cases and the prevalent cases were slight, the cases were combined. Adjusted for age, alcohol drinking and cigarette smoking. Possible partial overlap with Yokoyama *et al.* (2001)
		**1/*1*	41	1.00	
		**1/*2*	46	12.50 (7.23–21.61)	
Tanabe *et al.* (1999), Hokkaido, Japan, 1994–97	Squamous cell carcinoma	***ALDH2***		NS	Alcohol consumption and smoking did not differ between the cases and controls.
		**1/*1*	8		
		**1/*2*	11		
		**2/*2*	0		
Chao *et al.* (2000), Taipei, Taiwan, China, 1997–99	Oesophagus	***ALDH2***		Allele **2* was associated with risk ($P < 0.001$)	Alcoholics and non-alcoholic oesophageal cancer cases and alcoholic and non-alcoholic controls. No adjustment
		**1/*1*	22	Allele **1* was associated with risk ($P < 0.025$)	
		**1/*2*	37		
		**2/*2*	0		
		ADH1B		No significant difference in prevalence of alleles in alcoholics with different diseases and between alcoholic and non-alcoholic oesophageal cancer cases	
		**1/*1*	17		
		**1/*2*	26		
		**2/*2*	16		
		ADH1C			
		**1/*1*	38		
		**1/*2*	21		
		**2/*2*	0		

Table 2.73 (continued)

Reference, study location, period	Cancer site and/or type	Genes involved	No of cases/deaths	Relative risk (95% CI)[1]	Comments
Matsuo *et al.* (2001b), Aichi, Japan, 1999–2000 (cases were first diagnosed as having esophageal cancer between 1984–2000 and visited the study centre in 1999–2000)	Oesophagus NOS	***ALDH2***			Adjusted for age, sex, drinking, smoking. Heavy drinkers defined as those drinking 75 mL ethanol/d, ≥ 5 d/wk. "Other participants" refers to those who were not heavy drinker
		All participants			
		**1/*1*	35	1.00	
		**1/*2*	66	3.72 (1.88–7.36)	
		**2/*2*	1	0.80 (0.09–6.88)	
		Heavy drinkers			
		**1/*1*	22	1.00	
		**1/*2*	46	16.4 (4.41–61.2)	
		**2/*2*	0	–	
		Other participants			
		**1/*1*	13	1.00	
		**1/*2*	20	1.68 (0.78–3.62)	
		**2/*2*	1	0.42 (0.28–1.25)	
Yokoyama *et al.* (2001), Kanagawa, Japan, 1993–2000	Squamous cell carcinoma	***ALDH2***			Male alcoholics. Adjusted for age, drinking, smoking, *ALDH2* and *ADH1B* genotypes. Possible partial overlap with Yokoyama *et al.* (1998)
		**1/*1*	50	1.00	
		**1/*2*	62	13.50 (8.06–22.60)	
		ADH1B			
		**1/*2 + *2/*2*	56	1.00	
		**1/*1*	56	2.64 (1.62–4.31)	

Table 2.73 (continued)

Reference, study location, period	Cancer site and/or type	Genes involved	No of cases/deaths	Relative risk (95% CI)[1]	Comments
Boonyaphiphat *et al.* (2002), Songkhla, Thailand, 1997–2000	Squamous cell carcinoma	**By alcohol intake**			Unlike Japanese and Chinese studies, frequency of inactive *ALDH2* is low in the Thais: 20% in cases, 18% in controls. Adjusted for age, sex, smoking, betel chewing (drinking, *ALDH2* and *ADH1B* genotypes for overall)
		ALDH2			
		Non-drinker			
		**1/*1*	40	1.00	
		**1/*2*	12	1.56 (0.65–3.70)	
		≤ 60 g/d			
		**1/*1*	42	2.16 (1.11–4.21)	
		**1/*2*	8	2.52 (0.85–7.46)	
		> 60 g/d			
		**1/*1*	79	5.28 (2.70–10.32)	
		**1/*2*	20	10.83 (3.37–34.69) Interaction $P = 0.031$	
		ADH1B			
		Non-drinker			
		**1/*2*	35	1.00	
		**1/*1*	18	0.89 (0.41–1.93)	
		≤ 60 g/d			
		**1/*2*	28	2.00 (0.97–4.11)	
		**1/*1*	22	2.34 (1.06–5.11)	
		> 60 g/d			
		**1/*2*	38	3.35 (1.50–7.02)	
		**1/*1*	61	11.46 (5.16–25.45) Interaction $P = 0.064$	
Itoga *et al.* (2002), Chiba, Japan [study period NR]	Oesophagus NOS	Habitual drinkers			No adjustment was reported
		ALDH2*1	47	1.0	
		ALDH2*2	18	4.9 ($P < 0.0001$)	
Watanabe *et al.* (2002), Kagawa, Japan, 1998–2001	Squamous cell carcinoma	***ALDH2***		See comments	Prevalence of **2* allele was significantly higher in cases than in controls.
		**1/*1*	10		
		**1/*2*	18		
		**2/*2*	1		

Table 2.73 (continued)

Reference, study location, period	Cancer site and/or type	Genes involved	No of cases/deaths	Relative risk (95% CI)[1]	Comments
Yokoyama *et al.* (2002), Tokyo, Chiba, Kanagawa, Osaka, Japan, 2000–01	Squamous cell carcinoma	**By alcohol intake**			Only male participants. Multivariate odds ratio of *ALDH2*2/*2* in comparison with *ALDH2*1/*1* was 7.83 (1.33–46.08). However, most men with **2/*2* genotype drank rarely or never and the risk was evaluated based on a small sample size (2 cases/43 controls). For *ADH1C* genotype the relative risk was associated with less active *ADH1C*1/*1* versus active **1/*2* or **2/*2*. When the linkage disequilibrium between *ADH1B* and *ADH1C* was taken into consideration, the *ADH1C* genotype did not significantly affect the risk for cancer. Adjusted for age, strong alcoholic beverage, green-yellow vegetables and fruit (and alcohol drinking, *ALDH2*, *ADH1B* and *ADH1C* genotypes for overall association). Cases included in Yokoyama *et al.* (2001) were excluded from this study.
		ALDH2			
		**1/*1*			
		< 22 g/wk	0	0.0 (not calculable)	
		22–197 g/wk	3	1.00	
		198–395 g/wk	23	5.58 (1.54–20.25)	
		≥ 396 g/wk	33	10.38 (2.85–37.84)	
		Former drinker	4	8.81 (1.53–50.76)	
		**1/*2*			
		< 22 g/wk	3	0.75 (0.14–4.11)	
		22–197 g/wk	21	5.82 (1.59–21.38)	
		198–395 g/wk	63	55.84 (15.40–202.51)	
		≥ 396 g/wk	73	88.88 (23.97–329.57)	
		Former drinker	9	50.50 (9.18–277.95)	
		**2/*2*			
		< 22 g/wk	2	1.44 (0.22–9.54)	
		ADH1B			
		**1/*2 or *2/*2*			
		< 22 g/wk	4	0.21 (0.06–0.68)	
		22–197 g/wk	20	1.00	
		198–395 g/wk	68	4.09 (2.25–7.42)	
		≥ 396 g/wk	80	7.01 (3.77–13.04)	
		Former drinker	11	5.73 (2.03–16.20)	
		**1/*1*			

Table 2.73 (continued)

Reference, study location, period	Cancer site and/or type	Genes involved	No of cases/deaths	Relative risk (95% CI)[1]	Comments
Yokoyama *et al.* (2002) Contd.		< 22 g/wk	1	4.25 (0.41–43.82)	
		22–197 g/wk	4	3.97 (1.01–15.63)	
		198–395 g/wk	18	33.30 (11.14–99.50)	
		≥ 396 g/wk	26	38.64 (13.27–112.55)	
		Former drinker	2	19.63 (1.65–233.20)	
		ADH1C			
		**1/*1*			
		< 22 g/wk	5	0.23 (0.08–0.68)	
		22–197 g/wk	22	1.00	
		198–395 g/wk	69	3.66 (2.04–6.55)	
		≥ 396 g/wk	88	6.64 (3.66–12.05)	
		Former drinker	12	8.44 (2.94–24.25)	
		**1/*2 or *2/*2*			
		< 22 g/wk	0	Not calculable	
		22–197 g/wk	2	0.81 (0.17–3.99)	
		198–395 g/wk	17	13.32 (5.28–33.63)	
		≥ 396 g/wk	18	23.83 (7.67–74.06)	
		Former drinker	1	1.01 (0.09–11.93)	
Yang *et al.* (2005), Aichi, Japan, 2001–04	Oesophagus NOS	**Overall analyses**			Results from overall analyses were adjusted for age, sex, smoking and alcohol drinking. Results by alcohol intake were adjusted for smoking. *P* for interaction between alcohol intake and genotypes for *ALDH2* was 0.03 for ≤ 250 g/wk and < 0.01 for > 250 g/wk alcohol intake. *P* for interaction for *ADH1B* was 0.24 for ≤ 250 g/wk and 0.32 for > 250 g/wk alcohol intake
		ALDH2			
		**1/*1*		1.00	
		**1/*2*		6.43 (4.02–10.3)	
		**2/*2*		1.92 (0.23–15.7)	
		ADH1B			
		**2/*2*		1.00	
		**1/*2*		1.57 (1.04–2.36)	
		**1/*1*		0.62 (0.22–1.72)	
		By alcohol intake			
		ALDH2			
		**1/*1*			

Table 2.73 (continued)

Reference, study location, period	Cancer site and/or type	Genes involved	No of cases/deaths	Relative risk (95% CI)[1]	Comments
Yang *et al.* (2005), Contd.		Non drinker		1.00	
		≤ 250 g/wk		1.88 (0.42–8.37)	
		> 250 g/wk		4.62 (0.93–23.1)	
		**1/*2*			
		Non-drinker		1.00	
		≤ 250 g/wk		9.64 (3.23–28.8)	
		> 250 g/wk		95.4 (28.7–317)	
		ADH1B			
		**2/*2*			
		Non-drinker	38	1.00	
		< 1200 g/yr	126	5.03 (1.67–15.1)	
		≥ 1200 g/yr	1	25.8 (8.01–83.3)	
		**1/*2* or **1/*1*			
		Non-drinker	74	1.00	
		< 1200 g/yr	85	8.50 (1.90–38.0)	
		≥ 1200 g/yr	6	33.9 (7.34–157)	
Cai *et al.* (2006), Taixing, Jiangsu Province, China, 2000	Squamous cell carcinoma	***ALDH2***			Adjusted for age, sex, education level, body mass index, and history of smoking and alcohol drinking. An elevation of the risk for ESCC was pronounced most among carriers of *ALDH2* *2/*2 and *XRCC1* 399Gln/Gln or Gln/Arg who consumed a low level of dietary selenium (adjusted OR, 4.16; 95% CI: 1.14–15.12).
		**1/*1*	119	1.00	
		**1/*2*	61	0.76 (0.50–1.16)	
		**2/*2*	25	1.72 (0.85–3.48)	

Table 2.73 (continued)

Reference, study location, period	Cancer site and/or type	Genes involved	No of cases/deaths	Relative risk (95% CI)[1]	Comments
Yokoyama *et al.* (2006a), Tokyo, Chiba, Kanagawa, Osaka, Japan, 2000–04	Squamous cell carcinoma	**By alcohol intake**			Only female participants. Adjusted for age, smoking, green-yellow vegetables and fruit, hot food and beverages
		ALDH2*1/*1			
		< 22 g/wk	12	1	
		22–197 g/wk	5	0.80 (0.24–2.60)	
		198–395 g/wk	4	1.99 (0.52–7.68)	
		≥ 396 g/wk	4	3.16 (0.65–15.48)	
		ALDH2*1/*2			
		< 22 g/wk	8	0.5 (0.2–1.3)	
		22–197 g/wk	5	2.0 (0.5–7.1)	
		198–395 g/wk	2	4.7 (0.7–31)	
		≥ 396 g/wk	3	59 (4.7–750)	
		ADH1B		NS	
Hashibe *et al.* (2006), Romania, Poland, the Russian Federation, Slovakia, Czech Republic, 2000–02	Squamous cell carcinoma	***ADH1B** R48H*			*ALDH2* +82A > G, +348C > T and -261C > T showed linkage disequilibrium and were associated with risk for oesophageal squamous-cell carcinoma. Adjusted for age, sex, country, yr of alcohol drinking, pack-yr of tobacco smoking.
		*1/*1	163	1.00	
		*1/*2 + *2/*2	4	0.19 (0.07–0.53)	
		***ADH1C** I350V*			
		Ile/Ile (slow)	42	1.00	
		Ile/Val	92	1.61 (1.07–2.43)	
		Val/Val (fast; *1/*1)	30	1.74 (1.02–2.98)	
		***ADH1C** R272Q*			
		Arg/Arg (slow)	42	1.00	
		Arg/Gln	88	1.62 (1.07–2.44)	
		Gln/Gln (fast; *1/*1)	30	2.03 (1.18–3.47)	
		***ALDH2** +82A > G*			

Table 2.73 (continued)

Reference, study location, period	Cancer site and/or type	Genes involved	No of cases/deaths	Relative risk (95% CI)[1]	Comments
Hashibe *et al.* (2006), Contd.		A/A	82	1.00	
		A/G	69	2.11 (1.46–3.05)	
		G/G	15	4.14 (2.03–8.46)	
		ALDH2 *+348C > T*			
		T/T	83	1.00	
		T/C	71	2.29 (1.59–3.30)	
		C/C	12	3.71 (1.73–7.97)	
		ALDH2 *−261C > T*			
		T/T	85	1.00	
		T/C	71	2.32 (1.61–3.35)	
		C/C	12	3.85 (1.78–8.36)	
Homann *et al.* (2006), Germany, 1999–2003	Oesophagus NOS	*ADH1C*1/*1* in heavy drinkers		2.93 (1.84–4.67)	Study participants were heavy alcohol drinkers: 123 oesophageal cancer cases and 525 controls with benign tumours. Adjusted for age, sex and smoking. [The reference group was not reported: *ADH1C*2/*2* or *ADH1C*2/*2* + *ADH1C*1/*1*.]
Yang *et al.* (2007), Yanting, Sichuan Province, China, 2003–04	Oesophagus (96% squamous cell carcinoma)	***ADH1B***			Adjusted for age, sex, smoking, rapid food eating, quality of drinking-water, consumption of picked vegetables and fresh fruits, vegetables and eggs. Non-drinkers also included ex-drinkers.
		**2/*2*			
		Non-drinker	37	1.0	
		Current drinker	41	1.88 (0.86–4.15)	
		**1/*2 or *1/*1*			
		Non-drinker	43	1.21 (0.63–2.33)	
		Current drinker	70	3.94 (1.76–8.81)	
		ALDH2			
		**1/*1*			
		Non-drinker	33	1.0	
		Current drinker	57	3.15 (1.39–7.13)	
		**1/*2 or *2/*2*			
		Non-drinker	47	2.03 (1.03–3.99)	
		Current drinker	54	4.82 (2.06–11.27)	

Table 2.73 (continued)

Reference, study location, period	Cancer site and/or type	Genes involved	No of cases/deaths	Relative risk (95% CI)[1]	Comments
Terry *et al.* (2007a), Connecticut, New Jersey and Washington, USA, 1993–95	Squamous cell carcinoma	***ADH1C***			Adjusted for age, gender and geographic site
		**2/*2*	4	1.0	
		**1/*2*	10	1.0 (0.3–3.3)	
		**1/*1*	9	1.7 (0.5–5.9)	
	Oesophageal and gastric cardia adenocarcinoma	***ADH1C***			
		**2/*2*	17	1.0	
		**1/*2*	52	1.2 (0.6–2.5)	
		**1/*1*	45	2.0 (1.0–4.2)	
Guo *et al.* (2008), Lanzhou, Gansu Province, China, 2004–07	Squamous cell carcinoma	***ALDH2***			Variables for which the results were adjusted were NR
		**1/*1*	37	1.00	
		**1/*2*	43	2.89 (1.11–5.64)	
		**2/*2*	0	–	
		ADH1B			
		**1/*1*	17	1.00	
		**2/*1*	25	3.67 (1.26–8.73)	
		**2/*2*	38	1.46 (0.71–2.59)	
		By alcohol intake			
		ALDH2			
		**1/*1*			
		0–200 g/wk	7	1.00	
		> 200 g/wk	30	2.29 (0.91–5.57)	
		**1/*2*			
		0–200 g/wk	7	0.56 (0.20–1.59)	
		> 200 g/wk	36	8.58 (3.28–22.68)	
		**2/*2*			
		0–200 g/wk	0	–	
		ADH1B			
		**1/*2* or **2/*2*			
		0–200 g/wk	13	1.00	
		> 200 g/wk	50	4.75 (2.53–9.38)	
		**1/*1*			
		0–200 g/wk	1	1.00 (0.18–9.22)	
		> 200 g/wk	16	27.12 (8.52–70.19)	

Table 2.73 (continued)

Reference, study location, period	Cancer site and/or type	Genes involved	No of cases/deaths	Relative risk (95% CI)[1]	Comments
Lee *et al.* (2008b), Taipei and Kaohsiung, Taiwan, China, 2000–05	Squamous cell carcinoma	**By alcohol intake**			Adjusted for age, sex, study hospital, ethnicity, smoking, education, smoking, betel quid chewing, and consumption of fruits and vegetables. Another publication from this study (Lee *et al.*, 2009), reported that heterozygous ALDH2 increased the oesophageal cancer risk more prominently in younger population.
		ALDH2			
		**1/*1*			
		Non-drinker	17	1.0	
		0.1–30 g/d	45	2.2 (1.1–4.5)	
		> 30 g/d	49	7.2 (3.3–15.9)	
		**1/*2*			
		Non-drinker	38	1.1 (0.6–2.3)	
		0.1–30 g/d	114	14.5 (7.1–29.6)	
		> 30 g/d	129	102.6 (38.3–274.8)	
		**2/*2*			
		Non-drinker	8	1.2 (0.4–3.4)	
		0.1–30 g/d	3	17.3 (1.4–213.7)	
		> 30 g/d	3	– (0 control subject)	
		ADH1B			
		**2/*2*			
		Non-drinker	29	1.0	
		0.1–30 g/d	58	3.5 (1.9–6.5)	
		> 30 g/d	53	11.1 (5.0–24.4)	
		**1/*2*			
		Non-drinker	26	0.8 (0.4–1.6)	
		0.1–30 g/d	59	4.2 (2.2–7.9)	
		> 30 g/d	64	14.2 (6.6–30.6)	
		**1/*1*			
		Non-drinker	8	1.2 (0.4–3.6)	
		0.1–30 g/d	45	10.6 (4.7–23.7)	
		> 30 g/d	64	71.9 (22.6–228.5)	

Table 2.73 (continued)

Reference, study location, period	Cancer site and/or type	Genes involved	No of cases/deaths	Relative risk (95% CI)[1]	Comments
Ding *et al.* (2008), Taixing, Jiangsu Province, China, 2005–06	Oesophagus NOS	**By alcohol intake**			Adjusted for income
		ADH1B			
		Non-drinker			
		**2/*2*	50	1.00	
		**1/*2*	42	1.31 (0.70–2.46)	
		**1/*1*	4	2.10 (0.35–12.54)	
		**1/*2 or *1/*1*	46	1.37 (0.74–2.54)	
		Drinker			
		**2/*2*	56	1.00	
		**1/*2*	54	1.18 (0.64–2.16)	
		**1/*1*	15	2.90 (0.85–9.90)	
		**1/*2 or *1/*1*	69	1.36 (0.76–2.43)	
		ALDH2			
		Non-drinker			
		**1/*1*	26	1.00	
		**1/*2*	43	1.29 (0.65–2.55)	
		**2/*2*	27	4.67 (1.63–13.38)	
		**1/*2 or *2/*2*	70	1.78 (0.94–3.37)	
		Drinker			
		**1/*1*	64	1.00	
		**1/*2*	46	2.47 (1.27–4.82)	
		**2/*2*	15	8.63 (2.07–35.95)	
		**1/*2 or *2/*2*	61	3.08 (1.65–5.78)	
Li *et al.* (2008a), Cape Town, South Africa, 1997–2003	Squamous cell carcinoma	***ADH1B***			Results for participants from black racial groups (282 cases and 348 controls). All results for those with mixed ancestry (192 cases and 188 controls) were non-significant. Non-adjusted results.
		**1* allele	265	1.00	
		**2* allele	4	NS	
		**3* allele	13	NS	
		ADH1C			
		**1* allele	153	1.00	
		**2* allele	129	1.80 ($P = 0.0004$)	
		ALDH2			
		**1* allele	155	1.00	
		**2* allele	27	2.35 ($P = 0.008$)	

Table 2.73 (continued)

Reference, study location, period	Cancer site and/or type	Genes involved	No of cases/deaths	Relative risk (95% CI)[1]	Comments
Hashibe *et al.* (2008), Multicenter study (see Comments), 2000–05	Oesophagus	***ADH1B***			427 cases of oesophageal cancer. Pooled analysis of studies conducted in the Russian Federation (Moscow), Poland (Lodz), Romania (Bucharest), Czech Republic (Prague, Olomouc), Slovakia (Banska′ Bystrica), France (Paris), Greece (Athens), Italy (Aviano, Padova, Torino), Norway (Oslo), United Kingdom (Edinburgh, Manchester, Newcastle), Spain (Barcelona), Croatia (Zagreb), Cuba, Argentina (Buenos Aires) and Brazil (Goianna, Pelotas, Rio de Janeiro, Sao Paulo) Adjusted for age, sex, centre, cumulative alcohol consumption and smoking
		**1/*1*		1	
		**1/*2* or **2/*2*		0.34 (0.20–0.56)	
		ADH1C G > A was in linkage disequilibrium with *ADH1B*			
Cui *et al.* (2009), Japan (see Comments)	Squamous cell carcinoma	***ALDH2***			Case samples (n = 1070) were from BioBank Japan, a collaborative network of 66 hospitals in Japan. Control samples in the first stage (n = 938) were obtained from volunteers in Osaka, Japan. The control groups for the second stage and replication analysis consisted of 1898 individuals who were registered in BioBank Japan as subjects with diseases other than cancers. Adjusted for age, gender, alcohol and smoking. Heterozygous ALDH2 increased the oesophageal cancer risk more prominently in younger population.
		**1/*1*	314	1.00	
		**1/*2*	735	3.48 (2.99–4.06)	
		**2/*2*	17	0.47 (0.28–0.78)	
		ADH1B			
		**2/*2*	510	1.00	
		**1/*2*	363	1.17 (1.01–1.37)	
		**1/*1*	194	4.10 (3.24–5.18)	
		By alcohol intake			
		ALDH2			
		**2/*1* vs *1*1* + **2/*2*			
		0–96.5 g/wk		3.35 (2.66–4.22)	
		> 96.5 g/wk		6.20 (4.76–8.09)	
		ADH1B			
		**1/*1* vs **1/*2* + **2/*2*			
		0–96.5 g/wk		3.18 (2.28–4.43)	
		> 96.5 g/wk		4.74 (3.21–6.99)	

Table 2.73 (continued)

Reference, study location, period	Cancer site and/or type	Genes involved	No of cases/deaths	Relative risk (95% CI)[1]	Comments
Meta-analysis					
Lewis & Smith (2005)	Oesophagus NOS	*ALDH2*1/*1*		1.0	Meta-analysis of the studies: Hori *et al.* (1997), Matsuo *et al.* (2001b), Boonyaphiphat *et al.* (2002), Itoga *et al.* (2002), Yokoyama *et al.* (2002) [Reduced risk with *2/*2 likely due to markedly lower levels of alcohol consumption in *2/*2 versus *1/*1 homozygotes.]
		*ALDH2*1/*2*		3.19 (1.86–5.47)	
		*ALDH2*2/*2*		0.39 (0.16–0.80)	

*ALDH2 *1* is more active, *ADH1B *1* is less active, and *ADH1C *1* is more active alleles than the other allele in the respective genes.

ALDH, aldehyde dehydrogenase; *ADH*, alcohol dehydrogenase; CI, confidence intervall d, day or days; NOS, not otherwise specified; NR, not reported; NS, not significant; vs, versus; wk, week or weeks

Table 2.74 Cohort study of *ALDH2* and *ADH1B* genotype-associated risk for cancer of the oesophagus and upper aerodigestive tract

Reference, location	Cohort description	Exposure assessment	Cancer and site	Exposure categories	No. of subjects/ squamous-cell carcinoma	Hazard ratio (95% CI)	Adjustment factors	Comments
Yokoyama *et al.* (2006b), Kanagawa, Japan	808 Japanese alcoholic men confirmed cancer-free by endoscopic screening during 1993–2005; endoscopic follow-up from 1 to 148 mo (median, 31 mo)	*ALDH2*, *ADH1B* genotyping at baseline examination in 556 patients	Upper aerodigestive tract squamous-cell carcinoma	***ALDH2***			Age	
				**1/*1*	484/27	1		
				**1/*2*	72/26	11.6 (5.7–23.3)		
				ADH1B				
				**1/*2 + *2/*2*	381/28	1		
				**1/*1*	175/25	2.0 (1.02–4.0)		
			Oesophageal squamous-cell carcinoma	***ALDH2***				
				**1/*1*	484/14	1		
				**1/*2*	72/19	13.0 (5.2–32.1)		
				ADH1B				
				**1/*2 + *2/*2*	381/18	1		
				**1/*1*	175/15	1.6 (0.7–3.9)		
			Oropharyngolaryngeal squamous-cell carcinoma	***ALDH2***				
				**1/*1*	484/17	1		
				**1/*2*	72/13	11.7 (4.7–29.5)		
				ADH1B				
				**1/*2 + *2/*2*	381/16	1		
				**1/*1*	175/14	2.0 (0.8–5.0)		

ADH, alcohol dehydrogenase; *ALDH*, aldehyde dehydrogenase; CI, confidence interval; mo, month or months homodimer encoded by the *ADH1C*2* allele (Bosron & Li, 1986).

(a) Cancer of the oesophagus

Associations between *ADH1C* genotype and oesophageal cancer have been investigated in five studies in populations mainly composed of Caucasians. A higher *ADH1C*1/*1*-associated risk was found in four (Visapää *et al.*, 2004; Hashibe *et al.*, 2006; Homann *et al.*, 2006; Terry *et al.*, 2007a; Table 2.73), in one of which all UADT cancers were combined (Visapää *et al.*, 2004; Table 2.75). However, no association was observed when the linkage disequilibrium between *ADH1B*2* and *ADH1C*1* was taken into consideration in one study (Hashibe *et al.*, 2006). Both *ADH1B*2* and *ADH1C*1* were in linkage disequilibrium in an analysis by Hashibe *et al.* (2008).

In contrast to the overall direction in Caucasian populations, in two Japanese studies it was reported that the *ADH1C*2* allele increases the risk for oesophageal cancer (Yokoyama *et al.*, 2002; Muto *et al.*, 2005). Again, when the linkage disequilibrium between *ADH1B* and *ADH1C* was taken into consideration, no relationship was found between *ADH1C* genotype and UADT cancer risk (Yokoyama *et al.*, 2002). No significant associations were observed in a Chinese study (Chao *et al.*, 2000). An association between *ADH1C*2* allele and risk of oesophageal cancer was reported in an African population (Li *et al.*, 2008a).

(b) Other upper aerodigestive tract cancers

In six studies of Caucasians (Coutelle *et al.*, 1997; Harty *et al.*, 1997; Homann *et al.*, 2006; Hashibe *et al.*, 2006, 2008; Arndt *et al.*, 2008) increased risk of other upper aerodigestive tract cancer cancers associated with the *ADH1C*1/*1* genotype was reported (Table 2.75). In two other studies of Caucasians (Schwartz *et al.*, 2001; Peters *et al.*, 2005), two studies from Japan and India (Asakage *et al.*, 2007; Solomon *et al.*, 2008) and one Brazilian study of a mixed population (Nishimoto *et al.*, 2004) opposite results were reported, with the *ADH1C*2/*2* genotype increasing the risk. When the linkage disequilibrium between *ADH1B* and *ADH1C* was taken into consideration (Asakage *et al.*, 2007), no relationship was found between *ADH1C* genotype and cancer risk. No significant associations were observed in six other studies of Caucasians (Bouchardy *et al.*, 2000; Olshan *et al.*, 2001; Sturgis *et al.*, 2001; Zavras *et al.*, 2002; Risch *et al.*, 2003; Wang *et al.*, 2005), or in a study of Japan (Muto *et al.*, 2005).

(c) Cancers of the stomach and colorectum

In one study in the USA increased risk of gastric adenocarcinomas associated with the *ADH1C*1/*1* genotype was reported (Terry *et al.*, 2007a) but in a Polish study no significant effects of the *ADH1C* polymorphism on stomach cancer risk was found (Zhang *et al.*, 2007b) (Table 2.76 on-line).

Regarding the risk for cancer of the colorectum, in two European studies an increased risk in *ADH1C*1/*1* carriers compared with *ADH1C*2* subjects was found (Tiemersma *et al.*, 2003; Homann *et al.*, 2009). However, an increased risk with *ADH1C*2/*2* genotype was reported in another study (Giovannucci *et al.*, 2003). A trend with the *ADH1C*2/*2* genotype increasing the risk for cancer of the colorectum was also observed in another study of Caucasians [which was perhaps explained by higher alcohol consumption by those with **2/*2* genotype] (Jung *et al.*, 2008). In two other studies of primarily Caucasians (van der Logt *et al.*, 2006; Curtin *et al.*, 2007) and a study on Japanese subjects (Yin *et al.*, 2007) no significant associations between *ADH1C* polymorphism and cancer of the colorectum were found.

Table 2.75 Studies of *ALDH2, ADH1B* and *ADH1C* genotype-associated risk for cancers of the head and neck

Reference, study location, period	Cancer and site	Genes involved	Relative risk (95% CI)[1]	Comments
Coutelle *et al.* (1997), Bordeaux, France, study period NR	Oropharynx, larynx	***ADH1C***		Study participants were classified as alcoholics and consumed > 100 g ethanol per d for > 10 yr; 21 with oropharyngeal cancer, 18 with laryngeal cancer, and 37 controls with no cancer. ORs adjusted for age. Risk for laryngeal cancer in alcoholics who were *GSTμ*⁻ and *ADH3*1/*1* was 12.9 (95% 1.8–92) compared with those who were *GSTμ*⁻ and *ADH3*1/*2* or **2/*2*
	Both cancer sites	**1/*2, *2/*2*	1.0	
		**1/*1*	3.6 (0.7–10.0)	
	Oropharynx	**1/*2, *2/*2*	1	
		**1/*1*	2.6 (0.7–10.0)	
	Larynx	**1/*2, *2/*2*	1	
		**1/*1*	6.1 (1.3–28.6)	
Harty *et al.* (1997), Puerto Rico, 1992–95	Oral cavity and pharynx		**Alcohol intake**	Patients (n = 137) with histologically confirmed oral cancer, and 146 controls ORs adjusted for sex, age, cigarette use, other tobacco use, fruit and vegetable intake
		ADH1C	Non-drinkers	
		**1/*1*	1.0	
		**1/*2*	0.9 (0.2–3.7)	
		**2/*2*	–	
			0–14 drinks/wk	
		**1/*1*	1.2 (0.3–5.2)	
		**1/*2*	0.9 (0.2–4.2)	
		**2/*2*	1.0 (0.1–12.2)	
			15–56 drinks/wk	
		**1/*1*	3.5 (0.8–15.8)	
		**1/*2*	4.1 (0.9–18.7)	
		**2/*2*	6.3 (1.1–36.8)	
			≥ 57 drinks/wk	
		**1/*1*	40.1 (5.4–296.0)	
		**1/*2*	7.0 (1.4–35.0)	
		**2/*2*	4.4 (0.6–33.3)	
Yokoyama *et al.* (1998), Japan, 1987–97	Oropharynx-larynx		11.1 (5.1–24.4)	Adjusted for age, drinking, smoking. Because the differences in odds ratio between the incident cases and the prevalent cases were small, the cases were combined.
Katoh *et al.* (1999), Japan, 1992–98	Oral squamous-cell carcinoma	Overall *ALDH2*	 1.2 (0.7–2.1)	Alcoholic beverage drinking not significantly associated with the risk for oral cancer. Adjusted for age, sex, smoking.

Table 2.75 (continued)

Reference, study location, period	Cancer and site	Genes involved	Relative risk (95% CI)[1]	Comments
Bouchardy *et al.* (2000), France, 1988–92	UADT squamous-cell carcinoma	***ADH1C***		Hospital-based case–control study. Patients with oral cavity or pharyngeal cancer (n = 121), laryngeal cancer (n = 129), and 172 controls. Patients had histologically confirmed primary SCC. All were regular smokers. Adjusted for age, sex, alcohol drinking and smoking.
	All oral cavity and pharynx	**2/*2*	1.0	
		**1/*2*	1.1 (0.6–2.2)	
		**1/*1*	0.7 (0.4–1.4)	
	Oral cavity	**2/*2*	1.0	
		**1/*2*	0.9 (0.4–2.0)	
		**1/*1*	0.8 (0.4–1.8)	
	Pharynx	**2/*2*	1.0	
		**1/*2*	1.7 (0.7–4.3)	
		**1/*1*	0.8 (0.3–2.1)	
	Larynx	**2/*2*	1.0	
		**1/*2*	0.7 (0.4–1.4)	
		**1/*1*	1.0 (0.5–1.8)	
Nomura *et al.* (2000)	Oral squamous cell carcinoma	***ALDH2***		Hospital-based case–control study. Habitual drinking increased the risk for oral cancer (odd ratio [95%CI], 3.9 [2.4–6.3])
		Habitual drinkers	2.9 (1.1–7.8)	
Olshan *et al.* (2001), North Carolina, USA, 1994–96	UADT squamous cell carcinoma	***ADH1C***	**Alcohol intake**	Patients (n = 182), and 202 controls. Patients had pathologically confirmed SCC of oral cavity, pharynx, larynx. Adjusted for tobacco use, age, sex and race
			Non-drinkers	
		**1/*1 + *1/*2*	1.1 (0.3–4.8)	
		**2/*2*	1.0	
			1–19 drinks/wk	
		**1/*1 + *1/*2*	1.4 (0.3–5.8)	
		**2/*2*	1.5 (0.3–8.6)	
			20–59 drinks/wk	
		**1/*1 *1/*2*	2.8 (0.6–12.5)	
		**2/*2*	2.4 (0.2–29.2)	
			≥ 60 drinks/wk	
		**1/*1 + *1/*2*	5.2 (0.9–27.7)	
		**2/*2*	– (no controls)	

Table 2.75 (continued)

Reference, study location, period	Cancer and site	Genes involved	Relative risk (95% CI)[1]	Comments
Schwartz *et al.* (2001), Washington, USA, 1985–89	Oral squamous cell carcinoma	***ADH1C***	**Alcohol intake**	Population-based case–control study. Oral SCC cases (n = 333) and 541 controls Distribution of *ADH1C* among cases and controls: *ADH1C *1/*1*: 32.7% vs 36.5% *ADH1C *1/*2*: 49.0% vs 43.1% *ADH1C *2/*2*: 18.3% vs 20.3% ORs adjusted for age, race and cigarette smoking
			< 1 drinks/wk	
		**1/*1*	2.1 (0.8–5.9)	
		**1/*2*	1.7 (0.6–4.7)	
		**2/*2*	1.0	
			1–14 drinks/wk	
		**1/*1*	2.0 (0.8–5.3)	
		**1/*2*	2.1 (0.8–5.3)	
		**2/*2*	1.4 (0.5–4.1)	
			15–28 drinks/wk	
		**1/*1*	3.4 (1.1–10.8)	
		**1/*2*	3.9 (1.3–11.8)	
		**2/*2*	3.4 (1.0–11.5)	
			≥ 29 drinks/wk	
		**1/*1*	6.1 (1.9–19.5)	
		**1/*2*	8.7 (2.9–26.1)	
		**2/*2*	10.0 (2.5–40.2)	
			Overall	
		**1/*1*	1.3 (0.8–2.0)	
		**1/*2*	1.3 (0.9–2.0)	
		**2/*2*	1.0	

Table 2.75 (continued)

Reference, study location, period	Cancer and site	Genes involved	Relative risk (95% CI)[1]	Comments
Sturgis *et al.* (2001), Houston, TX, USA, 1995–2000	Oral cavity, pharynx	***ADH1C***		Cases (n = 229), histologically confirmed SCC of the oral cavity and pharynx, matched by age, sex and smoking status with 575 controls. ORs controlled for age, sex, and smoking status.
			Never drinkers	
		**1/*1*	1.0	
		**1/*2*	1.5 (0.7–3.1)	
		**2/*2*	1.2 (0.5–3.0)	
			Former drinkers	
		**1/*1*	2.9 (1.3–6.3)	
		**1/*2*	2.1 (1.0–4.4)	
		**2/*2*	3.4 (1.3–8.6)	
			Current drinkers	
		**1/*1*	2.6 (1.2–5.5)	
		**1/*2*	2.4 (1.2–4.9)	
		**2/*2*	3.6 (1.6–8.1)	
			Total	
		**1/*1*	1.0	
		**1/*2*	1.0 (0.7–1.4)	
		**2/*2*	1.2 (0.8–1.9)	

Table 2.75 (continued)

Reference, study location, period	Cancer and site	Genes involved	Relative risk (95% CI)[1]	Comments
Yokoyama *et al.* (2001), Kanagawa, Japan, 1993–2000	Oropharyngo-laryngeal squamous-cell carcinoma	***ALDH2***		Adjusted for age, drinking, smoking, *ALDH2* and *ADH1B* genotypes
		*1/*1	1.00	
		*1/*2	18.52 (7.72–44.44)	
		ADH1B		
		*1/*2 +*2/*2	1.00	
		*1/*1	6.68 (2.81–15.90)	
	Oral cavity/ oropharyngeal squamous-cell carcinoma	***ALDH2***		
		*1/*1	1.00	
		*1/*2	20.83 (6.62–65.49)	
		ADH1B		
		*1/*2 +*2/*2	1.00	
		*1/*1	5.48 (1.77–16.96)	
	Epilaryngeal/ hypolaryngeal squamous-cell carcinoma	***ALDH2***		
		*1/*1	1.00	
		*1/*2	20.83 (6.62–65.49)	
		ADH1B		
		*1/*2 +*2/*2	1.00	
		*1/*1	5.48 (1.77–16.96)	
Yokoyama et al. (2002a), Tokyo, Chiba, Japan, 1998–99	Multiple primary cancer with oesophageal squamous-cell carcinoma	***ALDH2*** *2/*2 or *1/*2 vs *1/*1	5.3 (1.1–51.1)	107 patients. Multiple cancers included both multiorgan cancer and multiple intra-oesophageal squamous-cell carcinoma. Adjusted for age, sex, drinking, smoking.
	Multiorgan primary cancer with head and neck squamous-cell carcinoma	***ALDH2*** *2/*2 or *1/*2 vs *1/*1	7.4 (1.3–80.1)	
	Oesophageal SCC	***ALDH2***		Desophageal cancer, $n = 48$; oropharyngolaryngeal cancer, $n = 29$; combination, $n = 30$ ORs for multiple cancer, adjusted for age, drinking, smoking
		*1/*1	1.0	
		*1/*2	5.26 (1.08–51.1)	
	Oropharyngolaryngeal SCC (alone or in combination)	*2/*2	7.36 (1.29–80.7)	

Table 2.75 (continued)

Reference, study location, period	Cancer and site	Genes involved	Relative risk (95% CI)[1]	Comments
Zavras *et al.* (2002), Athens, Greece, 1995–98	Oral cavity	***ADH1C***	**Alcohol intake**	93 cases and 99 controls. Adjusted for sex, smoking and referring hospital.
			Non-drinker	
		**1/*1*	1.0	
		**1/*2*	0.7 (0.3–2.0)	
		**2/*2*	0.4 (0.1–1.8)	
			1–28 drinks/wk	
		**1/*1*	1.7 (0.6–4.6)	
		**1/*2*	1.0 (0.3–3.0)	
		**2/*2*	3.4 (0.7–17.0)	
			> 28–42 drinks/wk	
		**1/*1*	1.9 (0.3–11.6)	
		**1/*2*	2.2 (0.4–12.3)	
		**2/*2*	– (no subjects)	
			> 42 drinks/wk	
		**1/*1*	3.0 (0.6–15.8)	
		**1/*2*	11.2 (1.1–112.1)	
		**2/*2*	– (no subjects)	

Table 2.75 (continued)

Reference, study location, period	Cancer and site	Genes involved	Relative risk (95% CI)[1]	Comments
Risch *et al.* (2003), Heidelberg, Germany, 1998–2000	Larynx	***ADH1C***	Low intake	Cases (n = 257) of histologically confirmed SCC of the larynx and 251 age- and sex-matched controls. Adjusted for tobacco use. Alcohol intake (gram/d): low, 0–16.95; medium, > 16.95–50.16; high, > 50.16.
		**1/*2 +*2/*2*	1.00	
		**1/*1*	1.14 (0.5–2.6)	
			Medium intake	
		**1/*2 +*2/*2*	0.85 (0.4–2.0)	
		**1/*1*	1.21 (0.6–2.5)	
			High intake	
		**1/*2 +*2/*2*	1.46 (0.7–3.1)	
		**1/*1*	1.14 (0.6–2.3)	
		ADH1B	Low intake	
		**1/*1*	1.00	
		**1/*2*	0.63 (0.2–2.8)	
			Medium intake	
		**1/*1*	0.94 (0.5–1.7)	
		**1/*2*	1.85 (0.2–14.3)	
			High intake	
		**1/*1*	1.16 (0.7–2.0)	
		**1/*2*	0.89 (0.3–2.5)	
Nishimoto *et al.* (2004), Sao Paulo, Brazil, 1995–2001	UADT (oral cavity, oropharynx, hypopharynx and larynx) cancers	***ADH1C***		Adjusted for age, sex and cancer in first-degree relative
			Lifetime alcohol intake	
			< 100 kg	
		**1/*1 + *1/*2*	1.0	
		**2/*2*	3.8 (1.5–9.7)	
			≤ 100 kg	
		**1/*1 + *1/*2*	1.0	
		**2/*2*	0.5 (0.2–1.2)	
Muto *et al.* (2005), Kashiwa, Japan, Japan, 1999–2001	Squamous-cell carcinoma, oesophagus and head and neck (multiple cancers only)	***ALDH2***		Male and female patients, development of multiple carcinomas, adjusted for age and sex
		**1* allele	1.0	
		**2* allele	5.45 (2.37 – 12.56)	
		ADH1C		
		**1* allele	1.0	
		**2* allele	2.08 (0.86–4.99)	

Table 2.75 (continued)

Reference, study location, period	Cancer and site	Genes involved	Relative risk (95% CI)[1]	Comments
Wang *et al.* (2005), Iowa, USA, 1994–97 and 2000–02	UADT (oral cavity, oropharynx, hypopharynx and larynx) squamous cell carcinoma	***ADH1C*1/*2***		Adjusted for age and tobacco pack-yr. "Total" were additionally adjusted for alcohol drinking. Reference group for each drinking level, *2/*2
		Never drinker	0.95 (0.4–2.0)	
		1–21 drinks/wk	0.5 (0.2–1.1)	
		≥ 22 drinks/wk	0.9 (0.4–2.1)	
		Total	0.8 (0.5–1.2)	
		ADH1C*1/*1		
		Never drinker	0.8 (0.4–1.8)	
		1–21 drinks/wk	0.6 (0.3–1.2)	
		≥ 22 drinks/wk	0.8 (0.3–1.9)	
		Total	0.7 (0.4–1.1)	
Peters *et al.* (2005), USA, 1999–2003	UADT (oral cavity, oropharynx, hypopharynx and larynx) squamous cell carcinoma	***ADH1C*1/*1 + *1/*2***		Adjusted for age, gender, race and smoking. Cutpoint for heavy alcohol is > 30 drinks per wk. Test for heavy drinking x ADH interaction, $P = 0.05$. *ADH1B* and *ADH1C* showed linkage disequilibrium.
		Non drinker	1.0	
		Light drinker	0.9 (0.6–1.3)	
		Heavy drinker	2.3 (1.4–3.8)	
		ADH1C*2/*2		
		Non drinker	0.8 (0.4–1.8)	
		Light drinker	0.9 (0.6–1.6)	
		Heavy drinker	7.1 (2.3–22.0)	
Hashimoto *et al.* (2006), Yamaguchi, Japan, 2002–04	UADT (oral cavity, oropharynx, hypopharynx and larynx) cancer	Case versus controls *ALDH2*	Not significantly different	More cases < 66 yr were drinkers than cases ≥ 66 yr.
		Case drinkers *ALDH2*	Significantly increased ($P < 0.009$) in cases < 66 yr compared with cases ≥ 66 yr	
Homann *et al.* (2006), Germany, 1999–2003	All tumours	***ADH1C*1/*1*** in heavy drinkers		818 patients with alcohol-associated esophageal ($n = 123$), head and neck ($n = 84$) and hepatocellular cancer ($n = 86$) as well as in patients with alcoholic pancreatitis ($n = 117$), alcoholic liver cirrhosis ($n = 217$), combined liver cirrhosis and pancreatitis ($n = 17$) and in alcoholics without gastrointestinal organ damage ($n = 174$). [The reference group was not reported: *ADH1C*2/*2* or *ADH1C*2/*2 + ADH1C*1/*1*.]
		Malignant versus benign tumour	2.77 (1.89–4.07)	
		Malignant vs benign tumour	2.2 (1.11–4.36)	

Table 2.75 (continued)

Reference, study location, period	Cancer and site	Genes involved	Relative risk (95% CI)[1]	Comments
Hashibe *et al.* (2006), Czech Republic, Poland Romania, the Russian Federation, Slovakia, 2000–02	UADT (oral cavity, oropharynx, hypopharynx and larynx) squamous cell carcinoma	***ADH1B*** *R48H *1/*2 + *2/*2*		Reference groups were as following: *ADH1B R48H*, *1/*1; *ADH1C I350V*, Ile/Ile; *ADH1C* R272Q, Arg/Arg; *ALDH2* +82A > G, A/A; *ALDH2* +348C > T, T/T; *ALDH2* –261C > T, T/T. Frequency of alcohol use was as following: Never/light drinkers, ≤ 2 times/wk; Medium/heavy ≥ 3 times/wk. Adjusted for age, sex, country, and pack-yr of tobacco smoking. Overall results were additionally adjusted for yr of alcohol drinking. Results for oral, pharyngeal, laryngeal and oesophageal cancers were also presented in the article. When results were analysed by subsite, strong main effects for *ALDH2* variants were observed for squamous cell carcinoma of the oesophagus; among other subsites, only the association between *ALDH2 +82A > G* (A/G versus A/A) and pharyngeal cancer remained statistically significant.
		Overall	0.47 (0.32–0.70)	
		Never/light alcohol use	0.57 (0.36–0.91)	
		Medium/heavy use	0.36 (0.17–0.77)	
		P for interaction	0.33	
		ADH1C *I350V*		
		Val/Val (*1/*1)		
		Overall	1.38 (1.01–1.88)	
		Never/light alcohol use	1.48 (1.02–2.15)	
		Medium/heavy use	1.48 (0.80–2.73)	
		P for interaction	0.52	
		ADH1C *R272Q*		
		Gln/Gln (*1/*1)		
		Overall	1.49 (1.08–2.05)	
		Never/light alcohol use	1.69 (1.15–2.46)	
		Medium/heavy use	1.42 (0.76–2.66)	
		P for interaction	0.30	
		ALDH2 *+82A > G*		
		G/G		
		Overall	1.63 (0.94–2.82)	
		Never/light alcohol use	1.70 (0.88–3.29)	
		Medium/heavy use	4.38 (1.32–14.5)	
		P for interaction	0.02	
		ALDH2 *+348C > T*		
		C/C		
		Overall	1.63 (0.92–2.89)	
		Never/light alcohol use	1.28 (0.65–2.55)	
		Medium/heavy use	5.79 (1.49–22.5)	
		P for interaction	0.009	

Table 2.75 (continued)

Reference, study location, period	Cancer and site	Genes involved	Relative risk (95% CI)[1]	Comments
Hashibe *et al.* (2006) Contd.		***ALDH2** −261C > T*		
		C/C		
		Overall	1.66 (0.93–2.95)	
		Never/light alcohol use	1.29 (0.65–2.58)	
		Medium/heavy use	5.79 (1.49–22.5)	
		P for interaction	0.007	
Asakage *et al.* (2007), Tokyo, Chiba, Kanagawa, Osaka, Japan 2000–03	Oral and hypo- and oropharynx		**Alcohol intake**	Patients with oropaharyngeal or oral/oropharynx cancer ($n = 53$) and with hypopharyngeal cancer ($n = 43$) and 642 cancer-free men. Moderate-to-heavy drinkers: 22 g/drink, ≥ 9 drinks/wk. Adjusted for age, strong alcoholic beverage use, smoking, green-yellow vegetable use, and subcategory of alcohol drinking. When the linkage disequilibrium between *ADH1B* and *ADH1C* was taken into consideration, no relationship was found between *ADH1C* genotype and cancer risk
		ALDH2	Never or light	
		**1/1*	1	
		**1/2*	0.56 (0.20–1.59)	
			Moderate-heavy	
		**1/1*	2.29 (0.94–5.57)	
		**1/2*	8.26 (3.30–20.68)	
		ADH1B	Never or light	
		**1/*2 + *2/*2*	1	
		**1/*1*	1.00 (0.10–10.22)	
			Moderate-heavy	
		**1/*2 + *2/*2*	4.75 (2.44–9.23)	
		**1/*1*	26.40 (9.57–72.84)	
		ADH1C	Never or light	
		**1/*1*	1	
		**1/*2 + *2/*2*	2.34 (0.58–9.48)	
			Moderate-heavy	
		**1/*1*	5.64 (2.82–11.31)	
		**1/*2 + *2/*2*	17.93 (6.43–50.00)	

Table 2.75 (continued)

Reference, study location, period	Cancer and site	Genes involved	Relative risk (95% CI)[1]	Comments
Hiraki *et al.* (2007), Aichi, Japan, 2001–04	Squamous cell carcinoma of the lip and oral cavity, pharynx, larynx	***ADH1B*** *His/His*		Adjusted for age, sex and smoking. No cases of heavy drinkers in *ALDH2 Lys/Lys* carriers. *P* trend for heavy drinkers for ADH1B, 0.002 *P* trend for heavy drinkers for ALDH2, 0.003
		Never drinker	1.0	
		Moderate drinker	1.08 (0.66–1.77)	
		Heavy drinker	1.98 (1.20–3.30)	
		P for trend	0.005	
		ADH1B *His/Arg*		
		Never drinker	1.22 (0.63–2.35)	
		Moderate drinker	1.06 (0.58–1.94)	
		Heavy drinker	1.66 (1.51–4.71)	
		P for trend drinker	0.056	
		ADH2 *Arg/Arg*		
		Never drinker	0.50 (0.06–4.11)	
		Moderate drinker	2.46 (0.89–6.73)	
		Heavy drinker	9.52 (3.89–23.3)	
		P for trend	0.008	
		ALDH2 *Glu/Glu*		
		Never drinker	1.0	
		Moderate drinker	0.66 (0.32–1.36)	
		Heavy drinker	1.41 (0.69–2.89)	
		P for trend	0.058	
		ALDH2 *Glu/Lys*		
		Never drinker	0.75 (0.37–1.53)	
		Moderate drinker	1.05 (0.50–2.20)	
		Heavy drinker	3.13 (1.46–6.72)	
		P for trend	< 0.001	
		ALDH2 *Lys/Lys*		
		Never drinker	0.56 (0.22–1.43)	
		Moderate drinker	3.14 (0.45–21.6)	
		Heavy drinker	n/a	
		P for trend	0.44	

Table 2.75 (continued)

Reference, study location, period	Cancer and site	Genes involved	Relative risk (95% CI)[1]	Comments
Visapää *et al.* (2004), Mannheim and Heidelberg, Germany, study period NR	UADT	***ADH1C***		Hospital-based case–control study. Cases (*n* = 107) of UADT cancer (99 smokers) and 103 control patients (95 smokers) with liver cirrhosis (*n* = 39), alcoholic pancreatitis (*n* = 38) or without organ injury (*n* = 26), whose alcohol intake was similar to that of the UADT patients. Adjusted for alcohol use, smoking, age, sex
		**2/*2*	1.00	
		**1/*1*	1.69 (1.12–2.56)	
Hashibe *et al.* (2008), Multicenter study (see Comments), 2000–05		***ADH1B***		Pooled analysis of studies conducted in the Russian Federation (Moscow), Poland (Lodz), Romania (Bucharest), Czech Republic (Prague, Olomouc), Slovakia (Banska´ Bystrica), France (Paris), Greece (Athens), Italy (Aviano, Padova, Torino), Norway (Oslo), United Kingdom (Edinburgh, Manchester, Newcastle), Spain (Barcelona), Croatia (Zagreb), Cuba, Argentina (Buenos Aires) and Brazil (Goianna, Pelotas, Rio de Janeiro, Sao Paulo). Mostly Caucasian populations, men and women, adjusted for age, gender, centre, alcohol and tobacco use. The OR (95% CI) for codominant model was 0.59 (0.50–0.69) for all four cancer sites combined.
	Oral/pharynx	**1/*1*	1.00	
		**1/*2+*2/*2*	0.45 (0.35–0.57)	
	Larynx	**1/*1*	1.00	
		**1/*2+*2/*2*	0.71 (0.57–0.88)	
	Oral, pharynx, larynx, and oesophagus	**1/*1*	1.00	
		**1/*2+*2/*2*	0.56 (0.47–0.66)	
		ADH7		
	Oral/pharynx	**1/*1*	1.00	
		**1/*2+*2/*2*	0.70 (0.59–0.84)	
	Larynx	**1/*1*	1.00	
		**1/*2+*2/*2*	0.78 (0.59–0.93)	
	Oral, pharynx, larynx, and oesophagus	**1/*1*	1.00	
		**1/*2+*2/*2*	0.68 (0.60–0.78)	
Solomon *et al.* (2008), Tamil Nadu, India, study period NR	Squamous-cell carcinoma, oral cavity	***ADH1B***	Heavy drinkers	
		**2/*1 + *2/*2*	1.00	
		**1/*1*	1.62 (1.08–2.14)	
		ADH1C		
		**1/*1 +*1/*2*	1	
		**2/*2*	2.65 (1.78–3.53)	
Arndt *et al.* (2008), Poznan, Poland, 2006–08	Laryngeal cancer	***ADH1C***		No adjustment was reported
		**2/*2*	1.00	
		**1/*2*	1.40 (0.68–2.85)	
		**1/*1*	1.53 (0.67–3.46)	

Table 2.75 (continued)

Reference, study location, period	Cancer and site	Genes involved	Relative risk (95% CI)[1]	Comments
Yokoyama *et al.* (2008), Japan	Development to multiple carcinomas in oropharyngolarynx	***ALDH2***		Prospective part of study
		**1/*1*	1.0	
		**1/*2*	4.3 (1.4–12.9)	
		ADH1B2		
		**1/*2 + *2/*2*	1.0	
		**1/*1*	0.8 (0.3–2.0)	
Meta-analysis				
Boccia *et al.* (2009)	Head and neck cancer	*ALDH2*1/*1*	1.0	Meta-analysis of six Japanese studies.
		*ALDH2*1/*2*	1.83 (1.21–2.77)	[Reduced risk with *2/*2 likely due to markedly lower levels of alcohol consumption in *2/*2 versus *1/*1 homozygotes.]
		*ALDH2*2/*2*	0.53 (0.28–1.00)	

*ALDH2 *1* is more active, *ADH1B *1* is less active, and *ADH1C *1* is more active alleles than the other allele in the respective genes.
ALDH, aldehyde dehydrogenase; *ADH*, alcohol dehydrogenase; CI, confidence interval; mo, month or months; NR, not reported; SCC, squamous cell carcinoma; vs, versus; wk, week or weeks

(d) Hepatocellular cancer

Two European studies investigated associations between *ADH1C* genotype and hepatocellular carcinoma. Covolo *et al.* (2005) reported negative results and Homann *et al.* (2006) found a positive association between *ADH1C*1/*1* and the risk for alcohol-associated hepatocellular carcinoma (Table 2.76 on-line).

(e) Cancer of the lung

No significant effect of the *ADH1C* polymorphism on the risk for cancer of the lung was found in one Japanese study (Minegishi *et al.*, 2007) and one study in the USA (Freudenheim *et al.*, 2003) (Table 2.76 on-line).

(f) Cancer of the female breast

Six studies conducted in Germany and the USA investigated the relationship between *ADH1C* genotype and the risk for cancer of the female breast. Three of them showed an increased risk in *ADH1C*1/*1* versus *ADH1C*1/*2* and *ADH1C*2/*2* carriers (Freudenheim *et al.*, 1999; Coutelle *et al.*, 2004; Terry *et al.*, 2006; Table 2.76 on-line). In two studies the association was more pronounced among premenopausal women (Freudenheim *et al.*, 1999; Terry *et al.*, 2006). No significant associations between *ADH1C* polymorphism and the risk for cancer of the female breast were observed in the three other studies (Hines *et al.*, 2000; Terry *et al.*, 2007b; Visvanathan *et al.*, 2007) as well as in one large pooled study (Breast Cancer Association Consortium, 2006).

(g) Cancer of the urinary bladder

An increased risk for cancer of the urinary bladder cancer in moderate drinkers of the *ADH1C*1/*1* genotype was reported from a Dutch study (van Dijk *et al.*, 2001) (Table 2.76 on-line).

2.18.3 Other ADHs

In a pooled study a rare allele of *ADH7* was found to be significantly protective against UADT cancer (Hashibe *et al.*, 2008). The role of this allele in the functional activity of the enzyme is not yet known.

2.18.4 CYP2E1

CYP2E1 is induced by chronic alcoholic beverage consumption and in addition to ethanol oxidation it plays a role in the metabolic activation of many carcinogens, including *N*-nitrosamines, benzene and aniline. The *CYP2E1* gene contains several single nucleotide polymorphisms, including C1053T (*CYP2E1*5*; also referred to as *Rsa*I polymorphism), G1293A (*CYP2E1*5*; also referred to as *Pst*I polymorphism), T7632TA (*CYP2E1*6*; also referred to as *Dra*I polymorphism) and G71T (*CYP2E1*7*).

(a) Cancer of the oesophagus

A *CYP2E1*5B* (earlier denoted **c2*; **1A* is the wild-type allele, earlier denoted **c1*) allele-associated risk of oesophageal cancer has been reported from one study of East-Asians (Tsutsumi *et al.*, 1993). Opposite results, with the **5B* allele decreasing the risk for oesophageal cancer, have been observed in four studies of East-Asians (Tan *et al.*, 2000; Lu *et al.*, 2005; Guo *et al.*, 2008; Qin *et al.*, 2008). The absence of significant results were reported from seven studies of East-Asians (Morita *et al.*, 1997; Hori *et al.*, 1997; Tanabe *et al.*, 1999; Chao *et al.*, 2000; Gao *et al.*, 2002; Yang *et al.*, 2005; Wang *et al.*, 2006b), and studies of Europeans (Lucas *et al.*, 1996), South Africans (Li *et al.*, 2005) and Brazilians (Rossini *et al.*, 2007) (Table 2.77 available at http://monographs.iarc.fr/ENG/Monographs/vol100E/100E-06-Table2.77.pdf).

(b) Other upper aerodigestive tract cancers combined

In seven studies from East-Asia, India, Brazil and Europe an increased risk for other upper aerodigestive tract cancer cancers in carriers of the *CYP2E1*5B* allele was found (Hildesheim *et al.*, 1997; Hung *et al.*, 1997; Bouchardy *et al.*, 2000; Gattás *et al.*, 2006; Sugimura *et al.*, 2006; Olivieri *et al.*, 2009; Ruwali *et al.*, 2009). In contrast, an inverse association between the **5B* allele and oral cancer has been reported in the USA (Liu *et al.*, 2001). No significant associations were reported from eight European studies (Jahnke *et al.*, 1996; Lucas *et al.*, 1996; González *et al.*, 1998; Matthias *et al.*, 1998; Zavras *et al.*, 2002; Boccia *et al.*, 2008), three Japanese studies (Katoh *et al.*, 1999; Morita *et al.*, 1999; Tanabe *et al.*, 1999), and two studies from USA (Buch *et al.*, 2008) and India (Soya *et al.*, 2008).

(c) Cancers of the stomach and colorectum

In three studies, two of Chinese (Cai *et al.*, 2001; Wu *et al.*, 2002) and one of Caucasians (Boccia *et al.*, 2007), increased risk for cancer of the stomach by polymorphic alleles of *CYP2E1* was found. Opposite results with the **5B* allele decreasing risk of cancer of the stomach were reported from one study from Brazil (Nishimoto *et al.*, 2000). Lack of significant associations between the **5B* allele and risk of cancer of the stomach has been reported from four studies of East-Asian populations (Kato *et al.*, 1995, 1997; Gao *et al.*, 2002; Nan *et al.*, 2005).

With regard to cancer of the colorectum, in two studies, one of Hungarians (Kiss *et al.*, 2000) and one study of Chinese (Gao *et al.*, 2007), an increased risk for cancer of the colorectum was demonstrated in carriers of the *CYP2E1*5B* allele. From one study in Hawaii, USA (Le Marchand *et al.*, 2002), and one study in Japan (Morita *et al.*, 2009) an increased risk of cancer of the colorectum with 5′ 96-bp insertion variant in *CYP2E1* was reported. In three other studies, one from China (Fan *et al.*, 2007) and two from Europe (Landi *et al.*, 2005; van der Logt *et al.*, 2006), significant associations between *CYP2E1* polymorphism and cancer of the colorectum were not reported. In one study in Japan a decreased risk for rectal cancer in carriers of the **5B* allele was found (Morita *et al.*, 2009).

(d) Hepatocellular cancer

A **5B* allele-associated increased risk for hepatocellular carcinoma was reported from three studies of Japanese and European populations (Ladero *et al.*, 1996; Koide *et al.*, 2000; Munaka *et al.*, 2003). No significant association was observed in four other East Asian populations (Lee *et al.*, 1997; Wong *et al.*, 2000; Yu *et al.*, 2002; Kato *et al.*, 2003). A decreased risk with **5B* allele was reported from a Taiwan, China study (Yu *et al.*, 1995).

(e) Cancer of the lung

An increased risk for cancer of the lung associated with the *CYP2E1*5B* allele was found in one Japanese study (Oyama *et al.*, 1997) and one study of mainly Caucasians (el-Zein *et al.*, 1997c). A similar association was reported in another Japanese study (Minegishi *et al.*, 2007), but the genotype distribution was not in Hardy–Weinberg equilibrium in the control population [so the finding of an association with cancer of the lung is most likely a false-positive result]. Opposite results with the **5B* allele decreasing risk for cancer of the lung have been obtained in studies from Sweden, USA and Republic of Korea (Persson, *et al.*, 1993; Wu *et al.*, 1997; Le Marchand *et al.*, 1998; Eom *et al.*, 2009). In eight studies, two of East Asians (Watanabe *et al.*, 1995; Persson *et al.*, 1999), four of mixed South and North American populations (Kato *et al.*, 1994; Hamada *et al.*, 1995; London *et al.*, 1996; Quiñones *et al.*, 2001), and one of Finns (Hirvonen *et al.*, 1993), no significant associations were observed.

(f) Cancer of the breast

In one Korean study a non-significant increased risk for cancer of the breast associated with the **5B/*5B* genotype was found (Choi *et al.*, 2003), while in a study from Taiwan, China, an inverse association between the **5B/*5B* genotype and breast cancer risk was found (Wu *et al.*, 2006).

(g) Other cancers

For cancer of the urinary bladder no significant associations to the **5B* allele were observed in an Egyptian (Anwar *et al.*, 1996) and a German population (Brockmöller *et al.*, 1996). Also for cancer of the kidney (renal cell) and urothelial cancer no significant associations were found in one study from Germany (Farker *et al.*, 1998a). Three studies on East-Asian populations demonstrated a decreased risk for cancer of the prostate associated with the **5B* allele (Murata *et al.*, 2001; Yang *et al.*, 2006a; Yang *et al.*, 2009). No association between polymorphism in *CYP2E1* and risk of cancer of the pancreas was observed in an East-Asian population (Lee *et al.* 2007).

2.18.5 ALDH2

The variant allele *2 that encodes an inactive subunit of *ALDH2* is prevalent among East Asians (28–45%; Goedde *et al.*, 1992), but is rare in most other populations. Individuals with inactive *ALDH2* generally abstain from heavy alcohol drinking due to subsequent acetaldehydaemia and alcoholic flushing responses. Most homozygotes for inactive *ALDH2*2/*2* are non-drinkers or occasional drinkers, but substantial percentages of East Asians who are habitual drinkers, including alcoholics, are heterozygous *ALDH2*1/*2*.

(a) Cancer of the oesophagus

The *ALDH2*2* allele has been found to be a risk factor for oesophageal cancer in 19 East-Asian studies (Hori *et al.*, 1997; Yokoyama *et al.*, 1998, 2001, 2002, 2006a, b; Tanabe *et al.*, 1999; Chao *et al.*, 2000; Matsuo *et al.*, 2001b; Boonyaphiphat *et al.*, 2002; Itoga *et al.*, 2002; Watanabe *et al.*, 2002; Yokoyama *et al.*, 2002; Yang *et al.*, 2005, 2007; Cai *et al.*, 2006; Guo *et al.*, 2008; Lee *et al.*, 2008b; Cui *et al.*, 2009; Ding *et al.*, 2009; Tables 2.73, 2.74). The magnitude of the *ALDH2*-associated risk depends on the extent of the association between oesophageal cancer and alcohol consumption. The risk was observed in light-to-moderate drinkers as well as heavy drinkers, but was higher among heavier drinkers including alcoholics than the other drinkers. The findings were also supported by a meta-analysis (Lewis & Smith, 2005). In two large case–control studies in Taiwan, China (Lee *et al.*, 2009) and Japan (Cui *et al.*, 2009) heterozygous *ALDH2* increased the oesophageal cancer risk more prominently in younger populations. Heterozygous *ALDH2* has been consistently reported to be a strong risk factor for multiple cancers in Japanese patients with oesophageal cancer (Yokoyama *et al.*, 2001, 2002; Muto *et al.*, 2005).

Case–control studies in high-risk rural regions in Mainland China showed modest-positive associations (Cai *et al.*, 2006; Yang *et al.*, 2007; Ding *et al.*, 2009; Guo *et al.*, 2008) between heterozygous *ALDH2* and oesophageal cancer risk. In these studies, the risks were more distinct where the impact of alcohol consumption on oesophageal cancer was more distinct and when only male populations were evaluated. Tian *et al.* (1998) reported no significant association between *ALDH2* polymorphism and oesophageal cancer, but this study included only cases of oesophageal squamous carcinoma and the *ALDH2* gene frequencies were compared just to other published data. In addition to the data on East-Asian populations, the association between oesophageal cancer and the *ALDH2*2* allele has been found in a study in South Africa (Li *et al.*, 2008a). In addition, the +82A > G, +348C > T and −261C > T variants of *ALDH2* (without known functional actions) have been related to oesophageal cancer in a large pooled European study (Hashibe *et al.*, 2006).

(b) Other upper aerodigestive tract cancer

In 10 Japanese studies, the *ALDH2*2* allele has been shown to be a risk factor for upper aerodigestive tract cancer (Yokoyama *et al.*, 1998, 2001, 2002, 2006b, 2008; Nomura *et al.*, 2000; Muto *et al.*, 2005; Hashimoto *et al.*, 2006; Asakage *et al.*, 2007; Hiraki *et al.*, 2007; Table 2.75). In one Japanese study significant associations between the **2* allele and oral cancer were not found (Katoh *et al.*, 1999); in this study a significant association between risk of oral cancer and consumption of alcoholic beverages was not found either. A meta-analysis of these Japanese studies showed that heterozygous *ALDH2* increased upper aerodigestive tract cancer risks more strongly in heavy drinkers including alcoholics than the other drinkers (Boccia *et al.*, 2009). In one Japanese study a higher frequency of heterozygous *ALDH2* in younger drinkers with upper aerodigestive tract cancer was found (Hashimoto *et al.*, 2006). Heterozygous *ALDH2* has been reported to be a strong risk factor for multiple cancers in Japanese patients with upper aerodigestive tract cancers (Yokoyama *et al.*, 2001, 2002, 2008; Muto *et al.*, 2005). The other *ALDH2* variants (reported by Hashibe *et al.*, 2006) did not significantly affect the risk of oral and other upper aerodigestive tract cancers (excluding oesophageal cancer).

(c) Cancers of the stomach, colorectum and pancreas

In two Japanese studies an increased risk for cancer of the stomach by the *ALDH2*2* allele has been reported (Yokoyama *et al.*, 1998, 2007b; Table 2.76 on-line). Such an association was reported from another Japanese study (Yokoyama *et al.*, 2001) when all gastric cancer cases, including gastric cancer alone or combined with upper aerodigestive tract cancers were considered. However, when only cases of cancer of the stomach alone were included in the analyses, there was no association with *ALDH2*. In a study of Polish consumers of alcoholic beverages an increased risk for cancer of the stomach by the *ALDH2 +82A > G* alleles was found (Zhang *et al.*, 2007b). No significant associations with the **2* allele were reported from a study from Republic of Korea (Nan *et al.*, 2005).

Increased risks of colon and/or rectal cancer have been associated with the **2* allele in three East-Asian studies (Yokoyama *et al.*, 1998; Murata *et al.*, 1999; Matsuo *et al.*, 2002). The **2* allele has also been associated with lower risk in one Chinese (Gao *et al.*, 2008) and a Japanese (Yin *et al.*, 2007) study. No significant differences were seen in four Japanese studies (Takeshita *et al.*, 2000a; Hirose *et al.*, 2005; Otani *et al.*, 2005; Matsuo *et al.*, 2006a).

In one of two Japanese studies Kanda *et al.* (2009) reported increased risk for the *ALDH2*2* allele for cancer of the pancreas; no significant associations were found by Miyasaka *et al.* (2005).

(d) Hepatocellular cancer

In four of 11 Japanese and Chinese studies an increased risk for hepatocellular carcinoma in carriers of the *ALDH2*2* allele has been found (Kato *et al.*, 2003; Munaka *et al.*, 2003; Sakamoto *et al.*, 2006; Ding *et al.*, 2008) (Table 2.76 on-line). Four Japanese (Shibata *et al.*, 1998; Yokoyama *et al.*, 1998; Koide *et al.*, 2000; Takeshita *et al.*, 2000b) and one Chinese (Yu *et al.*, 2002) study reported no significant associations between *ALDH2* polymorphism and hepatocellular cancer.

(e) Cancer of the lung

An increased risk for lung cancer associated with *ALDH2*2* alleles has been observed in three studies, two from Japan (Yokoyama *et al.*, 1998; Minegishi *et al.*, 2007) and one from Republic of Korea (Eom *et al.*, 2009) (Table 2.76 on-line).

(f) Cancer of the female breast

No significant association between *ALDH2* polymorphism and risk of cancer of the breast has been observed in a Korean (Choi *et al.*, 2003) and a Spanish population (Ribas *et al.*, 2008) (Table 2.76 on-line).

2.19 Synthesis

2.19.1 Oral cavity and pharynx

Data published since the previous *IARC monograph* (IARC, 2010) support the conclusion that consumption of alcoholic beverages is causally related to cancer of the oral cavity and pharynx. Increasing alcohol consumption increases risk in a dose-dependent manner, does not vary materially by beverage type or sex and the association is not due to chance, bias or confounding.

2.19.2 Larynx

Data published since the previous *IARC Monograph* (IARC, 2010) supports the conclusion that consumption of alcoholic beverages is causally related to cancer of the larynx. Increasing alcohol consumption increases risk in a dose-dependent manner, does not vary materially by beverage type or sex, and chance, bias and confounding can be ruled out.

2.19.3 Oesophagus

Data published since the previous *IARC Monograph* (IARC, 2010) supports the conclusion that consumption of alcoholic beverages is causally related to squamous cell carcinoma of the oesophagus. Increasing alcohol consumption increases risk in a dose-dependent manner, does not vary materially by beverage type or sex, and chance, bias and confounding can be ruled out. There is now a substantial body of evidence that alcoholic beverage consumption is not associated with adenocarcinoma of the oesophagus.

2.19.4 Upper aerodigestive tract combined

There is evidence that consumption of alcoholic beverages is causally related to cancer of the upper aerodigestive tract, as it is for cancer of the oral cavity and pharynx, larynx and oesophagus separately. Increasing alcohol consumption increases risk in a dose-dependent manner, does not vary materially by beverage type or sex and chance, bias and confounding can be ruled out.

2.19.5 Colon and rectum

Data published since the previous *IARC Monograph* (IARC, 2010) supports the conclusion that consumption of alcoholic beverages is causally related to cancer of the colorectum. Most of the evidence suggests that consumption of alcoholic beverages is positively associated with both cancer of the colon and cancer of the rectum, and is similar in men and women, although the data are not entirely consistent. Similarly, there is some evidence that risk may only be increased at relatively high levels of intake (i.e. > 30 g/d). There is consistent evidence that risk does not differ by beverage type; whether the risk associated with consumption of alcoholic beverages differs by smoking status or intake of dietary folate is inconsistent.

2.19.6 Liver

Data published since the previous IARC *Monograph* (IARC, 2010) support the previous conclusion that the consumption of alcoholic beverages is causally related to hepatocellular carcinoma. It is not possible to draw any conclusion concerning consumption of alcoholic beverages and risk of cholangiocarcinoma.

2.19.7 Stomach

Results on the association between consumption of alcoholic beverages and cancer of the stomach are difficult to interpret due to the lack of information on important confounders, such as possible dietary deficiencies.

2.19.8 Pancreas

There is accumulating evidence that high alcohol intake (i.e. ≥ 30 g/d) is associated with a small increased risk for cancer of the pancreas. However, the possibility that residual confounding by smoking may partly explain this association cannot be excluded. Whether the risk associated with heavy alcohol consumption differs by beverage type, smoking status or body mass index is unclear.

2.19.9 Lung

Available data are inadequate to determine a causal association between the consumption of alcoholic beverages and cancer of the lung. Although adjustment for tobacco smoking was attempted in many studies, residual confounding cannot be excluded for those analyses that found a positive association with consumption of alcoholic beverages. For those studies that attempted to evaluate risk for cancer of the lung from the consumption of alcoholic beverages in non-smokers, small numbers of cases, or few subjects with high consumption of alcoholic beverages, precluded detection of an association.

2.19.10 Breast

Occurrence of cancer of the female breast is causally associated with the consumption of alcoholic beverages. Cancer risk increases proportionately according to the amount of alcohol consumed, with an increase in risk of up to 12% for each additional drink consumed regularly each day (equivalent to about 10 g/d). The risk does not appear to vary significantly by beverage type or smoking status. It remains unclear whether the association of alcohol beverage consumption with risk for cancer of the female breast varies by use of hormone-replacement therapy or by tumour receptor status.

The evidence that alcoholic beverage consumption is associated with cancer of the male breast remains inconsistent.

2.19.11 Uterine cervix

The weak associations noted in some studies for consumption of alcoholic beverages and risk of cancer of the uterine cervix are sufficient to draw any conclusion on causality. Few studies were able to adjust for the known risk factors for the disease.

2.19.12 Endometrium

The evidence for an association between consumption of alcoholic beverages and risk for cancer of the endometrium is inconsistent. The majority of studies show no association; the few that show an inverse association were not able to adjust for tobacco smoking.

Among both the cohort and case–control studies, there was no consistent evidence of an interaction between consumption of alcoholic beverages and different variables known or suspected to be associated with cancer of the endometrium, such as use of hormone replacement therapy, body size, age, tobacco smoking, parity, education, physical activity, energy intake and other dietary aspects, oral contraceptive use or menopausal status.

2.19.13 Ovary

There is little evidence for an association between consumption of alcoholic beverages and risk for cancer of the ovary. The majority of studies show no association.

2.19.14 Prostate

There is little evidence for an association between consumption of alcoholic beverages and risk of cancer of the prostate. Although in some studies positive associations were found for advanced disease, the majority of studies show no association.

2.19.15 Kidney

There is no causal association between consumption of alcoholic beverages and cancer of the kidney.

2.19.16 Urinary bladder

Overall, the studies on cancer of the urinary bladder suggest no association with consumption of alcoholic beverages.

2.19.17 Haematopoietic malignancies

In cohort studies in the general population, most forms of lymphomas and leukaemias have shown no or inverse associations with consumption of alcoholic beverages; studies that assessed risk for non-Hodgkin lymphoma, the form of lymphomas and leukaemias most studied, generally found an inverse association.

There were consistent inverse associations in case–control studies investigating ever alcohol consumption and risk for Hodgkin lymphoma, with no significant differences between alcoholic beverage types. A large pooled study observed a lower risk of several histological subtypes, such as Burkitt, B-cell, follicular and T-cell lymphomas among ever drinkers.

No clear patterns of association between consumption of alcoholic beverages and risk of all leukaemias combined were shown in case–control studies. Two studies indicated increased risk of acute lymphocytic leukaemia with any or heavy alcohol drinking, and also increased risk of chronic lymphocytic leukaemia among wine drinkers, but there was no consistent pattern of association for different types of leukaemias. In most studies on multiple myeloma no consistent results were observed.

2.19.18 Other cancers

It is not possible to draw any conclusions regarding the association between intake of alcoholic beverages and risk for cancers of the brain and thyroid, melanoma and non-melanoma skin cancers.

2.19.19 Parental exposure and childhood cancers

Results for the association between maternal consumption of alcohol before or during pregnancy and risk of acute lymphocytic leukaemia, acute lymphocytic leukaemia and acute leukaemia in the offspring are inconsistent.

2.19.20 Polymorphisms and genetic susceptibility

(a) ADH1B

The available genetic epidemiological data suggest a positive association between *ADH1B*1/*1* polymorphism and cancer of the oesophagus, and cancers of the upper aerodigestive tract combined. The relationship between *ADH1B* genotype and cancer in other organs is inconclusive because of the small number of studies.

(b) ADH1C

The relationship between *ADH1C* genotype and cancer at any site is inconclusive, primarily because of the small number of studies.

(c) ALDH2

The available genetic epidemiological data provides ample evidence for a strong contribution of heterozygous *ALDH2* genotype to the development of alcohol-related cancer in the oesophagus and in the upper aerodigestive tract. While it is often difficult to differentiate clearly between exact locations of tumours in the oropharyngolaryngeal area based on the available published data, there is also strong evidence for a contribution of heterozygous *ALDH2* genotype to the development of alcohol-related cancer in the oropharyngolarynx as a whole, and especially in the hypopharynx. However, the epidemiological studies provide suggestive but inconclusive data for some association of heterozygous *ALDH2* genotype and alcohol-related cancers in the individual oropharyngolaryngeal subsites of the oral cavity, oropharynx and larynx.

The evidence for cancers of the stomach, colorectum, pancreas, liver, breast, bladder and prostate is inconclusive.

3. Cancer in Experimental Animals

Consumption of alcoholic beverages was evaluated in 2007 (IARC, 2010). The studies described below were considered; no new studies have been published since.

An issue in evaluating bioassays of ethanol is the nutritive value of this substance, which results in a hyperalimentation of alcohol-fed animals. For rigorous evaluation of the carcinogenicity of alcohol by ingestion in experimental animals, controls must be pair fed to equalize caloric intake.

3.1 Oral administration of ethanol in the drinking-water

Study design and results of studies of oral administration of ethanol in drinking-water are presented in Table 3.1.

3.1.1 Rat

Eight groups of 50 male and 50 female Sprague-Dawley rats received either 1% or 3% ethanol or an equicaloric amount of glucose in a semisynthetic liquid diet for 120 weeks (Holmberg & Ekström, 1995). Males were given 70 mL/day and females 60 mL/day of liquid diet. No tumours developed in male rats. There was a significant ($P < 0.05$) increase in pituitary tumours [not further specified] among 3% ethyl alcohol-treated females (80%) than among high-dose glucose-treated animals (58%). There was also an increase ($P < 0.05$) in mammary gland fibromas, fibroadenomas and adenomas combined, in the 1% ethyl alcohol-treated females compared with the low-dose glucose animals [no incidence provided].

Male Sprague-Dawley rats administered 5% ethanol in the drinking-water for 130 weeks developed hepatocellular carcinomas (8/79 versus 1/80 control rats). Additionally, the authors reported an increase in the incidence of hyperplastic liver nodules in the ethanol group. Pancreatic adenomas, adrenal gland adenomas, and pituitary adenomas occurred in the ethanol group in 18% (14/79), 18% (14/79), and 33% (26/79) of the animals, respectively. No tumours of the pancreas or adrenal gland were found in control rats. Pituitary adenomas were found in 8/80 control rats (Radike *et al.*, 1981).

In other experiments, the chronic administration of 5% or 10% ethanol had no effect on liver carcinogenesis of Wistar or F344 rats (Shibayama *et al.*, 1993; Yamagiwa *et al.*, 1994; Wanibuchi *et al.*, 2006).

Sprague-Dawley rats and their offspring received either 10% ethanol or no ethanol in the drinking-water *ad libitum* starting at 39 weeks of age, 7 days before mating or from embryo life (offspring) until death. The intake of fluid was lower in the treated group but no difference in body weight was noted. An increased incidence of total malignant tumours was noted in female

Table 3.1 Carcinogenicity studies on ethyl alcohol administered in the drinking-water to experimental animals

Species, strain (sex) Duration Reference	Dosing regimen, Animals/group at start	Incidence of tumours		Significance	Comments
Rat, Sprague-Dawley (M) 130 wk Radike *et al.* (1981)	5% 7 d/wk 79 animals 80 animals (controls)	Liver	Carcinoma Control (1/80) 5% Ethanol (8/79)	[$P < 0.05$]	
		Pituitary gland	Adenoma Control (8/80) 5% Ethanol (26/79)	[$P < 0.001$]	
		Adrenal gland	Adenoma Control (0/80) 5% Ethanol (14/79)	[$P < 0.0001$]	
		Pancreas	Adenoma Control (0/80) 5% Ethanol (14/79)	[$P < 0.0001$]	
		Testes	Seminoma Control (0/80) 5% Ethanol (3/79)	[NS]	
Rat, Sprague-Dawley (M) 140 wk Soffritti *et al.* (2002a)	10% 7 d/wk 110 animals 110 animals (controls)	Forestomach	Benign Control (1/110) 10% Ethanol (8/110)	[$P < 0.01$]	Animals were breeder
			Benign and malignant Control (1/110) 10% Ethanol (10/110)	[$P < 0.01$]	
		Head and other sites	Osteosarcoma Control (1/110) 10% Ethanol (12/110)	[$P = 0.0042$]	
		Oral cavity, lips and tongue	Carcinoma Control (3/110) 10% Ethanol (15/110)	$P < 0.01$	
		Testes	Interstitial cell adenoma Control (9/110) 10% Ethanol (23/110)	[$P = 0.013$]	
Rat, Sprague-Dawley (F) 140 wk Soffritti *et al.* (2002a)	10% 7 d/wk 110 animals 110 animals (controls)	Lymphomas and leukaemias	Control (17/110) 10% Ethanol (46/110)	[$P < 0.0001$]	
		Oral cavity, lips and tongue	Carcinoma Control (2/110) 10% Ethanol (12/110)	$P < 0.05$	

Table 3.1 (continued)

Species, strain (sex) Duration Reference	Dosing regimen, Animals/group at start	Incidence of tumours		Significance	Comments
Rat, Sprague-Dawley (M) 179 wk Soffritti *et al.* (2002a)	10% 7 d/wk 30 animals 49 animals (controls)	Oral cavity, lips and tongue	Carcinoma Control (2/49) 10% Ethanol (10/30)	$P < 0.01$	Animals were offspring
Rat, Sprague-Dawley (F) 179 wk Soffritti *et al.* (2002a)	10% 7 d/wk 39 animals/group 55 animals (controls)	Oral cavity, lips and tongue	Carcinoma Control (3/55) 10% Ethanol (16/39)	$P < 0.01$	Animals were offspring
Mouse B6C3F1 (M) 104 wk Beland *et al.* (2005)	0 (control), 2.5%, 5% 7 d/wk 48 animals/group	Liver	Adenoma or Carcinoma Control (12/46) 2.5% Ethanol (16/47) 5% Ethanol (25/48)	$P < 0.05$ dose-related trend, $P = 0.056$ (5% ethanol)	
			Adenoma Control (7/46) 2.5% Ethanol (12/47) 5% Ethanol (19/48)	$P < 0.05$ dose-related trend, $P < 0.05$ (5% Ethanol)	
Mouse, ICR (F) 106 wk Watabiki *et al.* (2000)	10–15% 7 d/wk 20 animals/group	Mammary gland	Adenocarcinoma Control (0/20) 10–15% Ethanol (9/20)	[$P = 0.012$]	
Mouse, C57/ BL6APCmin (M) 10 wk Roy *et al.* (2002)	15% alternating with 20% every other d 12 animals/group	Intestine	Adenoma Tumor multiplicity Control (26.8) 15–20% Ethanol (36.9)	$P < 0.05$	

d, day or days; F, female; M, male; NS, not significant; wk, week or weeks breeders and male offspring. This was due to a significant increase in the incidence of head and neck carcinomas (oral cavity, lips, tongue) in male and female breeders and male and female offspring; benign and combined benign and malignant tumours of the forestomach in male breeders; and combined lymphomas and leukemias in female breeders. Increases in the incidence of interstitial-cell adenomas of the testis and osteosarcomas of the head and other sites were also observed in male breeders (Soffritti *et al.*, 2002a). [The Working Group noted that some statements reporting increased incidence were not supported by statistical analyses performed by the Working Group].

3.1.2 Mouse

B6C3F$_1$ male and female mice received 2.5% or 5% of ethanol in drinking-water for 104 weeks. No significant difference in tumour incidence at any site was observed in females. There was a significant dose-related trend for the incidence of hepatocellular adenomas, and hepatocellular adenomas and carcinomas combined in male mice. The administration of 5% ethanol resulted in an increase in the incidence of hepatocellular adenomas ($P < 0.05$) and a marginal increase ($P = 0.056$) in the incidence of hepatocellular adenomas and carcinomas combined in male mice (NTP, 2004; Beland *et al.*, 2005).

ICR female mice received 10% ethanol in the drinking-water for 2 months and then 15% ethanol in the drinking-water for 23 months. Mammary gland tumours (papillary or medullary adenocarcinomas) were found in 9/20 mice given ethanol in drinking-water compared with 0/20 control mice [$P = 0.012$] (Watabiki *et al.*, 2000).

C57BL/6^{APCmin} male mice received ethanol in drinking-water at doses between 15 and 20% daily for 10 weeks. This treatment increased intestinal adenoma multiplicity (Roy *et al.*, 2002).

3.2 Oral administration of acetaldehyde in drinking-water

See Table 3.2.

Acetaldehyde was evaluated in 1984 (IARC, 1985), 1998 (IARC, 1999), and 2007 (IARC, 2010).

3.2.1 Rat

Sprague-Dawley male and female rats received acetaldehyde in the drinking-water at doses of 50, 250, 500, 1500 and 2500 mg/L for 161 weeks. With the exception of male rats treated with 1500 mg/L, the administration of acetaldehyde to male Sprague-Dawley rats resulted in a marginal dose-dependent increase in incidence of pancreatic islet cell adenomas. The incidence of pancreatic islet cell adenoma was significantly higher (18%; 9/50) in male rats exposed to the high dose of acetaldehyde (2500 mg/L) compared to 4% (2/50) in the control group. Acetaldehyde caused an increased incidence of head osteosarcomas in the 50 and 2500 mg/L groups. Additionally, ingestion of acetaldehyde resulted in a higher incidence of lymphomas and leukemias in male rats exposed to acetaldehyde at doses of 50 mg/L and 1500 mg/L. Acetaldehyde also caused an increase in lymphomas and leukemias in female rats, 16% in rats exposed to 250 mg/mL compared to 4% in control animals. A higher incidence of mammary gland adenocarcinomas and uterine adenocarcinomas was found in the groups of females exposed to 500 mg/L and 250 mg/L, respectively (Soffritti *et al.*, 2002b). [The Working Group noted that a variety of tumours were increased. However, no obvious dose–response relationship was observed.]

3.3 Co-carcinogenicity studies on alcohol administered in drinking-water

A comprehensive analysis of the studies on the co-carcinogenicity of ethanol was presented in the previous *IARC Monograph* (IARC, 2010). Simultaneous administration of alcohol with known carcinogens enhanced tumour development. A selection of positive studies is summarized below.

3.3.1 Rat

Chronic administration of ethanol potentiates the development of tumours in experimental animals induced by chemical agents.

Two groups of 80 Sprague-Dawley rats received either vinyl chloride or vinyl chloride and 5% ethanol in the drinking-water for 130 weeks. Increases in the incidence of liver carcinomas and liver angiosarcomas were observed in the vinyl chloride and ethanol group compared to the vinyl chloride treated control rats. In rats exposed to vinyl chloride and ethanol 15% developed pancreatic adenomas, whereas no tumours were found in control rats (Radike *et al.*, 1981).

Fischer 344/DuCrj rats were fed 200 ppm 2-amino-3,8-dimethylimidazo[4,5]quinoxaline (MeIQx). After 8 weeks, rats were subdivided to receive either drinking-water or 0.1, 0.3, 1, 3, or 10% ethanol in the drinking-water. In rats administered MeIQx in the diet, the incidence of hepatocellular adenoma, carcinoma and adenoma plus carcinoma was increased by ethanol consumption in a dose-dependent manner ($P < 0.001$) (Kushida *et al.*, 2005).

Chronic ethanol administration in drinking-water to male F344 rats for 55 weeks after treatment with the chemical carcinogens *N′*-nitrosonornicotine (NNN) or 4-(methylnitrosoamino)-1-(3-pyridyl)-1-butanone (NNK) increased the incidence of tumours of the oesophagus, oral cavity and lungs. NNK also induced liver tumours, which were significantly increased by ethanol ingestion (Nachiappan *et al.*, 1994). Similarly, administration of 5% ethanol to male Wistar rats enhanced the oesophageal tumourigenesis induced by *N*-nitrosomethylbenzylamine (Tsutsumi *et al.*, 2006). The enhancing effect of ethanol on *N*-nitrosodiethylamine (NDEA)-induced oesophageal carcinogenesis was also observed in male Fischer 344 rats. Two groups of Fischer 344 rats received either 50 ppm NDEA dissolved in 10% ethanol or 50 ppm NDEA solution in water, respectively, for 8 weeks. Rats were maintained on tap water and basal diet for 96 weeks. The incidence of oesophageal papillomas or carcinomas in rats that received NDEA dissolved in 10% ethanol was higher than in rats that received NDEA alone ($P < 0.01$) (Aze *et al.*, 1993).

Chronic intake of 10% ethanol for 56 weeks enhanced hepatocarcinogenesis induced by oral administration of combined ethinylestradiol and norethindrone acetate in male and especially female Wistar rats (Yamagiwa *et al.*, 1994). Long-term ethanol treatment had a similar effect in male rats on liver preneoplastic lesions induced by aflatoxin B_1 (Tanaka *et al.*, 1989), *N*-nitrosomorpholine (Tatsuta *et al.*, 1997), MeIQx (Wanibuchi *et al.*, 2006), and NDEA and 2-acetylaminofluorene (Pires *et al.*, 2008).

The administration of ethanol (15% in the drinking-water) during the initiation and promotion stages of mammary gland carcinogenesis, induced by *N*-methylnitrosourea in female Sprague-Dawley rats, increased the number of mammary adenocarcinomas compared to control rats. Likewise, ethanol intake during the promotion stage resulted in a greater number of mammary adenocarcinomas (Singletary *et al.*, 1995). The administration of ethyl alcohol to pregnant female Sprague-Dawley rats during gestation significantly increased mammary gland tumours induced by 7,12-dimethylbenz[*a*]anthracene (DMBA) in offspring, as evidenced

Table 3.2 Carcinogenicity studies on acetaldehyde administered with drinking-water to rats

Species, strain (sex) Duration Reference	Dosing regimen, Animals/group at start	Incidence of tumours		Significance	Comments
Rat, Sprague-Dawley (M) 161 wk Soffritti *et al.* (2002b)	50 mg/L 7 d/wk 50 animals/group	Head	Osteosarcoma Control (0/50) Acetaldehyde (5/50)	*P* < 0.05	
	2500 mg/L 7 d/wk 50 animals/group	Head	Osteosarcoma Control (0/50) Acetaldehyde (7/50)	*P* < 0.05	
	50 mg/L 7 d/wk 50 animals/group	Lymphomas and leukemias	Control (6/50) Acetaldehyde (14/50)	[*P* = 0.039]	
	1500 mg/L 7 d/wk 50 animals/group	Lymphomas and leukemias	Control (6/50) Acetaldehyde (15/50)	[*P* = 0.024]	
	2500 mg/L 7 d/wk 50 animals/group	Pancreas	Islet cell adenoma Control (2/50) Acetaldehyde (9/50)	[*P* = 0.026]	
Rat, Sprague-Dawley (F) 161 wk Soffritti *et al.* (2002b)	250 mg/L 7 d/wk 50 animals/group	Lymphomas and leukemias	Control (2/50) Acetaldehyde (8/50)	[*P* = 0.046]	
	500 mg/L 7 d/wk 50 animals/group	Mammary gland	Adenocarcinoma Control (3/50) Acetaldehyde (10/50)	[*P* = 0.036]	
	250 mg/L 7 d/wk 50 animals/group	Uterus	Adenocarcinoma Control (0/50) Acetaldehyde (5/50)	[*P* = 0.028]	

d, day or days; F, female; M, male; wk, week or weeks

by a greater tumour multiplicity (Hilakivi-Clarke *et al.*, 2004).

3.3.2 Mouse

Treatment of CF-1 male mice with 6% ethanol in the drinking-water increased development of invasive pancreatic adenocarcinoma induced by DMBA (Wendt *et al.*, 2007).

As part of the study to investigate the effect of ethanol on the carcinogenicity of NDEA, strain A male mice were administered NDEA in the drinking-water with or without 10% ethanol for 4 weeks and were maintained thereafter for 32 weeks on tap-water and basal diet. Ethanol strongly potentiated the tumorigenic effect of NDEA in the forestomach and the lung (Anderson *et al.*, 1993).

The effect of ethanol on the carcinogenicity of nitrosamines was comprehensively summarized in the previous *IARC Monographs* (IARC, 1988, 2010).

3.4 Synthesis

Administration of ethanol in the drinking-water increased the incidence of cancers of the head and neck and the liver, benign tumours of the adrenal glands, pituitary gland, testes, and pancreas, osteosarcomas of the head and other sites, forestomach tumours, and combined lymphomas and leukemias in rats and liver tumours and mammary gland adenocarcinomas in mice.

Administration of acetaldehyde in the drinking-water increased the incidence of pancreatic adenomas, combined lymphomas and leukaemias, uterine and mammary gland adenocarcinomas, and head osteosarcomas in rats.

Co-administration of ethanol in the drinking-water with several known carcinogens enhanced tumour development in rats and mice.

4. Other Relevant Data

The current knowledge on mechanistic and other data relevant to the carcinogenicity of alcoholic beverages was reported in the recent *IARC Monograph* (IARC, 2010). A synthesis of these data is presented below.

4.1 Absorption, distribution, metabolism and excretion

The biomedical effects of alcoholic beverages either originate from the properties of the ethanol major component, or from its metabolism. The metabolism of ethanol is depicted in Fig. 4.1. Ethanol is metabolized to acetaldehyde by three major pathways: the alcohol dehydrogenase (ADH) pathway, the microsomal ethanol oxidizing cytochrome P450 (CYP) pathway, and the catalase-H_2O_2 system. Acetaldehyde, to which many deleterious effects of ethanol can be attributed, is oxidized to acetate primarily by acetaldehyde dehydrogenases (ALDHs) (Vasiliou *et al.*, 2004). The four pharmacokinetic parameters, absorption, distribution, metabolism and excretion, that define the level of ethanol and/or its metabolites in different tissues, are relevant for consideration.

4.1.1 Ethanol

(a) Absorption and distribution

The absorption of orally ingested alcohol starts in the upper digestive mucosa and the stomach, but the bulk is absorbed by simple diffusion in the small intestine into the bloodstream. Hereafter, alcohol is distributed into the body water. The absorption, immediately followed by the distribution phase, largely determines the ascending part and the peak of the blood-alcohol curve. Food in conjunction with alcohol drinking lowers the rate of absorption and diminishes the peak alcohol concentration, while fasting and dehydration create opposite effects. The distribution process produces slightly lower ethanol levels in venous blood (Jones *et al.*, 2004) and urine (Jones 2006) compared with arterial blood levels during the absorption phase. More fat and less body water per unit body-mass create higher blood alcohol levels, which explains why women on average reach a 10–15% higher blood-alcohol concentration compared with the same amount of alcohol per body-mass ingested by men (Goist & Sutker, 1985).

(b) Metabolism and excretion

It is generally believed that more than 90% of the ingested alcohol is oxidized in the liver. The remaining extrahepatic alcohol oxidation and other modes of elimination take place in the gastrointestinal mucosa and bacteria, via oral bacteria, the kidneys and other peripheral tissues, by excretion of body fluids (urine and sweat) and via exhalation. First-pass metabolism, i.e. when the ethanol is oxidized at its first passage through the oral cavity, gut and liver, reduces the amount of ethanol that reaches target organs. The relative contribution of first-pass metabolism to alcohol oxidation is debatable (Lim *et al.*, 1993; Levitt & Levitt, 2000). However, the smaller the alcohol amount and the slower the alcohol absorption, the greater the relative contribution of first-pass oxidation in overall alcohol elimination (Levitt & Levitt, 1998).

(i) Endogenous alcohol formation

In addition to ingestion via consumption of alcoholic beverages, small amounts of ethanol are also produced endogenously in normal intermediary metabolism (Ostrovsky, 1986) and by microbial formation, especially in the gastrointestinal tract (Krebs & Perkins, 1970). The resulting concentrations in human venous blood are estimated to vary between 0–50 μM (Jones *et al.*, 1983; Watanabe-Suzuki *et al.*, 1999). Based on case reports (Kaji *et al.*, 1984; Spinucci *et al.*, 2006) and on data from experimental animals (Krebs & Perkins, 1970), it has been shown that considerably higher concentrations exist in the gastrointestinal tract. The relevance of endogenous metabolism is further discussed in Section 4.3.1.

(ii) Alcohol dehydrogenase pathway

The oxidation of ethanol is largely catalysed by cytosolic ADHs, primarily by the low-K_m variants in the liver. Because of the low K_m (0.05–4.2 mM) ADH quickly becomes saturated and the reaction follows zero-order kinetics with a constant rate for ethanol oxidation. In addition to the enzyme activity, the ADH-mediated ethanol oxidation rate is strictly regulated by the mitochondrial reoxidation of the reduced co-enzyme nicotinamide adenine dinucleotide (NADH) to the oxidized form, nicotinamide adenine nucleotide (NAD^+) (Zakhari, 2006). This explains why, in spite of huge variations in ADH activity, relatively small effects on the overall alcohol oxidation rate have been observed. The impact of the hepatic redox state is even more apparent under fasting conditions, which are well known to slow down the rate of alcohol oxidation (Rogers *et al.*, 1987), most likely due to limitations in the mitochondrial reoxidation of NADH (Lisander *et al.*, 2006). The less alcohol is ingested the larger the contribution of ADH activity in the regulation of the rate of alcohol oxidation (see Fig. 4.1).

Human ADHs

Three different nomenclature systems have been proposed for the human ADH genes (Table 4.1). The official nomenclature approved by the Human Genome Organization (HUGO) (www.gene.ucl.ac.uk/nomenclature) will be used here throughout.

Seven human ADHs have been isolated that are divided into five classes on the basis on similarities in their amino acid sequences and kinetic properties (Table 4.1). They are dimeric enzymes consisting of two 40kDa subunits named α, β, γ, π, χ and either σ or μ. Class I comprises three enzymes: ADH1A, which contains at least one α subunit (αα, αβ, or αγ), ADH1B (ββ or βγ), and ADH1C (γγ).Class II contains ADH4 (ππ). Class III contains ADH5 (χχ). Class IV contains ADH7 (μμ or σσ). Class V contains ADH6 for which there is no subunit designation (Parkinson & Ogilvie, 2008).

The low-K_m class I ADHs (α, β and γ subunits, formerly called ADH-1, -2, and -3) account for most of the ethanol-oxidizing capacity in the liver and gastrointestinal mucosa (Lee *et al.*, 2006). Class I *ADH* is also expressed in several other tissues, such as the upper and lower digestive tracts (Yin *et al.*, 1993; Seitz *et al.*, 1996; Yin *et al.*, 1997; Jelski *et al.*, 2002), pancreas (Chiang *et al.*, 2009), lungs (Engeland & Maret, 1993), breast (Triano *et al.*, 2003), blood vessels (Jelski *et al.*, 2009) and salivary glands (Visapää *et al.*, 2004). In brain no functionally significant class I ADH has been detected (Estonius *et al.*, 1996).

Allelic variants have been identified in the *ADH1B* and *ADH1C* genes that encode for the β1, β2, β3, γ1, and γ2 subunits, which can combine as homodimers or can form heterodimers with each other and with the α subunit. ADH1B enzymes that differ in the type of β subunit are known as allelozymes, as are ADH1C enzymes that differ in the type of γ subunit. Allelozymes

Fig. 4.1 Ethanol and acetaldehyde metabolism

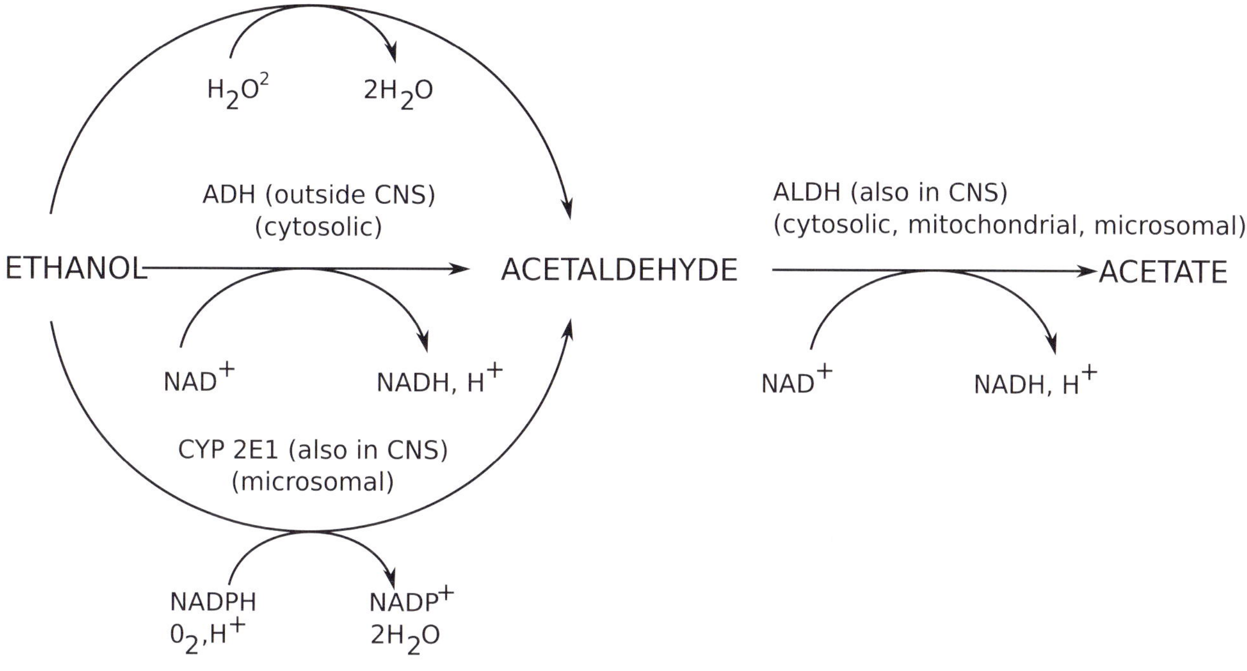

ADH, alcool dehydrogenase; ALDH, aldehyde dehydrogenase; CYP, cytochrome P450; CNS, central nervous system; NADPH, nicotinamide-adenine dinucleotide phosphate.
Adapted from Vasiliou *et al.* (2004).

present different kinetic properties (Table 4.1) and so differ in their capacity to oxidize ethanol. The allelozymes that are homodimers or heterodimers of β2 subunit (encoded by the *ADH1B*2* allele) are especially active ethanol oxidizing enzymes. The ADH1B*2 allelic variant is found in 90% of the Pacific Rim Asian population and is responsible for the unusually rapid conversion of ethanol to acetaldehyde in this population. ADH1B*2 is also more common in people of Jewish origin compared to people of other Caucasian descent (where it is found in 0 to < 20%) (Neumark *et al.* 1998). The ADH1B*1 allele is most common in Caucasians (up to 95%) and ADH1B*3 is found mostly in African and African Americans (~24%). These population differences in ADH1B alloenzyme expression potentially contribute to ethnic differences in alcohol consumption and toxicity. Unlike the ADH1B allelozymes, the ADH1C variants do not differ much in their ethanol oxidizing activities (Parkinson & Ogilvie, 2008).

The class II π-ADH (subunit encoded by *ADH4*) also contributes to hepatic ethanol oxidation, especially at higher concentrations (Edenberg 2007; Birley *et al.*, 2009; Kimura *et al.*, 2009). *ADH4* expression has been found in most epithelial tissues.

Little is known about the functional role of class III, IV and V ADHs (encoded by the genes *ADH5*, *7* and 6, respectively) in the oxidation of alcohol.

Microbial ADHs

There is a large population of microorganisms present in the gastrointestinal tract that may contribute to ethanol oxidation. Another local site for microbial alcohol oxidation is the oral cavity. Microorganisms express numerous forms of ADH, the role of which may become even more significant wherever microbial overgrowth occurs (Salaspuro, 2003).

Table 4.1 Major allele variants and biochemical properties of human alcohol dehydrogenases (ADHs)

Official nomenclature[a]	Former nomenclature[b]	Additional nonstandard nomenclature[c]	Sequence[d]	Allele	Amino Acid differences between alleles	Protein subunit	Class[e]	K_m (mM) [f]	V_{max} (min^{-1}) [g]
ADH1A	*ADH1*		NM_000667	*ADH1A*		α	I	4.0	30
ADH1B	*ADH2*		NM_000668	*ADH1B*1*	Arg48, Arg370	β1	I	0.05	4
				*ADH1B*2*	His48, Arg370	β2	I	0.9	350
				*ADH1B*3*	Arg48, Cys370	β3	I	40	300
ADH1C	*ADH3*		NM_000669	*ADH1C*1*	Arg272, Ile350	γ1	I	1.0	90
				*ADH1C*2*	Gln212, Val350	γ2	I	0.6	40
				*ADH1C*352Thr*	[h]Thr352	NR	I	NR	NR
ADH4	*ADH4*	*ADH2*	NM_000670	*ADH4*1*		π	II	30	40
				*ADH4*2*		π	II	NR	NR
ADH5	*ADH5*	*ADH3*	NM_000671			χ	III	> 1000	100
ADH6	*ADH6*	*ADH5*	NM_000672				V	NR	NR
ADH7	*ADH7*	*ADH4*	NM_000673			σ or μ	IV	30	1800

[a] Nomenclature approved by the Human Genome Organization (HUGO) Gene Nomenclature Committee (www.gene.ucl.ac.uk/nomenclature/), as used by the National Center for Biotechnology Information (NCBI)

[b] Former nomenclature

[c] Non-standard nomenclature proposed by Duester *et al.* (1999)

[d] Reference sequence number as listed in the NCBI RefSeq database (www.ncbi.nlm.nih.gov/RefSeq/)

[e] ADH proteins have been divided into five classes based on sequence and structural similarities

[f] V_{max} indicates how many molecules of ethanol the enzyme will convert to acetaldehyde in 1 minute at saturating ethanol concentrations.

[g] K_m indicates the concentration of ethanol at which the enzyme works at 50 percent capacity.

[h] *ADHIC*352Thr* has been found in Native Americans as an additional variation on chromosomes with the Val350 characteristics of ADH1C*2 (Osier *et al.*, 2002); the protein has not been isolated for study. The kinetic constants are noted for the homodiners of the ADH subunits listed (heterodimers behave as if the active sites were independent).

NR, not reported

Adapted from Edenberg (2007)

(iii) Cytochrome P450 oxidation pathway

See Fig. 4.1.

Cytochrome P450 2E1 (CYP2E1) is constitutively expressed in the endoplasmic reticulum of the liver and many other tissues including the brain, in contrast to the expression of ADHs. Its K_m for ethanol is about 10 mM; thus CYP2E1 may assume a greater role in the first-order oxidation reaction at high blood-alcohol levels. Other cytochrome enzymes, CYP1A2 and CYP3A4, also contribute to the oxidation of ethanol, albeit to a lesser extent (Lieber, 2004). CYP2E1 has the unique property of being induced as a result of chronic alcohol intake, which explains part of the increased alcohol elimination rate after chronic alcohol ingestion (Lieber, 2004). The CYP2E1-mediated ethanol oxidation is associated with nicotinamide-adenine dinucleotide phosphate (NADPH)-CYP reductase in the endoplasmic reticulum, and reduces molecular oxygen to water as ethanol is oxidized to acetaldehyde. CYP2E1 is unusually 'leaky' and generates reactive oxygen species including hydroxyl radical, superoxide anion, hydrogen peroxide and hydroxyethyl radical. Thus, CYP2E1 is a major source of alcohol-related oxidative stress (Caro & Cederbaum, 2004).

Genetic variants of *CYP2E1*

Several allele variants of *CYP2E1* have been described in humans (see Table 4.2).

The allele variant commonly denoted as c2, *CYP2E1*5B* according to the new recommended nomenclature, has been found more frequently in East Asian individuals (~40%) compared with Caucasians (~8%) (Garte *et al.*, 2001). Early studies showed an increased *CYP2E1* expression and activity in ethanol oxidation associated with the **5B* allele (Hayashi *et al.*, 1991; Tsutsumi *et al.*, 1994; Watanabe *et al.*, 1994), but this finding has not been confirmed in other studies (Carrière *et al.*, 1996; Kim *et al.*, 1996; Powell *et al.*, 1998; Kato *et al.*, 2003), and contrasting results have been reported (Huang *et al.*, 2003). So it is unclear to what extent the functional activities regarding ethanol oxidation differ from those of the corresponding wild types. Other variants of *CYP2E1* polymorphisms, such as *CYP2E1*6*, have also been shown to be more common in East Asians (ca. 52%) compared with Caucasian individuals (ca. 15%) (Garte *et al.*, 2001).

(iv) Ethanol oxidation by catalase (Fig. 4.1)

Catalase is constitutively expressed in the peroxisomal part of the endoplasmic reticulum in virtually all tissues. It is an important antioxidant enzyme that detoxifies H_2O_2 into oxygen and water and thus limits the deleterious effects of reactive oxygen species. The functional role of catalase in the oxidation of ethanol in humans is not known. Although catalase-mediated ethanol oxidation is very limited compared with ADH-mediated reactions, it may play a significant role in specific organs and tissues that lack the functional ADH. Based on experimental animal research, catalase seems to contribute to alcohol oxidation in the brain (Cohen *et al.*, 1980; Zimatkin *et al.*, 2006). As with CYP2E1, catalase also has a high K_m and, thus, the impact on alcohol oxidation would be higher at high alcohol levels. No functional polymorphism regarding alcohol oxidation or its effects has been reported.

(v) Non-oxidative ethanol metabolism

Ethanol can be non-oxidatively metabolized to form fatty-acid ethyl esters (FAEEs), which are toxic for cells (Laposata & Lange, 1986; Laposata *et al.*, 2002). These esters are formed during the hydrolysis of fatty-acid esters (e.g. triglycerides) in the presence of ethanol. Such esterification activity has been detected in humans mainly with the two high-K_m enzymes fatty-acid ethyl ester synthases (FAEEs) (Wright *et al.*, 1987) and acyl-coenzyme A:ethanol O-acyltransferase (AEAT) (Diczfalusy *et al.*, 2001). Highest activities have been located in the liver and pancreas, and in the liver and duodenum, for FAEEs and AEAT, respectively (Diczfalusy *et al.*, 2001).

Table 4.2 Major allelic variants and biochemical properties of humans cytochrome P450 2E1 (CYP2E1)

Recommended nomenclature[a]	Alternative nomenclature[a]	Protein	Nucleotide changes, Gene	RFLP	Effect	Enzyme activity	
						In_vivo	*In_vitro*
*CYP2E1*1A*	*CYP2E1*1*	CYP2E1.1	None			Normal	Normal
*CYP2E1*1B*	*CYP2E1*2*	CYP2E1.1	9896C > G	*Taq*I-			
*CYP2E1*1C*		CYP2E1.1	6 repeats in the 5′ flanking region				
*CYP2E1*1D*		CYP2E1.1	8 repeats in the 5′ flanking region	*Dra*I and *Xba*I		Incr. activity after alcohol exposure and in obese subjects	
*CYP2E1*2*		CYP2E1.2	1132G > A		R76H		Reduced
*CYP2E1*3*		CYP2E1.3	10023G > A		V389I		Normal
*CYP2E1*4*		CYP2E1.4	4768G > A		V179I		Normal
*CYP2E1*5A*		CYP2E1.1	−1293G > C; −1053C > T (c1 > c2); 7632T > A	*Pst*I+ *Rsa*I- *Dra*I-			
*CYP2E1*5B*	*CYP2E1*3*	CYP2E1.1	−1293G > C; −1053C > T (c1 > c2)	*Pst*I+ *Rsa*I-			
*CYP2E1*6*	*CYP2E1*4*	CYP2E1.1	7632T > A	*Dra*I-			
*CYP2E1*7A*		CYP2E1.1	−333T > A				
*CYP2E1*7B*		CYP2E1.1	−71G > T; −333T > A				
*CYP2E1*7C*		CYP2E1.1	−333T > A; −352A > G				
not included	*CYP2E1*5*						
not included	*CYP2E1*6*						

[a] Two different nomenclature systems were developed for the CYP2E1 alleles simultaneously. The authors of both nomenclature systems have agreed in July 2000 that the nomenclature system given in the first column should be the recommended one, see Ingelman-Sundberg *et al.* (2001); the other nomenclature that was proposed by Garte & Crosti (1999) is given in the second column.

RFLP, restriction fragment length polymorphism

Adapted from http://www.cypalleles.ki.se/cyp2e1.htm

Lower activities of both enzymes were found in heart, lung, adipose, gall bladder and gastric tissues. Although FAEE may be important in the etiology of alcohol-mediated cellular toxicity, especially in the case of long-term accumulation during chronic alcohol intake, the relative contribution to overall alcohol elimination is rather small. In addition to FAEEs, alcohol also forms other conjugates, such as ethyl glucuronide, often used as a marker for recent alcohol drinking (Wurst *et al.*, 2003).

4.1.2 Acetaldehyde

Acetaldehyde is the first metabolite in the oxidation of ethanol (Fig. 4.1). Interindividual variations of the acetaldehyde-mediated effects will depend on the genetic polymorphisms and other factors affecting the metabolism and levels of acetaldehyde, and the effects on the target organs.

(a) Origin of acetaldehyde

(i) Endogenous formation

Several degradation reactions are known to form endogenous acetaldehyde in the human body (Krebs & Perkins, 1970). Without external alcohol ingestion, acetaldehyde concentrations are below the level of detection, except in the gastrointestinal tract (Väkeväinen *et al.*, 2000). However, under conditions of inhibited acetaldehyde-oxidation capacity, endogenous acetaldehyde levels may be detected in the blood (Eriksson, 1985). The relevance of the endogenous acetaldehyde is further discussed in Section 4.3.1.

(ii) Acetaldehyde in alcoholic beverages

A small part of the total acetaldehyde to which the body is exposed comes directly from ingested alcoholic beverages. All alcoholic beverages contain acetaldehyde in variable amounts: average levels in different types vary between 60 to > 7000 µM (Lachenmeier & Sohnius, 2008). The magnitude and the significance of exposure to acetaldehyde from alcoholic beverages are further discussed in Section 4.3.1.

(iii) Acetaldehyde formation by oxidation of exogenous ethanol

The major part of the total acetaldehyde to which the body is exposed during alcohol ingestion originates from ethanol oxidation catalysed by the ADH, CYP2E1 and catalase enzymes. The liver and the gut are the primary sites of acetaldehyde formation to such an extent that the rate of alcohol oxidation exceeds the rate of acetaldehyde breakdown, which consequently leads to diffusion of the surplus acetaldehyde into the bloodstream. Under normal conditions, i.e. without reduced capacity for acetaldehyde oxidation or considerably increased acetaldehyde formation, the acetaldehyde produced at other sites is usually directly oxidized within the tissue. The exception is the aerodigestive tract, where acetaldehyde is produced at least partly by microbial alcohol oxidation. Consequently, acetaldehyde can be detected both in breath and saliva during alcohol intoxication (Eriksson, 2007).

(b) Metabolism

The bulk of the acetaldehyde formed in the liver is directly oxidized by NAD^+-dependent aldehyde dehydrogenases (ALDHs) to acetate. The efficacy of normal hepatic oxidation of the alcohol-derived acetaldehyde is estimated to be close to 99% (Eriksson & Fukunaga, 1993). In addition, a minor part of the acetaldehyde is probably oxidized by aldehyde oxidase and CYP2E1. In addition, acetaldehyde reacts with a variety of chemical compounds in the body.

(i) Aldehyde dehydrogenase pathway

Acetaldehyde is metabolized by ALDHs (Fig. 4.1), which are widely expressed in the mitochrondria (low-K_m enzyme) and cytosol (high-K_m enzyme) of most tissues (Crabb, 1995). Oxidation of acetaldehyde is regulated by the rate of acetaldehyde formation, ALDH activity and the cytosolic and mitochondrial redox states. Ethanol consumption is not known to induce *ALDH* expression. Chronic alcohol abuse, especially associated with liver disease, has been reported to reduce the ALDH activity (Nuutinen *et al.*, 1983).

The major allelic variants of human ALDHs, their respective K_m and their ethnical distribution are summarized in Table 4.3. The high-K_m ALDH1A1 accounts for most of the acetaldehyde-oxidizing capacity in the cytosolic compartment of the liver and other tissues. This enzyme is also abundant in the erythrocytes. Several variant alleles of *ALDH1A1* with potential functional relevance have recently been reported in the promoter (Spence *et al.*, 2003), intron and untranslated regions (Lind *et al.*, 2008) (Table 4.1).

The low-K_m (about 5 μM for acetaldehyde) ALDH2 is located in the mitochondria and is believed to be responsible for the bulk of the oxidation of the ethanol-derived acetaldehyde. This enzyme is not significantly expressed in the erythrocytes. Of all the polymorphisms in genes encoding enzymes that metabolize alcohol and acetaldehyde, the *ALDH2*2* allele has the greatest functional impact on the human phenotype. This allele is common in East-Asian populations, about 5–10% homozygotes and 30–40% heterozygotes (Brennan *et al.*, 2004). In these individuals the acetaldehyde levels are elevated, which creates several toxic effects and also euphoric reinforcing reactions (Eriksson, 2001). The relevance of the elevated acetaldehyde for the development of cancers is discussed in section 4.3.1. In addition to the **2* allele, promoter-region variants have been reported (Harada *et al.*, 1999). The functional significance of these other variants remains to be established. The relevance of other ALDHs, including ALDH1B1 and other classes of ALDH, also remains to be elucidated.

(ii) Other pathways in the metabolism and reactions of acetaldehyde

In addition to the ALDH-catalysed reactions, acetaldehyde may also be oxidized to a minor extent by CYP2E1 (Terelius *et al.*, 1991) and by different oxidases (Deitrich *et al.*, 2007).

Due to its chemical reactivity, most, if not all, of the ethanol-derived acetaldehyde that is not further oxidized binds to a variety of constituents. These interactions vary between easily reversible and firm covalent bonds. Different kinds of Schiff's base, which are formed by acetaldehyde and the free amino groups of amino acids, peptides and proteins, are the most common products (Eriksson & Fukunaga, 1993, Niemelä, 2007). Some of these unstable products become stable under reducing conditions, such as during alcohol intoxication. Although only a small fraction of all acetaldehyde formed during ethanol oxidation produces these adducts, they are important in some of the chronic toxic actions of alcohol. The role of the acetaldehyde adducts in the carcinogenic effects of alcohol is further discussed in Sections 4.2.2, 4.3.1 and 4.4.2.

(c) Levels of acetaldehyde in tissues

From the liver, where most of the ethanol-derived acetaldehyde is formed and oxidized, the remaining acetaldehyde, free and/or loosely bound, escapes into the *vena hepatica*, reaching concentrations of approximately 70 μM under normal conditions (Eriksson & Fukunaga, 1993). Thereafter, the concentration of acetaldehyde in the blood will be diluted by the *vena cava* blood and further reduced by the circulation in the heart and the lungs before reaching peripheral tissues. Human data show that acetaldehyde levels in pulmonary arterial blood are in the range of 0–4.4 μM, 30 and 60 minutes after ethanol consumption (DeMaster *et al.*, 1983) during normal alcohol oxidation. Acetaldehyde in peripheral arterial or venous blood is below the limit of detection (< 1 μM) during normal

Table 4.3 Major allelic variants, biochemical properties, and ethnical distribution of human acetaldehyde dehydrogenases (ALDHs)

Gene Locus	Allele	Km μM[a]	Ethnic/national distribution[b]	References
ALDH1A1		50	All	Vasiliou *et al.* (2000)
ALDH2	*ALDH2*1*	< 5	All	
	*ALDH2*2*		Asia	Crabb *et al.* (1989)
	*ALDH2*3*		Taiwan, People's Republic of China	Novoradovsky *et al.* (1995)
ALDH1B1	*ALDH1B1*1*	NR		
(ALDH5)	*ALDH1B1*2*	NR		Sherman *et al.* (1993)
ALDH9A1	*ALDH9A1*1*	30	All	Kurys *et al.* (1989)
	*ALDH9A1*2*			Lin (1996)

[a] Kinetic constant of the enzyme when acetaldehyde is the substrate
[b] The column labelled ethnic/national distribution indicates which populations have high allele frequencies for these variants. The alleles are not limited to those populations.
NR, not reported
Compiled by the Working Group

alcohol intoxication in Caucasian male populations (Eriksson & Fukunaga, 1993). However, in Caucasian women, acetaldehyde levels of 1–8 μM have been detected during the use of oral contraceptives and during the high-estradiol phase of the normal cycle (Eriksson *et al.*, 1996).

Except for the blood and the liver, in which acetaldehyde concentration should be approximately the same as in the *vena hepatica*, little is known about acetaldehyde levels in other tissues during normal alcohol oxidation in humans. Acetaldehyde levels should rise in tissues where the ethanol oxidation rate exceeds the capacity of acetaldehyde oxidation. Breath acetaldehyde concentrations of 10–20 and 20–40 nM at blood alcohol levels of about 10 and 20 mM, respectively, imply corresponding tissue acetaldehyde levels of 2–8 μM in the respiratory tract (Jones, 1995; Eriksson, 2007). Part of this acetaldehyde is derived by microbial ethanol oxidation (Pikkarainen *et al.*, 1980). Also, acetaldehyde levels in the saliva, which almost exclusively are derived from microbiological alcohol oxidation, correlate positively with the blood alcohol concentration (Väkeväinen *et al.*, 2001; Eriksson, 2007). Levels varying between 15 to 25 μM and 20 to 40 μM at corresponding blood ethanol concentrations of 10 to 20 mM, respectively, have been reported (Homann *et al.*, 1997; Eriksson, 2007). The role of the acetaldehyde concentrations in the upper aerodigestive tract in the carcinogenic effects of alcohol is discussed in Section 4.3.1.

Under certain conditions, such as chronic alcohol consumption especially in combination with increased alcohol oxidation rate and/or liver disease and genetically determined deficiency in the ALDHs, acetaldehyde levels are considerably elevated. Peripheral venous blood acetaldehyde concentrations of 14 μM have been detected during alcohol intoxication (after a dose of 0.8 g per kg) in alcoholics (Nuutinen *et al.*, 1984). In Asian subjects carrying the ALDH*2 allele, blood acetaldehyde levels above 200 μM have been reported (Eriksson & Fukunaga, 1993). In addition to ALDH2 polymorphism, the *ADH1B*2* and *ADH1C*1* variant alleles, which encode more active ADHs, in turn may elevate ethanol-derived acetaldehyde levels. This possibility was suggested by Visapää *et al.* (2004) who reported increased acetaldehyde concentrations in saliva of individuals with the *ADH1C*1/*1* genotype. The relevance of the *ALDH* and *ADH* genotypes for the etiology of cancer is further discussed in Section 4.3.1.

4.2 Genotoxicity

4.2.1 Humans

Studies of genotoxic effects of alcoholic beverages have been reviewed (Obe & Anderson, 1987; IARC, 1988, 2010).

(a) Genotoxic effects in alcoholics

Maffei *et al.* (2000, 2002) and Castelli *et al.* (1999) found that alcoholics had significantly more chromosomal aberrations and cells with micronuclei than either non-drinking controls or abstinent alcoholics. The three groups were matched for age, sex and smoking (Maffei *et al.*, 2002). When centromeric fluorescence in situ hybridization (FISH) was combined with the analysis of micronuclei, the alcoholics showed an increase in the number of lymphocytes with centromere-positive micronuclei, indicating an elevated formation of micronuclei harbouring whole chromosomes, ie, an aneugenic effect (Maffei *et al.*, 2000). In a combined analysis of three biomonitoring studies, Iarmarcovai *et al.* (2007) observed a small but significant increase in micronucleus frequency in alcoholic beverage users compared with controls (OR, 1.24; 95%CI: 1.01–1.53).

While the majority of published studies showed no increase in chromosomal alterations in alcoholics following abstinence from ethanol compared to non-drinkers, some studies reported positive results (De Torok, 1972; Matsushima, 1987). Gattás & Saldanha (1997) compared the frequency of structural or numerical chromosomal aberrations in lymphocytes of alcoholics who had been abstinent for 1 month to 32 years, with those in subjects not consuming alcoholic beverages. They noted a significant increase in the frequency of cells with structural chromosomal aberrations in the abstinent alcoholics. Burim *et al.* (2004) observed that the frequencies of chromosomal aberrations in lymphocytes of 29 chronic alcoholics and 11 alcoholics in abstinence were higher than those in 10 control individuals. The level of chromosomal aberrations was not statistically significantly different when smoking and non-smoking alcoholics were compared, which indicated a lack of interaction.

There is some indication that ethanol may lead to chromosomal aneuploidy in human sperm. Robbins *et al.* (1997) used FISH of the sex chromosomes and chromosome 18 to investigate the potential contribution of common lifestyle exposures to aneuploidy load in sperm from 45 healthy male volunteers. Consumption of alcoholic beverages was significantly associated with increased frequencies of aneuploidy XX18, XY18–18 apparent diploidy, or XX18–18 duplication phenotype, after controlling for caffeine, smoking and donor age.

Härkönen *et al.* (1999) reported a significant negative association between alcohol intake and sperm aneuploid for chromosomes 1 and 7 (1-1-7 and 1-7-7 constitutions and diploid sperm) among 30 agricultural workers before pesticide exposures, while no statistically significant findings were related to alcohol intake after the exposure. [These inconclusive findings may reflect moderate alcohol consumption (average 6 drinks/week).]

In a case–control study Kagan-Krieger *et al.* (2002) found no association between self-reported paternal or maternal alcohol consumption and Turner syndrome in offspring.

Pool-Zobel *et al.* (2004) used the comet assay to study DNA damage and repair in human rectal cells obtained from biopsies and found that male alcoholic beverage abusers had significantly less DNA strand-breaks than male controls. This may be the result of an enhancing effect on endogenous defence, e.g. through upregulation of DNA repair in response to damage. [Alternatively, a reduced amount of DNA in the comet tails could reflect DNA–protein crosslinks resulting from exposure to endogenous acetaldehyde.]

van Zeeland *et al.* (1999) and Lodovici *et al.* (2000) did not detect any increase in 8-hydroxy-deoxyguanosine (8-OHdG) levels [measure of oxidative DNA damage] in leukocyte DNA in relation to alcoholic beverage consumption. In a multicentre study in Europe, Bianchini *et al.* (2001) observed an inverse relationship between alcoholic beverage consumption and levels of 8-OHdG in leukocyte DNA. However, an increased level of 8-OHdG in leukocyte DNA was observed in ALDH2-deficient subjects who consumed alcoholic beverages (Nakajima *et al.*, 1996).

Frank *et al.* (2004) reported a significant increase in 1,N^6-ethenodeoxyadenosine DNA adducts in seven subjects diagnosed with alcoholic fatty liver and three diagnosed with alcoholic fibrosis. Patients with alcoholic fibrosis had a much higher level of these adducts than patients with alcoholic fatty liver. [No diagnostic criteria were provided for patients identified as 'alcoholic'.]

Wang *et al.* (2009) observed that protein-bound 4-hydroxynonenal [a major lipid peroxidation product] and both 1,N^6-ethenodeoxyadenosine and 3,N^4-ethenodeoxycytidine DNA adducts strongly correlated with CYP2E1 expression in fine-needle liver biopsy samples obtained from 14 German patients with alcoholic liver disease ($r = 0.97$, $P < 0.01$). [The results support the assumption that, particularly in non-Asian populations, ethanol-mediated induction of hepatic CYP2E1, leading to highly miscoding DNA lesions derived from lipid peroxidation, may play a central role in hepatocarcinogenesis in patients with alcoholic liver disease.]

A statistically significantly higher frequency of sister chromatid exchange in lymphocytes was observed in Japanese subjects deficient in *ALDH2* (at least one **2* allele) compared to those who were proficient in *ALDH2* (**1/*1* genotype) and drank alcohol almost daily; such an effect was not seen in subjects who drank less or did not drink at all (Morimoto & Takeshita, 1996).

(b) Effects of polymorphisms for metabolic enzymes

A significant difference in micronucleus frequency between the *ALDH2*2* allele carriers and the individuals carrying the *ALDH2*1/*1* genotype was found at all levels of alcohol consumption; the highest micronucleus levels were seen in the *ALDH2*2* allele carriers consuming more than 100 g of alcohol per week and more than 3 times a week (Ishikawa *et al.*, 2003).

In non-smoking regular or occasional Japanese drinkers, the frequency of micronuclei was shown to be higher in *ALDH2*2/*2* homozygotes versus *ALDH2*2/*1* heterozygotes and in *ADH1B*1/*1* homozygotes versus *ADH1B*1/*2* heterozygotes. The highest micronucleus levels were seen in regular drinkers carrying both the *ALDH2*2* and *ADH1B*1* alleles. Nonetheless, due to the low number of subjects, a statistically significant increase of micronuclei was only seen for regular drinkers who carry the more common combination, i.e. *ALDH2*2* and *ADH1B*2* alleles (Ishikawa *et al.*, 2007).

Regular drinkers with the *CYP2E1*1/*1* genotype showed a significantly higher micronucleus frequency than drinkers carrying the *CYP2E1*3* allele; and drinkers with combined *ALDH2*2* and *CYP2E1*1/*1* genotypes showed the highest micronucleus frequency (Ishikawa *et al.*, 2006).

4.2.2 Experimental systems

(a) Ethanol

The genotoxic potential of ethanol has been extensively evaluated in lower organisms, plants, mammalian systems and in human cells, as reviewed previously (IARC, 1988, 2010; Phillips & Jenkinson, 2001).

Ethanol gave negative results in bacterial mutagenicity tests, even in the presence of exogenous metabolic activation systems. These findings are consistent with the negative findings obtained with acetaldehyde, the primary *in vivo* metabolite of ethanol, in bacterial genotoxicity assays (IARC, 2010).

Positive results were reported for the induction of DNA strand breaks and chromosome malsegregation by ethanol in fungi and sister chromatid exchange in plants without exogenous metabolic activation. [These findings were obtained at very high concentrations (16000–39100 μg/ml) exceeding those usually recommended as the highest allowable concentrations in genotoxicity testing.]

In mammalian cells *in vitro*, ethanol was not usually able to produce gene mutations or chromosomal aberrations, but one study in mouse preimplantation embryos *in vitro* showed an induction of sister chromatid exchanges and chromosomal aberrations. In these experiments, sister chromatid exchange disappeared in the presence of 4-methylpyrazole, an inhibitor of alcohol dehydrogenase. This suggests that preimplantation embryos are able to convert ethanol to acetaldehyde.

A single study reported ethanol-induced DNA strand breaks in various types of human cells (Blasiak *et al.*, 2000). The majority of studies showed no induction of chromosome damage by ethanol in human lymphocytes and lymphoblastoid cells *in vitro*. [The Working Group noted that in most of the *in vitro* genotoxicity studies, external metabolic activation systems were not used, which reduces the value of the negative findings.]

Ethanol induced micronuclei in human lymphoblastoid cells without external metabolic activation (Kayani & Parry, 2010). This effect appeared to be independent of acetaldehyde, since the micronuclei mostly contained whole chromosomes, while those induced by acetaldehyde harboured chromosomal fragments. Thus, ethanol produced micronuclei *in vitro* by an aneugenic mechanism while acetaldehyde was clastogenic.

In animals *in vivo*, ethanol induced DNA adducts, DNA strand breaks, and sister chromatid exchanges and dominant lethal mutations. No effect of ethanol was seen in the micronucleus or chromosome aberration assays *in vivo*. In rats, exposure to ethanol increased mitochondrial DNA (mt DNA) oxidation and decreased the amount of mt DNA (Cahill *et al.*, 1997, 2005). Several studies showed that the administration of ethanol to rats and mice leads to changes in the activity and amount of DNA-repair proteins in the liver (Navasumrit *et al.*, 2001a; Bradford *et al.*, 2005).

The ethanol-induced DNA single-strand breaks in liver parenchymal cells of rat closely matched the timing of CYP2E1 induction and was inhibited by dietary antioxidants (Navasumrit *et al.*, 2000). Ethanol also increased the level of the lipid peroxidation-derived DNA adduct, ethenodeoxycytidine in rats (Navasumrit *et al.*, 2001b) and N^2-ethyl-2′-desoxyguanosine (N^2EtdG) adducts, not detectable in controls, were seen in liver DNA of ethanol-treated mice (Fang & Vaca, 1995). Rats and mice fed ethanol showed increased levels of oxidative DNA damage (abasic sites and 8-hydroxydeoxyguanosine) in the liver (Bradford *et al.* 2005); this effect was observed in transgenic mice that expressed human CYP2E1, but not in CYP2E1-knockout mice or in the presence of a CYP2E1 inhibitor. Increased levels of 1,N^6-ethenodeoxyadenosine and 3,N^4-ethenodeoxycytidine DNA adducts (measured by immunohistochemistry) were observed in the liver of ethanol-fed lean (Fa/Fa) and obese (fa/fa) Zucker rats (Wang *et al.*, 2009). The number of hepatocyte nuclei that stained positively for these etheno-DNA adducts correlated significantly with CYP2E1 expression.

(b) Acetaldehyde

Numerous *in vitro* studies have consistently shown that acetaldehyde causes DNA–protein crosslinks, DNA strand breaks, DNA adducts, sister chromatid exchanges, chromosomal aberrations, and micronuclei in eukaryotic cells *in vitro* (Speit *et al.*, 2008; Kayani & Parry, 2010; IARC, 2010). In comparison with other assays, the comet assay requires relatively high concentrations of acetaldehyde to show a positive result, probably reflecting the formation of crosslinks (Speit *et al.*, 2008).

Acetaldehyde induced also DNA protein crosslinks, sister chromatid exchanges, and chromosomal aberrations in rodents *in vivo* (IARC, 2010).

4.2.3 Genotoxicity of acetaldehyde

(a) DNA adduct formation

The structure of acetaldehyde-derived DNA adducts is depicted in Fig. 4.2.

(i) N^2-Ethyl-2′-deoxyguanosine (N^2EtdG)

The most abundant DNA adduct that results from the reaction of acetaldehyde is N^2-ethylidenedeoxyguanosine (N^2EtidG). This adduct is too unstable to be purified and isolated, but can be converted into the stable adduct N^2EtdG, by treatment with a reducing agent (sodium cyanoborohydride). The reduction step can also be carried out by a mixture of GSH and ascorbic acid, which may occur *in vivo* (Fang & Vaca, 1995; Wang *et al.*, 2006c).

Fang & Vaca (1997) examined the levels of the N^2EtdG adduct in a group of Swedish alcohol abusers compared to controls. They found that chronic alcoholics had higher levels of the N^2EtdG adduct in both lymphocytes and granulocytes compared with controls. The levels of adduct found in both cell types were on the order of one lesion/10^7 nucleotides. [The Working Group noted that the alcoholic subjects were also heavy smokers, whereas the control subjects were not. However, the authors reported that N^2EtdG levels were undetectable in the DNA sample from the one moderate smoker in the control group, and also stated that no adducts were detectable in samples obtained from five additional heavy smokers (> 20 cigarettes/week)].

Inclusion of a reducing agent (cyanoborohydride) in the DNA isolation and digestion solutions allowed N^2EtidG to be converted quantitatively to N^2EtdG. Wang *et al.* (2006c) concluded that N^2EtidG is in fact an endogenous DNA adduct that is present in every animal and human liver DNA at levels in the range of 0.1 lesion/10^6 normal nucleotides.

Balbo *et al.* (2008) measured the level of N^2-EtdG in blood leukocyte DNA of two groups of subjects, one consisting of alcohol drinkers and abstainers and the other of heavy drinkers. A significant trend between N^2-EtdG level and daily alcohol dose was found. In the first group, the mean level of N^2-EtdG was significantly higher in drinkers (5270 ± 8770 fmol/μmol dG) than in non-drinkers (2690 ± 3040 fmol/μmol dG; $P = 0.04$) after adjusting for potential confounders. Taking into account the dose, the adduct level was higher in younger than older drinkers.

Matsuda *et al.* (1999) reported that detectable levels of N^2EtdG were found in the urine of healthy Japanese individuals who had abstained from ethanol for at least 1 week. These authors proposed that the lesion resulted from endogenously formed acetaldehyde.

(ii) Other acetaldehyde-derived DNA adducts

In addition to the major adduct N^2EtidG, three acetaldehyde-derived DNA adducts have been identified. These are: N^2-(2,6-dimethyl-1,3-dioxan-4-yl) deoxyguanosine (N^2-Dio-dG); an interstrand crosslink, and two diastereisomers (R and S) of α-methyl-γ-hydroxy-1,N^2-propanodeoxyguanosine (α-Me-γ-OH-PdG) (Wang *et al.*, 2000).

Matsuda *et al.* (2006) analysed the levels of acetaldehyde-derived DNA adducts in DNA samples from peripheral white blood cells of Japanese alcoholic beverage abusers with two different *ALDH2* genotypes: **1/*1* versus **1/*2*. The groups were matched by age, smoking and alcoholic beverage consumption. These authors developed very sensitive and specific liquid chromatograph–mass spectrometry assays for the DNA adducts: N^2EtdG, α-Me-γ-OH-PdG (both R and S isomers) and N^2-Dio-dG. The N^2-Dio-dG adduct was not detected in any of the samples studied. Levels of the other three adducts were significantly higher in **1/*2* carriers than in **1/*1* genotypes.

The formation of the methyl-hydroxypropano-dG adducts can be facilitated by including basic amino acids, histones (which are rich in basic amino acids), or polyamines in the reaction mixture. In the presence of physiologically relevant polyamine concentrations, detectable amounts of these adducts were formed from concentrations as low as 100 μM acetaldehyde (Theruvathu *et al.*, 2005). Such concentrations are within the range of acetaldehyde concentrations formed in the saliva of human volunteers who drank alcoholic beverage in a laboratory setting (Homann *et al.*, 1997). Finally, acetaldehyde can react with malondialdehyde, and the resulting conjugate can form DNA adducts *in vitro* (Pluskota-Karwatka *et al.*, 2006).

(b) *Mutagenicity of acetaldehyde-derived DNA adducts*

The mutagenic potential of DNA adducts can be tested with single-stranded DNA vectors that contain a single adduct located within a reporter gene. These constructs can then be transfected into cells, allowed to replicate and the resulting replication products analysed for mutations in various ways, depending on the specific nature of the reporter gene. Using such an approach, the N^2EtdG adduct was only minimally mutagenic to the *supF* gene in the reporter plasmid pLSX (mean mutant fraction, 0.9 ± 0.2% for the adduct-containing construct versus 0.4 ± 0.2% for the lesion-free control) when replicated in *E. coli* ($P = 0.09$). When deoxyuridines were placed on the complementary strand at 5′ and 3′ positions flanking the adduct, the mutant fractions increased to 1.4 ± 0.5% for the lesion versus 0.6 ± 4% for the control ($P = 0.04$) (Upton *et al.*, 2006). The mutation spectrum generated by the N^2EtdG adduct included mainly G to T transversions and single base deletions three bases downstream from the adduct. [This study was carried out with N^2EtdG, whereas, *in vivo*, most probably N^2EtidG is formed predominantly.]

Two separate studies have shown that methylhydroxypropano-dG adducts result in mutant fractions of 5–11% when inserted into a shuttle vector and replicated in either monkey kidney cells (Fernandes *et al.*, 2005) or human xeroderma pigmentosum A (XPA) cells (Stein *et al.*, 2006). In both cases, the predominant mutagenic event observed was a G to T transversion, but G to A and G to C mutations were also found. In comparison, the ethenodeoxyadenosine adduct resulted in mutant fractions as a high as 70% in COS7 monkey kidney cells (Pandya & Moriya, 1996), but the mutant fraction was only 7–14% in human cells (Levine *et al.*, 2000). [Methodological differences, differences in the host cells used or in the local sequence in the shuttle vectors may be responsible for the results.]

An important feature of the methylhydroxypropano-dG adducts, which is not shared by N^2EtidG or N^2EtdG, is that these adducts can undergo ring-opening when located in double-stranded DNA (Mao *et al.*, 1999). The ring-opened forms of the methylhydroxypropano-dG adducts can react with proteins to generate DNA–protein crosslinks (Kurtz & Lloyd, 2003). With a deoxyguanosine residue in the opposite strand of the helix, a DNA-intrastrand crosslink can be formed (Wang *et al.*, 2000). Intrastrand crosslinks generated in this manner are also mutagenic (mutant fraction 3–6%) in mammalian cells, generating

Fig. 4.2 Structure of acetaldehyde-derived DNA adducts

a)

Reduction

N^2EtidG

N^2EtdG

b)

N^2-Dio-dG

α-*S*-Me-γ-OH-PdG

α-*R*-Me-γ-OH-PdG

c)

ICL-R

ICL-S

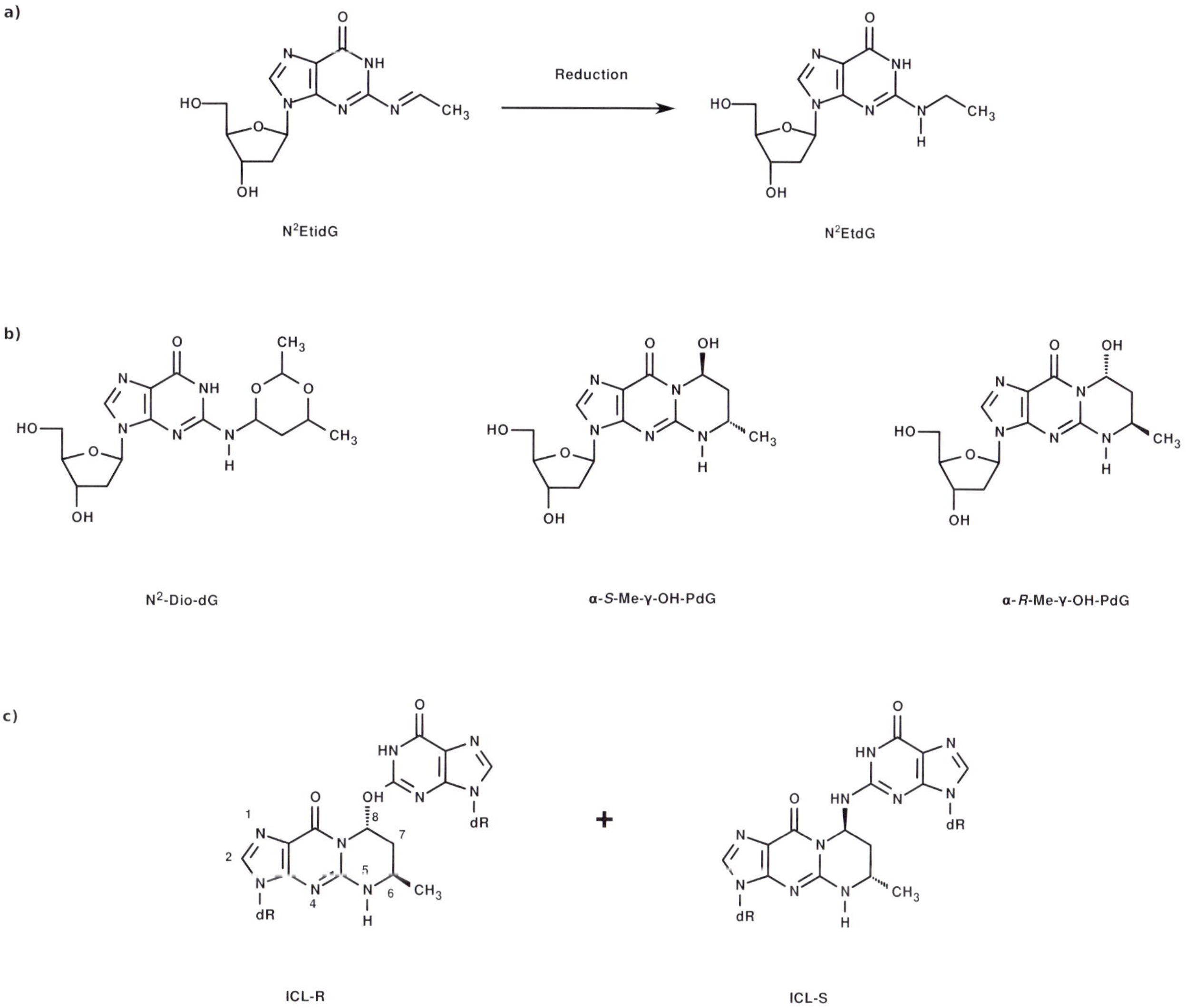

a) The immediate reaction of acetaldehyde with DNA is the unstable Schiff base adduct, N^2-ethylidene-2-deoxyguanosine (N^2EtidG). This adduct is reduced into the more stable N^2-ethyl-2-deoxyguanosine (N^2EtdG), the most abundant acetaldehyde-derived DNA adduct.
b) Three additional acetaldehyde-derived DNA adducts: N^2-(2,6-dimethyl-1,3-dioxan-4yl) deoxyguanosine (N^2-Dio-dG) and the two diastereisomers (R and S) of α-methyl-8-hydroxy-1,N^2-propanodeoxyguanosine (α-Me-γ-OH-PdG).
c) Structure of R and S interstrand crosslinks (ICL-R) and ICL-R).
Adapted from Wang *et al.* (2006c) and Matsuda *et al.* (2006).

primarily G to T transversions, as well as deletion and insertion mutations (Liu *et al.*, 2006). Matsuda *et al.* (1998) exposed plasmid DNA that contains a *supF* mutation reporter gene to acetaldehyde concentrations up to 1M, and allowed the plasmid to replicate in human XPA cells, which are deficient in nucleotide excision repair. In contrast to the results for the methylhydroxypropano-dG adducts, these authors observed specific tandem GG to TT mutations. The DNA lesions responsible for these mutations are most probably not propano-dG adducts, but the intrastrand crosslinks.

4.3 Synthesis: Mechanistic considerations

Although alcoholic beverages may contain several potentially carcinogenic compounds, this synthesis focuses on the role of ethanol and acetaldehyde in the carcinogenesis associated with alcoholic beverages.

4.3.1 Ethanol-related mechanisms of carcinogenesis

The role of ethanol metabolism in tumour initiation is implied by the associations observed between different forms of cancer and polymorphisms in genes involved in the oxidation of ethanol. Whether, or to what degree, these associations are explained by redox changes, formation of radicals, effects on intermediary metabolism and/or effects on other pro-carcinogens cannot be established from current findings.

(a) Oxidative stress

Ethanol-induced CYP2E1 produces various reactive oxygen species, which lead to the formation of lipid peroxidation products such as 4-hydroxy-nonenal and the condition of oxidative stress. Chronic tissue inflammation and increased iron content exacerbate these actions. The increased reactive oxygen species and oxidative stress, which damage the DNA and affect its repair, has been associated with ethanol-induced carcinogenesis in many organs, such as the breast, liver and pancreas.

(b) Cirrhosis

Ethanol causes hepatocellular injury that can lead to enhanced fibrogenesis and finally cirrhosis. Liver cirrhosis is strongly associated with an increased risk for developing hepatocellular carcinoma. Ethanol-related hepatocellular carcinoma without pre-existing cirrhosis is rare, which indicates that the pathogenic events that lead to cirrhosis precede those that cause cancer, or that the structural alterations in the liver during cirrhosis, together with other factors, favour the transformation of hepatocytes.

(c) Interaction between alcohol and tobacco smoking

This aspect is discussed in Section 4 of the *Monograph* on Tobacco Smoking in this Volume.

(d) Ethanol and sex hormones

Estrogens and androgens are well known activators of cellular proliferation, which is associated with an increased risk for carcinogenesis. Alcoholic beverage consumption in women causes an increase in the levels of estrogen and androgen, which has been suggested to contribute to the development of breast cancer. ADH-mediated alcohol oxidation, which increases the hepatic redox state, which in turn inhibits catabolism of sex steroids, has been suggested as the mechanism for the alcohol-mediated elevation in steroid levels.

(e) Folate metabolism and DNA methylation

Folate deficiency is associated with different forms of cancer, of which cancer of the colon is the most common. Ethanol per se, and an underlying unhealthy lifestyle associated with high alcoholic beverage consumption, cause folate deficiency. Several studies have shown interactions between alcohol use and polymorphisms of genes involved in folate metabolism in determining the risk for colon cancer and other cancers. The degree to which the relation between alcohol drinking, folate deficiency and cancer may be explained by the metabolism of ethanol is not known.

Other postulated modes of action of ethanol relevant to its carcinogenicity, such as tumour promotion, induction of the formation of polyunsaturated fatty acids, overproduction of mitogen-activated protein kinases, and effects on vitamin A (retinol) or insulin-like growth factors have not been rigorously established by published studies.

4.3.2 The role of acetaldehyde in alcohol-induced carcinogenesis

Over the past decade, epidemiological evidence of enhanced cancer risks among heterozygous carriers of the inactive ALDH enzyme has become much stronger, in particular for oesophageal cancer: practically all studies conducted in East-Asian populations who consumed alcoholic beverages show significantly increased odds ratios for carriers of the inactive ALDH allele. In addition, several studies have demonstrated associations between the polymorphism of ADH1B and upper aerodigestive tract cancers, which have been explained either by more active ADH producing more acetaldehyde or by less active ADH causing prolonged exposure to lower levels of ethanol-derived acetaldehyde. These data imply that acetaldehyde is the key compound in the development of cancers of the oesophagus and other upper aerodigestive tract cancers associated with alcoholic beverage consumption. The considerations that support this suggestion are:

1. there is an established causal relationship between alcoholic beverage consumption and cancers of the oesophagus, oral cavity, pharynx and larynx;
2. it is generally accepted that ethanol in alcoholic beverages is the principal ingredient that renders these beverages carcinogenic;
3. in the body, ethanol is converted by ADH and CYP2E1 to acetaldehyde, which is oxidized by ALDH to acetate;
4. the formation of acetaldehyde starts in the mouth, mediated mostly by oral bacteria, and continues along the digestive tract;
5. the main production of acetaldehyde occurs in the liver and in the gut. However, the highest levels of acetaldehyde after consumption of alcoholic beverages are found in the saliva of the oral cavity, which is in the vicinity of the target organ sites known to be susceptible to ethanol-induced cancer.
6. the upper digestive tract is also the site that is in first contact with the acetaldehyde content of the alcoholic beverages, which in turn are known to increase the salivary acetaldehyde levels;
7. acetaldehyde is a cytotoxic, genotoxic, mutagenic and clastogenic compound. It is carcinogenic in experimental animals;
8. after alcoholic beverage consumption, carriers of an inactive allele of the ALDH2 enzyme show accumulating levels of acetaldehyde in the peripheral blood, a direct consequence of their enzyme deficiency, and show increased levels of N^2EtdG and methylhydroxypropano-dG adducts in lymphocyte DNA. The latter adducts have been shown to be formed from acetaldehyde; during DNA replication, these methylhydroxypropano-dG adducts cause mutations;
9. consumers of alcoholic beverages have a higher frequency of chromosomal aberrations, sister chromatid exchange and micronucleus formation in the peripheral lymphocytes than non-consumers. These effects may be attributable to acetaldehyde, which is a clastogen;
10. several of the observations made in ALDH2-deficient individuals have been confirmed in ALDH2-knockout mice.

5. Evaluation

There is *sufficient evidence* in humans for the carcinogenicity of alcohol consumption. Alcohol consumption causes cancers of the oral cavity, pharynx, larynx, oesophagus, colorectum, liver (hepatocellular carcinoma) and female breast. Also, an association has been observed between alcohol consumption and cancer of the pancreas.

For cancer of the kidney and non-Hodgkin lymphoma, there is *evidence suggesting lack of carcinogenicity.*

There is *sufficient evidence* in humans for the carcinogenicity of acetaldehyde associated with the consumption of alcoholic beverages. Acetaldehyde associated with the consumption of alcoholic beverages causes cancers of the oesophagus and of upper aerodigestive tract combined.

There is *sufficient evidence* in experimental animals for the carcinogenicity of ethanol.

There is *sufficient evidence* in experimental animals for the carcinogenicity of acetaldehyde.

Alcohol consumption is *carcinogenic to humans (Group 1).*

Ethanol in alcoholic beverages is *carcinogenic to humans (Group 1).*

Acetaldehyde associated with the consumption of alcoholic beverages is *carcinogenic to humans (Group 1).*

In reaching the second and third evaluations, the Working Group took the following into consideration:

- The epidemiological evidence of the carcinogenicity of alcoholic beverage consumption shows little indication that the carcinogenic effects depend on the type of alcoholic beverage, with ethanol being the common ingredient.
- Upon ingestion of alcoholic beverages, ethanol is converted into acetaldehyde, which is then oxidized to acetate.
- Ethanol and acetaldehyde are both carcinogenic in experimental animals.
- There is sufficient epidemiological evidence showing that humans who are deficient in the oxidation of acetaldehyde to acetate have a substantially increased risk for development of alcohol-related cancers, in particular of the oesophagus and the upper aerodigestive tract.

References

Adami HO, McLaughlin JK, Hsing AW *et al.* (1992). Alcoholism and cancer risk: a population-based cohort study. *Cancer Causes Control*, 3: 419–425. doi:10.1007/BF00051354 PMID:1525322

Akhter M, Kuriyama S, Nakaya N *et al.* (2007). Alcohol consumption is associated with an increased risk of distal colon and rectal cancer in Japanese men: the Miyagi Cohort Study. *Eur J Cancer*, 43: 383–390. doi:10.1016/j.ejca.2006.09.020 PMID:17150353

Allen NE, Beral V, Casabonne D *et al.*Million Women Study Collaborators (2009). Moderate alcohol intake and cancer incidence in women. *J Natl Cancer Inst*, 101: 296–305. doi:10.1093/jnci/djn514 PMID:19244173

Altieri A, Bosetti C, Talamini R *et al.* (2002). Cessation of smoking and drinking and the risk of laryngeal cancer. *Br J Cancer*, 87: 1227–1229. doi:10.1038/sj.bjc.6600638 PMID:12439710

Anderson LM, Carter JP, Driver CL *et al.* (1993). Enhancement of tumorigenesis by N-nitrosodiethylamine, N-nitrosopyrrolidine and N6-(methylnitroso)-adenosine by ethanol. *Cancer Lett*, 68: 61–66. doi:10.1016/0304-3835(93)90220-4 PMID:8422650

Anderson LN, Cotterchio M, Gallinger S (2009). Lifestyle, dietary, and medical history factors associated with pancreatic cancer risk in Ontario, Canada. *Cancer Causes Control*, 20: 825–834. doi:10.1007/s10552-009-9303-5 PMID:19194662

Ansems TM, van der Pols JC, Hughes MC *et al.* (2008). Alcohol intake and risk of skin cancer: a prospective study. *Eur J Clin Nutr*, 62: 162–170. doi:10.1038/sj.ejcn.1602717 PMID:17392700

Anwar WA, Abdel-Rahman SZ, El-Zein RA *et al.* (1996). Genetic polymorphism of GSTM1, CYP2E1 and CYP2D6 in Egyptian bladder cancer patients. *Carcinogenesis*, 17: 1923–1929. doi:10.1093/carcin/17.9.1923 PMID:8824515

Arndt M, Rydzanicz M, Pabiszczak M *et al.* (2008). [Distribution of alcohol dehydrogenase (ADH1C) genotypes in subjects with tobacco smoke-associated laryngeal cancer] *Przegl Lek*, 65: 466–469. PMID:19189524

Asakage T, Yokoyama A, Haneda T *et al.* (2007). Genetic polymorphisms of alcohol and aldehyde dehydrogenases, and drinking, smoking and diet in Japanese men with oral and pharyngeal squamous cell carcinoma. *Carcinogenesis*, 28: 865–874. doi:10.1093/carcin/bgl206 PMID:17071628

Austin H, Drews C, Partridge EE (1993). A case-control study of endometrial cancer in relation to cigarette smoking, serum estrogen levels, and alcohol use. *Am J Obstet Gynecol*, 169: 1086–1091. PMID:8238164

Aze Y, Toyoda K, Furukawa F *et al.* (1993). Enhancing effect of ethanol on esophageal tumor development in rats by initiation of diethylnitrosamine. *Carcinogenesis*, 14: 37–40. doi:10.1093/carcin/14.1.37 PMID:8425269

Baglietto L, Severi G, English DR *et al.* (2006). Alcohol consumption and prostate cancer risk: results from the Melbourne collaborative cohort study. *Int J Cancer*, 119: 1501–1504. doi:10.1002/ijc.21983 PMID:16615108

Bagnardi V, Blangiardo M, La Vecchia C, Corrao G (2001). A meta-analysis of alcohol drinking and cancer risk. *Br J Cancer*, 85: 1700–1705. doi:10.1054/bjoc.2001.2140 PMID:11742491

Balbo S, Hashibe M, Gundy S *et al.* (2008). N2-ethyldeoxyguanosine as a potential biomarker for assessing effects of alcohol consumption on DNA. *Cancer Epidemiol Biomarkers Prev*, 17: 3026–3032. doi:10.1158/1055-9965.EPI-08-0117 PMID:18990745

Balder HF, Goldbohm RA, van den Brandt PA (2005). Dietary patterns associated with male lung cancer risk in the Netherlands Cohort Study. *Cancer Epidemiol Biomarkers Prev*, 14: 483–490. doi:10.1158/1055-9965.EPI-04-0353 PMID:15734976

Bandera EV, Freudenheim JL, Graham S *et al.* (1992). Alcohol consumption and lung cancer in white males. *Cancer Causes Control*, 3: 361–369. doi:10.1007/BF00146890 PMID:1617124

Bandera EV, Freudenheim JL, Marshall JR *et al.* (1997). Diet and alcohol consumption and lung cancer risk in the New York State Cohort (United States) *Cancer Causes Control*, 8: 828–840. doi:10.1023/A:1018456127018 PMID:9427425

Beji NK & Reis N (2007). Risk factors for breast cancer in Turkish women: a hospital-based case-control study. *Eur J Cancer Care (Engl)*, 16: 178–184. doi:10.1111/j.1365-2354.2006.00711.x PMID:17371428

Beland FA, Benson RW, Mellick PW *et al.* (2005). Effect of ethanol on the tumorigenicity of urethane (ethyl carbamate) in B6C3F1 mice. *Food Chem Toxicol*, 43: 1–19. doi:10.1016/j.fct.2004.07.018 PMID:15582191

Benedetti A, Parent ME, Siemiatycki J (2006). Consumption of alcoholic beverages and risk of lung cancer: results from two case-control studies in Montreal, Canada. *Cancer Causes Control*, 17: 469–480. doi:10.1007/s10552-005-0496-y PMID:16596299

Benedetti A, Parent ME, Siemiatycki J (2009). Lifetime consumption of alcoholic beverages and risk of 13 types of cancer in men: results from a case-control study in Montreal. *Cancer Detect Prev*, 32: 352–362. doi:10.1016/j.canep.2009.03.001 PMID:19588541

Bernstein JL, Thompson WD, Risch N, Holford TR (1992). Risk factors predicting the incidence of second primary breast cancer among women diagnosed with a first primary breast cancer. *Am J Epidemiol*, 136: 925–936. PMID:1456269

Berstad P, Ma H, Bernstein L, Ursin G (2008). Alcohol intake and breast cancer risk among young women. *Breast Cancer Res Treat*, 108: 113–120. doi:10.1007/s10549-007-9578-8 PMID:17468952

Bessaoud F & Daurès JP (2008). Patterns of alcohol (especially wine) consumption and breast cancer risk: a case-control study among a population in Southern France. *Ann Epidemiol*, 18: 467–475. doi:10.1016/j.annepidem.2008.02.001 PMID:18440826

Besson H, Brennan P, Becker N *et al.* (2006a). Tobacco smoking, alcohol drinking and Hodgkin's lymphoma: a European multi-centre case-control study (EPILYMPH). *Br J Cancer*, 95: 378–384. doi:10.1038/sj.bjc.6603229 PMID:16819547

Besson H, Brennan P, Becker N *et al.* (2006b). Tobacco smoking, alcohol drinking and non-Hodgkin's lymphoma: A European multicenter case-control study (Epilymph). *Int J Cancer*, 119: 901–908. doi:10.1002/ijc.21913 PMID:16557575

Bianchini F, Jaeckel A, Vineis P *et al.* (2001). Inverse correlation between alcohol consumption and lymphocyte levels of 8-hydroxydeoxyguanosine in humans. *Carcinogenesis*, 22: 885–890. doi:10.1093/carcin/22.6.885 PMID:11375894

Birley AJ, James MR, Dickson PA *et al.* (2009). ADH single nucleotide polymorphism associations with alcohol metabolism in vivo. *Hum Mol Genet*, 18: 1533–1542. doi:10.1093/hmg/ddp060 PMID:19193628

Blasiak J, Trzeciak A, Malecka-Panas E *et al.* (2000). In vitro genotoxicity of ethanol and acetaldehyde in human lymphocytes and the gastrointestinal tract mucosa cells. *Toxicol In Vitro*, 14: 287–295. doi:10.1016/S0887-2333(00)00022-9 PMID:10906435

Boccia S, Sayed-Tabatabaei FA, Persiani R *et al.* (2007). Polymorphisms in metabolic genes, their combination and interaction with tobacco smoke and alcohol consumption and risk of gastric cancer: a case-control study in an Italian population. *BMC Cancer*, 7: 206 doi:10.1186/1471-2407-7-206 PMID:17996038

Boccia S, Cadoni G, Sayed-Tabatabaei FA *et al.* (2008). CYP1A1, CYP2E1, GSTM1, GSTT1, EPHX1 exons 3 and 4, and NAT2 polymorphisms, smoking, consumption of alcohol and fruit and vegetables and risk of head and neck cancer. *J Cancer Res Clin Oncol*, 134: 93–100. doi:10.1007/s00432-007-0254-5 PMID:17611777

Boccia S, Hashibe M, Gallì P *et al.* (2009). Aldehyde dehydrogenase 2 and head and neck cancer: a meta-analysis implementing a Mendelian randomization approach. *Cancer Epidemiol Biomarkers Prev*, 18: 248–254. doi:10.1158/1055-9965.EPI-08-0462 PMID:19124505

Boffetta P, Stellman SD, Garfinkel L (1989). A case-control study of multiple myeloma nested in the American Cancer Society prospective study. *Int J Cancer*, 43: 554–559. doi:10.1002/ijc.2910430404 PMID:2703267

Boffetta P, Ye W, Adami H-O *et al.* (2001). Risk of cancers of the lung, head and neck in patients hospitalized for alcoholism in Sweden. *Br J Cancer*, 85: 678–682. doi:10.1054/bjoc.2001.1986 PMID:11531251

Bongaerts BW, de Goeij AF, van den Brandt PA, Weijenberg MP (2006). Alcohol and the risk of colon and rectal cancer with mutations in the K-ras gene. *Alcohol*, 38: 147–154. doi:10.1016/j.alcohol.2006.06.003 PMID:16905440

Bongaerts BW, van den Brandt PA, Goldbohm RA *et al.* (2008). Alcohol consumption, type of alcoholic beverage and risk of colorectal cancer at specific subsites. *Int J Cancer*, 123: 2411–2417. doi:10.1002/ijc.23774 PMID:18752250

Boonyaphiphat P, Thongsuksai P, Sriplung H, Puttawibul P (2002). Lifestyle habits and genetic susceptibility and the risk of esophageal cancer in the Thai population. *Cancer Lett*, 186: 193–199. doi:10.1016/S0304-3835(02)00354-3 PMID:12213289

Bosron WF & Li TK (1986). Genetic polymorphism of human liver alcohol and aldehyde dehydrogenases, and their relationship to alcohol metabolism and alcoholism. *Hepatology*, 6: 502–510. doi:10.1002/hep.1840060330 PMID:3519419

Bouchardy C, Hirvonen A, Coutelle C *et al.* (2000). Role of alcohol dehydrogenase 3 and cytochrome P-4502E1 genotypes in susceptibility to cancers of the upper aerodigestive tract. *Int J Cancer*, 87: 734–740. doi:10.1002/1097-0215(20000901)87:5<734::AID-IJC17>3.0.CO;2-E PMID:10925369

Bradford BU, Kono H, Isayama F *et al.* (2005). Cytochrome P450 CYP2E1, but not nicotinamide adenine dinucleotide phosphate oxidase, is required for ethanol-induced oxidative DNA damage in rodent liver. *Hepatology*, 41: 336–344. doi:10.1002/hep.20532 PMID:15660387

Breast Cancer Association Consortium (2006). Commonly studied single-nucleotide polymorphisms and breast cancer: results from the Breast Cancer Association Consortium. *J Natl Cancer Inst*, 98: 1382–1396. doi:10.1093/jnci/djj374 PMID:17018785

Brennan P, Lewis S, Hashibe M *et al.* (2004). Pooled analysis of alcohol dehydrogenase genotypes and head and neck cancer: a HuGE review. *Am J Epidemiol*, 159: 1–16. doi:10.1093/aje/kwh003 PMID:14693654

Breslow RA, Graubard BI, Sinha R, Subar AF (2000). Diet and lung cancer mortality: a 1987 National Health Interview Survey cohort study. *Cancer Causes Control*, 11: 419–431. doi:10.1023/A:1008996208313 PMID:10877335

Briggs NC, Levine RS, Bobo LD *et al.* (2002). Wine drinking and risk of non-Hodgkin's lymphoma among men in the United States: a population-based case-control study. *Am J Epidemiol*, 156: 454–462. doi:10.1093/aje/kwf058 PMID:12196315

Brinton LA, Carreon JD, Gierach GL *et al.* (2009). Etiologic factors for male breast cancer in the U.S. Veterans Affairs medical care system database. *Breast Cancer Res Treat*, In press PMID:19330525

Brinton LA, Richesson DA, Gierach GL *et al.* (2008). Prospective evaluation of risk factors for male breast cancer. *J Natl Cancer Inst*, 100: 1477–1481. doi:10.1093/jnci/djn329 PMID:18840816

Brockmöller J, Cascorbi I, Kerb R, Roots I (1996). Combined analysis of inherited polymorphisms in arylamine N-acetyltransferase 2, glutathione S-transferases M1 and T1, microsomal epoxide hydrolase, and cytochrome P450 enzymes as modulators of bladder cancer risk. *Cancer Res*, 56: 3915–3925. PMID:8752158

Brown LM, Gibson R, Burmeister LF *et al.* (1992). Alcohol consumption and risk of leukemia, non-Hodgkin's lymphoma, and multiple myeloma. *Leuk Res*, 16: 979–984. doi:10.1016/0145-2126(92)90077-K PMID:1405712

Brown LM, Gridley G, Wu AH *et al.* (2010). Low level alcohol intake, cigarette smoking and risk of breast cancer in Asian-American women *Breast Cancer Res Treat*, 120: 203–210. doi:10.1007/s10549-009-0464-4 PMID:19597702

Brown LM, Pottern LM, Silverman DT *et al.* (1997). Multiple myeloma among Blacks and Whites in the United States: role of cigarettes and alcoholic beverages. *Cancer Causes Control*, 8: 610–614. doi:10.1023/A:1018498414298 PMID:9242477

Buch SC, Nazar-Stewart V, Weissfeld JL, Romkes M (2008). Case-control study of oral and oropharyngeal cancer in whites and genetic variation in eight metabolic enzymes. *Head Neck*, 30: 1139–1147. doi:10.1002/hed.20867 PMID:18642288

Burim RV, Canalle R, Takahashi CS *et al.* (2004). Clastogenic effect of ethanol in chronic and abstinent alcoholics. *Mutat Res*, 560: 187–198. PMID:15157656

Byers T, Marshall J, Graham S *et al.* (1983). A case-control study of dietary and nondietary factors in ovarian cancer. *J Natl Cancer Inst*, 71: 681–686. PMID:6578362

Cahill A, Hershman S, Davies A, Sykora P (2005). Ethanol feeding enhances age-related deterioration of the rat hepatic mitochondrion. *Am J Physiol Gastrointest Liver Physiol*, 289: G1115–G1123. doi:10.1152/ajpgi.00193.2005 PMID:16020655

Cahill A, Wang X, Hoek JB (1997). Increased oxidative damage to mitochondrial DNA following chronic ethanol consumption. *Biochem Biophys Res Commun*, 235: 286–290. doi:10.1006/bbrc.1997.6774 PMID:9199183

Cai L, You NC, Lu H *et al.* (2006). Dietary selenium intake, aldehyde dehydrogenase-2 and X-ray repair cross-complementing 1 genetic polymorphisms, and the risk of esophageal squamous cell carcinoma. *Cancer*, 106: 2345–2354. doi:10.1002/cncr.21881 PMID:16639733

Cai L, Yu SZ, Zhan ZF (2001). Cytochrome P450 2E1 genetic polymorphism and gastric cancer in Changle, Fujian Province. *World J Gastroenterol*, 7: 792–795. PMID:11854903

Cao W, Cai L, Rao JY *et al.* (2005). Tobacco smoking, GSTP1 polymorphism, and bladder carcinoma. *Cancer*, 104: 2400–2408. doi:10.1002/cncr.21446 PMID:16240451

Caro AA & Cederbaum AI (2004). Oxidative stress, toxicology, and pharmacology of CYP2E1. *Annu Rev Pharmacol Toxicol*, 44: 27–42. doi:10.1146/annurev.pharmtox.44.101802.121704 PMID:14744237

Carpenter CL, Morgenstern H, London SJ (1998). Alcoholic beverage consumption and lung cancer risk among residents of Los Angeles County. *J Nutr*, 128: 694–700. PMID:9521630

Carrière V, Berthou F, Baird S *et al.* (1996). Human cytochrome P4502E1 (CYP2E1): from genotype to phenotype. *Pharmacogenetics*, 6: 203–211. doi:10.1097/00008571-199606000-00002 PMID:8807659

Carstensen JM, Bygren LO, Hatschek T (1990). Cancer incidence among Swedish brewery workers. *Int J Cancer*, 45: 393–396. doi:10.1002/ijc.2910450302 PMID:2407667

Cartwright RA, McKinney PA, O'Brien C *et al.* (1988). Non-Hodgkin's lymphoma: case control epidemiological study in Yorkshire. *Leuk Res*, 12: 81–88. doi:10.1016/S0145-2126(98)80012-X PMID:3357350

Casey R, Piazzon-Fevre K, Raverdy N *et al.* (2007). Case-control study of lymphoid neoplasm in three French areas: description, alcohol and tobacco consumption. *Eur J Cancer Prev*, 16: 142–150. doi:10.1097/01.cej.0000220629.00729.65 PMID:17297390

Castelli E, Hrelia P, Maffei F *et al.* (1999). Indicators of genetic damage in alcoholics: reversibility after alcohol abstinence. *Hepatogastroenterology*, 46: 1664–1668. PMID:10430317

Chalasani N, Baluyut A, Ismail A *et al.* (2000). Cholangiocarcinoma in patients with primary sclerosing cholangitis: a multicenter case-control study. Hepatology (Baltimore) *MD*, 31: 7–11.

Chang ET, Canchola AJ, Lee VS *et al.* (2007). Wine and other alcohol consumption and risk of ovarian cancer in the California Teachers Study cohort. *Cancer Causes Control*, 18: 91–103. doi:10.1007/s10552-006-0083-x PMID:17186425

Chang ET, Hedelin M, Adami HO *et al.* (2005). Alcohol drinking and risk of localized versus advanced and sporadic versus familial prostate cancer in Sweden. *Cancer Causes Control*, 16: 275–284. doi:10.1007/s10552-004-3364-2 PMID:15947879

Chang ET, Smedby KE, Zhang SM *et al.* (2004). Alcohol intake and risk of non-Hodgkin lymphoma in men and women. *Cancer Causes Control*, 15: 1067–1076. doi:10.1007/s10552-004-2234-2 PMID:15801490

Chao C (2007). Associations between beer, wine, and liquor consumption and lung cancer risk: a meta-analysis. *Cancer Epidemiol Biomarkers Prev*, 16: 2436–2447. doi:10.1158/1055-9965.EPI-07-0386 PMID:18006934

Chao C, Haque R, Van Den Eeden SK *et al.* (2010). Red wine consumption and risk of prostate cancer: the California men's health study. *Int J Cancer*, 126: 171–179. doi:10.1002/ijc.24637 PMID:19521962

Chao C, Slezak JM, Caan BJ, Quinn VP (2008). Alcoholic beverage intake and risk of lung cancer: the California Men's Health Study. *Cancer Epidemiol Biomarkers Prev*, 17: 2692–2699. doi:10.1158/1055-9965.EPI-08-0410 PMID:18843011

Chao YC, Wang LS, Hsieh TY *et al.* (2000). Chinese alcoholic patients with esophageal cancer are genetically different from alcoholics with acute pancreatitis and liver cirrhosis. *Am J Gastroenterol*, 95: 2958–2964. doi:10.1111/j.1572-0241.2000.02328.x PMID:11051375

Chiaffarino F, Gallus S, Negri E *et al.* (2002). Correspondence re: Weiderpass *et al.*, Alcoholism and risk of cancer of cervix uteri, vagina, and vulva. Cancer Epidemiol. Biomark. Prev., 10: 899–901, 2001. *Cancer Epidemiol Biomarkers Prev*, 11: 325–326. PMID:11895888

Chiang CP, Wu CW, Lee SP *et al.* (2009). Expression pattern, ethanol-metabolizing activities, and cellular localization of alcohol and aldehyde dehydrogenases in human pancreas: implications for pathogenesis of alcohol-induced pancreatic injury. *Alcohol Clin Exp Res*, 33: 1059–1068. doi:10.1111/j.1530-0277.2009.00927.x PMID:19382905

Chiu BC, Weisenburger DD, Cantor KP *et al.* (2002). Alcohol consumption, family history of hematolymphoproliferative cancer, and the risk of non-Hodgkin's lymphoma in men. *Ann Epidemiol*, 12: 309–315. doi:10.1016/S1047-2797(01)00259-9 PMID:12062917

Chiu BC-H, Cerhan JR, Gapstur SM *et al.* (1999). Alcohol consumption and non-Hodgkin lymphoma in a cohort of older women. *Br J Cancer*, 80: 1476–1482. doi:10.1038/sj.bjc.6690547 PMID:10424754

Chlebowski RT, Anderson GL, Lane DS *et al.*Women's Health Initiative Investigators (2007). Predicting risk of breast cancer in postmenopausal women by hormone receptor status. *J Natl Cancer Inst*, 99: 1695–1705. doi:10.1093/jnci/djm224 PMID:18000216

Cho E, Smith-Warner SA, Ritz J *et al.* (2004). Alcohol intake and colorectal cancer: a pooled analysis of

8 cohort studies. *Ann Intern Med*, 140: 603–613. PMID:15096331

Choi JY, Abel J, Neuhaus T *et al.* (2003). Role of alcohol and genetic polymorphisms of CYP2E1 and ALDH2 in breast cancer development. *Pharmacogenetics*, 13: 67–72. doi:10.1097/00008571-200302000-00002 PMID:12563175

Chow WH, Schuman LM, McLaughlin JK *et al.* (1992). A cohort study of tobacco use, diet, occupation, and lung cancer mortality. *Cancer Causes Control*, 3: 247–254. doi:10.1007/BF00124258 PMID:1610971

Cohen G, Sinet PM, Heikkila R (1980). Ethanol oxidation by rat brain in vivo. *Alcohol Clin Exp Res*, 4: 366–370. doi:10.1111/j.1530-0277.1980.tb04833.x PMID:7004234

Coutelle C, Höhn B, Benesova M *et al.* (2004). Risk factors in alcohol associated breast cancer: alcohol dehydrogenase polymorphism and estrogens. *Int J Oncol*, 25: 1127–1132. PMID:15375565

Coutelle C, Ward PJ, Fleury B *et al.* (1997). Laryngeal and oropharyngeal cancer, and alcohol dehydrogenase 3 and glutathione S-transferase M1 polymorphisms. *Hum Genet*, 99: 319–325. doi:10.1007/s004390050365 PMID:9050916

Covolo L, Gelatti U, Talamini R *et al.* (2005). Alcohol dehydrogenase 3, glutathione S-transferase M1 and T1 polymorphisms, alcohol consumption and hepatocellular carcinoma (Italy). *Cancer Causes Control*, 16: 831–838. doi:10.1007/s10552-005-2302-2 PMID:16132793

Cox A, Dunning AM, Garcia-Closas M *et al.*Kathleen Cunningham Foundation Consortium for Research into Familial Breast Cancer; Breast Cancer Association Consortium (2007). A common coding variant in CASP8 is associated with breast cancer risk. *Nat Genet*, 39: 352–358. doi:10.1038/ng1981 PMID:17293864

Crabb DW (1995). Ethanol oxidizing enzymes: roles in alcohol metabolism and alcoholic liver disease. *Prog Liver Dis*, 13: 151–172. PMID:9224501

Crabb DW, Edenberg HJ, Bosron WF, Li TK (1989). Genotypes for aldehyde dehydrogenase deficiency and alcohol sensitivity. The inactive ALDH2(2) allele is dominant. *J Clin Invest*, 83: 314–316. doi:10.1172/JCI113875 PMID:2562960

Cui R, Kamatani Y, Takahashi A *et al.* (2009). Functional variants in ADH1B and ALDH2 coupled with alcohol and smoking synergistically enhance esophageal cancer risk. *Gastroenterology*, 137: 1768–1775. doi:10.1053/j.gastro.2009.07.070 PMID:19698717

Curtin K, Slattery ML, Ulrich CM *et al.* (2007). Genetic polymorphisms in one-carbon metabolism: associations with CpG island methylator phenotype (CIMP) in colon cancer and the modifying effects of diet. *Carcinogenesis*, 28: 1672–1679. doi:10.1093/carcin/bgm089 PMID:17449906

Cusimano R, Dardanoni G, Dardanoni L *et al.* (1989). Risk factors of female cancers in Ragusa population (Sicily)–1. Endometrium and cervix uteri cancers. *Eur J Epidemiol*, 5: 363–371. doi:10.1007/BF00144839 PMID:2792311

De Stefani E, Correa P, Deneo-Pellegrini H *et al.* (2002). Alcohol intake and risk of adenocarcinoma of the lung. A case-control study in Uruguay. *Lung Cancer*, 38: 9–14. doi:10.1016/S0169-5002(02)00153-8 PMID:12367787

De Stefani E, Correa P, Fierro L *et al.* (1993). The effect of alcohol on the risk of lung cancer in Uruguay. *Cancer Epidemiol Biomarkers Prev*, 2: 21–26. PMID:8380549

De Stefani E, Deneo-Pellegrini H, Boffetta P *et al.* (2009). Dietary patterns and risk of cancer: a factor analysis in Uruguay. *Int J Cancer*, 124: 1391–1397. doi:10.1002/ijc.24035 PMID:19058195

De Stefani E, Fierro L, Barrios E, Ronco A (1995). Tobacco, alcohol, diet and risk of prostate cancer. *Tumori*, 81: 315–320. PMID:8804446

De Stefani E, Fierro L, Barrios E, Ronco A (1998). Tobacco, alcohol, diet and risk of non-Hodgkin's lymphoma: a case-control study in Uruguay. *Leuk Res*, 22: 445–452. doi:10.1016/S0145-2126(97)00194-X PMID:9652731

De Torok D (1972). Chromosomal irregularities in alcoholics. *Ann N Y Acad Sci*, 197: 1 Nature and Nu90–100. doi:10.1111/j.1749-6632.1972.tb28125.x PMID:4504611

Deandrea S, Bertuccio P, Chatenoud L *et al.* (2007). Reply to 'Alcohol consumption and risk of Hodgkin's lymphoma and multiple myeloma: a multicentre case-control study' by Gorini *et al. Ann Oncol*, 18: 1119–1121. doi:10.1093/annonc/mdm203 PMID:17586754

Deandrea S, Talamini R, Foschi R *et al.* (2008). Alcohol and breast cancer risk defined by estrogen and progesterone receptor status: a case-control study. *Cancer Epidemiol Biomarkers Prev*, 17: 2025–2028. doi:10.1158/1055-9965.EPI-08-0157 PMID:18708394

Deitrich RA, Petersen D, Vasiliou V (2007). Removal of acetaldehyde from the body. *Novartis Found Symp*, 285: 23–40, discussion 40–51, 198–199. doi:10.1002/9780470511848.ch3 PMID:17590985

DeMaster EG, Redfern B, Weir K *et al.* (1983). Elimination of artifactual acetaldehyde in the measurement of human blood acetaldehyde by the use of polyethylene glycol and sodium azide: normal blood acetaldehyde levels in the dog and human after ethanol. *Alcohol Clin Exp Res*, 7: 436–442. doi:10.1111/j.1530-0277.1983.tb05502.x PMID:6362469

Dennis LK (2000). Meta-analysis for combining relative risks of alcohol consumption and prostate cancer. *Prostate*, 42: 56–66. doi:10.1002/(SICI)1097-0045(20000101)42:1<56::AID-PROS7>3.0.CO;2-P PMID:10579799

Diczfalusy MA, Björkhem I, Einarsson C *et al.* (2001). Characterization of enzymes involved in formation of ethyl esters of long-chain fatty acids in humans. *J Lipid Res*, 42: 1025–1032. PMID:11441128

Ding J, Li S, Wu J *et al.* (2008). Alcohol dehydrogenase-2 and aldehyde dehydrogenase-2 genotypes, alcohol drinking and the risk of primary hepatocellular carcinoma in a Chinese population. *Asian Pac J Cancer Prev*, 9: 31–35. PMID:18439068

Ding JH, Li SP, Cao HX *et al.* (2009). Polymorphisms of alcohol dehydrogenase-2 and aldehyde dehydrogenase-2 and esophageal cancer risk in Southeast Chinese males. *World J Gastroenterol*, 15: 2395–2400. doi:10.3748/wjg.15.2395 PMID:19452585

Djoussé L, Dorgan JF, Zhang Y *et al.* (2002). Alcohol consumption and risk of lung cancer: the Framingham Study. *J Natl Cancer Inst*, 94: 1877–1882. doi:10.1093/jnci/94.24.1877 PMID:12488481

Doll R, Peto R, Hall E *et al.* (1994). Mortality in relation to consumption of alcohol: 13 years' observations on male British doctors. *BMJ*, 309: 911–918. doi:10.1136/bmj.309.6959.911 PMID:7950661

Dolle JM, Daling JR, White E *et al.* (2009). Risk factors for triple-negative breast cancer in women under the age of 45 years. *Cancer Epidemiol Biomarkers Prev*, 18: 1157–1166. doi:10.1158/1055-9965.EPI-08-1005 PMID:19336554

Donato F, Gelatti U, Tagger A *et al.* (2001). Intrahepatic cholangiocarcinoma and hepatitis C and B virus infection, alcohol intake, and hepatolithiasis: a case-control study in Italy. *Cancer Causes Control*, 12: 959–964. doi:10.1023/A:1013747228572 PMID:11808716

Dosemeci M, Gokmen I, Unsal M *et al.* (1997). Tobacco, alcohol use, and risks of laryngeal and lung cancer by subsite and histologic type in Turkey. *Cancer Causes Control*, 8: 729–737. doi:10.1023/A:1018479304728 PMID:9328195

Duester G, Farrés J, Felder MR *et al.* (1999). Recommended nomenclature for the vertebrate alcohol dehydrogenase gene family. *Biochem Pharmacol*, 58: 389–395. doi:10.1016/S0006-2952(99)00065-9 PMID:10424757

Duffy CM, Assaf A, Cyr M *et al.* (2009). Alcohol and folate intake and breast cancer risk in the WHI Observational Study. *Breast Cancer Res Treat*, 116: 551–562. doi:10.1007/s10549-008-0167-2 PMID:18785003

Edenberg HJ (2007). The genetics of alcohol metabolism: role of alcohol dehydrogenase and aldehyde dehydrogenase variants. *Alcohol Res Health*, 30: 5–13. PMID:17718394

el-Zein R, Zwischenberger JB, Wood TG *et al.* (1997c). Combined genetic polymorphism and risk for development of lung cancer. *Mutat Res*, 381: 189–200. doi:10.1016/S0027-5107(97)00166-8 PMID:9434875

Engeland K & Maret W (1993). Extrahepatic, differential expression of four classes of human alcohol dehydrogenase. *Biochem Biophys Res Commun*, 193: 47–53. doi:10.1006/bbrc.1993.1588 PMID:8503936

Engeset D, Dyachenko A, Ciampi A, Lund E (2009). Dietary patterns and risk of cancer of various sites in the Norwegian European Prospective Investigation into Cancer and Nutrition cohort: the Norwegian Women and Cancer study. *Eur J Cancer Prev*, 18: 69–75. doi:10.1097/CEJ.0b013e328305a091 PMID:19077568

Eom SY, Zhang YW, Kim SH *et al.* (2009). Influence of NQO1, ALDH2, and CYP2E1 genetic polymorphisms, smoking, and alcohol drinking on the risk of lung cancer in Koreans. *Cancer Causes Control*, 20: 137–145. doi:10.1007/s10552-008-9225-7 PMID:18798003

Ericson U, Sonestedt E, Gullberg B *et al.* (2007). High folate intake is associated with lower breast cancer incidence in postmenopausal women in the Malmö Diet and Cancer cohort. *Am J Clin Nutr*, 86: 434–443. PMID:17684216

Eriksson CJP (1985). Endogenous acetaldehyde in rats. Effects of exogenous ethanol, pyrazole, cyanamide and disulfiram. *Biochem Pharmacol*, 34: 3979–3982. doi:10.1016/0006-2952(85)90375-2 PMID:4062972

Eriksson CJP (2001). The role of acetaldehyde in the actions of alcohol (update 2000). *Alcohol Clin Exp Res*,, 25: 15S–32S.

Eriksson CJP (2007). Measurement of acetaldehyde: what levels occur naturally and in response to alcohol? *Novartis Found Symp*, 285: 247–255, discussion 256–260. PMID:17590999

Eriksson CJP & Fukunaga T (1993). Human blood acetaldehyde (update 1992). *Alcohol Alcohol Suppl*, 2: Suppl.29–25. PMID:7748353

Eriksson CJP, Fukunaga T, Sarkola T *et al.* (1996). Estrogen-related acetaldehyde elevation in women during alcohol intoxication. *Alcohol Clin Exp Res*, 20: 1192–1195. doi:10.1111/j.1530-0277.1996.tb01110.x PMID:8904969

Estonius M, Svensson S, Höög JO (1996). Alcohol dehydrogenase in human tissues: localisation of transcripts coding for five classes of the enzyme. *FEBS Lett*, 397: 338–342. doi:10.1016/S0014-5793(96)01204-5 PMID:8955375

Fan C, Jin M, Chen K *et al.* (2007). Case-only study of interactions between metabolic enzymes and smoking in colorectal cancer. *BMC Cancer*, 7: 115 doi:10.1186/1471-2407-7-115 PMID:17603900

Fan L & Cai L (2009). [Meta-analysis on the relationship between alcohol consumption and lung cancer risk] *Wei Sheng Yan Jiu*, 38: 85–89. PMID:19267084

Fan Y, Yuan JM, Wang R *et al.* (2008). Alcohol, tobacco, and diet in relation to esophageal cancer: the Shanghai Cohort Study. *Nutr Cancer*, 60: 354–363. doi:10.1080/01635580701883011 PMID:18444169

Fang J-L & Vaca CE (1995). Development of a 32P-postlabelling method for the analysis of adducts arising through the reaction of acetaldehyde with 2′-deoxyguanosine-3′-monophosphate and DNA. *Carcinogenesis*, 16: 2177–2185. doi:10.1093/carcin/16.9.2177 PMID:7554072

Fang J-L & Vaca CE (1997). Detection of DNA adducts of acetaldehyde in peripheral white blood cells of alcohol abusers. *Carcinogenesis*, 18: 627–632. doi:10.1093/carcin/18.4.627 PMID:9111191

Farker K, Lehmann MH, Kästner R *et al.* (1998a). CYP2E1 genotyping in renal cell/urothelial cancer patients in comparison with control populations. *Int J Clin Pharmacol Ther*, 36: 463–468. PMID:9760005

Fernandes PH, Kanuri M, Nechev LV *et al.* (2005). Mammalian cell mutagenesis of the DNA adducts of vinyl chloride and crotonaldehyde. *Environ Mol Mutagen*, 45: 455–459. doi:10.1002/em.20117 PMID:15690339

Ferrari P, Jenab M, Norat T *et al.* (2007). Lifetime and baseline alcohol intake and risk of colon and rectal cancers in the European prospective investigation into cancer and nutrition (EPIC). *Int J Cancer*, 121: 2065–2072. doi:10.1002/ijc.22966 PMID:17640039

Folsom AR, Demissie Z, Harnack LIowa Women's Health Study (2003). Glycemic index, glycemic load, and incidence of endometrial cancer: the Iowa women's health study. *Nutr Cancer*, 46: 119–124. doi:10.1207/S15327914NC4602_03 PMID:14690786

Frank A, Seitz HK, Bartsch H *et al.* (2004). Immunohistochemical detection of 1,N6-ethenodeoxyadenosine in nuclei of human liver affected by diseases predisposing to hepato-carcinogenesis. *Carcinogenesis*, 25: 1027–1031. doi:10.1093/carcin/bgh089 PMID:14742317

Freedman ND, Abnet CC, Leitzmann MF *et al.* (2007). A prospective study of tobacco, alcohol, and the risk of esophageal and gastric cancer subtypes. *Am J Epidemiol*, 165: 1424–1433. doi:10.1093/aje/kwm051 PMID:17420181

Freedman ND, Abnet CC, Leitzmann MF *et al.* (2007a). A prospective study of tobacco, alcohol, and the risk of esophageal and gastric cancer subtypes. *Am J Epidemiol*, 165: 1424–1433. doi:10.1093/aje/kwm051 PMID:17420181

Freedman ND, Schatzkin A, Leitzmann MF *et al.* (2007b). Alcohol and head and neck cancer risk in a prospective study. *Br J Cancer*, 96: 1469–1474. PMID:17387340

Freudenheim JL, Ambrosone CB, Moysich KB *et al.* (1999). Alcohol dehydrogenase 3 genotype modification of the association of alcohol consumption with breast cancer risk. *Cancer Causes Control*, 10: 369–377. doi:10.1023/A:1008950717205 PMID:10530606

Freudenheim JL, Ram M, Nie J *et al.* (2003). Lung cancer in humans is not associated with lifetime total alcohol consumption or with genetic variation in alcohol dehydrogenase 3 (ADH3). *J Nutr*, 133: 3619-3624. PMID:14608084

Freudenheim JL, Ritz J, Smith-Warner SA *et al.* (2005). Alcohol consumption and risk of lung cancer: a pooled analysis of cohort studies. *Am J Clin Nutr*, 82: 657–667. PMID:16155281

Friberg E & Wolk A (2009). Long-term alcohol consumption and risk of endometrial cancer incidence: a prospective cohort study. *Cancer Epidemiol Biomarkers Prev*, 18: 355–358. doi:10.1158/1055-9965.EPI-08-0993 PMID:19124521

Friborg JT, Yuan JM, Wang R *et al.* (2007). A prospective study of tobacco and alcohol use as risk factors for pharyngeal carcinomas in Singapore Chinese. *Cancer*, 109: 1183–1191. doi:10.1002/cncr.22501 PMID:17315158

Gajalakshmi V, Hung RJ, Mathew A *et al.* (2003). Tobacco smoking and chewing, alcohol drinking and lung cancer risk among men in southern India. *Int J Cancer*, 107: 441–447. doi:10.1002/ijc.11377 PMID:14506745

Gallagher RP, Spinelli JJ, Elwood JM, Skippen DH (1983). Allergies and agricultural exposure as risk factors for multiple myeloma. *Br J Cancer*, 48: 853–857. doi:10.1038/bjc.1983.277 PMID:6652026

Gallus S, Foschi R, Talamini R *et al.* (2007). Risk factors for prostate cancer in men aged less than 60 years: a case-control study from Italy. *Urology*, 70: 1121–1126. doi:10.1016/j.urology.2007.07.020 PMID:18158031

Ganesh B, Talole SD, Dikshit R (2009). A case-control study on diet and colorectal cancer from Mumbai, India. *Cancer Epidemiol*, 33: 189–193. doi:10.1016/j.canep.2009.07.009 PMID:19717354

Gao C, Takezaki T, Wu J *et al.* (2002). Interaction between cytochrome P-450 2E1 polymorphisms and environmental factors with risk of esophageal and stomach cancers in Chinese. *Cancer Epidemiol Biomarkers Prev*, 11: 29–34. PMID:11815398

Gao CM, Takezaki T, Wu JZ *et al.* (2007). CYP2E1 Rsa I polymorphism impacts on risk of colorectal cancer association with smoking and alcohol drinking. *World J Gastroenterol*, 13: 5725–5730. PMID:17963298

Gao CM, Takezaki T, Wu JZ *et al.* (2008). Polymorphisms of alcohol dehydrogenase 2 and aldehyde dehydrogenase 2 and colorectal cancer risk in Chinese males. *World J Gastroenterol*, 14: 5078–5083. doi:10.3748/wjg.14.5078 PMID:18763293

Gapstur SM, Potter JD, Sellers TA *et al.* (1993). Alcohol consumption and postmenopausal endometrial cancer: results from the Iowa Women's Health Study. *Cancer Causes Control*, 4: 323–329. doi:10.1007/BF00051334 PMID:8347781

Garavello W, Bosetti C, Gallus S *et al.* (2006). Type of alcoholic beverage and the risk of laryngeal cancer. *Eur J Cancer Prev*, 15: 69–73. doi:10.1097/01.cej.0000186641.19872.04 PMID:16374233

Garte S & Crosti F (1999). A nomenclature system for metabolic gene polymorphisms. *IARC Sci Publ*, 1485–12. PMID:10493244

Garte S, Gaspari L, Alexandrie AK *et al.* (2001). Metabolic gene polymorphism frequencies in control populations. *Cancer Epidemiol Biomarkers Prev*, 10: 1239–1248. PMID:11751440

Gattás GJ & Saldanha PH (1997). Chromosomal aberrations in peripheral lymphocytes of abstinent alcoholics. *Alcohol Clin Exp Res*, 21: 238–243. doi:10.1111/j.1530-0277.1997.tb03755.x PMID:9113258

Gattás GJF, de Carvalho MB, Siraque MS *et al.* (2006). Genetic polymorphisms of CYP1A1, CYP2E1, GSTM1, and GSTT1 associated with head and neck cancer. *Head Neck*, 28: 819–826. doi:10.1002/hed.20410 PMID:16721740

Genkinger JM, Spiegelman D, Anderson KE *et al.* (2009). Alcohol intake and pancreatic cancer risk: a pooled analysis of fourteen cohort studies. *Cancer Epidemiol Biomarkers Prev*, 18: 765–776. doi:10.1158/1055-9965.EPI-08-0880 PMID:19258474

Gibson LJ, Hery C, Mitton N *et al.* (2009). Risk factors for breast cancer among Filipino women in Manila *Int J Cancer*, PMID:19626603

Giovannucci E, Chen J, Smith-Warner SA *et al.* (2003). Methylenetetrahydrofolate reductase, alcohol dehydrogenase, diet, and risk of colorectal adenomas. *Cancer Epidemiol Biomarkers Prev*, 12: 970–979. PMID:14578131

Godard B, Foulkes WD, Provencher D *et al.* (1998). Risk factors for familial and sporadic ovarian cancer among French Canadians: a case-control study. *Am J Obstet Gynecol*, 179: 403–410. doi:10.1016/S0002-9378(98)70372-2 PMID:9731846

Goedde HW, Agarwal DP, Fritze G *et al.* (1992). Distribution of ADH2 and ALDH2 genotypes in different populations. *Hum Genet*, 88: 344–346. doi:10.1007/BF00197271 PMID:1733836

Goist KC Jr & Sutker PB (1985). Acute alcohol intoxication and body composition in women and men. *Pharmacol Biochem Behav*, 22: 811–814. doi:10.1016/0091-3057(85)90532-5 PMID:4011640

Gong Z, Kristal AR, Schenk JM *et al.* (2009). Alcohol consumption, finasteride, and prostate cancer risk: results from the Prostate Cancer Prevention Trial. *Cancer*, 115: 3661–3669. doi:10.1002/cncr.24423 PMID:19598210

González MV, Alvarez V, Pello MF *et al.* (1998). Genetic polymorphism of N-acetyltransferase-2, glutathione S-transferase-M1, and cytochromes P450IIE1 and P450IID6 in the susceptibility to head and neck cancer. *J Clin Pathol*, 51: 294–298. doi:10.1136/jcp.51.4.294 PMID:9659241

Goodman MT, Hankin JH, Wilkens LR *et al.* (1997). Diet, body size, physical activity, and the risk of endometrial cancer. *Cancer Res*, 57: 5077–5085. PMID:9371506

Goodman MT & Tung KH (2003). Alcohol consumption and the risk of borderline and invasive ovarian cancer. *Obstet Gynecol*, 101: 1221–1228. doi:10.1016/S0029-7844(03)00050-4 PMID:12798528

Gorini G, Stagnaro E, Fontana V *et al.* (2007a). Alcohol consumption and risk of leukemia: A multicenter case-control study. *Leuk Res*, 31: 379–386. doi:10.1016/j.leukres.2006.07.002 PMID:16919329

Gorini G, Stagnaro E, Fontana V *et al.* (2007b). Alcohol consumption and risk of Hodgkin's lymphoma and multiple myeloma: a multicentre case-control study. *Ann Oncol*, 18: 143–148. doi:10.1093/annonc/mdl352 PMID:17047000

Greving JP, Lee JE, Wolk A *et al.* (2007). Alcoholic beverages and risk of renal cell cancer. *Br J Cancer*, 97: 429–433. doi:10.1038/sj.bjc.6603890 PMID:17653076

Guo YM, Wang Q, Liu YZ *et al.* (2008). Genetic polymorphisms in cytochrome P4502E1, alcohol and aldehyde dehydrogenases and the risk of esophageal squamous cell carcinoma in Gansu Chinese males. *World J Gastroenterol*, 14: 1444–1449. doi:10.3748/wjg.14.1444 PMID:18322963

Gwack J, Hwang SS, Ko KP *et al.* (2007). [Fasting serum glucose and subsequent liver cancer risk in a Korean prospective cohort] *J Prev Med Pub Health*, 40: 23–28. doi:10.3961/jpmph.2007.40.1.23 PMID:17310595

Gwinn ML, Webster LA, Lee NC *et al.* (1986). Alcohol consumption and ovarian cancer risk. *Am J Epidemiol*, 123: 759–766. PMID:3962959

Hakulinen T, Lehtimäki L, Lehtonen M, Teppo L (1974). Cancer morbidity among two male cohorts with increased alcohol consumption in Finland. *J Natl Cancer Inst*, 52: 1711–1714. PMID:4834405

Hamada GS, Sugimura H, Suzuki I *et al.* (1995). The heme-binding region polymorphism of cytochrome P4501A1 (*CypIA1*), rather than the *RsaI* polymorphism of IIE1 (*CypIIE1*), is associated with lung cancer in Rio de Janeiro. *Cancer Epidemiol. Biomarkers Prev.*, 4: 63–67.

Hamajima N, Hirose K, Tajima K *et al.* Collaborative Group on Hormonal Factors in Breast Cancer (2002). Alcohol, tobacco and breast cancer–collaborative reanalysis of individual data from 53 epidemiological studies, including 58,515 women with breast cancer and 95,067 women without the disease. *Br J Cancer*, 87: 1234–1245. doi:10.1038/sj.bjc.6600596 PMID:12439712

Harada S, Okubo T, Nakamura T *et al.* (1999). A novel polymorphism (-357 G/A) of the ALDH2 gene: linkage disequilibrium and an association with alcoholism. *Alcohol Clin Exp Res*, 23: 958–962. doi:10.1111/j.1530-0277.1999.tb04212.x PMID:10397278

Härkönen K, Viitanen T, Larsen SB *et al.* (1999). Aneuploidy in sperm and exposure to fungicides and lifestyle factors. ASCLEPIOS. A European concerted action on occupational hazards to male reproductive capability. *Environ Mol Mutagen*, 34: 39–46. PMID:10462722

Harris RW, Brinton LA, Cowdell RH *et al.* (1980). Characteristics of women with dysplasia or carcinoma in situ of the cervix uteri. *Br J Cancer*, 42: 359–369. doi:10.1038/bjc.1980.246 PMID:7426342

Hartge P, Schiffman MH, Hoover R *et al.* (1989). A case-control study of epithelial ovarian cancer. *Am J Obstet Gynecol*, 161: 10–16. PMID:2750791

Harty LC, Caporaso NE, Hayes RB *et al.* (1997). Alcohol dehydrogenase 3 genotype and risk of oral cavity and pharyngeal cancers. *J Natl Cancer Inst*, 89: 1698–1705. doi:10.1093/jnci/89.22.1698 PMID:9390539

Hashibe M, Boffetta P, Zaridze D *et al.* (2006). Evidence for an important role of alcohol- and aldehyde-metabolizing genes in cancers of the upper aerodigestive tract. *Cancer Epidemiol Biomarkers Prev*, 15: 696–703. doi:10.1158/1055-9965.EPI-05-0710 PMID:16614111

Hashibe M, Brennan P, Benhamou S *et al.* (2007). Alcohol drinking in never users of tobacco, cigarette smoking in never drinkers, and the risk of head and neck cancer: pooled analysis in the International Head and Neck Cancer Epidemiology Consortium. *J Natl Cancer Inst*, 99: 777–789. doi:10.1093/jnci/djk179 PMID:17505073

Hashibe M, McKay JD, Curado MP *et al.* (2008). Multiple ADH genes are associated with upper aerodigestive cancers. *Nat Genet*, 40: 707–709. doi:10.1038/ng.151 PMID:18500343

Hashimoto T, Uchida K, Okayama N *et al.* (2006). ALDH2 1510 G/A (Glu487Lys) polymorphism interaction with age in head and neck squamous cell carcinoma. *Tumour Biol*, 27: 334–338. doi:10.1159/000096126 PMID:17033202

Hassan MM, Bondy ML, Wolff RA *et al.* (2007). Risk factors for pancreatic cancer: case-control study. *Am J Gastroenterol*, 102: 2696–2707. doi:10.1111/j.1572-0241.2007.01510.x PMID:17764494

Hassan MM, Spitz MR, Thomas MB *et al.* (2008). Effect of different types of smoking and synergism with hepatitis C virus on risk of hepatocellular carcinoma in American men and women: case-control study. *Int J Cancer*, 123: 1883–1891. doi:10.1002/ijc.23730 PMID:18688864

Hayashi S, Watanabe J, Kawajiri K (1991). Genetic polymorphisms in the 5⊠-flanking region change transcriptional regulation of the human cytochrome P450IIE1 gene. *J Biochem*, 110: 559–565. PMID:1778977

Hayes RB, Brown LM, Schoenberg JB *et al.* (1996). Alcohol use and prostate cancer risk in US blacks and whites. *Am J Epidemiol*, 143: 692–697. PMID:8651231

Heinen MM, Verhage BA, Ambergen TA *et al.* (2009). Alcohol consumption and risk of pancreatic cancer in the Netherlands cohort study. *Am J Epidemiol*, 169: 1233–1242. doi:10.1093/aje/kwp028 PMID:19318612

Herity B, Moriarty M, Daly L *et al.* (1982). The role of tobacco and alcohol in the aetiology of lung and larynx cancer. *Br J Cancer*, 46: 961–964. doi:10.1038/bjc.1982.308 PMID:7150489

Herrero R, Brinton LA, Reeves WC *et al.* (1989). Invasive cervical cancer and smoking in Latin America. *J Natl Cancer Inst*, 81: 205–211. doi:10.1093/jnci/81.3.205 PMID:2536087

Hilakivi-Clarke L, Cabanes A, de Assis S *et al.* (2004). In utero alcohol exposure increases mammary tumorigenesis in rats. *Br J Cancer*, 90: 2225–2231. PMID:15150620

Hildesheim A, Anderson LM, Chen CJ *et al.* (1997). CYP2E1 genetic polymorphisms and risk of nasopharyngeal carcinoma in Taiwan. *J Natl Cancer Inst*, 89: 1207–1212. doi:10.1093/jnci/89.16.1207 PMID:9274915

Hines LM, Hankinson SE, Smith-Warner SA *et al.* (2000). A prospective study of the effect of alcohol consumption and ADH3 genotype on plasma steroid hormone levels and breast cancer risk. *Cancer Epidemiol Biomarkers Prev*, 9: 1099–1105. PMID:11045794

Hiraki A, Matsuo K, Wakai K *et al.* (2007). Gene-gene and gene-environment interactions between alcohol drinking habit and polymorphisms in alcohol-metabolizing enzyme genes and the risk of head and neck cancer in Japan. *Cancer Sci*, 98: 1087–1091. doi:10.1111/j.1349-7006.2007.00505.x PMID:17489985

Hirayama T (1992). Life-style and cancer: from epidemiological evidence to public behavior change to mortality reduction of target cancers. *J Natl Cancer Inst Monogr*, 12: 65–74. PMID:1616813

Hirose M, Kono S, Tabata S *et al.* (2005). Genetic polymorphisms of methylenetetrahydrofolate reductase and aldehyde dehydrogenase 2, alcohol use and risk of colorectal adenomas: Self-Defense Forces Health Study. *Cancer Sci*, 96: 513–518. doi:10.1111/j.1349-7006.2005.00077.x PMID:16108833

Hirvonen A, Husgafvel-Pursiainen K, Anttila S *et al.* (1993). The human CYP2E1 gene and lung cancer: DraI and RsaI restriction fragment length polymorphisms in a Finnish study population. *Carcinogenesis*, 14: 85–88. doi:10.1093/carcin/14.1.85 PMID:8093864

Holmberg B & Ekström T (1995). The effects of long-term oral administration of ethanol on Sprague-Dawley rats–a condensed report. *Toxicology*, 96: 133–145. doi:10.1016/0300-483X(94)02917-J PMID:7886684

Homann N, Jousimies-Somer H, Jokelainen K *et al.* (1997). High acetaldehyde levels in saliva after ethanol consumption: methodological aspects and pathogenetic implications. *Carcinogenesis*, 18: 1739–1743. doi:10.1093/carcin/18.9.1739 PMID:9328169

Homann N, König IR, Marks M *et al.* (2009). Alcohol and colorectal cancer: the role of alcohol dehydrogenase 1C polymorphism. *Alcohol Clin Exp Res*, 33: 551–556. doi:10.1111/j.1530-0277.2008.00868.x PMID:19120062

Homann N, Stickel F, König IR *et al.* (2006). Alcohol dehydrogenase 1C*1 allele is a genetic marker for alcohol-associated cancer in heavy drinkers. *Int J Cancer*, 118: 1998–2002. doi:10.1002/ijc.21583 PMID:16287084

Honjo S, Srivatanakul P, Sriplung H *et al.* (2005). Genetic and environmental determinants of risk for cholangiocarcinoma via Opisthorchis viverrini in a densely infested area in Nakhon Phanom, northeast Thailand. *Int J Cancer*, 117: 854–860. doi:10.1002/ijc.21146 PMID:15957169

Hori H, Kawano T, Endo M, Yuasa Y (1997). Genetic polymorphisms of tobacco- and alcohol-related metabolizing enzymes and human esophageal squamous cell carcinoma susceptibility. *J Clin Gastroenterol*, 25: 568–575. doi:10.1097/00004836-199712000-00003 PMID:9451664

Hosgood HD 3rd, Baris D, Zahm SH *et al.* (2007). Diet and risk of multiple myeloma in Connecticut women. *Cancer Causes Control*, 18: 1065–1076. doi:10.1007/s10552-007-9047-z PMID:17694422

Hosono S, Matsuo K, Kajiyama H *et al.* (2008). Reduced risk of endometrial cancer from alcohol drinking in Japanese. *Cancer Sci*, 99: 1195–1201. doi:10.1111/j.1349-7006.2008.00801.x PMID:18422741

Hsing AW, Zhang M, Rashid A *et al.* (2008). Hepatitis B and C virus infection and the risk of biliary tract cancer: a population-based study in China. *Int J Cancer*, 122: 1849–1853. doi:10.1002/ijc.23251 PMID:18076042

Hu J, Mao Y, Dryer D, White KCanadian Cancer Registries Epidemiology Research Group (2002). Risk factors for lung cancer among Canadian women who have never smoked. *Cancer Detect Prev*, 26: 129–138. doi:10.1016/S0361-090X(02)00038-7 PMID:12102147

Huang YS, Chern HD, Su WJ *et al.* (2003). Cytochrome P450 2E1 genotype and the susceptibility to antituberculosis drug-induced hepatitis. *Hepatology*, 37: 924–930. doi:10.1053/jhep.2003.50144 PMID:12668988

Hung HC, Chuang J, Chien YC *et al.* (1997). Genetic polymorphisms of CYP2E1, GSTM1, and GSTT1; Environmental factors and risk of oral cancer. *Cancer Epidemiol. Biomarkers Prev.*, 6: 901–905.

Huxley RR, Ansary-Moghaddam A, Clifton P *et al.* (2009). The impact of dietary and lifestyle risk factors on risk of colorectal cancer: a quantitative overview of the epidemiological evidence. *Int J Cancer*, 125: 171–180. doi:10.1002/ijc.24343 PMID:19350627

IARC (1985). Allyl compounds, aldehydes, epoxides and peroxides. *IARC Monogr Eval Carcinog Risk Chem Hum*, 36: 1–369.

IARC (1988). Alcohol drinking. *IARC Monogr Eval Carcinog Risks Hum*, 44: 1–378. PMID:3236394

IARC (1999). Re-evaluation of some organic chemicals, hydrazine and hydrogen peroxide. *IARC Monogr Eval Carcinog Risks Hum*, 71: 1–315. PMID:10507919

IARC (2010). Alcohol consumption and ethyl carbamate. *IARC Monogr Eval Carcinog Risks Hum*, 96: 1–1428.

Iarmarcovai G, Bonassi S, Sari-Minodier I *et al.* (2007). Exposure to genotoxic agents, host factors, and lifestyle influence the number of centromeric signals in micronuclei: a pooled re-analysis. *Mutat Res*, 615: 18–27. PMID:17198715

Ide R, Mizoue T, Fujino Y *et al.*JACC Study Group (2008). Cigarette smoking, alcohol drinking, and oral and pharyngeal cancer mortality in Japan. *Oral Dis*, 14: 314–319. doi:10.1111/j.1601-0825.2007.01378.x PMID:18449960

Infante-Rivard C, Krajinovic M, Labuda D, Sinnett D (2002). Childhood acute lymphoblastic leukemia associated with parental alcohol consumption and polymorphisms of carcinogen-metabolizing genes. *Epidemiology*, 13: 277–281. doi:10.1097/00001648-200205000-00007 PMID:11964928

Ingelman-Sundberg M, Oscarson M, Daly AK *et al.* (2001). Human cytochrome P-450 (CYP) genes: a web page for the nomenclature of alleles. *Cancer Epidemiol Biomarkers Prev*, 10: 1307–1308. PMID:11751452

Ishiguro S, Sasazuki S, Inoue M *et al.*JPHC Study Group (2009). Effect of alcohol consumption, cigarette smoking and flushing response on esophageal cancer risk: a population-based cohort study (JPHC study). *Cancer Lett*, 275: 240–246. doi:10.1016/j.canlet.2008.10.020 PMID:19036500

Ishihara J, Otani T, Inoue M *et al.*Japan Public Health Center-based Prospective Study Group (2007). Low intake of vitamin B-6 is associated with increased risk of colorectal cancer in Japanese men. *J Nutr*, 137: 1808–1814. PMID:17585035

Ishikawa H, Ishikawa T, Yamamoto H *et al.* (2007). Genotoxic effects of alcohol in human peripheral lymphocytes modulated by ADH1B and ALDH2 gene polymorphisms. *Mutat Res*, 615: 134–142. doi:10.1016/j.mrfmmm.2006.11.026 PMID:17207821

Ishikawa H, Miyatsu Y, Kurihara K, Yokoyama K (2006). Gene-environmental interactions between alcohol-drinking behavior and ALDH2 and CYP2E1 polymorphisms and their impact on micronuclei frequency in human lymphocytes. *Mutat Res*, 594: 1–9. PMID:16126235

Ishikawa H, Yamamoto H, Tian Y *et al.* (2003). Effects of ALDH2 gene polymorphisms and alcohol-drinking behavior on micronuclei frequency in non-smokers. *Mutat Res*, 541: 71–80. PMID:14568296

Itoga S, Nomura F, Makino Y *et al.* (2002). Tandem repeat polymorphism of the CYP2E1 gene: an association study with esophageal cancer and lung cancer. *Alcohol Clin Exp Res*, 26: Suppl15S–19S. doi:10.1111/j.1530-0277.2002.tb02696.x PMID:12198369

Jahnke V, Matthias C, Fryer A, Strange R (1996). Glutathione S-transferase and cytochrome-P-450 polymorphism as risk factors for squamous cell carcinoma of the larynx. *Am J Surg*, 172: 671–673. doi:10.1016/S0002-9610(96)00298-X PMID:8988674

Jain MG, Howe GR, Rohan TE (2000b). Nutritional factors and endometrial cancer in Ontario, Canada. *Cancer Control*, 7: 288–296. PMID:10832115

Jelski W, Chrostek L, Szmitkowski M, Laszewicz W (2002). Activity of class I, II, III, and IV alcohol dehydrogenase isoenzymes in human gastric mucosa. *Dig Dis Sci*, 47: 1554–1557. doi:10.1023/A:1015871219922 PMID:12141816

Jelski W, Orywal K, Panek B *et al.* (2009). The activity of class I, II, III and IV of alcohol dehydrogenase (ADH) isoenzymes and aldehyde dehydrogenase (ALDH) in the wall of abdominal aortic aneurysms. *Exp Mol Pathol*, 87: 59–62. doi:10.1016/j.yexmp.2009.03.001 PMID:19332052

Jensen OM (1979). Cancer morbidity and causes of death among Danish brewery workers. *Int J Cancer*, 23: 454–463. doi:10.1002/ijc.2910230404 PMID:437924

Jiang X, Castelao JE, Groshen S *et al.* (2007). Alcohol consumption and risk of bladder cancer in Los Angeles County. *Int J Cancer*, 121: 839–845. doi:10.1002/ijc.22743 PMID:17440923

Jiao L, Silverman DT, Schairer C *et al.* (2009). Alcohol use and risk of pancreatic cancer: the NIH-AARP Diet and Health Study. *Am J Epidemiol*, 169: 1043–1051. doi:10.1093/aje/kwp034 PMID:19299403

Johansen D, Borgström A, Lindkvist B, Manjer J (2009). Different markers of alcohol consumption, smoking and body mass index in relation to risk of pancreatic cancer. A prospective cohort study within the Malmö Preventive Project. *Pancreatology*, 9: 677–686. doi:10.1159/000212088 PMID:19684432

Jones AW (1995). Measuring and reporting the concentration of acetaldehyde in human breath. *Alcohol Alcohol*, 30: 271–285. PMID:7545981

Jones AW (2006). Urine as a biological specimen for forensic analysis of alcohol and variability in the urine-to-blood relationship. *Toxicol Rev*, 25: 15–35. doi:10.2165/00139709-200625010-00002 PMID:16856767

Jones AW, Lindberg L, Olsson SG (2004). Magnitude and time-course of arterio-venous differences in blood-alcohol concentration in healthy men. *Clin Pharmacokinet*, 43: 1157–1166. doi:10.2165/00003088-200443150-00006 PMID:15568892

Jones AW, Mårdh G, Anggård E (1983). Determination of endogenous ethanol in blood and breath by gas chromatography-mass spectrometry. *Pharmacol Biochem Behav*, 18: Suppl 1267–272. doi:10.1016/0091-3057(83)90184-3 PMID:6634839

Jung AY, Poole EM, Bigler J *et al.* (2008). DNA methyltransferase and alcohol dehydrogenase: gene-nutrient interactions in relation to risk of colorectal polyps. *Cancer Epidemiol Biomarkers Prev*, 17: 330–338. doi:10.1158/1055-9965.EPI-07-2608 PMID:18268116

Kabat GC, Miller AB, Jain M, Rohan TE (2008). Dietary intake of selected B vitamins in relation to risk of major cancers in women. *Br J Cancer*, 99: 816–821. doi:10.1038/sj.bjc.6604540 PMID:18665162

Kabat GC & Wynder EL (1984). Lung cancer in nonsmokers. *Cancer*, 53: 1214–1221. doi:10.1002/1097-0142(19840301)53:5<1214::AID-CNCR2820530532>3.0.CO;2-8 PMID:6692309

Kagan-Krieger S, Selby P, Vohra S, Koren G (2002). Paternal alcohol exposure and Turner syndrome. *Alcohol Alcohol*, 37: 613–617. PMID:12414557

Kaji H, Asanuma Y, Yahara O *et al.* (1984). Intragastrointestinal alcohol fermentation syndrome: report of two cases and review of the literature. *J Forensic Sci Soc*, 24: 461–471. doi:10.1016/S0015-7368(84)72325-5 PMID:6520589

Kalandidi A, Tzonou A, Lipworth L *et al.* (1996). A case-control study of endometrial cancer in relation to reproductive, somatometric, and life-style variables. *Oncology*, 53: 354–359. doi:10.1159/000227587 PMID:8784467

Kanda J, Matsuo K, Suzuki T *et al.* (2009). Impact of alcohol consumption with polymorphisms in alcohol-metabolizing enzymes on pancreatic cancer risk in Japanese. *Cancer Sci*, 100: 296–302. doi:10.1111/j.1349-7006.2008.01044.x PMID:19068087

Kanteres F, Lachenmeier DW, Rehm J (2009). Alcohol in Mayan Guatemala: consumption, distribution, production and composition of cuxa. *Addiction*, 104: 752–759. doi:10.1111/j.1360-0443.2009.02507.x PMID:19215596

Kato I, Tominaga S, Terao C (1989). Alcohol consumption and cancers of hormone-related organs in females. *Jpn J Clin Oncol*, 19: 202–207. PMID:2810820

Kato S, Onda M, Matsukura N *et al.* (1995). Cytochrome P4502E1 (CYP2E1) genetic polymorphism in a case-control study of gastric cancer and liver disease. *Pharmacogenetics*, 5: Special IssueS141–S144. doi:10.1097/00008571-199512001-00016PMID:7581484

Kato S, Onda M, Matsukura N *et al.* (1997). Helicobacter pylori infection and genetic polymorphisms for cancer-related genes in gastric carcinogenesis. *Biomed Pharmacother*, 51: 145–149. doi:10.1016/S0753-3322(97)85581-3 PMID:9207980

Kato S, Shields PG, Caporaso NE *et al.* (1992). Cytochrome P450IIE1 genetic polymorphisms, racial variation, and lung cancer risk. *Cancer Res*, 52: 6712–6715. PMID:1423319

Kato S, Shields PG, Caporaso NE *et al.* (1994). Analysis of cytochrome P450 2E1 genetic polymorphisms in relation to human lung cancer. *Cancer Epidemiol Biomarkers Prev*, 3: 515–518. PMID:8000304

Kato S, Tajiri T, Matsukura N *et al.* (2003). Genetic polymorphisms of aldehyde dehydrogenase 2, cytochrome p450 2E1 for liver cancer risk in HCV antibody-positive japanese patients and the variations of CYP2E1 mRNA expression levels in the liver due to its polymorphism. *Scand J Gastroenterol*, 38: 886–893. doi:10.1080/00365520310004489 PMID:12940444

Katoh T, Kaneko S, Kohshi K *et al.* (1999). Genetic polymorphisms of tobacco- and alcohol-related metabolizing enzymes and oral cavity cancer. *Int J Cancer*, 83: 606–609. doi:10.1002/(SICI)1097-0215(19991126)83:5<606::AID-IJC6>3.0.CO;2-P PMID:10521794

Kawase T, Matsuo K, Hiraki A *et al.* (2009). Interaction of the effects of alcohol drinking and polymorphisms in alcohol-metabolizing enzymes on the risk of female breast cancer in Japan. *J Epidemiol*, 19: 244–250. doi:10.2188/jea.JE20081035 PMID:19667493

Kayani MA & Parry JM (2010). The in vitro genotoxicity of ethanol and acetaldehyde. *Toxicol In Vitro*, 24: 56–60. doi:10.1016/j.tiv.2009.09.003 PMID:19747536

Kelemen LE, Sellers TA, Vierkant RA *et al.* (2004). Association of folate and alcohol with risk of ovarian cancer in a prospective study of postmenopausal women. *Cancer Causes Control*, 15: 1085–1093. doi:10.1007/s10552-004-1546-6 PMID:15801492

Khurana V, Sheth A, Caldito G, Barkin JS (2007). Statins reduce the risk of pancreatic cancer in humans: a case-control study of half a million veterans. *Pancreas*, 34: 260–265. doi:10.1097/MPA.0b013e318030e963 PMID:17312467

Kim RB, Yamazaki H, Chiba K *et al.* (1996). In vivo and in vitro characterization of CYP2E1 activity in Japanese and Caucasians. *J Pharmacol Exp Ther*, 279: 4–11. PMID:8858968

Kimura Y, Nishimura FT, Abe S *et al.* (2009). Polymorphisms in the promoter region of the human class II alcohol dehydrogenase (ADH4) gene affect both transcriptional activity and ethanol metabolism in Japanese subjects. *J Toxicol Sci*, 34: 89–97. doi:10.2131/jts.34.89 PMID:19182438

Kiss I, Sándor J, Pajkos G *et al.* (2000). Colorectal cancer risk in relation to genetic polymorphism of cytochrome P450 1A1, 2E1, and glutathione-S-transferase M1 enzymes. *Anticancer Res*, 20: 1B519–522. PMID:10769717

Kjaerheim K & Andersen A (1994). Cancer incidence among waitresses in Norway. *Cancer Causes Control*, 5: 31–37. doi:10.1007/BF01830724 PMID:8123777

Klatsky AL, Friedman GD, Siegelaub AB (1981). Alcohol and mortality. A ten-year Kaiser-Permanente experience. *Ann Intern Med*, 95: 139–145. PMID:7258861

Klatsky AL, Li Y, Baer D *et al.* (2009). Alcohol consumption and risk of hematologic malignancies. *Ann Epidemiol*, 19: 746–753. doi:10.1016/j.annepidem.2009.03.005 PMID:19394864

Knight JA, Bernstein L, Largent J *et al.*WECARE Study Collaborative Group (2009). Alcohol intake and cigarette smoking and risk of a contralateral breast cancer: The Women's Environmental Cancer and Radiation Epidemiology Study. *Am J Epidemiol*, 169: 962–968. doi:10.1093/aje/kwn422 PMID:19211621

Kocić B, Petrovic B, Filipovic S (2008). Risk factors for breast cancer: a hospital-based case-control study. *J BUON*, 13: 231–234. PMID:18555470

Koide T, Ohno T, Huang XE *et al.* (2000). HBV/HCV infection, alcohol, tobacco and genetic polymorphisms for hepatocellular carcinoma in Nagoya, Japan. *Asian Pac J Cancer Prev*, 1: 237–243. PMID:12718671

Kolahdooz F, Ibiebele TI, van der Pols JC, Webb PM (2009). Dietary patterns and ovarian cancer risk. *Am J Clin Nutr*, 89: 297–304. doi:10.3945/ajcn.2008.26575 PMID:19056595

Kono S, Ikeda M, Tokudome S *et al.* (1986). Alcohol and mortality: a cohort study of male Japanese physicians. *Int J Epidemiol*, 15: 527–532. doi:10.1093/ije/15.4.527 PMID:3818161

Koo LC (1988). Dietary habits and lung cancer risk among Chinese females in Hong Kong who never smoked. *Nutr Cancer*, 11: 155–172. doi:10.1080/01635588809513983 PMID:2841651

Korte JE, Brennan P, Henley SJ, Boffetta P (2002). Dose-specific meta-analysis and sensitivity analysis of the relation between alcohol consumption and lung cancer risk. *Am J Epidemiol*, 155: 496–506. doi:10.1093/aje/155.6.496 PMID:11882523

Krebs HA & Perkins JR (1970). The physiological role of liver alcohol dehydrogenase. *Biochem J*, 118: 635–644. PMID:5481498

Kruk J (2007). Association of lifestyle and other risk factors with breast cancer according to menopausal status: a case-control study in the Region of Western Pomerania (Poland). *Asian Pac J Cancer Prev*, 8: 513–524. PMID:18260721

Kubík A, Zatloukal P, Tomásek L *et al.* (2004). Lung cancer risk among nonsmoking women in relation to diet and physical activity. *Neoplasma*, 51: 136–143. PMID:15190423

Kuper H, Lagiou P, Mucci LA *et al.* (2001). Risk factors for cholangiocarcinoma in a low risk Caucasian population. *Soz Praventivmed*, 46: 182–185. doi:10.1007/BF01324254 PMID:11565447

Kuper H, Titus-Ernstoff L, Harlow BL, Cramer DW (2000). Population based study of coffee, alcohol and tobacco use and risk of ovarian cancer. *Int J Cancer*, 88: 313–318. doi:10.1002/1097-0215(20001015)88:2<313::AID-IJC26>3.0.CO;2-5 PMID:11004686

Kurtz AJ & Lloyd RS (2003). 1,N2-deoxyguanosine adducts of acrolein, crotonaldehyde, and trans-4-hydroxynonenal cross-link to peptides via Schiff base linkage. *J Biol Chem*, 278: 5970–5976. doi:10.1074/jbc.M212012200 PMID:12502710

Kurys G, Ambroziak W, Pietruszko R (1989). Human aldehyde dehydrogenase. Purification and characterization of a third isozyme with low Km for gamma-aminobutyraldehyde. *J Biol Chem*, 264: 4715–4721. PMID:2925663

Kushi LH, Mink PJ, Folsom AR *et al.* (1999). Prospective study of diet and ovarian cancer. *Am J Epidemiol*, 149: 21–31. PMID:9883790

Kushida M, Wanibuchi H, Morimura K *et al.* (2005). Dose-dependence of promotion of 2-amino-3,8-dimethylimidazo[4,5-f]quinoxaline-induced rat hepatocarcinogenesis by ethanol: evidence for a threshold. *Cancer Sci*, 96: 747–757. doi:10.1111/j.1349-7006.2005.00110.x PMID:16271068

Kvåle G, Bjelke E, Gart JJ (1983). Dietary habits and lung cancer risk. *Int J Cancer*, 31: 397–405. doi:10.1002/ijc.2910310402 PMID:6832851

Kwan ML, Kushi LH, Weltzien E *et al.* (2009). Epidemiology of breast cancer subtypes in two prospective cohort studies of breast cancer survivors. *Breast Cancer Res*, 11: R31 doi:10.1186/bcr2261 PMID:19463150

La Vecchia C, Decarli A, Fasoli M, Gentile A (1986). Nutrition and diet in the etiology of endometrial cancer. *Cancer*, 57: 1248–1253. doi:10.1002/1097-0142(19860315)57:6<1248::AID-CNCR2820570631>3.0.CO;2-V PMID:3002600

La Vecchia C, Negri E, Franceschi S *et al.* (1992). Alcohol and epithelial ovarian cancer. *J Clin Epidemiol*, 45: 1025–1030. doi:10.1016/0895-4356(92)90119-8 PMID:1432017

Lachenmeier DW, Ganss S, Rychlak B *et al.* (2009b). Association between quality of cheap and unrecorded alcohol products and public health consequences in Poland. *Alcohol Clin Exp Res*, 33: Issue 101757–1769. doi:10.1111/j.1530-0277.2009.01013.x PMID:19572980

Lachenmeier DW, Kanteres F, Rehm J (2009a). Carcinogenicity of acetaldehyde in alcoholic beverages: risk assessment outside ethanol metabolism. *Addiction*, 104: 533–550. doi:10.1111/j.1360-0443.2009.02516.x PMID:19335652

Lachenmeier DW & Sohnius EM (2008). The role of acetaldehyde outside ethanol metabolism in the carcinogenicity of alcoholic beverages: evidence from a large chemical survey. *Food Chem Toxicol*, 46: 2903–2911. doi:10.1016/j.fct.2008.05.034 PMID:18577414

Ladero JM, Agúndez JAG, Rodríguez-Lescure A *et al.* (1996). RsaI polymorphism at the cytochrome P4502E1 locus and risk of hepatocellular carcinoma. *Gut*, 39: 330–333. doi:10.1136/gut.39.2.330 PMID:8977352

Lagiou P, Ye W, Wedrén S *et al.* (2001). Incidence of ovarian cancer among alcoholic women: a cohort study in Sweden. *Int J Cancer*, 91: 264–266. doi:10.1002/1097-0215(200002)9999:9999<::AID-IJC1027>3.3.CO;2-B PMID:11146456

Landi S, Gemignani F, Moreno V *et al.*Bellvitge Colorectal Cancer Study Group (2005). A comprehensive analysis of phase I and phase II metabolism gene polymorphisms and risk of colorectal cancer. *Pharmacogenet Genomics*, 15: 535–546. doi:10.1097/01.fpc.0000165904.48994.3d PMID:16006997

Laposata EA & Lange LG (1986). Presence of nonoxidative ethanol metabolism in human organs commonly damaged by ethanol abuse. *Science*, 231: 497–499. doi:10.1126/science.3941913 PMID:3941913

Laposata M, Hasaba A, Best CA *et al.* (2002). Fatty acid ethyl esters: recent observations. *Prostaglandins Leukot Essent Fatty Acids*, 67: 193–196. doi:10.1054/plef.2002.0418 PMID:12324241

Larsson SC, Giovannucci E, Wolk A (2007). Alcoholic beverage consumption and gastric cancer risk: a prospective population-based study in women. *Int J Cancer*, 120: 373–377. doi:10.1002/ijc.22204 PMID:17066442

Le Marchand L, Donlon T, Seifried A, Wikens LR (2002). Read meat intake, *CYP2E1* genetic polymorphisms, and colorectal cancer risk. *Cancer Epidemiol. Biomarkers Prev.*, 11: 1019–1024.

Le Marchand L, Sivaraman L, Pierce L *et al.* (1998). Associations of CYP1A1, GSTM1, and CYP2E1 polymorphisms with lung cancer suggest cell type specificities to tobacco carcinogens. *Cancer Res*, 58: 4858–4863. PMID:9809991

Lee CH, Lee JM, Wu DC *et al.* (2008b). Carcinogenetic impact of ADH1B and ALDH2 genes on squamous cell carcinoma risk of the esophagus with regard to the consumption of alcohol, tobacco and betel quid. *Int J Cancer*, 122: 1347–1356. doi:10.1002/ijc.23264 PMID:18033686

Lee CH, Wu DC, Lee JM *et al.* (2007). Carcinogenetic impact of alcohol intake on squamous cell carcinoma risk of the oesophagus in relation to tobacco smoking. *Eur J Cancer*, 43: 1188–1199. doi:10.1016/j.ejca.2007.01.039 PMID:17383866

Lee CH, Wu DC, Wu IC *et al.* (2009). Genetic modulation of ADH1B and ALDH2 polymorphisms with regard to alcohol and tobacco consumption for younger aged esophageal squamous cell carcinoma diagnosis. *Int J Cancer*, 125: 1134–1142. doi:10.1002/ijc.24357 PMID:19449376

Lee HC, Yoon YB, Kim CY (1997). Association between genetic polymorphisms of the cytochromes P-450 (1A1, 2D6, and 2E1) and the susceptibility to pancreatic cancer. *Korean J Intern Med*, 12: 128–136. PMID:9439147

Lee CH, Lee JM, Wu DC *et al.* (2005). Independent and combined effects of alcohol intake, tobacco smoking and betel quid chewing on the risk of esophageal cancer in Taiwan. *Int J Cancer*, 113: 475–482. doi:10.1002/ijc.20619 PMID:15455377

Lee SL, Chau GY, Yao CT *et al.* (2006). Functional assessment of human alcohol dehydrogenase family in ethanol metabolism: significance of first-pass metabolism. *Alcohol Clin Exp Res*, 30: 1132–1142. doi:10.1111/j.1530-0277.2006.00139.x PMID:16792560

Lee TY, Lee SS, Jung SW *et al.* (2008a). Hepatitis B virus infection and intrahepatic cholangiocarcinoma in Korea: a case-control study. *Am J Gastroenterol*, 103: 1716–1720. doi:10.1111/j.1572-0241.2008.01796.x PMID:18557716

Levi F, Franceschi S, Negri E, La Vecchia C (1993). Dietary factors and the risk of endometrial cancer. *Cancer*, 71: 3575–3581. doi:10.1002/1097-0142(19930601)71:11<3575::AID-CNCR2820711119>3.0.CO;2-0 PMID:8490907

Levine AJ, Siegmund KD, Ervin CM *et al.* (2000). The methylenetetrahydrofolate reductase 677C->T polymorphism and distal colorectal adenoma risk. *Cancer Epidemiol Biomarkers Prev*, 9: 657–663. PMID:10919734

Levitt MD & Levitt DG (1998). Use of a two-compartment model to assess the pharmacokinetics of human ethanol metabolism. *Alcohol Clin Exp Res*, 22: 1680–1688. PMID:9835281

Levitt MD & Levitt DG (2000). Appropriate use and misuse of blood concentration measurements to quantitate first-pass metabolism. *J Lab Clin Med*, 136: 275–280. doi:10.1067/mlc.2000.109100 PMID:11039847

Lew JQ, Freedman ND, Leitzmann MF *et al.* (2009). Alcohol and risk of breast cancer by histologic type and hormone receptor status in postmenopausal women: the NIH-AARP Diet and Health Study. *Am J Epidemiol*, 170: 308–317. doi:10.1093/aje/kwp120 PMID:19541857

Lewis SJ & Smith GD (2005). Alcohol, ALDH2, and esophageal cancer: a meta-analysis which illustrates the potentials and limitations of a Mendelian randomization approach. *Cancer Epidemiol Biomarkers Prev*, 14: 1967–1971. doi:10.1158/1055-9965.EPI-05-0196 PMID:16103445

Li CI, Daling JR, Malone KE *et al.* (2006). Relationship between established breast cancer risk factors and risk of seven different histologic types of invasive breast cancer. *Cancer Epidemiol Biomarkers Prev*, 15: 946–954. doi:10.1158/1055-9965.EPI-05-0881 PMID:16702375

Li CI, Daling JR, Porter PL *et al.* (2009a). Relationship between potentially modifiable lifestyle factors and risk of second primary contralateral breast cancer among women diagnosed with estrogen receptor-positive invasive breast cancer. *J Clin Oncol*, 27: 5312–5318. doi:10.1200/JCO.2009.23.1597 PMID:19738113

Li CI, Malone KE, Porter PL *et al.* (2003a). The relationship between alcohol use and risk of breast cancer by histology and hormone receptor status among women 65–79 years of age. *Cancer Epidemiol Biomarkers Prev*, 12: 1061–1066. PMID:14578143

Li CI, Malone KE, Porter PL, Daling JR (2003b). Epidemiologic and molecular risk factors for contralateral breast cancer among young women. *Br J Cancer*, 89: 513–518. doi:10.1038/sj.bjc.6601042 PMID:12888823

Li D, Dandara C, Parker MI (2005). Association of cytochrome P450 2E1 genetic polymorphisms with squamous cell carcinoma of the oesophagus. *Clin Chem Lab Med*, 43: 370–375. doi:10.1515/CCLM.2005.067 PMID:15899651

Li DP, Dandara C, Walther G, Parker MI (2008a). Genetic polymorphisms of alcohol metabolising enzymes: their role in susceptibility to oesophageal cancer. *Clin Chem Lab Med*, 46: 323–328. doi:10.1515/CCLM.2008.073 PMID:18254707

Li XM, Li J, Tsuji I *et al.* (2008b). Mass screening-based case-control study of diet and prostate cancer in Changchun, China. *Asian J Androl*, 10: 551–560. doi:10.1111/j.1745-7262.2008.00384.x PMID:18478158

Li Y, Baer D, Friedman GD *et al.* (2009b). Wine, liquor, beer and risk of breast cancer in a large population. *Eur J Cancer*, 45: 843–850. doi:10.1016/j.ejca.2008.11.001 PMID:19095438

Licciardone JC, Wilkins JR 3rd, Brownson RC, Chang JC (1989). Cigarette smoking and alcohol consumption in the aetiology of uterine cervical cancer. *Int J Epidemiol*, 18: 533–537. doi:10.1093/ije/18.3.533 PMID:2807654

Lieber CS (2004). The discovery of the microsomal ethanol oxidizing system and its physiologic and pathologic role. *Drug Metab Rev*, 36: 511–529. doi:10.1081/DMR-200033441 PMID:15554233

Lightfoot TJ, Barrett JH, Bishop T *et al.* (2008). Methylene tetrahydrofolate reductase genotype modifies the chemopreventive effect of folate in colorectal adenoma, but not colorectal cancer. *Cancer Epidemiol Biomarkers Prev*, 17: 2421–2430.

Lilla C, Koehler T, Kropp S *et al.* (2005). Alcohol dehydrogenase 1B (ADH1B) genotype, alcohol consumption and breast cancer risk by age 50 years in a German case-control study. *Br J Cancer*, 92: 2039–2041. doi:10.1038/sj.bjc.6602608 PMID:15886702

Lim HJ & Park BJ (2008). [Cohort study on the association between alcohol consumption and the risk of colorectal cancer in the Korean elderly] *J Prev Med Pub Health*, 41: 23–29. doi:10.3961/jpmph.2008.41.1.23 PMID:18250602

Lim RT Jr, Gentry RT, Ito D *et al.* (1993). First-pass metabolism of ethanol is predominantly gastric. *Alcohol Clin Exp Res*, 17: 1337–1344. doi:10.1111/j.1530-0277.1993.tb05250.x PMID:8116851

Lim U, Morton LM, Subar AF *et al.* (2007). Alcohol, smoking, and body size in relation to incident Hodgkin's and non-Hodgkin's lymphoma risk. *Am J Epidemiol*, 166: 697–708. doi:10.1093/aje/kwm122 PMID:17596266

Lim U, Weinstein S, Albanes D *et al.* (2006). Dietary factors of one-carbon metabolism in relation to non-Hodgkin lymphoma and multiple myeloma in a cohort of male smokers. *Cancer Epidemiol Biomarkers Prev*, 15: 1109–1114. doi:10.1158/1055-9965.EPI-05-0918 PMID:16775167

Lin HJ (1996). Smokers and breast cancer. 'Chemical individuality' and cancer predisposition. *JAMA*, 276: 1511–1512. doi:10.1001/jama.1996.03540180067035 PMID:8903264

Lind PA, Eriksson CJP, Wilhelmsen KC (2008). The role of aldehyde dehydrogenase-1 (ALDH1A1) polymorphisms in harmful alcohol consumption in a Finnish population. *Hum Genomics*, 3: 24–35. PMID:19129088

Linderborg K, Joly JP, Visapää JP, Salaspuro M (2008). Potential mechanism for Calvados-related oesophageal cancer. *Food Chem Toxicol*, 46: 476–479. doi:10.1016/j.fct.2007.08.019 PMID:17892909

Linet MS, Harlow SD, McLaughlin JK (1987). A case-control study of multiple myeloma in whites: chronic antigenic stimulation, occupation, and drug use. *Cancer Res*, 47: 2978–2981. PMID:3567914

Lisander B, Lundvall O, Tomner J, Jones AW (2006). Enhanced rate of ethanol elimination from blood after intravenous administration of amino acids compared with equicaloric glucose. *Alcohol Alcohol*, 41: 39–43. PMID:16087660

Liu S, Park JY, Schantz SP *et al.* (2001). Elucidation of CYP2E1 5′ regulatory RsaI/PstI allelic variants and their role in risk for oral cancer. *Oral Oncol*, 37: 437–445. doi:10.1016/S1368-8375(00)00099-3 PMID:11377232

Liu X, Lao Y, Yang IY *et al.* (2006). Replication-coupled repair of crotonaldehyde/acetaldehyde-induced guanine-guanine interstrand cross-links and their mutagenicity. *Biochemistry*, 45: 12898–12905. doi:10.1021/bi060792v PMID:17042508

Lodovici M, Casalini C, Cariaggi R *et al.* (2000). Levels of 8-hydroxydeoxyguanosine as a marker of DNA damage in human leukocytes. *Free Radic Biol Med*, 28: 13–17. doi:10.1016/S0891-5849(99)00194-X PMID:10656286

Loerbroks A, Schouten LJ, Goldbohm RA, van den Brandt PA (2007). Alcohol consumption, cigarette smoking, and endometrial cancer risk: results from the Netherlands Cohort Study. *Cancer Causes Control*, 18: 551–560. doi:10.1007/s10552-007-0127-x PMID:17437180

London SJ, Daly AK, Cooper J *et al.* (1996). Lung cancer risk in relation to the CYP2E1 Rsa I genetic polymorphism among African-Americans and Caucasians in Los Angeles County. *Pharmacogenetics*, 6: 151–158. doi:10.1097/00008571-199604000-00002 PMID:9156693

Lu Q-J, Yao S-Y, Huang C-Y *et al.* (2000[The cohort study on intake of alcohol and lung cancer risk in the Yunnan Tin Corporation (YTC) miners.]). *China Pub Health*, 16: 707–708.

Lu XM, Zhang YM, Lin RY *et al.* (2005). Relationship between genetic polymorphisms of metabolizing enzymes CYP2E1, GSTM1 and Kazakh's esophageal squamous cell cancer in Xinjiang, China. *World J Gastroenterol*, 11: 3651–3654. PMID:15968714

Lubin JH, Purdue M, Kelsey K *et al.* (2009). Total exposure and exposure rate effects for alcohol and smoking and risk of head and neck cancer: a pooled analysis of case-control studies. *Am J Epidemiol*, 170: 937–947. doi:10.1093/aje/kwp222 PMID:19745021

Lucas D, Ménez C, Floch F *et al.* (1996). Cytochromes P4502E1 and P4501A1 genotypes and susceptibility to cirrhosis or upper aerodigestive tract cancer in alcoholic caucasians. *Alcohol Clin Exp Res*, 20: 1033–1037. doi:10.1111/j.1530-0277.1996.tb01943.x PMID:8892524

Lucenteforte E, Scita V, Bosetti C *et al.* (2008). Food groups and alcoholic beverages and the risk of stomach cancer: a case-control study in Italy. *Nutr Cancer*, 60: 577–584. doi:10.1080/01635580802054512 PMID:18791920

Mabuchi K, Bross DS, Kessler II (1985). Epidemiology of cancer of the vulva. A case-control study. *Cancer*, 55: 1843–1848. doi:10.1002/1097-0142(19850415)55:8<1843::AID-CNCR2820550833>3.0.CO;2-M PMID:3978570

MacArthur AC, McBride ML, Spinelli JJ *et al.* (2008). Risk of childhood leukemia associated with parental smoking and alcohol consumption prior to conception and during pregnancy: the cross-Canada childhood leukemia study. *Cancer Causes Control*, 19: 283–295. doi:10.1007/s10552-007-9091-8 PMID:18283545

Madsen BS, Jensen HL, van den Brule AJ *et al.* (2008). Risk factors for invasive squamous cell carcinoma of the vulva and vagina–population-based case-control study in Denmark. *Int J Cancer*, 122: 2827–2834. doi:10.1002/ijc.23446 PMID:18348142

Maffei F, Fimognari C, Castelli E *et al.* (2000). Increased cytogenetic damage detected by FISH analysis on micronuclei in peripheral lymphocytes from alcoholics. *Mutagenesis*, 15: 517–523. doi:10.1093/mutage/15.6.517 PMID:11077004

Maffei F, Forti GC, Castelli E *et al.* (2002). Biomarkers to assess the genetic damage induced by alcohol abuse in human lymphocytes. *Mutat Res*, 514: 49–58. PMID:11815244

Mao H, Reddy GR, Marnett LJ, Stone MP (1999). Solution structure of an oligodeoxynucleotide containing the malondialdehyde deoxyguanosine adduct N2-(3-oxo-1-propenyl)-dG (ring-opened M1G) positioned in a (CpG)3 frameshift hotspot of the Salmonella typhimurium hisD3052 gene. *Biochemistry*, 38: 13491–13501. doi:10.1021/bi9910124 PMID:10521256

Marshall JR, Graham S, Byers T *et al.* (1983). Diet and smoking in the epidemiology of cancer of the cervix. *J Natl Cancer Inst*, 70: 847–851. PMID:6573528

Martin PM & Hill GB (1984). Cervical cancer in relation to tobacco and alcohol consumption in Lesotho, southern Africa. *Cancer Detect Prev*, 7: 109–115. PMID:6713445

Matsuda T, Kawanishi M, Yagi T *et al.* (1998). Specific tandem GG to TT base substitutions induced by acetaldehyde are due to intra-strand crosslinks between adjacent guanine bases. *Nucleic Acids Res*, 26: 1769–1774. doi:10.1093/nar/26.7.1769 PMID:9512551

Matsuda T, Terashima I, Matsumoto Y *et al.* (1999). Effective utilization of N2-ethyl-2′-deoxyguanosine triphosphate during DNA synthesis catalyzed by mammalian replicative DNA polymerases. *Biochemistry*, 38: 929–935. doi:10.1021/bi982134j PMID:9893988

Matsuda T, Yabushita H, Kanaly RA *et al.* (2006). Increased DNA damage in ALDH2-deficient alcoholics. *Chem Res Toxicol*, 19: 1374–1378. doi:10.1021/tx060113h PMID:17040107

Matsuo K, Hamajima N, Hirai T *et al.* (2002). Aldehyde dehydrogenase 2 (ALDH2) genotype affects rectal cancer susceptibility due to alcohol consumption. *J Epidemiol*, 12: 70–76. doi:10.2188/jea.12.70 PMID:12033531

Matsuo K, Hamajima N, Hirose K *et al.* (2001a). Alcohol, smoking, and dietary status and susceptibility to malignant lymphoma in Japan: results of a hospital-based case-control study at Aichi Cancer Center. *Jpn J Cancer Res*, 92: 1011–1017. doi:10.1111/j.1349-7006.2001.tb01054.x PMID:11676850

Matsuo K, Hamajima N, Shinoda M *et al.* (2001b). Gene-environment interaction between an aldehyde dehydrogenase-2 (ALDH2) polymorphism and alcohol consumption for the risk of esophageal cancer. *Carcinogenesis,* 22: 913–916. doi:10.1093/carcin/22.6.913 PMID:11375898

Matsuo K, Hiraki A, Hirose K *et al.* (2007). Impact of the alcohol-dehydrogenase (ADH) 1C and ADH1B polymorphisms on drinking behavior in nonalcoholic Japanese. *Hum Mutat*, 28: 506–510. doi:10.1002/humu.20477 PMID:17285601

Matsuo K, Wakai K, Hirose K *et al.* (2006a). A gene-gene interaction between ALDH2 Glu487Lys and ADH2 His47Arg polymorphisms regarding the risk of colorectal cancer in Japan. *Carcinogenesis*, 27: 1018–1023. doi:10.1093/carcin/bgi282 PMID:16332725

Matsuo K, Wakai K, Hirose K *et al.* (2006b). Alcohol dehydrogenase 2 His47Arg polymorphism influences drinking habit independently of aldehyde dehydrogenase 2 Glu487Lys polymorphism: analysis of 2,299 Japanese subjects. *Cancer Epidemiol Biomarkers Prev*, 15: 1009–1013. doi:10.1158/1055-9965.EPI-05-0911 PMID:16702384

Matsushima Y (1987). Chromosomal aberrations in the lymphocytes of alcoholics and former alcoholics. *Neuropsychobiology*, 17: 24–29. doi:10.1159/000118336 PMID:3627389

Matthias C, Bockmühl U, Jahnke V *et al.* (1998). Polymorphism in cytochrome P450 CYP2D6, CYP1A1, CYP2E1 and glutathione S-transferase, GSTM1, GSTM3, GSTT1 and susceptibility to tobacco-related cancers: studies in upper aerodigestive tract cancers. *Pharmacogenetics*, 8: 91–100. doi:10.1097/00008571-199804000-00001 PMID:10022746

Mayne ST, Janerich DT, Greenwald P *et al.* (1994). Dietary beta carotene and lung cancer risk in U.S. nonsmokers. *J Natl Cancer Inst*, 86: 33–38. doi:10.1093/jnci/86.1.33 PMID:8271280

McCann SE, Freudenheim JL, Marshall JR *et al.* (2000). Diet in the epidemiology of endometrial cancer in western New York (United States). *Cancer Causes Control*, 11: 965–974. doi:10.1023/A:1026551309873 PMID:11142531

McCann SE, Freudenheim JL, Marshall JR, Graham S (2003). Risk of human ovarian cancer is related to dietary intake of selected nutrients, phytochemicals and food groups. *J Nutr*, 133: 1937–1942. PMID:12771342

McKinney PA, Cartwright RA, Saiu JM *et al.* (1987). The inter-regional epidemiological study of childhood cancer (IRESCC): a case control study of aetiological factors in leukaemia and lymphoma. *Arch Dis Child*, 62: 279–287. doi:10.1136/adc.62.3.279 PMID:3646026

Menegaux F, Ripert M, Hémon D, Clavel J (2007). Maternal alcohol and coffee drinking, parental smoking and childhood leukaemia: a French population-based case-control study. *Paediatr Perinat Epidemiol*, 21: 293–299. doi:10.1111/j.1365-3016.2007.00824.x PMID:17564585

Menegaux F, Steffen C, Bellec S *et al.* (2005). Maternal coffee and alcohol consumption during pregnancy, parental smoking and risk of childhood acute leukaemia. *Cancer Detect Prev*, 29: 487–493. doi:10.1016/j.cdp.2005.06.008 PMID:16289502

Mettlin C (1989). Milk drinking, other beverage habits, and lung cancer risk. *Int J Cancer*, 43: 608–612. doi:10.1002/ijc.2910430412 PMID:2703270

Middleton Fillmore K, Chikritzhs T, Stockwell T *et al.* (2009). Alcohol use and prostate cancer: a meta-analysis. *Mol Nutr Food Res*, 53: 240–255. doi:10.1002/mnfr.200800122 PMID:19156715

Million Women Study Collaborators (2005). Endometrial cancer and hormone-replacement therapy in the Million Women Study. *Lancet*, 365: 1543–1551.

Millikan RC, Newman B, Tse CK *et al.* (2008). Epidemiology of basal-like breast cancer. *Breast Cancer Res Treat*, 109: 123–139. doi:10.1007/s10549-007-9632-6 PMID:17578664

Minegishi Y, Tsukino H, Muto M *et al.* (2007). Susceptibility to lung cancer and genetic polymorphisms in the alcohol metabolite-related enzymes alcohol dehydrogenase 3, aldehyde dehydrogenase 2, and cytochrome P450 2E1 in the Japanese population. *Cancer*, 110: 353–362. doi:10.1002/cncr.22795 PMID:17559142

Miyasaka K, Kawanami T, Shimokata H *et al.* (2005). Inactive aldehyde dehydrogenase-2 increased the risk of pancreatic cancer among smokers in a Japanese male population. *Pancreas*, 30: 95–98. doi:10.1097/01.mpa.0000147084.70125.41 PMID:15714130

Mizoue T, Inoue M, Wakai K *et al.*Research Group for Development and Evaluation of Cancer Prevention Strategies in Japan (2008). Alcohol drinking and colorectal cancer in Japanese: a pooled analysis of results from five cohort studies. *Am J Epidemiol*, 167: 1397–1406. doi:10.1093/aje/kwn073 PMID:18420544

Modugno F, Ness RB, Allen GO (2003). Alcohol consumption and the risk of mucinous and nonmucinous epithelial ovarian cancer. *Obstet Gynecol*, 102: 1336–1343. doi:10.1016/j.obstetgynecol.2003.08.008 PMID:14662224

Monnereau A, Orsi L, Troussard X *et al.* (2008). Cigarette smoking, alcohol drinking, and risk of lymphoid neoplasms: results of a French case-control study. *Cancer Causes Control*, 19: 1147–1160. doi:10.1007/s10552-008-9182-1 PMID:18781390

Mørch LS, Johansen D, Thygesen LC *et al.* (2007). Alcohol drinking, consumption patterns and breast cancer among Danish nurses: a cohort study. *Eur J Public Health*, 17: 624–629. doi:10.1093/eurpub/ckm036 PMID:17442702

Mori M, Harabuchi I, Miyake H *et al.* (1988). Reproductive, genetic, and dietary risk factors for ovarian cancer. *Am J Epidemiol*, 128: 771–777. PMID:3421242

Morimoto K & Takeshita T (1996). Low Km aldehyde dehydrogenase (ALDH2) polymorphism, alcohol-drinking behavior, and chromosome alterations in peripheral lymphocytes. *Environ Health Perspect*, 104: Suppl 3563–567. doi:10.2307/3432824 PMID:8781384

Morita M, Le Marchand L, Kono S *et al.* (2009). Genetic polymorphisms of CYP2E1 and risk of colorectal cancer: the Fukuoka Colorectal Cancer Study. *Cancer Epidemiol Biomarkers Prev*, 18: 235–241. doi:10.1158/1055-9965.EPI-08-0698 PMID:19124503

Morita S, Yano M, Shiozaki H *et al.* (1997). CYP1A1, CYP2E1 and GSTM1 polymorphisms are not associated with susceptibility to squamous-cell carcinoma of the esophagus. *Int J Cancer*, 71: 192–195. doi:10.1002/(SICI)1097-0215(19970410)71:2<192::AID-IJC11>3.0.CO;2-K PMID:9139841

Morita S, Yano M, Tsujinaka T *et al.* (1999). Genetic polymorphisms of drug-metabolizing enzymes and susceptibility to head-and-neck squamous-cell carcinoma. *Int J Cancer*, 80: 685–688. doi:10.1002/(SICI)1097-0215(19990301)80:5<685::AID-IJC9>3.0.CO;2-W PMID:10048967

Morton LM, Holford TR, Leaderer B *et al.* (2003). Alcohol use and risk of non-Hodgkin's lymphoma among Connecticut women (United States). *Cancer Causes Control*, 14: 687–694. doi:10.1023/A:1025626208861 PMID:14575367

Morton LM, Zheng T, Holford TR *et al.*InterLymph Consortium (2005). Alcohol consumption and risk of non-Hodgkin lymphoma: a pooled analysis. *Lancet Oncol*, 6: 469–476. doi:10.1016/S1470-2045(05)70214-X PMID:15992695

Munaka M, Kohshi K, Kawamoto T *et al.* (2003). Genetic polymorphisms of tobacco- and alcohol-related metabolizing enzymes and the risk of hepatocellular carcinoma. *J Cancer Res Clin Oncol*, 129: 355–360. doi:10.1007/s00432-003-0439-5 PMID:12759747

Murata M, Tagawa M, Watanabe S *et al.* (1999). Genotype difference of aldehyde dehydrogenase 2 gene in alcohol drinkers influences the incidence of Japanese colorectal cancer patients. *Jpn J Cancer Res*, 90: 711–719. doi:10.1111/j.1349-7006.1999.tb00805.x PMID:10470282

Murata M, Takayama K, Choi BCK, Pak AWP (1996). A nested case-control study on alcohol drinking, tobacco smoking, and cancer. *Cancer Detect Prev*, 20: 557–565. PMID:8939341

Murata M, Watanabe M, Yamanaka M *et al.* (2001). Genetic polymorphisms in cytochrome P450 (CYP) 1A1, CYP1A2, CYP2E1, glutathione S-transferase (GST) M1 and GSTT1 and susceptibility to prostate cancer in the Japanese population. *Cancer Lett*, 165: 171–177. doi:10.1016/S0304-3835(01)00398-6 PMID:11275366

Murtaugh MA, Curtin K, Sweeney C *et al.* (2007). Dietary intake of folate and co-factors in folate metabolism, MTHFR polymorphisms, and reduced rectal cancer. *Cancer Causes Control*, 18: 153–163. doi:10.1007/s10552-006-0099-2 PMID:17245555

Muto M, Takahashi M, Ohtsu A *et al.* (2005). Risk of multiple squamous cell carcinomas both in the esophagus and the head and neck region. *Carcinogenesis*, 26: 1008–1012. doi:10.1093/carcin/bgi035 PMID:15718256

Muwonge R, Ramadas K, Sankila R *et al.* (2008). Role of tobacco smoking, chewing and alcohol drinking in the risk of oral cancer in Trivandrum, India: a nested case-control design using incident cancer cases. *Oral Oncol*, 44: 446–454. doi:10.1016/j.oraloncology.2007.06.002 PMID:17933578

Nachiappan V, Mufti SI, Chakravarti A *et al.* (1994). Lipid peroxidation and ethanol-related tumor promotion in Fischer-344 rats treated with tobacco-specific nitrosamines. *Alcohol Alcohol*, 29: 565–574. PMID:7811340

Nakajima M, Takeuchi T, Takeshita T, Morimoto K (1996). 8-Hydroxydeoxyguanosine in human leukocyte DNA and daily health practice factors: effects of individual alcohol sensitivity. *Environ Health Perspect*, 104: 1336–1338. doi:10.2307/3432971 PMID:9118876

Nakaya N, Tsubono Y, Kuriyama S *et al.* (2005). Alcohol consumption and the risk of cancer in Japanese men: the Miyagi cohort study. *Eur J Cancer Prev*, 14: 169–174. doi:10.1097/00008469-200504000-00013 PMID:15785321

Nan HM, Song YJ, Yun HY *et al.* (2005). Effects of dietary intake and genetic factors on hypermethylation of the hMLH1 gene promoter in gastric cancer. *World J Gastroenterol*, 11: 3834–3841. PMID:15991278

Nandakumar A, Anantha N, Dhar M *et al.* (1995). A case-control investigation on cancer of the ovary in Bangalore, India. *Int J Cancer*, 63: 361–365. doi:10.1002/ijc.2910630310 PMID:7591232

Nasca PC, Liu S, Baptiste MS *et al.* (1994). Alcohol consumption and breast cancer: estrogen receptor status and histology. *Am J Epidemiol*, 140: 980–988. PMID:7985660

Navasumrit P, Margison GP, O'Connor PJ (2001a). Ethanol modulates rat hepatic DNA repair functions. *Alcohol Alcohol*, 36: 369–376. PMID:11524300

Navasumrit P, Ward TH, Dodd NJ, O'Connor PJ (2000). Ethanol-induced free radicals and hepatic DNA strand breaks are prevented in vivo by antioxidants: effects of acute and chronic ethanol exposure. *Carcinogenesis*, 21: 93–99. doi:10.1093/carcin/21.1.93 PMID:10607739

Navasumrit P, Ward TH, O'Connor PJ *et al.* (2001b). Ethanol enhances the formation of endogenously and exogenously derived adducts in rat hepatic DNA. *Mutat Res*, 479: 81–94. PMID:11470483

Nelson RA, Levine AM, Marks G, Bernstein L (1997). Alcohol, tobacco and recreational drug use and the risk of non-Hodgkin's lymphoma. *Br J Cancer*, 76: 1532–1537. doi:10.1038/bjc.1997.590 PMID:9400954

Neumark YD, Friedlander Y, Thomasson HR, Li TK (1998). Association of the ADH2*2 allele with reduced ethanol consumption in Jewish men in Israel: a pilot study. *J Stud Alcohol*, 59: 133–139. PMID:9500299

Newcomb PA, Nichols HB, Beasley JM *et al.* (2009). No difference between red wine or white wine consumption and breast cancer risk. *Cancer Epidemiol Biomarkers Prev*, 18: 1007–1010. doi:10.1158/1055-9965.EPI-08-0801 PMID:19273487

Newcomb PA, Trentham-Dietz A, Storer BE (1997). Alcohol consumption in relation to endometrial cancer risk. *Cancer Epidemiol Biomarkers Prev*, 6: 775–778. PMID:9332758

Newton R, Ziegler J, Casabonne D *et al.*Uganda Kaposi's Sarcoma Study Group (2007). A case-control study of cancer of the uterine cervix in Uganda. *Eur J Cancer Prev*, 16: 555–558. doi:10.1097/01.cej.0000243863.22137.b7 PMID:18090129

Nielsen NR & Grønbaek M (2008). Interactions between intakes of alcohol and postmenopausal hormones on risk of breast cancer. *Int J Cancer*, 122: 1109–1113. doi:10.1002/ijc.23195 PMID:17966122

Niemelä O (2007). Acetaldehyde adduct in circulation. *Novartis Found Symp*, 285: 19–197.

Nieters A, Deeg E, Becker N (2006). Tobacco and alcohol consumption and risk of lymphoma: results of a population-based case-control study in Germany. *Int J Cancer*, 118: 422–430. doi:10.1002/ijc.21306 PMID:16080191

Nishimoto IN, Hanaoka T, Sugimura H *et al.* (2000). Cytochrome P450 2E1 polymorphism in gastric cancer in Brazil: case-control studies of Japanese Brazilians and non-Japanese Brazilians. *Cancer Epidemiol. Biomarkers Prev.*, 9: 675–680.

Nishimoto IN, Pinheiro NA, Rogatto SR *et al.* (2004). Alcohol dehydrogenase 3 genotype as a risk factor for upper aerodigestive tract cancers. *Arch Otolaryngol Head Neck Surg*, 130: 78–82. doi:10.1001/archotol.130.1.78 PMID:14732773

Nishino Y, Wakai K, Kondo T *et al.*JACC Study Group (2006). Alcohol consumption and lung cancer mortality in Japanese men: results from Japan collaborative cohort (JACC) study. *J Epidemiol*, 16: 49–56. doi:10.2188/jea.16.49 PMID:16537984

Nomura T, Noma H, Shibahara T *et al.* (2000). Aldehyde dehydrogenase 2 and glutathione S-transferase M 1 polymorphisms in relation to the risk for oral cancer in Japanese drinkers. *Oral Oncol*, 36: 42–46. doi:10.1016/S1368-8375(99)00048-2 PMID:10889918

Novoradovsky A, Tsai SJ, Goldfarb L *et al.* (1995). Mitochondrial aldehyde dehydrogenase polymorphism in Asian and American Indian populations: detection of new ALDH2 alleles. *Alcohol Clin Exp Res*, 19: 1105–1110. doi:10.1111/j.1530-0277.1995.tb01587.x PMID:8561277

NTP (2004). *Toxicology and Carcinogenesis Studies of Urethane, Ethanol, and Urethane/ethanol (Urethane, CAS No.51-79-6; Ethanol, CAS No. 64-17-5) in B6C3F1 Mice (Drinking Water Studies).* Technical Report Series No. 510, Research Triangle Park, NC.

Nuutinen H, Lindros KO, Salaspuro M (1983). Determinants of blood acetaldehyde level during ethanol oxidation in chronic alcoholics. *Alcohol Clin Exp Res*, 7: 163–168. doi:10.1111/j.1530-0277.1983.tb05432.x PMID:6346918

Nuutinen HU, Salaspuro MP, Valle M, Lindros KO (1984). Blood acetaldehyde concentration gradient between hepatic and antecubital venous blood in ethanol-intoxicated alcoholics and controls. *Eur J Clin Invest*, 14: 306–311. doi:10.1111/j.1365-2362.1984.tb01186.x PMID:6434326

O'Neil MJ, editor (2001). *The Merck Index*, 13th ed. Whitehouse Station, NJ, Merck & Co., Inc., pp. 1818

Obe G & Anderson D (1987). International Commission for Protection against Environmental Mutagens and Carcinogens. ICPEMC Working Paper No. 15/1. Genetic effects of ethanol. *Mutat Res*, 186: 177–200. PMID:3313027

Ohishi W, Fujiwara S, Cologne JB *et al.* (2008). Risk factors for hepatocellular carcinoma in a Japanese population: a nested case-control study. *Cancer Epidemiol Biomarkers Prev*, 17: 846–854. doi:10.1158/1055-9965.EPI-07-2806 PMID:18398026

Olivieri EHR, da Silva SD, Mendonça FF *et al.* (2009). CYP1A2*1C, CYP2E1*5B, and GSTM1 polymorphisms are predictors of risk and poor outcome in head and neck squamous cell carcinoma patients. *Oral Oncol*, 45: e73–e79. doi:10.1016/j.oraloncology.2009.03.004 PMID:19442564

Olshan AF, Weissler MC, Watson MA, Bell DA (2001). Risk of head and neck cancer and the alcohol dehydrogenase 3 genotype. *Carcinogenesis*, 22: 57–61. doi:10.1093/carcin/22.1.57 PMID:11159741

Osier MV, Pakstis AJ, Goldman D *et al.* (2002). A proline-threonine substitution in codon 351 of ADH1C is common in Native Americans. *Alcohol Clin Exp Res*, 26: 1759–1763. doi:10.1111/j.1530-0277.2002.tb02481.x PMID:12500098

Ostrovsky YM (1986). Endogenous ethanol–its metabolic, behavioral and biomedical significance. *Alcohol*, 3: 239–247. doi:10.1016/0741-8329(86)90032-7 PMID:3530279

Otani T, Iwasaki M, Hanaoka T *et al.* (2005). Folate, vitamin B6, vitamin B12, and vitamin B2 intake, genetic polymorphisms of related enzymes, and risk of colorectal cancer in a hospital-based case-control study in Japan. *Nutr Cancer*, 53: 42–50. doi:10.1207/s15327914nc5301_5 PMID:16351505

Ough CS (1987). Chemicals used in making wine. *Chem Eng News*, 65: 19–28. doi:10.1021/cen-v065n001.p019

Oyama T, Kawamoto T, Mizoue T *et al.* (1997). Cytochrome P450 2E1 polymorphism as a risk factor for lung cancer: in relation to p53 gene mutation. *Anticancer Res*, 17: 1B583–587. PMID:9066584

Ozasa KJapan Collaborative Cohort Study for Evaluation of Cancer (2007). Alcohol use and mortality in the Japan Collaborative Cohort Study for Evaluation of

Cancer (JACC). *Asian Pac J Cancer Prev*, 8: Suppl81–88. PMID:18260706

Pacella-Norman R, Urban MI, Sitas F *et al.* (2002). Risk factors for oesophageal, lung, oral and laryngeal cancers in black South Africans. *Br J Cancer*, 86: 1751–1756. doi:10.1038/sj.bjc.6600338 PMID:12087462

Pandeya N, Williams G, Green AC *et al.* Australian Cancer Study (2009). Alcohol consumption and the risks of adenocarcinoma and squamous cell carcinoma of the esophagus. *Gastroenterology*, 136: 1215–1224, e1–e2. doi:10.1053/j.gastro.2008.12.052 PMID:19250648

Pandya GA & Moriya M (1996). 1,N6-ethenodeoxyadenosine, a DNA adduct highly mutagenic in mammalian cells. *Biochemistry*, 35: 11487–11492. doi:10.1021/bi960170h PMID:8784204

Parazzini F, La Vecchia C, D'Avanzo B *et al.* (1995a). Alcohol and endometrial cancer risk: findings from an Italian case-control study. *Nutr Cancer*, 23: 55–62. doi:10.1080/01635589509514361 PMID:7739915

Parazzini F, Moroni S, Negri E *et al.* (1995b). Selected food intake and risk of vulvar cancer. *Cancer*, 76: 2291–2296. doi:10.1002/1097-0142(19951201)76:11<2291::AID-CNCR2820761117>3.0.CO;2-W PMID:8635034

Parkin DM, Srivatanakul P, Khlat M *et al.* (1991). Liver cancer in Thailand. I. A case-control study of cholangiocarcinoma. *Int J Cancer*, 48: 323–328. doi:10.1002/ijc.2910480302 PMID:1645697

Parkin DM, Vizcaino AP, Skinner ME, Ndhlovu A (1994). Cancer patterns and risk factors in the African population of southwestern Zimbabwe, 1963–1977. *Cancer Epidemiol Biomarkers Prev*, 3: 537–547. PMID:7827583

Parkinson A, Ogilvie BW (2008). *Biotransformation of Xenobiotics.* In: *Casarett & Doull's Toxicology: The Basic Science of Poisons.* Klaassen CD, editor. Kansas City: McGraw Hill Medical, pp. 161–304.

Pelucchi C, Galeone C, Montella M *et al.* (2008). Alcohol consumption and renal cell cancer risk in two Italian case-control studies. *Ann Oncol*, 19: 1003–1008. doi:10.1093/annonc/mdm590 PMID:18187482

Pelucchi C, La Vecchia C, Negri E *et al.* (2002). Alcohol drinking and renal cell carcinoma in women and men. *Eur J Cancer Prev*, 11: 543–545. doi:10.1097/00008469-200212000-00006 PMID:12457106

Pelucchi C, Mereghetti M, Talamini R *et al.* (2005). Dietary folate, alcohol consumption, and risk of ovarian cancer in an Italian case-control study. *Cancer Epidemiol Biomarkers Prev*, 14: 2056–2058. doi:10.1158/1055-9965.EPI-05-0192 PMID:16103462

Pereira Serafim PV, Cotrim Guerreiro da Silva ID, Manoukias Forones N (2008). Relationship between genetic polymorphism of CYP1A1 at codon 462 (Ile462Val) in colorectal cancer. *Int J Biol Markers*, 23: 18–23. PMID:18409146

Persson I, Johansson I, Bergung H *et al.* (1993). Genetic polymorphism of cytochrome P4502E1 in a Swedish population. Relationship to incidence of lung cancer. *FEBS Lett*, 319: 207–211. doi:10.1016/0014-5793(93)80547-8 PMID:8096192

Persson I, Johansson I, Yue Q-Y *et al.* (1999). Genetic polymorphism of xenobiotic metabolizing enzymes among Chinese lung cancer patients. *Int J Cancer*, 81: 325–329. doi:10.1002/(SICI)1097-0215(19990505)81:3<325::AID-IJC2>3.0.CO;2-S PMID:10209943

Peters ES, McClean MD, Liu M *et al.* (2005). The ADH1C polymorphism modifies the risk of squamous cell carcinoma of the head and neck associated with alcohol and tobacco use. *Cancer Epidemiol Biomarkers Prev*, 14: 476–482. doi:10.1158/1055-9965.EPI-04-0431 PMID:15734975

Peterson NB, Trentham-Dietz A, Newcomb PA *et al.* (2006). Alcohol consumption and ovarian cancer risk in a population-based case-control study. *Int J Cancer*, 119: 2423–2427. doi:10.1002/ijc.22137 PMID:16921486

Petridou E, Koukoulomatis P, Dessypris N *et al.* (2002). Why is endometrial cancer less common in Greece than in other European Union countries? *Eur J Cancer Prev*, 11: 427–432. doi:10.1097/00008469-200210000-00004 PMID:12394239

Phillips BJ & Jenkinson P (2001). Is ethanol genotoxic? A review of the published data. *Mutagenesis*, 16: 91–101. doi:10.1093/mutage/16.2.91 PMID:11230549

Pierce RJ, Kune GA, Kune S *et al.* (1989). Dietary and alcohol intake, smoking pattern, occupational risk, and family history in lung cancer patients: results of a case-control study in males. *Nutr Cancer*, 12: 237–248. doi:10.1080/01635588909514023 PMID:2771801

Pikkarainen P, Baraona E, Seitz H, Lieber CS (1980). Breath acetaldehyde: evidence of acetaldehyde production by oropharynx microflora and by lung microsomes. *Adv Exp Med Biol*, 132: 469–474. PMID:7424726

Pires PW, Furtado KS, Justullin LA Jr *et al.* (2008). Chronic ethanol intake promotes double gluthatione S-transferase/transforming growth factor-alpha-positive hepatocellular lesions in male Wistar rats. *Cancer Sci*, 99: 221–228. doi:10.1111/j.1349-7006.2007.00677.x PMID:18271918

Platz EA, Leitzmann MF, Rimm EB *et al.* (2004). Alcohol intake, drinking patterns, and risk of prostate cancer in a large prospective cohort study. *Am J Epidemiol*, 159: 444–453. doi:10.1093/aje/kwh062 PMID:14977640

Pluskota-Karwatka D, Pawłowicz AJ, Kronberg L (2006). Formation of malonaldehyde-acetaldehyde conjugate adducts in calf thymus DNA. *Chem Res Toxicol*, 19: 921–926. doi:10.1021/tx060027h PMID:16841960

Pogoda JM, Nichols PW, Preston-Martin S (2004). Alcohol consumption and risk of adult-onset acute myeloid leukemia: results from a Los Angeles County case-control study. *Leuk Res*, 28: 927–931. doi:10.1016/j.leukres.2004.01.007 PMID:15234569

Pollack ES, Nomura AM, Heilbrun LK *et al.* (1984). Prospective study of alcohol consumption and cancer. *N Engl J Med*, 310: 617–621. doi:10.1056/NEJM198403083101003 PMID:6694673

Polychronopoulou A, Tzonou A, Hsieh CC *et al.* (1993). Reproductive variables, tobacco, ethanol, coffee and somatometry as risk factors for ovarian cancer. *Int J Cancer*, 55: 402–407. doi:10.1002/ijc.2910550312 PMID:8375923

Pool-Zobel BL, Dornacher I, Lambertz R *et al.* (2004). Genetic damage and repair in human rectal cells for biomonitoring: sex differences, effects of alcohol exposure, and susceptibilities in comparison to peripheral blood lymphocytes. *Mutat Res*, 551: 127–134. PMID:15225587

Potter JD, Sellers TA, Folsom AR, McGovern PG (1992). Alcohol, beer, and lung cancer in postmenopausal women. The Iowa Women's Health Study. *Ann Epidemiol*, 2: 587–595. doi:10.1016/1047-2797(92)90003-9 PMID:1342310

Powell H, Kitteringham NR, Pirmohamed M *et al.* (1998). Expression of cytochrome P4502E1 in human liver: assessment by mRNA, genotype and phenotype. *Pharmacogenetics*, 8: 411–421. doi:10.1097/00008571-199810000-00006 PMID:9825833

Prescott E, Grønbaek M, Becker U, Sørensen TI (1999). Alcohol intake and the risk of lung cancer: influence of type of alcoholic beverage. *Am J Epidemiol*, 149: 463–470. PMID:10067906

Prior P (1988). Long-term cancer risk in alcoholism. *Alcohol Alcohol*, 23: 163–171. PMID:3390240

Purdue MP, Hashibe M, Berthiller J *et al.* (2009). Type of alcoholic beverage and risk of head and neck cancer–a pooled analysis within the INHANCE Consortium. *Am J Epidemiol*, 169: 132–142. doi:10.1093/aje/kwn306 PMID:19064644

Putnam SD, Cerhan JR, Parker AS *et al.* (2000). Lifestyle and anthropometric risk factors for prostate cancer in a cohort of Iowa men. *Ann Epidemiol*, 10: 361–369. doi:10.1016/S1047-2797(00)00057-0 PMID:10964002

Qin JM, Yang L, Chen B *et al.* (2008). Interaction of methylenetetrahydrofolate reductase C677T, cytochrome P4502E1 polymorphism and environment factors in esophageal cancer in Kazakh population. *World J Gastroenterol*, 14: 6986–6992. doi:10.3748/wjg.14.6986 PMID:19058336

Quiñones L, Lucas D, Godoy J *et al.* (2001). CYP1A1, CYP2E1 and GSTM1 genetic polymorphisms. The effect of single and combined genotypes on lung cancer susceptibility in Chilean people. *Cancer Lett*, 174: 35–44. doi:10.1016/S0304-3835(01)00686-3 PMID:11675150

Rachtan J (2002). Alcoholic beverages consumption and lung cancer cell types among women in Poland. *Lung Cancer*, 35: 119–127. doi:10.1016/S0169-5002(01)00331-2 PMID:11804683

Rachtan J & Sokolowski A (1997). Risk factors for lung cancer among women in Poland. *Lung Cancer*, 18: 137–145. doi:10.1016/S0169-5002(97)00062-7 PMID:9316005

Radike MJ, Stemmer KL, Bingham E (1981). Effect of ethanol on vinyl chloride carcinogenesis. *Environ Health Perspect*, 41: 59–62. doi:10.1289/ehp.814159 PMID:6277614

Rauscher GH, Shore D, Sandler DP (2004). Alcohol intake and incidence of de novo adult acute leukemia. *Leuk Res*, 28: 1263–1265. doi:10.1016/j.leukres.2004.04.004 PMID:15475066

Rehm J, Patra J, Popova S (2007). Alcohol drinking cessation and its effect on esophageal and head and neck cancers: a pooled analysis. *Int J Cancer*, 121: 1132–1137. doi:10.1002/ijc.22798 PMID:17487833

Ribas G, Milne RL, Gonzalez-Neira A, Benítez J (2008). Haplotype patterns in cancer-related genes with long-range linkage disequilibrium: no evidence of association with breast cancer or positive selection. *Eur J Hum Genet*, 16: 252–260. doi:10.1038/sj.ejhg.5201953 PMID:18000525

Riman T, Dickman PW, Nilsson S *et al.* (2004). Some life-style factors and the risk of invasive epithelial ovarian cancer in Swedish women. *Eur J Epidemiol*, 19: 1011–1019. doi:10.1007/s10654-004-1633-8 PMID:15648594

Risch A, Ramroth H, Raedts V *et al.* (2003). Laryngeal cancer risk in Caucasians is associated with alcohol and tobacco consumption but not modified by genetic polymorphisms in class I alcohol dehydrogenases ADH1B and ADH1C, and glutathione-S-transferases GSTM1 and GSTT1. *Pharmacogenetics*, 13: 225–230. doi:10.1097/00008571-200304000-00007 PMID:12668919

Robbins WA, Vine MF, Truong KY, Everson RB (1997). Use of fluorescence in situ hybridization (FISH) to assess effects of smoking, caffeine, and alcohol on aneuploidy load in sperm of healthy men. *Environ Mol Mutagen*, 30: 175–183. doi:10.1002/(SICI)1098-2280(1997)30:2<175::AID-EM10>3.0.CO;2-A PMID:9329642

Robinette CD, Hrubec Z, Fraumeni JF Jr (1979). Chronic alcoholism and subsequent mortality in World War II veterans. *Am J Epidemiol*, 109: 687–700. PMID:453188

Rod NH, Hansen AM, Nielsen J *et al.* (2009). Low-risk factor profile, estrogen levels, and breast cancer risk among postmenopausal women. *Int J Cancer*, 124: 1935–1940. doi:10.1002/ijc.24136 PMID:19123466

Rogers J, Smith J, Starmer GA, Whitfield JB (1987). Differing effects of carbohydrate, fat and protein on the rate of ethanol metabolism. *Alcohol Alcohol*, 22: 345–353. PMID:3426763

Rohrmann S, Linseisen J, Boshuizen HC *et al.* (2006). Ethanol intake and risk of lung cancer in the European Prospective Investigation into Cancer and Nutrition (EPIC). *Am J Epidemiol*, 164: 1103–1114. doi:10.1093/aje/kwj326 PMID:16987924

Rohrmann S, Linseisen J, Key TJ *et al.* (2008). Alcohol consumption and the risk for prostate cancer in the European Prospective Investigation into Cancer and Nutrition. *Cancer Epidemiol Biomarkers Prev*, 17: 1282–1287. doi:10.1158/1055-9965.EPI-07-2888 PMID:18483352

Rohrmann S, Linseisen J, Vrieling A *et al.* (2009). Ethanol intake and the risk of pancreatic cancer in the European Prospective Investigation into Cancer and Nutrition (EPIC). *Cancer Causes Control*, 20: 785–794. doi:10.1007/s10552-008-9293-8 PMID:19145468

Rossini A, Rapozo DCM, Soares Lima SC *et al.* (2007). Polymorphisms of GSTP1 and GSTT1, but not of CYP2A6, CYP2E1 or GSTM1, modify the risk for esophageal cancer in a western population. *Carcinogenesis*, 28: 2537–2542. doi:10.1093/carcin/bgm222 PMID:17916905

Roy HK, Gulizia JM, Karolski WJ *et al.* (2002). Ethanol promotes intestinal tumorigenesis in the MIN mouse. Multiple intestinal neoplasia. *Cancer Epidemiol Biomarkers Prev*, 11: 1499–1502. PMID:12433735

Ruano-Ravina A, Figueiras A, Barros-Dios JM (2004). Type of wine and risk of lung cancer: a case-control study in Spain. *Thorax*, 59: 981–985. doi:10.1136/thx.2003.018861 PMID:15516476

Rudant J, Menegaux F, Leverger G *et al.* (2008). Childhood hematopoietic malignancies and parental use of tobacco and alcohol: the ESCALE study (SFCE). *Cancer Causes Control*, 19: 1277–1290. doi:10.1007/s10552-008-9199-5 PMID:18618277

Ruwali M, Khan AJ, Shah PP *et al.* (2009). Cytochrome P450 2E1 and head and neck cancer: interaction with genetic and environmental risk factors. *Environ Mol Mutagen*, 50: 473–482. doi:10.1002/em.20488 PMID:19334053

Sakamoto T, Hara M, Higaki Y *et al.* (2006). Influence of alcohol consumption and gene polymorphisms of ADH2 and ALDH2 on hepatocellular carcinoma in a Japanese population. *Int J Cancer*, 118: 1501–1507. doi:10.1002/ijc.21505 PMID:16187278

Salaspuro MP (2003). Acetaldehyde, microbes, and cancer of the digestive tract. *Crit Rev Clin Lab Sci*, 40: 183–208. doi:10.1080/713609333 PMID:12755455

Schmidt W & Popham RE (1981). The role of drinking and smoking in mortality from cancer and other causes in male alcoholics. *Cancer*, 47: 1031–1041. doi:10.1002/1097-0142(19810301)47:5<1031::AID-CNCR2820470534>3.0.CO;2-C PMID:7226036

Schouten LJ, Zeegers MPA, Goldbohm RA, van den Brandt PA (2004). Alcohol and ovarian cancer risk: results from the Netherlands Cohort Study. *Cancer Causes Control*, 15: 201–209. doi:10.1023/B:CACO.0000019512.71560.2b PMID:15017133

Schuurman AG, Goldbohm RA, van den Brandt PA (1999). A prospective cohort study on consumption of alcoholic beverages in relation to prostate cancer incidence (The Netherlands). *Cancer Causes Control*, 10: 597–605. doi:10.1023/A:1008925103542 PMID:10616828

Schwartz SM, Doody DR, Fitzgibbons ED *et al.* (2001). Oral squamous cell cancer risk in relation to alcohol consumption and alcohol dehydrogenase-3 genotypes. *Cancer Epidemiol Biomarkers Prev*, 10: 1137–1144. PMID:11700261

Seitz HK, Egerer G, Oneta C *et al.* (1996). Alcohol dehydrogenase in the human colon and rectum. *Digestion*, 57: 105–108. doi:10.1159/000201322 PMID:8785998

Sesso HD, Paffenbarger RS Jr, Lee IM (2001). Alcohol consumption and risk of prostate cancer: The Harvard Alumni Health Study. *Int J Epidemiol*, 30: 749–755. doi:10.1093/ije/30.4.749 PMID:11511598

Setiawan VW, Monroe KR, Goodman MT *et al.* (2008). Alcohol consumption and endometrial cancer risk: the multiethnic cohort. *Int J Cancer*, 122: 634–638. doi:10.1002/ijc.23072 PMID:17764072

Setiawan VW, Monroe KR, Wilkens LR *et al.* (2009). Breast cancer risk factors defined by estrogen and progesterone receptor status: the multiethnic cohort study. *Am J Epidemiol*, 169: 1251–1259. doi:10.1093/aje/kwp036 PMID:19318616

Severson RK, Buckley JD, Woods WG *et al.* (1993). Cigarette smoking and alcohol consumption by parents of children with acute myeloid leukemia: an analysis within morphological subgroups–a report from the Childrens Cancer Group. *Cancer Epidemiol Biomarkers Prev*, 2: 433–439. PMID:8220087

Shaib YH, El-Serag HB, Nooka AK *et al.* (2007). Risk factors for intrahepatic and extrahepatic cholangiocarcinoma: a hospital-based case-control study. *Am J Gastroenterol*, 102: 1016–1021. doi:10.1111/j.1572-0241.2007.01104.x PMID:17324130

Sharpe CR & Siemiatycki J (2001). Case-control study of alcohol consumption and prostate cancer risk in Montréal, Canada. *Cancer Causes Control*, 12: 589–598. doi:10.1023/A:1011289108040 PMID:11552706

Sherman D, Davé V, Hsu LC *et al.* (1993). Diverse polymorphism within a short coding region of the human aldehyde dehydrogenase-5 (ALDH5) gene. *Hum Genet*, 92: 477–480. doi:10.1007/BF00216454 PMID:8244338

Shibata A, Fukuda K, Nishiyori A *et al.* (1998). A case-control study on male hepatocellular carcinoma based on hospital and community controls. *J Epidemiol*, 8: 1–5. doi:10.2188/jea.8.1 PMID:9575688

Shibayama Y, Nishijima A, Asaka S, Nakata K (1993). Influence of chronic alcohol consumption on the development of altered hepatocellular foci in rats. *Exp Toxicol Pathol*, 45: 15–19. doi:10.1016/S0940-2993(11)80442-2 PMID:8467195

Shimazu T, Inoue M, Sasazuki S *et al.*Japan Public Health Center-based Prospective Study Group (2008). Alcohol and risk of lung cancer among Japanese men: data from a large-scale population-based cohort study, the

JPHC study. *Cancer Causes Control*, 19: 1095–1102. doi:10.1007/s10552-008-9173-2 PMID:18493860
Shin HR, Lee CU, Park HJ *et al.* (1996). Hepatitis B and C virus, Clonorchis sinensis for the risk of liver cancer: a case-control study in Pusan, Korea. *Int J Epidemiol*, 25: 933–940. doi:10.1093/ije/25.5.933 PMID:8921477
Shu XO, Brinton LA, Zheng W *et al.* (1991). A population-based case-control study of endometrial cancer in Shanghai, China. *Int J Cancer*, 49: 38–43. doi:10.1002/ijc.2910490108 PMID:1874568
Shu CC, Hoffman WE, Thomas C, Albrecht RF (1993). Sympathetic activity enhances glucose-related ischemic injury in the rat.). Sympathetic activity enhances glucose-related ischemic injury in the rat. *Anesthesiology*, 78: 1120–1125. doi:10.1097/00000542-199306000-00015 PMID:8099768
Shu XO, Ross JA, Pendergrass TW *et al.* (1996). Parental alcohol consumption, cigarette smoking, and risk of infant leukemia: a Childrens Cancer Group study. *J Natl Cancer Inst*, 88: 24–31. doi:10.1093/jnci/88.1.24 PMID:8847721
Sigvardsson S, Hardell L, Przybeck TR, Cloninger R (1996). Increased cancer risk among Swedish female alcoholics. *Epidemiology*, 7: 140–143. doi:10.1097/00001648-199603000-00006 PMID:8834552
Singletary K, Nelshoppen J, Wallig M (1995). Enhancement by chronic ethanol intake of N-methyl-N-nitrosourea-induced rat mammary tumorigenesis. *Carcinogenesis*, 16: 959–964. doi:10.1093/carcin/16.4.959 PMID:7728981
Soffritti M, Belpoggi F, Cevolani D *et al.* (2002a). Results of long-term experimental studies on the carcinogenicity of methyl alcohol and ethyl alcohol in rats. *Ann N Y Acad Sci*, 982: 46–69. doi:10.1111/j.1749-6632.2002.tb04924.x PMID:12562628
Soffritti M, Belpoggi F, Lambertin L *et al.* (2002b). Results of long-term experimental studies on the carcinogenicity of formaldehyde and acetaldehyde in rats. *Ann N Y Acad Sci*, 982: 87–105. doi:10.1111/j.1749-6632.2002.tb04926.x PMID:12562630
Solomon PR, Selvam GS, Shanmugam G (2008). Polymorphism in ADH and MTHFR genes in oral squamous cell carcinoma of Indians. *Oral Dis*, 14: 633–639. doi:10.1111/j.1601-0825.2007.01437.x PMID:18266839
Sørensen HT, Friis S, Olsen JH *et al.* (1998). Risk of liver and other types of cancer in patients with cirrhosis: a nationwide cohort study in Denmark. *Hepatology*, 28: 921–925. doi:10.1002/hep.510280404 PMID:9755226
Soya SS, Vinod T, Reddy KS *et al.* (2008). CYP2E1 polymorphisms and gene-environment interactions in the risk of upper aerodigestive tract cancers among Indians. *Pharmacogenomics*, 9: 551–560. doi:10.2217/14622416.9.5.551 PMID:18466102
Speit G, Fröhler-Keller M, Schütz P, Neuss S (2008). Low sensitivity of the comet assay to detect acetaldehyde-induced genotoxicity. *Mutat Res*, 657: 93–97. PMID:18755289
Spence JP, Liang T, Eriksson CJP *et al.* (2003). Evaluation of aldehyde dehydrogenase 1 promoter polymorphisms identified in human populations. *Alcohol Clin Exp Res*, 27: 1389–1394. doi:10.1097/01.ALC.0000087086.50089.59 PMID:14506398
Spinucci G, Guidetti M, Lanzoni E, Pironi L (2006). Endogenous ethanol production in a patient with chronic intestinal pseudo-obstruction and small intestinal bacterial overgrowth. *Eur J Gastroenterol Hepatol*, 18: 799–802. doi:10.1097/01.meg.0000223906.55245.61 PMID:16772842
Sriamporn S, Wiangnon S, Suwanrungruang K *et al.* (2007). Risk factors for colorectal cancer in northeast Thailand: lifestyle related. *Asian Pac J Cancer Prev*, 8: 573–577. PMID:18260731
Stein S, Lao Y, Yang IY *et al.* (2006). Genotoxicity of acetaldehyde- and crotonaldehyde-induced 1,N2-propanodeoxyguanosine DNA adducts in human cells. *Mutat Res*, 608: 1–7. PMID:16797223
Stemmermann GN, Nomura AMY, Chyou P-H, Yoshizawa C (1990). Prospective study of alcohol intake and large bowel cancer. *Dig Dis Sci*, 35: 1414–1420. doi:10.1007/BF01536750 PMID:2226103
Sturgeon SR, Ziegler RG, Brinton LA *et al.* (1991). Diet and the risk of vulvar cancer. *Ann Epidemiol*, 1: 427–437. doi:10.1016/1047-2797(91)90012-2 PMID:1669523
Sturgis EM, Dahlstrom KR, Guan Y *et al.* (2001). Alcohol dehydrogenase 3 genotype is not associated with risk of squamous cell carcinoma of the oral cavity and pharynx. *Cancer Epidemiol Biomarkers Prev*, 10: 273–275. PMID:11303599
Sugimura T, Kumimoto H, Tohnai I *et al.* (2006). Gene-environment interaction involved in oral carcinogenesis: molecular epidemiological study for metabolic and DNA repair gene polymorphisms. *J Oral Pathol Med*, 35: 11–18. doi:10.1111/j.1600-0714.2005.00364.x PMID:16393248
Sung NY, Choi KS, Park EC *et al.* (2007). Smoking, alcohol and gastric cancer risk in Korean men: the National Health Insurance Corporation Study. *Br J Cancer*, 97: 700–704. doi:10.1038/sj.bjc.6603893 PMID:17637680
Sutcliffe S, Giovannucci E, Leitzmann MF *et al.* (2007). A prospective cohort study of red wine consumption and risk of prostate cancer. *Int J Cancer*, 120: 1529–1535. doi:10.1002/ijc.22498 PMID:17211860
Suzuki R, Orsini N, Mignone L *et al.* (2008). Alcohol intake and risk of breast cancer defined by estrogen and progesterone receptor status — a meta-analysis of epidemiological studies. *Int J Cancer* 122: 1832–1841. EIN - *Int J Cancer*, 123: 981
Swanson CA, Wilbanks GD, Twiggs LB *et al.* (1993). Moderate alcohol consumption and the risk of endometrial cancer. *Epidemiology*, 4: 530–536. doi:10.1097/00001648-199311000-00009 PMID:8268282

Takeshita T, Morimoto K, Yamaguchi N *et al.* (2000a). Relationships between cigarette smoking, alcohol drinking, the ALDH2 genotype and adenomatous types of colorectal polyps in male self-defense force officials. *J Epidemiol*, 10: 366–371. doi:10.2188/jea.10.366 PMID:11210104

Takeshita T, Yang X, Inoue Y *et al.* (2000b). Relationship between alcohol drinking, ADH2 and ALDH2 genotypes, and risk for hepatocellular carcinoma in Japanese. *Cancer Lett*, 149: 69–76. doi:10.1016/S0304-3835(99)00343-2 PMID:10737710

Takezaki T, Inoue M, Kataoka H *et al.* (2003). Diet and lung cancer risk from a 14-year population-based prospective study in Japan: with special reference to fish consumption. *Nutr Cancer*, 45: 160–167. doi:10.1207/S15327914NC4502_04 PMID:12881009

Tan W, Song N, Wang GQ *et al.* (2000). Impact of genetic polymorphisms in cytochrome P450 2E1 and glutathione S-transferases M1, T1, and P1 on susceptibility to esophageal cancer among high-risk individuals in China. *Cancer Epidemiol Biomarkers Prev*, 9: 551–556. PMID:10868687

Tanabe H, Ohhira M, Ohtsubo T *et al.* (1999). Genetic polymorphism of aldehyde dehydrogenase 2 in patients with upper aerodigestive tract cancer. *Alcohol Clin Exp Res*, 23: Suppl17S–20S. doi:10.1111/j.1530-0277.1999.tb04527.x PMID:10235272

Tanaka T, Nishikawa A, Iwata H *et al.* (1989). Enhancing effect of ethanol on aflatoxin B1-induced hepatocarcinogenesis in male ACI/N rats. *Jpn J Cancer Res*, 80: 526–530. doi:10.1111/j.1349-7006.1989.tb01671.x PMID:2474524

Tatsuta M, Iishi H, Baba M *et al.* (1997). Enhancement by ethyl alcohol of experimental hepatocarcinogenesis induced by N-nitrosomorpholine. *Int J Cancer*, 71: 1045–1048. doi:10.1002/(SICI)1097-0215(19970611)71:6<1045::AID-IJC21>3.0.CO;2-B PMID:9185709

Tavani A, Gallus S, Dal Maso L *et al.* (2001a). Coffee and alcohol intake and risk of ovarian cancer: an Italian case-control study. *Nutr Cancer*, 39: 29–34. doi:10.1207/S15327914nc391_4 PMID:11588899

Tavani A, Gallus S, La Vecchia C, Franceschi S (2001b). Alcohol drinking and risk of non-Hodgkin's lymphoma. *Eur J Clin Nutr*, 55: 824–826. doi:10.1038/sj.ejcn.1601245 PMID:11593342

Tavani A, Pregnolato A, Negri E *et al.* (1997). Diet and risk of lymphoid neoplasms and soft tissue sarcomas. *Nutr Cancer*, 27: 256–260. doi:10.1080/01635589709514535 PMID:9101555

Terelius Y, Norsten-Höög C, Cronholm T, Ingelman-Sundberg M (1991). Acetaldehyde as a substrate for ethanol-inducible cytochrome P450 (CYP2E1). *Biochem Biophys Res Commun*, 179: 689–694. doi:10.1016/0006-291X(91)91427-E PMID:1822117

Terry MB, Gammon MD, Zhang FF *et al.* (2006). ADH3 genotype, alcohol intake and breast cancer risk. *Carcinogenesis*, 27: 840–847. doi:10.1093/carcin/bgi285 PMID:16344274

Terry MB, Gammon MD, Zhang FF *et al.* (2007a). Alcohol dehydrogenase 3 and risk of esophageal and gastric adenocarcinomas. *Cancer Causes Control*, 18: 1039–1046. doi:10.1007/s10552-007-9046-0 PMID:17665311

Terry MB, Knight JA, Zablotska L *et al.* (2007). Alcohol metabolism, alcohol intake, and breast cancer risk: a sister-set analysis using the Breast Cancer Family Registry. *Breast Cancer Res Treat*, 106: 281–288. doi:10.1007/s10549-007-9498-7 PMID:17268812

Terry MB, Knight JA, Zablotska L *et al.* (2007b). Alcohol metabolism, alcohol intake, and breast cancer risk: a sister-set analysis using the Breast Cancer Family Registry. *Breast Cancer Res Treat*, 106: 281–288. doi:10.1007/s10549-007-9498-7 PMID:17268812

Terry P, Baron JA, Weiderpass E *et al.* (1999). Lifestyle and endometrial cancer risk: a cohort study from the Swedish Twin Registry. *Int J Cancer*, 82: 38–42. doi:10.1002/(SICI)1097-0215(19990702)82:1<38::AID-IJC8>3.0.CO;2-Q PMID:10360818

Theruvathu JA, Jaruga P, Nath RG *et al.* (2005). Polyamines stimulate the formation of mutagenic 1,N2-propanodeoxyguanosine adducts from acetaldehyde. *Nucleic Acids Res*, 33: 3513–3520. doi:10.1093/nar/gki661 PMID:15972793

Thomas DB, Qin Q, Kuypers J *et al.* (2001b). Human papillomaviruses and cervical cancer in Bangkok. II. Risk factors for in situ and invasive squamous cell cervical carcinomas. *Am J Epidemiol*, 153: 732–739. doi:10.1093/aje/153.8.732 PMID:11296144

Thomas DB, Ray RM, Koetsawang A *et al.* (2001a). Human papillomaviruses and cervical cancer in Bangkok. I. Risk factors for invasive cervical carcinomas with human papillomavirus types 16 and 18 DNA. *Am J Epidemiol*, 153: 723–731. doi:10.1093/aje/153.8.723 PMID:11296143

Thun MJ, Hannan LM, DeLancey JO (2009). Alcohol consumption not associated with lung cancer mortality in lifelong nonsmokers. *Cancer Epidemiol Biomarkers Prev*, 18: 2269–2272. doi:10.1158/1055-9965.EPI-09-0361 PMID:19661085

Thygesen LC, Keiding N, Johansen C, Grønbaek M (2007). Changes in alcohol intake and risk of upper digestive tract cancer. *Acta Oncol*, 46: 1085–1089. doi:10.1080/02841860701441806 PMID:17851863

Thygesen LC, Mikkelsen P, Andersen TV *et al.* (2009). Cancer incidence among patients with alcohol use disorders–long-term follow-up. *Alcohol Alcohol*, 44: 387–391. PMID:19491282

Thygesen LC, Mørch LS, Keiding N *et al.* (2008a). Use of baseline and updated information on alcohol intake on risk for breast cancer: importance of latency. *Int*

J Epidemiol, 37: 669–677. doi:10.1093/ije/dyn060 PMID:18390878

Thygesen LC, Wu K, Grønbaek M *et al.* (2008b). Alcohol intake and colorectal cancer: a comparison of approaches for including repeated measures of alcohol consumption. *Epidemiology*, 19: 258–264. doi:10.1097/EDE.0b013e31816339e0 PMID:18300715

Tian D, Feng Z, Hanley NM *et al.* (1998). Multifocal accumulation of p53 protein in esophageal carcinoma: evidence for field cancerization. *Int J Cancer*, 78: 568–575. doi:10.1002/(SICI)1097-0215(19981123)78:5<568::AID-IJC7>3.0.CO;2-3 PMID:9808524

Tiemersma EW, Wark PA, Ocké MC *et al.* (2003). Alcohol consumption, alcohol dehydrogenase 3 polymorphism, and colorectal adenomas. *Cancer Epidemiol Biomarkers Prev*, 12: 419–425. PMID:12750236

Tønnesen H, Møller H, Andersen JR *et al.* (1994). Cancer morbidity in alcohol abusers. *Br J Cancer*, 69: 327–332. doi:10.1038/bjc.1994.59 PMID:8297729

Toriola AT, Kurl S, Laukanen JA *et al.* (2008). Alcohol consumption and risk of colorectal cancer: the Findrink study. *Eur J Epidemiol*, 23: 395–401. doi:10.1007/s10654-008-9244-4 PMID:18409007

Toriola AT, Kurl S, Laukkanen JA, Kauhanen J (2009). Does binge drinking increase the risk of lung cancer: results from the Findrink study. *Eur J Public Health*, 19: 389–393. doi:10.1093/eurpub/ckp049 PMID:19369490

Tramacere I, Scotti L, Jenab M *et al.* (2009). Alcohol drinking and pancreatic cancer risk: a meta-analysis of the dose-risk relation. *Int J Cancer*, In press PMID:19816941

Trentham-Dietz A, Newcomb PA, Nichols HB, Hampton JM (2007). Breast cancer risk factors and second primary malignancies among women with breast cancer. *Breast Cancer Res Treat*, 105: 195–207. doi:10.1007/s10549-006-9446-y PMID:17186360

Triano EA, Slusher LB, Atkins TA *et al.* (2003). Class I alcohol dehydrogenase is highly expressed in normal human mammary epithelium but not in invasive breast cancer: implications for breast carcinogenesis. *Cancer Res*, 63: 3092–3100. PMID:12810634

Trivers KF, Lund MJ, Porter PL *et al.* (2009). The epidemiology of triple-negative breast cancer, including race. *Cancer Causes Control*, 20: 1071–1082. doi:10.1007/s10552-009-9331-1 PMID:19343511

Tsong WH, Koh WP, Yuan JM *et al.* (2007). Cigarettes and alcohol in relation to colorectal cancer: the Singapore Chinese Health Study. *Br J Cancer*, 96: 821–827. doi:10.1038/sj.bjc.6603623 PMID:17311023

Tsutsumi M, George J, Ishizawa K *et al.* (2006). Effect of chronic dietary ethanol in the promotion of N-nitrosomethylbenzylamine-induced esophageal carcinogenesis in rats. *J Gastroenterol Hepatol*, 21: 805–813. doi:10.1111/j.1440-1746.2005.04040.x PMID:16704527

Tsutsumi M, Takase S, Takada A (1993). Genetic factors related to the development of carcinoma in digestive organs in alcoholics. *Alcohol Alcohol Suppl*, 1B: 21–26. PMID:8003125

Tsutsumi M, Wang JS, Takase S, Takada A (1994). Hepatic messenger RNA contents of cytochrome P4502E1 in patients with different P4502E1 genotypes. *Alcohol Alcohol Suppl*, 29: Suppl.29–32. PMID:9063815

Tworoger SS, Gertig DM, Gates MA *et al.* (2008). Caffeine, alcohol, smoking, and the risk of incident epithelial ovarian cancer. *Cancer*, 112: 1169–1177. doi:10.1002/cncr.23275 PMID:18213613

Tzonou A, Day NE, Trichopoulos D *et al.* (1984). The epidemiology of ovarian cancer in Greece: a case-control study. *Eur J Cancer Clin Oncol*, 20: 1045–1052. doi:10.1016/0277-5379(84)90107-X PMID:6540687

Upton DC, Wang X, Blans P *et al.* (2006). Mutagenesis by exocyclic alkylamino purine adducts in Escherichia coli. *Mutat Res*, 599: 1–10. doi:10.1016/j.mrfmmm.2005.12.014 PMID:16488449

Väkeväinen S, Tillonen J, Salaspuro M (2001). 4-Methylpyrazole decreases salivary acetaldehyde levels in aldh2-deficient subjects but not in subjects with normal aldh2. *Alcohol Clin Exp Res*, 25: 829–834. doi:10.1111/j.1530-0277.2001.tb02286.x PMID:11410717

Väkeväinen S, Tillonen J, Salaspuro M *et al.* (2000). Hypochlorhydria induced by a proton pump inhibitor leads to intragastric microbial production of acetaldehyde from ethanol. *Aliment Pharmacol Ther*, 14: 1511–1518. doi:10.1046/j.1365-2036.2000.00858.x PMID:11069323

van der Logt EMJ, Bergevoet SM, Roelofs HMJ *et al.* (2006). Role of epoxide hydrolase, NAD(P)H:quinone oxidoreductase, cytochrome P450 2E1 or alcohol dehydrogenase genotypes in susceptibility to colorectal cancer. *Mutat Res*, 593: 39–49. doi:10.1016/j.mrfmmm.2005.06.018 PMID:16039674

van Dijk BAC, van Houwelingen KP, Witjes JA *et al.* (2001). Alcohol dehydrogenase type 3 (ADH3) and the risk of bladder cancer. *Eur Urol*, 40: 509–514. doi:10.1159/000049827 PMID:11752857

van Duijn CM, van Steensel-Moll HA, Coebergh JW, van Zanen GE (1994). Risk factors for childhood acute non-lymphocytic leukemia: an association with maternal alcohol consumption during pregnancy? *Cancer Epidemiol Biomarkers Prev*, 3: 457–460. PMID:8000294

van Zeeland AA, de Groot AJ, Hall J, Donato F (1999). 8-Hydroxydeoxyguanosine in DNA from leukocytes of healthy adults: relationship with cigarette smoking, environmental tobacco smoke, alcohol and coffee consumption. *Mutat Res*, 439: 249–257. PMID:10023075

Vasiliou V, Pappa A, Estey T (2004). Role of human aldehyde dehydrogenases in endobiotic and xenobiotic

metabolism. *Drug Metab Rev*, 36: 279–299. doi:10.1081/DMR-120034001 PMID:15237855
Vasiliou V, Pappa A, Petersen DR (2000). Role of aldehyde dehydrogenases in endogenous and xenobiotic metabolism. *Chem Biol Interact*, 129: 1–19. doi:10.1016/S0009-2797(00)00211-8 PMID:11154732
Vaughan TL, Shapiro JA, Burt RD *et al.* (1996). Nasopharyngeal cancer in a low-risk population: defining risk factors by histological type. *Cancer Epidemiol Biomarkers Prev*, 5: 587–593. PMID:8824359
Velicer CM, Kristal A, White E (2006). Alcohol use and the risk of prostate cancer: results from the VITAL cohort study. *Nutr Cancer*, 56: 50–56. doi:10.1207/s15327914nc5601_7 PMID:17176217
Vioque J, Barber X, Bolumar F *et al.*PANESOES Study Group (2008). Esophageal cancer risk by type of alcohol drinking and smoking: a case-control study in Spain. *BMC Cancer*, 8: 221 doi:10.1186/1471-2407-8-221 PMID:18673563
Visapää JP, Götte K, Benesova M *et al.* (2004). Increased cancer risk in heavy drinkers with the alcohol dehydrogenase 1C*1 allele, possibly due to salivary acetaldehyde. *Gut*, 53: 871–876. doi:10.1136/gut.2003.018994 PMID:15138216
Visvanathan K, Crum RM, Strickland PT *et al.* (2007). Alcohol dehydrogenase genetic polymorphisms, low-to-moderate alcohol consumption, and risk of breast cancer. *Alcohol Clin Exp Res*, 31: 467–476. doi:10.1111/j.1530-0277.2006.00334.x PMID:17295732
Wakabayashi I, Sakamoto K, Masui H *et al.* (1994). A case-control study on risk factors for leukemia in a district of Japan. *Intern Med*, 33: 198–203. doi:10.2169/internalmedicine.33.198 PMID:8069013
Wakai K, Nagata C, Mizoue T *et al.*Research Group for the Development and Evaluation of Cancer Prevention Strategies in Japan (2007). Alcohol drinking and lung cancer risk: an evaluation based on a systematic review of epidemiologic evidence among the Japanese population. *Jpn J Clin Oncol*, 37: 168–174. doi:10.1093/jjco/hyl146 PMID:17332056
Walker AR, Walker BF, Tsotetsi NG *et al.* (1992). Case-control study of prostate cancer in black patients in Soweto, South Africa. *Br J Cancer*, 65: 438–441. doi:10.1038/bjc.1992.89 PMID:1558801
Wang D, Ritchie JM, Smith EM *et al.* (2005). Alcohol dehydrogenase 3 and risk of squamous cell carcinomas of the head and neck. *Cancer Epidemiol Biomarkers Prev*, 14: 626–632. doi:10.1158/1055-9965.EPI-04-0343 PMID:15767341
Wang J, Gajalakshmi V, Jiang J *et al.* (2006a). Associations between 5,10-methylenetetrahydrofolate reductase codon 677 and 1298 genetic polymorphisms and environmental factors with reference to susceptibility to colorectal cancer: a case-control study in an Indian population. *Int J Cancer*, 118: 991–997. doi:10.1002/ijc.21438 PMID:16152599
Wang M, McIntee EJ, Cheng G *et al.* (2000). Identification of DNA adducts of acetaldehyde. *Chem Res Toxicol*, 13: 1149–1157. doi:10.1021/tx000118t PMID:11087437
Wang M, Yu N, Chen L *et al.* (2006c). Identification of an acetaldehyde adduct in human liver DNA and quantitation as N2-ethyldeoxyguanosine. *Chem Res Toxicol*, 19: 319–324. doi:10.1021/tx0502948 PMID:16485909
Wang Y, Millonig G, Nair J *et al.* (2009). Ethanol-induced cytochrome P4502E1 causes carcinogenic etheno-DNA lesions in alcoholic liver disease. *Hepatology*, 50: 453–461. doi:10.1002/hep.22978 PMID:19489076
Wang Z, Tang L, Sun G *et al.* (2006b). Etiological study of esophageal squamous cell carcinoma in an endemic region: a population-based case control study in Huaian, China. *BMC Cancer*, 6: 287 doi:10.1186/1471-2407-6-287 PMID:17173682
Wanibuchi H, Wei M, Karim MR *et al.* (2006). Existence of no hepatocarcinogenic effect levels of 2-amino-3,8-dimethylimidazo[4,5-f]quinoxaline with or without coadministration with ethanol. *Toxicol Pathol*, 34: 232–236. doi:10.1080/01926230600713632 PMID:16698719
Watabiki T, Okii Y, Tokiyasu T *et al.* (2000). Long-term ethanol consumption in ICR mice causes mammary tumor in females and liver fibrosis in males. *Alcohol Clin Exp Res*, 24: Suppl117S–122S. PMID:10803793
Watanabe J, Hayashi S, Kawajiri K (1994). Different regulation and expression of the human CYP2E1 gene due to the RsaI polymorphism in the 5⊠-flanking region. *J Biochem*, 116: 321–326. PMID:7529759
Watanabe J, Yang JP, Eguchi H *et al.* (1995). An Rsa I polymorphism in the CYP2E1 gene does not affect lung cancer risk in a Japanese population. *Jpn J Cancer Res*, 86: 245–248. doi:10.1111/j.1349-7006.1995.tb03046.x PMID:7744693
Watanabe S, Sasahara K, Kinekawa F *et al.* (2002). Aldehyde dehydrogenase-2 genotypes and HLA haplotypes in Japanese patients with esophageal cancer. *Oncol Rep*, 9: 1063–1068. PMID:12168074
Watanabe-Suzuki K, Seno H, Ishii A *et al.* (1999). Ultra-sensitive method for determination of ethanol in whole blood by headspace capillary gas chromatography with cryogenic oven trapping. *J Chromatogr B Biomed Sci Appl*, 727: 89–94. doi:10.1016/S0378-4347(99)00063-8 PMID:10360426
Webb PM, Purdie DM, Bain CJ, Green AC (2004). Alcohol, wine, and risk of epithelial ovarian cancer. *Cancer Epidemiol Biomarkers Prev*, 13: 592–599. PMID:15066924
Webster LA & Weiss NSCancer and Steroid Hormone Study Group (1989). Alcoholic beverage consumption and the risk of endometrial cancer. *Int J Epidemiol*, 18: 786–791. doi:10.1093/ije/18.4.786 PMID:2695474
Wei YS, Lu JC, Wang L *et al.* (2009). Risk factors for sporadic colorectal cancer in southern Chinese. *World J Gastroenterol*, 15: 2526–2530. PMID:19469004

Weiderpass E & Baron JA (2001). Cigarette smoking, alcohol consumption, and endometrial cancer risk: a population-based study in Sweden. *Cancer Causes Control*, 12: 239–247. doi:10.1023/A:1011201911664 PMID:11405329

Weiderpass E, Ye W, Tamimi R *et al.* (2001). Alcoholism and risk for cancer of the cervix uteri, vagina, and vulva. *Cancer Epidemiol Biomarkers Prev*, 10: 899–901. PMID:11489758

Weikert C, Dietrich T, Boeing H *et al.* (2009). Lifetime and baseline alcohol intake and risk of cancer of the upper aero-digestive tract in the European Prospective Investigation into Cancer and Nutrition (EPIC) study. *Int J Cancer*, 125: 406–412. doi:10.1002/ijc.24393 PMID:19378340

Weinstein SJ, Stolzenberg-Solomon R, Pietinen P *et al.* (2006). Dietary factors of one-carbon metabolism and prostate cancer risk. *Am J Clin Nutr*, 84: 929–935. PMID:17023722

Wendt LR, Osvaldt AB, Bersch VP *et al.* (2007). Pancreatic intraepithelial neoplasia and ductal adenocarcinoma induced by DMBA in mice: effects of alcohol and caffeine. *Acta Cir Bras*, 22: 202–209. doi:10.1590/S0102-86502007000300008 PMID:17546293

West RO (1966). Epidemiologic study of malignancies of the ovaries. *Cancer*, 19: 1001–1007. doi:10.1002/1097-0142(196607)19:7<1001::AID-CNCR2820190714>3.0.CO;2-S PMID:5939299

Whittemore AS, Wu ML, Paffenbarger RS Jr *et al.* (1988). Personal and environmental characteristics related to epithelial ovarian cancer. II. Exposures to talcum powder, tobacco, alcohol, and coffee. *Am J Epidemiol*, 128: 1228–1240. PMID:3195564

WHO (2000). *International Guide for Monitoring Alcohol Consumption and Related Harm*. Geneva, World Health Organization,.

WHO (2004). *Global Status Report on Alcohol*. Geneva, World Health Organization.

WHO (2007). Expert Committee on Problems Related to Alcohol Consumption Second Report. WHO.

WHO (2008). *Global Information System on Alcohol and Health*. Available at http://apps.who.int/globalatlas/default.asp

Willett EV, O'Connor S, Smith AG, Roman E (2007). Does smoking or alcohol modify the risk of Epstein-Barr virus-positive or -negative Hodgkin lymphoma? *Epidemiology*, 18: 130–136. doi:10.1097/01.ede.0000248899.47399.78 PMID:17099321

Willett EV, Smith AG, Dovey GJ *et al.* (2004). Tobacco and alcohol consumption and the risk of non-Hodgkin lymphoma. *Cancer Causes Control*, 15: 771–780. doi:10.1023/B:CACO.0000043427.77739.60 PMID:15456990

Williams RR & Horm JW (1977). Association of cancer sites with tobacco and alcohol consumption and socio-economic status of patients: interview study from the Third National Cancer Survey. *J Natl Cancer Inst*, 58: 525–547. PMID:557114

Wong NACS, Rae F, Simpson KJ *et al.* (2000). Genetic polymorphisms of cytochrome p4502E1 and susceptibility to alcohol liver disease and hepatocellular carcinoma in a white population: a study and literature review, including meta-analysis. *J. Clin. Pathol. Mol. Pathol*, 53: 88–93. doi:10.1136/mp.53.2.88

Woodson K, Albanes D, Tangrea JA *et al.* (1999). Association between alcohol and lung cancer in the alpha-tocopherol, beta-carotene cancer prevention study in Finland. *Cancer Causes Control*, 10: 219–226. doi:10.1023/A:1008911624785 PMID:10454067

Wright M, Bieser KJ, Kinnunen PM, Lange LG (1987). Nonoxidative ethanol metabolism in human leukocytes: detection of fatty acid ethyl ester synthase activity. *Biochem Biophys Res Commun*, 142: 979–985. doi:10.1016/0006-291X(87)91510-5 PMID:3827909

Wu IC, Lee CH, Kuo CH *et al.* (2009). Consumption of cigarettes but not betel quid or alcohol increases colorectal cancer risk. *J Formos Med Assoc*, 108: 155–163. doi:10.1016/S0929-6646(09)60046-2 PMID:19251551

Wu MS, Chen CJ, Lin MT *et al.* (2002). Genetic polymorphisms of cytochrome p450 2E1, glutathione S-transferase M1 and T1, and susceptibility to gastric carcinoma in Taiwan. *Int J Colorectal Dis*, 17: 338–343. doi:10.1007/s00384-001-0383-2 PMID:12172927

Wu SH, Tsai SM, Hou MF *et al.* (2006). Interaction of genetic polymorphisms in cytochrome P450 2E1 and glutathione S-transferase M1 to breast cancer in Taiwanese woman without smoking and drinking habits. *Breast Cancer Res Treat*, 100: 93–98. doi:10.1007/s10549-006-9226-8 PMID:16758119

Wu X, Shi H, Jiang H *et al.* (1997). Associations between cytochrome P4502E1 genotype, mutagen sensitivity, cigarette smoking and susceptibility to lung cancer. *Carcinogenesis*, 18: 967–973. doi:10.1093/carcin/18.5.967 PMID:9163682

Wurst FM, Skipper GE, Weinmann W (2003). Ethyl glucuronide–the direct ethanol metabolite on the threshold from science to routine use. *Addiction*, 98: Suppl 251–61. doi:10.1046/j.1359-6357.2003.00588.x PMID:14984242

Yamagiwa K, Mizumoto R, Higashi S *et al.* (1994). Alcohol ingestion enhances hepatocarcinogenesis induced by synthetic estrogen and progestin in the rat. *Cancer Detect Prev*, 18: 103–114. PMID:8025892

Yamamoto S, Kubo S, Hai S *et al.* (2004). Hepatitis C virus infection as a likely etiology of intra-hepatic cholangiocarcinoma. *Cancer Sci*, 95: 592–595. doi:10.1111/j.1349-7006.2004.tb02492.x PMID:15245596

Yang CX, Matsuo K, Ito H *et al.* (2005). Esophageal cancer risk by ALDH2 and ADH2 polymorphisms and alcohol consumption: exploration of gene-environment and

gene-gene interactions. *Asian Pac J Cancer Prev*, 6: 256–262. PMID:16235983
Yang J, Gu M, Song NH *et al.* (2009). [Correlation of prostate cancer susceptibility with genetic polymorphism of cytochrome P450 2E1, smoking and drinking: a case-control study in the population of Nanjing area] *Zhonghua Nan Ke Xue*, 15: 7–11. PMID:19288740
Yang J, Qian LX, Wu HF *et al.* (2006a). Genetic polymorphisms in the cytochrome P450 1A1 and 2E1 genes, smoking, drinking and prostate cancer susceptibility: a case-control study in a Han nationality population in Southern China. *Int J Urol*, 13: 773–780. doi:10.1111/j.1442-2042.2006.01401.x PMID:16834659
Yang SJ, Wang HY, Li XQ *et al.* (2007). Genetic polymorphisms of ADH2 and ALDH2 association with esophageal cancer risk in southwest China. *World J Gastroenterol*, 13: 5760–5764. PMID:17963305
Yen ML, Yen BL, Bai CH, Lin RS (2003). Risk factors for ovarian cancer in Taiwan: a case-control study in a low-incidence population. *Gynecol Oncol*, 89: 318–324. doi:10.1016/S0090-8258(03)00088-X PMID:12713998
Yen TT, Lin WD, Wang CP *et al.* (2008). The association of smoking, alcoholic consumption, betel quid chewing and oral cavity cancer: a cohort study. *Eur Arch Otorhinolaryngol*, 265: 1403–1407. doi:10.1007/s00405-008-0659-z PMID:18389268
Yin G, Kono S, Toyomura K *et al.* (2007). Alcohol dehydrogenase and aldehyde dehydrogenase polymorphisms and colorectal cancer: the Fukuoka Colorectal Cancer Study. *Cancer Sci*, 98: 1248–1253. doi:10.1111/j.1349-7006.2007.00519.x PMID:17517051
Yin SJ, Chou FJ, Chao SF *et al.* (1993). Alcohol and aldehyde dehydrogenases in human esophagus: comparison with the stomach enzyme activities. *Alcohol Clin Exp Res*, 17: 376–381. doi:10.1111/j.1530-0277.1993.tb00779.x PMID:8488982
Yin SJ, Liao CS, Wu CW *et al.* (1997). Human stomach alcohol and aldehyde dehydrogenases: comparison of expression pattern and activities in alimentary tract. *Gastroenterology*, 112: 766–775. doi:10.1053/gast.1997.v112.pm9041238 PMID:9041238
Yokoyama A, Kato H, Yokoyama T *et al.* (2002). Genetic polymorphisms of alcohol and aldehyde dehydrogenases and glutathione S-transferase M1 and drinking, smoking, and diet in Japanese men with esophageal squamous cell carcinoma. *Carcinogenesis*, 23: 1851–1859. doi:10.1093/carcin/23.11.1851 PMID:12419833
Yokoyama A, Kato H, Yokoyama T *et al.* (2006a). Esophageal squamous cell carcinoma and aldehyde dehydrogenase-2 genotypes in Japanese females. *Alcohol Clin Exp Res*, 30: 491–500. doi:10.1111/j.1530-0277.2006.00053.x PMID:16499490
Yokoyama A, Muramatsu T, Ohmori T *et al.* (1998). Alcohol-related cancers and aldehyde dehydrogenase-2 in Japanese alcoholics. *Carcinogenesis*, 19: 1383–1387. doi:10.1093/carcin/19.8.1383 PMID:9744533
Yokoyama A, Muramatsu T, Omori T *et al.* (2001). Alcohol and aldehyde dehydrogenase gene polymorphisms and oropharyngolaryngeal, esophageal and stomach cancers in Japanese alcoholics. *Carcinogenesis*, 22: 433–439. doi:10.1093/carcin/22.3.433 PMID:11238183
Yokoyama A, Omori T, Yokoyama T *et al.* (2006b). Risk of squamous cell carcinoma of the upper aerodigestive tract in cancer-free alcoholic Japanese men: an endoscopic follow-up study. *Cancer Epidemiol Biomarkers Prev*, 15: 2209–2215. doi:10.1158/1055-9965.EPI-06-0435 PMID:17119048
Yokoyama A, Omori T, Yokoyama T *et al.* (2008). Risk of metachronous squamous cell carcinoma in the upper aerodigestive tract of Japanese alcoholic men with esophageal squamous cell carcinoma: a long-term endoscopic follow-up study. *Cancer Sci*, 99: 1164–1171. doi:10.1111/j.1349-7006.2008.00807.x PMID:18429959
Yokoyama A, Yokoyama T, Omori T *et al.* (2007b). Helicobacter pylori, chronic atrophic gastritis, inactive aldehyde dehydrogenase-2, macrocytosis and multiple upper aerodigestive tract cancers and the risk for gastric cancer in alcoholic Japanese men. *J Gastroenterol Hepatol*, 22: 210–217. doi:10.1111/j.1440-1746.2006.04377.x PMID:17295873
Yong L-C, Brown CC, Schatzkin A *et al.* (1997). Intake of vitamins E, C, and A and risk of lung cancer. The NHANES I epidemiologic followup study. First National Health and Nutrition Examination Survey. *Am J Epidemiol*, 146: 231–243. PMID:9247007
Yu MW, Gladek-Yarborough A, Chiamprasert S *et al.* (1995). Cytochrome P450 2E1 and glutathione S-transferase M1 polymorphisms and susceptibility to hepatocellular carcinoma. *Gastroenterology*, 109: 1266–1273. doi:10.1016/0016-5085(95)90587-1 PMID:7557094
Yu SZ, Huang XE, Koide T *et al.* (2002). Hepatitis B and C viruses infection, lifestyle and genetic polymorphisms as risk factors for hepatocellular carcinoma in Haimen, China. *Jpn J Cancer Res*, 93: 1287–1292. doi:10.1111/j.1349-7006.2002.tb01236.x PMID:12495467
Zakhari S (2006). Overview: how is alcohol metabolized by the body? *Alcohol Res Health*, 29: 245–254. PMID:17718403
Zang EA & Wynder EL (2001). Reevaluation of the confounding effect of cigarette smoking on the relationship between alcohol use and lung cancer risk, with larynx cancer used as a positive control. *Prev Med*, 32: 359–370. doi:10.1006/pmed.2000.0818 PMID:11304097
Zaridze D, Brennan P, Boreham J *et al.* (2009). Alcohol and cause-specific mortality in Russia: a retrospective case-control study of 48,557 adult deaths. *Lancet*, 373: 2201–2214. doi:10.1016/S0140-6736(09)61034-5 PMID:19560602
Zavras AI, Wu T, Laskaris G *et al.* (2002). Interaction between a single nucleotide polymorphism in the alcohol dehydrogenase 3 gene, alcohol consumption

and oral cancer risk. *Int J Cancer*, 97: 526–530. doi:10.1002/ijc.1642 PMID:11802217

Zhang FF, Hou L, Terry MB *et al.* (2007b). Genetic polymorphisms in alcohol metabolism, alcohol intake and the risk of stomach cancer in Warsaw, Poland. *Int J Cancer*, 121: 2060–2064. doi:10.1002/ijc.22973 PMID:17631643

Zhang SM, Lee IM, Manson JE *et al.* (2007a). Alcohol consumption and breast cancer risk in the Women's Health Study. *Am J Epidemiol*, 165: 667–676. doi:10.1093/aje/kwk054 PMID:17204515

Zhou YM, Yin ZF, Yang JM *et al.* (2008). Risk factors for intrahepatic cholangiocarcinoma: a case-control study in China. *World J Gastroenterol*, 14: 632–635. doi:10.3748/wjg.14.632 PMID:18203300

Zimatkin SM, Pronko SP, Vasiliou V *et al.* (2006). Enzymatic mechanisms of ethanol oxidation in the brain. *Alcohol Clin Exp Res*, 30: 1500–1505. doi:10.1111/j.1530-0277.2006.00181.x PMID:16930212

Zintzaras E, Stefanidis I, Santos M, Vidal F (2006). Do alcohol-metabolizing enzyme gene polymorphisms increase the risk of alcoholism and alcoholic liver disease? *Hepatology*, 43: 352–361. doi:10.1002/hep.21023 PMID:16440362

CHINESE-STYLE SALTED FISH

Chinese-style salted fish was considered by a previous IARC Working Group in 1992 (IARC, 1993). Since that time, new data have become available, these have been incorporated in the *Monograph*, and taken into consideration in the present evaluation.

1. Exposure Data

1.1 Mode of production

In southern China, about 20 different fish, such as red snapper, threadfin, Spanish mackerel, croaker, Japanese mackerel, are used to prepare salted fish (Armstrong & Eng, 1983; Poirier *et al.*, 1987). Procedures for preparation of salted fish have been described in detail previously (IARC, 1993). Briefly, salted fish are prepared by salting, brining, dry-salting, pickle curing, or a combination of these treatments. In brining, fish are placed in a solution of crude salt in water until the fish tissue has absorbed the required amount of salt. For dry-salting, fish are mixed with dry salt and the resultant brine (from dissolution of the salt in the water present in the fish) is allowed to drain away. When pickling or pickle curing the fish is mixed with salt and stored under the brine (pickle) formed when the salt dissolves in the water extracted from the fish.

In southern China, fish are generally not gutted before salting, and only when bigger fish such as red snapper are salted are the guts drawn out through the throat, without making an incision in the belly of the fish. Salting is done with crude salt in wooden vats. After a few days, the fish are immersed in brine and weights (often large stones placed on top of grass mats) are placed on the surface to prevent the fish from floating, for one to five days. After this the fish are dried under the sun for one to seven days, depending on the size of the fish and the weather. Salted fish prepared in this way are called 'tough' or 'hard meat' salted fish. Sometimes, fish is allowed to soften by decomposition before salting, to produce 'soft meat' salted fish (Poirier *et al.*, 1989; Yu *et al.*, 1989a). During drying salted fish, insect infestation can be a serious problem, especially in damp weather. In southern China, the average annual temperature and humidity are high and are favourable for the growth of bacteria such as *Staphylococci* (Armstrong & Eng, 1983; Zou *et al.*, 1994). Salted fish are stored for 4 to 5 months before being consumed.

1.2 Compounds present in salted fish

The previous *IARC Monograph* (IARC, 1993) reviewed levels of *N*-nitrosamines reported for uncooked salted fish obtained from different countries. The levels of *N*-nitrosodimethylamine in uncooked salted fish ranged from not detected to 388 μg/kg (Poirier *et al.*, 1989). Some other volatile nitrosamines such as *N*-nitrosodiethylamine, *N*-nitrosopyrrolidine and *N*-nitrosopiperidine were also reported, their levels ranged between not detected and about 30 µg/kg (Poirier *et al.*, 1989). Twenty samples of salted fish purchased in high- and low-risk areas for nasopharyngeal carcinoma (NPC) were analysed for four volatile *N*-nitrosamines; the highest levels of the sum of the four *N*-nitrosamines (373 µg/kg) were found in samples from the area with the highest NPC mortality (Zou *et al.*, 1992). Salted fish samples were also analysed for total *N*-nitroso compounds determined as the amount of nitric oxide (NO) released from the compounds after treatment with bromhydric acid (HBr) (Haorah *et al.*, 2001). Six types of dried salted fish purchased in the Fujian province of China, on the coast ~500 miles south of Shanghai, contained 3.9 ± 2.0 (range: 1.8–6.0) µmol/kg *N*-nitroso compounds. Upon steaming *N*-nitrosodiethylamine was detected in more samples than in uncooked or fried fish; *N*-nitrosodimethylamine was detected in all of the samples, whether cooked or uncooked (Huang *et al.*, 1981). The average levels of *N*-nitrosamines in steam-cooked salted fish collected from areas with high NPC mortality (1.51 ± 0.23 mg/kg) were significantly higher than those from areas with lower NPC mortality (0.60 ± 0.14–0.83 ± 0.18) (Zou *et al.*, 1994).

Fish are rich sources of secondary and tertiary amines, and nitrate and possibly nitrite occur in the crude salt used to pickle them. Steam-cooked, salted fish purchased in various areas in China have been found to contain nitrites (0.15 ± 0.24 mg/kg) and nitrates (6.54 ± 0.43 mg/kg) (Zou *et al.*, 1994). No differences were found in the levels of nitrites or nitrates between areas with different NPC mortality rates.

N-nitroso compounds, including *N*-nitrosamines, can form during the preparation of salted fish. Several factors may affect the levels of *N*-nitroso compounds, including levels of nitrites and nitrates in crude salt, those of nitrogen oxide in the air (when the preparation took place in open air), the growth of nitrate-reducing bacteria and pH. *N*-Nitroso compounds can also be formed after ingestion of foods by chemical nitrosation under acidic conditions in the stomach (IARC, 2010).

Aqueous food extracts of 116 samples of salted fish from China were analysed for four volatile *N*-nitrosamines before and after strong acid-catalysed nitrosation *in vitro*. After nitrosation, *N*-nitrosodimethylamine levels were increased about 70-fold, while *N*-nitrosopiperidine levels were increased nearly 200-fold (Zou *et al.*, 1994). Six types of dried salted fish purchased in the Fujian province of China contained 6000 ± 3200 (range: 4200–12300) µmol/kg precursors of total *N*-nitroso compounds determined as the amount of NO released after HBr treatment (Haorah *et al.*, 2001). These results confirm that salted fish contains high concentrations of precursors of *N*-nitroso compounds.

1.3 Prevalence of use of Chinese-style salted fish

Chinese-style salted fish is popular in Chinese populations along the south China coast and South-eastern Asian countries, where it is often used as an accompaniment to other dishes or rice. Although the amount consumed at any one time is small (not more than 10 g), the dish may appear at every meal; some people prefer the spoiled parts (Fong & Chan, 1973). Salted fish mixed with rice has also been used as a traditional weaning food, and was often given to infants early and frequently in their life (Topley, 1973; Yu *et al.*, 1981, 1989b). In three studies, 6–53% of individuals reported use during weaning; use in the post-weaning period was slightly lower in each subsequent study (Yu *et al.*, 1986, 1988, 1989b).

Data on prevalence of use are mainly derived from studies on the association with NPC, but in most studies the type of salted fish is not specified. Prevalence of use varies significantly (Table 1.1); in southern Chinese populations 4 to 48% of the adult population have reported eating

Table 1.1 Prevalence of salted fish consumption once weekly or more in Chinese populations[a]

Reference	Region or country	Data collection	Number of adult controls[b]	Consumption of salted fish	
				Childhood[c]	Adulthood
Armstrong & Eng (1983)	Malaysia	1980	100	[47%]	[20%]
Yu *et al.* (1986)	Hong Kong Special Administrative Region	1981–NR	250	[16%]	[8%]
Yu *et al.* (1988)	Guangxi, Southern China	1984–86	174	4%	NR
Yu *et al.* (1989b)	Guangzhou, Southern China	1983–85	304	47%	33%
Ning *et al.* (1990)	Tianjin, Northern China	1985–86	300	3%	NR
Zheng *et al.* (1994a)	Guangzhou, Southern China	1985–88	195	10%	1–3%
Lee *et al.* (1994)	Singapore	1988–90	369	16%	4%
Yuan *et al.* (2000)	Shanghai	1988–91	1032	NR	2%
Zou *et al.* (2000)	Yangjiang, Southern China	1987–95	192	NR	48%
Ward *et al.* (2000)	Taiwan, China	1991–94	327	NR	< 5%
			110	31%	NR
Yang *et al.* (2005)	Taiwan, China	1996–NR	1636	2%	NR
Guo *et al.* (2009)	Guangxi, Southern China	2004–05	758	NR	4%

[a] Prevalence in the control groups from the studies
[b] Number of controls with information on salted fish consumption
[c] Age 10 years, except Armstrong & Eng (1983) ('Childhood'); Zheng *et al.* (1994a) (0–3 years). Childhood and adulthood population are the same but were asked their consumption at different time points.
NR, not reported

salted fish more than once weekly. Comparing earlier and later studies shows a decreasing trend in the prevalence of use. Consumption of salted fish in Chinese populations has been declining since the second half of the 20th century, and consumption in weaning and early childhood is now rare (Zheng *et al.*, 1994a; Yu & Yuan, 2002). Both cultural changes and other methods of preserving food may be responsible for the decrease.

2. Cancer in Humans

2.1 Nasopharyngeal carcinoma

2.1.1 Overview of studies

Ho (1967) estimated that the Tankas (boat people), who consumed Chinese-style salted fish in their daily diet, had twice the incidence of nasopharyngeal carcinoma (NPC) compared with the land-dwelling Cantonese in Hong Kong Special Administrative Region. Subsequent studies demonstrated that the distinct pattern of NPC incidence among different ethnic or dialect groups in southern China coincided with the prevalence of their consumption of salted fish (Ho, 1978; Yu *et al.*, 1981), and that high incidence rates of NPC were retained in the Chinese who continued consuming salted fish after they migrated to Malaysia (Armstrong *et al.*, 1979; Armstrong & Eng, 1983). The peak in incidence rates at ages 45–54 years and decline thereafter suggested that the consumption of salted fish occurred early in life. [Salted fish mixed with soft rice was commonly fed to infants in the weaning and post-weaning period.]

Eight case–control studies on the association of salted fish with NPC, conducted between the 1970s and 1980s, were reviewed in the previous *IARC Monograph* (IARC, 1993) and are summarized in Table 2.1 (available at http://monographs.iarc.fr/ENG/Monographs/vol100E/100E-07-Table2.1.pdf) (Henderson *et al.*, 1976; Henderson & Louie, 1978; Geser *et al.*, 1978; Armstrong & Eng, 1983; Yu *et al.*, 1986, 1988, 1989b; Ning *et al.*, 1990; Sriamporn *et al.*, 1992). All but one were conducted on Chinese subjects and consistently demonstrated that consumption of Chinese salted fish was associated with increased risk for NPC. There was a dose-dependent relationship between frequency and duration of consumption and NPC risk. The association was stronger for intake of salted fish during childhood up to 10 years of age compared with intake at older ages.

Since the publication of the previous *IARC Monograph* (IARC, 1993), an additional 11 case–control studies on the association of Chinese-style salted fish with NPC association have been published in English or Chinese-language articles, all but one in Chinese populations (see Table 2.1 on-line). No cohort studies have been performed. In six studies a significant association between salted fish and NPC was observed (Huang *et al.*, 1993; Zheng *et al.*, 1994a, b; Armstrong *et al.*, 1998; Zou *et al.*, 2000; Guo *et al.*, 2009), in two the association was of borderline significance (Yuan *et al.*, 2000; Yang *et al.*, 2005), while lack of an association was observed in three studies (West *et al.*, 1993; Lee *et al.*, 1994; Ward *et al.*, 2000). Two of the negative studies were performed in populations with a low consumption of Chinese-style salted fish (West *et al.*, 1993; Ward *et al.*, 2000). In the positive studies, the strongest association was seen for intake in early childhood and during weaning, while the association with adult consumption was weaker. Only modestly increased risks were found in the majority of studies, and in the three largest studies (with more than 500 cases), increased risks were only observed for the most exposed individuals.

There are several possible reasons for the smaller risk observed in more recent studies. First, the consumption of salted fish by Chinese populations, especially feeding young children, has declined in parallel with economic development (Lee *et al.*, 1994; Zheng *et al.*, 1994b). While NPC incidence in certain areas of Southern China has remained stable in recent decades (Jia *et al.*, 2006), the incidence of NPC has declined significantly in Hong Kong Special Administrative Region and Singapore, and a preceding decrease in salted fish consumption may be a contributing factor (Yu & Yuan, 2002). Second, in recent decades the consumption of commercially produced salted fish and other preserved foods has increased and the consumption of home-preserved foods with possible higher nitrite and nitrosamine levels has declined (Ward *et al.*, 2000). Third, compared with later studies (Yuan *et al.*, 2000; Guo *et al.*, 2009; Yang *et al.*, 2005), the cases in some of the earlier studies were younger (Yu *et al.*, 1986, 1988). This is relevant as the effect of salted fish on the risk of NPC seems to be most pronounced in younger onset cases (Yang *et al.*, 2005).

2.1.2 Interaction with other risk factors

(a) Genetic risk factors

The involvement of a genetic factor in the development of NPC is likely and the familial risk of NPC in endemic areas is among the highest of any malignancy (IARC, 1997; Ung *et al.*, 1999) compared to those reported for other cancers (Goldgar *et al.*, 1994). Yang *et al.* (2005) found that the risk of NPC associated with salted fish consumption was strongest in families with three or more affected members in Taiwan, China; however, both genetic factors and shared environment could be responsible. In a study from Guangzhou comparing familial cases of NPC with sporadic cases, no significant differences in salted fish consumption between the two case groups were found (Luo *et al.*, 2009).

(b) Epstein-Barr virus

The association between Epstein-Barr virus (EBV) and undifferentiated NPC is firmly established and EBV is found in all tumour cells from NPC in endemic areas (Hjalgrim *et al.*, 2007). A synergistic effect between EBV and salted fish intake on the risk of NPC is suggested from a study where the association between salted fish and NPC was stronger in EBV VCA IgA positive individuals (Zheng *et al.*, 1994a). In a study of Caucasian NPC patients in the USA, intake of preserved meats with high levels of added nitrites increased the risk of undifferentiated NPC, while the risk of differentiated NPC was unaffected (Farrow *et al.*, 1998). In areas with low NPC incidence, undifferentiated, but not differentiated, NPC is associated with EBV (Hjalgrim *et al.*, 2007).

In studies attempting to control for EBV-infection status, the association between Chinese-style salted fish and NPC remained (Zheng *et al.*, 1994a; Guo *et al.*, 2009).

2.2 Cancer of the stomach

2.2.1 Overview of studies

A total of five case–control studies have investigated the association between Chinese-style salted fish and development of stomach cancer (Table 2.2 available at http://monographs.iarc.fr/ENG/Monographs/vol100E/100E-07-Table2.2.pdf). Two of the studies were conducted in Southern Chinese populations (Ye *et al.*, 1998; Cai *et al.*, 2003), two studies in Northern Chinese populations (You *et al.*, 1988; Takezaki *et al.*, 2001a) and one study in Malaysia (33% of the controls were Chinese) (Goh *et al.*, 2007). In the two largest studies, with 564 and 272 cases, modest increased risks around 1.4–1.6 were found in the most exposed group (You *et al.*, 1988; Ye *et al.*, 1998). However, the amount of fish consumed in the study from Shandong was small (You *et al.*, 1988). Higher risks were found in two of the smaller studies (Cai *et al.*, 2003; Goh *et al.*, 2007). A dose–response relationship was found in two smaller studies, with odds ratios ranging from 3.4 to 5.7 in the most exposed individuals (salted fish at least three times/week) (Takezaki *et al.*, 2001a; Cai *et al.*, 2003). Adjustments for smoking and alcohol were missing in two studies (You *et al.*, 1988; Ye *et al.*, 1998), while adjustment for *Helicobacter pylori* status was only performed in one study (Goh *et al.*, 2007).

An increased risk for stomach cancer associated with intake of highly salty foods has been observed in other populations (You *et al.*, 1988; Tsugane & Sasazuki, 2007).

2.2.2 Histology and topography

In the single study reporting histology, all cases were adenocarcinomas (Goh *et al.*, 2007). An equal effect of salted fish consumption was observed on cardia and non-cardia stomach cancer (Cai *et al.*, 2003).

2.2.3 Interactions

Interactions between salted fish consumption and other risk factors for stomach cancer have not been reported. The possible significance of early age at consumption and risk for stomach cancer has not been investigated. Growing evidence has associated EBV infection with a subset (5–10%) of all gastric carcinomas globally (Hjalgrim *et al.*, 2007). Analogous to nasopharyngeal carcinoma, the virus in EBV-positive gastric carcinomas is found in all tumour cells (Imai *et al.*, 1994), and EBV-antibodies are elevated in patients before diagnosis (Levine *et al.*, 1995). However, no studies have investigated the association between salted fish and EBV-positive gastric carcinomas. Nor has a possible interaction between salted fish intake and *Helicobacter pylori* infection been investigated.

2.3 Cancer of the oesophagus

Three studies have investigated the association between Chinese-style salted fish and cancer of the oesophagus (see Table 2.2 on-line). In Hong Kong Special Administrative Region, frequent consumption of salted fish, especially early in life, was associated with an increased risk for oesophageal cancer in univariate analyses, but was much weakened when alcohol and other confounders were taken into account (Cheng *et al.*, 1992). In a Northern Chinese population consumption of salted fish more than once weekly (the most exposed individuals) was associated with a non-significant 80% increased risk, and there was no significant trend (Takezaki *et al.*, 2001a). In a Southern Chinese population an increased risk for oesophageal cancer was associated with adult salted fish consumption in women, but not in men, and there was no dose–response relationship from both sexes combined (Li *et al.*, 2001). In the one study reporting histology, 85% of tumours were squamous cell carcinomas (Cheng *et al.*, 1992). Information on topography was not provided.

2.4 Other cancers

Consumption of salted fish in Chinese populations has also been associated with an increased risk for cancer of the lung (Wang *et al.*, 1996; Lu *et al.*, 2003), brain (Hu *et al.*, 1999), and prostate (Jian *et al.*, 2004); no such association was seen for lung cancer in two studies in Japan (Takezaki *et al.*, 2001b, 2003). Studies at these sites are too sparse to allow for a systematic evaluation.

2.5 Synthesis

In all five case–control studies salted fish consumption in adulthood is associated with an increased risk for stomach cancer. However, the effect in the largest studies is modest, and adjustment for important confounding risk factors (including smoking, alcohol and *Helicobacter pylori* status) were missing in several of the studies.

3. Cancer in Experimental Animals

Cantonese-style salted fish and salted fish extracts have been tested for carcinogenicity in three studies in rats and in one study in Syrian golden hamsters. Investigators administered specifically Cantonese-style salted fish to experimental animals (Table 3.1).

3.1 Oral administration

3.1.1 Rat

In one study, carcinomas of the nasal or paranasal regions developed in 4/10 [not significant] female rats fed steamed Cantonese-style salted fish for six months followed by extract of Cantonese-style salted fish heads as drinking-water for 1–2 years. No such tumours developed in similarly treated males (0/10) or in controls of either sex (0/3 and 0/3) (Huang *et al.*, 1978). [The working group noted the small number of animals.] In a larger study, malignant nasal cavity tumours of various kinds developed in male and female rats (4/148) fed Cantonese-style salted fish mixed in powdered diet for 18 months and observed until three years of age, but not in controls (0/73) (Yu *et al.*, 1989a).

Groups of 40–41 offspring (male and female) of rats were exposed to Cantonese-style salted fish mixed in the dams' diet during pregnancy and lactation and were themselves fed Cantonese-style salted fish mixed in diet after weaning for two years; 5 rats of both sexes developed malignant nasal and nasopharyngeal tumours of various kinds. Two offspring of rats exposed to control diet during pregnancy and lactation that were given Cantonese-style salted fish-containing diet after weaning also developed

Table 3.1 Carcinogenicity studies of oral administration of Cantonese-style salted fish in experimental animals

Species, strain (sex) Duration Reference	Dosing regimen, Animals/group at start	Incidence of tumours	Significance	Comments
Rat, Inbred WA albino (M, F) up to 24 mo Huang *et al.* (1978)	Steamed salted fish (30 g/d) for 6 mo, 5 d/wk, followed by salted fish soup (20 mL, 0.2 g fish/mL), 5 d/wk, for 1–2 yr 10 M, 10 F 3 M, 3 F (controls)	Adenocarcinoma of the nasal cavity: M–0/10 F–2/10 Undifferentiated carcinoma of the paranasal sinus: M–0/10 F–1/10 Highly invasive squamous carcinoma in the upper posterior part of the right buccoalveolar sulcus: M–0/10 F–1/10	NR [NS]	Small number of animals
		No nasal cavity tumours in controls (0/6)	-	
Rat, Inbred Wistar-Kyoto (M, F) 3 yr Yu *et al.* (1989a)	Steamed Cantonese-style salted fish (48% soft- & 52% hard-type):rat chow, 1:3 or 1:5, for 18 mo Controls given rat chow only 36–37 F or 37 M	Undifferentiated carcinoma in the mid-and left portions of the nasal cavity: (M–1/37) high dose diet Moderately differentiated squamous cell carcinoma in the left lateral nasal cavity: (F–1/37) high dose diet		Positive (one sided $P = 0.02$), 4/148 vs historical controls.
		Spindle cell carcinoma in the left lateral nasal cavity: (F–1/37) high dose diet Spindle cell tumour in the left posterior nasal cavity: (M–1/37) low dose diet No tumours in 73 controls	NS	
Rat, Sprague-Dawley (M, F) 2 yr Zheng *et al.* (1994c)	Steamed & dried Cantonese-style salted fish (50% soft- & 50% hard-type), 0, 5 or 10% in the diet 40–41 M, F		Positive (P for trend = 0.041)	Positive, 7/122 vs historical controls (one tailed, $P = 0.004$)
	Pregnant rats fed 10% salted fish, 41 new born rats fed 10% salted fish (Group 1)	One squamous cell carcinoma (M) and 1 poorly differentiated carcinoma (F) of the nasopharynx; 1 adenocarcinoma (F) and 1 fibrosarcoma (M) of the nasal cavity		
	Pregnant rats fed control pellets, 41 new born rats fed 10% salted fish (Group 2)	One squamous cell carcinoma (M) of the nasopharynx and 1 rhabdomyosarcoma (F) of the nasal cavity		
	Pregnant rats fed 5% salted fish, 40 new born rats fed 5% salted fish (Group 3)	One soft tissue sarcoma (F) of the nasal cavity		
	40 untreated controls	No nasal cavity or nasopharygeal tumours in controls	-	

d, day or days; F, female; M, male; mo, month or months; NR, not reported; NS, not significant; vs, versus; wk, week or weeks; yr, year or years malignant nasal or nasopharyngeal tumours. No nasal or nasopharyngeal tumours were found in control offspring born to untreated dams and fed regular pelleted diet throughout life (Zheng *et al.*, 1994c).

3.1.2 Hamster

No nasal or paranasal tumours were observed in eight male and six female Syrian golden hamsters fed steamed Cantonese-style salted fish for six months and then an extract of Cantonese-style salted fish heads as drinking-water five times per week for 1–2 years (Huang *et al.*, 1978).

3.2 Synthesis

In three studies in rats fed Cantonese-style salted fish, there was a consistent increased frequency of nasal cavity tumours, which are uncommon neoplasms in rats.

4. Other Relevant Data

4.1 Absorption, distribution, metabolism and excretion

No data were available to the Working Group.

4.2 Genetic and related effects

4.2.1 Humans

No data were available to the Working Group.

4.2.2 Experimental systems

The genotoxicity and mutagenicity of Chinese-style salted fish in experimental systems has been reviewed in detail (IARC, 1993).

(a) Genotoxicity and mutagenicity in bacteria

DMSO extracts of 4 samples of different species of salted fish and 2 samples of dried shrimps were mutagenic in *Salmonella typhimurium* TA 100 and TA 98 in the presence of a metabolic activation system (Fong *et al.*, 1979). However, n-hexane and ethyl acetate extracts of hard and soft salted dried fish samples obtained in a high risk area for NPC in China were not mutagenic in *S. typhimurium* TA 100 and TA 98 in the absence or presence of rat liver metabolic activation system. Nevertheless, these salted fish samples contained high levels of precursors that upon nitrosation *in vitro* with sodium nitrite under acidic conditions yielded directly-acting genotoxic (probably *N*-nitroso) compounds (Tannenbaum *et al.*, 1985; Poirier *et al.*, 1989). Mutagenicity on *S. typhimurium* TA 100 of salted fish obtained from Hong Kong Special Administrative Region increased with increasing nitrite concentration (Weng *et al.*, 1992).

In one study, urine samples collected from WA rats fed Chinese-style salted fish showed mutagenic activity on *S. typhimurium* TA 100 and TA 98 (Fong *et al.*, 1979).

(b) Genotoxicity and mutagenicity in experimental animals

(i) DNA adduct

In one study, the levels of 7-methylguanine in the liver and nasopharynx of rats fed 5% or 10% steamed and dried Chinese-style salted fish were analysed by a post-labelling method. There was no significant difference in adduct levels between exposed and control animals, the levels ranging between 3.2–1.2 and 3.3–1.4 per 10^7 nucleotides, respectively (Widlak *et al.*, 1995).

(ii) EBV-activation activity

Aqueous extracts of Cantonese-style salted dried fish from China showed a strong activity in EBV reactivation when assayed in Raji cells (Shao *et al.*, 1988). EBV-reactivation activity was decreased or showed no change after chemical nitrosation, but it was not correlated with the genotoxicity or nitrosamine levels of the samples (Poirier *et al.*, 1989).

4.3 Mechanistic considerations

The mechanisms by which consumption of Cantonese-style salted fish induces NPC remain unresolved.

NPC has been classified into three histologic types: keratinizing squamous cell carcinoma (class I), nonkeratinizing carcinoma (class II) and basaloid squamous-cell carcinoma (class III) (Chan *et al.*, 2005). Distinct etiological factors could be responsible for the three types of NPC. In high incidence areas such as southern China, 99% of NPC are class II whereas class I NPC is predominant in low-incidence regions. The etiological factors of NPC in high incidence areas include EBV, environmental risk factors and genetic susceptibility.

EBV has been classified as a Group 1 carcinogen by IARC, based on sufficient evidence for its carcinogenicity in humans, namely for NPC (IARC, 1997, 2012). EBV infects primarily B lymphocytes, but also epithelial cells such as oropharyngeal cells, essentially in the lymphoepithelium of the palatine tonsils from Waldeyers ring. The etiological association of NPC with EBV was first suggested on the basis of serological evidence (Old *et al.*, 1966). Circulating cell-free EBV DNA is detected in the plasma and serum of NPC patients, but not in healthy individuals, and its levels are positively correlated with disease stage and prognosis (Lin *et al.*, 2004). EBV DNA, RNA and gene products are also present in most tumour cells (zur Hausen *et al.*, 1970). EBV is detected in cancer cells of virtually all cases of class II NPC in endemic regions. In addition, NPC tumour cells were shown to be clonal expansions of a single EBV-infected progenitor cell (Raab-Traub & Flynn, 1986). EBV infection alone is, however, not a sufficient cause of NPC: the ubiquitous EBV infects and persists latently in over 90% of the world population, yet only a small proportion of individuals develop NPC. Although there is little variation in the prevalence of infection or the age at primary infection with EBV throughout China, risk for NPC is more than 20-fold higher in three provinces in southern China (Zeng, 1985). Therefore environmental and/or genetic factors may also contribute to NPC risk.

On the basis of studies on the natural history of NPC from southern Chinese populations, the following pathogenesis model for NPC has been proposed (Lo & Huang, 2002; Young & Rickinson, 2004). Clonal cell proliferation with 3p and 9p deletion is frequently detected in dysplastic lesions and even in histologically normal nasopharyngeal epithelia in the absence of EBV infection; loss of heterozygosity (LOH) appear to be an early event in the pathogenesis of NPC in this high-risk area (allelic loss may confer growth advantage and cells may expand to form multiple clonal population within the nasopharynx). These genetic events could result from the consumption of Cantonese-style salted fish and other traditional foods. Samples of Chinese-style salted fish contain high concentrations of several *N*-nitrosamines and their precursors such as *N*-nitrosodimethylamine, *N*-nitrosodiethylamine, *N*-nitrosopyrroline and *N*-nitrosopiperidine (see Section 1.2) which were all shown to be carcinogenic in animals (IARC, 1978, 1993; Tricker & Preussmann, 1991). In addition, increased formation of *N*-nitrosamines occurs after endogenous chemical nitrosation of salted fish with nitrite under acidic conditions (see Section 1.2). *N*-nitrosamino acids excreted in the urine were shown to be increased in subjects living in the high-risk areas of NPC in southern China, compared to those living in the low-risk areas (Yi *et al.*, 1993). These results suggest exposure to carcinogenic *N*-nitroso compounds, preformed in salted fish or formed endogenously by nitrosation of their precursors.

Polymorphisms in *cytochrome P450* (CYP) *2E1* (*CYP2E1*) (Hildesheim *et al.*, 1995, 1997; Kongruttanachok *et al.*, 2001) and *CYP2A6* (Tiwawech *et al.*, 2006) and the absence of *glutathione-S-transferase M1* (*GSTM1*) and/or *GSTT1* (Guo *et al.*, 2008; Zhuo *et al.*, 2009) have been associated with increased risk of NPC in Southern China. Polymorphisms in genes encoding for enzymes involved in *N*-nitrosamine metabolism and detoxification could affect carcinogenesis but exact mechanisms have not been elucidated.

Aqueous extracts of Cantonese-style salted dried fish from China can activate EBV-reactivation (Shao *et al.*, 1988). This is important, since EBV can persist benignly in the body unless it is reactivated. Active EBV can induce many different cellular processes that may lead to carcinogenesis (IARC, 2012). It can for instance, induce genomic instability (Fang *et al.*, 2009) and activation of the NADPH oxidase (Gruhne *et al.*, 2009) and increased expression of inducible nitric oxide synthase (Yu *et al.*, 2002). These enzymes produce reactive oxygen and nitrogen species that damage DNA through formation of 8-oxo-deoxyguanosine and 8-nitroguanine in NPC (Ma *et al.*, 2008; Segawa *et al.*, 2008; Gruhne *et al.*, 2009). Increased lipid peroxidation product (malondialdehyde) was also detected in the blood of NPC patients (Gargouri *et al.*, 2009). These findings indicate that reactivation by Chinese-style salted fish of latent EBV in infected cells may play a substantial role in NPC, by promoting genomic instability via induction of oxidative and nitrative DNA damage. Interestingly, epidemiological data showed that both EBV and Chinese-style salted fish are also associated with gastric carcinoma.

4.4 Synthesis

Possible mechanisms for the association of consumption of Cantonese-style salted fish with risk of NPC are the formation endogenously of *N*-nitroso compounds in the human body and/or their formation due to the processing of the fish — i.e. a reaction between secondary and tertiary amines in the fish and nitrate/nitrite in the crude salt used — and activation of the oncogenic Epstein-Barr virus. These two mechanisms are not mutually exclusive.

5. Evaluation

There is *sufficient evidence* in humans for the carcinogenicity of Chinese-style salted fish. Chinese-style salted fish causes cancer of the nasopharynx. Also, a positive association has been observed between consumption of Chinese-style salted fish and cancer of the stomach.

There is *sufficient evidence* in experimental animals for the carcinogenicity of Cantonese-style salted fish.

Chinese-style salted fish *is carcinogenic to humans (Group 1).*

References

Armstrong RW & Eng AC (1983). Salted fish and nasopharyngeal carcinoma in Malaysia. *Soc Sci Med*, 17: 1559–1567. doi:10.1016/0277-9536(83)90100-4 PMID:6635717

Armstrong RW, Imrey PB, Lye MS *et al.* (1998). Nasopharyngeal carcinoma in Malaysian Chinese: salted fish and other dietary exposures. *Int J Cancer*, 77: 228–235. doi:10.1002/(SICI)1097-0215(19980717)77:2<228::AID-IJC11>3.0.CO;2-7 PMID:9650558

Armstrong RW, Kannan Kutty M, Dharmalingam SK, Ponnudurai JR (1979). Incidence of nasopharyngeal carcinoma in Malaysia, 1968–1977. *Br J Cancer*, 40: 557–567. doi:10.1038/bjc.1979.221 PMID:497106

Cai L, Zheng ZL, Zhang ZF (2003). Risk factors for the gastric cardia cancer: a case–control study in Fujian Province. *World J Gastroenterol*, 9: 214–218. PMID:12532434

Chan JKC, Bray F, McCarron P *et al.* (2005). *Nasopharyngeal carcinoma.* In: *World Health Organization Classification of Tumours – Pathology and genetics of head and neck tumours*. Barnes EL, Eveson JW, Reichart P *et al.*, editors. Lyon, France: IARC Press, pp. 85–97.

Cheng KK, Day NE, Duffy SW *et al.* (1992). Pickled vegetables in the aetiology of oesophageal cancer in Hong Kong Chinese. *Lancet*, 339: 1314–1318. doi:10.1016/0140-6736(92)91960-G PMID:1349991

Fang CY, Lee CH, Wu CC *et al.* (2009). Recurrent chemical reactivations of EBV promotes genome instability and enhances tumor progression of nasopharyngeal carcinoma cells. *Int J Cancer*, 124: 2016–2025. doi:10.1002/ijc.24179 PMID:19132751

Farrow DC, Vaughan TL, Berwick M *et al.* (1998). Diet and nasopharyngeal cancer in a low-risk population. *Int J Cancer*, 78: 675–679. doi:10.1002/(SICI)1097-0215(19981209)78:6<675::AID-IJC2>3.0.CO;2-J PMID:9833758

Fong LY, Ho JH, Huang DP (1979). Preserved foods as possible cancer hazards: WA rats fed salted fish have mutagenic urine. *Int J Cancer*, 23: 542–546. doi:10.1002/ijc.2910230416 PMID:374286

Fong YY & Chan WC (1973). Dimethylnitrosamine in Chinese marine salt fish. *Food Cosmet Toxicol*, 11: 841–845. PMID:4768880

Gargouri B, Lassoued S, Ayadi W *et al.* (2009). Lipid peroxidation and antioxidant system in the tumor and in the blood of patients with nasopharyngeal carcinoma. *Biol Trace Elem Res*, 132: 27–34. PMID: 19436958 doi:10.1007/s12011-009-8384-z PMID:19436958

Geser A, Charnay N, Day NE *et al.* (1978). Environmental factors in the etiology of nasopharyngeal carcinoma: report on a case–control study in Hong Kong. *IARC Sci Publ*, 20: 213–229. PMID:730191

Goh KL, Cheah PL, Md N *et al.* (2007). Ethnicity and H. pylori as risk factors for gastric cancer in Malaysia: A prospective case control study. *Am J Gastroenterol*, 102: 40–45. doi:10.1111/j.1572-0241.2006.00885.x PMID:17100981

Goldgar DE, Easton DF, Cannon-Albright LA, Skolnick MH (1994). Systematic population-based assessment of cancer risk in first-degree relatives of cancer probands. *J Natl Cancer Inst*, 86: 1600–1608. doi:10.1093/jnci/86.21.1600 PMID:7932824

Gruhne B, Sompallae R, Marescotti D *et al.* (2009). The Epstein-Barr virus nuclear antigen-1 promotes genomic instability via induction of reactive oxygen species. *Proc Natl Acad Sci USA*, 106: 2313–2318. doi:10.1073/pnas.0810619106 PMID:19139406

Guo X, Johnson RC, Deng H *et al.* (2009). Evaluation of nonviral risk factors for nasopharyngeal carcinoma in a high-risk population of Southern China. *Int J Cancer*, 124: 2942–2947. doi:10.1002/ijc.24293 PMID:19296536

Guo X, O'Brien SJ, Zeng Y *et al.* (2008). GSTM1 and GSTT1 gene deletions and the risk for nasopharyngeal carcinoma in Han Chinese. *Cancer Epidemiol Biomarkers Prev*, 17: 1760–1763. doi:10.1158/1055-9965.EPI-08-0149 PMID:18628429

Haorah J, Zhou L, Wang X *et al.* (2001). Determination of total N-nitroso compounds and their precursors in frankfurters, fresh meat, dried salted fish, sauces, tobacco, and tobacco smoke particulates. *J Agric Food Chem*, 49: 6068–6078. doi:10.1021/jf010602h PMID:11743810

Henderson BE & Louie E (1978). Discussion of risk factors for nasopharyngeal carcinoma. *IARC Sci Publ*, 20: 251–260. PMID:730193

Henderson BE, Louie E, SooHoo Jing J *et al.* (1976). Risk factors associated with nasopharyngeal carcinoma. *N Engl J Med*, 295: 1101–1106. doi:10.1056/NEJM197611112952003 PMID:980005

Hildesheim A, Anderson LM, Chen CJ *et al.* (1997). CYP2E1 genetic polymorphisms and risk of nasopharyngeal carcinoma in Taiwan. *J Natl Cancer Inst*, 89: 1207–1212. doi:10.1093/jnci/89.16.1207 PMID:9274915

Hildesheim A, Chen CJ, Caporaso NE *et al.* (1995). Cytochrome P4502E1 genetic polymorphisms and risk of nasopharyngeal carcinoma: results from a case–control study conducted in Taiwan. *Cancer Epidemiol Biomarkers Prev*, 4: 607–610. PMID:8547826

Hjalgrim H, Friborg J, Melbye M (2007). *Epstein-Barr virus and malignant disease*. In: *Human Herpesviruses: Biology, therapy and immunoprophylaxis*. Arvin A, Campadelli-Fiume G, Moore P *et al.*, editors. Cambridge: Cambridge University Press, pp. 929–959.

Ho JH (1967). *Nasopharyngeal carcinoma in Hong Kong*. In: *Cancer of the nasopharynx*. Muir CS, Shanmugaratnam K, editors. Copenhagen: Munksgaard, pp. 58–63.

Ho JH (1978). An epidemiologic and clinical study of nasopharyngeal carcinoma. *Int J Radiat Oncol Biol Phys*, 4: 182–198. PMID:640889

Hu J, La Vecchia C, Negri E *et al.* (1999). Diet and brain cancer in adults: a case–control study in northeast China. *Int J Cancer*, 81: 20–23. doi:10.1002/(SICI)1097-0215(19990331)81:1<20::AID-IJC4>3.0.CO;2-2 PMID:10077146

Huang DP, Ho JH, Saw D, Teoh TB (1978). Carcinoma of the nasal and paranasal regions in rats fed Cantonese salted marine fish. *IARC Sci Publ*, 20315–328. PMID:730197

Huang DP, Ho JH, Webb KS *et al.* (1981). Volatile nitrosamines in salt-preserved fish before and after cooking. *Food Cosmet Toxicol*, 19: 167–171. doi:10.1016/0015-6264(81)90353-9 PMID:7286866

Huang TB, Yu MC, Zhu JH (1993). Diet and nasopharyngeal carcinoma: a case–control study in Guangzhou, China. *Chinese Journal of Cancer*, 12: 7–10.

IARC (1978). Some N-nitroso compounds. *IARC Monogr Eval Carcinog Risk Chem Man*, 17: 1–349. PMID:150392

IARC (1993). Some naturally occurring substances: food items and constituents, heterocyclic aromatic amines and mycotoxins. *IARC Monogr Eval Carcinog Risks Hum*, 56: 1–599.

IARC (1997). Epstein-barr virus and Kaposi's sarcoma herpesvirus/Human herpesvirus 8. *IARC Monogr Eval Carcinog Risks Hum*, 70: 1–492. PMID:9705682

IARC (2010). Ingested nitrate and nitrite, and cyanobacterial peptide toxins. *IARC Monogr Eval Carcinog Risks Hum*, 94: 1–448.

IARC (2012). Biological Agents. *IARC Monogr Eval Carcinog Risk Chem Man*, 100B: 1–475.

Imai S, Koizumi S, Sugiura M *et al.* (1994). Gastric carcinoma: monoclonal epithelial malignant cells expressing Epstein-Barr virus latent infection protein. *Proc Natl Acad Sci USA*, 91: 9131–9135. doi:10.1073/pnas.91.19.9131 PMID:8090780

Jia WH, Huang QH, Liao J *et al.* (2006). Trends in incidence and mortality of nasopharyngeal carcinoma over a 20–25 year period (1978/1983–2002) in Sihui and Cangwu counties in southern China. *BMC Cancer*, 6: 178 doi:10.1186/1471-2407-6-178 PMID:16822324

Jian L, Zhang DH, Lee AH, Binns CW (2004). Do preserved foods increase prostate cancer risk? *Br J Cancer*, 90: 1792–1795. doi:10.1038/sj.bjc.6601755 PMID:15208621

Kongruttanachok N, Sukdikul S, Setavarin S *et al.* (2001). Cytochrome P450 2E1 polymorphism and nasopharyngeal carcinoma development in Thailand: a correlative study. *BMC Cancer*, 1: 4 doi:10.1186/1471-2407-1-4 PMID:11389775

Lee HP, Gourley L, Duffy SW *et al.* (1994). Preserved foods and nasopharyngeal carcinoma: a case-control study among Singapore Chinese. *Int J Cancer*, 59: 585–590. doi:10.1002/ijc.2910590502 PMID:7960230

Levine PH, Stemmermann G, Lennette ET *et al.* (1995). Elevated antibody titers to Epstein-Barr virus prior to the diagnosis of Epstein-Barr-virus-associated gastric adenocarcinoma. *Int J Cancer*, 60: 642–644. doi:10.1002/ijc.2910600513 PMID:7860138

Li K, Yu P, Zhang ZX *et al.* (2001). Food components and risk of esophageal cancer in Chaoshan region of China, a high-risk area of esophageal cancer. *Chinese Journal of Cancer*, 20: 160–163.

Lin JC, Wang WY, Chen KY *et al.* (2004). Quantification of plasma Epstein-Barr virus DNA in patients with advanced nasopharyngeal carcinoma. *N Engl J Med*, 350: 2461–2470. doi:10.1056/NEJMoa032260 PMID:15190138

Lo KW & Huang DP (2002). Genetic and epigenetic changes in nasopharyngeal carcinoma. *Semin Cancer Biol*, 12: 451–462. doi:10.1016/S1044579X02000883 PMID:12450731

Lu JC, Shi LY, Wu ZL *et al.* (2003). Case-control study of human lung cancers in Guangzhou *China J Cancer Prev Treat*, 10: 673–676.

Luo XY, Liu WS, Chen LZ *et al.* (2009). [Comparative study on risk factors and family history of familial and sporadic nasopharyngeal carcinoma patients] *Zhonghua Yu Fang Yi Xue Za Zhi*, 43: 293–298. PMID:19534949

Ma N, Kawanishi M, Hiraku Y *et al.* (2008). Reactive nitrogen species-dependent DNA damage in EBV-associated nasopharyngeal carcinoma: the relation to STAT3 activation and EGFR expression. *Int J Cancer*, 122: 2517–2525. doi:10.1002/ijc.23415 PMID:18307254

Ning J-P, Yu MC, Wang Q-S, Henderson BE (1990). Consumption of salted fish and other risk factors for nasopharyngeal carcinoma (NPC) in Tianjin, a low-risk region for NPC in the People's Republic of China. *J Natl Cancer Inst*, 82: 291–296. doi:10.1093/jnci/82.4.291 PMID:2299678

Old LJ, Boyse EA, Oettgen HF *et al.* (1966). Precipitating antibody in human serum to an antigen present in cultured burkitt's lymphoma cells. *Proc Natl Acad Sci USA*, 56: 1699–1704. doi:10.1073/pnas.56.6.1699 PMID:16591407

Poirier S, Bouvier G, Malaveille C *et al.* (1989). Volatile nitrosamine levels and genotoxicity of food samples from high-risk areas for nasopharyngeal carcinoma before and after nitrosation. *Int J Cancer*, 44: 1088–1094. doi:10.1002/ijc.2910440625 PMID:2558079

Poirier S, Ohshima H, de-Thé G *et al.* (1987). Volatile nitrosamine levels in common foods from Tunisia, south China and Greenland, high-risk areas for nasopharyngeal carcinoma (NPC). *Int J Cancer*, 39: 293–296. doi:10.1002/ijc.2910390305 PMID:3818121

Raab-Traub N & Flynn K (1986). The structure of the termini of the Epstein-Barr virus as a marker of clonal cellular proliferation. *Cell*, 47: 883–889. doi:10.1016/0092-8674(86)90803-2 PMID:3022942

Segawa Y, Oda Y, Yamamoto H *et al.* (2008). Overexpression of inducible nitric oxide synthase and accumulation of 8-OHdG in nasopharyngeal carcinoma. *Histopathology*, 52: 213–223. doi:10.1111/j.1365-2559.2007.02920.x PMID:18184270

Shao YM, Poirier S, Ohshima H *et al.* (1988). Epstein-Barr virus activation in Raji cells by extracts of preserved food from high risk areas for nasopharyngeal carcinoma. *Carcinogenesis*, 9: 1455–1457. doi:10.1093/carcin/9.8.1455 PMID:2841048

Sriamporn S, Vatanasapt V, Pisani P *et al.* (1992). Environmental risk factors for nasopharyngeal carcinoma: a case-control study in northeastern Thailand. *Cancer Epidemiol Biomarkers Prev*, 1: 345–348. PMID:1305465

Takezaki T, Gao CM, Wu JZ *et al.* (2001a). Dietary protective and risk factors for esophageal and stomach cancers in a low-epidemic area for stomach cancer in Jiangsu Province, China: comparison with those in a high-epidemic area. *Jpn J Cancer Res*, 92: 1157–1165. doi:10.1111/j.1349-7006.2001.tb02135.x PMID:11714439

Takezaki T, Hirose K, Inoue M *et al.* (2001b). Dietary factors and lung cancer risk in Japanese: with special reference to fish consumption and adenocarcinomas.

Br J Cancer, 84: 1199–1206. doi:10.1054/bjoc.2001.1722 PMID:11336471

Takezaki T, Inoue M, Kataoka H *et al.* (2003). Diet and lung cancer risk from a 14-year population-based prospective study in Japan: with special reference to fish consumption. *Nutr Cancer*, 45: 160–167. doi:10.1207/S15327914NC4502_04 PMID:12881009

Tannenbaum SR, Bishop W, Yu MC, Henderson BE (1985). Attempts to isolate N-nitroso compounds from Chinese-style salted fish. *Natl Cancer Inst Monogr*, 69: 209–211. PMID:3834334

Tiwawech D, Srivatanakul P, Karalak A, Ishida T (2006). Cytochrome P450 2A6 polymorphism in nasopharyngeal carcinoma. *Cancer Lett*, 241: 135–141. doi:10.1016/j.canlet.2005.10.026 PMID:16377082

Topley M (1973). *Cultural and social factors related to Chinese infants feeding and weaning*. In: *Growing up in Hong Kong*. Field CE, Barber FM, editors. Hong Kong: University Press, pp. 56–65.

Tricker AR & Preussmann R (1991). Carcinogenic N-nitrosamines in the diet: occurrence, formation, mechanisms and carcinogenic potential. *Mutat Res*, 259: 277–289. doi:10.1016/0165-1218(91)90123-4 PMID:2017213

Tsugane S & Sasazuki S (2007). Diet and the risk of gastric cancer: review of epidemiological evidence. *Gastric Cancer*, 10: 75–83. doi:10.1007/s10120-007-0420-0 PMID:17577615

Ung A, Chen CJ, Levine PH *et al.* (1999). Familial and sporadic cases of nasopharyngeal carcinoma in Taiwan. *Anticancer Res*, 19: 1B661–665. PMID:10216473

Wang SY, Hu YL, Wu YL *et al.* (1996). A comparative study of the risk factors for lung cancer in Guangdong, China. *Lung Cancer*, 14: Suppl 1S99–S105. doi:10.1016/S0169-5002(96)90215-9 PMID:8785673

Ward MH, Pan WH, Cheng YJ *et al.* (2000). Dietary exposure to nitrite and nitrosamines and risk of nasopharyngeal carcinoma in Taiwan. *Int J Cancer*, 86: 603–609. doi:10.1002/(SICI)1097-0215(20000601)86:5<603::AID-IJC1>3.0.CO;2-H PMID:10797279

Weng YM, Hotchkiss JH, Babish JG (1992). N-nitrosamine and mutagenicity formation in Chinese salted fish after digestion. *Food Addit Contam*, 9: 29–37. doi:10.1080/02652039209374045 PMID:1397390

West S, Hildesheim A, Dosemeci M (1993). Non-viral risk factors for nasopharyngeal carcinoma in the Philippines: results from a case-control study. *Int J Cancer*, 55: 722–727. doi:10.1002/ijc.2910550504 PMID:7503957

Widlak P, Zheng X, Osterdahl BG *et al.* (1995). N-nitrosodimethylamine and 7-methylguanine DNA adducts in tissues of rats fed Chinese salted fish. *Cancer Lett*, 94: 85–90. doi:10.1016/0304-3835(95)03828-K PMID:7621449

Yang XR, Diehl S, Pfeiffer R *et al.*Chinese and American Genetic Epidemiology of NPC Study Team (2005). Evaluation of risk factors for nasopharyngeal carcinoma in high-risk nasopharyngeal carcinoma families in Taiwan. *Cancer Epidemiol Biomarkers Prev*, 14: 900–905. doi:10.1158/1055-9965.EPI-04-0680 PMID:15826929

Ye WM, Yi YN, Luo RX *et al.* (1998). Diet and gastric cancer: a casecontrol study in Fujian Province, China. *World J Gastroenterol*, 4: 516–518. PMID:11819359

Yi Z, Ohshima H, Bouvier G *et al.* (1993). Urinary excretion of nitrosamino acids and nitrate by inhabitants of high- and low-risk areas for nasopharyngeal carcinoma in southern China. *Cancer Epidemiol Biomarkers Prev*, 2: 195–200. PMID:8318871

You WC, Blot WJ, Chang YS *et al.* (1988). Diet and high risk of stomach cancer in Shandong, China. *Cancer Res*, 48: 3518–3523. PMID:3370645

Young LS & Rickinson AB (2004). Epstein-Barr virus: 40 years on. *Nat Rev Cancer*, 4: 757–768. doi:10.1038/nrc1452 PMID:15510157

Yu JS, Tsai HC, Wu CC *et al.* (2002). Induction of inducible nitric oxide synthase by Epstein-Barr virus B95-8-derived LMP1 in Balb/3T3 cells promotes stress-induced cell death and impairs LMP1-mediated transformation. *Oncogene*, 21: 8047–8061. doi:10.1038/sj.onc.1205990 PMID:12439755

Yu MC, Ho JH, Lai SH, Henderson BE (1986). Cantonese-style salted fish as a cause of nasopharyngeal carcinoma: report of a case-control study in Hong Kong. *Cancer Res*, 46: 956–961. PMID:3940655

Yu MC, Ho JH, Ross RK, Henderson BE (1981). Nasopharyngeal carcinoma in Chinese — salted fish or inhaled smoke? *Prev Med*, 10: 15–24. doi:10.1016/0091-7435(81)90002-5 PMID:7232343

Yu MC, Huang TB, Henderson BE (1989b). Diet and nasopharyngeal carcinoma: a case-control study in Guangzhou, China. *Int J Cancer*, 43: 1077–1082. doi:10.1002/ijc.2910430621 PMID:2732001

Yu MC, Mo CC, Chong WX *et al.* (1988). Preserved foods and nasopharyngeal carcinoma: a case-control study in Guangxi, China. *Cancer Res*, 48: 1954–1959. PMID:3349469

Yu MC, Nichols PW, Zou XN *et al.* (1989a). Induction of malignant nasal cavity tumours in Wistar rats fed Chinese salted fish. *Br J Cancer*, 60: 198–201. doi:10.1038/bjc.1989.250 PMID:2765365

Yu MC & Yuan JM (2002). Epidemiology of nasopharyngeal carcinoma. *Semin Cancer Biol*, 12: 421–429. doi:10.1016/S1044579X02000858 PMID:12450728

Yuan JM, Wang XL, Xiang YB *et al.* (2000). Preserved foods in relation to risk of nasopharyngeal carcinoma in Shanghai, China. *Int J Cancer*, 85: 358–363. doi:10.1002/(SICI)1097-0215(20000201)85:3<358::AID-IJC11>3.0.CO;2-E PMID:10652427

Zeng Y (1985). Seroepidemiological studies on nasopharyngeal carcinoma in China. *Adv Cancer Res*, 44: 121–138. doi:10.1016/S0065-230X(08)60027-5 PMID:2994402

Zheng X, Luo Y, Christensson B, Drettner B (1994c). Induction of nasal and nasopharyngeal tumours in Sprague-Dawley rats fed with Chinese salted fish. *Acta Otolaryngol*, 114: 98–104. doi:10.3109/00016489409126024 PMID:7510449

Zheng X, Yan L, Nilsson B *et al.* (1994a). Epstein-Barr virus infection, salted fish and nasopharyngeal carcinoma. A case–control study in southern China. *Acta Oncol*, 33: 867–872. doi:10.3109/02841869409098448 PMID:7818917

Zheng YM, Tuppin P, Hubert A *et al.* (1994b). Environmental and dietary risk factors for nasopharyngeal carcinoma: a case–control study in Zangwu County, Guangxi, China. *Br J Cancer*, 69: 508–514. doi:10.1038/bjc.1994.92 PMID:8123482

Zhuo X, Cai L, Xiang Z *et al.* (2009). GSTM1 and GSTT1 polymorphisms and nasopharyngeal cancer risk: an evidence-based meta-analysis. *J Exp Clin Cancer Res*, 28: 46 doi:10.1186/1756-9966-28-46 PMID:19338664

Zou J, Sun Q, Akiba S *et al.* (2000). A case–control study of nasopharyngeal carcinoma in the high background radiation areas of Yangjiang, China. *J Radiat Res (Tokyo)*, 41: Suppl53–62. doi:10.1269/jrr.41.S53 PMID:11142212

Zou X, Li J, Lu S *et al.* (1992). Volatile N-nitrosamines in salted fish samples from high- and low-risk areas for NPC in China. *Chin Med Sci J*, 7: 201–204. PMID:1307494

Zou XN, Lu SH, Liu B (1994). Volatile N-nitrosamines and their precursors in Chinese salted fish–a possible etological factor for NPC in china. *Int J Cancer*, 59: 155–158. doi:10.1002/ijc.2910590202 PMID:7927911

zur Hausen H, Schulte-Holthausen H, Klein G *et al.* (1970). EBV DNA in biopsies of Burkitt tumours and anaplastic carcinomas of the nasopharynx. *Nature*, 228: 1056–1058. doi:10.1038/2281056a0 PMID:4320657

INDOOR EMISSIONS FROM HOUSEHOLD COMBUSTION OF COAL

Indoor combustion of coal was considered by a previous IARC Working Group in 2006 (IARC, 2010a). Since that time, new data have become available, these have been incorporated into the *Monograph*, and taken into consideration in the present evaluation.

1. Exposure Data

1.1 Constituents of coal emissions from household use of coal

1.1.1 Types and forms of coal

Coal is a highly variable fuel, which ranges from high heating-value anthracite through various forms of bituminous coal to intermediates in coal formation, viz. lignite and peat. Each of these types of fuel can contain different levels of moisture, non-combustible inorganic material (ash), sulfur, and sometimes significant levels of other impurities, e.g. arsenic, fluorine, lead and mercury.

Raw coal may be used in many forms, from lumps and briquettes to fine powders. Processing of coal may be as simple as forming coal balls or cakes by hand followed by sun-drying, or it may be a sophisticated procedure, blending coal into a uniform mixture with binders to reduce sulfur and particulate emissions and formed into briquettes designed to burn efficiently and cleanly in special stoves.

1.1.2 Constituents of coal emissions

When using small and simple combustion devices such as household cooking and heating stoves, coals are difficult to burn without substantial emission of pollutants principally due to the difficulty of completely pre-mixing the fuel and air during burning. Consequently, a substantial fraction of the fuel carbon is converted to products of incomplete combustion. For example, typical household coal stoves in China and India divert between more than 10% and up to ~30% of their fuel carbon into products of incomplete combustion (Smith *et al.*, 2000; Zhang *et al.*, 2000a).

The products that are formed can be present in the gas phase, the particle phase, or both, depending on their volatility. Hence, they represent a complex mixture of particulate and gaseous chemical species, including carbon monoxide, nitrogen dioxide and particulate matter (PM). Products of incomplete combustion include polycyclic aromatic hydrocarbons (PAHs) and a large number of compounds that are precursor components of photochemical smog, such as aldehydes (Chuang *et al.*, 1992a; Tsai *et al.*, 2003). In addition, many types of coal contain intrinsic contaminants from their mineral deposits, such as sulfur, arsenic, silica, fluorine, lead or mercury. During combustion, these contaminants are released into the air in their original or oxidized form. In households that use sulfur-rich coals, for example, sulfur dioxide is present at elevated levels. The high temperature of coal combustion leads to emission of large amounts of nitrogen oxides (Zhang *et al.*, 2000a).

The chemical constituents of coal emissions have been reported as individual chemical compounds (e.g. carbon monoxide, benzene, formaldehyde, PAHs), groups of compounds (e.g. total non-methane hydrocarbon, total organic carbon), elements (e.g. carbon, arsenic), or ions (e.g. fluoride, sulfate) (IARC, 2010a). The constituents identified to date are summarized in Table 1.1 by compound class, element and ion, respectively. Selected chemicals that are associated with carcinogenicity are discussed below.

(a) Particles and particle components

Particles emitted from coal combustion are fine and ultra-fine in size (well below 1 µm in diameter) (Kleeman *et al.*, 1999; Hays *et al.*, 2002). Fresh coal emissions contain a large number of ultra-fine particles that condense rapidly as they cool and age. The emissions may include larger particles resulting from suspension of ash and solid fuel debris. Combustion-generated particles and ash/debris particles have different chemical composition and particle size. For this reason, there has been a switch in recent studies from measuring total suspended particles (TSP) to measuring inhalable particles (< 10 µm, referred to as PM_{10}) or respirable particles (< 2.5 µm, referred to as $PM_{2.5}$).

A large number of chemical species are found in combustion-generated particles and many of these are not stable (Rogge *et al.*, 1998). Elemental carbon has a characteristic core onto which many metals and organic compounds can be readily adsorbed or absorbed.

Earlier studies also focused on different solvent extracts of particles (soot) emitted from coal combustion. For example, in Xuanwei County, China, particles released from smoky-coal combustion contained the highest amount of organic compounds extractable with dichloromethane, followed by particles released from anthracite (smokeless) coal combustion (Mumford *et al.*, 1987). Some particles carry stabilized free radicals (Tian, 2005).

Analytical techniques such as ion chromatography can measure chemicals in the extracts of combustion particles in their dissociated form (ions). The most abundant commonly identified ions in coal emissions are shown in Table 1.1.

(b) PAHs and substituted PAHs

Polycyclic aromatic hydrocarbons are formed during incomplete combustion of all carbon-based fuels and organic materials, including coal. At typical ambient temperature, lower molecular-weight PAHs (with 2–4 aromatic rings) are present predominantly in the gas phase while higher molecular-weight PAHs are present predominantly in the particle phase. Because PAHs of higher cancer potency are predominantly present in the particle phase (IARC, 2010a), combustion particles have often been subject to compositional analysis for PAHs and PAH derivatives. A detailed analysis of PAHs in dichloromethane extracts of soot deposits from coal-burning stoves in several homes of Hunan Province, China, has identified 32 individual PAHs ranging in size from three to eight fused aromatic rings. The PAHs found in the soot deposits included 20 benzenoid PAHs, six fluoranthene benzologues, one cyclopenta-fused PAH, one indene benzologue, three oxygenated PAHs and one ring-sulfur-containing aromatic compound (Table 1.1; Wornat *et al.*, 2001). Carcinogenic PAHs, methylated PAHs and nitrogen-containing heterocyclic aromatics were detected in the particles emitted from smoky coal combustion, as typically found

Table 1.1 Constituents of coal emissions, by chemical class

Compound	Species	
Inorganic compounds	CO, SO_2, NO_x	
Hydrocarbons		
Alkanes	C_1–C_{10}	
Alkenes	C_2–C_{10} (including 1,3-butadiene)	
Aromatics	Benzene, Xylene, Toluene, Styrene	
PAHs and substituted PAHs	Acenaphthene	Cyclopenta[*bc*]coronene
	Acenaphthylene	Cyclopenta[*cd*]fluoranthrene
	Acephenanthrylene	Cyclopenta[*cd*]pyrene
	Anthracene	Dibenz[*a,c*]anthracene
	Benz[*a*]anthracene	Dibenz[*a,h*]anthracene
	Benzanthrone	Dibenz[*a,j*]anthracene
	Benzo[*b*]chrysene	Dibenzo[*a,e*]pyrene
	Benzo[*a*]coronene	Dibenzo[*e,l*]pyrene
	Benzo[*b*]fluoranthene	Dibenzo[*b,k*]fluoranthene
	Benzo[*k*]fluoranthene	Dicyclopenta[*cd,mn*]pyrene
	Benzo[*b+j+k*]fluorene	Dicyclopenta[*cd,jk*]pyrene
	Benzo[*a*]fluorine	Fluoranthene
	Benzo[*b*]naphtha[2,1-*d*]thiophene	Fluorene
	Benzo[*pqr*]naphtha[8,1,2-*bcd*]perylene	Indeno[123-*cd*]pyrene
	Benzo[*ghi*]perylene	Naphtho[1,2-*b*]fluoranthene
	Benzo[*a*]pyrene	Naphtho[2,1-*a*]pyrene
	Benzo[*e*]pyrene	Phenanthrene
	Chrysene	Picene
	Coronene	Pyrene
	Cyclopenta[*def*]chrysene-4-one	Triphenylene
	Cyclopent[*hi*]acephenanthrylene	Tribenzo[*e,ghi,k*]perylene
	Cyclopenta[*cd*]benzo[*ghi*]perylene	4-Oxa-benzo[*cd*]pyrene-3,5-dione
Aldehydes and ketones	Acetaldehyde	Isobutyraldehyde
	Acetone	Isovaleraldehyde
	Acrolein	*meta,para*-Tolualdehyde
	Benzaldehyde	*ortho*-Tolualdehyde
	Butyraldehyde	Propionaldehyde
	Crotonaldehyde	Valeraldehyde
	Formaldehyde	2-Butanone
	Hexaldehyde	2,4-Dimethylbenzaldehyde
Carbon	Elemental and organic	
Metals	Na, Mg, Al, K, Ca, Ti, V, Cr, Mn, Fe, Co, Ni, Cu, Zn, Ga, As, Se, Br, Rb, Sr, Yt, Zr, Mo, Pd, Ag, In, Sn, Sb, Ba, La, Au, Hg, Tl, Pb	
Non-metals	S, P, Si, Cl, Br	
Anions	SO_4^{2-}, Cl^-, NO_3^-	
Cations	NH_4^+, K^+	

From Kauppinen & Pakkanen (1990), Chuang *et al.* (1992a), Miller *et al.* (1994), Zhang & Smith (1999), Watson *et al.* (2001), Wornat *et al.* (2001), Ross *et al.* (2002), Yan *et al.* (2002), Tsai *et al.* (2003), Chen *et al.* (2004, 2005), Ge *et al.* (2004), Lee *et al.* (2005)

in numerous households in Xuanwei County, Yunnan Province, China (Mumford *et al.*, 1987; Chuang *et al.*, 1992a). In the aromatic fraction, coal combustion particles appeared to contain high concentrations and many species of methylated PAHs (Chuang *et al.*, 1992a). However, profiles of specific PAHs and their abundance vary largely, depending on the fuel types and combustion conditions (Tian, 2005).

(c) Hydrocarbons and partially oxidized organic compounds

Hydrocarbons identified in coal emissions include alkanes with 1–10 carbons, alkenes with 2–10 carbons (including 1,3-butadiene) and aromatic compounds (e.g. benzene, xylenes, toluene, styrene) (Table 1.1). Partially oxidized organic compounds identified in coal emissions include alkanols, aldehydes and ketones (carbonyls), carboxylic acids, alkyl esters and methoxylated phenolic compounds (Rogge *et al.*, 1998).

(d) Metals

Some carcinogenic substances were found to be released during the combustion of lignites used in Shenyang City in northern China and smoky coals used in Xuanwei County, China. Lignites from a local Shenyang coal field had very high concentrations of nickel (75 ppm) and chromium (79 ppm) (Ren *et al.*, 1999, 2004) when compared with the levels reported elsewhere in the world (0.5–50 ppm for nickel and 0.5–60 ppm for chromium) (Swaine, 1990). Microfibrous quartz has been found in some smoky coals from Xuanwei County and the resulting coal emissions (Tian, 2005). In Guizhou Province of China and other areas, particles emitted from burning coal have been reported to contain high levels of chemicals like fluorine, arsenic and mercury (Gu *et al.*, 1990; Yan, 1990; Shraim *et al.*, 2003).

1.1.3 Emission factors of some carcinogens

The emission factor of a particular chemical species can be measured as the mass of the species emitted per unit mass of fuel combusted or the mass of the species emitted per unit energy produced or delivered through combustion. Few studies conducted to date have quantified emission factors of common pollutants from household stoves used in developing countries.

The available data for several known human carcinogens (benzene, 1,3-butadiene, formaldehyde and benzo[*a*]pyrene) are summarized in Table 1.2. The sum of PAHs, when ≥14 individual PAHs were measured, is also shown. The cited studies measured the PAHs that are most commonly reported in the literature: acenaphthene, acenaphthylene, anthracene, benz[*a*]anthracene, benzo[*b*]fluoranthene, benzo[*a*]pyrene, benzo[*ghi*]perylene, benzo[*k*]fluoranthene, chrysene, dibenz[*a,h*]anthracene, fluoranthene, fluorene, indeno[1,2,3-*cd*]pyrene, naphthalene, phenanthrene and pyrene.

Burning four types of household coal fuel (honeycomb coal briquette, coal briquette, coal powder and water-washed coal powder) in three different coal stoves generated a very wide range of benzene (2.71–1050 mg/kg fuel) (Tsai *et al.*, 2003) and 1,3-butadiene emission factors (Table 1.2). The range of emission factors for formaldehyde was smaller.

These patterns of emission factors measured under experimental conditions are, in general, consistent with indoor air concentration profiles measured in households using coal stoves.

1.2 Prevalence of use and exposure

1.2.1 China

(a) Use and determinants of use of coal

In China, coal accounts for 70–75% of energy consumption (Millman *et al.*, 2008).

Table 1.2 Emission factors of carcinogenic compounds from household stoves

Compound	Fuel type	Fuel source	Emission factor[a] (mg/kg fuel)	Emission factor[a, b] (mg/MJ)	Reference
Benzene	Coal (4 types)	China	2.71–1050	0.9–390	Tsai *et al.* (2003)
1,3-Butadiene	Coal (4 types)	China	ND–21.3	ND–7.9	Tsai *et al.* (2003)
Styrene	Coal (4 types)	China	ND	ND	Tsai *et al.* (2003)
Formaldehyde	Coal (3 types)	China	2–51	0.9–12	Zhang & Smith (1999)
Acetaldehyde	Coal (3 types)	China	0.8–81	0.3–20	Zhang & Smith (1999)
Naphthalene	Coal briquettes	Viet Nam	44.5		Kim Oanh *et al.* (1999)
Benzo[*a*]pyrene	Coal briquettes	Viet Nam	0.30		Kim Oanh *et al.* (1999)
Benz[*a*]anthracene	Coal briquettes	Viet Nam	0.11		Kim Oanh *et al.* (1999)
Dibenz[*a*,*h*]anthracene	Coal briquettes	Viet Nam	ND		Kim Oanh *et al.* (1999)
Sum of PAHs (≥14 individual PAHs)	Coal briquettes	Viet Nam	102	4.4	Kim Oanh *et al.* (1999)

[a] The values are ranges of the means reported in individual studies.
[b] Denotes milligrams per megajoule of energy delivered to the pot
ND, not detected (below method detection limit)

Although in-home coal use is banned in all Chinese cities, about 10% of urban households still use coal as their primary source of fuel. In 2004, this corresponded to 27 million tonnes of coal. The use of coal is associated with access to local fuel sources and household income; a greater percentage of households in rural areas tend to use coal than in urban areas. In rural regions with ample and inexpensive coal supplies, virtually all households depend upon coal as their domestic fuel. In aggregate, about 40% of all households in rural China rely on coal for heating or cooking (National Bureau of Statistics, 2005).

According to the National Bureau of Statistics (2005, 2006), household energy use from coal (raw coal, washed coal and briquettes) in China represented 21% of total energy use in urban areas, and 12.8% in rural areas. An earlier publication by the Ministry of Agriculture (EBCREY, 1999), by contrast, reported a corresponding value of 34% in rural households.

Occasionally, use of coal for heating does not equate with use of coal for cooking. For example, some households that use coal for heating may use wood for cooking. A recent survey evaluated the specific types of fuels used for cooking throughout rural China. Overall, about 30% of rural households cook with coal. This distribution varied by geographic region, with coal being used for cooking in 19% of homes in Eastern China, 38% in Central China, 27% in Western China, and 7% in North-eastern China (National Bureau of Statistics, 2008).

The use of coal varies largely by geographical conditions and socioeconomic status. Coal and other commercial fuels in generally associated with higher incomes. Where coal resources are highest – predominantly in the north – coal use is highest. In a 2003–04 winter survey of rural areas near Xi'an, 16% and 33% of the households, located in a small village, depended mainly on coal for heating and cooking, respectively (Tonooka *et al.*, 2006). In a study in Shaanxi, Hubei and Zhejiang in China, most households (64%) in Shaanxi reported that they heated with coal in winter, compared to 0.2% in Zhejiang and 28.5% in Hubei (Sinton *et al.*, 2004). Similarly, 70% of the households in Shaanxi used coal for heating, compared to 1.5% in Zhejiang and 6% in Hubei (Sinton *et al.*, 2004).

Table 1.3 Levels of indoor air pollutants from coal emissions in Chinese homes

Pollutant	Urban (mg/m^3)	Rural (mg/m^3)
TSP	0.21–2.8	0.01–20
PM_{10}	0.16–2.7	0.12–26
CO	0.58–97	0.7–87
SO_2	0.01–5.8	0.01–23
NO_x	0.01–1.8	0.01–1.7
B[*a*]P	0.3–190	5.3–19000

B[*a*]P, benzo[*a*]pyrene; PM, particulate matter; TSP, total suspended particles
From Sinton *et al.* (1995)

(b) Pollutant levels and exposures

Since the 1980s, many studies of indoor air quality in China have been published, measuring particulate matter, benzo[*a*]pyrene, sulfur dioxide, nitrogen oxide and carbon monoxide (Table 1.3). The three-province survey (Sinton *et al.*, 2004) found that in summer when stove use was dominantly for cooking, households that used coal experienced high particulate (PM_4) levels, and traditional stoves emitted higher particulate levels than improved stoves.

Kitchens may not be the sites with the highest average particulate matter levels. In the three-province study (Sinton *et al.*, 2004), those households that used coal had higher particulate levels in living rooms than in kitchens; heating, smoking and perhaps other factors can result in levels over time that are higher in living rooms than in kitchens, despite the peaks associated with cooking. In another study (Jin *et al.*, 2005), differences between rooms with and without stoves were small.

A large number of studies monitored benzo[*a*]pyrene in households in Xuanwei County, Yunnan Province, others reported measurements taken elsewhere (IARC, 2010a). Indoor levels of benzo[*a*]pyrene were in a range spanning four orders of magnitude, from 1 ng/m^3 to over 10 000 ng/m^3 in some of the studies in Xuanwei County, in which bituminous coal led to much higher indoor levels than anthracite coal. In studies performed in other parts of the country, household averages rarely exceeded 40 ng/m^3.

A recent study examined winter levels of PM_4 in households in Guizhou and Shaanxi, in areas where coal in contaminated with fluorine, and found that average levels in kitchen and living areas were from about 200 $\mu g/m^3$ to 2000 $\mu g/m^3$ (He *et al.*, 2005).

1.2.2 Ouside China

There is little literature about coal use outside China.

A few measurements of particulate size fractions have been made in households of peri-urban Gujarat (in western India) that use coal (Aggarwal *et al.*, 1982; Raiyani *et al.*, 1993). During cooking, the proportion of total suspended particulates < 9 µm in aerodynamic diameter was 92%, and 70% were particles < 2 µm in aerodynamic diameter. Particulate PAH size distributions measured in these same indoor environments showed that in houses that used coal, 76% of the PAH mass was contained in particulates < 2 µm aerodynamic diameter (Raiyani *et al.*, 1993).

In one study, conducted in winter on households in urban Santiago in Chile, levels of PM_{10} were 250 $\mu g/m^3$ in the kitchen, and 295 ppb SO_2 (Cáceres *et al.*, 2001).

2. Cancer in Humans

The Working Group evaluated studies that focused on exposure to coal emissions only without exposure to other solid fuels.

2.1 Studies in China

2.1.1 *Cancer of the lung*

(a) Overview of studies

Since the previous *IARC Monograph* (IARC, 2010a), two new case–control studies (Galeone *et al.*, 2008; Lan *et al.*, 2008) and a re-analysis of a previously published cohort (Hosgood *et al.*, 2008) were published.

A retrospective cohort study carried out in Xuanwei, China, evaluated the association between lung cancer risk and in-home coal use (Lan *et al.*, 2002). Among lifetime smoky coal users, households that changed to stoves with chimneys experienced a significantly decreased risk of lung cancer in both men and women compared to individuals that used fire pits. Reduction in lung cancer mortality was also observed among lifetime smoky coal users that changed to portable stoves compared to those that used fire pits, both in men and women (Hosgood *et al.*, 2008). Both analyses were adjusted for average tons of fuel used annually, years of tobacco smoking, years of cooking, history of spousal lung cancer, family history of lung cancer, as well as other potential confounders.

Several case–control studies (Koo *et al.*, 1983; Xu *et al.*, 1989; Wu-Williams *et al.*, 1990; Liu *et al.*, 1991; Huang *et al.*, 1992; Sun, 1992; Ger *et al.*, 1993; Lan *et al.*, 1993; Liu *et al.*, 1993; Dai *et al.*, 1996; Du *et al.*, 1996; Lei *et al.*, 1996; Luo *et al.*, 1996; Shen *et al.*, 1996; Wang *et al.*, 1996; Ko *et al.*, 1997; Shen *et al.*, 1998; Zhong *et al.*, 1999; Lan *et al.*, 2000; Zhou *et al.*, 2000; Le *et al.*, 2001; Kleinerman *et al.*, 2002; Galeone *et al.*, 2008; Lan *et al.*, 2008), have evaluated the association of lung cancer risk with in-home coal use in China (Table 2.1 available at http://monographs.iarc.fr/ENG/Monographs/vol100E/100E-08-Table2.1.pdf). Four evaluated the effects by histology of lung cancer (Ger *et al.*, 1993; Luo *et al.*, 1996; Shen *et al.*, 1996; Le *et al.*, 2001). While these studies assessed exposure with different questionnaires and methodologies, in the aggregate, almost every study found in-home coal use to be associated with lung cancer risk in China by some measure of exposure. Notably, lung cancer has been associated with years of coal stove use (Xu *et al.*, 1989; Wu-Williams *et al.*, 1990; Dai *et al.*, 1996), years of kang use (heated by coal) (Wu-Williams *et al.*, 1990; Dai *et al.*, 1996), years of cooking or heating with coal as the fuel source (Xu *et al.*, 1989; Wu-Williams *et al.*, 1990; He *et al.*, 1991; Liu *et al.*, 1991 Lan *et al.*, 2002; Hosgood *et al.*, 2008), amount of coal used (Lan *et al.*, 1993; Lan *et al.*, 2000; Kleinerman *et al.*, 2002; Hosgood *et al.*, 2008), and quality of ventilation in homes that use coal (Liu *et al.*, 1993; Ko *et al.*, 1997; Le *et al.*, 2001). The studies were from different areas in China, including northern, southern, Xuanwei and the rest of central China, and Taiwan, China.

(b) Exposure–response evidence

All studies reporting an exposure–response association between coal use and lung cancer controlled for tobacco smoking. Lan *et al.* (1993) reported a significant exposure–response relationship according to the amount of smoky coal used per year in Xuanwei, China (P for trend < 0.001). Duration of cooking with coal was significantly and positively associated with the risk for lung cancer among women (Lan *et al.*, 2002; Hosgood *et al.*, 2008). In Gansu, individuals who use coal as their main fuel source were also found to experience higher lung cancer risk, with a significant exposure–response relationship among men (P for trend = 0.04) (Kleinerman *et al.*, 2002) but not among women. In northern China, lung cancer risk increased in an exposure–response manner according to the duration of use of heated kang (Xu *et al.*, 1989). Galeone *et al.* (2008) constructed an index of indoor air pollution due to solid fuel use (mainly coal) and found a significant exposure–response relationship.

(c) Type of coal

Various smoky coal types were associated with a range of lung cancer risks with substantial heterogeneity ($P < 0.001$) in Xuanwei, China (Lan *et al.*, 2008). The risk for lung cancer ranged from 24.8 (95%CI: 12.4–49.6) for using smoky coal from the Laibin mine to 0.7 (95%CI: 0.2–3.1) from the Yangliu mine, compared to use of smokeless coal or wood. In this study, indoor benzo[*a*]pyrene concentrations were highly correlated with the risk for lung cancer.

(d) Histology

In-home coal use has been associated with both adenocarcinomas and squamous-cell carcinomas of the lung (Ger *et al.*, 1993; Luo *et al.*, 1996; Shen *et al.*, 1996; Le *et al.*, 2001); however these studies are based on small sample sizes.

(e) Population characteristics

Most studies have focused on women, as they tend to spend more time at home and consequently have greater exposures to coal combustion products than men. Six studies enrolled only women (Dai *et al.*, 1996; Wang *et al.*, 1996; Ko *et al.*, 1997; Shen *et al.*, 1998; Zhong *et al.*, 1999; Zhou *et al.*, 2000), of which three (Dai *et al.* 1996; Wang *et al.*, 1996; Shen *et al.*, 1998) were also restricted to non-smokers. [Fuel type was not specified in Zhou *et al.* (2000) but both cases and controls had 'high level' of exposure to coal emissions.] In-home coal was associated with lung cancer risk in three studies (Dai *et al.*, 1996; Shen *et al.*, 1998; Zhong *et al.*, 1999). In study populations including men, the risks associated with in-home coal use was generally greater among women than among men (He *et al.*, 1991; Liu *et al.*, 1991; Liu *et al.*, 1993).

(f) Interactions

The most notable genetic interaction with in-home coal use involves the *GSTM1* null genotype. A meta-analysis found the *GSTM1* null genotype to be associated with lung cancer risk (OR, 1.64; 95%CI: 1.25–2.14; 4 studies) among studies carried out in regions of China that use coal for heating and cooking (Hosgood *et al.*, 2007).

2.2 Studies outside China

2.2.1 Indoor exposures

Two case–control studies that adequately separated the effect of coal from wood or other biomass products evaluated the association of coal use for heating or cooking and cancers of the lung, hypopharynx and larynx (Lissowska *et al.*, 2005; Sapkota *et al.*, 2008; Table 2.2 available at http://monographs.iarc.fr/ENG/Monographs/vol100E/100E-08-Table2.2.pdf).

In a multicenter study conducted in seven European countries (Czech republic, Hungary, Poland, Romania, the Russian Federation, Slovakia and the United Kingdom), Lissowska *et al.* (2005) evaluated the association of heating and cooking with solids fuels with risk of lung cancer. The study included 2861 cases and 3118 matched population-based controls. In an analysis that evaluated coal use specifically, ever use of coal (either as a cooking or heating fuel) was not significantly related to the risk of lung cancer, after adjusting for tobacco smoking and other factors.

Sapkota *et al.* (2008) conducted a multicenter hospital-based case–control study in India to investigate lifetime fuel usage as risk factors for three different cancer types (1042 hypopharyngeal/laryngeal and 635 lung) and 718 matched controls. Compared with never users, among those who always used coal for cooking the odds ratios for cancer was 1.92 (95%CI: 0.67–5.54) for the hypopharynx, 2.42 (95%CI: 0.94–6.25) for the larynx, and 3.76 (95%CI: 1.64–8.63) for the lung after adjusting for tobacco smoking and other factors. Among never smokers, the risk for lung cancer was 7.46 (95%CI: 2.15–25.94; based on 11 cases). The risk increased with years of coal usage for cancers of the hypopharynx (P for trend = 0.06), larynx (P for trend = 0.05) and lung (P for trend < 0.01).

2.2.2 Ambient coal smoke exposure from ecological studies

Two ecological studies evaluated the association of coal emissions with lung cancer. A study conducted in Dublin (Kabir *et al.*, 2007) evaluated the impact of coal burning (black smoke outdoor concentration) on lung cancer mortality using data from 1981 to 2000. In 1990 the use of coal was banned in Dublin. A strong decline in black smoke was noted between the pre- and post-ban periods, from 46.4 μg/m^3 in 1981–90 (pre-ban) to 18.2 μg/m^3 in 1991–2000 (post-ban). After adjusting for age, sex and smoking, annual mean black smoke concentration was not related to annual death rates from lung cancer. [The Working Group noted that the post-ban period was too short to see any changes in lung cancer mortality.]

Another study evaluated the impact of industrial installations involving combustion of coal and other fuels on the mortality due to lung, laryngeal and bladder cancer in the population of 8073 Spanish towns in 1994–2003 (García-Pérez *et al.*, 2009). Mortality data were obtained form the National Statistics Institute and population exposure was evaluated by the distance of the centroid of the town to the closest combustion facility. Installations using coal only as the fuel source, within a vicinity of 5 km, was related to an increased risk for lung cancer overall (OR, 1.10; 95%CI: 1.02–1.18) with higher risk in men (OR, 1.13; 95%CI: 1.05–1.22), for bladder cancer overall (OR, 1.18; 95%CI: 1.01–1.37) and 1.22 (95%CI: 1.03–1.44) in men and for laryngeal cancer (OR, 1.46; 95%CI: 1.21–1.77 in men) after adjusting for smoking and sociodemographic variables. The authors noted that there was no other industry nearby that could bias the risk estimates.

2.3 Synthesis

Several case–control studies from China and a study from India have demonstrated an increased risk for lung cancer associated with exposure to emissions from coal burning, after accounting for potential confounders, including smoking and in analyses restricted to non-smokers. There were higher risks in women than men, and exposure–response relationships were found. A European case–control study did not find a significant effect of indoor coal use for cooking or heating. An ecological study from Europe provided further evidence of an increased risk for lung cancer in the vicinity of coal plants. No major effect was observed on lung cancer mortality after the ban of coal use in Dublin, probably because there was insufficient latency to see a change. Other cancer sites have been studied (larynx, bladder, hypopharynx); however there is not enough evidence to evaluate carcinogenicity with exposure to coal emissions.

In conclusion, there is convincing evidence based on multiple studies, mainly from different parts of China and one in India, that indoor emissions from household combustion of coal (used for heating and cooking) are causally linked to lung cancer in humans.

3. Cancer in Experimental Animals

Soots have been evaluated previously (IARC, 1985, 2010a).

Coal soot has been tested for carcinogenicity to mice by whole body exposure and coal emissions have been tested by inhalation in both mice and rats. Extracts of coal soot and smoke particles have also been tested by intratracheal, dermal, and subcutaneous administration to mice. A veterinary case–control study has studied sinonasal cancer in pet dogs from households with indoor use of coal.

3.1 Coal emissions and coal soot

3.1.1 Whole-body and inhalation exposure

In one study, whole-body exposure of Buffalo strain mice to coal soot mixed with bedding caused eight lung adenocarcinomas in 100 exposed mice compared to one in 50 controls [not significant] (Seeling & Benignus, 1936). In a second study, no increase in lung or skin tumours resulted from repeated exposure of mice to a 'moderate' cloud of soot in an inhalation chamber for a period of one year (Campbell, 1939).

Inhalation exposure to coal emissions for periods of 15 to 24 months caused markedly increased incidence of lung cancer in two studies in mice (Liang *et al.*, 1988; Lin *et al.*, 1995) and one study in rats (Liang *et al.*, 1988; Table 3.1). Squamous cell lung carcinomas occurred in exposed animals in one of the studies in mice and the study in rats (Liang *et al.*, 1988).

3.2 Extracts of coal soot

3.2.1 Intratracheal administration

Intratracheal administration of an aqueous detergent extract of coal soot once every 10 days for about 100 days increased lung adenocarcinoma incidence (29/72 versus 7/43, $P < 0.01$) in Kumming mice compared to controls after 18 months (Yin *et al.*, 1984).

3.2.2 Dermal application

Coal-soot extracts applied repeatedly to mouse skin increased the incidence of skin tumours including squamous cell carcinomas in four studies (Passey, 1922; Passey & Carter-Braine, 1925; Campbell, 1939; Mumford *et al.*, 1990).

Smoky coal-soot extracts applied to mouse skin followed by repeated dermal applications of the skin tumour promoter 12-*O*-tetradecanoylphorbol-13-acetate initiated skin tumours in mice in two studies (Liang & Wang, 1987; Mumford *et al.*, 1990; Table 3.2).

3.2.3 Subcutaneous injection

In one study, a low incidence (17%) of injection-site subcutaneous tumours [histology not specified] developed after 55 weeks in 30 (C57BpxCBA)F_1 male mice given five subcutaneous injections of extracts of brown coal. No tumours were observed in controls (Khesina *et al.*, 1977).

In two experiments, repeated subcutaneous injections for 10 weeks of extracts of coal soot collected from Xuanwei County, China, increased the incidence of lung cancer (adenocarcinomas, adenosquamous and squamous cell carcinomas) in Kumming mice after 10 months (Liang *et al.*, 1983, 1984; Table 3.3).

3.3 Veterinary epidemiology

A case–control study in pet dogs found that indoor use of coal was a strong risk factor for sinonasal cancers (adjusted odds ratio, 4.24; 95% confidence interval: 1.30–16.52) (Bukowski *et al.*, 1998).

Table 3.1 Carcinogenicity studies of inhalation exposure to coal emissions in experimental animals

Species, strain (sex) Duration Reference	Dosing regimen, Animals/group at start	Incidence of tumours	Significance	Comments
Mouse, Kunming (M, F) 2 yr Lin *et al.* (1995)	Control air Smoke, 60 g coal, daily Smoke, 105 g coal, daily Smoke, 160 g coal, daily 30 M + 30 F	Lung cancer, 3.6% Lung cancer, 9.4% Lung cancer, 12.8% Lung cancer, 24.3%	– NS $P < 0.05$ $P < 0.05$	Purity NR; Age at start NR (weight, 13 ± 1 g) Amounts of coal chosen to simulate normal indoor air conditions for humans in Harbin City, China Exposure assumed to be daily exposure
Mouse, Kunming (M, F) 15 mo Liang *et al.* (1988)	Control air Coal smoke 113 M + 58 F (control) 160 M + 50 F	29/171, total lung cancer (all adenocarcinomas) 188/210, total lung cancer (including: 119/210, adenocarcinoma; 45/210 adenosquamous carcinoma; 24/210 squamous-cell carcinoma)	– $P < 0.001$	Age at start NR (weight, 21 g) Total suspended particles, 0.91 mg/m^3 (control air) vs 14.38 mg/m^3 (coal smoke). B[*a*]P, 0.15 µg/m^3 (control air), 50.5 µg/m^3 (coal smoke) Bituminous coal incompletely burned to simulate normal indoor air in Xuanwei County, China
Rat, Wistar (M, F) 19 mo Liang *et al.* (1988)	Control air Coal smoke 59 M + 51 F (control) 62 M + 63 F	1/110, total lung tumours (1 adenocarcinoma) 84/125, total lung carcinomas (all squamous cell carcinomas)	– $P < 0.001$	Age at start NR (weight, 105 g) Total suspended particles, 0.91mg/m^3 (control air) vs 14.38 mg/m^3 (coal smoke). B[*a*]P, 0.15 µg/m^3 (control air), 50.5 µg/m^3 (coal smoke) Bituminous coal incompletely burned to simulate normal indoor air in Xuanwei County, China

B[*a*]P, Benzo[*a*]pyrene; F, female; M, male; mo, month or months; NR, not reported; NS, not significant; yr, year or years

Table 3.2 Carcinogenicity studies of dermal exposure to coal-soot extracts in mice

Species, strain (sex) Duration Reference	Dosing regimen, Animals/group at start	Incidence of tumours	Significance	Comments
Mouse, SENCAR (F) 77 wk Mumford *et al.* (1990)	0.2 ml, Acetone twice/wk, 52 wk (control)	No skin carcinomas at 52 wk (100% survival) or at 77 wk (78% survival)	–	Exposure to organic extracts of indoor air particles from burned smoky coal in Xuanwei County, China. B[*a*]P content, 19.3 µg/m³ air
	1 mg smoky coal extract, twice/wk, 52 wk	38% carcinomas[a] (1.3 per tumour bearing mouse) at 52 wk (88% survival), 88%[a] (1.1 per tumour bearing mouse) at 77 wk (10% survival)	NR [significant]	
	40 animals			
Mouse, SENCAR (F) 27 wk Mumford *et al.* (1990)	Initiation with smoky coal extract, followed one wk after by promotion with TPA (2 µg/mouse in 0.2 ml acetone, twice/wk, 26 wk). Initiation doses:			Exposure to organic extracts of indoor air particles from burned smoky coal in Xuanwei County, China. B[*a*]P content, 19.3 µg/m³ air Tumour incidence and numbers estimated from graphical presentation of data.
	0 mg	15% with skin papillomas	–	
	1 mg	80% with papillomas	NR [significant]	
	2 mg	90% with papillomas	NR [significant]	
	5 mg	> 90% with papillomas	NR [significant]	
	10 mg	> 90% with papillomas	NR [significant]	
	20 mg	100% with papillomas	NR [significant]	
	40 animals			
Mouse, Kunming (M) 26 wk Liang & Wang (1987)	Initiation with 0, 1, 5, 10, 20 mg smoky coal soot; promotion with TPA (repeated application of 2 µg/mouse) 40 animals	Skin tumours: 10, 25, 54, 60, 40%	[$P < 0.05$], 5–20 mg coal soot	Age at start NR (weight, 28.7 g) Extracts of smoky coal soot from Xuanwei County, China

[a] mainly squamous cell carcinomas

B[*a*]P, benzo[*a*]pyrene; F, female; M, male; NR, not reported; TPA, 12-*O*-tetradecanoylphorbol-13-acetate; wk, week or weeks

Table 3.3 Carcinogenicity studies of subcutaneous injections of coal soot extracts in mice

Species, strain (sex) Duration Reference	Dosing regimen, Animals/group at start	Incidence of tumours	Significance	Comments
		Lung cancer[a]		
Mouse, Kunming (M) 10 mo Liang *et al.* (1983)	Once/wk, 10 wk: 0 mg (control) 500 mg soot extract (total dose) 1000 mg soot extract (total dose) 38–57 animals	1/38 44/57 36/56	- $P < 0.001$ $P < 0.001$	Age at start NR (weight, 18–26 g) Exposure to cyclohexane extracts of coal soot from Xuanwei County, China.
Mouse, Kunming (M) 311 d Liang *et al.* (1984)	Once/wk, 10 wk: 0 mg (control) 119 mg soot extract (total dose) 400 mg soot extract (total dose) ~60 animals	6/60, all adenocarcinomas 52/58 39/59	- $P < 0.001$ $P < 0.001$	Age at start NR (weight, 18–22 g) Exposure to Tween 80 – saline extracts of coal soot from Xuanwei County, China.

[a] Lung cancers included squamous cell carcinomas, adenosquamous carcinomas, and adenocarcinomas.
d, day or days; M, male; mo, month or months; NR, not reported; wk, week or weeks

3.4 Synthesis

There is convincing evidence for the carcinogenicity of coal smoke and coal soot in experimental animals, based on the consistent induction of lung cancers in mice and rats exposed to coal emissions by inhalation, and in mice given subcutaneous injections of coal soot extract, and induction of malignant tumours of the skin in mice given repeated dermal applications of coal soot extract.

4. Other Relevant Data

4.1 Inhalable particles

The primary mechanisms for deposition of airborne particles in the respiratory tract are sedimentation, impaction and diffusion (see IARC (2010b) for a review). Deposition by sedimentation and impaction depends on the aerodynamic diameter of the particle, whereas deposition by diffusion depends on its thermodynamic diameter (ICRP, 1994). Following inhalation, particles may either deposit in the extrathoracic, tracheobronchial or pulmonary airways or remain in the air stream and be eliminated upon exhalation. The deposition of particles in the respiratory tract depends primarily on the size of the inhaled particle, the route of breathing (i.e. through the nose and/or mouth) and the breathing pattern (e.g. volume and frequency) (Bailey *et al.*, 1985; Freedman & Robinson, 1988; ICRP, 1994).

Particles are frequently aggregates or agglomerates of smaller primary particles. The aerodynamic and thermodynamic properties of these aggregates (rather than the primary particles) affect their behaviour in the air and the probability of deposition in the respiratory tract. Once deposited, properties such as the size and surface area of both the aggregate and the primary particle can potentially affect the kinetics of clearance (ICRP, 1994; Oberdörster, 1996).

The deposition and clearance of particles vary among individuals for several reasons, including age, sex, tobacco smoking status and health status. Pre-existing lung diseases or conditions such as asthma or chronic obstructive pulmonary disease can influence the efficiency and pattern of deposition within the respiratory tract. Deposition and retention determine the initial and retained dose of particles in each region of the respiratory tract and may, therefore, influence the risk for developing diseases specific to those regions of the respiratory tract (Oberdörster, 1988; ICRP, 1994).

All animal species that are routinely used in particle toxicology, as well as humans, are susceptible to impairment of clearance of poorly soluble particles from the lungs. In rats, impaired clearance is probably one of the first steps necessary to initiate a sequence of events that may lead to lung cancer. Different animal species exhibit differences in particle-induced impairment of clearance, which can result in different lung burdens (expressed as mass or surface area) following exposures to the same particle concentration (Brown *et al.*, 2005; IARC, 2010b). In cancer bioassays in rats exposed to various types of poorly soluble particles of fine or ultrafine size, the surface area of the particles may be a better predictor of lung tumours than particle mass (Oberdörster & Yu, 1990; Driscoll *et al.*, 1996).

Inhaled and deposited particles are cleared more rapidly from the normal lungs of healthy rats than from those of humans. However, at high lung burdens, macrophage-mediated clearance from the rat lung can be impaired and in time, clearance effectively ceases. This phenomenon (termed 'overload') is observed with poorly soluble particles generally considered to have low toxicity (Morrow, 1988). Several studies have shown that rats, but not mice or hamsters, develop excess incidence of lung cancer after chronic inhalation of 'overloading' doses of poorly soluble particles. Several authors have discussed this phenomenon and the challenges it poses for the extrapolation of chronic effects in rats to humans (Morrow, 1994; Levy, 1995; Watson & Valberg, 1996; ILSI, 2000; Miller, 2000; Oberdörster 2002; Hext *et al.*, 2005; IARC, 2010b).

The events proposed to describe the biological process that starts with particle deposition on critical target cells (e.g. alveolar epithelial cells type II) or tissues within the rat lung and results in lung tumours include:

- sustained inflammation, where the cell population (dominated by activated and probably persistent polymorphonuclear neutrophils) secretes a collection of pro-/anti-inflammatory cytokines, proteases, cytotoxins, fibrogenic and other growth factors;

- production of reactive oxygen species by particle effects or intracellular formation, which may gradually deplete the antioxidant defences; damage DNA directly and potentially induce mutations, promote cell turnover and cell proliferation; events that may enhance the risk for DNA replication error and/or expand a mutated or transformed cell to initiate a tumour (Castranova, 2000; Knaapen *et al.*, 2004).

Some of these events have been demonstrated in humans exposed to poorly soluble particles, but it is not known to what extent they are operative in humans and whether humans are eventually susceptible to particle-induced lung cancer. Species differences such as breathing conditions, respiratory tract structure and pulmonary defences must be considered when extrapolating toxicological findings from rodents to humans (Castranova, 2000; Knaapen *et al.*, 2004; Brown *et al.*, 2005). Clear differences in antioxidant defence mechanisms in the lungs also exist between humans and rats, and there is evidence that humans overall are relatively deficient in some of these mechanisms compared with rats (IARC, 2010b). Studies in rats have shown that, depending on the concentration and duration of exposure, the long-term retention of particles in humans can be greater than that predicted from rodent studies that used lower concentrations or shorter durations of exposure (Morrow, 1988, 1992; ILSI, 2000).

Although the degree of sustained inflammation experienced by rats at high lung burdens is not observed in humans, humans may experience sustained inflammation under certain disease conditions, including late-stage interstitial pulmonary fibrosis. Patients who have interstitial pulmonary fibrosis have a high incidence of lung tumours (Daniels & Jett, 2005).

4.2 Polycyclic aromatic hydrocarbons

Polycyclic aromatic hydrocarbons are important components of coal emissions (see IARC (2010c) for a review). These compounds are absorbed through the respiratory tract – from where, as adsorbed particulates, they can also be swept back up and swallowed into the gastrointestinal tract and even reach the skin. Smaller molecules (2–3-ring) are absorbed more rapidly than larger ones (IARC, 2010c).

The rate and extent of absorption by the respiratory tract of PAHs from particles onto which they are adsorbed is generally dependent on particle size, which determines regional deposition in the respiratory tract and the rate of release of PAHs from the particle. Highly lipophilic PAHs released from particles deposited in the conducting and bronchial airways are largely retained for several hours and absorbed slowly by a diffusion-limited process. In contrast, PAHs that are released from particles in alveolar airways are generally absorbed within minutes (Gerde & Scott, 2001; IARC, 2010c).

Once absorbed, PAHs are distributed widely to most organs and tissues and tend to accumulate in fatty tissue (WHO, 1998; IARC, 2010c). They are metabolized rapidly to more soluble metabolites, e.g. phenols, dihydrodiols, and phenol dihydrodiols, and in some cases to more reactive species like epoxides, dihydrodiol epoxides, quinones and tetrols. At least three main pathways of metabolism are involved:

- the cytochrome P450 (CYP) pathway, where PAHs may be (1) metabolized to their bay- and fjord-region diol epoxides with the involvement of epoxide hydrolase (Xue & Warshawsky, 2005) or (2) undergo cyclopenta-ring oxidation (IARC, 2010c).
- the cytochrome P450/peroxidase pathway, where removal of one electron from the π system by CYPs or peroxidases generates a radical cation (Cavalieri & Rogan, 1992; Xue & Warshawsky, 2005).
- the cytochrome P450/aldo-keto reductase (oxidative) pathway where, following metabolization to dihydrodiols by CYPs and epoxide hydrolase, formation of *ortho*-quinones and generation of reactive oxygen species is ensured by aldo-keto reductases (Penning *et al.*, 1999; Xue & Warshawsky, 2005; Penning & Drury, 2007).

Many of the above-mentioned metabolites are electrophilic and bind to DNA and proteins, which results in genotoxic effects — primarily through the formation of DNA adducts (Xue & Warshawsky, 2005). Beyond these phase-I metabolic pathways, PAH metabolites may be eliminated in a conjugated form with either glutathione, sulfate or glururonic acid via the phase-II metabolism (WHO, 1998; IARC, 2010c).

Ample evidence, summarized in IARC (2010c), supports a role for PAHs in lung cancer due to exposure to indoor emissions from coal combustion.

A general genotoxic mechanism has emerged in which PAHs such as benzo[*a*]pyrene are metabolized to electrophilic compounds (e.g. benzo[*a*]pyrene-7,8-diol-9,10-epoxide) that form adducts in DNA (Xue & Warshawsky, 2005; IARC, 2010c). If these adducts are not repaired, misreplication converts them primarily into G→T transversion mutations in the *TP53* gene in the lung. An over-representation of G→T transversions has been found on the non-transcribed strand of DNA in the *TP53* gene in lung tumours from smoky coal-exposed women in China, which is consistent with exogenous exposure and the lack of transcription-coupled DNA repair on that strand, resulting in mutations (DeMarini *et al.*, 2001). A preference for G→T transversions in the methylated CpG dinucleotides in human lung tumours has been found, in agreement with in-vitro studies that show the same dinucleotide as a target of benzo[*a*]pyrene diol epoxide (Casale *et al.*, 2001; DeMarini *et al.*, 2001; Hainaut & Pfeifer, 2001; Pfeifer & Hainaut, 2003).

A study by Sun *et al.* (2007) found that coal emission-exposed subjects carrying an exon-3 mutation in the microsomal epoxide hydrolase gene had a nearly 2-fold increased risk for lung cancer compared to those with the wild type version of the gene. Thus, metabolism to PAH-epoxides plays an important role in lung cancer associated with coal emissions.

A role for the aldo-keto reductase (AKR) pathway in the formation of mutagenic/carcinogenic metabolites of PAHs has also been found among smoky coal emission-exposed lung cancer patients in China. Lan *et al.* (2004) found that subjects who had the *AKR1C3-Gln/Gln* genotype had a 1.84-fold increased risk for lung cancer compared with those without the polymorphism. In subjects having the *OGG1-Cys/Cys* or the *OGG1-Ser/Cys* polymorphism, the risk for lung cancer was increased about 1.9-fold relative to *OGG1-Ser/Ser*. Indeed, AKRs convert trans-dihydrodiols to *ortho*-quinones, and Park *et al.* (2008) have used a yeast system to show that the pattern of *ortho*-quinone-induced mutations in *TP53* in this system is driven by 8-oxo-dGuo formation, whereas the spectrum of mutations is driven by biological selection for dominance. Park *et al.* (2009) have shown recently that the aryl-hydrocarbon receptor shuttles the AKR-generated *ortho*-quinones into the nucleus.

Consistent with a role for PAHs, studies in smoky coal-exposed women in China have shown that a polymorphism in nucleotide excision repair (*ERCC2 Gln* at codon 751) reduced lung cancer risk by 60%. A similar reduction was also found for subjects with a particular haplotype in *ERCC2*. A 2-fold increased risk for lung cancer was found for subjects having 1 or 2 copies of the *RAD23B* gene with Val at codon 249 (Shen *et al.*, 2005).

In addition, accumulation of mutations in other key genes (e.g. *KRAS*; Mass *et al.*, 1993; DeMarini *et al.*, 2001; Keohavong *et al.*, 2003), production of reactive oxygen species (Xue & Warshawsky, 2005), photomutagenicity (Yan *et al.*, 2004), together with interruption of gap-junctional intercellular communication (Bláha *et al.*, 2002), cell-cycle dysregulation, increase in cell proliferation, tumour promotion (Tannheimer *et al.*, 1998, 1999; Burdick *et al.*, 2003; Oguri *et al.*, 2003; Plísková *et al.*, 2005), and induction of apoptosis (Ko *et al.*, 2004) can result in tumour formation. PAHs can also have immunosuppressive and haematological effects (Burchiel & Luster, 2001; Booker & White, 2005). Several of the above effects are partly mediated by activation of the aryl-hydrocarbon receptor to which many PAHs can bind (IARC, 2010c).

4.3 Biomarkers and mutagenicity

The available information on the mutagenicity and genotoxicity of smoky-coal emissions from Xuanwei County, China, includes a wide range of end-points that encompass mutations in *KRAS* and *TP53* genes in lung tumours from non-smokers who were exposed to smoky-coal emissions (Li *et al.*, 1997; DeMarini *et al.*, 2001; Keohavong *et al.*, 2003, 2004, 2005). In addition, studies show that such exposures result in the excretion of several PAHs and their metabolites, e.g. methylated- and hydroxyl-PAHs (Mumford *et al.*, 1995; Siwińska *et al.*, 1999) and that exposed individuals exhibit elevated levels of DNA adducts (Gallagher *et al.*, 1993; Mumford *et al.*, 1993; Xu *et al.*, 1997; Casale *et al.*, 2001) and accumulation of *TP53* protein (Feng *et al.*, 1999; Lan *et al.*, 2001). Recently, mitochondrial DNA content, which is associated with production of reactive oxygen species through oxidative phosphorylation, was found to be elevated in smoky coal-exposed subjects (Bonner *et al.*, 2009).

It was also reported that exposure to coal emissions in Guizhou Province, China, is associated with increased levels of DNA–protein cross-links, unscheduled DNA synthesis (Zhang *et al.*, 2000b), sister chromatid exchange, chromosomal aberrations, micronucleus formation (Zhang *et al.*, 2007a) and *p16* gene deletion and hypermethylation (Zhang *et al.*, 2007b) in peripheral blood lymphocytes. Mutated P53 protein was also elevated in the skin (Hu *et al.*, 2001). [Some of the observed cytogenetic damage were probably due to the elevated levels of arsenic present in this coal].

In many studies, extracts or condensates of coal emissions were found to be mutagenic in *Salmonella* with or without metabolic activation: in strain TA98 in the presence of S9 the potency for smoky-coal could reach 60000 revertants per cubic metre of air (Mumford *et al.*, 1987) and 3000 revertants per milligram of particle (Nakanishi *et al.*, 1997). Bioassay-directed fractionation studies with *Salmonella* have identified that, for smoky-coal, most of the mutagenic activity is due to PAHs and alkylated PAHs (Chuang *et al.*, 1992a, b). Evaluation of the mutation spectrum produced by smoky coal extract in *Salmonella* showed a similar percentage of GC to TA mutations (≈77–86%) as found in the *TP53* (76%) and *KRAS* (86%) genes in lung tumours from smoky coal-exposed women (Granville *et al.*, 2003).

Several studies evaluated populations who are exposed to indoor air pollution from coal for associations between polymorphisms in genes that are involved in xenobiotic metabolism and risk for lung cancer. However, multiple comparisons and generally small sample sizes could have resulted in both false-positive and false-negative findings. There is some evidence that the *GSTM1*-null genotype was associated with increased risk for lung cancer in some studies in which at least part of the study population was definitely or probably exposed to indoor coal emissions, particularly where exposure to PAHs was suspected to be a contributing agent (Lan *et al.*, 2000; Chen *et al.*, 2006). However, results for polymorphisms in other genes are inconsistent or have been analysed in only one study. Therefore, no conclusion can be made regarding the effect of polymorphisms of genes other than possibly *GSTM1* on risk for lung cancer in these populations.

4.4 Synthesis

Chemical analyses and bioassay-directed fractionation of smoky coal emissions have identified PAHs as an important chemical class that accounts for much of their mutagenicity and carcinogenicity. The epidemiological link between exposure to smoky coal emissions and an increased risk for lung cancer is strengthened mechanistically by the fact that the mutation spectra of the *P53* tumour-suppressor gene and the *KRAS* oncogene in the lung tumours from non-smokers exposed to smoky coal esmissions reflect an exposure to PAHs and differs from the mutation spectra found in these genes in lung tumours from cigarette smokers. Thus, the mutation spectra in lung tumours from non-smokers whose cancers are linked to smoky coal emissions reflect the primary DNA damage induced by the most prominent class of mutagens/carcinogens in these emissions.

5. Evaluation

There is *sufficient evidence* in humans for the carcinogenicity of indoor emissions from household combustion of coal. Indoor emissions from household combustion of coal cause cancer of the lung.

There is *sufficient evidence* in experimental animals for the carcinogenicity of coal-derived soot extract.

There is *sufficient evidence* in experimental animals for the carcinogenicity of emissions from combustion of coal.

Indoor emissions from household combustion of coal are *carcinogenic to humans (Group 1).*

References

Aggarwal AL, Raiyani CV, Patel PD *et al.* (1982). Assessment of exposure to benzo(a)pyrene in air for various population groups in Ahmedabad. *Atmos Environ*, 16: 867–870. doi:10.1016/0004-6981(82)90405-X

Bailey MR, Fry FA, James AC (1985). Long-term retention of particles in the human respiratory tract. *J Aerosol Sci*, 16: 295–305. doi:10.1016/0021-8502(85)90037-0

Bláha L, Kapplová P, Vondrácek J *et al.* (2002). Inhibition of gap-junctional intercellular communication by environmentally occurring polycyclic aromatic hydrocarbons. *Toxicol Sci*, 65: 43–51. doi:10.1093/toxsci/65.1.43 PMID:11752684

Bonner MR, Shen M, Liu CS *et al.* (2009). Mitochondrial DNA content and lung cancer risk in Xuan Wei, China. *Lung Cancer*, 63: 331–334. doi:10.1016/j.lungcan.2008.06.012 PMID:18691788

Booker CD & White KL Jr (2005). Benzo(a)pyrene-induced anemia and splenomegaly in NZB/WF1 mice. *Food Chem Toxicol*, 43: 1423–1431. doi:10.1016/j.fct.2005.03.018 PMID:15936865

Brown JS, Wilson WE, Grant LD (2005). Dosimetric comparisons of particle deposition and retention in rats and humans. *Inhal Toxicol*, 17: 355–385. doi:10.1080/08958370590929475 PMID:16020034

Bukowski JA, Wartenberg D, Goldschmidt M (1998). Environmental causes for sinonasal cancers in pet dogs, and their usefulness as sentinels of indoor cancer risk. *J Toxicol Environ Health A*, 54: 579–591. doi:10.1080/009841098158719 PMID:9726781

Burchiel SW & Luster MI (2001). Signalling by environmental polycyclic aromatic hydrocarbons in human lymphocytes. *Clin Immunol*, 98: 2–10. doi:10.1006/clim.2000.4934 PMID:11141320

Burdick AD, Davis JW 2nd, Liu KJ *et al.* (2003). Benzo(a)pyrene quinones increase cell proliferation, generate reactive oxygen species, and transactivate the epidermal growth factor receptor in breast epithelial cells. *Cancer Res*, 63: 7825–7833. PMID:14633709

Cáceres D, Adonis L, Retarnal C *et al.* (2001). Contaminación intradomiciliaria en un sector de extrema pobreza de la comuna de La Pintana. (Indoor air pollution in a zone of extreme poverty of La Pintana, Santiago-Chile) *Rev Med Chil*, 129: 33–42. PMID:11265203

Campbell JA (1939). Carcinogenic agents present in the atmosphere and incidence of primary tumours in mice. *Br J Exp Pathol*, 20: 122–132.

Casale GP, Singhal M, Bhattacharya S *et al.* (2001). Detection and quantification of depurinated benzo[a]pyrene-adducted DNA bases in the urine of cigarette smokers and women exposed to household coal smoke. *Chem Res Toxicol*, 14: 192–201. doi:10.1021/tx000012y PMID:11258968

Castranova V (2000). From coal mine dust to quartz: Mechanisms of pulmonary pathogenicity. *Inhal Toxicol*, 12: Suppl. 37–14. doi:10.1080/08958370050164842

Cavalieri EL & Rogan EG (1992). The approach to understanding aromatic hydrocarbon carcinogenesis. The central role of radical cations in metabolic activation. *Pharmacol Ther*, 55: 183–199. doi:10.1016/0163-7258(92)90015-R PMID:1289900

Chen HC, Cao YF, Hu WX *et al.* (2006). Genetic polymorphisms of phase II metabolic enzymes and lung cancer susceptibility in a population of Central South China. *Dis Markers*, 22: 141–152. PMID:16788248

Chen Y, Bi XH, Mai B *et al.* (2004). Emission characterization of particulate/gaseous phases and size association for polycyclic aromatic hydrocarbons from residential coal combustion. *Fuel*, 83: 781–790. doi:10.1016/j.fuel.2003.11.003

Chen YJ, Sheng GY, Bi XH *et al.* (2005). Emission factors for carbonaceous particles and polycyclic aromatic hydrocarbons from residential coal combustion in China. *Environ Sci Technol*, 39: 1861–1867. doi:10.1021/es0493650 PMID:15819248

Chuang JC, Cao SR, Xian YL *et al.* (1992a). Chemical characterization of indoor air of homes from communes in Xuan Wei, China, with high lung cancer mortality rate. *Atmos Environ*, 26: 2193–2201. doi:10.1016/0960-1686(92)90408-D

Chuang JC, Wise S, Cao S, Mumford JL (1992b). Chemical characterization of mutagenic fractions of particles from indoor coal combustion - a study of lung-cancer in Xuan-Wei, China. *Environ Sci Technol*, 26: 999–1004. doi:10.1021/es00029a020

Dai XD, Lin CY, Sun XW *et al.* (1996). The etiology of lung cancer in nonsmoking females in Harbin, China. *Lung Cancer*, 14: Suppl 1S85–S91. doi:10.1016/S0169-5002(96)90213-5 PMID:8785670

Daniels CE & Jett JR (2005). Does interstitial lung disease predispose to lung cancer? *Curr Opin Pulm Med*, 11: 431–437. doi:10.1097/01.mcp.0000170521.71497.ba PMID:16093818

DeMarini DM, Landi S, Tian D *et al.* (2001). Lung tumor KRAS and TP53 mutations in nonsmokers reflect exposure to PAH-rich coal combustion emissions. *Cancer Res*, 61: 6679–6681. PMID:11559534

Driscoll KE, Carter JM, Howard BW *et al.* (1996). Pulmonary inflammatory, chemokine, and mutagenic responses in rats after subchronic inhalation of carbon black. *Toxicol Appl Pharmacol*, 136: 372–380. doi:10.1006/taap.1996.0045 PMID:8619246

Du YX, Cha Q, Chen XW *et al.* (1996). An epidemiological study of risk factors for lung cancer in Guangzhou, China. *Lung Cancer*, 14: Suppl 1S9–S37. doi:10.1016/S0169-5002(96)90208-1 PMID:8785671

EBCREY; Editorial Board of the China Rural Energy Yearbook (1999). *Zhongguo Nongcun Nengyuan Nianjian 1998–1999* [China Rural Energy Yearbook 1998–1999]. Beijing: Zhongguo Nongye Chubanshe

Feng Z, Tian D, Lan Q, Mumford JL (1999). A sensitive immunofluorescence assay for detection of p53 protein accumulation in sputum. *Anticancer Res*, 19: 5B3847–3852. PMID:10628322

Freedman AP, Robinson K (1988). *Noninvasive magnetopneumographic studies of lung dust retention and clearance in coal miners.* In: *Respirable Dust in the Mineral Industries: Health Effects, Characterization and Control.* Frantz RL, Ramani RV, editors. University Park, PA: Penn State University Press, pp. 181–186.

Galeone C, Pelucchi C, La Vecchia C *et al.* (2008). Indoor air pollution from solid fuel use, chronic lung diseases and lung cancer in Harbin, Northeast China. *Eur J Cancer Prev*, 17: 473–478. doi:10.1097/CEJ.0b013e328305a0b9 PMID:18714191

Gallagher J, Mumford J, Li X *et al.* (1993). DNA adduct profiles and levels in placenta, blood and lung in relation to cigarette smoking and smoky coal emissions. *IARC Sci Publ*, 124: 283–292. PMID:8225497

García-Pérez J, Pollán M, Boldo E *et al.* (2009). Mortality due to lung, laryngeal and bladder cancer in towns lying in the vicinity of combustion installations. *Sci Total Environ*, 407: 2593–2602. doi:10.1016/j.scitotenv.2008.12.062 PMID:19187950

Ge S, Xu X, Chow JC *et al.* (2004). Emissions of air pollutants from household stoves: honeycomb coal versus coal cake. *Environ Sci Technol*, 38: 4612–4618. doi:10.1021/es049942k PMID:15461170

Ger LP, Hsu WL, Chen KT, Chen CJ (1993). Risk factors of lung cancer by histological category in Taiwan. *Anticancer Res*, 13: 5A1491–1500. PMID:8239527

Gerde P & Scott BR (2001). A model for absorption of low-volatile toxicants by the airway mucosa. *Inhal Toxicol*, 13: 903–929. doi:10.1080/089583701752378160 PMID:11696866

Granville CA, Hanley NM, Mumford JL, DeMarini DM (2003). Mutation spectra of smoky coal combustion emissions in Salmonella reflect the TP53 and KRAS mutations in lung tumors from smoky coal-exposed individuals. *Mutat Res*, 525: 77–83. PMID:12650907

Gu SL, Ji RD, Cao SR (1990). The physical and chemical characteristics of particles in indoor air where high fluoride coal burning takes place. *Biomed Environ Sci*, 3: 384–390. PMID:2096842

Hainaut P & Pfeifer GP (2001). Patterns of p53 G->T transversions in lung cancers reflect the primary mutagenic signature of DNA-damage by tobacco smoke. *Carcinogenesis*, 22: 367–374. doi:10.1093/carcin/22.3.367 PMID:11238174

Hays MD, Geron CD, Linna KJ *et al.* (2002). Speciation of gas-phase and fine particle emissions from burning of foliar fuels. *Environ Sci Technol*, 36: 2281–2295. doi:10.1021/es0111683 PMID:12075778

He G, Ying B, Liu J *et al.* (2005). Patterns of household concentrations of multiple indoor air pollutants in China. *Environ Sci Technol*, 39: 991–998. doi:10.1021/es049731f PMID:15773470

He XZ, Chen W, Liu ZY, Chapman RSCase-control Study on Lung Cancer and Cooking Fuel (1991). An epidemiological study of lung cancer in Xuan Wei County, China: current progress. Case-control study on lung cancer and cooking fuel. *Environ Health Perspect*, 94: 9–13. doi:10.2307/3431286 PMID:1954946

Hext PM, Tomenson JA, Thompson P (2005). Titanium dioxide: inhalation toxicology and epidemiology. *Ann Occup Hyg*, 49: 461–472. doi:10.1093/annhyg/mei012 PMID:15790613

Hosgood HD 3rd, Berndt SI, Lan Q (2007). GST genotypes and lung cancer susceptibility in Asian populations with indoor air pollution exposures: a meta-analysis. *Mutat Res*, 636: 134–143. doi:10.1016/j.mrrev.2007.02.002 PMID:17428724

Hosgood HD 3rd, Chapman R, Shen M *et al.* (2008). Portable stove use is associated with lower lung cancer mortality risk in lifetime smoky coal users. *Br J Cancer*, 99: 1934–1939. doi:10.1038/sj.bjc.6604744 PMID:19034286

Hu C, Zhang A, Huang X (2001). [Study on expression of P53mt protein in skin of patient with arseniasis caused by coal-burning] *Zhonghua Yu Fang Yi Xue Za Zhi*, 35: 23–25. PMID:11860954

Huang C, Zhang X, Qiao Z *et al.* (1992). A case-control study of dietary factors in patients with lung cancer. *Biomed Environ Sci*, 5: 257–265. PMID:1333225

IARC (1985). Polynuclear aromatic compounds, Part 4, bitumens, coal-tars and derived products, shale-oils and soots. *IARC Monogr Eval Carcinog Risk Chem Hum*, 35: 1–247. PMID:2991123

IARC (2010a). Household use of solid fuels and high-temperature frying. *IARC Monogr Eval Carcinog Risks Hum*, 95: 1–424. PMID:18756632

IARC (2010b). Carbon black, titanium dioxide, and talc. *IARC Monogr Eval Carcinog Risks Hum*, 93: 1–452. PMID:21449489.

IARC (2010c). Some non-heterocyclic polycyclic aromatic hydrocarbons and some related exposures. *IARC Monogr Eval Carcinog Risks Hum*, 92: 1–853. PMID:21141735 PMID:18756632

ICRP; International Commission on Radiological Protection (1994). *Human Respiratory Tract Model for Radiological Protection. A Report of a Task Group of the International Commission on Radiological Protection*. Oxford: Pergamon, ICRP Publication 66.

ILSI; Risk Science Institute Workshop Participants (2000). The relevance of the rat lung response to particle overload for human risk assessment: a workshop consensus report. *Inhal Toxicol*, 12: 1–17. doi:10.1080/08958370050029725 PMID:10715616

Jin Y, Zhou Z, He G *et al.* (2005). Geographical, spatial, and temporal distributions of multiple indoor air pollutants in four Chinese provinces. *Environ Sci Technol*, 39: 9431–9439. doi:10.1021/es0507517 PMID:16475318

Kabir Z, Bennett K, Clancy L (2007). Lung cancer and urban air-pollution in Dublin: a temporal association? *Ir Med J*, 100: 367–369. PMID:17432813

Kauppinen EI & Pakkanen TA (1990). Coal Combustion Aerosols - A Field-Study. *Environ Sci Technol*, 24: 1811–1818. doi:10.1021/es00082a004

Keohavong P, Gao WM, Zheng KC *et al.* (2004). Detection of K-ras and p53 mutations in sputum samples of lung cancer patients using laser capture microdissection microscope and mutation analysis. *Anal Biochem*, 324: 92–99. doi:10.1016/j.ab.2003.09.030 PMID:14654050

Keohavong P, Lan Q, Gao WM *et al.* (2003). K-ras mutations in lung carcinomas from nonsmoking women exposed to unvented coal smoke in China. *Lung Cancer*, 41: 21–27. doi:10.1016/S0169-5002(03)00125-9 PMID:12826308

Keohavong P, Lan Q, Gao WM *et al.* (2005). Detection of p53 and K-ras mutations in sputum of individuals exposed to smoky coal emissions in Xuan Wei County, China. *Carcinogenesis*, 26: 303–308. doi:10.1093/carcin/bgh328 PMID:15564291

Khesina AIa, Gaevaia TIa, Linnik AB (1977). Polycyclic aromatic hydrocarbon content and carcinogenic activity of soot extracts from the heating systems *Gig Sanit*, 8107–109. PMID:590784

Kim Oanh NT, Reutergardh LB, Dung NT (1999). Emission of polycyclic aromatic hydrocarbons and particulate matter from domestic combustion of selected fuels. *Environ Sci Technol*, 33: 2703–2709. doi:10.1021/es980853f

Kleeman MJ, Schauer JJ, Cass GR (1999). Size and composition distribution of fine particulate matter emitted from wood burning, meat charbroiling and cigarettes. *Environ Sci Technol*, 33: 3516–3523. doi:10.1021/es981277q

Kleinerman RA, Wang Z, Wang L *et al.* (2002). Lung cancer and indoor exposure to coal and biomass in rural China. *J Occup Environ Med*, 44: 338–344. doi:10.1097/00043764-200204000-00014 PMID:11977420

Knaapen AM, Borm PJ, Albrecht C, Schins RP (2004). Inhaled particles and lung cancer. Part A: Mechanisms. *Int J Cancer*, 109: 799–809. doi:10.1002/ijc.11708 PMID:15027112

Ko CB, Kim SJ, Park C *et al.* (2004). Benzo(a)pyrene-induced apoptotic death of mouse hepatoma Hepa1c1c7 cells via activation of intrinsic caspase cascade and mitochondrial dysfunction. *Toxicology*, 199: 35–46. doi:10.1016/j.tox.2004.01.039 PMID:15125997

Ko YC, Lee CH, Chen MJ *et al.* (1997). Risk factors for primary lung cancer among non-smoking women in Taiwan. *Int J Epidemiol*, 26: 24–31. doi:10.1093/ije/26.1.24 PMID:9126500

Koo LC, Lee N, Ho JH (1983). Do cooking fuels pose a risk for lung cancer? A case–control study of women in Hong Kong. *Ecol Dis*, 2: 255–265. PMID:6681156

Lan Q, Chapman RS, Schreinemachers DM *et al.* (2002). Household stove improvement and risk of lung cancer in Xuanwei, China. *J Natl Cancer Inst*, 94: 826–835. PMID:12048270

Lan Q, Chen W, Chen H, He XZ (1993). Risk factors for lung cancer in non-smokers in Xuanwei County of China. *Biomed Environ Sci*, 6: 112–118. PMID:8397894

Lan Q, Feng Z, Tian D *et al.* (2001). p53 gene expression in relation to indoor exposure to unvented coal smoke in Xuan Wei, China. *J Occup Environ Med*, 43: 226–230. doi:10.1097/00043764-200103000-00010 PMID:11285870

Lan Q, He X, Costa DJ *et al.* (2000). Indoor coal combustion emissions, GSTM1 and GSTT1 genotypes, and lung cancer risk: a case–control study in Xuan Wei, China. *Cancer Epidemiol Biomarkers Prev*, 9: 605–608. PMID:10868696

Lan Q, He X, Shen M *et al.* (2008). Variation in lung cancer risk by smoky coal subtype in Xuanwei, China. *Int J Cancer*, 123: 2164–2169. PMID:18712724

Lan Q, Mumford JL, Shen M *et al.* (2004). Oxidative damage-related genes AKR1C3 and OGG1 modulate risks for lung cancer due to exposure to PAH-rich coal combustion emissions. *Carcinogenesis*, 25: 2177–2181. doi:10.1093/carcin/bgh240 PMID:15284179

Le CH, Ko YC, Cheng LS *et al.* (2001). The heterogeneity in risk factors of lung cancer and the difference of histologic distribution between genders in Taiwan. *Cancer Causes Control*, 12: 289–300. doi:10.1023/A:1011270521900 PMID:11456224

Lee RG, Coleman P, Jones JL *et al.* (2005). Emission factors and importance of PCDD/Fs, PCBs, PCNs, PAHs and PM10 from the domestic burning of coal and wood in the U.K. *Environ Sci Technol*, 39: 1436–1447. doi:10.1021/es048745i PMID:15819195

Lei YX, Cai WC, Chen YZ, Du YX (1996). Some lifestyle factors in human lung cancer: a case–control study of 792 lung cancer cases. *Lung Cancer*, 14: Suppl 1S121–S136. doi:10.1016/S0169-5002(96)90218-4 PMID:8785658

Levy LS (1995). Review: Inhalation toxicology and human risk assessment of carbon black. *Indoor and Built Environment*, 4: 263 280. doi:10.1177/1420326X9500400504

Li J, Li X, Quan X (1997). [Studies on serum regulatory protein for cell growth in patients with lung cancer exposed to indoor coal-burning] *Zhonghua Yu Fang Yi Xue Za Zhi*, 31: 92–94. PMID:9812620

Liang CK, Guan NY, Ma F *et al.* (1983). Carcinogenicity in mice of soot extract collected from Xuan Wei County *Zhongguo Yi Xue Ke Xue Yuan Xue Bao*, 5: 307–310. PMID:6329534

Liang CK, Guan NY, Yin XR *et al.* (1984). Extracts from Xuan Wei coal and wood smoke induce lung cancer in mice. *Wei Sheng Yan Jiu*, 13: 19–23.

Liang CK, Quan NY, Cao SR *et al.* (1988). Natural inhalation exposure to coal smoke and wood smoke induces lung cancer in mice and rats. *Biomed Environ Sci*, 1: 42–50. PMID:3268107

Liang CK & Wang W (1987). Kunming mouse skin tumor-initiating activity of extracts of inhalable particles in indoor air *Zhonghua Yu Fang Yi Xue Za Zhi*, 21: 316–318. PMID:3452506

Lin C, Dai X, Sun X (1995). Expression of oncogene and anti-oncogene in mouse lung cancer induced by coal-burning smoke *Zhonghua Zhong Liu Za Zhi*, 17: 432–434. PMID:8697995

Lissowska J, Bardin-Mikolajczak A, Fletcher T *et al.* (2005). Lung cancer and indoor pollution from heating and cooking with solid fuels: the IARC international multicentre case–control study in Eastern/Central Europe and the United Kingdom. *Am J Epidemiol*, 162: 326–333. doi:10.1093/aje/kwi204 PMID:16014775

Liu Q, Sasco AJ, Riboli E, Hu MX (1993). Indoor air pollution and lung cancer in Guangzhou, People's Republic of China. *Am J Epidemiol*, 137: 145–154. PMID:8452118

Liu ZY, He XZ, Chapman RS (1991). Smoking and other risk factors for lung cancer in Xuanwei, China. *Int J Epidemiol*, 20: 26–31. doi:10.1093/ije/20.1.26 PMID:2066232

Luo RX, Wu B, Yi YN *et al.* (1996). Indoor burning coal air pollution and lung cancer–a case–control study in Fuzhou, China. *Lung Cancer*, 14: Suppl 1S113–S119. doi:10.1016/S0169-5002(96)90217-2 PMID:8785657

Mass MJ, Jeffers AJ, Ross JA *et al.* (1993). Ki-ras oncogene mutations in tumors and DNA adducts formed by benz[j]aceanthrylene and benzo[a]pyrene in the lungs of strain A/J mice. *Mol Carcinog*, 8: 186–192. doi:10.1002/mc.2940080309 PMID:8216737

Miller C, Srivastava RK, Ryan JV (1994). Emissions Of Organic Hazardous Air-Pollutants From The Combustion Of Pulverized Coal In A Small-Scale Combustor. *Environ Sci Technol*, 28: 1150–1158. doi:10.1021/es00055a028

Miller FJ (2000). Dosimetry of particles in laboratory animals and humans in relationship to issues

surrounding lung overload and human health risk assessment: a critical review. *Inhal Toxicol*, 12: 19–57. doi:10.1080/089583700196536 PMID:10715617
Millman A, Tang D, Perera FP (2008). Air pollution threatens the health of children in China. *Pediatrics*, 122: 620–628. doi:10.1542/peds.2007-3143 PMID:18762533
Morrow PE (1988). Possible mechanisms to explain dust overloading of the lungs. *Fundam Appl Toxicol*, 10: 369–384. doi:10.1016/0272-0590(88)90284-9 PMID:3286345
Morrow PE (1992). Dust overloading of the lungs: update and appraisal. *Toxicol Appl Pharmacol*, 113: 1–12. doi:10.1016/0041-008X(92)90002-A PMID:1553742
Morrow PE (1994). *Mechanisms and significance of "particle overload"*. In: *Toxic and carcinogenic effects of solid particles in the respiratory tract. [Proceedings of the 4th international inhalation symposium, March 1993]*. Mohr U, editor-in-chief. Hannover, Germany: International Life Sciences Institute Press, pp. 17–25.
Mumford JL, He XZ, Chapman RS *et al.* (1987). Lung cancer and indoor air pollution in Xuan Wei, China. *Science*, 235: 217–220. doi:10.1126/science.3798109 PMID:3798109
Mumford JL, Helmes CT, Lee XM *et al.* (1990). Mouse skin tumorigenicity studies of indoor coal and wood combustion emissions from homes of residents in Xuan Wei, China with high lung cancer mortality. *Carcinogenesis*, 11: 397–403. doi:10.1093/carcin/11.3.397 PMID:2311182
Mumford JL, Lee X, Lewtas J *et al.* (1993). DNA adducts as biomarkers for assessing exposure to polycyclic aromatic hydrocarbons in tissues from Xuan Wei women with high exposure to coal combustion emissions and high lung cancer mortality. *Environ Health Perspect*, 99: 83–87. doi:10.1289/ehp.939983 PMID:8319664
Mumford JL, Li X, Hu F *et al.* (1995). Human exposure and dosimetry of polycyclic aromatic hydrocarbons in urine from Xuan Wei, China with high lung cancer mortality associated with exposure to unvented coal smoke. *Carcinogenesis*, 16: 3031–3036. doi:10.1093/carcin/16.12.3031 PMID:8603481
Nakanishi Y, Chen S, Inutsuka S *et al.* (1997). Possible role of indoor environment and coal combustion emission in lung carcinogenesis in Fuyuan County, China. *Neoplasma*, 44: 69–72. PMID:9201284
National Bureau of Statistics (2005). *China Energy Statistical Yearbook 2005*. Beijing: China Statistics Press.
National Bureau of Statistics (2006). *China Statistical Yearbook 2006*. Beijing: China Statistics Press.
National Bureau of Statistics (2008). *The Major Statistics of the 2nd National Survey for Agriculture*. Beijing: China Statistics Press.
Oberdörster G (1988). Lung clearance of inhaled insoluble and soluble particles. *J Aerosol Med*, 1: 289–330. doi:10.1089/jam.1988.1.289
Oberdörster G (1996). Significance of particle parameters in the evaluation of exposure-dose-response relationships of inhaled particles. *Inhal Toxicol*, 8: Suppl73–89. PMID:11542496
Oberdörster G (2002). Toxicokinetics and effects of fibrous and nonfibrous particles. *Inhal Toxicol*, 14: 29–56. doi:10.1080/089583701753338622 PMID:12122559
Oberdörster G & Yu PP (1990). The carcinogenic potential of inhaled diesel exhaust: a particle effect? *J Aerosol Sci*, 21: S397–S401. doi:10.1016/0021-8502(90)90265-Y
Oguri T, Singh SV, Nemoto K, Lazo JS (2003). The carcinogen (7R,8S)-dihydroxy-(9S,10R)-epoxy-7,8,9,10-tetrahydrobenzo[a]pyrene induces Cdc25B expression in human bronchial and lung cancer cells. *Cancer Res*, 63: 771–775. PMID:12591724
Park JH, Gelhaus S, Vedantam S *et al.* (2008). The pattern of p53 mutations caused by PAH o-quinones is driven by 8-oxo-dGuo formation while the spectrum of mutations is determined by biological selection for dominance. *Chem Res Toxicol*, 21: 1039–1049. doi:10.1021/tx700404a PMID:18489080
Park JH, Mangal D, Frey AJ *et al.* (2009). Aryl hydrocarbon receptor facilitates DNA strand breaks and 8-oxo-2′-deoxyguanosine formation by the aldo-keto reductase product benzo[a]pyrene-7,8-dione. *J Biol Chem*, 284: 29725–29734. doi:10.1074/jbc.M109.042143 PMID:19726680
Passey RD (1922). Experimental soot Cancer. *BMJ*, ii: 1112–1113.
Passey RD & Carter-Braine J (1925). Experimental soot cancer. *J Pathol Bacteriol*, 28: 133–144. doi:10.1002/path.1700280202
Penning TM, Burczynski ME, Hung CF *et al.* (1999). Dihydrodiol dehydrogenases and polycyclic aromatic hydrocarbon activation: generation of reactive and redox active o-quinones. *Chem Res Toxicol*, 12: 1–18. doi:10.1021/tx980143n PMID:9894013
Penning TM & Drury JE (2007). Human aldo-keto reductases: Function, gene regulation, and single nucleotide polymorphisms. *Arch Biochem Biophys*, 464: 241–250. doi:10.1016/j.abb.2007.04.024 PMID:17537398
Pfeifer GP & Hainaut P (2003). On the origin of G -> T transversions in lung cancer. *Mutat Res*, 526: 39–43. PMID:12714181
Plísková M, Vondrácek J, Vojtesek B *et al.* (2005). Deregulation of cell proliferation by polycyclic aromatic hydrocarbons in human breast carcinoma MCF-7 cells reflects both genotoxic and nongenotoxic events. *Toxicol Sci*, 83: 246–256. doi:10.1093/toxsci/kfi040 PMID:15548639
Raiyani CV, Jani JP, Desai NM *et al.* (1993). Assessment of indoor exposure to polycyclic aromatic hydrocarbons for urban poor using various types of cooking fuels.

Bull Environ Contam Toxicol, 50: 757–763. doi:10.1007/BF00194673 PMID:8490282

Ren D, Zhao F, Wang Y *et al.* (1999). Distributions of minor and trace elements in Chinese coals. *Int J Coal Geol*, 40: 109–118. doi:10.1016/S0166-5162(98)00063-9

Ren DY, Xu DW, Zhao FH (2004). A preliminary study on the enrichment mechanism and occurrence of hazardous trace elements in the Tertiary lignite from the Shenbei coalfield, China. *Int J Coal Geol*, 57: 187–196. doi:10.1016/j.coal.2003.10.001

Rogge W, Hildemann LM, Mazurek MA, Cass GR (1998). Sources of fine organic aerosol. 9. Pine, oak and synthetic log combustion in residential fireplaces. *Environ Sci Technol*, 32: 13–22. doi:10.1021/es960930b

Ross AB, Jones JM, Chaiklangmuang S *et al.* (2002). Measurement and prediction of the emission of pollutants from the combustion of coal and biomass in a fixed bed furnace. *Fuel*, 81: 571–582. doi:10.1016/S0016-2361(01)00157-0

Sapkota A, Gajalakshmi V, Jetly DH *et al.* (2008). Indoor air pollution from solid fuels and risk of hypopharyngeal/laryngeal and lung cancers: a multicentric case–control study from India. *Int J Epidemiol*, 37: 321–328. doi:10.1093/ije/dym261 PMID:18234740

Seeling MG & Benignus EL (1936). Coal smoke soot and tumors of the lung and mice. *Am J Cancer*, 28: 96–111.

Shen M, Berndt SI, Rothman N *et al.* (2005). Polymorphisms in the DNA nucleotide excision repair genes and lung cancer risk in Xuan Wei, China. *Int J Cancer*, 116: 768–773. doi:10.1002/ijc.21117 PMID:15849729

Shen XB, Wang GX, Huang YZ *et al.* (1996). Analysis and estimates of attributable risk factors for lung cancer in Nanjing, China. *Lung Cancer*, 14: Suppl 1S107–S112. doi:10.1016/S0169-5002(96)90216-0 PMID:8785656

Shen XB, Wang GX, Zhou BS (1998). Relation of exposure to environmental tobacco smoke and pulmonary adenocarcinoma in non-smoking women: a case control study in Nanjing. *Oncol Rep*, 5: 1221–1223. PMID:9683839

Shraim A, Cui X, Li S *et al.* (2003). Arsenic speciation in the urine and hair of individuals exposed to airborne arsenic through coal-burning in Guizhou, PR China. *Toxicol Lett*, 137: 35–48. doi:10.1016/S0378-4274(02)00379-X PMID:12505431

Sinton JE, Smith KR, Hu HS, Liu JZ (1995). *Indoor Air Pollution Database for China*. WHO/EHG/95.8. Geneva: World Health Organization.

Sinton JE, Smith KR, Peabody J *et al.* (2004). An assessment of programs to promote improved household stoves in China. *Energy for sustainable development*, 8: 33–52. doi:10.1016/S0973-0826(08)60465-2

Siwińska E, Mielzyńska D, Bubak A, Smolik E (1999). The effect of coal stoves and environmental tobacco smoke on the level of urinary 1-hydroxypyrene. *Mutat Res*, 445: 147–153. PMID:10575425

Smith KR, Uma R, Kishore V *et al.* (2000). Greenhouse implications of household stoves. *Annu Rev Energy Environ*, 25: 741–763. doi:10.1146/annurev.energy.25.1.741

Sun XW (1992). Heating fuels and respiratory diseases in the risks of female lung cancer. *Zhonghua Zhong Liu Za Zhi*, 13: 413–415. PMID:1576905

Sun XW, Ma YY, Wang B *et al.* (2007). The interaction between microsomal epoxide hydrolase polymorphisms and indoor pollution in non small cell lung cancer. *Chinese*, 41: 130–34. PMID:17767854.

Swaine D (1990). *Trace Elements in Coal.* Boston, MA: Butterworth Press.

Tannheimer SL, Ethier SP, Caldwell KK, Burchiel SW (1998). Benzo[a]pyrene- and TCDD-induced alterations in tyrosine phosphorylation and insulin-like growth factor signalling pathways in the MCF-10A human mammary epithelial cell line. *Carcinogenesis*, 19: 1291–1297. doi:10.1093/carcin/19.7.1291 PMID:9683191

Tannheimer SL, Lauer FT, Lane J, Burchiel SW (1999). Factors influencing elevation of intracellular Ca2+ in the MCF-10A human mammary epithelial cell line by carcinogenic polycyclic aromatic hydrocarbons. *Mol Carcinog*, 25: 48–54. doi:10.1002/(SICI)1098-2744(199905)25:1<48::AID-MC6>3.0.CO;2-6 PMID:10331744

Tian L (2005). *Coal combustion emissions and lung cancer in Xuan Wei, China* [PhD Thesis]. Berkeley, CA: University of California.

Tonooka Y, Liu J, Kondou Y *et al.* (2006). A survey on energy consumption in rural households in the fringes of Xian city. *Energy Build*, 38: 1335–1342. doi:10.1016/j.enbuild.2006.04.011

Tsai SM, Zhang JJ, Smith KR *et al.* (2003). Characterization of non-methane hydrocarbons emitted from various cookstoves used in China. *Environ Sci Technol*, 37: 2869–2877. doi:10.1021/es026232a PMID:12875388

Wang TJ, Zhou BS, Shi JP (1996). Lung cancer in nonsmoking Chinese women: a case–control study. *Lung Cancer*, 14: Suppl 1S93–S98. doi:10.1016/S0169-5002(96)90214-7 PMID:8785672

Watson AY, Valberg PA (1996). *Particle-induced lung tumors in rats: evidence for species specificity in mechanisms.* In: *Particle overload in the rat lung and lung cancer: Implications for human risk assessment.* Taylor and Francis, editors. Washington, DC: pp. 227–257.

Watson JG, Chow JC, Houck JE (2001). PM2.5 chemical source profiles for vehicle exhaust, vegetative burning, geological material, and coal burning in Northwestern Colorado during 1995. *Chemosphere*, 43: 1141–1151. doi:10.1016/S0045-6535(00)00171-5 PMID:11368231

WHO (1998). *Selected Non-heterocyclic Polycyclic Aromatic Hydrocarbons.* Geneva: International Programme on Chemical Safety, No. Environmental Health Criteria 202.

Wornat MJ, Ledesma EB, Sandrowitz AK *et al.* (2001). Polycyclic aromatic hydrocarbons identified in soot extracts from domestic coal-burning stoves of Henan Province, China. *Environ Sci Technol*, 35: 1943–1952. doi:10.1021/es001664b PMID:11393972

Wu-Williams AH, Dai XD, Blot W *et al.* (1990). Lung cancer among women in north-east China. *Br J Cancer*, 62: 982–987. doi:10.1038/bjc.1990.421 PMID:2257230

Xu K, Li X, Hu F (1997). [A study on polycyclic aromatic hydrocarbon-DNA adduct in lung cancer patients exposed to indoor coal-burning smoke] *Zhonghua Yu Fang Yi Xue Za Zhi*, 31: 95–98. PMID:9812621

Xu ZY, Blot WJ, Xiao HP *et al.* (1989). Smoking, air pollution, and the high rates of lung cancer in Shenyang, China. *J Natl Cancer Inst*, 81: 1800–1806. doi:10.1093/jnci/81.23.1800 PMID:2555531

Xue W & Warshawsky D (2005). Metabolic activation of polycyclic and heterocyclic aromatic hydrocarbons and DNA damage: a review. *Toxicol Appl Pharmacol*, 206: 73–93. doi:10.1016/j.taap.2004.11.006 PMID:15963346

Yan J, Wang L, Fu PP, Yu H (2004). Photomutagenicity of 16 polycyclic aromatic hydrocarbons from the US EPA priority pollutant list. *Mutat Res*, 557: 99–108. PMID:14706522

Yan L (1990). [Epidemiological survey of endemic fluorosis in Xiou Shan and Bao Jing areas] *Zhonghua Liu Xing Bing Xue Za Zhi*, 11: 302–306. PMID:2261621

Yan R, Zhu H, Zheng C, Xu M (2002). Emissions of organic hazardous air pollutants during Chinese coal combustion. *Energy*, 27: 485–503. doi:10.1016/S0360-5442(02)00003-8

Yin XR, Guan N, Liang C *et al.* (1984). Study on lung cancer in mice by intra-bronchial injection of Xuan Wei coal fumes extracts. *Wei sheng Yan Jui*, 13(3): 21–25.

Zhang A, Feng H, Yang G *et al.* (2007a). Unventilated indoor coal-fired stoves in Guizhou province, China: cellular and genetic damage in villagers exposed to arsenic in food and air. *Environ Health Perspect*, 115: 653–658. doi:10.1289/ehp.9272 PMID:17450239

Zhang AH, Bin HH, Pan XL, Xi XG (2007b). Analysis of p16 gene mutation, deletion and methylation in patients with arseniasis produced by indoor unventilated-stove coal usage in Guizhou, China. *J Toxicol Environ Health A*, 70: 970–975. doi:10.1080/15287390701290808 PMID:17479413

Zhang AH, Yang GH, Li J *et al.* (2000b). The situation of DNA synthesis DNA damage and DNA repair in arsenism patients blood cells caused by coal burning. *Carcinogen Teratogen Mutagen*, 12: 76–78.

Zhang J & Smith KR (1999). Emissions of carbonyl compounds from various cookstoves in China. *Environ Sci Technol*, 33: 2311–2320. doi:10.1021/es9812406

Zhang J, Smith KR, Ma Y *et al.* (2000a). Greenhouse gases and other airborne pollutants from household stoves in China: a database for emission factors. *Atmos Environ*, 34: 4537–4549. doi:10.1016/S1352-2310(99)00450-1

Zhong L, Goldberg MS, Gao YT, Jin F (1999). Lung cancer and indoor air pollution arising from Chinese-style cooking among nonsmoking women living in Shanghai, China. *Epidemiology*, 10: 488–494. doi:10.1097/00001648-199909000-00005 PMID:10468420

Zhou BS, Wang TJ, Guan P, Wu JM (2000). Indoor air pollution and pulmonary adenocarcinoma among females: a case-control study in Shenyang, China. *Oncol Rep*, 7: 1253–1259. PMID:11032925

LIST OF ABBREVIATIONS

α-Me-γ-OH-PdG	α-Methyl-γ-hydroxy-1,$\underline{N}^2$-propanodeoxyguanosine
16α-OHE1	16-α-hydroxyestrone
1-OHP or 1-HOP	1-hydroxypyrene
ADH	alcohol dehydrogenase
AEAT	acyl-coenzyme A: ethanol O-acyltransferase
AFRO	WHO African Region
AhR	aryl-hydrocarbon receptor
AIDS	acquired immunodeficiency syndrome
AKR	aldo-keto reductase
ALDH	aldehyde dehydrogenase
AMRO	WHO Region of the Americas
Apc	adenomatous polyposis coli
BaP	benzo[*a*]pyrene
BMI	body mass index
CalEPA	California Environmental Protection Agency
CDH1	E-cadherin 1
CHEK	checkpoint
CI	confidence interval
CIMP	CpG island methylator phenotype
CML	chronic myeloid leukaemia
COX-2	cyclooxygenase-2
CPS-I	American Cancer Society Cancer Prevention Study I
CPS-II	American Cancer Society Cancer Prevention Study II
CYP	cytochrome P450
DMBA	7,12-dimethylbenz[*a*]anthracene
DMSO	dimethyl sulfoxide
DRR	direct reversal repair
EBV	Epstein-Barr virus
EGFR	Epidermal growth factor receptor
EHPX	Microsomal epoxide hydrolase
ELISA	enzyme linked immunosorbent assay
EMRO	Eastern Mediterranean Region
EPIC	European Prospective Investigation into Cancer and Nutrition
ERCC	excision repair cross-complementing protein
ER	estrogen receptor
EURO	WHO European Region
FAEE	fatty-acid ethyl ester

FAEES	fatty-acid ethyl ester synthases
FISH	fluorescence in situ hybridization
GSHS	Global School based Student Health Survey
GST	glutathione-*S*-transferase
GYTS	Global Youth Tobacco Survey
Hb	haemoglobin
HBSC	Health Behaviour in School Aged Children
HCS	high dose cigarette smoke
HEMA	2-hydroxyethyl mercapturic acid
HER	human epidermal growth factor receptor
HPB	4-hydroxy-1-(3-pyridyl)-1-butanone
HPLC	high pressure liquid chromatography
HPMA	3-hydroxypropyl mercapturic acid
HPV	human papillomavirus
HR	hazard ratio
HRT	hormone replacement therapy
IGF-2	insulin-like growth factor-2
iso-NNAC	4-(methylnitrosamino)-4-(3-pyridyl)butyric acid
LC-MS/MS	liquid chromatography-tandem mass spectrometry
LCS	low dose cigarette smoke
LOH	loss of heterozygosity
MA	mercapturic acid
MGMT	O^6-methylguanine DNA methyl-transferase
MHBMA	monohydroxybutyl mercapturic acid
MHL1	mutL homologue 1
MINT	methylation in tumour
MNBA	4-(methylnitrosamino)butyric acid
MNPA	3-(methylnitrosamino)propionic acid
MNPhPA	2-(methylnitrosamino)-3-phenylpropionic acid
MNTCA	N-nitroso-2-methylthiazolidine-4-carboxylic acid
MPO	myeloperoxidase
N^2 EtdG	N^2-ethyl-2'-deosygnanosine
N^2 EtidG	N^2-ethylidene-2'-deosygnanosine
N^2-Dio-dG	N^2-(2,6-demethyl-1,3-dioxan-4-yl)deoxyguanosine
NAA	N-nitrosamino acid
NADH	nicotinamide adenine dinucleotide
NADPH	nicotinamide adenine dinucleotide phosphate
NAT	N-acetyltransferase
NAzCA	N-nitrosoazetidine-4-carboxylic acid
NDEA	N-nitrosodiethylamine
NDMA	N-nitrosodimethylamine
NER	nucleotide excision repair
NHL	non-Hodgkin lymphoma
NHPRO	N-nitrosohydroxyproline
NIH-AARP	National Institutes of Health American Association of Retired People
NNAL	4-(methylnitrosamino)-1-(3-pyridyl)-1-butanol
NNK	4-(methylnitrosamino)-1-(3-pyridyl)-1-butanone
NNN	N'-nitrosonornicotine
NO	nitric oxide
NPIC	N-nitrosopipecolic acid

NPIP	N-nitrosopiperidine
NPRO	N-nitrosoproline
NPYR	N-nitrosopyrrolidine
NQO	NAD(P)H quinone oxidoreductase
NTCA	N-nitrosothiazolidine- 4-carboxylic acid
OR	odds ratio
PAHs	polycyclic aromatic hydrocarbons
PGE2	prostaglandin
PheT	*r*-1,*t*-2,3,*c*-4-tetrahydroxy-1,2,3,4-tetrahydrophenanthrene
PhIP	2-amino-1-methyl-6-phenylimidazo[4,5,6]pyridine
PM	particulate matter
PM_{10}	inhalable particles <10 µm
$PM_{2.5}$	respirable particles <2.5 µm
POB	pyridyloxobutyl
PR	progestogen receptor
RFLP	restriction fragment lenght polymorphism
RR	relative risk
SEARO	WHO South-East Asian Region
SEER	National Cancer Institute's Surveillance, Epidemiology, and End Results program
SFRP	soluble Frizzled receptor protein
SIR	standardized incidence ratio
SNPs	Single Nucleotide Polymorphisms
SPMA	S-phenyl mercapturic acid
SULT	sultotransferase
TGF-α	transforming growth factor- α
total NNAL	NNAL and its glucuronides
total NNN	NNN and its glucuronides
TSNA	tobacco-specific N-nitrosamines
TSP	total suspended particles
UDP	uridine diphosphate
UGT	Uridine-5'-diphosphate glucuronosyl transferase (also called uridine-5'-diphosphate glycosyltransferase)
WHO FCTC	WHO Framework Convention on Tobacco Control
WLM	work-level-months
WPRO	WHO Western Pacific Region
XP	Xeroderma pigmentosum
XRCC	X-ray repair cross-complementing protein

CUMULATIVE CROSS INDEX TO *IARC MONOGRAPHS*

The volume, page and year of publication are given. References to corrigenda are given in parentheses.

A

B

C

D

E

F

G

H

I

J

K

L

M

N

O

P

Q

R

S

T

U

V

W

X

Y

Z

LIST OF *IARC MONOGRAPHS*

Volume 1

Some Inorganic Substances, Chlorinated Hydrocarbons, Aromatic Amines, N-Nitroso Compounds, and Natural Products

1972; 184 pages (out-of-print)

Volume 2

Some Inorganic and Organometallic Compounds

1973; 181 pages (out-of-print)

Volume 3

Certain Polycyclic Aromatic Hydrocarbons and Heterocyclic Compounds

1973; 271 pages (out-of-print)

Volume 4

Some Aromatic Amines, Hydrazine and Related Substances, N-Nitroso Compounds and Miscellaneous Alkylating Agents

1974; 286 pages (out-of-print)

Volume 5

Some Organochlorine Pesticides

1974; 241 pages (out-of-print)

Volume 6

Sex Hormones

1974; 243 pages (out-of-print)

Volume 7

Some Anti-Thyroid and Related Substances, Nitrofurans and Industrial Chemicals

1974; 326 pages (out-of-print)

Volume 8

Some Aromatic Azo Compounds

1975; 357 pages (out-of-print)

Volume 9

Some Aziridines, N-, S- and O-Mustards and Selenium

1975; 268 pages (out-of-print)

Volume 10

Some Naturally Occurring Substances

1976; 353 pages (out-of-print)

Volume 11

Cadmium, Nickel, Some Epoxides, Miscellaneous Industrial Chemicals and General Considerations on Volatile Anaesthetics
1976; 306 pages (out-of-print)

Volume 12

Some Carbamates, Thio- carbamates and Carbazides
1976; 282 pages (out-of-print)

Volume 13

Some Miscellaneous Pharmaceutical Substances
1977; 255 pages

Volume 14

Asbestos
1977; 106 pages (out-of-print)

Volume 15

Some Fumigants, the Herbicides 2,4-D and 2,4,5-T, Chlorinated Dibenzodioxins and Miscellaneous Industrial Chemicals
1977; 354 pages (out-of-print)

Volume 16

Some Aromatic Amines and Related Nitro Compounds—Hair Dyes, Colouring Agents and Miscellaneous Industrial Chemicals
1978; 400 pages

Volume 17

Some N-Nitroso Compounds
1978; 365 pages

Volume 18

Polychlorinated Biphenyls and Polybrominated Biphenyls
1978; 140 pages (out-of-print)

Volume 19

Some Monomers, Plastics and Synthetic Elastomers, and Acrolein
1979; 513 pages (out-of-print)

Volume 20

Some Halogenated Hydrocarbons
1979; 609 pages (out-of-print)

Volume 21

Sex Hormones (II)
1979; 583 pages

Volume 22

Some Non-Nutritive Sweetening Agents
1980; 208 pages

Volume 23

Some Metals and Metallic Compounds
1980; 438 pages (out-of-print)

Volume 24
Some Pharmaceutical Drugs
1980; 337 pages

Volume 25
Wood, Leather and Some Associated Industries
1981; 412 pages

Volume 26
Some Antineoplastic and Immunosuppressive Agents
1981; 411 pages (out-of-print)

Volume 27
Some Aromatic Amines, Anthraquinones and Nitroso Compounds, and Inorganic Fluorides Used in Drinking-water and Dental Preparations
1982; 341 pages (out-of-print)

Volume 28
The Rubber Industry
1982; 486 pages (out-of-print)

Volume 29
Some Industrial Chemicals and Dyestuffs
1982; 416 pages (out-of-print)

Volume 30
Miscellaneous Pesticides
1983; 424 pages (out-of-print)

Volume 31
Some Food Additives, Feed Additives and Naturally Occurring Substances
1983; 314 pages (out-of-print)

Volume 32
Polynuclear Aromatic Compounds, Part 1: Chemical, Environmental and Experimental Data
1983; 477 pages (out-of-print)

Volume 33
Polynuclear Aromatic Compounds, Part 2: Carbon Blacks, Mineral Oils and Some Nitroarenes
1984; 245 pages (out-of-print)

Volume 34
Polynuclear Aromatic Compounds, Part 3: Industrial Exposures in Aluminium Production, Coal Gasification, Coke Production, and Iron and Steel Founding
1984; 219 pages (out-of-print)

Volume 35
Polynuclear Aromatic Compounds, Part 4: Bitumens, Coal-tars and Derived Products, Shale-oils and Soots
1985; 271 pages

Volume 36
Allyl Compounds, Aldehydes, Epoxides and Peroxides
1985; 369 pages

Volume 37
Tobacco Habits Other than Smoking; Betel-Quid and Areca-Nut Chewing; and Some Related Nitrosamines
1985; 291 pages (out-of-print)

Volume 38
Tobacco Smoking
1986; 421 pages

Volume 39
Some Chemicals Used in Plastics and Elastomers
1986; 403 pages (out-of-print)

Volume 40
Some Naturally Occurring and Synthetic Food Components, Furocoumarins and Ultraviolet Radiation
1986; 444 pages (out-of-print)

Volume 41
Some Halogenated Hydrocarbons and Pesticide Exposures
1986; 434 pages (out-of-print)

Volume 42
Silica and Some Silicates
1987; 289 pages

Volume 43
Man-Made Mineral Fibres and Radon
1988; 300 pages (out-of-print)

Volume 44
Alcohol Drinking
1988; 416 pages

Volume 45
Occupational Exposures in Petroleum Refining; Crude Oil and Major Petroleum Fuels
1989; 322 pages

Volume 46
Diesel and Gasoline Engine Exhausts and Some Nitroarenes
1989; 458 pages

Volume 47
Some Organic Solvents, Resin Monomers and Related Compounds, Pigments and Occupational Exposures in Paint Manufacture and Painting
1989; 535 pages (out-of-print)

Volume 48
Some Flame Retardants and Textile Chemicals, and Exposures in the Textile Manufacturing Industry
1990; 345 pages

Volume 49
Chromium, Nickel and Welding
1990; 677 pages

Volume 50
Pharmaceutical Drugs
1990; 415 pages

Volume 51
Coffee, Tea, Mate, Methylxanthines and Methylglyoxal
1991; 513 pages

Volume 52
Chlorinated Drinking-water; Chlorination By-products; Some Other Halogenated Compounds; Cobalt and Cobalt Compounds
1991; 544 pages

Volume 53
Occupational Exposures in Insecticide Application, and Some Pesticides
1991; 612 pages

Volume 54
Occupational Exposures to Mists and Vapours from Strong Inorganic Acids; and Other Industrial Chemicals
1992; 336 pages

Volume 55
Solar and Ultraviolet Radiation
1992; 316 pages

Volume 56
Some Naturally Occurring Substances: Food Items and Constituents, Heterocyclic Aromatic Amines and Mycotoxins
1993; 599 pages

Volume 57
Occupational Exposures of Hairdressers and Barbers and Personal Use of Hair Colourants; Some Hair Dyes, Cosmetic Colourants, Industrial Dyestuffs and Aromatic Amines
1993; 428 pages

Volume 58
Beryllium, Cadmium, Mercury, and Exposures in the Glass Manufacturing Industry
1993; 444 pages

Volume 59
Hepatitis Viruses
1994; 286 pages

Volume 60
Some Industrial Chemicals
1994; 560 pages

Volume 61
Schistosomes, Liver Flukes and Helicobacter pylori
1994; 270 pages

Volume 62
Wood Dust and Formaldehyde
1995; 405 pages

Volume 63
Dry Cleaning, Some Chlorinated Solvents and Other Industrial Chemicals
1995; 551 pages

Volume 64
Human Papillomaviruses
1995; 409 pages

Volume 65
Printing Processes and Printing Inks, Carbon Black and Some Nitro Compounds
1996; 578 pages

Volume 66
Some Pharmaceutical Drugs
1996; 514 pages

Volume 67
Human Immunodeficiency Viruses and Human T-Cell Lymphotropic Viruses
1996; 424 pages

Volume 68
Silica, Some Silicates, Coal Dust and para-Aramid Fibrils
1997; 506 pages

Volume 69
Polychlorinated Dibenzo-para-Dioxins and Polychlorinated Dibenzofurans
1997; 666 pages

Volume 70
Epstein-Barr Virus and Kaposi's Sarcoma Herpesvirus/Human Herpesvirus 8
1997; 524 pages

Volume 71
Re-evaluation of Some Organic Chemicals, Hydrazine and Hydrogen Peroxide
1999; 1586 pages

Volume 72
Hormonal Contraception and Post-menopausal Hormonal Therapy
1999; 660 pages

Volume 73
Some Chemicals that Cause Tumours of the Kidney or Urinary Bladder in Rodents and Some Other Substances
1999; 674 pages

Volume 74
Surgical Implants and Other Foreign Bodies
1999; 409 pages

Volume 75
Ionizing Radiation, Part 1, X-Radiation and γ-Radiation, and Neutrons
2000; 492 pages

Volume 76
Some Antiviral and Antineoplastic Drugs, and Other Pharmaceutical Agents
2000; 522 pages

Volume 77
Some Industrial Chemicals
2000; 563 pages

Volume 78
Ionizing Radiation, Part 2, Some Internally Deposited Radionuclides
2001; 595 pages

Volume 79
Some Thyrotropic Agents
2001; 763 pages

Volume 80
Non-Ionizing Radiation, Part 1: Static and Extremely Low-Frequency (ELF) Electric and Magnetic Fields
2002; 429 pages

Volume 81
Man-made Vitreous Fibres
2002; 418 pages

Volume 82
Some Traditional Herbal Medicines, Some Mycotoxins, Naphthalene and Styrene
2002; 590 pages

Volume 83
Tobacco Smoke and Involuntary Smoking
2004; 1452 pages

Volume 84
Some Drinking-Water Disinfectants and Contaminants, including Arsenic
2004; 512 pages

Volume 85
Betel-quid and Areca-nut Chewing and Some Areca-nut-derived Nitrosamines
2004; 334 pages

Volume 86
Cobalt in Hard Metals and Cobalt Sulfate, Gallium Arsenide, Indium Phosphide and Vanadium Pentoxide
2006; 330 pages

Volume 87
Inorganic and Organic Lead Compounds
2006; 506 pages

Volume 88
Formaldehyde, 2-Butoxyethanol and 1-tert-Butoxypropan-2-ol
2006; 478 pages

Volume 89

Smokeless Tobacco and Some Tobacco-specific N- Nitrosamines
2007; 626 pages

Volume 90

Human Papillomaviruses
2007; 670 pages

Volume 91

Combined Estrogen- Progestogen Contraceptives and Combined Estrogen-Progestogen Menopausal Therapy
2007; 528 pages

Volume 92

Some Non-heterocyclic Polycyclic Aromatic Hydrocarbons and Some Related Exposures
2010; 853 pages

Volume 93

Carbon Black, Titanium Dioxide, and Talc
2010; 452 pages

Volume 94

Ingested Nitrate and Nitrite, and Cyanobacterial Peptide Toxins
2010; 450 pages

Volume 95

Household Use of Solid Fuels and High-temperature Frying
2010; 430 pages

Volume 96

Alcohol Consumption
2010; 1431 pages

Volume 97

1,3-Butadiene, Ethylene Oxide and Vinyl Halides (Vinyl Fluoride, Vinyl Chloride and Vinyl Bromide)
2008; 510 pages

Volume 98

Painting, Firefighting, and Shiftwork
2010; 806 pages

Volume 99

Some Aromatic Amines, Organic Dyes, and Related Exposures
2010; 692 pages

Volume 100A

Pharmaceuticals
2012; 435 pages

Volume 100B

Biological Agents
2012; 475 pages

Volume 100C
Arsenic, metals, fibres, and dusts
2012; 501 pages

Volume 100D
Radiation
2012; 341 pages

Volume 100E
Personal habits and indoor combustions
2012; 575 pages

Volume 100F
Chemical agents and related occupations
2012; 599 pages

Supplement No. 1
Chemicals and Industrial Processes Associated with Cancer in Humans (IARC Monographs, Volumes 1 to 20)
1979; 71 pages (out-of-print)

Supplement No. 2
Long-term and Short-term Screening Assays for Carcinogens: A Critical Appraisal
1980; 426 pages (out-of-print)
(updated as IARC Scientific Publications No. 83, 1986)

Supplement No. 3
Cross Index of Synonyms and Trade Names in Volumes 1 to 26 of the IARC Monographs
1982; 199 pages (out-of-print)

Supplement No. 4
Chemicals, Industrial Processes and Industries Associated with Cancer in Humans (IARC Monographs, Volumes 1 to 29)
1982; 292 pages (out-of-print)

Supplement No. 5
Cross Index of Synonyms and Trade Names in Volumes 1 to 36 of the IARC Monographs
1985; 259 pages (out-of-print)

Supplement No. 6
Genetic and Related Effects: An Updating of Selected IARC Monographs from Volumes 1 to 42
1987; 729 pages (out-of-print)

Supplement No. 7
Overall Evaluations of Carcinogenicity: An Updating of IARC Monographs Volumes 1–42
1987; 440 pages (out-of-print)

Supplement No. 8
Cross Index of Synonyms and Trade Names in Volumes 1 to 46 of the IARC Monographs
1990; 346 pages (out-of-print)